# BMA

## Oxford Specialty Training
## Training in Medicine

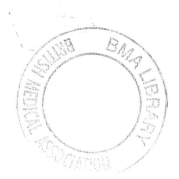

# Oxford Specialty Training: Training in Medicine

## Edited by

### Elaine Jolly

Specialist Registrar in Nephrology and General Internal Medicine
Department of Medicine
Addenbrooke's Hospital
Cambridge University Hospitals NHS Foundation Trust
Cambridge, UK

### Andrew Fry

Consultant in Nephrology and Acute Medicine
Addenbrooke's Hospital
Cambridge University Hospitals NHS Foundation Trust
Cambridge, UK

### Afzal Chaudhry

Chief Medical Information Officer
Consultant Physician
Associate Lecturer
Addenbrooke's Hospital
Cambridge University Hospitals NHS Foundation Trust
Cambridge, UK

## Series Editor

### Matthew D. Gardiner

Specialty Trainee in Plastic Surgery
Imperial College London

Honorary Clinical Lecturer in Plastic Surgery
Kennedy Institute of Rheumatology
University of Oxford

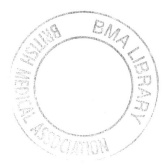

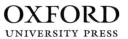

OXFORD
UNIVERSITY PRESS

**OXFORD**
UNIVERSITY PRESS

Great Clarendon Street, Oxford, OX2 6DP,
United Kingdom

Oxford University Press is a department of the University of Oxford.
It furthers the University's objective of excellence in research, scholarship,
and education by publishing worldwide. Oxford is a registered trade mark of
Oxford University Press in the UK and in certain other countries

First Edition published in 2016

Impression: 1

Published in the United States of America by Oxford University Press
198 Madison Avenue, New York, NY 10016, United States of America

British Library Cataloguing in Publication Data
Data available

Library of Congress Control Number: 2015956497

ISBN 978–0–19–923045–7

Printed in Italy by
L.E.G.O. S.p.A.

# Contents

# Detailed contents

vii

# Symbols and abbreviations

| | |
|---|---|
| 🛈 | warning |
| ► | important |
| ↓ | decreased |
| ↑ | increased |
| ↔ | normal |
| ♂ | male |
| ♀ | female |
| ~ | approximately |
| ± | plus/minus |
| 2,3-DPG | 2,3-diphosphoglycerate |
| 2D | two-dimensional |
| 3D | three-dimensional |
| 5ASA | 5-aminosalicylic acid |
| α | alpha |
| A&E | accident and emergency department |
| A1AT | alpha-1 antitrypsin |
| AA | aplastic anaemia |
| AAA | abdominal aortic aneurysms |
| AAFB | acid and alcohol-fast bacilli |
| AASV | ANCA-associated systemic vasculitis |
| ABG | arterial blood gas |
| ABPA | allergic bronchopulmonary aspergillosis |
| ABPI | ankle–brachial pressure index |
| ACA | anticentromere antibody |
| ACA | anterior cerebral artery |
| ACE | angiotensin-converting enzyme |
| ACh | acetylcholine |
| ACL | anticardiolipin antibody |
| ACLE | acute cutaneous lupus erythematosus |
| ACLF | acute on chronic liver failure |
| ACR | albumin:creatinine ratio |
| ACS | acute coronary syndromes |
| ACS | abdominal compartment syndrome |
| ACTH | adrenocorticotrophic hormone |
| AD | Alzheimer dementia |
| AD | autosomal dominant |
| ADH | antidiuretic hormone |
| ADP | adenosine diphosphate |
| AE | atopic eczema |
| AED | antiepileptic drug |
| AF | atrial fibrillation |
| AHA | acquired haemophilia-A |
| AI | adrenal incidentaloma |
| AICA | anterior inferior cerebral artery |
| AIDS | acquired immunodeficiency syndrome |
| AIH | autoimmune hepatitis |
| AKI | acute kidney injury |
| ALCL | anaplastic large cell lymphoma |
| ALD | alcoholic liver disease |
| ALF | acute liver failure |

| | |
|---|---|
| ALL | acute lymphoblastic leukaemia |
| AMI | acute myocardial infarction |
| AML | acute myeloid leukaemia |
| AN | acanthosis nigricans |
| ANA | antinuclear antibody |
| ANCA | antineutrophil cytoplasmic antibody |
| aO$_2$ | arterial oxygen content |
| APC | activated protein C |
| APD | automated peritoneal dialysis |
| aPL | antiphospholipid antibody |
| APS | antiphospholipid syndrome |
| aPTT | activated partial thromboplastin time |
| AR | autosomal recessive |
| AR | aortic regurgitation |
| ARAS | ascending reticular activating system |
| ARB | angiotensin receptor blocker |
| ARDS | adult respiratory distress syndrome |
| ARF | cute renal failure |
| ARR | absolute risk reduction |
| ART | antiretroviral therapy |
| AS | Angelman syndrome |
| AS | ankylosing spondylitis |
| ASA | anterior spinal artery |
| ASD | atrial septal defect |
| ASH | alcoholic steatohepatitis |
| AT | antithrombin |
| ATD | antithyroid drug |
| ATG | antithymocyte globulin |
| ATIN | acute interstitial nephritis |
| ATLL | adult T-cell leukaemia/lymphoma |
| ATP | adenosine triphosphate |
| AV | atrioventricular |
| AVF | arteriovenous fistula |
| AVM | arteriovenous malformation |
| AVNRT | atrioventricular nodal re-entry tachycardia |
| AVP | arginine vasopressin |
| AVRT | atrioventricular re-entry tachycardia |
| AWS | alcohol withdrawal syndrome |
| AXR | abdominal X-ray |
| AZT | zidovudine |
| β | beta |
| B2M | beta-2-microglobulin |
| BAL | bronchoalveolar lavage |
| BASHH | British Association for Sexual Health and HIV |
| BBB | bundle branch block |
| BBBB | blood–brain barrier breakdown |
| BBV | blood-borne virus |
| BCG | Bacillus Calmette–Guérin |
| BD | twice a day |
| BDA | Blackman–Diamond anaemia |

| | |
|---|---|
| BHIVA | British HIV Association |
| BHS | British Hypertension Society |
| BIPAP | bilevel positive airway pressure |
| BL | Burkitt lymphoma |
| BMD | bone mineral density |
| BMI | body mass index |
| BNF | *British National Formulary* |
| BP | blood pressure |
| B-PLL | B-prolymphocytic leukaemia |
| BPPV | benign paroxysmal positional vertigo |
| C&S | culture and sensitivity |
| CA | cancer antigen |
| CADASIL | cerebral autosomal dominant arteriopathy with subcortical infarcts and leucoencephalopathy |
| CAL | café-au-lait |
| cANCA | cytoplasmic antineutrophil cytoplasmic antibody |
| CAPD | continuous ambulatory peritoneal dialysis |
| CAS | cold agglutinin disease |
| CASS | continuous aspiration of subglottic secretions |
| CBD | corticobasal degeneration |
| CBG | cortisol binding globulin |
| CCP | cyclic citrullinated peptide |
| CCU | critical care unit |
| CD | cluster of differentiation |
| CD | Cushing disease |
| CDAD | Clostridium difficile-associated diarrhoea |
| CDK | cyclin-dependent kinase |
| CEA | carcinoembryonic antigen |
| CFU | colony-forming unit |
| CGH | comparative genomic hybridization |
| CHF | chronic heart failure |
| CHL | classical Hodgkin lymphoma |
| CHOP | cyclophosphamide, doxorubicin, vincristine, and prednisolone |
| CHOP | carbohydrate |
| CIDP | chronic inflammatory demyelinating polyneuropathy |
| CIN | contrast-induced nephropathy |
| CIN | chronic interstitial nephritis |
| CK | creatine kinase |
| CLL | chronic lymphocytic leukaemia |
| CLP | common lymphoid precursor |
| CML | chronic myeloid leukaemia |
| CMML | chronic myelomonocytic leukaemia |
| CMP | common myeloid precursor |
| CMT | Charcot–Marie–Tooth |
| CMV | Cytomegalovirus |
| CN | cranial nerve |
| CNS | central nervous system |
| CO | carbon monoxide |
| CO | cardiac output |
| $CO_2$ | carbon dioxide |
| COHb | carboxyhaemoglobin |
| CoNS | coagulase-negative staphylococci |
| CoW | Circle of Willis |
| COX | cyclo-oxygenase |
| CPAP | continuous positive airway pressure |
| CPP | cerebral perfusion pressure |

| | |
|---|---|
| CPR | cardiopulmonary resuscitation |
| CR | complete remission |
| CRBSI | catheter-related bloodstream infection |
| CRC | colorectal cancer |
| CrCl | creatinine clearance |
| CRH | corticotropin-releasing hormone |
| CRP | C-reactive protein |
| CRP | complement receptor |
| CS | Cushing syndrome |
| CS | carcinoid syndrome |
| CSA | ciclosporin |
| CSF | cerebrospinal fluid |
| CSII | continuous subcutaneous insulin infusion |
| CSM | Committee on Safety of Medicines |
| CSS | Churg–Strauss syndrome |
| CT | computed tomography |
| CTPA | computed tomography pulmonary angiogram |
| CV | cardiovascular |
| CVA | cerebrovascular accident |
| CVC | central venous catheter |
| CVID | common variable immunodeficiency |
| CVP | central venous pressure |
| CVS | chorionic villus sample |
| CVVH | continuous veno-venous haemofiltration |
| CVVHDF | continuous veno-venous diafiltration |
| CXR | chest X-ray |
| DAD | diffuse alveolar damage |
| DAT | direct antiglobulin test |
| DBP | diastolic blood pressure |
| DC | dyskeratosis congenita |
| DCM | dilated cardiomyopathy |
| dcSS | diffuse cutaneous systemic sclerosis |
| DDx | differential diagnosis |
| DeE | dementia elderly |
| DEET | diethyl toluamide |
| DFS | disease-free survival |
| DG | diglyceride |
| DHAP | cisplatin, cytarabine, and dexamethasone |
| DHEAS | dehydroepiandrosterone sulphate |
| DI | diabetes insipidus |
| DIC | disseminated intravascular coagulation |
| DKA | diabetic ketoacidosis |
| DLB | dementia with Lewy bodies |
| DLBCL | diffuse large B-cell lymphoma |
| DLE | discoid lupus erythematosus |
| DM | diabetes mellitus |
| DN | diabetic nephropathy |
| DNAR | do not attempt resuscitation |
| $DO_2$ | oxygen delivery |
| dsDNA | double stranded deoxyribonucleic acid |
| DVT | deep vein thrombosis |
| DWI | diffusion-weighted imaging |
| DXA | dual-energy X-ray absorptiometry |
| EAA | extrinsic allergic alveolitis |
| EAS | ectopic ACTH syndrome |
| EBUS | endobronchial ultrasound |
| EBV | Epstein–Barr virus |

| | |
|---|---|
| ECG | electrocardiogram |
| ECM | extracellular matrix |
| ECMO | extracorporeal membrane oxygenation |
| ED | emergency department |
| ED | erectile dysfunction |
| EDS | Ehlers–Danlos syndrome |
| EDTA | ethylenediaminetetraacetic acid |
| EDV | end-diastolic volume |
| EEG | electroencephalogram |
| EGDT | early goal-directed therapy |
| EGFR | epidermal growth factor receptor |
| ELISA | enzyme-linked immunosorbent assay |
| EM | erythema multiforme |
| EMA | European Medicines Agency |
| EMG | electromyogram |
| EMI | elderly mentally infirm |
| EMR | endoscopic mucosal resection |
| ENA | extractable nuclear antigen |
| ENS | enteric nervous system |
| ENT | ear, nose, and throat |
| EPO | erythropoietin |
| ERCP | endoscopic retrograde cholangiopancreatography |
| ESBL | extended-spectrum beta-lactamase |
| ESR | erythrocyte sedimentation rate |
| ESRF | end-stage renal failure |
| ESV | end-systolic volume |
| ET | essential thrombocythaemia |
| ET | endotracheal tube |
| FA | Fanconi anaemia |
| FA | fatty acid |
| FAB | French–American–British |
| FBC | full blood count |
| FCHL | familial combined hyperlipidaemia |
| FDA | Food and Drug Administration |
| FDG | 2-fluoro-2-deoxy-D-glucose |
| FEV1 | forced expiratory volume in 1 second |
| FFP | fresh frozen plasma |
| FHH | familial hypocalciuric hypercalcaemia |
| FISH | fluorescent in situ hybridization |
| FLAIR | fluid attenuated inversion recovery |
| FNA | fine needle aspiration |
| FRC | functional residual capacity |
| FSH | follicle-stimulating hormone |
| FT3 | free triiodothyronine |
| FT4 | free thyroxine |
| FVC | forced vital capacity |
| γ | gamma |
| G6PD | glucose-6-phosphate dehydrogenenase |
| GABA | gamma-aminobutyric acid |
| GBM | glomerular basement membrane |
| GBS | Guillain–Barré syndrome |
| GCA | giant cell arteritis |
| GCS | Glasgow Coma Scale |
| G-CSF | granulocyte colony stimulating factor |
| GDM | gestational diabetes mellitus |
| GFR | glomerular filtration rate |
| GGT | gamma-glutamyl transferase |

| | |
|---|---|
| GH | growth hormone |
| GHRH | growth hormone-releasing hormone |
| GHS | growth hormone secretagogue |
| GI | gastrointestinal |
| GM | grey matter |
| GM-CSF | granulocyte macrophage colony-stimulating factor |
| GN | glomerulonephritis |
| GnRH | gonadotropin-releasing hormone |
| GORD | gastro-oesophageal reflux disease |
| GP | glycoprotein |
| GPI | glycosylphosphatidylinositol |
| GTN | glyceryl trinitrate |
| GVHD | graft-versus-host disease |
| H&E | haematoxylin and eosin |
| HAART | highly active antiretroviral therapy |
| HAV | hepatitis A virus |
| HbA1c | glycated haemoglobin |
| HBC | hepatitis B virus |
| HBcAG | hepatitis B core antigen |
| HBeAg | hepatitis B e antigen |
| HBGM | home blood glucose monitoring |
| HBIG | hepatitis B immune globulin |
| HBsAg | hepatitis B surface antigen |
| HBV | hepatitis B virus |
| HCC | hepatocellular cancer |
| hCG | human chorionic gonadotropin |
| HCL | hairy cell leukaemia |
| Hct | haematocrit |
| HCV | hepatitis C virus |
| HDL | high-density lipoprotein |
| HDM | house dust mite |
| HDU | high dependency unit |
| HDV | hepatitis D virus |
| HE | hereditary elliptocytosis |
| HER | human epidermal growth factor receptor |
| HEV | hepatitis E virus |
| HFOV | high-frequency oscillation ventilation |
| HH | hereditary haemochromatosis |
| HHS | hyperosmolar hyperglycaemic state |
| HIGM | X-linked hyper IgM |
| HIT | heparin-induced thrombocytopenia |
| HIV | human immunodeficiency virus |
| HL | Hodgkin lymphoma |
| HLA | human leucocyte antigen |
| HMSN | hereditary motor and sensory neuropathy |
| HMW | high molecular weight |
| HMWK | high-molecular-weight kininogen |
| HNPCC | hereditary non-polyposis colorectal cancer |
| HNPP | hereditary neuropathy and liability to pressure palsies |
| HOCM | hypertrophic obstructive cardiomyopathy |
| HPA | Health Protection Agency |
| HPA | hypothalamic–pituitary–adrenal |
| HPV | human papilloma virus |
| HRCT | high-resolution computed tomography |
| HRS | Hodgkin and Reed/Sternberg |
| HRS | hepatorenal syndrome |

| | |
|---|---|
| HS | hereditary spherocytosis |
| HSC | hepatic stellate cell |
| HSC | haematopoietic stem cell |
| HSCT | haematopoietic stem cell transplantation |
| HSE | herpes simplex encephalitis |
| HSP | Henoch–Schönlein purpura |
| HSV | herpes simplex virus |
| HTLV | human T-cell leukaemia virus |
| HUS | haemolytic uraemic syndrome |
| IAH | intra-abdominal hypertension |
| IAT | indirect antiglobulin test |
| IBD | inflammatory bowel disease |
| IBN | inclusion body myositis |
| IBS | irritable bowel syndrome |
| ICB | intracerebral bleed |
| ICD | implantable cardioverter defibrillators |
| ICP | intracranial pressure |
| ICU | intensive care unit |
| IDF | International Diabetes Federation |
| IDSA | Infectious Diseases Society of America |
| IDT | intradermal testing |
| IE | infective endocarditis |
| IF | intrinsic factor |
| IF | immunofluorescence |
| IF | intrinsic factor |
| IFN | interferon |
| IFRT | involved field radiotherapy |
| Ig | immunoglobulin |
| IgAN | immunoglobulin A nephropathy |
| IGF | insulin-like growth factor |
| IGT | impaired glucose tolerance |
| IHA | immune haemolytic anaemia |
| IHD | ischaemic heart disease |
| IIH | idiopathic intracranial hypertension |
| IJV | internal jugular vein |
| IL | interleukin |
| IM | intramuscular |
| INO | internuclear opthalmoplegia |
| INR | international normalized ratio |
| IPF | idiopathic pulmonary fibrosis |
| IPI | International Prognostic Index |
| IPSS | international prognostic scoring system |
| ITP | idiopathic thrombocytopenic purpura |
| ITT | insulin tolerance test |
| IV | intravenous |
| IVCD | intraventricular conduction defect |
| IVDU | intravenous drug use |
| IVIG | intravenous immunoglobulin |
| Ix | investigation |
| JGA | juxtaglomerular apparatus |
| JME | juvenile myoclonic epilepsy |
| JVP | jugular venous pulse/pressure |
| KF | Kayser–Fleischer |
| KS | Kaposi sarcoma |
| KUB | kidneys/ureter/bladder |
| LA | lupus anticoagulant |
| LA | left atrial/atrium |

| | |
|---|---|
| LACS | lacunar syndrome |
| LBBB | left bundle branch block |
| LBC | liquid-based cytology |
| lcSS | limited cutaneous systemic sclerosis |
| LCV | leucocytoclastic vasculitis |
| LDH | lactate dehydrogenase |
| LDL | low-density lipoprotein |
| LEMS | Lambert–Eaton myasthenic syndrome |
| LFT | liver function test |
| LH | luteinizing hormone |
| LIDCO | lithium dilution cardiac output |
| LMN | lower motor neurone |
| LMWH | low-molecular-weight heparin |
| LOC | loss of consciousness |
| LP | lumbar puncture |
| LP | lichen planus |
| LQTS | long QT syndrome |
| L-T3 | levo-triiodothyronine |
| L-T4 | levo-thyroxine |
| LTG | lamotrigine |
| LUQ | left upper quadrant |
| LV | left ventricular/ventricle |
| LVD | left ventricular dysfunction |
| LVEDD | left ventricular end-diastolic diameter |
| LVEF | left ventricular ejection fraction |
| LVESD | left ventricular end-systolic diameter |
| LVH | left ventricular hypertrophy |
| LVSD | left ventricular systolic dysfunction |
| MAC | *Mycobacterium avium* complex |
| MAG3 | mercaptoacetyltriglycine |
| MAHA | microangiopathic haemolytic anaemia |
| MAI | *Mycobacterium avium-intracellulare* |
| MALT | mucosa-associated lymphoid tissue |
| MAOI | monoamine oxidase inhibitor |
| MAP | mean arterial pressure |
| MCA | middle cerebral artery |
| MCD | minimal change disease |
| MCGN | mesangiocapillary glomerulonephritis |
| MCH | mean cell haemoglobin |
| MCHC | mean cell haemoglobin concentration |
| MCI | mass casualty incident |
| MCL | mantle cell lymphoma |
| MCTD | mixed connective tissue disease |
| MDR | multidrug-resistant |
| MDR-TB | multidrug-resistant tuberculosis |
| MDS | myelodysplastic syndromes |
| MDS-U | myelodysplastic syndrome unclassified |
| MDT | multidisciplinary team |
| MELD | model for end-stage liver disease |
| MEN | multiple endocrine neoplasia |
| MF | mycosis fungoides |
| MG | monoglyceride |
| MG | myasthenia gravis |
| MGUS | monoclonal gammopathy of uncertain significance |
| MHC | major histocompatibility complex |
| MHC | major histocompatibility complex |

| | |
|---|---|
| MHRA | Medicines and Healthcare products Regulatory Agency |
| MI | myocardial infarction |
| MIBG | metaiodobenzylguanidine |
| MIC | minimum inhibitory concentration |
| MIMMS | major incident management and support |
| MIT | multiple injection therapy |
| MLF | medial longitudinal fasciculus |
| MLPA | multiplex ligation-dependent probe amplification |
| MM | multiple myeloma |
| MMF | mycophenolate mofetil |
| MMSE | Mini Mental State Examination |
| MND | motor neurone disease |
| MND | membranous nephropathy |
| MOF | multi-organ failure |
| MP | mercaptopurine |
| MR | mitral regurgitation |
| MR | mineralocorticoid receptor |
| MRCP | magnetic resonance cholangiopancreatography |
| MRI | magnetic resonance imaging |
| MRSA | methicillin-resistant *Staphylococcus aureus* |
| MRV | magnetic resonance venography |
| MS | multiple sclerosis |
| MSM | men who have sex with men |
| MSSA | methicillin-sensitive *Staphylococcus aureus* |
| MTB | *Mycobacterium tuberculosis* |
| MTCT | mother-to-child transmission |
| mtDNA | mitochondrial DNA |
| MV | mitral valve |
| $MVO_2$ | myocardial oxygen demand |
| NAC | N-acetylcysteine |
| Nad | noradrenaline |
| NADPH | nicotinamide adenine dinucleotide phosphate |
| NAFLD | non-alcoholic fatty liver disease |
| NASH | non-alcoholic steatohepatitis |
| NBM | nil by mouth |
| NEA | non-epileptic attack |
| NET | neuroendocrine tumour |
| NF | neurofibromatosis |
| NHL | non-Hodgkin lymphoma |
| NHS | National Health Service |
| NICE | National Institute for Health and Care Excellence |
| NINDS | National Institute of Neurological Disorders and Stroke |
| NIV | non-invasive ventilation |
| NK | natural killer |
| NL | necrobiosis lipoidica |
| NMDA | N-methyl-D-aspartate |
| NNRTI | non-nucleoside reverse transcriptase inhibitor |
| NNT | number needed to treat |
| NO | nitric oxide |
| NPV | negative predictive value |
| NREM | non-rapid eye movement |
| NRTI | nucleoside reverse transcriptase inhibitor |
| NS | nephrotic syndrome |
| NSAID | non-steroidal anti-inflammatory drug |
| NSCLC | non-small cell lung cancer |

| | |
|---|---|
| NSF | national service framework |
| NSTEACS | non-ST elevation acute coronary syndromes |
| NSTEMI | non-ST elevation myocardial infarction |
| NTM | non-tuberculous mycobacteria |
| NYHA | New York Heart Association |
| O/E | on examination |
| $O_2$ | oxygen |
| OA | osteoarthritis |
| OCP | oral contraceptive pill |
| OD | once a day |
| OGTT | oral glucose tolerance test |
| OHGA | oral hypoglycaemic agent |
| OR | odds ratio |
| OS | overall survival |
| PAC | pulmonary artery catheter |
| $PaCO_2$ | arterial partial pressure of carbon dioxide |
| PACS | partial anterior circulation syndrome |
| PAH | pulmonary arterial hypertension |
| PAMP | pathogen-associated molecular pattern |
| PAN | polyarteritis nodosa |
| $PaO_2$ | arterial partial pressure of oxygen |
| PAR | patient at risk |
| PAS | periodic acid–Schiff |
| PBC | primary biliary cirrhosis |
| PBP | penicillin binding protein |
| PCA | posterior cerebral artery |
| PCH | paroxysmal cold haemoglobinuria |
| PCI | percutaneous coronary intervention |
| PCOS | polycystic ovarian syndrome |
| PCP | Pneumocystis pneumonia |
| PCR | polymerase chain reaction |
| PCT | porphyria cutanea tarda |
| PCWP | pulmonary capillary wedge pressure |
| PD | Parkinson disease |
| PD | peritoneal dialysis |
| PDT | photodynamic therapy |
| PEA | pulseless electrical activity |
| PEEP | positive end- expiratory pressure |
| PEFR | peak expiratory flow rate |
| PEG | percutaneous endoscopic gastroscopy |
| PEP | post-exposure prophylaxis |
| PET | positron emission tomography |
| PF | platelet factor |
| PFS | progression-free survival |
| Ph | Philadelphia |
| PHA | primary hyperaldosteronism |
| PHG | portal hypertensive gastropathy |
| PHY | phenytoin |
| PI | protease inhibitor |
| PICA | posterior inferior cerebral artery |
| PiCCo | pulse-induced contour cardiac output |
| PK | pyruvate kinase |
| PKU | phenylketonuria |
| PMC | pseudomembranous colitis |
| PM | primary myelofibrosis |
| PML | progressive multifocal leucoencephalopathy |
| pmp | per million population |

| | |
|---|---|
| PMR | polymyalgia rheumatica |
| PN | parenteral nutrition |
| PNES | psychogenic non-epileptic seizures |
| PNH | paroxysmal nocturnal haemoglobinuria |
| PO | *per os* (orally) |
| pO$_2$ | partial pressure of oxygen |
| POCS | posterior circulation syndrome |
| POMC | pro-opiomelanocortin |
| PPI | proton-pump inhibitor |
| PPMS | primary progressive multiple sclerosis |
| PPRF | paramedian pontine reticular formation |
| PPV | positive predictive value |
| PR | per rectum (rectally) |
| PSA | prostate-specific antigen |
| PsA | psoriatic arthritis |
| PSA | prostate-specific antigen |
| PSC | primary sclerosing cholangitis |
| PSP | progressive supranuclear palsy |
| PT | prothrombin time |
| PTH | parathyroid hormone |
| PTLD | post-transplant lymphoproliferative disorder |
| PUD | peptic ulcer disease |
| PUJ | pelviureteric junction |
| PUO | pyrexia of unknown origin |
| PUVA | psoralen and ultraviolet A |
| PV | polycythaemia vera |
| PVS | persistent vegetative state |
| PWS | Prader–Willi syndrome |
| Px | prognosis |
| QID | four times a day |
| QOF | Quality Outcome Framework |
| RA | rheumatoid arthritis |
| RA | refractory anaemia |
| RA | right atrial/atrium |
| RAA | renin–angiotensin–aldosterone |
| RAEB | refractory anaemia with excess of blasts |
| RAI | radioiodine |
| RARS | refractory anaemia with ringed sideroblasts |
| RAST | radioallergosorbent test |
| RBBB | right bundle branch block |
| RBC | red blood cell |
| RCC | renal cell carcinoma |
| R-CHOP | rituximab, cyclophosphamide, doxorubicin, vincristine, and prednisolone |
| RCMD | refractory cytopenia with multilineage dysplasia |
| RCT | randomized controlled trial |
| RCUD | refractory cytopenias with unilineage dysplasia |
| RDW | red cell distribution width |
| ReA | reactive arthritis |
| REM | rapid eye movement |
| RF | rheumatoid factor |
| RhF | rheumatoid factor |
| RIC | reduced intensity conditioning |
| RIPA | ristocetin-induced platelet aggregation |
| RN | refractory neutropenia |
| ROC | receiver operating characteristic |
| RPE | retinal pigment epithelium |

| | |
|---|---|
| RPGN | rapidly progressive glomerulonephritis |
| RR | relative risk |
| RRT | renal replacement therapy |
| RSV | respiratory syncytial virus |
| RT | refractory thrombocytopenia |
| RTA | renal tubular acidosis |
| rTPA | recombinant tissue plasminogen activator |
| RT-PCR | reverse transcription polymerase chain reaction |
| RUQ | right upper quadrant |
| RV | residual volume |
| RV | right ventricular/ventricle |
| Rx | treatment |
| SA | sinoatrial |
| SAGH | subclinical autonomous glucocorticoid hypersecretion |
| SAH | subarachnoid haemorrhage |
| SARS | severe acute respiratory syndrome |
| SBP | systolic blood pressure |
| SC | subcutaneous |
| SCC | squamous cell carcinoma |
| SCD | sudden cardiac death |
| SCLC | small cell lung cancer |
| SCLE | subacute cutaneous lupus erythematosus |
| SD | standard deviation |
| SHBG | sex hormone binding globulin |
| SIADH | syndrome of inappropriate antidiuretic hormone secretion |
| SIRS | systemic inflammatory response syndrome |
| SJS | Stevens–Johnson syndrome |
| SK | seborrhoeic keratosis |
| SLE | systemic lupus erythematosus |
| SLR | straight leg raise |
| SOB | shortness of breath |
| SOL | space-occupying lesion |
| SPD | storage pool disease |
| SPECT | single-photon emission computed tomography |
| SPT | skin prick testing |
| SS | systemic sclerosis |
| SS | Sézary syndrome |
| SSPE | subacute sclerosing panencephalitis |
| SSRI | selective serotonin re-uptake inhibitor |
| SST | short Synacthen® test |
| STEMI | ST-elevation myocardial infarction |
| SUDEP | sudden unexplained death in epilepsy |
| SVC | superior vena cava |
| SVCO | superior vena cava obstruction |
| SVR | systematic vascular resistance |
| SVT | supraventricular tachycardia |
| Sx | symptoms |
| $t_{1/2}$ | half-life |
| T1DM | type 1 diabetes mellitus |
| T2DM | type 2 diabetes mellitus |
| T3 | triiodothyronine |
| T4 | thyroxine |
| TACS | total anterior circulation syndrome |
| TAVI | transcutaneous aortic valve implantation |
| TB | tuberculosis |

| | |
|---|---|
| TBG | thyroid binding globulin |
| TBI | traumatic brain injury |
| Tc | technetium |
| TCA | tricyclic antidepressant |
| TCC | transitional cell carcinoma |
| TEDS | thromboembolic deterrent stockings |
| TF | tissue factor |
| TFPI | tissue factor pathway inhibitor |
| TfR | transferrin receptor |
| TFT | thyroid function test |
| TG | triglyceride |
| TG | thyroglobulin |
| Th | T helper |
| TIA | transient ischaemic attack |
| TIBC | total iron binding capacity |
| TID | three times a day |
| TIPSS | transjugular intrahepatic portosystemic stent shunt |
| TKI | tyrosine kinase inhibitor |
| TLC | total lung capacity |
| TLCO | transfer factor of carbon monoxide |
| TNF | tumour necrosis factor |
| TOE | transoesophageal echocardiography |
| TPMT | thiopurine S-methyltransferase |
| TPMT | thiopurine methyl transferase |
| TPN | total parenteral nutrition |
| TPO | thrombopoietin |
| TPO | thyroid peroxidase |
| TR | tricuspid regurgitation |
| TRAb | TSH receptor antibody |
| TRH | thyrotropin-releasing hormone |
| TRM | transplant-related mortality |
| TSC | tuberous sclerosis complex |
| TSH | thyroid stimulating hormone |
| TSS | toxic shock syndrome |
| TTE | transthoracic echocardiography |
| TTP | thrombotic thrombocytopenic purpura |
| TZD | thiazolidinedione |
| U&Es | urea and electrolytes |
| UC | ulcerative colitis |
| UFH | unfractionated heparin |
| UMN | upper motor neurone |

| | |
|---|---|
| UO | urinary output |
| UPD | uniparental disomy |
| URTI | upper respiratory tract infection |
| USS | ultrasound scan |
| UTI | urinary tract infection |
| UV | ultraviolet |
| V/Q | ventilation/perfusion |
| VA | alveolar ventilation |
| VAP | ventilator-associated pneumonia |
| VATS | video-assisted thoracoscopic |
| VC | vital capacity |
| Vd | volume of distribution |
| VDLD | very low-density lipoprotein |
| VDRL | Venereal Disease Research Laboratory |
| VEGF | vascular endothelial growth factor |
| VF | ventricular fibrillation |
| VHF | viral haemorrhagic fever |
| VILI | ventilator-induced lung injury |
| $vO_2$ | venous oxygen content |
| VOR | vestibulo-ocular reflex |
| VPA | valproate |
| VRE | vancomycin-resistant enterococci |
| VSD | ventricular septal defect |
| VT | ventricular tachycardia |
| VTE | venous thromboembolism |
| VWD | von Willebrand disease |
| VWF | von Willebrand factor |
| VZV | varicella zoster virus |
| WBC | white blood cell |
| WCC | white cell count |
| WG | granulomatosis with polyangiitis (Wegener) |
| WHO | World Health Organization |
| WM | Waldenström macroglobulinaemia |
| WM | white matter |
| WPW | Wolff–Parkinson–White |
| XLA | X-linked agammaglobulinaemia |
| XP | xeroderma pigmentosum |
| ZF | zona fasciculata |
| ZG | zona glomerulosa |
| ZN | Ziehl–Neelsen |
| ZR | zona reticularis |

# Contributors

**Victoria Allgar**
Senior Lecturer in Medical Statistics
Hull and York Medical School/Health Sciences
University of York
York, UK

**Anand Kumar Annamalai**
Speciality Registrar in Endocrinology
Metabolic Research Laboratories
Wellcome Trust-MRC Institute of Metabolic Science
Addenbrooke's Hospital
Cambridge Biomedical Campus
Cambridge, UK

**John Martin Bland**
Professor of Health Statistics
Department of Health Sciences
University of York
York, UK

**Timothy J Burton**
Clinical Pharmacology
University of Cambridge
Addenbrooke's Hospital
Cambridge University Hospitals NHS Foundation Trust
Cambridge, UK

**Aristeidis Chaidos**
Consultant Haematologist
Imperial College Healthcare NHS Trust
London, UK

**Afzal N Chaudhry**
Chief Medical Information Officer
Consultant Physician
Associate Lecturer
Addenbrooke's Hospital
Cambridge University Hospitals NHS Foundation Trust
Cambridge, UK

**John Connelly**
Wellcome Trust Senior Clinical Fellow and Consultant Hepatologist
MRC Centre for Inflammation Research
Queen's Medical Research Institute
University of Edinburgh
Edinburgh, UK

**Paul A Corris**
Professor of Thoracic Medicine and Honorary Consultant
Institute of Cellular Medicine
Newcastle University and Department of Respiratory Medicine
Freeman Hospital
Newcastle upon Tyne, UK

**Francesco Dazzi**
Professor of Regenerative and Haematological Medicine
KHP Lead for Cellular Therapies
King's College
London, UK

**Anthony De Soyza**
Senior Lecturer and Honorary Consultant
Institute of Cellular Medicine
Newcastle University and Department of Respiratory medicine
Freeman Hospital
Newcastle upon Tyne, UK

**Giles Dunnill**
Consultant Dermatologist
Department of Dermatology
Bristol Royal Infirmary
Bristol, UK

**Spencer Ellis**
Consultant Rheumatologist and General Physician
Department of Rheumatology
East and North Herts NHS Trust
Lister Hospital
Stevenage, UK

**Nikos Evangelou**
Division of Neurosciences
Queen's Medical Centre
Nottingham University Hospitals
University of Nottingham
England, UK

**Professor TJ Evans**
Institute of Infection, Immunity and Inflammation
University of Glasgow
Glasgow, UK

**John Forrester**
Section of Immunology and Infection
Division of Applied Medicine
School of Medicine and Dentistry
Institute of Medical Science, Foresterhill
University of Aberdeen
Scotland, UK
  *and*
Ocular Immunology Program
Centre for Ophthalmology and Visual Science
The University of Western Australia
Australia
  *and*
Centre for Experimental Immunology
Lions Eye Institute
Nedlands, Australia

**Andrew Fry**
Consultant in Nephrology and Acute Medicine
Addenbrooke's Hospital
Cambridge University Hospitals NHS Foundation Trust
Cambridge, UK

**Christopher P Gilmore**
Department of Neurology
Queens Medical Centre NHS Trust
Nottingham University Hospitals
Nottingham, UK

**Paul A Glynne**
Consultant Physician
University College London NHS Foundation Trust
London, UK

**Eleanor Gurnell**
Consultant Diabetologist
Addenbrooke's Hospital
Cambridge University Hospitals NHS Foundation Trust
Cambridge, UK

**Mark Gurnell**
Clinical SubDean
University of Cambridge School of Clinical Medicine
Senior Lecturer in Endocrinology
*and*
Honorary Consultant Physician
University of Cambridge
*and*
Metabolic Research Laboratories
Wellcome Trust-MRC Institute of Metabolic Science
Addenbrooke's Hospital
Cambridge Biomedical Campus
Cambridge, UK

**Neil Henderson**
Wellcome Trust Senior Clinical Fellow and Consultant Hepatologist
MRC Centre for Inflammation Research
Queen's Medical Research Institute
University of Edinburgh
Edinburgh, UK

**David CJ Howell**
Divisional Clinical Director
Critical Care Unit
University College London NHS Foundation Trust
London, UK

**John Iredale**
Regius Professor of Medical Science
MRC Centre for Inflammation Research
Queen's Medical Research Institute
University of Edinburgh
Edinburgh, UK

**Elaine C Jolly**
Specialist Registrar in Nephrology and General Internal Medicine
Department of Medicine
Addenbrooke's Hospital
Cambridge University Hospitals NHS Foundation Trust
Cambridge, UK

**Dinakantha Kumararatne**
Consultant Clinical Immunologist
Immunology Department
Addenbrooke's Hospital
Cambridge University Hospitals NHS Foundation Trust
Cambridge, UK

**Jeffrey Lee**
Consultant Rheumatologist & General Physician
Department of Rheumatology
Barnet Hospital
Royal Free Foundation NHS Trust
Hertfordshire, UK

**John McMurray**
Professor of Medical Cardiology
Institute of Cardiovascular & Medical Sciences
University of Glasgow
*and*
Honorary Consultant Cardiologist
Queen Elizabeth University Hospital
Glasgow, UK

**Claire L Meek**
Metabolic Physician
Metabolic Research Laboratories
Wellcome Trust-MRC Institute of Metabolic Science
Addenbrooke's Hospital
Cambridge Biomedical CampusCambridge, UK

**Agnieszka Michael**
Consultant Medical Oncologist
Royal Surrey County Hospital
*and*
Senior Lecturer
University of Surrey
Surrey, UK

**Brian Murphy**
Consultant Cardiologist
Queen Elizabeth University Hospital
Glasgow, UK

**Claire Nicholl**
Consultant Geriatrician
Department of Medicine for the Elderly
Cambridge University Hospitals NHS Foundation Trust
Cambridge, UK

**Hardev Pandha**
Professor of Medical Oncology
Targeted Cancer Therapy, Faculty of Health and Medical Sciences
University of Surrey
Guildford, UK

**Dayangku Siti Nur Ashikin Pengiran Tengah**
Consultant Neurologist
Neurology Division
Raja Isteri Pengiran Anak Saleha Hospital
Bandar Seri Begawan
Brunei

**Andrew Powlson**
Clinical Research Associate and Honorary Specialist Registrar
Metabolic Research Laboratories
Institute of Metabolic Science
University of Cambridge
Addenbrooke's Hospital
Cambridge Biomedical Campus Cambridge, UK

**Rachel Quail**
Consultant in Acute Medicine
East and North Herts NHS Trust
Lister Hospital
Stevenage, UK

**Shefali Rajpopat**
Consultant Dermatologist
Barts Health NHS Trust
London, UK

**Kate Relph**
Research Fellow
Targeted Cancer Therapy
Faculty of Health and Medical Sciences
University of Surrey
Guildford, UK

**Paul Robertson**
Specialty Registrar in Medical Microbiology
Department of Microbiology
Glasgow Royal Infirmary
Glasgow, UK

**Anand Saggar**
Consultant in Clinical Genetics
St George's University of London
London, UK

**Jack Satsangi**
Professor of Gastroenterology
University of Edinburgh
Edinburgh, UK

**Suranjit Seneviratne**
Consultant in Clinical Immunology and Allergy
Department of Clinical Immunology and UCL Centre
for Immunodeficiency
Institute of Immunity and Transplantation
Royal Free Hospital
London, UK

**Jonathan Silverman**
Honorary Visiting Senior Fellow
School of Clinical Medicine
University of Cambridge
Cambridge, UK

**Sumeet Singal**
Consultant Neurologist
Queen's Medical Centre
Nottingham University Hospitals
Nottingham, UK

**Derek Soon**
Consultant Neurologist
National University Health System
Singapore, Singapore
    *and*
Undergraduate Education Director for Medicine
Yong Loo Lin School of Medicine
National University of Singapore
Singapore, Singapore

**Chris Strey**
Facharzt Innere Medizin
Spez. Endokrinologie
eSwiss Medical Center
St. Gallen, Switzerland

**Ravi Suchak**
Department of Dermatology
Basildon University Hospital
Essex, UK

**Emma Tallantyre**
Post-CCT Research Fellow
Department of Clinical Neurology
University Hospital of Wales
Cardiff, UK

**Jennifer Thomson**
Consultant in Clinical Genetics
Leeds Teaching Hospitals NHS Trust
Chapel Allerton Hospital
Leeds, UK

**Antoinette Tuthill**
Consultant Endocrinologist and Lecturer
Cork University Hospital
Cork, Ireland

**Stephen Wallis**
Consultant Geriatrician
Department of Medicine for the Elderly
Addenbrooke's Hospital
Cambridge University Hospitals NHS Foundation Trust
Cambridge, UK

**David Watts**
Gastroenterologist and Clinical Lead
Gastrointestinal Unit
NHS Forth Valley
Forth Valley Royal Hospital
Larbert, UK

**Robin AP Weir**
Department of Cardiology
Hairmyres Hospital
Scotland, UK

**Ian B Wilkinson**
Professor of Therapeutics
Department of Medicine, EMIT Division
Addenbrooke's Hospital
Cambridge University Hospitals NHS Foundation Trust
Cambridge, UK

**Lisa C Willcocks**
Consultant Nephrologist
Department of Medicine
Addenbrooke's Hospital
Cambridge University Hospitals NHS Foundation Trust
Cambridge, UK

**Graeme J Williams**
Consultant Medical Ophthalmologist
Gartnavel General Hospital
Glasgow, UK

**Katie Wood**
Consultant Clinical Oncologist
Royal Surrey County Hospital
Guildford, UK
    *and*
Clinical Oncologist
The Royal Surrey County Hospital NHS Foundation Trust
Surrey, UK

# Chapter 1

## Acute medical emergencies and practical procedures

1

# 1.1 Cardiorespiratory arrest

## Definitions

- Respiratory arrest = lack of spontaneous respiratory effort.
- Cardiac arrest = absence of effective cardiac output.

Within 3 minutes of cardiorespiratory arrest, cerebral hypoxia develops resulting in brain damage, necessitating urgent cardiopulmonary resuscitation (CPR) and restoration of circulation where possible.

## Presentation

Identified in patients who are unconscious, apnoeic, and with absent central pulses (carotid and/or femoral pulses).

## Basic life support

Aiming to maintain adequate ventilation and circulation to preserve cerebral perfusion (Fig. 1.1).

### Management

- Ensure personal safety in approach to patient.
- Shout for help.
- Check patient response.
- Turn patient onto their back.
- Open airway using head tilt and chin lift—use C-spine precautions if at risk of injury.
- Check airway—foreign body/debris (remove with forceps/suction).
- Look, listen, and feel for respiration whilst checking carotid pulsation—no longer than 10 seconds.
- If no sign of life, no respiratory effort, and no pulse: call cardiac arrest team.
- Commence CPR immediately (instigate if any doubt).
- 30 chest compressions followed by 2 ventilations.
- Hand position for chest compressions is the middle of the lower half of the sternum.
- Depth of 4–5cm with a rate of 100/minute.
- A palpable pulse should not be used to guide effectiveness of compressions.
- Ventilation (aiming inspiratory phase of 1 second) through pocket mask if a bag mask not immediately available—mouth-to-mouth if no adjunctive equipment available.
- If ventilation not possible or contraindicated if no equipment available (corrosives/poisons), continue uninterrupted chest compressions.
- Once defibrillator arrives immediately place pads/electrodes in position.
- Respiratory arrest only—ventilate, checking for carotid pulsation every 10 breaths.

## Advanced life support

Provides a structured algorithm to follow in the case of cardiac arrest to facilitate treatment with the aim of restoring cardiac output (Fig. 1.2).

Improved survival has been shown for early defibrillation of shockable rhythms and effective CPR.

### Shockable rhythms: ventricular fibrillation/tachycardia (VF/VT)

- Commonest rhythm seen in adult cardiac arrest—may be preceded by cardiac history or other arrhythmia.

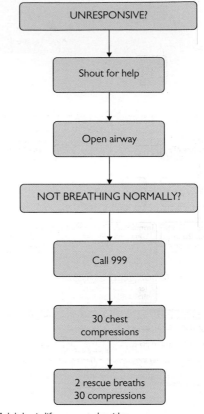

**Fig. 1.1** Adult basic life support algorithm.
Reproduced with the kind permission of the Resuscitation Council (UK).

*Management*

- As for basic life support.
- In the case of witnessed and monitored cardiac arrest a precordial thump may be attempted—deliver a quick, sharp, recoiled impact to the lower half of the sternum from approximately 20cm.
- Confirmation of rhythm.
- Immediate defibrillation with 1 shock 150J biphasic (360J monophasic).
- Immediately resume chest compressions at 30:2.
- Continue CPR for 2 minutes.
- Establish IV access and consider intubation.
- Check monitor for rhythm.
- Persistent VF/VT: 1 shock 150J biphasic, with immediate recommencement of CPR for 2 minutes.
- Check monitor for rhythm.
- Persistent VF/VT: give 1mg IV adrenaline immediately followed by 1 shock (150J biphasic) and resumption of CPR for 2 minutes.
- Persistent VF/VT: give amiodarone 300mg IV immediately followed by 1 shock (150J) and commencement of CPR for 2 minutes.
- Continue to give further shocks if persistent VF/VT every 2 minutes.
- 1mg IV adrenaline prior to alternate shocks.
- Do not check for a pulse after delivery of a shock as this delays effective cardiac compressions and risks further myocardial damage.
- Drugs given should be flushed through with 20mL normal saline.

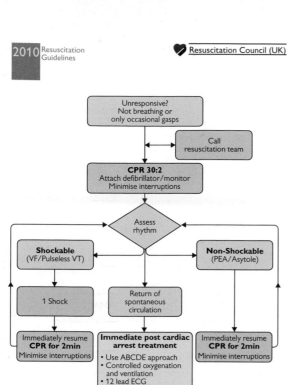

**During CPR**
- Ensure high-quality CPR: rate, depth, recoil
- Plan actions before interrupting CPR
- Give oxygen
- Consider advanced airway and capnography
- Continuous chest compressions when advanced airway in place
- Vascular access (intravenous, intraosseous)
- Give adrenaline every 3–5min
- Corret reversible causes

**Reversible Causes**
- Hypoxia
- Hypovolaemia
- Hypo-/hyperkalaemia/metabolic
- Hypothermia
- Thrombosis - coronary or pulmonary
- Tamponade - cardiac
- Toxins
- Tension pneumothorax

**Fig. 1.2** Adult advanced life support algorithm.
Reproduced with the kind permission of the Resuscitation Council (UK).

- Lidocaine 100mg IV can be used as an alternative to amiodarone if contraindicated (not to be given concurrently).
- Magnesium sulphate (2g IV) if risk of hypomagnesaemia—patients on diuretic therapy.
- Check pad position and contacts. Consider change to anteroposterior position.
- If doubt over VF or asystole treat as non-shockable—continued shocks to possible fine VF is unlikely to prove successful with increased myocardial injury due to chest compression interruptions and direct electrical current.
- If patient's rhythm changes to PEA/asystole move to non-shockable rhythms.

### Non-shockable rhythms: asystole/pulseless electrical activity (PEA)
- PEA is the absence of palpable pulsation in the presence of organized electrical activity.
- In the presence of asystole check carefully for present of p waves and ventricular standstill (option for pacing).
- Potential reversible causes should be identified and treated quickly, without which survival is unlikely.

*Management*
- As for basic life support.
- Establish IV access and consider intubation.
- Immediately give 1mg IV adrenaline.
- For PEA <60/minute: give 3mg IV atropine.

- Continue CPR at a rate of 30:2 (continuous cardiac compressions if intubated).
- Continue CPR for 2 minutes.
- Check monitor for rhythm.
- If organized electrical activity is seen, check for signs of life and pulse.
- If no pulse (PEA) or asystole: continue CPR for 2 minutes.
- Check monitor for rhythm.
- If organized electrical activity present check for signs of life and pulse.
- If no pulse or asystole: continue CPR for 2 minutes.
- 1mg IV adrenaline every alternate cycle.
- Intubation (tracheal) to protect the patient's airway and provide continuous cardiac compressions (during ventilation, cardiac perfusion pressure is severely reduced and takes time on resumption of compressions to be restored). Expert personnel only—each attempt should take no longer than 30 seconds.
- Assessment of tube placement is made by observing chest rise and auscultation in all areas.
- Ventilate at a rate of 10/minute.

## Reversible causes

Survival from cardiac arrest is higher in the presence of a number of reversible causes, identified using the '4 Hs and 4 Ts' technique:
- **H**ypoxia—adequate ventilation with airway adjuncts and high-flow oxygen.
- **H**ypovolaemia—IV fluids to restore volume and stop haemorrhage—surgery etc.
- **H**yperkalaemia, hypokalaemia, hypoglycaemia—IV replacement (e.g. calcium chloride, IV glucose).
- **H**ypothermia—usually given from the history (e.g. drowning)—rapid re-warming to temp >30°C (drugs withheld until above this temperature).
- **T**ension pneumothorax—clinical diagnosis with urgent needle thoracocentesis (2nd intercostal space, midclavicular line).
- **T**amponade—consider in penetrating chest trauma, obtain emergency echo, needle pericardiocentesis or thoracotomy may be required.
- **T**hromboembolic—massive pulmonary embolism or myocardial infarct, consider thrombolytic therapy.
- **T**oxic—review of history may reveal toxic exposures. Antidotes for some drugs exist (naloxone, flumazenil) but should not be used speculatively.

## Post-resuscitation care

Following return of spontaneous circulation, further intervention is required in order to stabilize cardiac function as much as possible.

Ongoing treatment of the airway, breathing, and circulation are important for maintaining haemodynamic stability and specialist care should be sought throughout this period.

## Do not resuscitate decisions

Decisions should involve the patient and their families if possible. Of note, relatives do **not** have the power to make decisions on medical care on behalf of another person, but their opinion should be considered during any decision-making process.

These are difficult decisions and should take into account:
- Underlying condition makes successful outcome unlikely.
- Resuscitation is not in the patient's best interest in terms of poorer quality of life.
- A competent patient's stated or prior advance directive wish not for resuscitation.

# 1.2 Shock

## Definition

Shock is the medical emergency of profound circulatory collapse resulting in reduced organ and tissue perfusion, requiring immediate intervention to prevent end-organ damage and ultimately cardiac arrest.

## Types of shock

- Anaphylactic
- Cardiogenic
- Hypovolaemic
- Septic.

## Examination

- Tachypnoea.
- Hypotension: systolic blood pressure (BP) <90mmHg.
- Tachycardia: heart rate (HR) >100/minute (care if taking β-blockers).
- Reduced capillary return: >2 seconds.
- Cool peripheries and cyanosis.
- Pallor.
- Confusion (cerebral hypoxia).
- Reduced urine output: <0.5mL/kg/hour.

## Anaphylactic shock

Severe systemic allergic reaction with hypotension and/or respiratory problems.

### Presentation
- Angio-oedema.
- Erythema.
- Urticaria.
- Pruritis.
- Swelling of upper airways (lips to epiglottis) and stridor.
- Shortness of breath and wheeze.

### Management
- Immediate management = airway protection, administration of adrenaline (epinephrine), and fluid resuscitation.
- Discontinue causative agent if possible.
- Airway protection: severe laryngeal oedema may require intubation or surgical airway (needle cricothyroidotomy, tracheostomy).
- Oxygen delivery to maintain saturations >95%.
- IM adrenaline (epinephrine) 0.5mL of 1 in 1000.
- Repeat in 5 minutes if no clinical response.
- Continuous electrocardiograph (ECG) monitoring.
- Large-bore IV cannula (>18G/green).
- IV fluid resuscitation (colloid or crystalloid).
- IV antihistamine (e.g. chlorpheniramine 10mg).
- IV steroids (e.g. hydrocortisone 100mg).
- Salbutamol nebulizers (5mg) if wheeze present.
- Admit for 24 hours to observe for delayed reaction.
- Continue oral antihistamine for 24–72 hours.
- Supply preloaded adrenaline syringe to patients at risk of recurrence. Consider referral to local allergy/immunology service.

## Cardiogenic shock

- Cardiogenic shock results from cardiac dysfunction impairing the ability to maintain adequate tissue perfusion.
- Mortality can range from 50–75% even with treatment.
- Defined clinically as reduced cardiac output and poor tissue perfusion in the presence of euvolaemia.

### Presentation
- As for clinical definition, plus signs and symptoms of cause:
  - Myocardial infarction (MI).
  - Acute coronary syndrome (ACS).
  - Acute mitral regurgitation (MR; papillary muscle rupture).
  - Rupture of interventricular septum.
  - Myocardial suppressants, e.g. calcium antagonist overdose.
- Raised jugular venous pressure (JVP) and signs of pulmonary oedema.
- Pansystolic murmur of MR or ventricular septal defect (VSD).
- Evidence of endocarditis—splinter haemorrhages, etc.

### Investigation
- Full blood count (FBC)—anaemia or raised white cell count (WCC; infection).
- Urea and electrolytes (U&Es)—renal dysfunction.
- Cardiac enzymes—troponin for MI.
- Lactate—evidence of poor tissue perfusion.
- Arterial blood gas (ABG) analysis.
- ECG—ischaemia, arrhythmia.
- Chest X-ray (CXR)—pulmonary oedema.
- Urgent echocardiography.

### Management
- Aim: increase tissue perfusion to prevent end-organ damage and treat the cause.
- Early specialist cardiology input is imperative and these patients will require CCU/HDU/ITU support.
- Ensure patients have adequate fluid resuscitation (care with pulmonary oedema). Fluid resuscitation in right-sided myocardial infarctions may improve blood pressure, but **do not** overload as this may worsen symptoms.
- Continuous cardiac monitoring.
- Treatment of coronary ischaemia/infarction: antiplatelets, heparin, glycoprotein (GP)-IIb/IIIa inhibitors, thrombolysis, or primary percutaneous coronary intervention (PCI).
- Treatment of arrhythmia—DC cardioversion or pacing as indicated.
- Central venous access for fluid balance monitoring (and drugs) is often essential—beware of potential cardiac irritability (if myocardial ischaemia) during line insertion.

If persistent hypotension:
- Inotropic support (through central venous access) should be considered, aiming for a mean arterial pressure (MAP) of 60mmHg if possible:
  - Dopamine 5–10mcg/kg/min.
  - Noradrenaline 0.5mcg/kg/min (if dopamine fails to effect response).
  - Adrenaline.
- Placement of an intra-aortic balloon pump (to stabilize prior to definitive treatment, usually at a tertiary centre).
- Left ventricular assist device or urgent coronary artery bypass surgery may be required.

# Hypovolaemic shock

Severe blood/fluid loss causing haemodynamic compromise.

## Presentation
- Cause for hypovolaemic shock can often be identified by history—i.e. trauma, melaena, fresh bleeding, diarrhoea & vomiting.
- Degree of volume loss can often be estimated from the haemodynamic status of the patient (Table 1.1).

## Investigation
- FBC and coagulation screen.
- U&Es—renal failure, raised urea with normal creatinine may indicate gastrointestinal (GI) haemorrhage.
- Group and save—haemorrhage should instigate a cross-match request for 4–6 units.
- ABG (or venous gas)—lactic acidosis indicates poor tissue perfusion.

## Management
- Immediate management should involve fluid replacement, prevention of further fluid loss, and identification/treatment of the cause. Management should then focus on stabilization of the patient pending definitive management, i.e. surgery for ruptured abdominal aortic aneurysms (AAAs), embolization, endoscopy, etc.
- Airway protection if reduced Glasgow Coma Scale (GCS) score.
- Oxygen delivery—15L via non-rebreathe mask.
- Pressure on any open bleeding points.
- 2 × large-bore IV cannula (≥18G/green).
- IV fluid resuscitation—colloid/crystalloid, rapidly.
- Blood transfusion if haemoglobin (Hb) <10g/dL or massive haemorrhage (activate 'massive blood transfusion' protocol)
- Correction of coagulopathy if indicated: fresh frozen plasma (FFP), cryoprecipitate, Beriplex®, vitamin K.
- Consider central venous access for monitoring central venous pressure (CVP) to guide fluid replacement. Caution with central venous access (subclavian, jugular) if hypovolaemic, and remember ability to fluid resuscitate is limited through central access due to line gauge.

### Urgent investigations
- Imaging:
  - Focused abdominal scan (ultrasound) for intra-abdominal bleeding ('rule in, not rule out', i.e. AAA).
  - Computed tomography (CT).
- Angiography: identify (and potentially embolize) source.
- Endoscopy (gastroscopy/colonoscopy): potential to inject/ligate bleeding point.

- Continued haemorrhage with persistent hypotension should precipitate **urgent** surgical referral.

# Septic shock

- Sepsis = the presence of infection associated with a systemic inflammatory reaction.
- A set of clinical criteria, known as systemic inflammatory response syndrome (SIRS), provides a helpful indicator for the severity of sepsis:
  - Meeting two or more criteria should alert to the possibility of development of end-organ dysfunction and potential for septic shock.

| Temperature: | <36°C | >38°C |
|---|---|---|
| Pulse: | >90/min | |
| Respiratory rate: | >20/min | pCO$_2$ <3.2 |
| WCC: | >14 | <4 |

- Septic shock = severe infection with associated hypotension despite adequate fluid resuscitation.

## Presentation
- Pyrexia, flushed appearance.
- Rigors.
- Bounding pulse.
- Focal signs of localizing infection: i.e. meningism, cellulitis.
- Be aware: patients may present as flushed and warm, or cold and peripherally shut down.

## Investigation
- FBC—raised WCC.
- U&Es—renal failure.
- Clotting—disseminated intravascular coagulation (DIC).
- C-reactive protein (CRP).
- Liver function test—possible biliary source?
- Blood cultures: prior to antibiotics if at all possible.
- Urinalysis and culture.
- Sputum/stool cultures, wound swabs (as indicated).
- ABG or venous gas (measure lactate).
- CXR—pneumonia, adult respiratory distress syndrome (ARDS).

## Management
- Immediate management involves fluid resuscitation, administration of antibiotics, and removal of any septic foci.
- Administer oxygen to maintain saturations >95%.
- IV access and bloods.
- Administer broad-spectrum antibiotics as per local policy.
- Fluid resuscitation with colloid/crystalloid.
- Maintain Hb >10g/dL.
- Catheterization and hourly urine output monitoring.
- CVP monitoring—for fluid management and inotropes.
- Early specialist intensive care input.
- Continued hypotension after adequate fluid resuscitation (CVP 10–12mmHg) should necessitate inotropic use:
  - Noradrenaline 1–12mcg/min.
  - Adrenaline 1–12mcg/min.
  - Dobutamine 2.5–15mcg/kg/min.
  - Vasopressin.
- Further investigation as indicated to define infective source.

| Table 1.1 Classification of hypovolaemic shock | | | | |
|---|---|---|---|---|
| **Classification** | **1** | **2** | **3** | **4** |
| Blood loss | <750mL | 0.75–1.5L | 1.5–2L | >2L |
| % | 0–15 | 15–30 | 30–40 | >40 |
| Systolic BP | No change | No change | Reduced | Much reduced |
| Diastolic BP | No change | Increased | Reduced | Unrecordable |
| Pulse/minute | Increased | 100–120 | 120 | >120 + thready |
| Respiratory rate | Normal | Normal | Increased | Increased |
| Mental state | Normal | Anxious | Drowsy | Confused |
| | | Thirsty | Aggressive | Unconscious |

# 1.3 Acute coronary syndromes

## Definitions

### Acute coronary syndromes (ACS)

Symptoms consistent with myocardial ischaemia, including:
- ST-elevation myocardial infarction (STEMI).
- Non-ST elevation myocardial infarction (NSTEMI).
- Unstable angina.

### Definition of MI (European Society of Cardiology)

- Elevated cardiac biomarkers (troponins).

With one or more of the following:
- New pathological Q waves.
- New or dynamic ST or T changes.
- New left bundle branch block (LBBB).
- Imaging of new myocardial dysfunction.
- Symptoms of ischaemia for >20 minutes.

In the patient presenting with symptoms suggestive of ACS (see also Section 3.3):

## Initial assessment

- Airway, breathing, circulation.
- Ensure that airway is safe; commence high-flow oxygen therapy through a non-rebreathe mask.
- Check respiratory rate and oxygen saturations.
- Check HR and BP in both arms, attach continuous cardiac monitor, and obtain 12-lead ECG.
- Brief history—think about the differential diagnosis.
- Analgesia if required (e.g. diamorphine 2.5–10mg IV) + anti-emetic.

| Differential diagnosis of chest pain |
| --- |
| - Acute coronary syndrome |
| - Pericarditis |
| - Myocarditis |
| - Arrhythmias |
| - Pulmonary embolism |
| - Pneumonia |
| - Chest wall pathology |
| - Costochondritis (Tietze syndrome) |
| - Aortic dissection |
| - Gastro-oesophageal spasm or rupture |
| - Odynophagia |
| - Reflux disease |
| - Gallstones and biliary disease |
| - Herpes zoster |

## Investigations

### ECG

ECG is fundamental to the diagnosis of ACS—a good quality tracing is required. Check the ambulance rhythm strip for paroxysmal arrhythmias which may be missed on a single ECG.

In a STEMI, look for:
- ST elevation of >2mm in more than two adjacent chest leads **or** >1mm in two adjacent limb leads.
- Concomitant ST depression in another area indicates reciprocal changes or multivessel disease.
- New LBBB (prolonged QRS duration, M pattern in V5–V6)—may need to check previous ECGs.
- Q waves may develop after several hours or days.
- T wave inversion develops over days to weeks.

Other conditions which may cause similar ECG changes include pericarditis, myocarditis, myocardial contusion, pulmonary embolism, hyperkalaemia, pancreatitis, and intracranial haemorrhage.

### Cardiac enzymes

Troponins are the most sensitive and specific markers of myocardial ischaemia. Troponin levels begin to rise 3 hours after an event and may be elevated for 14 days. Troponin may also rise in pericarditis, pulmonary emboli, and arrhythmias.

### Chest radiograph

Look for mediastinal widening and pulmonary oedema.

## NSTEMI

- More common than STEMIs and tend to occur in older, comorbid, or hospitalized patients.
- Mortality at 6 months is similar to that of STEMI patients.
- Initial management is similar to that of STEMIs but there is no proven role for reperfusion therapy.

### Initial assessment (see Fig. 1.3)

As listed earlier:
- Cardiac monitoring and regular ECGs to check for new changes.
- Measure troponin at 12 hours after onset of symptoms. Check potassium and magnesium and replace if low.

### Anticoagulant and antiplatelet therapy

- Give aspirin 300mg and clopidogrel 300mg.
- Anticoagulate with low-molecular-weight heparin (LMWH; enoxaparin 1mg/kg 12-hourly), or unfractionated heparin (UFH) if risks of bleeding are high. Reduce dose if significant renal impairment.
- GPIIb/IIIa inhibitors such as abciximab, tirofiban, and eptifibatide are useful in patients with intermediate/high-risk features, concurrent diabetes, ST depression, or preceding angiography.
- Abciximab 0.25mg/kg IV bolus, then infuse 0.125mcg/kg/min (max. 10mcg/min) for 12–24 hours.
- Eptifibatide 180mcg/kg IV bolus (repeat bolus in 10min prior to PCI) then infuse 2mcg/kg/min for 3–4 days.
- Tirofiban 0.4mcg/kg/min IV over 30 minutes then infuse at 0.1mcg/kg/min for 2–4 days.

### Other agents

- Nitrates—standard symptomatic therapy but no evidence of benefit in mortality. Give as glyceryl trinitrate (GTN) spray, buccal nitrate, or a GTN infusion (1 mg/hour: titrate to response).
- Beta-blockers—no proven role but give if no contraindication—e.g. metoprolol 50mg PO 8-hourly.
- Calcium channel blockers may be given with beta-blockers especially for ongoing pain. In the longer term, diltiazem may reduce event rate.
- Start high-intensity statin therapy.

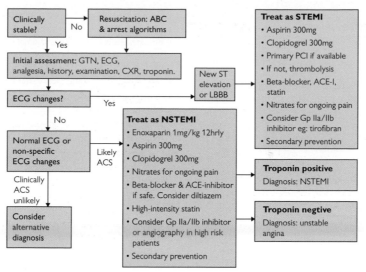

**Fig. 1.3** Summary: management of patients presenting with ACS.

### Invasive evaluation

- Consider angiography in patients with profound or dynamic ECG changes, life-threatening heart failure or arrhythmias, or with severe ongoing angina.
- Angiography within 72 hours of symptom onset followed by revascularization (PCI or coronary artery bypass graft (CABG)) is recommended.
- Many patients may be unsuitable due to comorbidities.

### Afterwards

- Give lifestyle and driving advice (see under 'STEMI'). Refer for cardiac rehabilitation. Give anti-anginals if required.

---

## STEMI

For patients presenting with symptoms and an ECG suggestive of STEMI:

- Initial management as for NSTEMI (see Fig. 1.3).
- Give oxygen, analgesia (+ anti-emetic), nitrates, and aspirin 300mg plus clopidogrel 300mg PO.
- Hypotensive patients should receive cautious 100–500mL boluses of fluid—if hypotension is prolonged, insert central access and consider inotropes.
- Auscultate for the murmur of acute MR.

### Beta-blockers

- Early beta-blockade reduces mortality, infarct size, and complications.
- Especially useful if there is ongoing pain, hypertension, tachycardia, or tachyarrhythmias such as atrial fibrillation (AF).
- Avoid in: HR <60bpm, systolic blood pressure (SBP) <100mmHg, atrioventricular (AV) block, moderate to severe heart failure (negatively inotropic), peripheral vascular disease with ischaemic limb. Caution in inferior infarcts affecting the right ventricle.
- Start with metoprolol 2.5–5mg IV every 1–2 minutes (max. 15–20mg) to achieve a SBP of ~100 110mmHg with a HR of 60–100bpm. If this is tolerated well, start 50mg PO 8-hourly.

### Angiotensin-converting enzyme (ACE) inhibitors

- ACE inhibitors also offer a mortality benefit—high-risk patients, the elderly, and those with large infarcts or concomitant heart failure benefit most.

> **Box 1.1 Reperfusion therapy in STEMI**
>
> *Primary PCI*
> - Gold standard: reduces mortality, reduces further events, and confers better long-term left ventricular function and improved anginal symptoms compared to patients treated with thrombolysis.
> - Indications: all patients with chest pain and ECG changes suggestive of STEMI are potentially suitable.
> - Complications occur in ~1%: stroke, significant bleeding at puncture site, recurrent infarct, emergency CABG, death.
> - Consider discharge in 72 hours.
>
> *Thrombolysis*
> - Indications: symptoms suggestive of myocardial ischaemia for <12 hours with typical ECG changes.
> - Absolute contraindications: active internal bleeding, suspected aortic aneurysm, brain tumour, haemorrhagic stroke (ever), ischaemic stroke (within 1 year), recent head trauma, surgery within 2 weeks with bleeding risk.
> - Relative contraindications: surgery >2 weeks previously, severe hypertension (SBP >180mmHg), warfarin use with INR >2, prolonged CPR (>10 minutes), previous ischaemic stroke >1 year previously, menstruation, liver or renal impairment.
> - Complications (10%): bleeding, intracranial haemorrhage, allergic reactions to older agents, arrhythmias, embolization of plaque.
> - Doses:
>   - Alteplase: 15mg IV bolus then 0.75mg/kg for 30 minutes, then 0.5mg/kg for 60 minutes. Max. 35mg.
>   - Reteplase: 10mg IV bolus. Repeat after 10 minutes.
>   - Tenecteplase: give a bolus of 0.5mg/kg over 10 seconds. Max. 50mg.
>   - Anistreplase: give a bolus of 30mg over 2–5 minutes IV.
> - Consider discharge in 5–7 days.

- Start ramipril 1.25mg PO. The dose can be up-titrated over several days if tolerated. Monitor renal function.

### Reperfusion therapy

- Reperfusion treatment must be carried out as soon as possible after symptom onset—ideally within 4 hours, when 50–70% patients are successfully reperfused with thrombolysis, and 70–90% with primary PCI (Box 1.1).
- Primary PCI is the treatment of choice but is not available in all areas.

### Afterwards

- Consider enoxaparin 1mg/kg 12-hourly, especially post-thrombolysis.
- Consider GPIIb/IIIa inhibitors post-PCI—check local protocol.

- Continue daily aspirin 75mg, clopidogrel 75mg, ACE inhibitor, and beta-blocker.
- Risk stratification with submaximal exercise test, stress echo, or angiography particularly in high-risk patients with further chest pain, arrhythmias, or poor LV function.
- Start a high-dose statin (atorvastatin 80mg).
- Discuss lifestyle factors, exercise, smoking cessation, and dietary advice.
- Avoid driving for 1 week after successful PCI, 4 weeks after MI with no/unsuccessful PCI, or for 6 weeks for group 2 licence holders.

# 1.4 Tachycardia

## Definition

Tachycardia is a fast heart rate, >100 beats per minute (bpm) (see Section 3.4). This may be symptomatic or asymptomatic. Not all tachycardias are pathological: sinus tachycardia can be normal.

## History

- Ask about associated chest pain, syncope/pre-syncope, or breathlessness.
- Ask about caffeine, alcohol, and illicit drug use.
- Check for family history of arrhythmias and sudden death.

## Examination

- Auscultate for murmurs, added heart sounds, and pulmonary oedema.
- Listen for a carotid bruit.
- Look for features of systemic disease: exophthalmos in Graves disease, malar flush, chronic liver disease.

## Investigations (in the acute setting)

- ECG.
- Investigation should include potassium, magnesium, and thyroid function. Check Hb (anaemia).
- In acute symptomatic disease, consider CXR and ABG.

## Sinus tachycardia

Heart rate can be increased in exercise, fever, anaemia, pregnancy, thyrotoxicosis, and acute pulmonary embolism.
  Identify the cause and treat if required.

## Narrow complex tachycardia

These arrhythmias arise from the atria or nodal areas and include atrial fibrillation/flutter, supraventricular tachycardia (SVT), and junctional rhythms. The QRS duration is <120ms.

## Atrial fibrillation/flutter

- Some or all beats can be conducted giving 1:1 to 3:1 AV blocks. On other occasions the block can be variable.
- In fibrillation, beats are erratic and the ECG may show absent or variably sized p waves (Fig. 1.4).
- In flutter, there are regular 'saw-tooth' waves (Fig. 1.5).
- AF may present as acute, paroxysmal, or chronic disease.

*Treatment of atrial fibrillation/flutter*

*Acute management*

- Resuscitation—'ABC', IV access, monitoring.

*Stable (SBP >90mmHg)*

- If BP is adequate, give a beta-blocker—slows rate and helps reversion to sinus rhythm, e.g. metoprolol 50mg, two to three times daily. Caution in patients with pulmonary oedema.
- An alternative is amiodarone, given through a large-bore venous access, ideally a central line: 5mg/kg (usually around 300mg) IV over 1 hour, then 900mg over 24 hours.
- In young patients, or those without ischaemic heart disease, flecainide (2mg/kg IV over 25 minutes or 300mg orally) may be helpful. In patients who respond, it can be used as a 'pill in the pocket' regimen for paroxysmal AF. Flecainide is not advised in atrial flutter as it can provoke a 1:1 block and worsening tachycardia.
- If BP poor (SBP 90–110mmHg), consider digoxin (a weak inotrope). Dose according to weight—give two loading doses of 250–500mcg PO/IV 6 hours apart, then start daily dosing at 125–250mcg. Check levels after several days. Reduce maintenance doses with renal impairment.

*Unstable (SBP <90mmHg)*

- DC cardioversion may be appropriate if decompensated.
- Ask for anaesthetic help: patients need sedation or a brief general anaesthetic. Cardiovert with 120–150J biphasic (synchronized); deliver two further shocks at higher energy levels if initially unsuccessful.
- Use lower energy levels (e.g. start at 70–120J biphasic) in atrial flutter.
- IV amiodarone if unsuccessful.

## Supraventricular tachycardia (SVT)

This arrhythmia is commonly paroxysmal and occurs at ~140–250bpm.

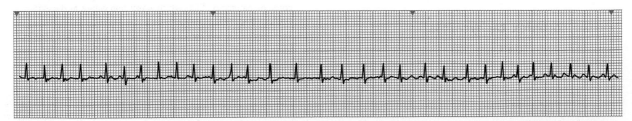

**Fig. 1.4** Fast atrial fibrillation with a ventricular response of 236bpm. Reproduced with the kind permission of Dr. med. Oliver Meyer, MME.

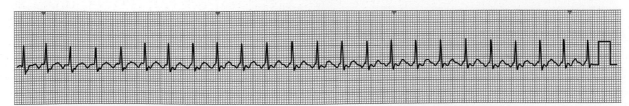

**Fig. 1.5** Atrial flutter with sawtooth pattern and 2:1 block. Reproduced with the kind permission of Dr. med. Oliver Meyer, MME.

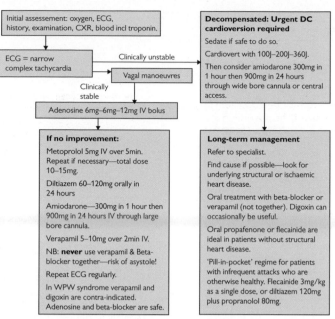

| Initial assessement: oxygen, ECG, history, examination, CXR, blood incl troponin. | | **Decompensated: Urgent DC cardioversion required**<br>Sedate if safe to do so.<br>Cardiovert with 100J–200J–360J.<br>Then consider amiodarone 300mg in 1 hour then 900mg in 24 hours through wide bore cannula or central access. |
|---|---|---|

ECG = narrow complex tachycardia — Clinically unstable →

Vagal manoeuvres

Clinically stable

Adenosine 6mg–6mg–12mg IV bolus

**If no improvement:**
Metoprolol 5mg IV over 5min. Repeat if necessary—total dose 10–15mg.

Diltiazem 60–120mg orally in 24 hours

Amiodarone—300mg in 1 hour then 900mg in 24 hours IV through large bore cannula.

Verapamil 5–10mg over 2min IV.

NB: **never** use verapamil & Beta-blocker together—risk of asystole!

Repeat ECG regularly.

In WPW syndrome verapamil and digoxin are contra-indicated. Adenosine and beta-blocker are safe.

**Long-term management**
Refer to specialist.

Find cause if possible—look for underlying structural or ischaemic heart disease.

Oral treatment with beta-blocker or verapamil (not together). Digoxin can occasionally be useful.

Oral propafenone or flecainide are ideal in patients without structural heart disease.

'Pill-in-pocket' regime for patients with infrequent attacks who are otherwise healthy. Flecainide 3mg/kg as a single dose, or diltiazem 120mg plus propranolol 80mg.

**Fig. 1.6** Summary: management of patients presenting with supraventricular tachycardia (SVT).

*Treatment*
- Vagal manoeuvres (e.g. Valsalva manoeuvre, carotid sinus massage) may occasionally restore sinus rhythm (Fig. 1.6).
- Adenosine: initially, give 6mg quickly through a large-bore cannula: elevate arm, and immediately flush with 10mL saline. This will cardiovert some patients, and allows identification of underlying rhythm in others. If unsuccessful, give up to three further bolus doses in 3mg increments (up to 12mg). Patients experience a sense of impending doom due to transient AV block: warn them!
- If this does not work, consider beta-blockers, verapamil, diltiazem, or amiodarone.
- Avoid beta-blockers and adenosine in patients with significant asthma, and IV verapamil in patients already taking beta-blockers.
- As with patients in AF, if the patient is unstable or deteriorating, consider urgent DC cardioversion.

### Wolff–Parkinson–White (WPW) syndrome
- When treating patients with WPW syndrome, avoid digoxin and verapamil. Beta-blockers and adenosine are safe.

## Broad complex tachycardia

These arrhythmias have QRS >120ms and usually arise from the ventricles.

### Ventricular tachycardia (VT)
- Patients with VT (Fig. 1.7) may present with a spectrum of clinical effects, from palpitations and breathlessness to cardiac arrest. Some patients attend outpatient clinics with a history of episodic collapse.
- Treatment—see Fig. 1.8.
- Those in peri-arrest situations with hypotension, cardiac failure, and severe symptoms should be assessed for urgent DC cardioversion. Conscious patients should be sedated prior to cardioversion if it is safe to do so.
- A minority of patients presenting with VT are relatively stable. These patients could be treated with amiodarone intravenously.
- Untreated, VT can result in VF and cardiac arrest. All patients should receive continuous cardiac monitoring usually in a coronary care unit setting.
- Consider the cause: check troponin in case of myocardial infarction, check electrolytes and replace if necessary. If the cause is not clear, refer for investigation.

### Torsades de pointes
- Torsades de pointes is a variation of VT causing a regular broad complex pattern on ECG which waxes and wanes as the axis changes (Fig. 1.9).
- Torsades de pointes can occur when there is prolonged ventricular repolarization, with a long QT interval on ECG (Box 1.2).
- Treat (see Fig. 1.8) and address the underlying cause.

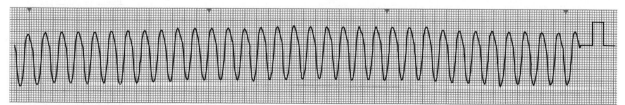

**Fig. 1.7** Ventricular tachycardia (VT): regular broad complex tachycardia. Reproduced with the kind permission of Dr. med. Oliver Meyer, MME.

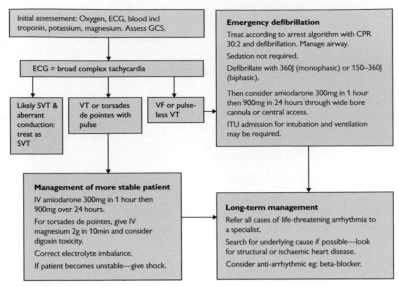

**Fig. 1.8** Management of broad complex tachycardia.

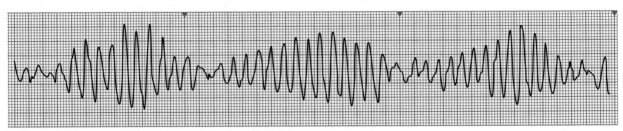

**Fig. 1.9** Torsades de pointes: regular rotating broad complex tachycardia. Reproduced with the kind permission of Dr. med. Oliver Meyer, MME.

---

### Box 1.2 Causes of prolonged QT interval and torsades de pointes

**Congenital:**
- Romano–Ward syndrome
- Jervell and Lange–Nielson syndrome.

**Drugs:**
- Class Ia anti-arrhythmics, e.g. quinidine, procainamide
- Class III anti-arrhythmics, e.g. amiodarone, sotalol
- Tricyclic antidepressants, e.g. amitriptyline
- Macrolides, e.g. erythromycin

**Electrolyte disturbance:**
- Hypokalaemia
- Hypomagnesaemia
- Hypocalcaemia

**Pathological/physiological:**
- Prolonged fasting
- Mitral valve prolapse
- Acute myocardial infarction
- CNS disease

### Ventricular fibrillation (VF)

VF is not compatible with life: patients present with cardiac arrest. There may be occasional fibrillation pulse beats felt, but there is an absence of a regular, functional pulse.

- In VF, the ECG shows irregularly sized broad complexes of chaotic ventricular activity (Fig. 1.10).
- VF should be treated according to the cardiac arrest algorithms with prompt defibrillation and CPR.
- A common cause of VF is myocardial infarction. With prompt successful defibrillation, the prognosis for these patients is reasonably good.

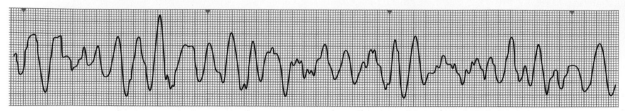

**Fig. 1.10** Ventricular fibrillation (VF): irregular broad complex tachycardia. Reproduced with the kind permission of Dr. med. Oliver Meyer, MME.

# 1.5 Bradycardia

## Definition

- Bradycardia is a slow HR, <60bpm.
- For some patients, this represents normal variation between individuals.
- At night, the HR can drop to 50bpm.
- Consider treating patients with HR <40bpm or with symptoms of bradycardia (see Section 3.4).

## History and examination

- Ask about palpitations, dizziness, collapse, chest pain, ankle oedema, breathlessness, and family history of sudden death.
- Ask about medication—any changes recently?
- Look for signs of cardiac failure, cardiomegaly, or previous cardiac surgery.
- Auscultate for murmurs.
- Look for features of hypothyroidism or connective tissue diseases such as systemic lupus erythematosus (SLE) and rheumatoid arthritis (RA).

## Investigations

- Observations including BP, HR, and temperature are fundamental to the initial assessment.
- ECG and rhythm strip—repeat regularly.
- Blood tests including FBC, U&Es (especially K$^+$), calcium, magnesium, thyroid function, and possibly troponin.
- CXR—to check for pulmonary oedema and cardiac size.
- Haemodynamically unstable patients should receive continuous cardiac monitoring.

## Sinus bradycardia

There is a P wave prior to every QRS complex but rate <60bpm. Causes include:
- Normal variation.
- Medications such as beta-blockers and digoxin.
- Sick sinus syndrome.
- Hypothyroidism.
- Hypothermia.

This rhythm does not always need treatment, particularly if the patient is asymptomatic. If medication is the cause, consider reducing the dose or changing to an alternative agent.

## Heart block

### First-degree heart block
Long PR interval (>0.2 seconds), can be normal variation (Fig. 1.11).

### Second-degree heart block
Mobitz I (Wenkebach)—PR interval increases over several beats with eventual absent QRS (Fig. 1.12).
Mobitz II—unconducted P waves which can have a regular pattern (e.g. 3:1 or 2:1). PR interval remains constant (Fig. 1.13).

### Third-degree (complete) heart block
Complete dissociation of atrial and ventricular beats. P waves are not followed by QRS complexes (Fig. 1.14).

## Treatment of bradycardias

Treat all patients with symptoms or HR <40bpm.
- Medications such as beta-blockers and digoxin should be stopped or doses reduced.
- Oxygen if hypoxic or unstable.
- Atropine 0.6–1.2mg IV repeated to maximum dose of 3mg.
- Isoprenaline 0.2mg IV. If patient remains unstable, start an infusion at 1mg in 100mL saline and infuse at 1mcg/min. Titrate up according to HR response.
- Secure good venous access in all patients—many may require central access.
- In stable but symptomatic patients, admit and consider pacemaker insertion.
- In severely compromised patients (cardiac arrest, asystole, hypotensive (SBP <90mmHg), confused, or hypoxic due to pulmonary oedema), consider pacing to maintain output.
- Consider external pacing in an emergency setting or post-infarct/thrombolysis. External pacing is uncomfortable and should be used as a temporary measure only until a pacing wire can be inserted. Patients may require sedation to tolerate external pacing.
- A transvenous pacing wire is a more comfortable option for patients but is a more challenging procedure. Central access is

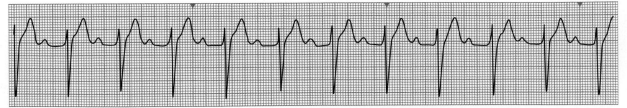

**Fig. 1.11** First-degree heart block. Reproduced with the kind permission of Dr. med. Oliver Meyer, MME.

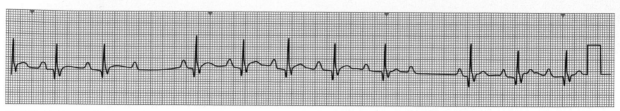

**Fig. 1.12** Mobitz type I (Wenckebach) second-degree heart block. Reproduced with the kind permission of Dr. med. Oliver Meyer, MME.

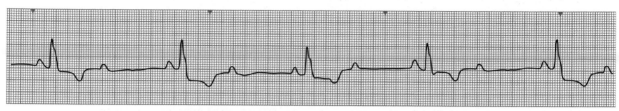

**Fig. 1.13** Mobitz type II second-degree heart block. Reproduced with the kind permission of Dr. med. Oliver Meyer, MME.

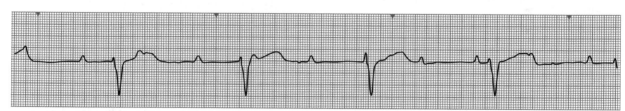

**Fig. 1.14** Third-degree (complete) heart block. Reproduced with the kind permission of Dr. med. Oliver Meyer, MME.

obtained, usually via the left internal jugular vein, and a pacing wire is fed carefully into the right atrium and through the tricuspid valve. The pacing wire is then manoeuvred to place the tip of the wire at the tip of the right ventricle. Position and pacing effect are checked. Once the wire is in a satisfactory position, pacing can commence at around 70bpm. Check the rhythm strip to ensure there is successful capture. Risks of the procedure include perforation, pneumothorax, tamponade, diaphragmatic pacing, and arrhythmias.

## Permanent pacemakers

- The definitive treatment for persistent or symptomatic bradycardias.
- Consider a pacemaker for patients with:
  - Complete AV block
  - Mobitz type II block
  - Persistent AV block post-infarct
  - Sick sinus syndrome
  - Symptomatic bradycardias
- The pacemaker is usually inserted just under the skin around the left pectoral area. The procedure is straightforward and done under local anaesthetic with few major complications. Prophylactic antibiotics may be given.
- Suspect pacemaker malfunction if there is bradycardia with no pacing spikes, if there are spikes with no capture, or if there are inappropriate spikes.
- Pacemakers can last up to 15 years and require an annual pacing check.

# 1.6 Hypertensive emergencies

## Definitions

- A hypertensive **crisis** constitutes an acute, severe elevation in arterial blood pressure (typically SBP >200mmHg, DBP >130mmHg) with significant threat of microvascular damage, if the rate of change is rapid.
- A hypertensive **emergency** implies the presence of end-organ damage, which will become irreversible within a matter of hours if sustained. Examples include encephalopathy, retinal haemorrhages, papilloedema, and acute kidney injury (AKI).
- A hypertensive **urgency** may have 'softer' symptoms, without demonstrable end-organ damage, but threatens the same within days if left untreated.
- Classifications are ultimately somewhat academic and a general approach to evaluation and management is presented here. If in any doubt seek senior/specialist support early. In specialist centres, clinical pharmacologists offer expert advice.

## Presentation

- May be asymptomatic.
- Non-specific symptoms, e.g. mild headache, epistaxis.
- Features of renal damage (hypertensive nephrosclerosis):
  - Haematuria
  - Proteinuria
  - AKI
- Neurological complications/encephalopathy:
  - Severe headache
  - Nausea and vomiting
  - Focal neurological deficits
  - Fits
  - Confusion
  - Coma
  - Intracranial haemorrhage
- Visual symptoms/signs:
  - Retinopathy/papilloedema
- Cardiovascular symptoms/associations:
  - Chest pain
  - Myocardial infarction
  - Left ventricular failure with pulmonary oedema
  - Aortic dissection
- Features of precipitating condition:
  - Phaeochromocytoma
  - Pregnancy (eclampsia/pre-eclampsia)
  - Chronic renal disease
  - Rheumatological conditions
- In the context of acute withdrawal of antihypertensive therapy.

Ask about/look for previous history of hypertension to help determine the rate of elevation.

## Examination

- Fundi (looking in particular for grade 3 or 4 retinopathy with progression to bilateral retinal haemorrhages, exudates, and papilloedema).
- BP in both arms.
- Cardiomegaly.
- Left ventricular function.
- Peripheral pulses.

- Renal masses.
- Focal neurology.

## Investigations

- FBC: microangiopathic haemolytic anaemia (MAHA).
- U&Es: renal failure/hypokalaemia.
- Clotting: disseminated intravascular coagulation (DIC).
- CXR: cardiomegaly, pulmonary oedema, widened mediastinum.
- Urinalysis: blood/protein/casts.
- Glucose: always important to check if encephalopathy.

Consider:
- Urine albumin:creatinine ratio (ACR).
- Urinary/plasma metanephrines.
- Plasma renin/aldosterone.
- Echo: left ventricular hypertrophy (LVH)/dissection.
- Renal ultrasound scan (USS): renal size.
- Magnetic resonance (MR) renal angiogram: renal artery stenosis.
- CT aortography: aortic dissection.
- CT head: intracranial haemorrhage.
- Toxicology screen: cocaine, amphetamines.

## Admission criteria

- DBP persistently >120mmHg.
- Retinal haemorrhages or papilloedema.
- Encephalopathy or focal neurology.
- AKI.
- Suspicion of dissection, phaeochromocytoma, pre-eclampsia, eclampsia, or cardiac disease.

## Management principles

In general, the cardinal rule is that rapid reduction of BP is dangerous and should be avoided. Cerebral blood flow autoregulation is disturbed in severe hypertension and local flow can drop precipitously leading to watershed infarcts. Cortical blindness, myocardial infarction, and death may also ensue.

The main focus of treatment is thus to lower BP in a controlled manner. Normality is **not** the desired endpoint. This is more important than the choice of agent. Longer-acting antihypertensives are favoured and oral medications have a better side effect profile. Short-acting oral and sublingual agents should be avoided. Beta-blockers and long-acting calcium channel blockers are reasonable first-line treatments with a reduction target of ~20mmHg BP per day.

More rapid reversal of extreme hypertension is, however, mandated in aortic dissection and myocardial infarction.

A comprehensive discussion of available antihypertensive agents and their properties is beyond the scope of this chapter. Local guidelines may exist or consult the BNF.

## Acute management of the hypertensive emergency

- Transfer the patient to a high dependency setting.
- Consider arterial and central venous monitoring.
- Catheterize and monitor urine output.
- If early features: use oral therapy (e.g. amlodipine 5mg).

- Parenteral treatment is indicated with late symptoms or deterioration. Titratable medications given as continuous infusions are preferred. Suggested first-line approaches in specific presentations are discussed as follows.

### Hypertensive emergency with retinopathy

- Beta-blockade (e.g. labetalol bolus followed by infusion, aiming for reduction to 100mmHg DBP or 20–25mmHg/day, whichever is the lesser reduction).

### Hypertensive emergency with encephalopathy

- Sodium nitroprusside/GTN as first line, aiming for 25% reduction in diastolic BP over 1–2 hours.

### Hypertensive emergency in context of stroke/intracranial haemorrhage

- Only treat, and then with caution, if DBP >130mmHg *and* clinical signs of cerebral oedema. Neurology/neurosurgery input advised.

### Hypertensive emergency with acute LVF

- Opiates, furosemide, and sodium nitroprusside/GTN.

### Hypertensive emergency with AKI

- Treat AKI as per Sections 1.11 and 17.6.
- Nephrology input advised.

### Hypertensive emergency in context of phaeochromocytoma

- Alpha-blockade with phentolamine and/or phenoxybenzamine.

### Hypertensive emergency in context of aortic dissection

- Beta-blockade (e.g. labetalol), sodium nitroprusside/GTN.
- Aim to reduce SBP to 100–120mmHg rapidly. Cardiology/cardiothoracic input advised.

### Hypertensive emergency in eclampsia/pre-eclampsia

- Deliver the baby.
- Magnesium sulphate/hydralazine.

## Summary

Management should usually be in a high-dependency setting with early specialist input. After the acute phase, BP should be gradually and cautiously normalized under the care of a specialist cardiology or clinical pharmacology team.

# 1.7 Pulmonary oedema

## Definition

- The extravasation of fluid from the pulmonary circulation into the interstitial spaces and alveoli of the lung.
- Causes acute or chronic breathlessness and may be accompanied by wheeze and expectoration of pink, frothy sputum.

## Aetiology and diagnosis

Pulmonary oedema has many causes, although it is most commonly due to cardiac disease. Causes include:

- Cardiac failure with inadequate left ventricular function.
- Obstructed flow through the left heart: tamponade, cardiomyopathy, myxoma, or valvular disease.
- High output states: anaemia, thyrotoxicosis, or shunts.
- Renal causes: acute or chronic renal failure or renal artery stenosis with hypertension.
- Hypoalbuminaemia of any cause such as liver failure, nephrotic syndrome, or a systemic inflammatory response.
- Infection, including aspiration.
- ARDS.
- DIC.
- Lymphangitis carcinomatosis: blockage of lymphatic ducts.
- Other causes: including prescribed medication (e.g. NSAIDs, beta-blockers), eclampsia, alcohol, altitude, heroin, and drug overdoses.

## Immediate management for acute cardiac failure

- Give oxygen to maintain saturations >95% (>90% in chronic obstructive pulmonary disease (COPD) patients). Monitor with ABGs.
- IV access, continuous ECG monitoring and regular measurement of BP.
- Diuretic treatment should be initiated promptly. Give 40–100mg furosemide IV and reassess. Many patients require repeated doses.
- Give IV diamorphine 2.5–5mg IV (and IV anti-emetic).
- If SBP >90mmHg give sublingual GTN (two puffs) or buccally (2mg or 5mg buccal tablet).
- Reassess patient—is pulmonary oedema the correct diagnosis and is the underlying cause apparent?—see Box 1.3. Send blood samples and arrange urgent CXR.
- If SBP>100 mmHg commence nitrate infusion (caution may be required to maintain BP): start with 0.5–10mL/hour (start at 1mL/hour) of 50mg GTN in 50mL of saline and titrate carefully to achieve symptom control while maintaining SBP >90mmHg.
- Consider further doses of diuretic if not improving.
- Non-invasive ventilation such as continuous positive airway pressure (CPAP) improves left ventricular function by reducing afterload. Start with a positive end-expiratory pressure of 5cmH$_2$O and titrate up to 10cmH$_2$O with a FiO$_2$ of >40%.
- Consider referral to ITU and invasive ventilation in patients with insufficient oxygenation despite high-flow oxygen administration. Early referral improves survival.
- If SBP <100mmHg then consider inotropic support and ITU/HDU level care, especially if hypotension, cardiogenic shock, and evidence of tissue hypoperfusion, such as acidosis, clammy

---

### Box 1.3  Clinical features of pulmonary oedema

- Breathlessness, exertional or constant.
- Cough, productive of pink, frothy sputum in severe disease.
- Basal coarse crepitations.
- Cyanosis.
- Fluid overload with pleural effusions.

*Look for the underlying cause—clinically*
- Take a careful history, particularly of medication use.
- Orthopnoea and paroxysmal nocturnal dyspnoea are typically cardiac symptoms.
- S3 gallop rhythm indicates left ventricular failure or fluid overload states.
- Listen for features of valvular disease.
- Look for signs of right heart failure (pulsatile hepatomegaly, raised JVP, peripheral oedema) which would indicate congestive cardiac failure.
- Conjunctival pallor in anaemia.
- Goitre, tremor, lid lag, or proptosis in thyrotoxicosis.
- Signs of alcohol use: parotid swelling, spider naevi, and other stigmata of chronic liver disease.
- Petechial rash with bruising or ecchymosis in DIC.

*Look for the underlying cause—investigations*
- Do an ECG to check for arrhythmias or MI.
- CXR is essential to confirm a clinical diagnosis.
- FBC, clotting, U&Es, LFT, TFT.
- Check troponin to identify ACS.
- CT may be indicated where the diagnosis is unclear, and is useful for lymphangitis carcinomatosis.
- Consider echocardiography.

*CXR evidence of pulmonary oedema*
- Blunting of costophrenic angle or frank pleural effusions, usually bilateral (see Fig. 1.15).
- Fluid in the horizontal fissure (Fig. 1.15: right mid-zone).
- Kerley B lines (horizontal lines).
- Upper lobe diversion.
- Fluffy-looking infiltrates throughout lung fields in severe disease.
- Think about cause: look for cardiomegaly, valve replacements, and sternotomy wires.

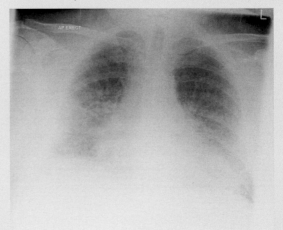

Fig. 1.15 Antero-posterior chest radiograph of patient with pulmonary oedema showing bilateral fluffy infiltrates, fluid in the horizontal fissure, and upper lobe blood vessel diversion.

peripheries, or confusion. Consider dobutamine (2–3mcg/kg/min) or dopamine (2–3mg/kg/min) with continuous cardiac monitoring.

Also:

- Catheterize patients to measure fluid output.
- Renal function must be carefully monitored as most treatments have a nephrotoxic effect.

- Haemodialysis or haemofiltration may be required for patients with concomitant cardiac and renal failure.
- *In extremis*, venesection (e.g. 500mL) is an option but rarely undertaken in practice.
- Address the underlying cause: e.g. patients with a new ischaemic event may require treatment for acute coronary syndrome.

# 1.8 Acute asthma

## Background

Acute, severe asthma is a medical emergency and a common cause of morbidity and mortality in children and young adults (see Section 18.12).

## Classification according to British Thoracic Society guidelines

### Moderate exacerbation of asthma
- Peak expiratory flow rate (PEFR) 50–75% best or predicted.
- Increasing symptoms.
- No features of acute severe asthma.

### Acute severe asthma
One of the following:
- PEFR 33–50% best or predicted.
- Respiratory rate >25/minute.
- Heart rate >110/minute.
- Unable to complete sentences in one breath.

### Life-threatening asthma
One of the following:
- PEFR <33% best or predicted.
- Oxygen saturation <92%.
- $PaO_2$ <8kPa.
- Silent chest.
- Cyanosis.
- Poor respiratory effort.
- Arrhythmia.
- Exhaustion or reduced conscious level.

### Near-fatal asthma
One of the following:
- Rising $PaCO_2$ levels.
- Requiring mechanical ventilation.

## Investigations
- CXR if there is suspected infection, pneumothorax, or features of life-threatening asthma. Do **NOT** send the patient to the radiology department.
- Pulse oximetry—concerns develop if saturations <92%.
- ABGs—show type 1 respiratory failure initially. A low $PaCO_2$ suggests that the patient is not yet tiring. A rising $PaCO_2$, even into the reference range, should prompt consideration of treatment escalation.

## Management
- Involve senior colleagues early (including anaesthetists).
- Oxygen therapy (at least 60% with a high-flow mask) to maintain saturations >94%.
- Inhaled or nebulized $\beta_2$ agonist bronchodilator, e.g. salbutamol 2.5–5mg nebs 4–6-hourly and additionally as required (up to every 15 minutes).
- Nebulized ipratropium bromide (0.5mg 4–6-hourly) in patients with acute severe or life-threatening asthma or in those with inadequate response to previous therapies.
- Nebulizers should be oxygen-driven.
- Steroids are essential—give IV hydrocortisone 100–200mg initially or oral prednisolone (30–50mg) if able to swallow. Continue either 100mg IV four times a day or prednisolone 30–50mg for at least 5 days. Oral steroids are preferred after the initial presentation as they have a longer duration of action than intravenous alternatives.
- Magnesium sulphate 1.2–2g infused IV over 20 minutes is used in patients who are not improving after initial measures (single dose only).
- Consider an IV salbutamol and/or aminophylline infusion in those with severe asthma or when there is clinical deterioration in spite of other treatments.
- Do not give a loading dose of aminophylline in those taking oral theophyllines and check levels daily. Reduce the dose in those with cirrhosis or congestive heart failure and in those taking erythromycin or ciprofloxacin.
- Patients should not be given antibiotics routinely unless there is convincing evidence of infection, e.g. fever, raised CRP, raised WCC, or consolidation on CXR.
- Repeated and regular clinical assessment is warranted including ABGs and PEFR measurements.
- Ensure that the patient is properly hydrated. Remember that $\beta_2$ agonists may lower serum potassium levels.
- In the longer term, patients with severe or life-threatening asthma should receive respiratory outpatient follow-up.
- Check inhaler technique in patients with frequent exacerbations.

### Which patients may be suitable to send home?
- Patients with no features of life-threatening asthma or no features of acute severe asthma following initial treatment.
- Patients with PEFR ≥75% predicted 1 hour after treatment.

### Which patients require referral to ITU?
- Those with severe and life-threatening asthma, failing to respond to therapy.
- Hypoxia, $PaO_2$ <8kPa despite 60% inhaled $O_2$.
- Hypercapnia, rising or $PaCO_2$ > 6kPa.
- Exhaustion, deteriorating conscious level, or coma.

## Differential diagnosis—is it really asthma?

Other diagnoses to consider:
- Pulmonary embolism—may present with wheeze.
- COPD—ask about smoking history and look for type 2 respiratory failure.
- Foreign body—can cause wheeze and stridor particularly common in children.
- Cystic fibrosis—often presents in childhood with persistent cough, wheeze and recurrent infections.
- Eosinophilic granulomatosis with polyangiitis (EGPA, formerly known as Churg-Strauss syndrome)—systemic vasculitis causing eosinophilic asthma, pulmonary haemorrhage with haemoptysis, and renal impairment.
- Tracheomalacia—softening of the tracheal cartilage causes airways obstruction, wheeze, and stridor.
- Alpha-1 antitrypsin deficiency—often misdiagnosed as asthma in early stages. Check liver function.
- Gastro-oesophageal reflux disease—recurrent minor aspiration of acid may cause chronic cough, wheeze, and mild breathlessness. Consider a trial of a proton pump inhibitor.

# 1.9 Massive pulmonary embolism

## Background

Pulmonary embolism (PE) is diagnosed in around 1 in 1000 patients per year and is an important unrecognized cause of death with a prevalence of 1–8% in postmortem studies (see Section 18.14).

## Clinical features of massive PE

- Pleuritic chest pain, dyspnoea, and palpitations may be present, as in non-massive PE.
- Collapse and/or loss of consciousness.
- Sudden cardiovascular instability.
- Hypotension (SBP <90mmHg, or BP fallen >40mmHg).
- Tachycardia.
- Cardiac arrest—PEA is common and has a very poor outlook.

## Risk factors

- Immobility
- Recent surgery/fracture
- Pregnancy/postpartum
- Stroke
- Spinal cord injury
- Air travel
- Varicose veins
- Metastatic malignancy
- Pelvic mass
- Chemotherapy
- Thrombotic tendency
- Oral oestrogens

## Investigations

- In unstable patients, investigations must be arranged quickly and safely. The gold standard is computed tomography pulmonary angiography (CTPA) scanning which shows filling defects in the central pulmonary circulation.
- Echocardiography is a very useful bedside test which can demonstrate right ventricular (RV) strain and may even visualize the emboli.
- ECG: right ventricular strain pattern, right axis deviation, or tachycardia.
- ABGs: type 1 respiratory failure.

## Initial treatment and resuscitation

- ABC.
- High-flow oxygen, regular observations, regular ABGs.

| Poor prognostic factors | |
| --- | --- |
| - Hypotension | - Cardiac arrest |
| - Altered mental state | - Cardiogenic shock |
| - Hypoxia | - RV dilatation |
| - Malignancy | - Brain natriuretic peptide (BNP) elevated. |

- Cardiac monitoring is essential—patients with massive PE are prone to arrhythmias (Fig. 1.16).

### Treat hypotension

- Consider rapid 0.5–1L crystalloid fluids to improve preload and RV end-diastolic volume.

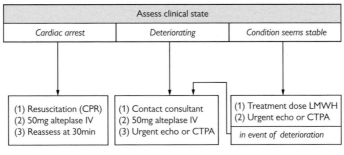

Comments

1. Massive PE is highly likely if:
    - collapse/hypotension, and
    - unexplained hypoxia, and
    - engorged neck veins, and
    - right ventricular gallop (often)

2. In stable patients where massive PE has been confirmed, iv dose of alteplase is 100mg in 90min (i.e. accelerated myocardial infarction regimen).

3. Thrombolysis is followed by unfractionated heparin after 3 hours, preferably weight-adjusted.

4. A few units have facilities for clot fragmentation via pulmonary artery catheter. Elsewhere, contraindications to thrombolysis should be ignored in life-threatening PE.

5. "Blue light" patients with out-of-hospital cardiac arrest due to PE rarely recover.

**Fig. 1.16** Management of patient presenting with probable massive pulmonary embolus (PE).
Reproduced from 'British Thoracic Society guidelines for the management of suspected acute pulmonary embolism', 58, 2003, with permission from BMJ Publishing Group Ltd.

- If hypotension persists, consider insertion of a central line or Swan–Ganz catheter with vascular pressure monitoring to guide fluid administration. Giving more fluids without invasive monitoring risks exacerbating RV stress and may worsen cardiac output.
- Inotropes should be considered early to maintain BP that has not responded to initial fluids.
- First-line agents include dopamine (2.5–10mcg/kg/min) and dobutamine (2–5mcg/kg/min). Noradrenaline may be used additionally, or as an alternative.
- Involve senior colleagues and ITU/CCU teams.

### Thrombolysis in massive PE

- Indications include suspected or confirmed PE with cardiovascular instability and significant hypotension or pending cardiac arrest.
- Absolute contraindications to thrombolysis include recent haemorrhage, haemorrhagic stroke, and current GI haemorrhage.
- Relative contraindications include surgery within 7 days, history of peptic ulcer or other GI or urological bleeding, pancreatitis, endocarditis, and prolonged CPR.
- Thrombolysis with alteplase is first-line treatment for massive PE. It may be given on clinical grounds alone if there is concern about imminent cardiac arrest.
- Start alteplase with a 10mg IV bolus over 1–2 minutes, then an infusion of 90mg over 2 hours. In patients <65kg, total dose should be reduced to 1.5mg/kg.

- Alternative agents for thrombolysis include reteplase (unlicensed for PE), streptokinase, and urokinase (less effective in trials, older agents).
- Massive PE in pregnancy requires specialist obstetric involvement. British Thoracic Society guidelines suggest that thrombolysis is advisable in massive PE but not within 6 hours of delivery or in the early postpartum period due to bleeding risks.
- If thrombolysis fails in a deteriorating patient, consider surgical embolectomy.

### Anticoagulate

- In massive PE, heparin is generally used after thrombolysis as an infusion without a bolus.
- If thrombolysis is contraindicated or in non-massive PE, treatment with LMWH is standard. UFH is an alternative where rapid reversal of effect is desired.
- LMWH, e.g. enoxaparin: give 1.5mg/kg in a single daily dose. Adjust dose in renal failure to 1mg/kg/day and monitor anti-Xa levels.
- Heparin: start with an IV bolus of 5000–10,000 units then infuse at 400–600 units/kg/day. Monitor APPT aiming to keep the ratio between 1.5 and 2.5.

### Once stable

- Start oral anticoagulants (target INR 2.5 in uncomplicated cases) and continue LMWH until INR >2.
- Consider investigating for malignancy or thrombophilia.

# 1.10 Acute upper gastrointestinal haemorrhage

## Background

Acute upper GI haemorrhage is a life-threatening emergency in which clinical diagnosis is based on the history, and early intensive resuscitation with emergency access to an endoscopy service is the key to effective management (see Section 8.5).

## Presentation

- Fresh haematemesis or coffee-ground vomit.
- Melaena.
- Collapse.
- Hypovolaemic shock.
- Rectal bleeding.
- Complications of anaemia—chest pain, dyspnoea.

## Examination

- HR, BP (including postural), peripheral perfusion—evidence of hypovolaemia and shock.
- Evidence of chronic liver disease—raises suspicion of variceal bleed.
- Rectal examination for melaena.

## Investigations

- FBC—anaemia (specifically Hb drop >2g/dL).
- U&Es—increased urea levels (relative to creatinine) due to digested blood, renal function.
- LFT and coagulation screen.
- Group and save sample—haematemesis complicated by shock should initiate a 4–6 unit cross-match.
- ABGs—lactic acidosis indicates poor tissue perfusion.
- CXR—perforation (subdiaphragmatic air) and aspiration.
- ECG—cardiac ischaemia.

### Rockall scoring
Used to risk stratify—very effective at predicting risk of:
(a) Death
(b) Re-bleeding (Table 1.2)

## Management: massive haemorrhage and Rockall score ≥1

- Immediate management should involve protection of airway from risk of aspiration, fluid resuscitation, correction of coagulopathy, and emergency access to endoscopy.

Table 1.2 Rockall scoring

| Variable | 0 | 1 | 2 | 3 |
|---|---|---|---|---|
| Age (years) | <60 | 60–79 | >80 | |
| Shock | None | HR >100bpm | SBP <100bpm | |
| Comorbidity | None | | CCF/IHD | Liver/renal failure |
| | | | Other major disease | Disseminated malignancy |

Reproduced from *Gut*, T A Rockall, R F Logan, H B Devlin, T C Northfield, 'Risk assessment after acute upper gastrointestinal haemorrhage', 38, 3, pp. 316–321, Copyright 1996, with permission from BMJ Publishing Group Ltd.

- Airway protection: avoid supine position due to risk of aspiration. Improve cerebral perfusion by head-down position in hypotension.
- Intubation—required if low GCS.
- Oxygen delivery to maintain saturations ≥95%—care with mask due to vomiting.
- Minimum 2 × large-bore IV cannulae (>18G/green).
- Rapid fluid resuscitation (colloid or crystalloid).

After 1–2L use blood or plasma expanders (if necessary):

- Transfusion of packed red cells if massive bleed, Hb <8g/dL, or Hb <10g/dL with postural hypotension.
- Correct coagulopathy if active bleeding and INR >1.5 or PT >3 seconds prolonged. Use FFP/vitamin K/Beriplex® (Beriplex® and vitamin K if warfarinized).
- Give platelets if count < 50 × 10⁹/L and active bleeding.
- Urinary catheter—hourly urine output aiming >0.5mL/kg/hour.
- High dependency monitoring.
- The aim is to resuscitate patients such that they are cardiovascularly stable by the point of endoscopy, i.e. euvolaemic with normal BP (and no postural drop), minimal tachycardia and normal urine output.

Urgent referral for endoscopy:

- Emergency endoscopy is indicated in:
  - Shocked patients (once resuscitated).
  - Continued bleeding, or re-bleeding.
  - Variceal bleeds (known or suspected).
- Endoscopy significantly reduces probability of re-bleeding/surgery/death if there is active bleeding, or a non-bleeding vessel visible. It allows the distinction to be made between variceal and non-variceal bleeding, and gives information regarding the underlying pathology.
- Warn the surgical team pre-endoscopy: performing endoscopy in the operating theatre may be a sensible precaution.

## Variceal bleeding

- Involve anaesthetic colleagues early for airway protection.
- Early specialist gastroenterology input.
- IV vasopressin analogue (e.g. terlipressin IV 2g four times a day).
- IV antibiotic therapy: third-generation cephalosporin.
- Early endoscopy—sclerotherapy, injection, and banding.
- Consideration of balloon tamponade (Sengstaken–Blakemore tube) and transjugular intrahepatic portosystemic shunt (TIPSS).

## Peptic ulcer disease (post-endoscopy)

- IV proton pump inhibitor—stat dose then 72-hour infusion to reduce risk of re-bleed (e.g. omeprazole 80mg IV stat then 8mg/hour IVI).
- 12–24 hours nil by mouth prior to reintroduction of clear fluids if no signs of re-bleed.
- Discontinue any contributing risk factors.
- *Helicobacter pylori* eradication where required.
- Repeat endoscopy in 4–6 weeks.

## Management: Rockall score 0

- Consideration of early discharge if no evidence of ongoing haematemesis or melaena.
- Follow-up out-patient endoscopy.
- Discontinuation of any risk factors (e.g. NSAIDs).

# 1.11 Acute kidney injury

## Background

- Acute kidney injury (AKI; see Section 17.6), previously termed acute renal failure (ARF), occurs in 5–10% of medical admissions.
- It is most often a biochemical diagnosis as evidenced by increasing concentrations of serum urea and creatinine.
- Many patients have few symptoms, but may report reduced urine output, general malaise, and fatigue.

## Causes

### Pre-renal

- Hypovolaemia, shock, decreased cardiac output.
- Renovascular disease, such as renal artery stenosis, or hypoxic injury through vessel clamping during aneurysm surgery.
- Iatrogenic agents interfering with renal blood flow autoregulation.

### Renal

- Glomerulonephritis.
- Tubular damage—including rhabdomyolysis, ischaemia, myeloma (cast nephropathy), hypercalcaemia, nephrotoxins.
- Interstitial renal disease—infection, infiltrations, drugs.

### Post-renal

- Bladder or ureteric obstruction—prostatism, stones, clots, tumours, retroperitoneal fibrosis.

## History and examination

- Take a careful history, particularly of medications which have recently been started or doses amended.
- Ask about onset of symptoms: is this acute, subacute, or a first presentation of chronic renal failure? A baseline creatinine level is very helpful (contact their GP).
- Fluid status: check BP, JVP, oedema, bibasal crepitations. Is the patient hypovolaemic, euvolaemic, or overloaded? Document this in the notes.
- Features of systemic disease, such as systemic lupus erythematosus or vasculitis.
- Abdominal examination: renal mass or renal angle tenderness.
- Is there urinary retention? Catheterize if any doubt.
- Conscious level and general condition: is the patient critically unwell with multi-organ failure and new-onset cognitive dysfunction? Consider ITU referral.

## Priorities of management

### Investigations

- Blood tests; U&Es, bicarbonate, calcium, CRP, creatine kinase (CK), FBC, and coagulation are essential. LFT, troponin, erythrocyte sedimentation rate (ESR), myeloma screen, blood cultures, antinuclear antibody (ANA), antineutrophil cytoplasmic antibody (ANCA), glomerular basement membrane (GBM), and complement levels may also be indicated.
- Urgent ultrasound of the urinary tract: excludes many obstructive or post-renal causes.

- Urinalysis: heavy protein and blood ('active' urinary sediment) may reflect a glomerular cause. Nitrites and leucocytes indicate possible infection.
- Identify and treat any precipitating cause. Common precipitants include infection; nephrotoxic medication such as ACE inhibitors, diuretics, NSAIDs, antibiotics, and chemotherapeutics; surgery or cardiac events with hypoperfusion. Do a CXR.
- What is the underlying renal cause? Many patients with infection, hypovolaemia, and AKI develop acute tubular necrosis. Where the renal diagnosis is unclear, or where renal function does not recover, consider renal biopsy.

### Practical steps: fluids and medications

- Insert urinary catheter and keep strict hourly input/output charts.
- Withhold nephrotoxins such as ACE inhibitors, diuretics, and NSAIDs during the acute illness. These medications can be reviewed prior to discharge.
- Be cautious with prescribing—antibiotic doses may need to be adjusted.
- If the patient is clinically hypovolaemic, rehydrate with Normal saline (try 1L over 4–8 hours and reassess). Profoundly hypovolaemic patients may benefit from more aggressive initial rehydration. In all patients, particularly those with cardiac failure, repeated review of volume status prevents significant fluid overload.
- Patients with fluid overload should not be given additional fluid, particularly if this is compromising respiratory status. Diuretics should be used with extreme caution in this situation: involve senior or specialist colleagues.

### Practical steps: management of potassium

- Hyperkalaemia results from acidosis and reduced glomerular filtration rate: all patients with AKI are at risk.
- ECG: check for hyperkalaemic changes. If present, urgent action is required. Medical management of moderate hyperkalaemia (K >6–6.5mmol/L) includes:
  - Calcium gluconate—10mL of 10% given over 2–3 minutes stabilizes the myocardium. Buys time to prepare the next step.
  - Insulin and dextrose: give 10–15 units of insulin in 50mL 50% dextrose over 30 minutes (and repeat if necessary).
  - Calcium resonium 15mg three times a day orally—works over several days, unpleasant taste, constipating effect (give laxatives concurrently).
  - Acidosis drives potassium out of cells. If present consider treating with sodium bicarbonate 1g three times a day PO.
- Severe hyperkalaemia with K >7mmol/L and resistant to medical management requires renal replacement therapy.

### Dialysis or haemofiltration

- Life-threatening fluid overload or hyperkalaemia.
- Unresolving AKI with uraemic symptoms.
- Requires placement of a dialysis line and specialist services.
- Ensure platelet count and coagulation are satisfactory prior to line placement.
- Generally, haemodialysis (intermittent therapy) is provided by nephrological services, and is used if patients are cardiovascularly stable with single-organ failure. If multiple-organ failure, or unstable, consider haemofiltration (continuous therapy)—usually provided in an ITU setting.

# 1.12 Coma

## Background

- Coma refers to a state of 'unrousable unresponsiveness' and most usually and perhaps accurately refers to a patient who scores as '3' on the Glasgow Coma Scale (GCS; see Section 14.2).
- The approach to the patient in a comatose state also applies to patients with a diminution of responsiveness, corresponding with a reduced GCS score, and imprecisely described as lethargy, stupor, or obtundation.
- Coma represents both an acute medical emergency and a considerable challenge to diagnose the underlying cause. Immediate management should focus on resuscitation and empirical treatment at the same time as looking for clues as to the specific aetiology.

## Causes

Can be crudely classified as:

| | |
|---|---|
| • Metabolic | • Toxic |
| • Infective | • Structural |

Coma may present with or without focal brainstem signs, lateralizing cerebral signs, or meningism. Toxic and metabolic causes rarely have such lateralizing signs, while infective and structural precipitants do, due to brainstem or cerebral dysfunction. Meningism suggests meningitis, encephalitis, or subarachnoid haemorrhage (SAH).

### Usually without lateralizing/focal signs

- Metabolic causes such as hypo/hyperglycaemia (diabetic ketoacidosis (DKA) or hyperosmolar hyperglycaemic state (HHS), previously known as HONK), acid–base disturbances, electrolyte disturbances (usually Na or Ca), renal failure (uraemia), liver failure.
- Toxic causes such as alcohol, opiates, benzodiazepines, tricyclic antidepressants, neuroleptic medications, lithium, barbiturates, carbon monoxide.
- Hypoxia, $CO_2$ narcosis (retention, e.g. in COPD).
- Endocrine causes—hypothyroidism, Addisonian crisis, hypopituitarism.
- Temperature—hypothermia or malignant hyperthermia.
- Epilepsy.
- Hypertensive emergency with encephalopathy.
- Profound hypoperfusion secondary to systemic sepsis.

### Usually with lateralizing or focal signs

- Ischaemic or haemorrhagic stroke.
- Space-occupying lesions: tumour, haematoma, or abscess—either within the brainstem or with sufficient mass effect to compress it.

### With meningism

- Meningitis or encephalitis.
- SAH.

## Immediate management

Prompt resuscitation, regardless of cause.
- ABC, $O_2$ (caution if $CO_2$ retention suspected).
- Any suggestion of 'brainstem' breathing patterns requires early involvement of critical care and consideration of early intubation.
- IV access.
- Capillary blood glucose.
- Circulatory support with IV fluids.
- If possibility of trauma, stabilize the cervical spine.
- Control any seizure activity—beware of over-sedation.
- Consider giving IV glucose to correct any hypoglycaemia, though there is the potential for this to precipitate Wernicke encephalopathy in malnourished patients. In this case, IV thiamine (100–200mg, or as Pabrinex®) should be given first.
- Naloxone (IV/IM/endotracheal tube (ET)) should be given for suspected opiate toxicity (as a slow titration series of boluses up to a maximum total dose of 10mg). If effective, a maintenance infusion may be required: give 2/3 of the initial dose required (to achieve reversal) per hour.
- Flumazenil should be given if there is a probability of benzodiazepine intoxication and breathing is compromised, but not where there is a suspicion of a mixed overdose. It may precipitate seizures, especially in tricyclic antidepressant overdose, and is contraindicated in epileptics who have received prolonged benzodiazepine therapy. Initial dose 200mcg given over 15 seconds then further 100mcg doses at 1-minute intervals up to a maximum of 1mg.

## Initial investigations

- ABGs, U&Es, LFT, calcium, phosphate, clotting, CRP, ESR.
- Paracetamol and salicylate levels, urine toxicology, ethanol.
- Septic screen: CXR, blood culture, urine culture, serology, (malaria film).
- Further imaging and investigations after history, examination, and empirical management.

## History

This is often lacking but a brief and pertinent history can greatly inform subsequent examination, investigation, and management by narrowing the differential diagnosis. Family members, witnesses, and ambulance crews are all likely sources. Key lines of enquiry include:

- **Timecourse**—abrupt suggests a vascular event such as SAH or seizure, gradual may suggest structural lesion, fluctuating suggests recurrent seizures, metabolic causes, subdural bleed.
- **Preceding symptoms/signs/illnesses**—focal signs or symptoms, weakness, visual symptoms, fever, nausea, vomiting, headaches, confusion, delirium.
- **Past medical history**—is there a MedicAlert bracelet? Any recent falls, previous stroke, or TIA? Any old notes available? Electronic records can be particularly useful. Any diabetes, adrenal insufficiency, epilepsy? Recent travel?
- **Psychiatric history**—any suggestion of depression, previous suicide attempts, suspicious circumstances, or a note left?
- **Drug history**—prescription drugs, illicit drugs, alcohol, toxins?

## General examination

- **Core temperature**—hyperthermia usually suggests infection but may also occur with anticholinergic medications, heatstroke, or diencephalic lesions. Hypothermia can be due to exposure, hypothalamic dysfunction, hypothyroidism, adrenal insufficiency, sepsis, alcohol intoxication.
- **BP**—extreme hypertension suggests hypertensive encephalopathy, intracerebral haemorrhage, or posterior reversible encephalopathy syndrome (PRES).

Hypotension can lead to anoxia and cerebral ischaemia and thus coma. Cardiac failure, sepsis, hypovolaemia, adrenal insufficiency and drugs should be considered as precipitants.

- **Cardiac**—HR, rhythm, ECG may suggest an underlying dysrhythmic cause for poor cerebral perfusion.
- **Respiratory pattern**—hypoventilation can suggest drug intoxication, hyperventilation may be a feature of metabolic abnormalities, such as Kussmaul breathing in acidosis. Specific breathing patterns can be seen in brainstem lesions.
- **Breath**—alcohol, ketosis, hepatic foetor, uraemia.
- **Skin**—look for signs of head trauma, such as periorbital bruising, Battle's sign (bruising over the mastoid), or blood in the ears suggesting skull base trauma. Rashes can suggest meningococcal or other infection or coagulopathic conditions such as DIC. Are there signs of liver or renal disease? Intravenous drug users may have track marks. Sweating is common in hypoglycaemia and sepsis. Cherry red mucous membranes suggest carbon monoxide poisoning. Fingerprick marks suggest diabetes on insulin.
- **Chest**—breath sounds, consolidation, rub, wheeze.
- **Heart**—murmurs may suggest endocarditis.
- **Abdomen**—organomegaly. Peritonism suggestive of bleed, perforation, aneurysmal rupture.
- **Chronic disease**—stigmata of alcoholism, liver disease, diabetes, myxoedema.
- **Infection**—any local focus of infection.
- **Pupils**—may localize intracranial lesions. Pinpoint pupils suggest opiate toxicity.
- **Fundi**—papilloedema suggests, but is not required for, raised intracranial pressure (ICP). May also see diabetic or hypertensive changes.
- **Meningism**—neck stiffness, photophobia, etc.

## Neurological examination

Full discussion of a comprehensive neurological examination is beyond the scope of this chapter but the fundamental elements to consider are outlined. Remember to look for any *change* in neurological status.

**Conscious level**
- Establish GCS score and continue to monitor along with vital signs.

**Motor responses**
- Muscle tone.
- Spontaneous and elicited movements.
- Reflexes.
- Asymmetry—lateralizing lesion.
- Decorticate or decerebrate posturing.
- Myoclonus/asterixis—suggests metabolic aetiology.
- Cranial nerves—localizing lesion.

**Brainstem function**
- Pupillary reactivity (usually reactive in metabolic coma).
- Corneal reflex.
- Eye position/spontaneous movements.
- Doll's head manoeuvre/vestibulo-ocular response.
- Swallowing.
- Respiratory pattern.

Brainstem lesions may be structural (intrinsic or extrinsic compression) or due to metabolic dysfunction. The latter tends to have a better prognosis; the former is more likely to give focal brainstem dysfunction.

## Further management

If brainstem function is intact, proceed to CT head. If a potentially operable lesion is identified (e.g. subdural, subarachnoid/intracerebral bleed, or ischaemic stroke with oedema), then refer to neurosurgery. A lumbar puncture (LP) should be considered if the CT is normal to exclude infection (although if a high degree of suspicion exists, proceed to treat for meningitis).

If brainstem function is compromised, then compressive brain shift should be considered and treatment for suspected raised ICP, such as mannitol and surgical referral, instigated (see Section 1.13). An urgent CT should be performed when able, and LP, again, considered if the CT is normal. An MRI may be helpful if the CT/LP fail to identify a cause for coma.

At all stages, seek senior and specialist input where appropriate.

# 1.13 Traumatic brain injury

## Background

Head injury, or traumatic brain injury (TBI), is a significant cause of mortality and lifelong disablement in young and middle-aged patients (see Section 13.3).

## Approach

- Patients with head injury often have other injuries (e.g. fractures, pneumothorax, myocardial contusion, internal haemorrhage) requiring involvement of many specialties.
- These injuries can contribute to hypoxia and hypotension, which are poor prognostic markers.

### Hospital care

- 'ABC' and resuscitation as needed.
- Disability: examine thoroughly to assess extent of the injuries, including neurological assessment and GCS score.
- Observations—take baseline and monitor regularly.
- Investigations: ABGs, glucose, FBC, U&Es, coagulation, and blood alcohol concentration. Urinary toxicology.
- Neuroimaging with CT scanning in all patients with GCS score <14 or if clinical deterioration. Urgent CT is also recommended in patients with focal neurological abnormalities, coagulopathy, suspected skull fracture, or amnesia. CT will identify an intracranial haematoma, cerebral oedema, and skull fractures. Image the spine with CT or X-rays.
- Admit all patients who are difficult to assess, with neurological signs or symptoms of raised ICP.

### Neurosurgical input

- Contact neurosurgeons early.
- Operative therapy is recommended for patients with:
  - Large extradural haematoma (>30mL volume), or a smaller haematoma associated with reduced GCS score or pupillary abnormalities.
  - Subdural haematoma >10mm in diameter or with evidence of midline shift.
  - Cerebral haemorrhage involving the posterior fossa with mass effect, or in other areas if large and GCS score of 6–8.
  - Depressed open skull fracture with haemorrhage or pneumocephalus.
  - Base of skull fracture or cerebrospinal fluid (CSF) leak.

### Intensive care

- Patients benefit from management in a specialized neurocritical care department with a multidisciplinary approach.
- Principles of management are to avoid further brain injury by treating hypoxia, seizures, and raised ICP and by maintaining cerebral perfusion.
- Airway management with intubation, sedation, and ventilation is often required. Ventilate all patients with GCS score <8, $PaO_2$ <9kPa on air, or $PaCO_2$ <3.5 or >6kPa, and consider ventilating patients with seizures and reducing GCS score.
- Check electrolytes and glucose and correct as required. Tight glycaemic control may improve outcomes.
- Consider prophylaxis for deep vein thrombosis (DVT).
- Nutritional support is important.

### Seizures

- In severe head injury, treat prophylactically for seizures: phenytoin is ideal. Monitor carefully for seizure activity and for non-convulsive seizures and treat aggressively.

### Neuroprotective treatments

- Induced hypothermia can reduce ICP and improve long-term neurological function and has been employed in the clinical trial setting in patients with TBI.
- Glucocorticoids result in a worse outcome after TBI: avoid (unless indicated for coexistent conditions).

## Raised intracranial pressure

- Raised ICP may occur following intracranial haemorrhage or TBI. Other causes include intracranial tumour, ischaemic stroke, hydrocephalus, venous sinus thrombosis, and hepatic encephalopathy. Prompt identification and treatment are essential to improve survival.

### Clinical features

- Headache with vomiting.
- Reduced consciousness. Listless, irritable behaviour.
- Papilloedema.
- False localizing cranial nerve signs may be present.

### Signs suggesting impending herniation—need *urgent* treatment

- Unilaterally or bilaterally fixed and dilated pupils.
- Decerebrate posturing.
- Cushing triad (bradycardia, respiratory depression, hypertension) indicates likely brainstem compression and impending herniation.

### Management of raised ICP

- Treat the underlying cause.
- The insertion of an intraventricular catheter allows monitoring of ICP. In adults, an ICP <15mmHg is normal: >20mmHg is considered raised and requires treatment.
- Patients with GCS score <8 with signs suggestive of impending herniation need urgent treatment.
- Elevate the head of the bed to 20 –30°. Keep the neck in the neutral position to optimize venous drainage.
- Osmotic therapy (e.g. mannitol).
- Dexamethasone is useful to reduce cerebral oedema in patients with intracranial tumours.
- Surgical decompressive craniectomy removes part of the skull to reduce ICP.
- Avoid giving excess fluid; aim for euvolaemia. Fluid restriction to 1.5L per day is occasionally required.
- Treat pyrexia and seizures aggressively.
- Hyperventilation reduces $CO_2$ levels, promoting cerebral vasoconstriction and reducing ICP. Unfortunately it can also lead to cerebral ischaemia and so must be undertaken with caution.
- Sedation is thought to reduce metabolic demands, and hence reduce ICP. In practice, most patients with severe TBI who are ventilated will require some sedation. Propofol or barbiturates are recommended.

## Prognosis after severe TBI

- 30% die.
- 45% survive with disability.
- 25% achieve independence.

## Poor prognostic factors

| | |
|---|---|
| • Increasing age | • GCS score at presentation |
| • Multiple pre-existing medical conditions | • Pupillary function |
| • Multiple associated injuries | • Hypotension |
| • Raised ICP | • Hypoxaemia |
| • Severity of the brain injury | • Bleeding diathesis |
| • CT findings—midline shift, SAH | • Pyrexia |

# 1.14 Status epilepticus

## Definition

- Status epilepticus is a potentially fatal medical emergency requiring prompt treatment to avoid both neurological and metabolic complications.
- It is defined as continuous seizures for >30 minutes or failure to regain full consciousness between seizures.

## Presentation

- Generalized tonic–clonic seizures.
- Complex partial seizures.
- Non-convulsive status—confusion, psychosis, automatisms, and in known epileptics a prolonged post-ictal phase.
- Continuing symptoms for >30 minutes despite initial intervention with benzodiazepines.

## Investigations

- Blood glucose measurement to detect hypoglycaemia.
- U&Es, calcium, and magnesium to detect potential reversible causes.
- Blood levels of antiepileptic medications for compliance review.
- Toxicology screen if possible.
- Prolactin levels may be useful in the differential of non-epileptiform seizures.
- ABGs—respiratory failure prompting treatment escalation, lactic acidosis.
- CXR for signs of aspiration or causative infection.
- Electroencephalogram (EEG)—differential diagnosis and distinguish non-epileptiform seizures.

## Management

- Immediate management should involve the protection of the patient from risks (injury, aspiration, and hypoxia) and correction of reversible causes.
- Involve senior colleagues early, including anaesthetists for airway protection.
- Airway protection: recovery position, nasopharyngeal or Guedel airway (do not force between clenched teeth).
- Oxygen delivery via mask to maintain saturations ≥95%.
- Benzodiazepine—current recommendation is IV lorazepam 1mg IV in increments to a maximum of 4mg over 10 minutes (care with patients of low weight and known type II respiratory failure). Use of rectal diazepam is not recommended in hospital settings due to slow rate of absorption.
- IV phenytoin should be used if these measures fail to control seizures within 30 minutes—give loading dose of 18mg/kg at a rate of 50mg per minute.

- Continue phenytoin at 100mg IV 6–8-hourly.
- Patients should be cardiac monitored throughout all phenytoin infusions.
- Failure to control seizures despite the outlined management and certainly if seizures are still evident after 60 minutes, prompt referral for anaesthetic review should be made. The patient may require intubation, sedation, and paralysing in the ITU setting.
- Once control of seizures has been gained, investigation for potential cause should be undertaken.
- Repeated and regular clinical assessment is warranted in a monitored higher-level dependency setting.

## Further management and investigation

- Hypoglycaemia should be corrected with IV glucose (100mL of 10% dextrose).
- Consideration of IV thiamine (Pabrinex®) in patients suspected of having malnutrition (e.g. alcohol abuse)—prior to correction of hypoglycaemia.
- Hyponatraemia: correct if severe (usually <115mmol/L to cause seizures)—exercise caution with rate/degree of correction (see Section 7.21).
- Cerebral infections—consider meningitis and/or encephalitis if previous history suggestive and treat initially with high-dose IV medications as per local policy (e.g. 2g IV cefotaxime ± 10mg/kg IV aciclovir).
- CT head to detect cause (haemorrhage, cerebrovascular accident (CVA), space-occupying lesion, raised ICP).
- Lumbar puncture if symptoms/signs suggestive of intracerebral infection (and no contraindication on CT).
- IV fluids for rehydration and maintenance: remember that excessive fluid losses occur during active seizures.
- Continuation of patient's usual anti-epileptic medications (oral or nasogastric).
- Referral to specialist neurology team for inpatient review and follow-up on discharge from hospital.

## Non-convulsive and non-epileptiform status

- Non-convulsive status is less common then generalized tonic–clonic seizures.
- Treatment should include use of EEG for diagnosis, benzodiazepines, and early specialist input.
- Non-epileptiform seizures (pseudo-seizures) should be considered in patients with atypical limb movements, active resistance to passive movement, absence of metabolic complications, gaze aversion, and in the absence of a post-ictal phase.
- Early specialist referral and EEG are beneficial in this diagnosis—if any doubt, treat as status epilepticus initially.

# 1.15 Adrenal crisis

## Background

- Acute adrenal crisis can occur either in those with known disease on maintenance steroid therapy, or in those with subclinical disease not yet diagnosed.
- Acute adrenal crisis can result from stressful precipitants such as infection, surgery, trauma, or other systemic disease.
- Such a crisis may also be the initial presentation and constitutes an acute life-threatening medical emergency, in which treatment should be instigated on clinical suspicion.
- Suspicion should be raised in any critically ill patient with no clear alternative diagnosis.

## Presentation

Often varied and non-specific. The trigger for adrenal crisis (e.g. pneumonia) may be the most apparent feature:

- Hypotension and cardiovascular shock.
- Postural symptoms.
- Nausea and vomiting.
- Abdominal pain.
- Dehydration.
- Anorexia, weight loss, fatigue, myalgia.
- Diarrhoea.
- Psychiatric features.
- Hypoglycaemia.
- Hyponatraemia and hyperkalaemia.
- Hyperpigmentation in chronic primary disease.

## Aetiology of adrenal insufficiency

- Autoimmune.
- Tuberculosis.
- Malignant adrenal secondaries.
- Adrenal haemorrhage (e.g. meningococcal septicaemia—Waterhouse–Friderichsen syndrome).
- Traumatic shock.
- Fungal infection.
- Hypopituitarism.
- Drugs (metyrapone, aminoglutethimide).
- Adrenoleucodystrophy.
- Congenital adrenal hyperplasia.
- Familial glucocorticoid deficiency.

## Crisis precipitants in stable disease

- Infection and sepsis.
- Trauma.
- Severe burns.
- Anaesthesia and surgery (especially if there is a failure to continue or increase steroid therapy to cover the period of physiological stress).
- Drugs (ketoconazole, etomidate, rifampicin, phenytoin, phenobarbitone).
- Liver failure.
- Later stages of pregnancy and parturition.

## Investigations

- U&Es: hyponatraemia, hyperkalaemia, dehydration (may be less pronounced in secondary disease with preserved mineralocorticoid activity).
- FBC: normocytic anaemia.
- Glucose: hypoglycaemia.
- Calcium: elevated.
- Cortisol: note 'normal' level in illness should be ~1000nmol/L.
- ACTH: High or low, depending on the cause of adrenal insufficiency.
- ABGs: metabolic acidosis.
- Full septic screen including CXR (in case of past tuberculosis).

## Acute management

- Treat on clinical suspicion.
- Resuscitation ('ABC').
- Involve intensive care and manage in high dependency setting with CVP monitoring and catheter for urine output.
- Fluid resuscitation for shock—may require several litres of 0.9% saline but exercise caution if chronic hyponatraemia as rapid correction can precipitate central pontine myelinolysis. Seek endocrine advice if severe hyponatraemia at presentation.
- Carefully monitor U&Es and fluid balance.
- Hydrocortisone 100mg IV/IM bolus and then 150–400mg/24 hours in divided doses.
- Correct hypoglycaemia.
- Investigate and treat precipitant (such as infection). Broad-spectrum antibiotic cover may be indicated.

## Subsequent management

- A full endocrine review of the likely aetiology is mandated including paired ACTH and cortisol, Synacthen testing, adrenal autoantibodies, etc. (see Section 7.13).
- Steroid replacement can be transitioned to oral hydrocortisone once stable at a minimum of double replacement dose (i.e. 20/10/10mg daily). This can then be weaned under supervision to a maintenance regimen of 10/5/5mg daily as tolerated. At total daily hydrocortisone doses of <40mg, fludrocortisone must be added in primary adrenal disease (50–200mcg daily) to provide sufficient mineralocorticoid activity.
- Steroid sick day rules should be reviewed in patients with existing disease and taught to newly diagnosed patients.
- Endocrine follow-up must be arranged.

# 1.16 Thyroid emergencies

## Background

Thyroid disease usually manifests insidiously and when symptoms develop, there is ample time to make the diagnosis before the situation becomes critical. There are, however, occasions when dysthyroid states present as acute medical emergencies, requiring prompt recognition and action.

## Thyroid storm/thyrotoxic crisis

See Section 7.3.

## Myxoedema/myxoedema coma

- This represents severe hypothyroidism and can occur in the context of severe long-standing disease with inadequate treatment or be precipitated by an acute event.
- Coma and ultimately death may ensue.
- Collateral history to establish previous thyroid status, progressive symptoms, and potential precipitants is important.
- Other causes of coma should be considered.

### Presentation

*Neurological features*
- Altered mental status/confusion.
- Lethargy.
- Decreased conscious level, coma.
- Psychosis, depression.
- Encephalopathy, seizures.
- Cerebellar ataxia.
- Slow-relaxing reflexes (symmetrical).

*Other features*
- Cardiac failure, pericardial effusion.
- Bradycardia, hypotension.
- Hypothermia.
- Hypoglycaemia, hyponatraemia.
- Hypoventilation (hypoxia and hypercapnia).
- Intestinal obstruction.

### Precipitants
- Any untreated cause of hypothyroidism.
- Drugs (especially sedatives, opiates).
- Cold exposure.
- Trauma, infection, stroke.

### Investigations
- U&Es, glucose, FBC, CK, thyroid stimulating hormone (TSH) and free thyroxine (FT4), cortisol, ABGs.
- Septic screen, CXR, ECG.

### Management
- Do not wait for thyroid function results.
- Treat any precipitants (e.g. antibiotics after culture).
- Support ventilation/circulation (HDU/ITU) as appropriate.
- Correct hypoglycaemia/hyponatraemia.
- Correct core temperature (by 0.5°C/hour).
- Cardiac monitoring.
- Hydrocortisone 50–100mg IV 6–8-hourly until adrenal sufficiency demonstrated.
- Thyroid hormone replacement as per local specialist endocrine advice—e.g. 300–500mcg levothyroxine (L-T4) NG/IV as a bolus then 50–100mcg daily. If no improvement within 48 hours, liothyronine (L-T3) can be given IV at 10–25mcg/8 hours.

# 1.17 Acute poisoning

## Background

Accounting for 10% of hospital admissions, acute poisoning is an important cause of coma and cardiac arrest, especially in younger people. It may occur both deliberately and accidentally, with many different routes of exposure.

Despite the many and varied potential poisons, initial management follows the same 'ABC' approach, stabilize the patient, prevent further drug absorption, and increase toxin clearance.

## Routes of exposure

- Inhalation
- Ingestion
- Absorption
- Injection (IV, IM, SC)

## Approach to management

- Personal safety is extremely important to avoid self-exposure.
- If the patient is unconscious, obtain a collateral history from friends or relatives.
- **A**irway: clear and maintain the airway, use adjuncts as necessary, and consider endotracheal intubation if GCS score <8 (aspiration risk).
- **B**reathing: if absent or inadequate use bag-mask ventilation. Avoid mouth- to-mouth respiration due to risk of contamination. Administer $O_2$ to maintain saturations 95%. Check ABGs.
- **C**irculation: cardiac compressions and full advanced life support if indicated. Hypotension requires fluid resuscitation with inotropic support if failure to respond. Cardiac monitoring should be commenced. Send routine bloods including paracetamol and salicylate levels.
- **D**: reduced GCS score should warrant ITU review. Check blood glucose.
- **E**: examine for specific signs related to individual poisons.

### Prevention of further drug absorption

- Remove patient from the source.
- Activated charcoal (50g) should be given to fully conscious patients within 1 hour of ingestion of a poison known to be absorbed by charcoal. Repeated doses may be helpful.
- Gastric lavage followed by activated charcoal may be considered within 1 hour of ingestion for intubated patients.

### Increased elimination

- Urine alkalinization by giving IV 1.4% sodium bicarbonate may be used in severe salicylate poisoning (see Section 5.8).

- Haemodialysis may be used for lithium, methanol, ethylene glycol, and salicylate poisoning.
- Haemoperfusion is rarely required.

## Specific antidotes/therapies

The more common specific antidotes are listed as follows. This list is not exhaustive and each individual case should be reviewed on its own merits:

- Naloxone: opioids—400mcg IV with repeated doses to max. 10mg if no response. Caution: short half-life so may require further doses or infusion. (A rough guide is to use 2/3 of the naloxone dose needed initially as an infusion per hour, titrating according to response.)
- Flumazenil: benzodiazepine—200mcg IV with repeated doses (severe cases only). Should not be given in mixed overdoses or as a diagnostic test.
- N-acetylcysteine: paracetamol—IV infusion: first dose 150mg/kg in 200mL 5% dextrose over 15 minutes, then 50mg/kg in 500mL over 4 hours, followed by 100mg/kg in 1L over 16 hours. Repeated third doses may be required. Use nomograms to assess whether serum paracetamol level requires treating (see Section 5.7).
- Oxygen: carbon monoxide poisoning (paraquat lung injury is worsened by high oxygen concentrations) (see Section 5.11).
- Vitamin K and Beriplex®: warfarin.
- Ethanol: methanol/ethylene glycol (see Section 5.12).
- Glucagon: beta-blockers—5–10mg IV (may precipitate severe vomiting).
- Digoxin antibodies: severe digoxin toxicity (see Section 5.10).
- Sodium bicarbonate: tricyclic antidepressants with cardiac arrhythmia (see Section 5.13).

## Follow-up

- Patients presenting with deliberate self-poisoning should be referred for a psychiatric review.

## Further information

- MIMS Colour Index, British National Formulary (BNF), and Data Sheet Compendium may aid in the identification of tablets.
- UK National Poisons Information Service (NPIS) offers 24-hour phone advice to clinicians: Telephone: 0844 892 0111.
- TOXBASE® (<http://www.toxbase.org>) is an Internet database of specific poisons, available in the UK.

# 1.18 Burns

## Background

- Burns constitute a significant cause of accidental morbidity and, when severe, mortality.
- Whilst emergency medicine departments, intensivists, and plastic surgeons shoulder much of the burden of care for these patients, there is a role for the physician to play in managing the multisystem sequelae of moderate and severe burns.
- Full use of appropriate specialist teams should be sought and referral to a tertiary burns unit made in severe cases.
- This section focuses on thermal burns. Chemical or electrical burns require expert input.

## Assessment of patient

### Airway

- Be vigilant for airway burns from inhalation of hot gases, which can lead to progressive or delayed upper airway obstruction. This represents the most common cause of death in burn victims and is present in 2/3 of patients with >70% burns.
- Signs include visible burns peri-orally, oedema or blistering of the oropharynx, hoarseness, dysphagia, stridor, singeing of facial or nasal hair, and soot-staining of the oral and nasal cavities. Such patients may be obtunded.
- Flexible laryngoscopy or bronchoscopy should be considered for assessment and to guide placement of airway adjuncts or intubation, which may well be life-saving if done early. Anaesthetic input is valuable in this situation. The cervical spine should be assessed and protected as appropriate if injury is suspected.

### Breathing

- Severe burns may restrict chest wall movement and there may be coexistent rib injuries or pneumothorax. Decompression may prove necessary.
- Carbon monoxide (CO) poisoning (cherry-red skin, raised carboxyhaemoglobin) or inhalational cyanide toxicity (dizziness, headaches, seizures, raised lactate) should be suspected. CO poisoning mandates the use of high-flow $O_2$ via a non-rebreathe mask and the consideration of hyperbaric $O_2$ therapy. Suspected cyanide toxicity should precipitate specialist referral. Treatment options include sodium thiosulphate and hydroxycobalamin.
- ABG analysis, peak flow readings, and chest radiography may inform management. Pulse oximetry should be interpreted with caution in the context of inhalational injury. Alongside supplementary $O_2$ and airway adjuncts, bronchodilators may have a role. Where mechanical ventilation is required, low tidal volumes should be used to reduce mechanical lung injury.

### Circulation

- Fluid resuscitation is paramount in management of burns patients. Hypovolaemic shock results from large fluid shifts due to increased capillary permeability and impaired cardiac function. Rapid repletion of intravascular volume is crucial for maintenance of end-organ perfusion and function. Losses can be severe but over-correction can result in pulmonary oedema and increased risk of compartment syndrome. As such, arterial line monitoring and catheterization for accurate fluid balance assessment is mandatory. A urine output of 0.5mL/kg/hour is optimal. Two large-bore IV cannulae or a central line should be sited and resuscitation commenced with 0.9% saline or Hartmann solution. Colloid has not been proven to be superior.
- A number of calculators for fluid requirements in burns exist, and hospitals may have local guidelines. The commonly used Parkland formula advises 4 × (weight in kg) × (% total body surface affected) mL Hartmann per 24 hours, with half to be given in the first 8 hours. Changes in rate of infusion should be minimized to avoid vascular collapse and major fluid shifts but adjust input according to vital signs, urine output, and fluid status.
- It must be remembered that any suggested regimen is only a starting point; age, comorbidities, and severity of burn and injury will affect requirements. Electrolytes must be monitored. Serum lactate may be a useful monitoring tool—elevated lactate implies insufficient organ perfusion.
- Cautious blood transfusion may be indicated in severe burns, e.g. where there is a risk of acute coronary syndrome. Haemoconcentration is frequently evident in the early stages.

## Assessment of circumstances

A collateral history should be taken alongside immediate resuscitation measures and should address:
- Material burned (chemical/textile/plastic)?
- Was there an explosion (blast injury)?
- Was there associated trauma?
- Duration of exposure.
- Confinement in enclosed space (risk of CO poisoning).
- Any loss of consciousness.
- Past medical history.
- Coexisting use of alcohol or drugs.

## Assessment of burn severity and extent

### Burn depth
Assessment informs the need for surgical intervention.

**Superficial** burns involve the epidermal layer of the skin and manifest as painful blanching erythema. They usually heal in a matter of days without significant scarring.

**Superficial partial-thickness burns** involve the epidermis and superficial dermis, are painful, erythematous, and may not blanch under pressure. Often associated with blistering, they heal in weeks not days, although scarring is again unusual.

**Deep partial-thickness** burns extend to the deeper dermis and are often insensate except under pressure, do not blanch and have extensive blistering. They usually scar, sometimes extensively, and take several weeks to heal.

**Full-thickness** burns extend through the dermis, are usually painless, and can appear white or grey/black with no blanching. They will not heal without plastic surgery intervention.

**Fourth-degree** burns extend into underlying tissues and are life-threatening.

### Burn area
Assessment of the surface area involved informs fluid resuscitation, influencing the magnitude of the inflammatory response and subsequent fluid shift. A variety of ways of estimating total body surface area (TBSA) exist, the most familiar of which are the rule of 'nines', which apportions 9% for the head, and each arm, 18% for the each leg and the front and back of the trunk, and 1% for the perineum, and the Lund and Browder chart (Fig. 1.17).

## Burn treatment

- Burned clothing, jewellery, and foreign material should be removed.
- Wounds should be irrigated. Water is acceptable, disinfectants should be avoided. Cool fluid may minimize the zone of injury but excessive exposure to very cold solutions can exacerbate tissue

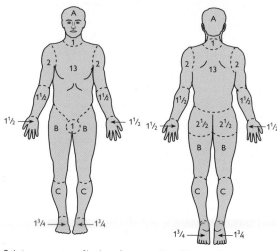

Relative percentage of body surface area affected by growth

| Area | Age | 0 | 1 | 5 | 10 | 15 | Adult |
|---|---|---|---|---|---|---|---|
| A: half of head | | $9\frac{1}{2}$ | $8\frac{1}{2}$ | $6\frac{1}{2}$ | $5\frac{1}{2}$ | $4\frac{1}{2}$ | $3\frac{1}{2}$ |
| B: half of thigh | | $2\frac{3}{4}$ | $3\frac{1}{4}$ | 4 | $4\frac{1}{4}$ | $4\frac{1}{2}$ | $4\frac{3}{4}$ |
| C: half of leg | | $2\frac{1}{2}$ | $2\frac{1}{2}$ | $2\frac{3}{4}$ | 3 | $3\frac{1}{4}$ | $3\frac{1}{2}$ |

**Fig. 1.17** Lund and Browder chart for calculating the percentage of body surface area.

Reproduced from *British Medical Journal*, 'ABC of burns: Initial management of a major burn: II—assessment and resuscitation', Shehan Hettiaratchy and Remo Papini, 529, p. 101, 2004, with permission from BMJ Publishing Group Ltd.

damage and precipitate systemic shock. Some authors advocate the use of warmed fluids to avoid this.

- Blisters should be left intact.

- The burn site should be protected with cling-film or dry sterile sheets. More extensive dressing should be held until after assessment by a specialist.
- Escharotomy may be required in compartment syndrome or constriction of the thorax by circumferential full-thickness burns.
- Partial-thickness burns may be dressed with a variety of biological or synthetic dressings, or with silver sulfadiazine cream. Full-thickness burns should be assessed for early split-skin grafting.

## Adjunctive measures

- Analgesia is important. Large doses of IV opiates may be required, with appropriate anti-emetic cover. There may be a case for anxiolytics such as benzodiazepines.
- Tetanus status should be established and immunization administered accordingly.
- Antibiotic prophylaxis is indicated in partial and full-thickness burns. In addition to the obvious portal of entry for pathogenic organisms, burns patients are rendered immunosuppressed. Topical antibiotics can be used at burn sites in addition to systemic administration.
- The gross elevation of stress hormones predisposes to hyperglycaemia and insulin administration should be considered.
- Beta-blockade can be used judiciously to mitigate tachycardia and the catabolic effect of severe burns.

## Special circumstances

Electrical burns can cause deep tissue damage with limited superficial entry and exit wounds. Muscle necrosis can precipitate renal failure. Cardiac function should be assessed fully.

Chemical and radiation burns require decontamination and the input of a specialist burns team.

# Chapter 2

# Allergy

37

# 2.1 Basic science

## Host defence mechanisms

### Innate immunity
- First line of host defence.
- Immediately active.
- **Non-specific**.

### Mechanisms
- **Physical:** epithelial cells.
- **Chemical:** gastric acid, defensins (small proteins which act mainly by penetrating microbial cell wall and forming pores).
- **Immune:**
  - Soluble: acute-phase reactants, complement, cytokines.
  - Cellular: phagocytes—neutrophils, macrophages, eosinophils, mast cells, basophils, NK (natural killer) cells (Fig. 2.1).

### Acute-phase reactants
- CRP.
- Serum amyloid P protein.
- Mannose-binding lectin.

### Complement
- Series of plasma proteins.
- Nine basic complement components.
- Activators: classical, alternative, and lectin pathways (Fig. 2.2).
- Activates C3, a key component required to switch on the effectors.
- Effectors: anaphylatoxins, complement receptors, and membrane attack complex.
- Main effects:
  - Opsonization.
  - Chemotaxis and inflammation.
  - B-cell stimulation.
  - Immune complex clearance.
  - Cell lysis.
- Complement regulators: C1 inhibitor, C4 binding protein, complement receptor 1 (CR1), decay accelerating factor (DAF), factor H, factor I, and cluster of differentiation 59 (CD59).

### Cytokines
- Small soluble intercellular messengers.

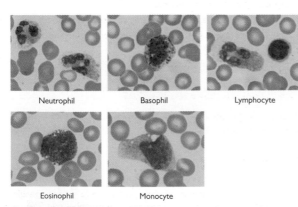

**Fig. 2.1** Cells involved in host defence.
With permission from Dr Donald J. Innes, Jr., M.D.

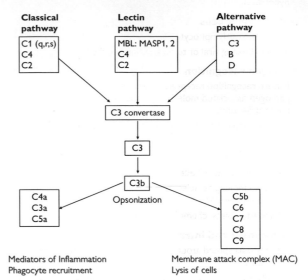

**Fig. 2.2** The complement pathways.
The classical, lectin, and alternate pathways of complement activation. MBL: mannose-binding lectin; MASP: mannose-binding lectin-associated serine protease.

*Interferons (IFNs)*
- Type I—alpha and beta:
  - Produced by fibroblasts, monocytes, and virus-infected cells.
  - Antiviral, anti-proliferative.
- Type II—gamma:
  - Produced by activated T cells and NK cells.
  - Activate macrophage/neutrophil killing.
  - Stimulate NK cells.
  - Increase MCH class II expression.

*Interleukins (ILs)*
- IL-6, IL-8 (chemoattractant).

*Chemokines*
- Chemoattractant cytokines.

### Neutrophils
- The principal phagocytic cells in the body.
- Without neutrophils survival is not possible.
- Released from bone marrow into the bloodstream in response to infection.
- Important role in phagocytosis and destruction of extracellular bacteria and some fungi.
- Surface receptors for immunoglobulin (Ig)-G, IgA, and complement components.

### Eosinophils
- Important in parasite control and allergy.
- Produces: major basic protein, eosinophil cationic protein.
- Surface receptors for IgG, C3, and C5.

### Basophils and mast cells
- Basophils circulate in blood, mast cells are tissue bound.
- Surface receptors for C3, C5, and IgE.

- Produce: histamine, prostaglandins, leukotrienes, platelet-activating factor, cytokines.
- Involved in the immune response to parasites.
- Interaction of antigen with bound IgE produces immediate hypersensitivity.

### Natural killer cells

- Large granular lymphocytes.
- Kill cells bearing viral or tumour surface markers.

### Pathogen recognition

- Pattern recognition receptors on immune cells recognize pathogen-associated molecular patterns (PAMPs) on micro-organisms.
- PAMPs: bacterial lipopolysaccharides (LPS), dsRNA, CpG, peptidoglycan.
- The main group of receptors for PAMPs are called Toll receptors.

### Cell adhesion and recruitment

- Adhesion molecules: selectins, integrins, cadherins, intercellular adhesion molecules.
- Chemoattractants: chemokines, leukotriene B4, FMLP.

### Phagocytosis and intracellular killing

- Pseudopodia spread around the organism or particle to form a phagosome.
- Phagolysosome: phagosome fuses with cytoplasmic granules. This exposes the microbe to the action of bactericidal components contained within lysosomes.
- Opsonization (coating of bacteria with specific antibody and complement) increases efficiency of phagocytosis.

### Killing mechanisms operating within phagocytes

- Nicotinamide adenine dinucleotide phosphate (NADPH) oxidase-*dependent* mechanisms: depend on the generation of reactive oxygen molecules.
- NADPH oxidase-*independent* mechanisms act via proteolytic enzymes contained within lysosomes, e.g. cathepsin and elastase.

### Adaptive immunity

- **Specific**.
- Depends on generation of specific antibodies and antigen-specific effector T cells.
- Takes time to develop.
- Characterized by development of immunological memory (generation of a pool of memory T and B cells).
- Hallmark of immune systems of higher animals.

### CD molecules

- CD3: present on all T-cells; accessory molecule required for signalling via T-cell receptor.
- CD4: present on T-helper cells and monocytes; interacts with MHC class II antigens on antigen-presenting cells.
- CD8: present on cytotoxic T-cells, recognizes MHC class I antigens on target cells.

### T lymphocytes

- 70–80% of total lymphocyte population (Fig. 2.3).
- Important role in intracellular infections, tumour surveillance, and graft rejection.
- Precursors formed in the bone marrow, undergo maturation in the thymus.

### CD4+ T cells

- Helper T cells (Th).
- 60% of circulating T-cell population.
- Recognizes antigen when presented with class II MHC antigens.
- Provides help for B cells.

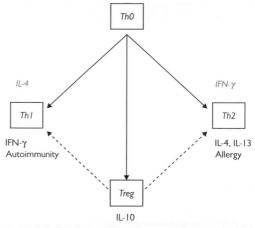

**Fig. 2.3** CD4+ T-cell subsets. Subsets of CD4+ T cells and the prototype cytokines they produce. Treg: regulatory T cell; broken line refers to suppression of effect.

- Involved in type IV hypersensitivity.
- Th0 cells—naïve mature T cells which can differentiate into either Th1 or Th2 cells upon activation.

### Th1-type CD4+ T cells

- When activated secrete IL-2 and IFN-γ.
- Are suppressed by IL-10.
- Produce cell-mediated immunity and type IV hypersensitivity reactions.

### Th2-type CD4+ T cells

- When activated secrete IL-4, IL-5, IL-6, and IL-10.
- Are suppressed by IFN-γ.
- Cause B-lymphocyte proliferation and differentiation.
- Stimulate secretion of IgG, IgA, or IgE.
- Contribute to generation of antibody-mediated hypersensitivity reactions.

### CD8+ T cells

- Cytotoxic T cells.
- 40% of circulating T-cell population.
- Recognize antigen presented by MHC class I antigens.
- Important in eliminating cells infected by viruses.

### B lymphocytes

- Produced in the bone marrow, final maturation occurs in the spleen and lymph nodes.
- Express Igs on their cell surface.
- Differentiate into plasma cells; plasma cells secrete antibody.
- Activation of B cells by protein antigens needs both antigen and helper CD4+ T cells.
- Polysaccharides can produce B-cell activation without T-cell help.

## Hypersensitivity reactions

### What is hypersensitivity?

- Immune responses with excessive or undesirable consequences (Table 2.1).
- Can cause tissue or organ damage.

### Type I: anaphylactic or immediate

- These reactions are initiated by antigen binding to antigen-specific IgE located on the surface of mast cells and basophils (Fig. 2.4).
- Cross-linking of mast cell-bound IgE molecules by antigen results in the activation of a signal cascade. This leads to the release of

| Table 2.1 Details of the four different types of hypersensitivity reaction | | | | |
|---|---|---|---|---|
| | Type I Anaphylactic/ immediate | Type II Antibody-dependent cytotoxicity | Type III Immune complex mediated | Type IV Cell mediated or delayed type |
| Onset | Seconds | Seconds | Hours | 2–3 days |
| Effectors | IgE Mast cells Eosinophils | IgG Complement Phagocytes | IgG Complement Neutrophils | T cells (CD4+) Macrophages |
| Clinical examples | Anaphylaxis Hay fever Asthma | Transfusion reactions Goodpasture syndrome | SLE EAA (extrinsic allergic alveolitis) | Contact dermatitis |

preformed mediators stored within secretory granules contained within mast cells (e.g. histamine, eosinophil cationic protein) as well as newly synthesized mediators derived from membrane phospholipids (**leukotrienes**).

- Reactions usually start within 30 minutes of antigen exposure.
- **Clinical significance:** type 1 hypersensitivity is responsible for anaphylaxis and also contributes to the pathogenesis of asthma and hay fever.

## Type II: antibody-dependent cytotoxicity

- Initiated by binding of circulating IgM or IgG antibody to antigen located on cells or basement membranes.
- Tissue breakdown is due to complement activation and by activation of phagocytes attracted to the site by complement breakdown products (C5a).
- **Clinical significance:** type II hypersensitivity is responsible for Goodpasture syndrome, idiopathic thrombocytopenic purpura (ITP), myasthenia gravis, pemphigus, and pemphigoid (this is not an exhaustive list).

## Type III: immune complex-mediated or Arthus reaction

- This is initiated by circulating antigen–antibody complexes which get deposited on endothelial surfaces of affected organs.
- Tissue damage is produced by complement activation and the attraction and activation of phagocytes by the immune complexes.
- **Clinical significance:** multi-organ damage in SLE is initiated by deposition of immune complexes of nuclear antigens and antinuclear antibodies. Immune complex deposition initiates pathology in extrinsic allergic alveolitis, allergic bronchopulmonary aspergillosis, and many forms of glomerulonephritis.

## Type IV: cell-mediated or delayed type hypersensitivity

- This is produced by the activation of CD4+ T cells by antigen presented by antigen-presenting cells. The activated T cells

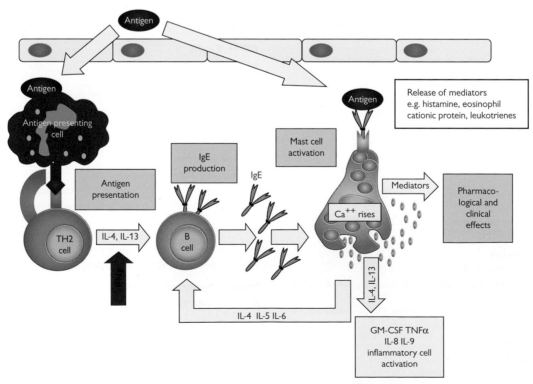

**Fig. 2.4** Diagrammatic representation of events during a type 1 hypersensitivity reaction. Reproduced with permission of Dr. Richard Hunt, University of South Carolina.

produce cytokines which attract and activate monocytes producing granulomatous inflammation.
- Takes 48–72 hours to develop following antigen exposure; hence called delayed hypersensitivity.
- **Clinical significance:** this type of hypersensitivity is responsible for contact dermatitis, tuberculin reaction, tissue damage in mycobacterial disease. Sarcoid and Crohn disease are examples of granulomatous inflammation where the initiating antigen is unknown.

## Autoimmunity

### What is autoimmunity?
- State when antibodies and T cells recognize normal components of the body.

### Autoimmune disease
- Occurs when the immune system fails to recognize the body's own tissues as 'self' and attacks itself.
- Mediated by type II, III, and IV hypersensitivity reactions.
- Tends to run in families.
- There is often a female preponderance.
- Individuals with one autoimmune disease are more likely to develop another.

### Mechanisms of autoimmunity

*Immunological tolerance*
- During T-cell development in the thymus, self-reactive T cells are identified and undergo apoptosis or programmed cell death.

- Autoimmune B cells are generally deleted or rendered unresponsive during development in the bone marrow.
- Any autoreactive lymphocytes that reach the periphery are held in check by the action of a population of CD4+CD25+ T cells called T-regulatory cells.
- Autoimmunity arises when immunological tolerance breaks down.

*Breakdown of thymic tolerance*
- Inheritance of a human leucocyte antigen (HLA) allele that does not bind self-antigen. Autoreactive T cells are not deleted.
- Inheritance of gene polymorphisms that reduces thymic expression of normal peptide antigens. T cells that recognize these peptide antigens are not deleted.
- Release of sequestered/cryptic antigens to which the immune system is not tolerant. Examples of such antigens are ocular antigens.

*Breakdown of peripheral tolerance*
- Activation of the immune system by microbial PAMPs may reverse autoreactive T-cell anergy. This may occur during microbial infections.
- Cross reactivity and molecular mimicry between microbial antigens and self antigens of the host may lead to a breakdown of self-tolerance. Initiation of cardiac damage following infection with *Streptococcus pyogenes* as occurs in rheumatic fever is an example of this mechanism.
- Failure of T-suppressor cell function has been postulated to produce autoimmunity.

## 2.2 Atopy

### Definition

- Genetic susceptibility to allergy—manifestations: allergic rhinitis, atopic eczema, allergic asthma.

### Genetic susceptibility

- If one parent is atopic, a child has 25–40% chance of being atopic.
- Both parents atopic: risk rises to 70–80%.
- HLA associations with atopy: HLA-A1, -B8, -DR3, -A3.
- Other gene associations: IL-4, IL-5, IL-13, high-affinity IgE receptor β-subunit, IL-4 receptor α-subunit, ADAM33 metalloproteinase.

### Mechanisms of allergy

- Allergen-specific IgE binds high-affinity FcεR1 receptors on mast cells.
- On subsequent allergen exposure, surface IgE molecules are cross-linked initiating a cascade of intravascular events.
- Mast cells degranulate liberating preformed mediators (Fig. 2.5).
- Synthesis and release of newly-formed mediators including leukotrienes.
- Action of mediators results in:
  - Increased vascular permeability (swelling).
  - Increased airway reactivity (bronchoconstriction).
  - Increased mucosal secretion contributing to airway narrowing.
  - Dilatation of post-capillary venules leading to reduced venous return and secondary hypotension during severe reactions.

### History

- Most important aspect for making the correct diagnosis.
- Tests are ordered based on the history.

### Skin prick testing (SPT)

- Used to detect *in vivo* antigen-specific IgE antibodies.
- Done by pricking skin through a drop of diluted antigen placed on the skin; positive reaction produces a wheal >3mm in diameter (or 2mm more than negative control).
- Advantages: rapid, relatively cheap, more clinically informative (*in vivo* test) (Fig. 2.6).
- Disadvantages: limited availability of standardized reagents, anaphylaxis (very rare), trained staff needed to interpret test.

42

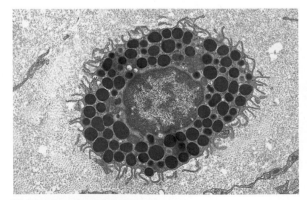

**Fig. 2.5** Mast cell containing multiple granules.
Reproduced from Vaughan DW, *A Learning System in Histology: CD-ROM and Guide*, 2002, by permission of Oxford University Press, USA, www.oup.com

Drugs such as anti-histamines/steroids/calcium channel blockers/antidepressants may interfere with the test.

### Measurement of specific IgE in blood: radioallergosorbent test (RAST)

- Semi-quantitative, six grades (0–6) or fully quantitative (expressed as kUA/L (kilounits of allergen per litre)).
- Levels usually do not correlate with severity of clinical disease.
- Preferred in the following settings:
  - Severe and extensive eczema.
  - Very young child.
  - Patients being treated with antihistamines.
  - Patients with significant risk of anaphylaxis.

### Total IgE

- Not always raised in allergic individuals with elevated antigen-specific IgE antibody levels.
- Levels can be significantly raised in: parasitic infections, atopic dermatitis, hyper IgE syndrome (typically >2000IU/L).
- Of little value in the assessment of patients with suspected allergy.

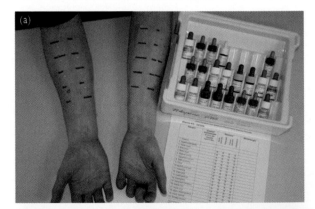

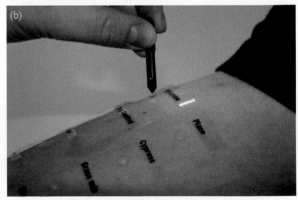

**Fig. 2.6** (a) Preparation for skin prick test on forearm. (b) Prick testing with lancet through a drop of allergen extract.
Reproduced from Heinzerling et al., 'The skin prick test: European Standards', *Clinical and Translational Allergy*, 3, 3, February 2013, © 2013 Heinzerling et al.; licensee BioMed Central Ltd. This is an Open Access article distributed under the terms of the Creative Commons Attribution License (http://creativecommons.org/licenses/by/2.0), which permits unrestricted use, distribution, and reproduction in any medium, provided the original work is properly cited.

## Challenge tests

- Open challenge by administering suspected allergen with resuscitation measures to hand; should only be done by an experienced physician.
- Double-blind placebo controlled challenge: is the gold standard but rarely used in practice.

## Allergic rhinitis

- **Seasonal** symptoms due to allergy to pollen/moulds.
- **Perennial** (year-round) symptoms due to allergy to house dust mite (HDM), cat or dog.

- History:
  - Red, itchy, runny nose.
  - Itchy, swollen watery eyes.
- Investigation:
  - Skin prick test.
  - Measurement of allergen-specific IgE.
- Management:
  - Allergen avoidance: pets, HDM.
  - Pharmacological.
  - Non-sedating antihistamines.
  - Nasal corticosteroids (use regularly for at least 2–3 weeks for noticeable benefit).
  - Allergen desensitization: good evidence for the efficacy of desensitization to a number of antigens including grass.

# 2.3 Food, drug, latex, and venom allergy

## Food allergy

- A group of disorders caused by an immune response to proteins in food.
- Need to distinguish between IgE-mediated food allergy and food intolerance (due to non-immunological and psychogenic causes).
- Most reactions are caused by a limited number of foods:
  - In children: milk, egg, peanuts, tree nuts, wheat, and soy.
  - In adults: peanuts, tree nuts, fish, and shellfish.

### IgE-mediated food allergy

- Common in children—0.5% allergic to cows' milk.
- Most food allergens: heat stable (resist cooking), acid stable (resist stomach acid).
- Signs and symptoms occur within minutes to a couple of hours of food consumption.
- May cause local symptoms affecting the gastrointestinal tract, skin, and respiratory tract. Can rarely cause systemic life-threatening reactions.
- Diagnosis is based on history of reactions occurring on exposure; sensitivity is confirmed by skin tests or RAST tests.

### Cows' milk allergy

- Common (especially among children).
- Usually disappears by the age of 5 years.
- Major milk allergens: β-lactoglobulin, α-lactalbumin, casein, bovine serum albumin, and bovine Igs.

### Egg allergy

- Common in children <5 years; also relevant for adults.
- Often disappears with age.
- Major egg allergens: ovomucoid and ovalbumin.
- Anaphylactic responses may occur.

### Fish and shellfish allergy

- Shellfish: crustacea (prawns, crabs, and lobsters); molluscs (mussels, scallops, and oysters).
- May be severe.
- Usually permanent.

### Peanut allergy

- Major cause of severe allergic reactions.
- May not be declared on labels.
- Avoidance may be difficult.
- Sensitization may occur through the use of groundnut oil in formula milks and emollient creams.
- Most cases start during infancy and can be long-lasting.
- Most affected individuals are atopic.

### Tree nut allergy

- Walnut, almond, brazil, and hazel nuts are the most common causes but reactions to all types of tree nuts are documented.
- Can give rise to anaphylaxis.

### Cereal allergy

- Wheat, barley, and rye are closely related.
- Can cause: IgE-mediated allergic response, gluten intolerance (coeliac disease), or occupational asthma.
- Rice and maize allergies are rare.

## Oral allergy syndrome

- Pollen-allergic individuals may develop allergic reactions to soft fruits (plum, peach, apples) or vegetables due to the presence of antigenically similar proteins in the fruit or vegetable.
- Heat-labile allergens—allergy is produced by *raw* fruit but not cooked or canned fruit.
- Fresh extract of suspected food required for skin testing.
- Reported cross reactivities:
  - Birch pollen: hazelnut, almonds, apple, peach, pear, plums, cherries, carrot.
  - Grass pollen: melon, tomato.
  - Ragweed pollen: melon, banana.

## Food intolerance

- Pharmacological: tyramine (headaches, hypertension in patients on monoamine oxidase inhibitors (MAOIs)), caffeine, alcohol.
- Enzyme deficiencies: lactase deficiency (common in Asian people).
- Toxic: scombotoxin (spoiled mackerel/tuna), *Bacillus cereus* food poisoning, monosodium glutamate (Chinese restaurant syndrome).
- Bowel disorders: irritable bowel syndrome, coeliac disease, Crohn disease, infections (*Giardia*, *Yersinia*).
- Pancreatic insufficiency: cystic fibrosis.
- Psychogenic.

## Drug allergy

Allergic reactions to drugs represent 5–10% of all adverse reactions to drugs.
Mechanisms of drug allergic reactions include:
- Hypersensitivity: types I, II, III, or IV.
- Direct histamine release (opiates, radiocontrast media).
- Undue sensitivity to the pharmacological effect (NSAIDs).
- Direct complement activation.

### Penicillin allergy

- Common.
- Severe reactions are rare.
- Major antigenic determinants—benzylpenicilloyl nucleus.
- Minor antigenic determinants—benzylpenicillin, benzyl penicilloate, and others.
- Both capable of causing severe immediate reactions.

*Clinical manifestations*
- Anaphylaxis (type I).
- Haemolytic anaemia (type II).
- Serum sickness (type III).
- Interstitial nephritis, contact dermatitis (type IV).
- Stevens–Johnson syndrome (unknown mechanism).

*Investigation*
- RAST and SPT/intradermal testing (IDT):
  - Detects type I hypersensitivity.
  - Not predictive of other types of reactions.
There are no reliable laboratory tests that can detect other types of hypersensitivity reactions to penicillin or other drugs.
Difficulties with obtaining skin test reagents containing minor determinants.

- Up to 5% of SPT positive penicillin-allergic patients may react to cephalosporins.
- High level of cross-reactivity with carbapenems and the mono-bactams (β-lactam ring semisynthetic penicillins).
- IgE can be directed at shared side-chain (aztreonam and ceftazidime).

*Management*

- Avoid penicillin and other semi-synthetic β-lactam antibiotics.
- Desensitization for patients with IgE-mediated allergy if penicillin is essential:
  - No lasting tolerance.
  - Not to be attempted if patient had a Stevens–Johnson reaction.

**Insulin allergy**

- The tertiary structure of human insulin is changed during manu-facturing process.
- Protamine and zinc may cause reactions.

*Manifestations*

- Urticaria/induration at the injection site.
- Systemic reactions (rare).

*Treatment*

- Difficult.
- Local reaction: antihistamines, hydrocortisone with the insulin.
- Try using a different insulin preparation.
- Desensitization.

**Anaesthetic allergy**

- Royal College of Anaesthesia guidelines available.
- Mechanisms: IgE-mediated, direct mast cell degranulation (opi-oids), complement activation (solvents).

*Causes*

- Muscle relaxants (suxamethonium, rocuronium).
- Latex.
- Antibiotics.
- Plasma expanders/blood products.
- Less commonly reactions may occur to other anaesthetic agents.

*Management*

- Mast cell tryptase: at time of reaction, 3 and 24 hours later.
- Refer to a specialist centre for investigation with a copy of drug chart and observation chart kept during the anaesthetic procedure.
- Most patients will need skin tests with diluted drugs to identify the agent responsible for the allergic reaction; this should only be done by experienced investigators.
- RAST tests currently limited to suxamethonium and thiopentone.

# Latex allergy

- Increasing problem in hospitals: 20% of staff in theatres or ITU may become sensitized.

*Presentation*

- Type I reactions:
  - Anaphylaxis, asthma, angio-oedema, rhinoconjunctivitis, contact urticaria.
- Materials: gloves, condoms, clothing, bungs of drug vials.

- Food cross-reactivity: bananas, avocado, kiwi fruit, potato, tomato, chestnut, lettuce, pineapple, papaya.
- Type IV reactions:
  - Contact hypersensitivity to additives used in processing rubber.

*Diagnosis*

- Type I reactions:
  - Based on history and confirmation of latex sensitization.
  - RAST: 60–80% sensitive.
  - SPT: 95% sensitive.
  - Use standardized commercial latex reagents for skin test.
- Type IV reactions:
  - Identified by patch testing.

*Management*

- Type I reactions:
  - Avoidance of contact with rubber-containing articles essential (Table 2.2).
  - Education of patient, healthcare professionals, and employers is essential; provide written information.
  - Occupational issues can be difficult.
  - Hospitals and dental surgeries: latex-free equipment must be available in key areas (theatres, A&E, Medical Admissions).
- Hospital trusts need latex policy (Health and Safety Executive requirement).
- Latex allergy support group: information on latex content of products (<www.lasg.org.uk>).
- Pharmacy: advice on latex content of drugs.

# Insect venom allergy

- Bee or wasp venom.
- High risk: bee keepers, forestry workers.
- Reactions can be: minor/limited or major/systemic (potentially fatal).

*Treatment*

- Depends on severity of previous reaction, risk of future stings.
- Emergency kit: antihistamines, injectable adrenaline.
- Desensitization: vaccines made from venom induce long-term tolerance to the allergen; refer for specialist advice.

| Table 2.2 List of products containing latex |
| --- |
| **Dipped products** |
| Gloves |
| Balloons |
| Tourniquets |
| Catheters |
| Condoms |
| **Dry rubber** |
| Tyres |
| Syringe plungers |
| Vial stoppers |
| Shoe soles |

# 2.4 Urticaria and angio-oedema

## Urticaria

This term is used to describe an elevated papular or plaque-like eruption that is intensely pruritic; each lesion lasts for <24 hours.

- Affects 10–20% of individuals at some time.
- Swelling involves superficial dermis.
- May occur alone or with angio-oedema (swelling involving the deeper dermis and subcutaneous tissue).
- Acute urticaria: symptoms of short duration.
- Chronic urticaria: symptoms lasting >6 weeks.

### Acute urticaria

- Cause usually obvious from history and include:
  - Food.
  - Drugs.
  - Contact with allergies (e.g. latex, plants, foods).
  - Viral infections.
  - Parasitic infections.
  - Insect bites.

### Physical urticarias (~10%)

- Cold: induced by exposure to cold; rare familial form due to mutation of cryopyrin gene; acquired form due to cryoglobulins or infections.
- Cholinergic: induced by exercise or heat.
- Pressure: produced by physical pressure on skin.
- Vibration: induced by vibration in contact with skin.
- Solar: produced by sun exposure; exclude porphyria.

### Chronic urticaria

- Cause is not evident in >90% patients (Fig. 2.7).
- Autoantibodies to FcεR1 and IgE are found in serum of 30–40% of patients.
- ~5–10% of patients have associated autoimmune thyroid disease (treatment of thyroid disease does not, however, cure urticaria).

### Special categories of urticaria

- Urticaria pigmentosa: cutaneous manifestation of systemic mastocytosis.

### Urticarial vasculitis

- Lesions persist >24 hours.
- Brown stain left when lesions fade.
- Biopsy: leucocytoclastic vasculitis.
- Associated with reduced serum C3, C4, and C1q levels.
- Various aetiologies including SLE and auto-antibodies to C1q.

### Pathogenesis

- Mast cell activation with local release of mediators.
- Activation of the complement and kinin pathways.
- Autoantibodies against IgE and the IgE receptor (FcεR1).
- Perivascular leucocytic infiltrates.

### Diagnosis

- History is very important.
- Look for dermatographism, appearance of lesions.
- Physical causes: pressure tests, ice cube test.
- Allergy testing: usually of no value in chronic urticaria.
- Laboratory investigations are not usually helpful.
- In chronic urticaria check thyroid function and FBC.
- Cold urticaria: check for family history, check for cryoglobulins.
- Autoantibodies useful in cases of suspected urticarial vasculitis (ANA, extractable nuclear antigen (ENA), dsDNA, rheumatoid factor (RF)).
- Complement studies indicated in suspected urticarial vasculitis: C3, C4, C1q level.
- Skin biopsy: if urticarial vasculitis suspected.

### Treatment

- Acute urticaria readily responds to antihistamines.
- Chronic urticaria may last up to 2–3 years before going into remission.
- First-line treatment comprises non-sedative, long-acting antihistamines (e.g. cetirizine, levocetirizine, fexofenadine, loratadine).
- May need higher than average dose.
- Prescribe daily treatment for 3 months and then try to withdraw therapy.
- If non-sedative antihistamines alone are not effective, add sedative antihistamine (e.g. hydroxyzine).
- Some patients not responding to H1 receptor antagonists alone respond to addition of H2 receptor blockers or leukotriene antagonists.
- Third-line treatment in patients not responding to above: omalizumab, ciclosporin, sulphasalazine. In these circumstances refer to specialist centre.

## Angio-oedema

Deep tissue swelling. May occur alone or be associated with urticaria.

### Epidemiology

- Idiopathic: 15% of general population.
- Sex: ♂>♀.

### Aetiology

- Allergic.
- Physical (pressure, vibration, cold).
- Drugs (ACE inhibitors, NSAIDs, statins, proton-pump inhibitors (PPIs)).

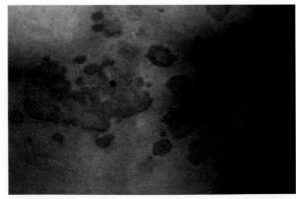

Fig. 2.7 Widespread ordinary urticaria. The smooth erythematous papules and plaques may expand into annular shapes.

Reproduced from Burge S. and Wallis D., *Oxford Handbook of Medical Dermatology*, 2010, Figure 11.1, page 215, with permission from Oxford University Press.

- Hereditary C1 inhibitor deficiency.
- Acquired C1 inhibitor deficiency: SLE, lymphoma.
- Idiopathic: diagnosis made when other causes excluded; this is the **most common** condition.

## Pathogenesis

- Fluid leaks from post-capillary venules.
- Activation of the kinin system with bradykinin production.
- ACE inhibitors inhibit bradykinin breakdown.
- C1 inhibitor protein has a role in complement and clotting systems. It is also a control protein for the kinin cascade.

## Clinical presentation

- Rarely itchy.
- Tends to give discomfort from pressure.
- Premonitory tingling before the swelling occurs in C1 inhibitor deficiency.
- Severe abdominal pain due to angio-oedema of intestinal tissue; these attacks may mimic an acute abdomen.

## History

- Accompanied by urticaria or anaphylaxis (allergic).
- Association with:
  - Physical stimuli.
  - Drug exposure.
- Family history (hereditary C1 inhibitor deficiency).
- Connective tissue disease.
- Lymphoma (may be occult).
- Angio-oedema **with** urticaria will not be due to hereditary angio-oedema.
- Angio-oedema **without** urticaria: exclude C1 esterase inhibitor deficiency.

## Diagnosis

Allergen-specific IgE: skin prick tests or RAST tests.
C1 inhibitor deficiency:
- C4 will be low (even between attacks).
- C1 inhibitor level is reduced in 85% of patients.
- C1 inhibitor function is very low/absent in 100% of cases.

If acquired C1 inhibitor deficiency is suspected: check for a paraprotein in serum and seek advice from an immunologist regarding further investigation.

## Management

Treatment is dependent on the cause:
- Avoid trigger: allergen, NSAIDs, ACE inhibitors.

- Antihistamines comprise the mainstay of treatment.
- Short courses of steroids are indicated for severe attacks.
- Airway compromise is very uncommon except in C1 inhibitor deficiency and ACE-inhibitor induced angio-oedema.

## Hereditary C1 inhibitor deficiency

- Prevention of angio-oedema achieved by use of modified **androgens** (stanozolol 2.5–10mg/day; danazol 200–800mg/day). Monitor LFTs every 4–6 months and consider annual ultrasound scan of liver.
- **Antifibrinolytics** (tranexamic acid 2–4g/day) can prevent attacks but may be less effective. Main indication is to treat symptomatic children before linear growth is complete.
- **Purified C1 inhibitor** is the treatment of choice for angio-oedema with risk of respiratory obstruction or in patients with severe abdominal pain. An alternative is **fresh frozen plasma**.
- **Icatibant (Firazyr®)**: synthetic oligopeptide, Bradykinin receptor antagonist, blocks bradykinin type 2 receptor, approved in the EU for treatment of acute attacks, subcutaneous injection (pre-filled syringe).
- Major surgery or dental extraction should be covered by prophylactic infusions of C1 inhibitor concentrate.
- This is an autosomal dominant trait, therefore genetic counselling and family studies are important.

## Acquired C1 inhibitor deficiency

- Improved by effective treatment of the underlying disease.
- Treatment is difficult; seek specialist advice.

## Complications/prognosis

- Sudden death may occur due to laryngeal oedema in C1 inhibitor deficiency. Before androgenic steroids were used for prophylaxis, the condition had high mortality due to respiratory obstruction.
- Respiratory obstruction can also occur in ACE-inhibitor induced angio-oedema but is very rare in **idiopathic** angio-oedema.
- Recurrent abdominal pain (GI involvement) can occur in C1 inhibitor deficiency; it may be mistaken for an acute abdomen and lead to exploratory laparotomy.
- Increased incidence of SLE in C1 inhibitor deficiency.

## Prevention

- Patients with a history of angio-oedema for any reason should **never** be given ACE inhibitors or oestrogen-containing contraceptive agents. These drugs may precipitate life-threatening angio-oedema.

# 2.5 Anaphylaxis

## Definition

- Severe systemic allergic reaction involving respiratory difficulty and/or hypotension.

## Incidence

- 1:2300 attendees at emergency departments (EDs).
- Incidence at hospital discharge with a primary diagnosis of anaphylaxis:
  - 5.6/100,000 (1991/92).
  - 10.2/100,000 (1994/95).
- 214 deaths attributed to anaphylaxis in the UK between 1992 and 2001.

## Mechanism

- Anaphylactic reactions are IgE-mediated.
- Similar reactions which are non-IgE mediated are called **anaphylactoid** reactions.
- The sequence of events is as follows:
  - Production of IgE in susceptible individual (sensitization).
  - IgE sensitized mast cells and basophils.
  - Exposure to allergen leads to mast cell degranulation and release of chemical mediators including histamine, leukotrienes, and platelet activating factor.
- Mediators act on blood vessels to cause leakage of fluid from the circulation and also cause vasodilatation which further reduces venous return to the heart.
- Mediators also cause bronchoconstriction.

## Causes

- Foods: peanuts, tree nuts (e.g. almonds, walnuts), fish, shrimps, shellfish, egg, milk, sesame, gelatin.
- Drugs.
- Latex.
- Insect venom.
- Radiocontrast media (mainly anaphylactoid reactions).
- Vaccinations.
- Biological fluids (e.g. seminal fluid and biological therapeutic agents).
- Anaesthetic agents and muscle relaxants.
- Exercise (rare).
- Idiopathic (rare).

## Clinical manifestations

- Erythema.
- Pruritus—generalized.
- Urticaria, angio-oedema.
- Laryngeal oedema.
- Difficulty in swallowing or speaking.
- Rhinitis.
- Conjunctivitis.
- Severe asthma/tightness of the chest.
- Nausea, vomiting, abdominal pain, diarrhoea.

- Sense of impending doom.
- Palpitations.
- Fainting, dizziness.
- Collapse, loss of consciousness.

All these features may not be evident in all cases.

## Diagnosis

- Based on clinical grounds and should be made in the presence of hypotension and/or respiratory compromise together with any of the other features listed under 'Clinical manifestations'.
- Obtain any records from acute event.
- Detailed history including suspected inducing agent, route, dose, sequence of symptoms, treatment, associated factors (exercise, medications).

## Differential diagnosis

- Vasovagal syncope.
- Syndromes associated with flushing (e.g. carcinoid).
- Angio-oedema secondary to ACE inhibition.
- Panic attacks.
- Scromboid poisoning.

## Laboratory confirmation

- Serum mast cell **tryptase** (not elevated in all cases).
- Collect serial blood samples at 30-minute intervals for 2 hours ideally (or a single sample with a later baseline).
- Allergen-specific IgE (SPT, RAST): useful to confirm antigen specificity but not to be performed at the time of an active episode.

## Treatment

### Immediate

**ABC** approach (see Section 1.1 and Fig. 2.8):

- Maintain airway, administer oxygen, treat hypotension (IV fluids, vasopressors).
- Adrenaline: 0.5mg 1:1000 solution IM (not IV unless cardiac monitoring available and drug highly diluted).
- Chlorpheniramine IV.
- Hydrocortisone IV (for preventing late phase effects).
- Treat bronchospasm.
- Once recovered observe for 24 hours for possible late-phase relapse.

### Long term

- Identify and train patient to avoid responsible agent (specialist referral is ideal).
- Teach patient/carers how to identify and treat anaphylactic reaction.
- Issue pre-loaded adrenaline injection kits and training in their use: EpiPen®, Anapen®.
- Doses: adult (300mcg, more may be needed in a large adult), child (150mcg).
- Recommend a MedicAlert bracelet.
- Patient information from The Anaphylaxis Campaign (<http://www.anaphylaxis.org.uk>).

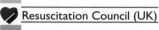

Resuscitation Council (UK)

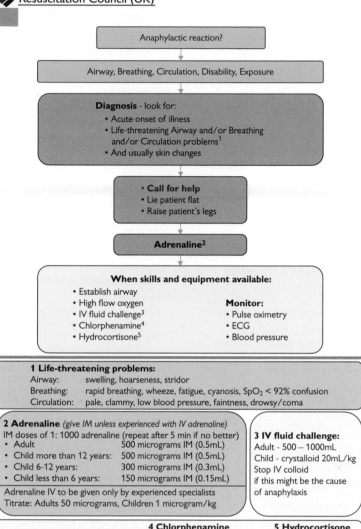

Anaphylactic reaction?

Airway, Breathing, Circulation, Disability, Exposure

**Diagnosis** - look for:
• Acute onset of illness
• Life-threatening Airway and/or Breathing
  and/or Circulation problems[1]
• And usually skin changes

• **Call for help**
• Lie patient flat
• Raise patient's legs

**Adrenaline[2]**

**When skills and equipment available:**
• Establish airway
• High flow oxygen
• IV fluid challenge[3]          **Monitor:**
• Chlorphenamine[4]          • Pulse oximetry
• Hydrocortisone[5]          • ECG
                                          • Blood pressure

**1 Life-threatening problems:**
Airway:          swelling, hoarseness, stridor
Breathing:     rapid breathing, wheeze, fatigue, cyanosis, $SpO_2$ < 92% confusion
Circulation:    pale, clammy, low blood pressure, faintness, drowsy/coma

**2 Adrenaline** (give IM unless experienced with IV adrenaline)
IM doses of 1: 1000 adrenaline (repeat after 5 min if no better)
• Adult                                  500 micrograms IM (0.5mL)
• Child more than 12 years:   500 micrograms IM (0.5mL)
• Child 6-12 years:                300 micrograms IM (0.3mL)
• Child less than 6 years:        150 micrograms IM (0.15mL)

Adrenaline IV to be given only by experienced specialists
Titrate: Adults 50 micrograms, Children 1 microgram/kg

**3 IV fluid challenge:**
Adult - 500 – 1000mL
Child - crystalloid 20mL/kg
Stop IV colloid
if this might be the cause
of anaphylaxis

|  | **4 Chlorphenamine**<br>(IM or slow IV) | **5 Hydrocortisone**<br>(IM or slow IV) |
|---|---|---|
| Adult or child more than 12 years | 10mg | 200mg |
| Child 6-12 years | 5mg | 100mg |
| Child 6 months: 6 years | 2.5mg | 250mg |
| Child less than 6 months | 250 micrograms/kg | 25mg |

**Fig. 2.8** Resuscitation treatment algorithm for first medical responders to anaphylactic reactions in adults.
IM: intramuscular; IV: intravenous.
Reproduced with the kind permission of the Resuscitation Council (UK).

## Warning signs of immunodeficiency

- Failure to thrive during infancy.
- Eight or more new infections in a year.
- Two or more serious sinus infections in a year.
- Two or more episodes of pneumonia in a year.
- Recurrent deep skin or organ abscesses.
- Two or more deep-seated infections (osteomyelitis, liver abscess).
- Persistent oral or cutaneous thrush >1 year old.
- Antibiotics for 2 months without effect.
- Surgical intervention for chronic infection (e.g. lobectomy, recurrent drainage of abscess).
- Family history of primary immunodeficiency.

## Suspect underlying immunodeficiency if infections are:

- **S**erious: e.g. meningococcal septicaemia.
- **P**ersistent: e.g. oral candidiasis resistant to local therapy.
- **U**nusual: organism, e.g. *Aspergillus*, non-tuberculous mycobacteria (NTM), *Pneumocystis*.
- **S**ite: e.g. liver or bone.
- **R**ecurrent:
  - Recurrent upper or lower respiratory tract infection.
  - Two major infections in 1 year.
  - One major and recurrent minor infections in 1 year.

## Investigation for suspected immunodeficiency

### History

- Infections (site, severity, need for antibiotics, hospital admissions).
- Failure to thrive.
- Surgical operations (grommets, lobectomies).
- Chronic diarrhoea: severe combined immunodeficiency (SCID), antibody deficiencies.
- Autoimmunity: common variable immunodeficiency (CVID), hyper-IgM syndrome.
- Immunization history.
- Childhood infections.
- Family history (consanguinity, unexplained sudden deaths).
- Risk factors for human immunodeficiency virus (HIV).
- Immunosuppressive therapy.

### Examination

- Failure to thrive (weight/height).
- Ears, sinuses, lungs.
- Lymph node hyperplasia.
- Mouth ulceration: neutropaenia.
- Signs of autoimmunity: vitiligo, alopecia.
- Skin rash (atypical eczema): Wiskott–Aldrich syndrome, hyper-IgE syndrome, Omenn syndrome.
- Chronic osteomyelitis/deep seated abscesses: chronic granulomatous disease (CGD).
- Hepatosplenomegaly: CVID, Omenn syndrome.

### Laboratory

Specialized investigations always required; seek advice of immunologist and infectious disease specialist first.

### Microbiology

- Microscopy and culture as appropriate.
- Molecular techniques: PCR for microbes.
- In patients with immunodeficiency, serology is unreliable for diagnosis of infection.

### Immunology

- The microbial pathogen and site of infection may be the first pointer to the probability and type of immune defect (Table 2.3).
- The more virulent the organism (e.g. measles), the less likely that there is an immune defect, whereas infections with organisms of low-grade virulence (e.g. *Pneumocystis*) should arouse suspicion.

Patients with disorders of the immune system tend to present in one of five ways, depending on the nature of the defect:

*Presentation 1*

- Recurrent, severe, unusual **pyogenic** infections, most commonly of the upper or lower **respiratory tract**, usually by encapsulated bacteria.
- Infants with failure to thrive (sometimes).

Investigate for **antibody** defect (sometimes complement deficiency): serum IgG, IgA and IgM levels.

Immunoglobulin levels vary with age. Antibody deficiency is present if levels are below the 5th centile confidence limits for age.

*Presentation 2*

- Recurrent **pyogenic skin** sepsis (cellulitis, abscesses) without explanation (i.e. eczema, excoriation) or visceral abscesses (lung, liver, lymph nodes), often caused by *Staphylococcus aureus*.
- Invasive fungal infection.
- Recurrent or persistent oral/mucocutaneous ulceration.
- Unexplained granulomatous inflammation.

Investigate for abnormality in **phagocytosis**:

- Absolute neutrophil count (may need repeating to exclude cyclical neutropaenia).
- Phagocyte oxidase function (to exclude CGD).
- Neutrophil and lymphocyte surface marker analysis to exclude leucocyte adhesin deficiency.

For serious/recurrent encapsulated bacterial sepsis exclude asplenia by splenic ultrasonography and blood film for red cell inclusions (Howell–Jolly bodies).

Table 2.3  Nature of organisms as a guide to the immunodeficiency state

| Category of organism | Types of defect |
| --- | --- |
| Encapsulated bacteria, e.g. *S. pneumoniae*, Hib | Antibody Complement (rare) Asplenia (anatomical or functional) Innate immune deficiency |
| *S. aureus* Gram-negative bacteria Invasive fungal infection | Phagocytic Innate immune deficiency |
| Viral infections (especially reactivation of latent viruses e.g. CMV) Intracellular bacteria, e.g. mycobacteria Fungi, e.g. mucocutaneous candidiasis pneumocystis Protozoa, e.g. *Toxoplasma*, cryptosporidium | Cell-mediated immunity (caused by primary and secondary immunodeficiency; think of HIV) Innate immune deficiency |

*Presentation 3*

- Failure to thrive from early **infancy**, especially if associated with intracellular pathogens (viruses—cytomegalovirus (CMV), *Herpes simplex*, bacteria—mycobacteria, fungi—*Candida, Pneumocystis*).
- Sometimes features of graft-versus-host reaction from materno-fetal or postnatal blood transfusions (skin rash, diarrhoea, hepatomegaly, lymphadenopathy) are observed.
- Infants with HIV may present in this way.

Investigate for defective **cell-mediated immunity**:

- Absolute lymphocyte count.
- Lymphocyte surface marker analysis to enumerate T, B, and NK cells.
- Lymphocyte function tests.

(Note: poor antibody production may also be a consequence of T-cell deficiency and patients may present with pyogenic bacterial infections.)

*Presentation 4*

Patients with infections caused by one or more of the following micro-organisms:

- Viruses (especially reactivation of latent viruses e.g. CMV), persistent *Molluscum contagiosum*, extensive human papilloma virus infection.
- Intracellular bacteria (*Mycobacterium tuberculosis* or disseminated NTM infection, *Listeria, Salmonella*).
- Fungi (mucocutaneous candidiasis or invasive aspergillosis, *Pneumocystis* pneumonia).
- Protozoa (*Toxoplasma, Cryptosporidium*).

*Presentation 5*

- Immunodeficient patients can present with *autoimmune* or *chronic inflammatory* diseases. It is thought that the basic abnormality leading to immunodeficiency may also lead to faulty discrimination between self and non-self, and thus to autoimmune disease.
- The manifestations of these disorders may be limited to a single target cell or organ (e.g. autoimmune haemolytic anaemia, thrombocytopenia, or thyroiditis), or may involve a number of different target organs (e.g. vasculitis, SLE or rheumatoid arthritis (RA)).
- The autoimmune and inflammatory diseases are more commonly seen in:
  - CVID.
  - Selective IgA deficiency.
  - Chronic mucocutaneous candidiasis.
  - Deficiencies of early components of the classical complement pathway (C1–C4).
- Occasionally a disorder that appears to be autoimmune in nature may, in fact, be due to an infectious agent. For example, the dermatomyositis that is sometimes seen in patients with X-linked agammaglobulinaemia is really a manifestation of chronic enterovirus infection and not an autoimmune disease.

# 2.7 Immunodeficiency

## Definition

- Immune system unable to respond appropriately and effectively to infectious micro-organisms.

## Causes of immunodeficiency

- **Primary immunodeficiency:**
  - Due to an intrinsic defect in a component of the immune system.
  - Usually due to a single gene defect and is therefore heritable.
- **Secondary immunodeficiency** (more common):
  - Drugs: corticosteroids.
  - Infection: HIV, Epstein–Barr virus (EBV).
  - Malignancy: lymphoproliferative disease.
  - Malnutrition.
  - Systemic disease: liver/renal failure, diabetes.
  - Splenectomy.

## Primary antibody deficiency

### X-linked agammaglobulinaemia (XLA)

- Mutation in Bruton tyrosine kinase, *BTK* gene (X chromosome).
- B-cell maturation arrest (pro-B to pre-B stages).
- Recurrent infections: sinus, pulmonary, ears.
- Main pathogens: *Streptococcus pneumoniae* and *Haemophilus influenza*.
- Recurrent infections lead to bronchiectasis and chronic sinus damage.
- Diarrhoea and malabsorption may occur (due to overgrowth of commensal bacteria in small intestine) or chronic infections with enteric pathogens.
- Meningoencephalitis: *Enterovirus*.
- Arthritis: *Ureaplasma/Mycoplasma*.

*Diagnosis*

- All immunoglobulins absent or low.
- B-cell lymphopenia with normal numbers of T and NK cells.
- A defect in the *BTK* gene or expression is confirmed (by DNA, mRNA, or protein analysis).

*Management*

- Ig replacement therapy by intravenous or subcutaneous route.
- Antibiotics.
- No live vaccines.
- Genetic counselling.

### IgA deficiency

- **Most common UK primary immunodeficiency, 1:600**.
- IgA 0.05g/L.
- Majority are asymptomatic and healthy.
- A small proportion may be associated with an increased risk of sino-pulmonary infections; this is causally associated with poor specific antibody responses to bacterial capsular polysaccharides.
- Increased incidence of atopy, coeliac disease, and other autoimmune diseases.

### Common variable immunodeficiency (CVID)

- Commonest *symptomatic* antibody deficiency.
- May present at any age.

- Peak age of presentation: early childhood/adulthood.
- Recurrent respiratory infections and gastrointestinal complications (as for X-linked antibody deficiency).
- ~1/5 develop autoimmune disorders (cytopenias, endocrinopathies, chronic hepatitis).
- Sarcoid-like systemic granulomatous disease can affect lungs, liver, and spleen.
- Lymphopenia: reduction of naïve T and B cells common.
- Complications: bronchiectasis/chronic sinus disease, malabsorption, increased risk of malignancy (lymphoma/gastric carcinoma).

*Diagnosis*

- Reduction of serum immunoglobulins below 5th centile for age.
- Associated with absent specific antibodies to routine childhood vaccines (if testing vaccine responses avoid live vaccines).

*Management*

- Immunoglobulins and antibiotics as for XLA.
- Systemic granulomatous disease may need steroids.

### Specific antibody deficiency

- Clinical history suggestive of antibody deficiency.
- Total IgG and IgG subclasses normal.
- Pathogen-specific IgG levels and immunization responses deficient.
- Treat with appropriate immunizations, antibiotics, and immunoglobulin replacement.

### IgG subclass deficiency

- Serum IgG is comprised of four subclasses: IgG1, IgG2, IgG3, and IgG4.
- IgG subclass deficiency—low IgG subclasses, more than two standard deviations below the mean value for age.
- Many individuals with IgG subclass deficiencies are asymptomatic (similar to IgA deficiency).
- Some with IgG subclass deficiencies exhibit reduced antibody responses to bacterial capsular polysaccharides and are prone to recurrent sino-pulmonary infections. This is most often seen in individuals with **IgG2** subclass deficiency with or without concomitant IgA deficiency.
- Most patients with recurrent infections can be managed with antibiotics alone.

### Transient hypogammaglobulinaemia of infancy

- Gap between disappearance of maternally acquired Igs and production of own Igs.
- Low IgG levels at 3–12 months of age.
- Bacterial infections.
- Retrospective diagnosis (when antibody levels return to normal).
- Exclude diagnosis of SCID, XLA, and early-onset CVID.

### X-linked hyper IgM (HIGM) syndrome

- Due to CD40 ligand deficiency; CD40L is a T-cell costimulatory molecule.
- Develop clinical features of antibody deficiency (see under XLA).
- Also develop infections characteristic of T-cell deficiency (*Pneumocystis* pneumonia, cryptosporidial infection—diarrhoea, ascending cholangitis, chronic liver impairment).
- Autoimmune diseases.
- Malignancy: lymphoma.
- IgG and IgA low, IgM high or normal.
- Neutropaenia is common.

- Treatment of antibody deficiency (as for XLA).
- Due to the high incidence of severe liver damage, allogeneic haematopoietic stem cell transplantation (HSCT), which is curative, should be considered in affected children.
- Rare autosomal recessive HIGM syndromes also exist.

### Consequences of antibody deficiency

- Lung damage due to recurrent infections is the main cause of morbidity and mortality.
- There is also an increased incidence of autoimmunity and malignancy as described earlier.

### Management of patients with antibody deficiency

Due to the occurrence of pathologies affecting multiple systems, patients are best managed in specialist immunology centres.

Lifelong immunoglobulin replacement is required—intravenous or subcutaneous.

Extent of associated pulmonary and gastrointestinal pathology needs to be assessed by appropriate investigation.

*Replacement intravenous immunoglobulins (IVIG)*

- 0.4g/kg every 3 weeks.
- Maintain pre-infusion trough IgG >8g/L.
- Higher doses may be required in those with structural lung damage and poor clinical response.
- Donor screening and viral inactivation steps used during manufacture help to ensure safety of Ig preparations.
- Nonetheless, Ig is a biological product which is associated with the theoretical risk of transmission of blood-borne infections.
- Many patients can be established on home therapy with Igs. Licensed subcutaneously infused Ig preparations are also now available.

*Ancillary therapy*

- Prompt treatment of infections with antibiotics is essential; higher doses and longer courses may be required.
- Inhalers and postural drainage may be required in those with chronic lung disease.

# Primary T-cell immunodeficiency

### DiGeorge syndrome

- One of the chromosome 22q deletion syndromes (hemizygous deletion 22q11.2).
- Has an incidence of 1/2500 live births, but the clinical phenotype is highly variable.
- Causes a complex inherited syndrome characterized by:
  • Learning difficulties.
  • Cardiac malformations.
  • Thymic hypoplasia.
  • Palato-pharyngeal abnormalities with associated velopharyngeal dysfunction.
  • Hypoparathyroidism (manifesting as hypocalcaemia).
  • Facial dysmorphism.
- About 20% of individuals with 22q deletion have thymic aplasia resulting in T-cell lymphopenia and impaired cell mediated immunity.
- In most, the degree of T lymphopenia is modest and complete recovery of the T-cell repertoire occurs by 2 years of age.
- Infections characteristic of T-cell deficiency are rare in these individuals.

*Investigation*

- CXR: absent thymic shadow, abnormal cardiac outline.
- Immunological deficiency: variable.
- T cell numbers: reduced.

- Lymphocyte proliferation: reduced.
- Chromosomal defect is detected by the technique called fluorescent *in-situ* hybridization (FISH).

### Chronic mucocutaneous candidiasis

- Rare, both sexes affected.
- Chronic candida infection (skin, mucous membranes, nails).
- Autoimmune endocrine deficiency (hypoparathyroidism, Addison disease).
- T-cell responses to: *Candida*—poor; mitogens—normal.
- Antifungal therapy: regular, high dose, long periods.

# Combined immunodeficiency

### Severe combined immunodeficiency (SCID)

- Typically presents in first few weeks of life.
- Failure to thrive.
- Multiple severe infections caused by a broad range of microbial pathogens.
- **Absent lymphoid tissue**.
- Hypogammaglobulinaemia.
- Lymphopenia (absolute lymphocyte count <2.5 × 10$^9$/L in 1st year of life is pathognomonic).
- Inheritance can be autosomal recessive or X-linked recessive.
- SCID can be caused by a large range of molecular defects.

*Investigation*

- Seek the advice of an immunologist.
- Determine absolute lymphocyte count.
- Enumerate T, B, and NK cells.
- Measure serum Igs.
- Rare cases without severe lymphopenia may need tests of lymphocyte function and assessment of lymphocyte clonality.

*Management*

- Invariably fatal in early infancy unless rescued by HSCT.
- The diagnosis constitutes a medical emergency needing urgent referral to a specialist centre which can confirm diagnosis and undertake bone marrow transplantation.
- HSCT with HLA-matched **sibling** donor can achieve cure rates of >80% (60% with matched **unrelated** donor).
- While awaiting referral to a specialist centre, the following steps are important:
  1. Investigate and treat infections.
  2. Barrier nursing.
  3. Avoid live vaccines (e.g. Bacillus Calmette–Guérin (BCG)).
  4. Commence treatment with IVIG.
  5. Start prophylaxis for *Pneumocystis.*
  6. Blood transfusions should be **irradiated** (to prevent graft-versus-host disease (GVHD) and from CMV-negative donors).

### Wiscott–Aldrich syndrome

- X-linked disorder—loss of function of the WAS protein gene located at Xp11.22–23.
- Thrombocytopenia (small volume platelets).
- Eczema.
- Recurrent infections.
- Increased incidence of lymphoid malignancies.
- Low IgM, normal IgG and IgA.
- Poor response to polysaccharide antigens (e.g. pneumococcal capsular polysaccharide).
- Treatment of choice is HSCT.

### Ataxia telangiectasia

- Autosomal recessive due to mutation in *ATM* (ataxia telangiectasia mutated) gene encoding a protein required for DNA repair.
- Defective DNA repair.
- Increased radiosensitivity.
- Neurological features: cerebellar ataxia, nystagmus.
- Telangiectases: conjunctiva, ear-lobes.
- Lymphoid malignancy: common in 2nd–3rd decade.
- Low IgA and IgG2.
- No curative therapy available.
- Needs management by multidisciplinary team in specialist centres.

## Phagocytic disorders

### Chronic granulomatous disease (CGD)

- Congenital defect of bacterial killing by phagocytic cells (neutrophils and monocytes).
- Oxidative pathway of microbial killing severely impaired due to defect in NADPH-oxidase complex.
- Develop subcutaneous, lymph node, pulmonary, and liver abscesses (Fig. 2.9).
- The spectrum of micro-organisms which cause infections in CGD include: *Staphylococcus aureus*, Gram-negative bacteria (*Burkholderia cepacea, Salmonella, Serratia*) and fungi (*Aspergillus* spp.)
- The formation of chronic granulomata in various tissues is a typical feature of CGD. In critical locations, granuloma formation may cause pathology (e.g. obstruction of the gastrointestinal or genitourinary tract).

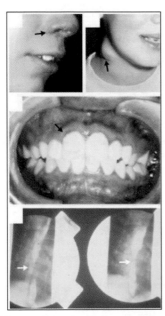

**Fig. 2.9** Clinical features of chronic granulomatous disease (arrows indicate localized abscesses).

*Top and middle figures:* From *The New England Journal of Medicine*, Lekstrom-Himes, JA, and Gallin, JI, Immunodeficiency Diseases Caused by Defects in Phagocytes, 343 (23), Copyright © (2000) Massachusetts Medical Society. Reprinted with permission from Massachusetts Medical Society.

*Bottom figure:* Reprinted from *The Journal of Pediatrics*, 111, 3, Chin TW et al., 'Corticosteroids in treatment of obstructive lesions of chronic granulomatous disease', pp. 349–352, Copyright (1987), with permission from Elsevier.

- Hepatosplenomegaly may occur (granulomatous infiltration).
- A granulomatous colitis resembling Crohn disease occurs in about 15%.

#### Investigation

- Test for phagocyte oxidase activity of blood neutrophils using nitro-blue tetrazolium test or equivalent flow-cytometric method.

#### Management

- Prophylactic antimicrobial therapy (bacteria, fungi).
- Usually treated with co-trimoxazole and itraconazole.
- IFN-γ therapy also reduces incidence of serious infections.
- Prompt and aggressive investigation and treatment of infections with bacteriological guidance important.

### Cyclical neutropaenia

- Recurrent abscesses, mouth ulcers and fever at 3-weekly intervals.
- Neutrophil count $<1 \times 10^9$/L at time of infection.

#### Investigation

- Neutrophil count on alternate days for 4 weeks.

#### Management

- Prophylactic antibiotics (when neutrophil count is low).
- GM-CSF therapy (maintains normal neutrophil count).

### Leucocyte adhesion deficiency

- Caused by defects in surface molecules on leucocytes (required for normal migration from the blood into the sites of infection).
- Patients typically present in **early childhood** with recurrent pyogenic infection of skin, respiratory, and gastrointestinal tracts.
- Older children have severe gingivitis and periodontal disease.
- Poor wound healing and delayed umbilical cord separation are typical.
- Due to impaired neutrophil migration, these patients develop a leucocytosis and pus fails to form at sites of infection.
- These inherited disorders are rare.

#### Investigation

- Flow cytometry of blood leucocytes for expression of leucocyte adhesion molecules (CD18 or rarely CD15).

#### Management

- Prognosis is poor without HSCT.

### Type 1 cytokine pathway defects

- Some bacterial species (*Mycobacteria, Salmonella*) can grow and multiply within macrophages. The elimination of these organisms depends on activation of bactericidal mechanisms operating within macrophages by the cytokine IFN-γ.
- On exposure to these pathogens, macrophages and dendritic cells secrete the cytokine IL-12 which in turn stimulates T cells and NK cells to secrete IFN-γ.
- Patients with defects in the IL-12-dependent IFN-γ axis develop disseminated infections caused by mycobacterial species of low-grade virulence (NTM, BCG) or *Salmonella*.
- Such patients may have a defect in IL-12, IL-12 receptors or IFN-γ receptors.

#### Investigation

- The functional integrity of the IL-12 dependent IFN-γ pathway needs to be assessed in patients with disseminated NTM/BCG or *Salmonella* infections.
- Seek the advice of an immunologist.

#### Management

- Patients with **complete** IFN-γ receptor defects present in early infancy with NTM or BCG infections. Prognosis is poor unless treated with a bone marrow transplant.

- **Partial** IFN-γ receptor defects and defects in IL-12 or IL-12 receptors usually present later in life and usually respond to prolonged courses of antibiotics.
- If response to antibiotics is poor, they can be treated with recombinant IFN-γ.

# Complement pathway deficiencies

See Table 2.4.

| Table 2.4 Complement pathway deficiencies | |
|---|---|
| Complement deficiency | Clinical association |
| C1q, C1r, C1s, C4, C2 | SLE, immune complex disorders |
| C3 properdin, membrane attack complex proteins (C5, C6, C7, C8, C9) | Neisserial infection |
| C1 inhibitor | Angio-oedema |
| CD59 | Haemolysis, thrombosis |
| C3 | Pyogenic bacterial infections (may be accompanied by distinctive rash) Membranoproliferative glomerulonephritis |
| Factor H and factor I | Haemolytic uraemic syndrome Membranoproliferative glomerulonephritis |

From *The New England Journal of Medicine*, Walport M.J, Com plement, 344 (14), Copyright © (2001) Massachusetts Medical Society. Reprinted with permission from Massachusetts Medical Society.

# Splenectomy

- Main indications:
  - Splenic trauma.
  - Hypersplenism.
  - Autoimmune haemolysis.
  - ITP.
  - Congenital haemolytic anaemia.
- Post-splenectomy blood film: Howell–Jolly bodies, target cells.
- Lifelong increased risk from infection: mainly from **encapsulated** organisms which are normally cleared from the circulation by the spleen (*Streptococcus pneumoniae, Haemophilus influenzae, Neisseria meningitides, Capnocytophaga canimorsus*, the latter almost exclusively after dog bites or dog scratches).

*Management*
- Vaccinations:
  - Pneumococcal (every 5–10 years, or when antibodies fall below protective level).
  - *Haemophilus influenzae* type b.
  - Meningococcal C.
  - Influenza (yearly).
- MedicAlert bracelet.
- Prophylactic oral antibiotics (lifelong), phenoxymethyl-penicillin (erythromycin if penicillin allergic).
- Seek urgent medical attention if signs of infection.
- International travel—risk of severe malaria (appropriate malaria prophylaxis and mosquito avoidance measures advised).

# 2.8 Immunology investigations

## Immunoassays

### ELISA (enzyme-linked immunosorbent assay)

*Method*
- Antigen bound to solid phase (bead/plate).
- Reacted with serum.
- React with anti-serum against human Ig coupled to enzyme.
- React with substrate (direct or amplification).
- Spectrophotometric reading taken.
- Pros: more sensitive, can automate.
- Cons: may lose specificity, pure antigen required (recombinant), commercial kit based assays may be costly.

### Radioimmunoassay
- Highly sensitive.
- Requires pure antigen/radioisotopes.
- Laboratories are moving away from using this technique.

### Fluoroimmunoassay

*Method*
- Antigen bound to solid phase (bead/plate).
- Reacted with serum.
- React with anti-serum against human Ig coupled to fluorescent dye or its precursor.
- React with substrate (direct or amplification).
- Fluorescence readout.

## Immunochemistry

### Examples of assays
- Serum immunoglobulins and electrophoresis.
- Urinary protein analysis.
- Specific antibodies.
- Total and allergen-specific IgE.
- Assays for complement components.
- Measurement of acute-phase reactants.

### Serum immunoglobulins
- Levels vary according to age.
- Polyclonal elevation: chronic infection/inflammatory disorders, liver disease, autoimmune disease.
- Monoclonal elevation: myeloma/monoclonal gammopathy of uncertain significance (MGUS), Waldenström macroglobulinae-mia, lymphoma.

### Serum electrophoresis
- Separates proteins according to electrical charge.
- Main use is to detect paraproteinaemia.
- Densitometry: measures size of paraprotein band.

### Urinary protein analysis
- Urine electrophoresis: concentrated urine used.
- Urinary free light chains: spot morning urine or 24-hour sample (no preservative).

### Immunoblotting

*Method*
- Antigens electrophoresed in a matrix or applied to a matrix.

- Incubate with dilutions of serum.
- Enzyme-conjugated anti-serum added.
- Substrate added.
- Read out: coloured band.
- Pros: quick, can automate.
- Examples: ENA/PR3/MPO/M2 mitochondrial assays.

### Immunoprecipitation assay

*Principle*
- Antigen meets antibody at optimum concentration.
- Forms insoluble immune complex.
- Solid phase:
  - Double diffusion (DD).
  - Counter-current immunoelectrophoresis (CCIE).
- Liquid phase:
  - Nephelometry/turbidometry (automated analysis possible).

## Immunofluorescence

### Indirect immunofluorescence

*Method*
- Tissue substrate on glass slide (rodent/human).
- Patient serum incubated with slide.
- Conjugated anti-human Ig added.
- Read using a fluorescence microscope.

*Examples*
- Autoantibodies (ANA (see Fig. 2.10), AMA, SMA, endomysial, adrenal).

### Direct immunofluorescence

*Method*
- Tissue biopsy on slide (renal or skin).
- Conjugated anti-human Ig.
- Read using a fluorescence microscope.

## Cellular immunology

### Lymphocyte phenotyping
- Flow cytometric assay.
- Lymphocyte sub-populations (T, B, and NK cells).
- Panel of monoclonal antibodies directed at CD markers.
- Age-appropriate ranges.
- Immunodeficiency and lymphoid malignancy panels.
- Serial CD4+ measurements, e.g. HIV monitoring—**not** to be used as a surrogate for HIV diagnosis.

### Lymphocyte proliferation tests

*Method*
- Heparinized blood.
- Incubate for 3–5 days with: mitogens or antigens (*Candida*, tetanus).
- Cell proliferation detected by 3H-thymidine incorporation or equivalent non-isotopic test.

*Indications*
- SCID/DiGeorge syndrome.

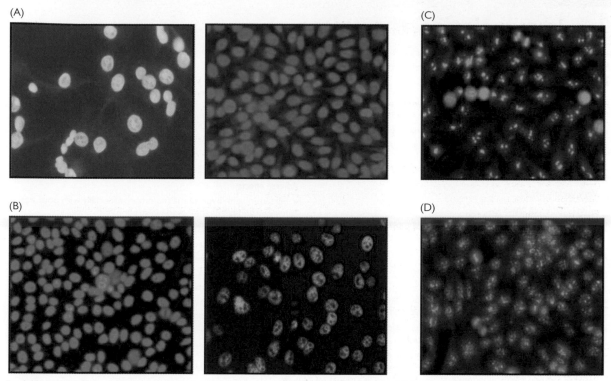

**Fig. 2.10** Antinuclear antibody patterns (ANA). (A) Homogeneous. (B) Speckled. (C) Nucleolar. (D) Centromere.

## Neutrophil function tests
*Indications*
- Recurrent skin infections.
- Chronic gingivitis.
- Recurrent deep-seated bacterial/fungal infections.

*Types of assays*
- Oxidative burst test assays.
- Nitro blue tetrazolium assay.
- Flow cytometric assay: di-hydro rhodamine test.
- Adhesion molecule assay.
- CD18 and CD15 expression by flow cytometry.

# 2.9 Immunological therapies

## Immunosuppressive drugs

- Used in the treatment of autoimmunity, allergy, and transplant rejection.
- Most also suppress immune responses to pathogens.
- Specific tolerance not possible resulting in an increased infection risk.

### Corticosteroids

- Very widely used.
- Affect many cell types.
- Cause a wide range of side effects including metabolic, cardiovascular, musculoskeletal, and neurological disturbance.

### Azathioprine

- Inhibits purine synthesis which is essential for proliferation of many cell types (especially T cells).
- Converted in the body to the active metabolites 6-mercaptopurine (6-MP) and 6-thioinosinic acid.
- Used alone in many disorders and in combination with other immunosuppressants in organ transplantation.
- Side effects are uncommon but include: nausea, rash, haemolytic anaemia, and bone marrow suppression (remember to avoid co-administration with allopurinol).
- Thiopurine S-methyltransferase (TPMT) deactivates 6-MP and genetic polymorphisms can lead to drug toxicity. Serum TPMT assays may be useful to prevent this complication.

### Mycophenolate mofetil (MMF)

- Also inhibits purine synthesis essential for the proliferation of T and B lymphocytes.
- Increasingly being used in favour of azathioprine in organ transplantation, and in the treatment of various autoimmune diseases.

### Cyclophosphamide

- Alkylating agent cross-links DNA.
- Especially toxic to B cells.

*Indications*

- Malignancy.
- Severe autoimmune disease (SLE, vasculitis).

*Adverse effects*

- Neutropaenia, lymphopenia.
- Alopecia, infertility (especially ♀).
- Haemorrhagic cystitis (to prevent: increase fluid intake and consider mesna).

### Methotrexate

- Inhibit dihydrofolate reductase (folic acid not converted to active form—tetrahydrofolate).

*Indications*

- Malignancy: leukaemia.
- Inflammatory disorders: RA, psoriasis, polymyositis.
- GVHD.
- Steroid-dependent asthma.

*Adverse effects*

- Bone marrow suppression, megaloblastic anaemia.
- Mucositis, pneumonitis.
- Hepatic impairment.
- Folinic acid rescue for acute adverse effects.

### Ciclosporin

- Interacts with immunophilins.
- Prevents signalling following T-cell receptor activation.
- Narrow therapeutic range: therapeutic drug monitoring required to assess risk of toxicity.
- Reduces incidence of transplant rejection.
- Significantly improves graft survival.

*Adverse effects*

- Hirsutism, gum hyperplasia (common: especially with poor oral hygiene and nifedipine co-administration).
- Hypertension, nephrotoxicity (dose-dependent).
- Liver dysfunction, fluid and potassium retention.
- Burning hands and feet (especially during the first week of therapy).
- Skin and lymphoid malignancy (with long-term therapy).
- Grapefruit or grapefruit juice should not be taken for 1 hour before the dose of ciclosporin.

### Tacrolimus

- Macrolide.
- Binds cytosolic FK506 binding protein (FKBP).
- Prevents *IL-2* gene activation.

*Indications*

- Renal and liver transplantation.
- Autoimmune disease.
- Atopic dermatitis (topical).

*Adverse effects*

- Similar to ciclosporin.
- Most common adverse events associated with topical tacrolimus includes: sensation of skin burning, itching, flu-like symptoms, and headache.

### Sirolimus

- Binds specific protein tyrosine kinase.
- Inhibits signals after IL-2 has bound to its receptor.

## Monoclonal antibodies

### Infliximab

- Chimeric monoclonal antibody to tumour necrosis factor alpha (TNF-α).
- Uses: Crohn disease, RA, ankylosing spondylitis.
- Dose: 3mg/kg IV infusion, repeated at intervals of 2–8 weeks.

*Adverse effects*

- Increase risk of tuberculosis (screening important).
- Production of ANA.
- Production of human anti-chimaeric antibody (HACA) which reduces the therapeutic effect minimized by combined use with methotrexate.

### Adalimumab

- Human monoclonal antibody to TNF-α.
- Often co-administered with methotrexate.
- 40mg subcutaneous dose on alternate weeks.
- Indications and side effects: similar to infliximab.

### Etanercept

- Soluble fusion protein of TNFR2 and Fc portion of human IgG1.
- Binds TNF-α, TNF-β.
- Synergistic with methotrexate.
- Indications: RA, psoriatic arthritis.
- Subcutaneous administration.
- Increased risk of infection (including varicella zoster).

### Rituximab

- Humanized anti-CD20 monoclonal antibody.
- Depletes B cells.
- IV infusion administration.

*Uses*

- Advanced follicular lymphoma (and other types).
- Inflammatory disease: RA, SLE, systemic vasculitis.
- Adjunctive therapy in ABO-incompatible organ transplantation.

*Adverse effects*

- Cytokine release syndrome.
- Arrhythmia, heart failure.
- Pre-medicate: antihistamines, steroids.

### Anakinra

- Recombinant IL-1R antagonist.
- Blocks action of IL-1.
- 100mg/day, subcutaneous administration.
- Indications: RA, auto-inflammatory disorders.
- Adverse effects: neutropaenia, headaches.

### Omalizumab

- Murine anti-human IgE monoclonal antibody.
- Inhibits IgE binding to its receptor.
- Blocks IgE mediated release of inflammatory mediators from mast cells.
- Indications: moderate-severe asthma, allergic conjunctivitis and rhinitis, food allergy.

### Basiliximab

- Monoclonal antibody against the IL-2 receptor on T cells.
- T cells are unable to proliferate.
- Used as induction therapy for organ transplantation (especially renal) to prevent rejection.

## Immunoglobulin therapy (IVIG)

### Replacement therapy for antibody deficiency

- Dose: 0.2–0.6g/kg body weight every 4 weeks.

### High-dose IVIG therapy

*Mechanism of action*

- Fc receptor blockade.
- Inhibits macrophage activation.
- Inhibits T-cell activation.
- Alters networks pertinent to autoreactivity and induction of tolerance to self.
- Dose: 1–2g/kg.

*Uses*

- Autoimmune thrombocytopenia.

- Kawasaki disease.
- Guillain–Barré syndrome.
- Dermatomyositis.
- Multifocal motor neuropathy.

*Adverse effects*

- Aseptic meningitis.
- Acute haemolysis.
- Deterioration in renal function.

## Cytokine therapy

### Interferon-α

*Indications*

- Lymphoma, leukaemia.
- AIDS-related Kaposi sarcoma.
- Renal cell carcinoma.
- Chronic hepatitis B and C infection.
- Administered subcutaneously.

*Adverse effects*

- Influenza-like syndrome.
- Bone marrow suppression.
- Hepatic/renal toxicity.

### Interferon-β

*Indications*

- Relapsing-remitting multiple sclerosis (MS)—benefits some, may cause deterioration in others.
- Administered subcutaneously.

*Adverse effects*

- Local irritation at injection site.
- Influenza-like symptoms.
- Hypersensitivity reaction (anaphylaxis, urticaria).

### Interferon-γ

*Indications*

- CGD.
- IFN-γ/IL-12 pathway defects.
- Administered subcutaneously, three times a week.
- Dose based on body surface area.

*Adverse effects*

- Influenza-like symptoms.
- Anaemia.
- Abnormalities in liver/renal function.

### Granulocyte macrophage colony-stimulating factor (GM-CSF)

- Increases the production of mature neutrophils.

*Indications*

- Chemotherapy/neutropaenic sepsis.
- To mobilize stem cells (stem cell harvest).
- Congenital neutrophil disorders (cyclical neutropaenia).

*Adverse effects*

- Increased risk of myeloid malignancy.
- Bone pain.

# Chapter 3

# Cardiovascular medicine

# 3.1 Basic science

## Introduction

Cardiovascular disease remains the most common cause of death worldwide. Despite advances in primary and secondary preventive treatment, mortality from ischaemic heart disease remains high in the developed world and is increasing in developing countries. There is wide geographical variation in other cardiac disorders, such as rheumatic fever and endomyocardial fibrosis. A precise understanding of normal cardiac structure and function is essential to understanding the pathophysiology and treatment of cardiovascular disorders (Fig. 3.1).

## Normal cardiac rhythm

The cardiac cycle begins with atrial depolarization, originating in the normal heart in the sinoatrial (SA) node.

Normal cardiac conduction depends on the integrity of:

- SA node.
- Internodal fibres.
- Atrioventricular (AV) node.
- AV bundle (of His).
- Ventricular Purkinje fibres.

## The cardiac cycle

The cardiac cycle can be represented graphically as the pressure–volume relationship of the left ventricle (Fig. 3.2).

### Notable points

- Atrial systole ('a' on Fig. 3.2) boosts left ventricular (LV) filling at the end of diastole, and is particularly advantageous in impaired ventricular filling (e.g. when the left ventricle fails to relax normally, such as in LVH).
- Isovolumetric contraction begins when LV pressure exceeds atrial pressure, and continues until it exceeds aortic pressure.
- **Physiological** systole lasts from the start of isovolumetric contraction to the peak of the ejection phase.
- **Cardiological** systole lasts from closure of the mitral valve to closure of the aortic valve (i.e. between heart sounds S1 and S2).

## Heart sounds

The timing of the heart sounds in relation to the cardiac cycle is shown in Fig. 3.2:

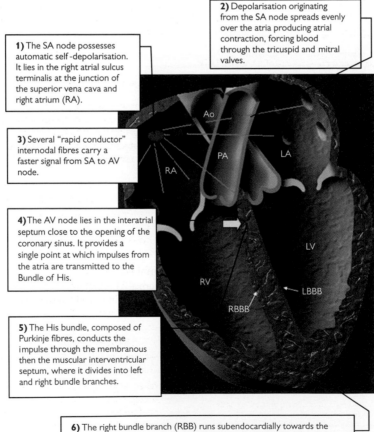

**1)** The SA node possesses automatic self-depolarisation. It lies in the right atrial sulcus terminalis at the junction of the superior vena cava and right atrium (RA).

**2)** Depolarisation originating from the SA node spreads evenly over the atria producing atrial contraction, forcing blood through the tricuspid and mitral valves.

**3)** Several "rapid conductor" internodal fibres carry a faster signal from SA to AV node.

**4)** The AV node lies in the interatrial septum close to the opening of the coronary sinus. It provides a single point at which impulses from the atria are transmitted to the Bundle of His.

**5)** The His bundle, composed of Purkinje fibres, conducts the impulse through the membranous then the muscular interventricular septum, where it divides into left and right bundle branches.

**6)** The right bundle branch (RBB) runs subendocardially towards the apex, and breaks up to supply the right ventricle (RV). The left bundle branch (LBB) runs down the left border of the septum, dividing earlier than the RBB to supply the left ventricle (LV) and papillary muscles. This delivery of the cardiac impulse allows contraction from the base of the heart directing blood upwards through the aortic and pulmonary valves

**Fig. 3.1** Anatomy of the cardiac conducting system.

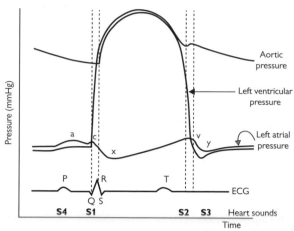

**Fig. 3.2** The cardiac cycle. The changes in left ventricular (LV), aortic, and left atrial pressures during the cardiac cycle (timed against the ECG), and the timing of the heart sounds (including S3 and S4 if present). Atrial depolarization ('P' wave on ECG) is closely followed by atrial contraction at the end of diastole ('a' wave—see section on JVP). Systole begins with a brief period of isovolumetric ventricular contraction (between first set of dotted vertical lines) followed by ejection of blood into the aorta (once LV pressure exceeds aortic). The ejection phase ends when LV pressure falls below aortic pressure and the aortic valve closes; a brief period of isovolumetric ventricular relaxation (between second set of dotted vertical lines) follows, until the atrioventricular valves open and passive ventricular filling resumes.

- S1 corresponds with closure of the mitral and tricuspid valves, while closure of the aortic and pulmonary valves corresponds with the A2 (aortic) and P2 (pulmonary) components of S2 respectively.
- The interval between A2 and P2 is caused by the variation of venous return to the right heart with respiration.
- Wider separation ('splitting') of A2 and P2 can occur in certain pathological states.
- S3 is caused by passive ventricular filling as soon as the mitral and tricuspid valves open. S3 can be normal in those <40 years old, but can also occur in LV dilatation, significant mitral or tricuspid regurgitation, constrictive pericarditis, or ventricular septal defects.
- S4 is caused by atrial systole, propelling blood into a stiff left ventricle. Any cause of decreased LV elasticity (e.g. LVH, infiltrative diseases) can cause an audible S4; rarely, it can be heard in the acute myocardial infarction (MI) setting.

See Box 3.1 for abnormalities of S1 and S2.

## Arterial pulse

Abnormalities of arterial pulse character are common MRCP (membership of the royal colleges of physicians) questions. In summary: An exaggeration of the normal drop in systolic (and pulse) pressure during inspiration; >10mmHg is pathological.

| | |
|---|---|
| Slow rising | Aortic stenosis. |
| Collapsing | Aortic incompetence, patent ductus arteriosus, hyperdynamic circulation (e.g. anaemia, thyrotoxicosis). |
| Bisferiens | Mixed aortic valve disease (aka biphasic—the pulse has a palpable double peak). |
| Alternans | Alternating strong and weak beats: severe LV failure, can occur in tachyarrhythmias in a normal heart. |
| Bigeminus | Premature ectopic after each sinus beat (benign in the absence of ischaemic or structural heart disease). |
| Jerky | LV outflow tract obstruction. |
| Paradoxus | Asthma, constrictive pericarditis, tamponade. |

### Box 3.1 Abnormalities of S1 and S2

**S1**

| Loud | Soft |
|---|---|
| Short P–R interval | Long P–R interval |
| Mitral stenosis (mobile) | Mitral stenosis (immobile) |
| Tachycardic states | Mitral regurgitation |
| Hyperdynamic states | Hypodynamic states |

*Tachycardia*

S1 can be split on normal inspiration; pathological causes of splitting of S1 include: right (RBBB) and left bundle branch block (LBBB), ventricular tachycardia.

**S2**

| Loud | Soft |
|---|---|
| Systemic hypertension Pulmonary hypertension Atrial septal defect Tachycardia | Advanced aortic stenosis |

Physiological splitting of S2 occurs on inspiration and is normal. Abnormal splitting can occur:
- **Fixed:** atrial septal defect.
- **Wide:** RBBB, deep inspiration, pulmonary stenosis, mitral regurgitation.
- **Reverse** (i.e. splitting increases on expiration): systemic hypertension, LBBB, aortic stenosis, patent ductus arteriosus, right ventricular pacing lead.

## Jugular venous pulse

The jugular venous pulse (JVP) acts as a 'manometer' of right atrial pressure. As there are no valves between the internal jugular system and the right atrium, the JVP directly reflects pressure changes within the right atrium. Examination of the JVP is an essential component of clinical cardiovascular assessment and is outlined in Fig. 3.3 and Box 3.2.

The external jugular vein may be distended when the central venous pressure is elevated, but it is an unreliable marker as it not only contains valves, but also may be kinked as it passes through the deep fascia of the neck.

An abnormally low JVP—usually caused by severe hypovolaemia—cannot be measured clinically.

### Normal waveform

The normal JVP waveform consists of three peaks (*a*, *c*, and *v* waves) and two troughs (*x* and *y* waves; see Fig. 3.3). These coincide with specific events in the cardiac cycle (Fig. 3.2):
- *a* **wave:** atrial systole (may cause an audible S4 if prominent); absent in atrial fibrillation.
- *x* **descent:** drop in JVP that begins as soon as atrial contraction has ceased.
- *c* **wave:** very difficult to see—no more than a flicker during the *x* descent. Caused by rapid increase in right ventricular pressure just before tricuspid valve closes, transmitted retrogradely up the internal jugular vein. In practice, the *c* wave signifies closure of the tricuspid valve.
- *v* **wave:** passive filling of the right atrium during ventricular systole (tricuspid valve closed) leads to a gradual increase in right atrial pressure, the peak of which corresponds to the *v* wave.
- *y* **descent:** passive draining of blood from right atrium to ventricle through the tricuspid valve; if prominent, an S3 may be audible.

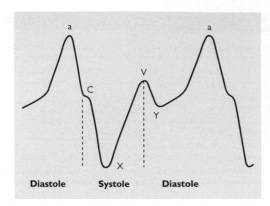

**Fig. 3.3** Jugular venous pulse waveform.

## Causes of a raised JVP

The JVP may be raised with a normal waveform, or else individual components of the waveform may be abnormal. An elevated JVP that paradoxically rises with inspiration is termed Kussmaul sign, caused by cardiac tamponade, constrictive pericarditis, or right ventricular infarction. Superior vena cava obstruction (e.g. by tumour) causes a highly elevated, pulseless JVP with no respiratory variation.

*Raised JVP with normal waveform*

- Fluid overload.
- Right heart failure.
- Marked bradycardia.

*Raised JVP with abnormal waveform*

*a waves can be:*

- **Giant:** tricuspid stenosis (although often in atrial fibrillation hence no *a* waves), pulmonary stenosis, pulmonary hypertension. Marked hypertrophy of the ventricular septum (e.g. hypertrophic cardiomyopathy) can encroach on the right ventricular cavity, obstructing right ventricular filling (Bernheim effect).
- **Cannon:** occur when the right atrium contracts against a closed tricuspid valve; the high pressure generated causes a rapid rising—and larger—*a* wave, e.g. complete heart block, ventricular

extrasystoles, ventricular tachycardia, 2:1 2nd-degree heart block, junctional rhythms.

- **Absent:** atrial fibrillation.

*x descent*
In states of extrinsic myocardial compression (e.g. constrictive pericarditis, tamponade), passive filling of the right atrium can only occur during ventricular systole; a steep *x* descent ensues.

*Giant v waves*
Tricuspid regurgitation (TR): throughout ventricular systole right ventricular pressure is transmitted directly to the right atrium/IJV. With mild-moderate TR, elevated or giant v waves are seen, becoming a single sinusoidal waveform (systolic *cv* waves) with severe TR. Associated with pulsatile hepatomegaly.

*y descent can be:*

- **Rapid:** rapid flow through the tricuspid valve as soon as it opens (tricuspid regurgitation, cardiac tamponade).
- **Slow:** tricuspid stenosis.

## Normal cardiac function and exercise

Changes in both systolic and diastolic function occur during exercise. The effects of exercise on LV pressure and volume are shown in Fig. 3.4.

### Systolic function

- Vagal withdrawal causes the initial increase in heart rate.
- Sympathetic nervous system promotes a further increase in heart rate and increases contractility.
- Left and right ventricular end-diastolic volumes (EDVs) rise slightly while end-systolic volumes (ESVs) decrease.
- Stroke volume, ejection fraction, and cardiac output (CO) increase.
- Mild exercise—CO increase is due to increases in both heart rate and stroke volume; more severe exercise—CO increase is driven predominantly by increase in heart rate.

### Diastolic function

- Less well studied than systolic function.
- LV ESV is smaller in exercise, but rate of LV relaxation in diastole is increased.

---

**Box 3.2 Examination of the JVP**

- Maximal pulsation of the internal jugular vein (IJV) (usually) occurs when the trunk is inclined at 45° to the horizontal; therefore this angulation is most commonly used in clinical examination.
- If central venous pressure is highly elevated, sit the patient up further.
- Patient must be allowed to relax; the IJV runs deep to the strap muscles on anterior neck and is difficult to see if they are tensed.
- Ask the patient to turn their head slightly to the left or right. Shining a light (bedside lamp) tangentially across the skin overlying the IJV makes pulsation more obvious.
- The contralateral carotid pulse can be palpated simultaneously to allow timing against events of the cardiac cycle (*a* wave occurs just before carotid pulse; *v* wave accompanies carotid pulse).
- Vertical height of the JVP column (from the sternal angle ('angle of Louis') which provides a fixed reference point to the midpoint of the right atrium) is measured.
- The JVP should be ≤4cm above the angle of Louis in health; corresponds to the JVP being just visible above the clavicle.
- CVP = JVP + 5cmH$_2$O.

*Venous or arterial pulse?*
The following features help differentiate the JVP from carotid pulse:

- It is not palpable.
- It is obliterated by finger pressure.
- The pulsation is upwards rather than outwards.
- Rises transiently with pressure applied to the abdomen below the right costal margin (hepatojugular re*flux* (not reflex)).
- Alters with posture (falls as patient sits up) and respiration (falls with deep inspiration).
- Double waveform for every arterial pulse.

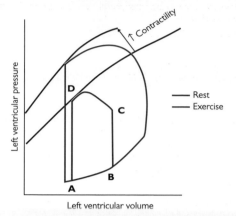

Left ventricular pressure (y-axis)

Left ventricular volume (x-axis)

↑ Contractility

D

C

A

B

—— Rest
—— Exercise

**Fig. 3.4** Left ventricular volume/pressure curve at rest and during exercise.

• The 'elastic recoil' of the left ventricle is therefore increased in exercise.
• This creates a 'diastolic suction effect' which allows more rapid LV filling during diastole—one-third of the stroke volume may enter the left ventricle while the LV pressure is still falling.

Abnormalities of systolic or diastolic function may lead to the syndrome of heart failure (see Section 3.5).

During ventricular diastole, passive filling of the left ventricle results in a gradual increase in LV volume and mild increase in pressure (AB in Fig. 3.4). Once the atrioventricular valves close, there is a period of isovolumetric ventricular contraction during which LV pressure rises steeply (BC); once the aortic and pulmonary valves open, LV pressure continues to rise but volume falls as blood is ejected into the aorta (systole—CD). At the end of systole, these two valves close and there is a period of isovolumetric ventricular relaxation (DA). The increased stroke volume, enhanced contractility, and higher LV pressures that occur during exercise in a normal heart are shown in Fig. 3.4.

## 3.2 Cardiovascular investigation

## Electrocardiology

### The electrocardiogram (ECG)

The recording of an ECG is a simple, cheap, non-invasive means of providing immediate information about the cardiac status of a patient, yet the ECG contains more information than is appreciated by most physicians. A structured methodology in ECG interpretation, which is beyond the scope of this book, is required, together with knowledge of key 'checklists' of causes of common ECG abnormalities.

#### Cardiac intervals

##### PR interval

- Normal range 120–200ms.
- Can be abnormally short or long.
- Short PR interval usually indicates pre-excitation via an accessory pathway (e.g. Wolff–Parkinson–White (WPW) syndrome) but may also be caused by low atrial rhythms, nodal rhythms, ventricular extrasystoles; rarely Duchenne muscular dystrophy and glycogen storage disorders.
- Prolongation of the PR interval suggests first-degree heart block (see Section 3.4).

##### QRS complex duration

- Normal if <120ms.
- Prolongation of the QRS duration suggests a conduction defect within the ventricles.
- Most commonly, the typical left or right bundle branch block (BBB) pattern will be present (Table 3.1).
- If QRS >120ms but the typical RBBB or LBBB pattern is not present, a non-specific intraventricular conduction defect (IVCD) is said to be present.
- Incomplete or 'partial' BBB present if the QRS complexes display the typical BBB morphology but QRS <120ms.
- R wave dominance in V1 is a common MRCP question (Box 3.3)

##### QT interval

- Affected by heart rate hence usually corrected for this.
- Bazett formula corrects QT (QTc) using interval between the peaks of successive R waves (the RR interval):
  $$QTc = QT/\sqrt{RR}$$
- Normal QTc = 380–420ms.
- Prolongation can be congenital or acquired (see Box 3.4 and Fig. 3.5).

#### Cardiac axis

Can be deviated to the left (LAD) or right (RAD). See Table 3.2 for causes.

---

**Box 3.3 R wave dominance in lead V1**

More common in examinations than in clinical practice!
  Causes include:

- True posterior myocardial infarction.
- WPW type A syndrome.
- RBBB.
- RVH.
- Duchenne muscular dystrophy.
- Hypertrophic cardiomyopathy.
- Dextrocardia.
- Dextroposition (e.g. due to right basal atelectasis).

---

#### ST segment

The ST segment deviation is measured as the vertical shift of the ST segment from the isoelectric line, at a point 80ms beyond the J point (where the QRS complex ends) (Box 3.5).

Early repolarization or 'high take-off' often confuses junior and senior doctors alike. It typically occurs in healthy young males. The T wave begins early, resulting in elevation of the ST segment at the J point. It is best seen in leads V1–V3 and is benign (Fig. 3.6). It is very difficult to differentiate from ST elevation due to acute infarction, hence it is safer to assume the latter if the patient has a chest pain history.

### Ambulatory ECG recording

While many dysrhythmias are relatively benign, several are malignant yet cause only intermittent symptoms. Ambulatory ECG monitoring is a key component of the investigation of arrhythmias, syncope/ presycnope, and response of arrhythmias to treatment. Four main categories:

##### Holter monitors (Inventor: Dr Norman Holter)

- Continuous ECG recording (24–48 hours).
- Requires the continuous attachment of recorder via three or more electrodes to skin.

---

**Box 3.4 Causes of long QT syndrome (LQTS)**

*Congenital*

*Drug-induced*

- Quinidine, procainamide, N-acetylprocainamide, disopyramide
- Amiodarone, bretylium, sotalol
- Amitriptyline and other tricyclics
- Erythromycin and other macrolides
- Chlorpromazine and other phenothiazines
- Cisapride
- Non-sedating antihistamines (astemizole, terfenadine)
- Probucol

*Metabolic/electrolyte disturbances*

- Hypokalaemia
- Hypocalcaemia
- Hypomagnesaemia
- Hypothermia

*Other*

- Starvation
- CNS lesions (e.g. subarachnoid haemorrhage (SAH))
- Cardiac ganglionitis
- Mitral valve prolapse

**Note:** <http://www.sads.org.uk/drugs_to_avoid.htm> provides an extensive list of causative medications

---

| Table 3.1  Causes of bundle-branch block | |
|---|---|
| **LBBB** | **RBBB** |
| Ischaemic heart disease | Normal variant |
| Acute MI | Idiopathic |
| Severe coronary disease* | Coronary artery disease* |
| LV outflow tract obstruction | RV strain |
| Aortic stenosis | Atrial septal defect (ASD) |
| Severe LVH | Myocarditis |
| Myocarditis | RV cardiomyopathy |
| Cardiomyopathy | |
| RV pacemaker lead | |

\* LBBB and RBBB suggest more severe coronary disease.

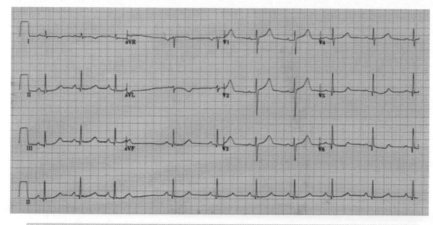

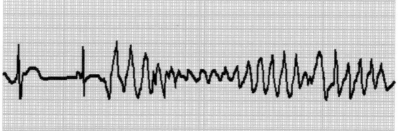

**Fig. 3.5** Long QT syndrome: QTc = 510ms.

- Tape recorder, or in modern systems solid-state storage systems (flash cards) used to store data prior to analysis.
- Useful if daily symptoms but low detection rate if symptoms infrequent.

*Event recorders*
- Can be used for up to 30 days so useful if patient's symptoms weekly/monthly.
- Do not have to be worn constantly but patients encouraged to wear as much as possible.
- Older devices need activation during symptoms and then 'phoned-in' to cardiology department for analysis.
- Not useful if symptoms very brief, or if patient experiences syncope without premonitory symptoms.

*External loop recorders*
- Can be used for up to 30 days.
- Continuously record and delete ECG; activation (by pressing button) will 'freeze' recording and store ECG from 1–4 minutes before activation until 30–60 seconds afterwards.
- Newer models can be programmed to store ECG automatically if heart rate outside pre-set parameters.

*Implantable loop recorders*
- Can be used for up to 24–30 months dependent on model.
- Involves implantation of recorder (Fig. 3.7) in subcutaneous pocket on left anterior chest wall.

- Reserved for those with infrequent but severe symptoms who have undergone unrevealing Holter/event monitors.
- Can be activated by patient but also activate automatically.
Certain pacemakers, and implantable cardioverter defibrillators, can record significant rhythm disturbances also.

*Congenital LQTS*
- Two major forms of congenital LQTS: Romano–Ward (autosomal dominant) and Jervell–Lange–Nielsen (autosomal recessive, associated with deafness) syndromes.
- >250 mutations in multiple genes have been described in congenital LQTS (numbered LQTS 1–13; LQTS 1–3 account for most disease cases).
- Presents as syncope or sudden cardiac death (SCD), often during physical exertion; other triggers include emotion and sudden 'startling' or loud noises, e.g. alarms.
- Higher risk of SCD: those with family members who died suddenly at an early age; those with syncope.
- Variation in 'risk' between mutations—LQTS 1 and 2 have highest risk of arrhythmias. LQTS 3 is associated with fewer cardiac events but they are more likely to be lethal.
- LQTS 1 and 2 events are associated with sympathetic activation (e.g. exercise); LQTS 3 events with sleep.

**Table 3.2** Causes of left and right axis deviation

| LAD | RAD |
| --- | --- |
| Left anterior hemiblock | Left posterior hemiblock |
| LBBB | RBBB (rarely LBBB*) |
| LVH | RVH |
| Primum ASD | Secundum ASD |
| Tricuspid atresia | Infancy |

*LBBB can rarely be associated with right axis deviation.

**Box 3.5 Causes of ST shift on 12-lead ECG**

| ST elevation | ST depression |
| --- | --- |
| Acute MI<br>Myopericarditis<br>LV aneurysm | Normal variant: fixed change;<br>sinus tachycardia-induced<br>J-point depression |
| Variant angina (formerly<br>Prinzmetal—coronary artery<br>spasm) | Ischaemia: acute myocardial<br>ischaemia; reciprocal changes<br>in acute MI |
| Early repolarization<br>Hyperkalaemia<br>Takotsubo cardiomypathy | Non-ischaemic: LVH/RVH with<br>strain, digoxin effect, hypo-<br>kalaemia, mitral valve prolapse, |
| Brugada syndrome | CNS disease e.g. SAH |

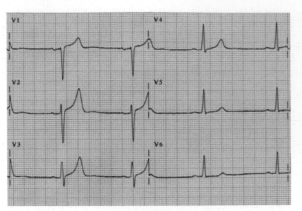

**Fig. 3.6** ECG demonstrating high take-off. Praecordial leads of resting ECG in a 23-year-old fit male; note the early commencement of the T wave resulting in elevation of the ST segment at the J-point. This is 'high take-off'.

- Any child or young adult presenting with an unexplained collapse **must** undergo an ECG to exclude LQTS; in up to 12% QTc will be within normal limits on the resting ECG.
- Treatment aims to reduce the effects of sudden sympathetic stimulation of the cardiac conducting system, hence β-blockers are first-line therapy. If these drugs induce AV block or profound bradycardia, consider permanent pacemaker implantation (allows continued ß-blockade).
- Cervical sympathectomy is an option.
- Implantable cardioverter defibrillators are indicated in patients with recurrent ventricular arrhythmias despite heavy β-blockade.

Short QT syndrome also exists (QTc ≤300ms, unaffected by heart rate). It is a rare autosomal dominant potassium channelopathy associated with palpitations and syncope. Atrial fibrillation is common, and increased risk of SCD.

## Exercise testing

Most frequently used in the evaluation of patients with suspected ischaemic heart disease (IHD; see Section 3.3) but also used to assess prognosis after MI and in multivessel disease, assessment of exercise tolerance, exercise-induced arrhythmias, response to treatment and building patient confidence (e.g. following MI) (see Boxes 3.6 and 3.7). Performed according to:

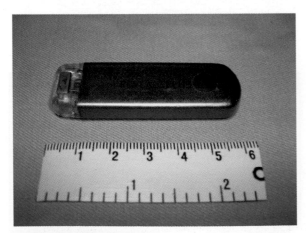

**Fig. 3.7** Implantable loop recorder.

*Full Bruce protocol*
Patient walks on uphill treadmill in a graded exercise test; every 3 minutes the speed and inclination of the treadmill increase (five stages).

*Modified Bruce protocol*
Treadmill initially horizontal; for first three stages inclination increases but speed remains constant.

Specificity is low in the following situations:

| | |
|---|---|
| LVH | Hyperventilation |
| LBBB | Mitral valve prolapse |
| Anaemia | Pre-excitation syndrome |
| Hypokalaemia | Young ♀ with atypical chest pain |
| Digitalis use | |

# Non-invasive imaging

Cardiac imaging is an expanding field. Most if not all of these investigations are performed and interpreted by cardiologists, specialist radiologists, or experienced cardiac physiologists. The general physician requires knowledge of indications for each test, suitability for individual patients, and whether the clinical question will be answered by the test. This should limit inappropriate requests.

## Echocardiography (echo)

*Transthoracic echo (TTE)*
With the patient in the left lateral position, the transducer (probe) is placed on the left anterior chest in certain standard positions (Fig. 3.8); ultrasound jelly augments contact between skin and probe. Varying frequency ultrasound waves are transmitted by and reflected back to the probe, allowing real-time images to be visualized.

While TTE is rarely impossible, image acquisition can be difficult in obesity, chest wall deformities, and chronic lung disease (e.g. emphysema).

There are no specific British or European guidelines for indications for echo, although American guidelines exist (Cheitlin et al., 2003). The specific clinical question should be clearly stated on the request card.

Common indications in clinical practice include:
- LV mass/function (systolic and diastolic function; tissue Doppler imaging provides quantitative data concerning myocardial function), e.g. heart failure, post-MI.
- Murmurs/valvular assessment and follow-up.
- Arrhythmias (exclusion of structural abnormality).
- Endocarditis investigation (to detect vegetations).
- Stroke/TIA/arterial embolism (intracardiac clot/masses).
- Hypertension (assessment of LVH, myocardial mass).
- Pericardial disease (including effusion/tamponade).
- Aortic disease (e.g. dissection).
- Congenital heart disease.
- Pulmonary disease and pulmonary hypertension.

*Stress echo*
Aids in the diagnosis of IHD, particularly if there is a contraindication to treadmill testing or if the treadmill has been equivocal. Also used to assess infarct size, hibernating myocardium, and dynamic LV outflow tract gradients.

Stress is either physical (e.g. exercise bike, treadmill) or pharmacological (e.g. dobutamine, dipyridamole, adenosine infusion). Contrast agents are often used to delineate endocardial contours and assess myocardial perfusion more precisely. Complications include provocation of tachyarrhythmias and side effects of drugs used.

**Box 3.6 Indicators of a positive exercise test**

- Moderate to severe angina.
- Failure of BP to rise with exercise; a drop in systolic BP of >10mmHg despite an increase in workload is an indication to stop test.
- Failure to achieve target heart rate (allowing for β-blockade if applicable).
- Arrhythmia with exercise (particularly ventricular).
- ST segment elevation in non-infarct leads without Q waves.
- ST segment depression (>1mm) planar or down-sloping.
- Failure to achieve predicted time due to any of previous listed points.

**Box 3.7 Contraindications to exercise testing**

*Absolute*
- Acute MI (within 2 days).
- High-risk unstable angina.
- Severe symptomatic aortic stenosis.
- Uncontrolled cardiac arrhythmias (causing symptoms or haemodynamic compromise).
- Acute (myo)pericarditis.
- Acute pulmonary embolus.
- Acute aortic dissection.

*Relative*
- Left main coronary disease.
- Moderate aortic stenosis/other valvular disease.
- Hypertrophic cardiomyopathy/other forms of LV outflow tract obstruction.
- Severe hypertension (systolic >200mmHg and/or diastolic >100mmHg).
- High-degree atrioventricular block.
- Electrolyte abnormalities (e.g. hypokalaemia).

*Transoesophageal echo (TOE)*

Transducer attached to angulated tip of modified gastroscopy probe, which can be advanced to varying depths within oesophagus and stomach. Pros/cons:

- Transducer closer to the heart (no intervening tissue/air in lungs); higher-frequency waves can be used: clearer images acquired.

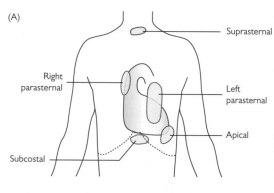

Standard echo windows

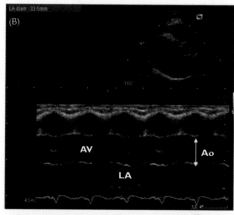

M-mode through aorta and left atrium

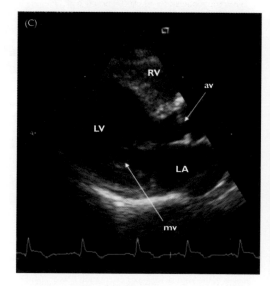

Parasternal long axis view

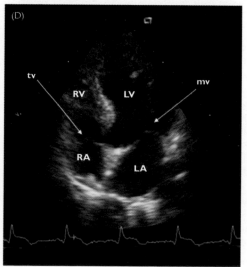

Apical 4 chamber view

**Fig. 3.8** (A) Standard probe positions in transthoracic echo. (B) M-mode with cursor through aorta (Ao) and left atrium (LA); aortic valve (av) leaflets seen. (C) Parasternal long axis view showing LA, mitral valve (mv), left and right ventricles (LV, RV). (D) Apical 4-chamber view showing both ventricles and atria.

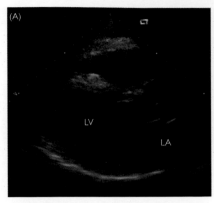

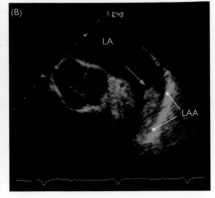

Transthoracic echo (parasternal long axis)  Transoesophageal echo

**Fig. 3.9** Transthoracic echo (A) showing left atrium (LA) clear of thrombus while transoesophageal echo in the same patient (B) shows thrombus (arrowed) in left atrial appendage (LAA).

- Posterior structures (e.g. left atrial appendage, descending aorta, pulmonary veins) well visualized (Fig. 3.9).
- Invasive test, requires mild sedation and does have (small) risk (oesophageal damage, reflux, risks of sedation) so should only be performed if there is a specific indication (by experienced operator).

*Specific indications for TOE*
- Aortic dissection.
- Endocarditis (vegetations of 1–2mm can be detected); paravalvular abscess.
- Intracardiac masses/thrombus (e.g. pre-DC cardioversion).
- Prosthetic valvular function/anatomy.
- Native valvular assessment (particularly mitral and aortic valves*); note: tricuspid valve not particularly well-visualised on TOE, but transthoracic views often provide sufficient information.
- Septal defects (bubble contrast study during TOE can highlight small patent foramen ovale or ASD).
- Intraoperative assessment of valve repairs/replacements.
- Congenital heart disease (Section 3.6).

*TOE can aid in decisions such as whether to repair or replace a leaking mitral valve, or whether valvotomy is feasible in mitral stenosis.

### Nuclear cardiology
Most common imaging is myocardial perfusion scintigraphy.
- Most common indication is measurement of LV ejection fraction (more reproducible than echo).
- Useful also in the assessment of patients with possible IHD who have 'unhelpful' treadmill tests (e.g. unable to walk on treadmill, abnormal resting ECG, atypical pain with non-specific ECG changes); also used to assess response to revascularization and assess hibernating myocardium in patients being considered for revascularization.
- Involves injection of radiolabelled tracer (thallium-201 or technetium-99m ($^{99m}$Tc)) to provide physiological data on myocardial function during rest and exercise.
- Stress can be physical (treadmill, exercise bike) or pharmacological (e.g. dobutamine, dipyridamole, adenosine).
- Single-photon emission computed tomography (SPECT) images acquired and compared during rest and stress.
- Perfusion defects can be fixed (e.g. infarct) or reversible (e.g. flow-limiting stenosis in coronary artery that supplies territory affected by defect)—see Fig. 3.10.

- $^{99m}$Tc provides higher quality images, and has a shorter $t_{1/2}$ (6 vs. 73 hours for thallium)—less radiation exposure

### Computed tomography (CT) angiography
CT angiography is a new technique that is being increasingly utilized clinically. It is the best non-invasive means of assessing coronary circulation (Fig. 3.11). Scan time is significantly shorter than CMR, but CT does involve (relatively high dose) X-rays and iodine-based contrast agents. Used in:
- Assessing anatomy of coronary arteries/great vessels, and identifying coronary lesions (at present used mainly in patients labelled high risk for angiography).
- Assessing aneurysms/detecting dissection of great vessels.
- Pericardial assessment in possible constrictive pericarditis.
- Calculating a 'calcium score' (linked to development of atherosclerosis—identifies at-risk patients).

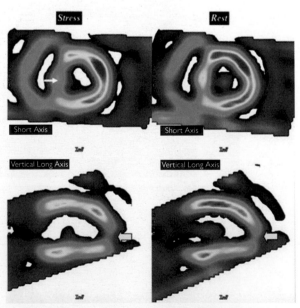

**Fig. 3.10** Nuclear myocardial perfusion scintigraphy in a patient with known coronary artery disease unsuitable for treadmill testing. Rest images in the vertical long axis orientation (lower right) reveal an apical perfusion defect (block arrow) that remains unchanged with stress—this represents an old infarct. On the short axis images (upper panel) there is a perfusion defect in the septum (line arrow) that is present only on stress—this represents reversible myocardial ischaemia.

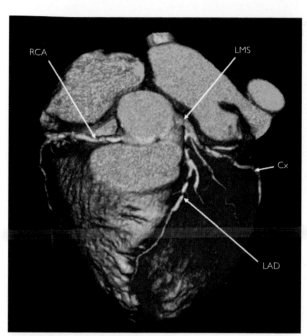

**Fig. 3.11** Cardiac CT image, showing gross anatomy of coronary arteries and their epicardial course. Diffuse stenoses in the left anterior descending (LAD) and circumflex (Cx) arteries are visible. LMS: left main stem; RCA: right coronary artery.

## Cardiac magnetic resonance imaging (CMR)

CMR has revolutionized non-invasive cardiac imaging. Cine images are acquired in standard planes and allow precise calculation of LV and RV mass, volumes, and ejection fraction. The anatomy of the great vessels is also clearly defined. CMR aids in the assessment of:

- Aortic disease
- Cardiomyopathy
- Congenital heart disease
- Contrast enhancement
- Coronary artery disease
- Intracardiac masses/thrombi
- Myocardial viability
- Pericardial disease
- Pulmonary vessel anatomy
- Right ventricular function
- Valvular disease

*Contrast enhancement*
*First-pass imaging*

- Images acquired in real time as gadolinium (a water-soluble extracellular contrast agent) is infused into peripheral vein.
- Gadolinium shows up as white dye, seen initially in the blood pool of the RV then in the blood pool of the LV.
- It then rapidly perfuses through the LV myocardium (from endocardium to epicardium).
- Gadolinium will initially fail to penetrate any area of non-perfused myocardium (e.g. infarct, fibrosis) thus a 'black defect' will be seen on the first pass images—this is a resting perfusion defect (see Fig. 3.12).

*Delayed enhancement imaging*

- After a delay, gadolinium will be 'held up' in the non-perfused area: a white area of 'late gadolinium uptake' will be seen—Fig. 3.12.

**Caution:** gadolinium should be avoided in significant renal dysfunction—linked to nephrogenic fibrosing dermopathy.

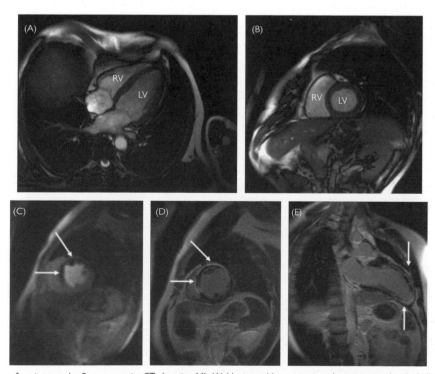

**Fig. 3.12** CMR images of patient on day 3 post anterior ST elevation MI. (A) Horizontal long axis view shows precise detail of all 4 cardiac chambers. (B) Short axis view allows LV and RV mass, volumes, and ejection fractions to be calculated. (C) First-pass image (note light blood pool in LV and RV due to gadolinium) reveals extensive perfusion defect in septum/anterior wall, (D, E) Show extensive late gadolinium uptake in septum, anterior wall, apex, and apical inferior wall (arrowed); microvascular obstruction is also present.

*Advantages of CMR*

No radiation used; body habitus less relevant (but patient must fit in scanner!); highly reproducible.

*Disadvantages of CMR*

Claustrophobia; metallic implants (including certain implantable cardiac devices) are currently contraindications to CMR; long scan time (up to 60 minutes in some cases); scan quality dependent on patient comprehension of instructions.

**Note:** coronary stents are safe, as are most metallic valves (although valve magnetic safety MUST be ascertained prior to scan).

## Invasive studies

Cardiac catheterization involves the insertion of certain pre-shaped catheters through a peripheral artery or vein, from where they are manipulated manually to the appropriate position within the heart/ great vessels. Coronary angiography is the most important product of cardiac catheterization, but pressure measurements, blood sampling, oxygen saturation analysis, and ventriculography can all be performed.

Specific guidelines for coronary angiography exist (Scanlon et al., 1999); indications for and outcomes of angiography are discussed in Section 3.3.

### Intracardiac electrophysiological studies

Specialized catheters inserted through neck or groin veins allow access to cardiac chambers. Used in provoking and assessing arrhythmias, identifying and ablating accessory pathways, cardiac mapping, and assessing response to treatment.

Important complications of diagnostic coronary angiography in an otherwise healthy patient:

- Vascular access complications:
  - Bruising.
  - Bleeding.
  - Haematoma (including retroperitoneal).
  - Femoral arterial (intimal) dissection.
  - Pseudoaneurysm formation.
- Coronary dissection.
- Acute MI (risk <0.03%).
- Stroke (risk around 0.06%).
- Arrhythmias (atrial/ventricular); note: selective injection of the conus branch of the right coronary can provoke VF.
- Contrast allergy/nephropathy.
- Air embolism.
- Death (risk <1:1000).

## References

Cheitlin MD, Armstrong WF, Aurigemma GP, *et al*. ACC/AHA/ASE 2003 guideline update for the clinical application of echocardiography. *J Am Coll Cardiol* 2003; *42*(5): 954–70.

Scanlon PJ, Faxon DP, Audet A-M, *et al*. ACC/AHA guidelines for coronary angiography: executive summary and recommendations. *Circulation* 1999; *99*(17): 2345–57.

# 3.3 Ischaemic heart disease

## Background

With the increase in life expectancy, atherogenic diet, and sedentary lifestyle in the developed world, ischaemic heart disease has become the leading cause of death, being responsible for a quarter of all deaths in the UK (Box 3.8).

## Pathophysiology

### Normal arterial wall

This is typically a three-layer structure:

*Intima*

Endothelial monolayer and underlying basement membrane with a variable degree of intimal thickening. The endothelium plays a pivotal role in vascular homeostasis (Box 3.9).

*Media*

Separated from the intima by the internal elastic membrane. Smooth muscle layer.

*Adventitia*

Separated from the media by the external elastic membrane. Loose array of collagen fibrils, sparsely cellular. Contains vasa vasorum and nerve endings.

### Atherosclerosis

This process underlies all the manifestations of ischaemic heart disease. In recent years, great advances have been made in understanding the pathogenesis of atherosclerosis, and it is now apparent that it is a chronic inflammatory condition.

The process begins at an early age with evidence of atherosclerosis in the second and third decades of life. It appears that an atherogenic diet leads to an accumulation of low-density lipoprotein (LDL) particles in the intima, which are oxidized to produce oxidized LDL (ox-LDL).

This is accompanied by the development of endothelial dysfunction. Rather than predominantly anti-inflammatory and anticoagulant functions, the endothelium becomes pro-inflammatory and procoagulant. Cellular adhesion molecules (such as vascular cell adhesion molecule-1 (VCAM-1) and intercellular adhesion molecule-1 (ICAM-1)) are expressed on the surface of the endothelium allowing leucocyte binding and migration into the intima (Fig. 3.13).

In the vessel wall monocytes mature into macrophages which ingest ox-LDL to become lipid laden foam cells. In combination with activated T lymphocytes, macrophages elaborate numerous cytokines. These cytokines stimulate vascular smooth muscle cell (VSMC) migration from the media. Plaque growth occurs with accumulation of lipids and VSMC, which also produce extracellular matrix (ECM).

Mature plaque morphology is heterogeneous for reasons which are incompletely understood. It may be a result of variable cytokine production by foam cells and T lymphocytes. In some plaques there is only a small lipid layer, with predominant smooth muscle and ECM production. In other areas there may be a large lipid core covered by a very thin fibrous cap of smooth muscle and ECM.

---

**Box 3.8 Major risk factors for atherosclerosis**

- Cigarette smoking.
- Hyperlipidaemia.
- Hypertension.
- Diabetes.
- Family history of premature coronary disease.
- Obesity.
- Sedentary lifestyle.

---

**Box 3.9 Endothelial vascular homeostatic function**

- Anticoagulant: heparin sulphate glycoproteins and thrombomodulin expressed on surface and nitric oxide, prostacyclin, and tissue plasminogen activator (tPA) secreted into arterial lumen prevent thrombus formation.
- Procoagulant: tissue factor, von Willebrand factor and plasminogen activator inhibitor (PAI-1) stimulate thrombus formation.
- Anti-inflammatory: nitric oxide, resists leucocyte adherence.
- Pro-inflammatory: cellular adhesion molecules (e.g. ICAM-1) can be expressed on endothelial cell surface to promote leucocyte adhesion.
- Vasodilatory: nitric oxide.
- Vasoconstrictor: endothelin, angiotensin II.

---

Although atherosclerosis is a diffuse process which occurs throughout the arterial tree, there is a predilection for certain areas. In the coronary circulation this appears to be in proximal arteries and branch points. Normal laminar blood flow in the coronary arteries leads to shear stress on the endothelium which stimulates nitric oxide production. This has vasodilatory and anti-inflammatory properties. At branch points there is more turbulent flow, so less shear stress and nitric oxide production. There may be a greater degree of endothelial dysfunction in these areas leading to more aggressive plaque growth.

A substantial volume of plaque is present before luminal narrowing becomes apparent. Initially the arterial wall expands outwards to accommodate plaque growth—so-called positive remodelling. Only once plaque occupies ~40% of the volume of the arterial wall does luminal narrowing occur. This has important implications for the understanding of the manifestations of atherosclerosis.

Until recently it was believed that plaque growth occurred gradually, and though this is often the case, there is evidence that it may occur in a stepwise fashion with episodes of sudden plaque expansion. This may occur due to subclinical plaque rupture and incorporation of thrombus into the arterial wall. Similarly there may be intra-plaque haemorrhage due to rupture of the small feeder arteries which develop in the mature plaque. Both of these processes stimulate a more vigorous inflammatory response from the T lymphocytes and macrophages in the intima leading to more cytokine production and a period of VSMC expansion and ECM production.

### Acute manifestations of atherosclerosis

*Acute coronary syndromes and sudden cardiac death*

The pathophysiology is rupture or erosion of the endothelial lining, exposing the procoagulant intimal plaque. This initially causes platelet thrombus production which in turn triggers the coagulation cascade leading to fibrin formation. It has been shown that certain plaque types are more prone to rupture. Plaques with a large lipid core and thin fibrous cap are so-called 'vulnerable plaques,' because they are particularly prone to rupture. The consequences of plaque rupture depend on the pre-existing luminal stenosis, the thrombogenicity of the exposed intima, the extent of luminal obstruction caused by the thrombus, and the location of the plaque rupture in the coronary tree.

### Chronic manifestations of atherosclerosis

*Chronic stable angina*

Gradual luminal narrowing leads to angina. This occurs when there is a flow-limiting stenosis in an epicardial coronary artery. Historically a 70% luminal stenosis on angiography was considered to be functionally significant, although recent technological advances including coronary pressure wire studies have challenged this notion.

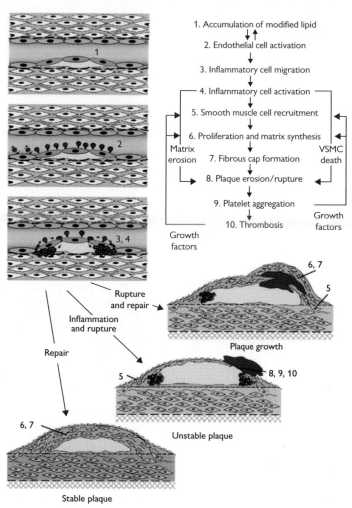

1. Accumulation of modified lipid
2. Endothelial cell activation
3. Inflammatory cell migration
4. Inflammatory cell activation
5. Smooth muscle cell recruitment
6. Proliferation and matrix synthesis
7. Fibrous cap formation
8. Plaque erosion/rupture
9. Platelet aggregation
10. Thrombosis

Matrix erosion

VSMC death

Growth factors

Growth factors

Rupture and repair

Inflammation and rupture

Repair

Plaque growth

Unstable plaque

Stable plaque

**Fig. 3.13** Cellular interactions in the development and progression of atherosclerosis. VSMC, vascular smooth muscle cells.
Reproduced from *Heart*, Weissberg PL, 'Atherogenesis: current understanding of the causes of atheroma', 83, pp. 247–252, 2000, with permission from BMJ Publishing Group Ltd.

### Coronary blood flow and myocardial ischaemia

The myocardium relies almost exclusively on aerobic metabolism. Under resting conditions, the ability of the myocardium to extract oxygen from the blood is near maximal. Therefore in order to meet increased oxygen demand under conditions of stress, myocardial blood flow must increase.

Myocardial ischaemia occurs when myocardial oxygen demand ($MVO_2$) exceeds oxygen supply by the coronary arteries (Box 3.10).

Increased $MVO_2$ results in vasodilation and increased blood flow (Box 3.11). If there is a stenosis in an epicardial artery, when a patient undertakes exercise and the $MVO_2$ increases, the epicardial stenosis prevents the necessary increase in blood flow to maintain oxygen supply and myocardial ischaemia ensues.

### Box 3.10 Determinants of myocardial oxygen demand ($MVO_2$)

- Heart rate—most important.
- Contractility.
- Wall tension—dependent on aortic pressure, LV volume, and myocardial fibril length.

# Angina

### Pathophysiology

Angina is the symptom of chest pain or discomfort caused by myocardial ischaemia. It is a result of a mismatch between myocardial oxygen demand and oxygen supply as described earlier. Although most commonly due to stenoses of the epicardial arteries, when assessing the patient with angina one must always consider other potential causes

### Box 3.11 Regulation of coronary blood flow

- Epicardial arteries—capacitance vessels which in the absence of atherosclerosis offer no resistance to blood flow. Responsive to flow-mediated dilatation.
- Prearterioles—offer considerable resistance to blood flow. Key role is autoregulation. They are very responsive to changes in pressure and main purpose is to maintain a constant pressure at the origin of the arterioles.
- Arterioles—main site of metabolic regulation of blood flow. High resting tone. Vasodilate in response to the release of metabolites by the myocytes due to increased oxygen consumption.

of a myocardial oxygen supply/demand mismatch especially anaemia, thyrotoxicosis, and left ventricular outflow tract obstruction.

## Clinical assessment

### History

This is crucial to the diagnosis. The following aspects of a chest pain history are typical of angina:

- Central chest pain, discomfort, tightness or heaviness.
- Radiation to arm(s), neck, and jaw.
- Provocation by exertion or emotion.
- Rapid relief with rest or nitrolingual spray.
- Duration typically <10 minutes.

The nature and location of the pain may vary from the classical description, but the exacerbating and relieving factors are essential to reliably make the diagnosis of chronic stable angina. The severity of symptoms may be classified according to the Canadian Cardiovascular Society classification (Box 3.12).

The history should also identify the presence of any risk factors.

### Examination

Most often normal. Particular attention should be paid to any signs of hypercholesterolaemia, e.g. xanthelasma, tendon xanthomata and corneal arcus, blood pressure, and signs of aortic stenosis or hypertrophic cardiomyopathy.

### Investigation

Full blood count, thyroid function tests, glucose and lipid profile. Resting 12-lead ECG—particular attention should be paid to evidence of prior MI or left ventricular hypertrophy. An abnormal resting ECG is a marker of increased clinical risk.

## Non-invasive stress testing

### Treadmill exercise testing

This is the first-line investigation of choice in patients who are able to exercise. The full Bruce protocol is commonly used which increases both the speed and the gradient every 3 minutes. Interpretation of the test should take into account:

- Exercise time.
- Maximal heart rate.
- Blood pressure response.
- ST segment change—>2mm horizontal or downsloping ST depression at 80ms after the J point is significant (Fig. 3.14).
- Symptoms.
- Arrhythmias.

High-risk features are described in Box 3.13. The value of exercise testing is linked to the pre-test likelihood of significant coronary disease. Overall sensitivity is 68% and specificity is 77%. False positive tests are more common in females at low risk.

### Stress echocardiography/myocardial perfusion imaging

Useful for patients who are unable to exercise or those in whom treadmill exercise testing is equivocal. Dobutamine or dipyridamole is used to stress the myocardium pharmacologically.

## Non-invasive imaging techniques

### CT coronary angiography

This is emerging as an alternative to diagnostic coronary angiography. At the present time it is useful for patients in whom the likelihood of significant coronary disease is low, or for assessing bypass graft patency.

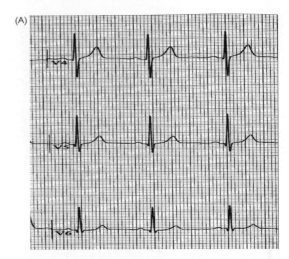

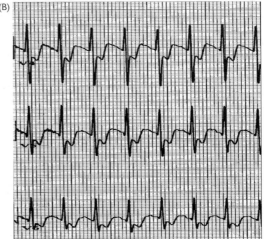

**Fig. 3.14** (A) Resting and (B) peak exercise tracings from the leads V4–V6 of a patient undergoing exercise tolerance testing using the Bruce protocol. The test was terminated at the start of stage II (3 minutes 6 seconds) due to chest pain and 4mm downsloping ST depression. This is a strongly positive test. The patient went on to have coronary angiography which demonstrated severe three vessel coronary disease.

## Invasive investigation

### Coronary angiography

This is the gold standard investigation for coronary artery disease (Fig. 3.15). It is used selectively because of a 1 in 500 procedures risk of serious complications such as death, non-fatal MI, or stroke.

### Indications

- High-risk features on non-invasive stress testing.
- Ongoing anginal symptoms in spite of appropriate anti-anginal therapy.

| Box 3.12 | Canadian Cardiovascular Society Classification of anginal symptoms | |
|---|---|---|
| Class I | Angina only on strenuous exertion, not on ordinary physical activity | |
| Class II | Slight limitation of ordinary activity | |
| Class III | Marked limitation of ordinary activity | |
| Class IV | Angina comes on with any exertion, and may be present at rest | |
| Data from Canadian Cardiovascular Society | | |

**Box 3.13 Adverse prognostic indicators on exercise tolerance testing**

- Poor exercise tolerance.
- Failure to increase systolic BP >120mmHg, or a sustained decrease>10mmHg.
- ST-segment depression >2mm in stage I or II (full Bruce).
- ST-segment elevation.
- Angina at low workload.
- Sustained or symptomatic ventricular tachycardia.

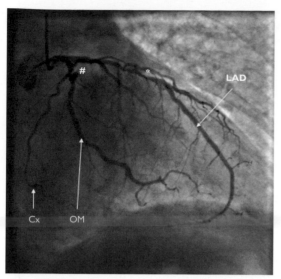

**Fig. 3.15** Coronary angiogram of the left coronary artery of a male with exertional angina and a positive exercise test. This is taken from the right anterior oblique projection. The left anterior descending artery (LAD) has a long segment of severe disease in the mid vessel (*). The true circumflex (Cx) is a small vessel, but there is a severe stenosis (#) in the large obtuse marginal (OM) branch which is partially hidden in this projection, emphasizing the importance of taking views in multiple projections.

- In cases of diagnostic uncertainty where other investigations have been inconclusive.
- Adverse prognostic features such as crescendo symptoms, abnormal resting ECG, or left ventricular dysfunction.

### Medical therapy
This can be divided into disease-modifying therapy and symptomatic treatment (Box 3.14).

Unless there are high-risk features on stress testing, a trial of medical therapy should be given before deciding to undertake coronary angiography.

### Revascularization

#### CABG
This is a very effective operation for long-term relief of anginal symptoms and freedom from the need for repeat revascularization. It has also been shown to improve survival compared with medical therapy in the following circumstances:
- Left main stem stenosis.
- Three-vessel disease.
- Two-vessel disease including proximal left anterior descending artery disease.

---

**Box 3.14 Anti-anginal therapy**

*Disease-modifying agents*
- Antiplatelets—aspirin or clopidogrel (**not** both).
- Lipid-lowering agents—statins.
- ACE inhibitors.

*Symptomatic treatments*
- Sublingual glyceryl trinitrate.
- β-blockers.
- Calcium channel blockers.
- Long-acting oral nitrates.
- Potassium channel activators (nicorandil).
- $Ik_f$ ('funny') channel blockers (ivabradine).
- Late $I_{Na}$ channel blockers (ranolazine).

---

especially in the context of left ventricular dysfunction, severe symptoms, or positive stress test.

#### PCI
No prognostic benefit has been demonstrated over medical therapy, though it is more effective at reducing anginal symptoms.

There is no evidence to suggest that PCI is superior to CABG in multi-vessel coronary disease, and in fact long-term outcomes are better with CABG in the high-risk subsets described previously.

Current evidence would favour coronary artery bypass surgery for prognostically important disease, and PCI for other circumstances where symptoms are not controlled by medical therapy alone, or where CABG is not feasible or appropriate.

### Prognosis in chronic stable angina
Annual incidence of death or MI in stable patients is of the order of 4%.

## Acute coronary syndromes

### Definition
Ischaemic chest pain occurring at rest or on minimal exertion associated with ECG changes, biochemical markers of myocyte necrosis, and/or known or subsequently proven coronary disease. This definition covers a spectrum of conditions ranging from unstable angina to ST-segment elevation myocardial infarction which share the common pathophysiology of thrombus formation on a ruptured or eroded atheromatous plaque (Fig. 3.16).

### Classification
Acute coronary syndromes (ACS) are divided into ST elevation myocardial infarction (STEMI) and non-ST elevation acute coronary syndromes (NSTEACS) based on the presence or absence of ST-segment elevation on the presenting ECG. This is crucially important, as patients with ST elevation should be considered for urgent reperfusion therapy. NSTEACS can be further subdivided according to the presence of elevated cardiac biomarkers.

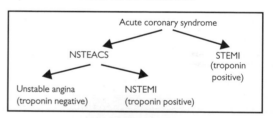

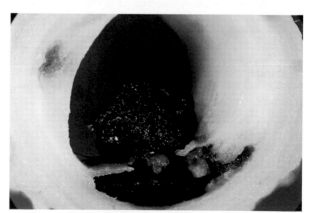

**Fig. 3.16** Pathological specimen demonstrating a ruptured atherosclerotic plaque with superimposed non-occlusive thrombus in a coronary artery of a patient who experienced sudden cardiac death. This is the typical lesion responsible for non ST-segment elevation acute coronary syndromes.

Reproduced from *Heart*, Davies MJ, 'The pathophysiology of acute coronary syndromes', 83, pp. 361–366, 2000 with permission from BMJ Publishing Group Ltd.

## NSTEACS

*Initial assessment*

- History—pattern of symptoms, risk factors, prior cardiac history.
- Clinical examination—often normal. Look for signs of cardiac failure or valvular heart disease
- 12-lead ECG—exclude ST elevation. Definite signs of ischaemia are new ST depression or T-wave inversion.
- Cardiac biomarkers—troponin I (TnI) on admission and at 12 hours. Troponin elevation should be interpreted in the clinical context (see Boxes 3.15 and 3.16).

### Treatment

This is based on our understanding of the pathophysiology.

*Antiplatelet therapy*

*Aspirin*

A cyclo-oxygenase inhibitor. The first therapy shown to be of prognostic benefit in NSTEACS, aspirin resulted in a 5–11% absolute reduction in cardiovascular death and non-fatal MI compared with placebo in four randomized trials. Aspirin 300mg orally should be administered immediately followed by 75mg once daily thereafter.

*Clopidogrel*

A thienopyridine platelet adenosine diphosphate receptor antagonist. A single RCT comparing aspirin and clopidogrel versus aspirin and placebo resulted in a 2.1% absolute risk reduction in the primary end point of cardiovascular death, non-fatal MI, and non-fatal CVA. In patients with a definite NSTEACS associated with ECG changes or elevated troponin, clopidogrel 300mg orally should be administered immediately followed by 75mg daily for 3–12 months.

*Prasugrel*

A thienopyridine adenosine diphosphate receptor antagonist. A single RCT has demonstrated the benefit of prasugrel over clopidogrel in combination with aspirin in patients with ACS undergoing PCI with a 2.2% reduction in cardiovascular death, non-fatal MI and non-fatal stroke at the expense of an increase in major bleeding, including fatal bleeding.

*Ticagrelor*

A pyrimidine derivative, ticagrelor is a more potent adenosine diphosphate inhibitor than clopidogrel. A single RCT has shown the benefit of ticagrelor over clopidogrel in combination with aspirin

---

> **Box 3.15  Third universal definition of myocardial infarction—criteria for acute MI**
>
> 1. Detection of a rise and/or fall in biomarkers of myocyte necrosis (usually troponin) plus one of the following:
>    - Symptoms of ischaemia.
>    - New ST–T changes or new LBBB.
>    - Development of pathological Q waves.
>    - Imaging evidence of new regional wall motion abnormality.
>    - Intracoronary thrombus detected by angiography or autopsy.
> 2. Cardiac death, with symptoms of myocardial ischaemia and new ECG changes, before elevated cardiac biomarkers could be detected.
> 3. PCI-related MI—troponin levels >5 × 99th percentile ULR and one of:
>    - Symptoms of ischaemia.
>    - New ECG changes.
>    - Angiographic findings consistent with procedural complication.
>    - Imaging studies showing new wall motion abnormality.
> 4. Stent thrombosis associated MI— detected by angiography or autopsy in the setting of myocardial ischaemia and elevated markers of myocyte necrosis.
> 5. CABG-related MI—troponin levels >10 × 99th percentile ULR and one of:
>    - New pathological Q waves/LBBB.
>    - New graft or native artery occlusion on angiography.
>    - New regional WMA on imaging studies.

---

> **Box 3.16  Alternative causes of an elevated troponin**
>
> - Tachyarrhythmia
> - Bradyarrhythmia
> - Acute pulmonary oedema
> - Heart failure
> - Pulmonary embolism
> - Myocarditis
> - Pericarditis
> - Sepsis
> - Hypoxia
> - Hypotension
> - Cardioversion/ablation/pacing/endomyocardial biopsy
> - Trauma
> - Aortic dissection
> - Renal dysfunction
> - Hypertensive crisis
> - Takotsubo cardiomyopathy
> - Hypothyroidism
> - Acute neurological event
> - Infiltrative disease

with a 1.9% reduction in vascular death, MI or stroke at the expense of an increase in major non-procedural bleeding. A significant 1.4% reduction in all-cause mortality was a secondary endpoint. A loading dose of 180mg ticagrelor is followed by 90mg twice daily for up to 12 months. Many guidelines now recommend ticagrelor as the antiplatelet of choice in combination with aspirin 75mg.

*Glycoprotein IIb/IIIA inhibitors*

A meta-analysis of RCTs of these agents in NSTEACS has demonstrated a 1% absolute risk reduction in the primary endpoint of death or non-fatal MI. The benefit was seen only if troponin +ve, particularly those undergoing PCI. They should be considered for patients with refractory ischaemia on otherwise maximal therapy, and those undergoing PCI.

*Antithrombotic therapy*

*Heparin*

Early trials demonstrated the benefit of unfractionated heparin (UFH) in unstable angina. More recent studies have compared UFH with low-molecular-weight heparins (LMWH). There is a minor reduction in the combined endpoint of death/non-fatal MI with enoxaparin (LMWH) compared with UFH. LMWH are now the heparin of choice in ACS as they are easy to administer and no APTT monitoring is required.

*Fondaparinux*

This is a selective Factor Xa antagonist which has similar efficacy to LMWH with less bleeding complications. It is administered at a fixed dose of 2.5mg once a day (contraindicated if eGFR <20mL/min).

*Anti-ischaemic therapy*

*Beta-blockers*

Effective anti-anginal agents. A meta-analysis of five small randomized trials in NSTEACS demonstrated a 13% relative reduction in the risk of recurrent MI.

*Intravenous nitrates*

No clear prognostic benefit but good treatment for ischaemia.

*Rate-limiting calcium channel blockers (verapamil, diltiazem)*

An alternative to β-blockers if intolerant.

### Risk stratification

The short-term risk of death, recurrent MI, or urgent revascularization in NSTEACS varies from 4.7% in the lowest-risk patients to 40% in those at highest risk. The importance of risk stratification in NSTEACS has clearly been demonstrated in clinical trials where the benefit of therapy is greatest in the highest-risk groups. This is of particular importance in selecting patients for a routine invasive strategy (see later). Several trials have demonstrated that this strategy was most beneficial in patients at highest risk.

A number of risk scores have been developed to predict individual patient risk. The TIMI risk score (Box 3.17) has been the most widely used, with patients at intermediate to high risk being selected for a routine invasive strategy. The GRACE risk predictor is gaining popularity since it is derived from 'real-world' patients rather than a clinical trial population. It can be downloaded from <http://www.outcomes-umassmed.org>. It has been suggested that an invasive strategy should be undertaken in patients with a Grace score >140, or <140 if there are other high risk features (e.g. troponin rise, ST depression, diabetes, impaired LV function).

### Invasive investigation

Several large-scale clinical trials have compared the strategy of routine coronary angiography and revascularization as necessary, with a conservative strategy of invasive investigation only if there is either recurrent spontaneous or provoked ischaemia (on stress testing). A routine invasive strategy has proven superior, although the major effect is a reduction in non-fatal MI and recurrent ischaemia requiring revascularization. 5-year follow up of the RITA-3 study has, however, demonstrated a mortality reduction with the routine invasive strategy. Patients at highest risk are more likely to benefit and should be risk stratified as previously described.

Box 3.18 Indications for reperfusion therapy

History consistent with acute MI within 12 hours of onset (primary PCI may be considered if ongoing ischaemia >12 hours after symptom onset)
**AND**
1mm ST elevation in two or more adjacent limb leads or
2mm ST elevation in two or more adjacent chest leads or
New LBBB

### Non-invasive investigation

*Treadmill exercise testing*

This still has a role in improving risk stratification in patients initially deemed as low risk, who do not undergo routine invasive investigation.

## STEMI

A patient with chest pain and ST-segment elevation or new LBBB (Box 3.18) must be urgently considered for reperfusion therapy.

### Initial assessment

A 12-lead ECG should be obtained within 10 minutes of first medical contact (Figs 3.17 and 3.18).

Concise history including potential contraindications to thrombolytic therapy if appropriate (Box 3.19).

Aspirin 300mg and clopidogrel 600mg or ticagrelor 180mg should be administered.

IV access should be obtained and opiate analgesia given.

Clinical examination should be brief and focus particularly on signs of haemodynamic compromise, heart failure, and murmurs. See Box 3.20 for complications of STEMI.

### Reperfusion therapy

The most crucial issue is that reperfusion therapy should be delivered as quickly as possible. There is a clear inverse correlation between time from symptom onset to reperfusion therapy and myocardial salvage and survival.

### Choice of reperfusion strategy

Primary PCI is the reperfusion strategy of choice as it has been demonstrated to be superior to thrombolysis. A meta-analysis of clinical trials comparing primary PCI to thrombolysis demonstrated

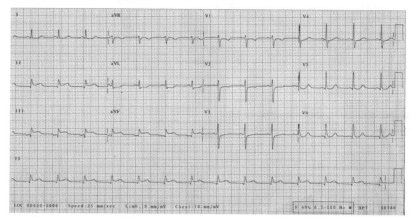

**Fig. 3.17** Acute inferoposterior STEMI. ST elevation is present in leads II, III, and aVf as well as V6. The ST depression in V1–V3 represents posterior 'ST elevation'. © Glen Larson. http://en.wikipedia.org/wiki/Image:ECG_001.jpg. This file is licensed under the Creative Commons Attribution-Share Alike 3.0 Unported (//creativecommons.org/licenses/by-sa/3.0/deed.en) license.

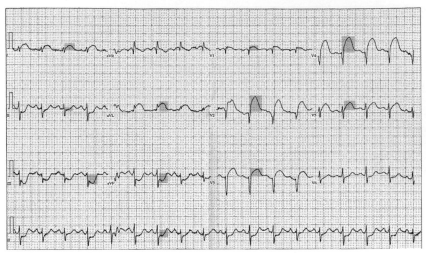

**Fig. 3.18** Acute anterior STEMI. Extensive anterior and high lateral ST elevation with reciprocal ST depression inferiorly. This image has been released into the public domain: https://commons.wikimedia.org/wiki/File:12_Lead_EKG_ST_Elevation_tracing_color_coded.jpg

that primary PCI is associated with a significant 2% absolute mortality reduction, a 3% absolute reduction in recurrent non-fatal MI, and a 1% absolute reduction in stroke.

## Primary PCI

Primary PCI is the strategy of immediate coronary angiography and percutaneous revascularization for patients with STEMI, without any prior thrombolysis. This requires a structured clinical pathway, usually at a regional level, where patients are identified as having a STEMI in the ambulance or in accident and emergency and are then transferred to a high-volume PCI centre with 24/7 PCI cover. The aim is to have a delay of <90 minutes from presentation to balloon inflation (door-to-balloon time). Primary PCI is the reperfusion strategy of choice in almost all circumstances, with particular benefit over thrombolysis in patients presenting >6 hours after symptom onset, and in the presence of cardiogenic shock.

However, thrombolysis may be as effective as primary PCI if administered within 3 hours of **symptom** onset, or in circumstances where the door-to-balloon time will be >90 minutes.

If primary PCI cannot be undertaken within 120 minutes of presentation the initial reperfusion therapy should be thrombolysis with a view to immediate transfer to a PCI centre for 'rescue' PCI (if failed reperfusion) or delayed (3–24 hours) angiography with PCI to the infarct-related artery if indicated.

Whereas thrombolysis has not been shown to be of benefit outside 12 hours from symptom onset, primary PCI can be considered in these circumstances if there is evidence of ongoing ischaemia or a 'stuttering' presentation.

---

### Box 3.19 Contraindications to thrombolysis

Absolute:
Active bleeding or bleeding diathesis.
Significant closed head or facial trauma within 3 months.
Ischaemic stroke within 3 months.
Any prior intracerebral haemorrhage.
Known cerebral vascular lesion.
Known malignant intracranial neoplasm.
Relative:
Uncontrolled hypertension (systolic >200mmHg, diastolic >110mmHg).
Ischaemic stroke >3 months.
Prolonged or traumatic CPR.
Major surgery <3 weeks, internal bleeding 2–4 weeks.
Recent non-compressible vascular punctures.
Pregnancy.
Concurrent anticoagulant therapy.

---

## Thrombolysis

The use of thrombolytic therapy for reperfusion in STEMI is associated with a highly significant 2.5% absolute mortality reduction (NNT 40 to save one life).

### Thrombolytic agents

#### Streptokinase

This is an enzyme obtained from haemolytic streptococci. It works by binding plasminogen leading to the activation of plasmin which lyses fibrin.

---

### Box 3.20 Complications of STEMI

#### Bradyarrhythmias

Inferior STEMI—temporary pacing only required if haemodynamic compromise.

Anterior STEMI—poor prognosis. Temporary pacing indicated for alternating bundle branch block or second- or third-degree AV block.

#### Tachyarrhythmias

Atrial fibrillation is most common.

Ventricular arrhythmias in the first 24 hours are not associated with an adverse prognosis. Late ventricular arrhythmias usually occur in the context of impaired LV function and ICD implantation should be considered.

#### Heart failure

IV nitrates and diuretics, ACE inhibitors should be introduced early and an aldosterone antagonist should also be given if LVEF <40%.

#### Cardiogenic shock

Systolic blood pressure <90mmHg with signs of impaired organ perfusion (oliguria, cool clammy skin, confusion).

Urgent echocardiography (exclude 'mechanical complications'). IABP is the most useful therapy, and inotropic support with dobutamine is likely to be required.

#### RV infarction

Most often associated with an inferior STEMI. Suggested by hypotension, a raised JVP, and ST elevation >0.1mV in RV leads. Unless there are also signs of pulmonary oedema, initial treatment is a fluid challenge.

#### Mechanical complications

**Free wall rupture**—usually presents with circulatory collapse or cardiac arrest. May present as tamponade. Almost invariably fatal.
**Intraventricular septal rupture**—can complicate anterior or inferior MI. Presents with acute pulmonary oedema and a new harsh pansystolic murmur. Often there is haemodynamic compromise. IABP is helpful, but mortality 90% without surgical repair.
**Papillary muscle rupture**—causes acute, severe mitral regurgitation with pulmonary oedema and often haemodynamic embarrassment. Stabilization with IABP, but again mortality 90% without surgical repair.

*Tissue plasminogen activator (tPA) and derivatives*

These agents are recombinant forms of human tPA. They also activate plasminogen, but are thought to be more specific for fibrin-bound plasminogen leading to less systemic fibrinolysis.

*Choice of thrombolytic*

Fibrin-specific agents are preferred. This is driven by their increased early patency rates and shorter half-life than streptokinase.

*Failed thrombolysis*

Failed thrombolysis is diagnosed if the ST-segment elevation in the lead with the maximum ST-segment elevation pre-thrombolysis has not fallen by at least 50% 90 minutes after administration. The ST-segment is measured at 80ms after the J-point. All patients diagnosed with failed thrombolysis should be considered for rescue angioplasty.

## Further management in STEMI

- CCU monitoring.
- Secondary prevention.
- Echocardiography.
- Cardiac rehabilitation.

Early discharge should be considered in patients who have undergone primary PCI. Otherwise length of hospital stay will usually be 5–7 days. In patients who reperfused with thrombolysis, or indeed received no reperfusion therapy, further risk stratification should be undertaken prior to discharge.

## Secondary prevention in all ACS

- A antiplatelet, ACE inhibitor.
- B β-blocker, blood pressure control.
- C cholesterol reduction, cigarette cessation.
- D diet, diabetes (diagnosis and treatment).
- E exercise, eplerenone.
- F fish oils (omega-3 fatty acids).

*Aspirin*

All patients unless intolerant.

*Beta-blocker*

All patients without a contraindication, **especially** if the acute event is complicated by heart failure/left ventricular dysfunction.

*Statins*

All patients. There is some evidence suggesting a small benefit of high-dose statins after acute coronary syndromes.

*ACE inhibitors*

Should be considered in all patients. Largest benefit if MI complicated by LV dysfunction or heart failure.

*Aldosterone antagonists*

Patients who have clinical evidence of heart failure and LVEF <40%, or diabetic patients with LVEF <40%.

*Clopidogrel/ticagrelor/prasugrel*

For 3–12 months in patients with unstable angina and ECG change/ NSTEMI/STEMI.

# 3.4 Arrhythmias

## Making a diagnosis

This should be on the basis of a 12-lead ECG. A structured approach to the ECG allows at least an accurate description, and often a confident diagnosis:

- What is the rate?
- Is it regular or irregular?
- Are P waves present?
- Is there any organized atrial activity?
- What is the relationship between the atrial and the ventricular activity?
- Are the QRS complexes narrow or broad?

## Tachyarrhythmias

### Definition
A heart rate >100 beats per minute (bpm). Can be classified according to QRS duration (narrow or broad complex) or site of origin of tachycardia (supraventricular or ventricular).

### Narrow complex tachycardias
These are tachycardias which originate above the ventricles, and although usually narrow complex, they may be broad complex in the presence of pre-existing bundle branch block, aberrant conduction, or antegrade conduction over an accessory pathway.

*Sinus tachycardia*

An underlying cause should be sought. Always consider the possibility of atrial flutter with 2:1 block if there is a 'sinus tachycardia' of around 150 bpm.

*Atrial fibrillation (AF)*

An irregular, usually narrow complex, tachycardia (Fig. 3.19). The most common tachyarrhythmia, affecting 5–10% of the population >65 years. AF is often initiated by ectopic foci in the ostia of the pulmonary veins and sustained by multiple micro-re-entry circuits within the atria leading to chaotic electrical activity and the loss of atrial contraction. See Box 3.21 for causes of AF.

*Treatment*

New-onset AF

- Treat precipitating factors, if present. Check thyroid function.
- Commence anticoagulation with heparin.
- Cardioversion—can be attempted if clear onset of arrhythmia within 48 hours.
- Pharmacological cardioversion—amiodarone or flecainide.
- Electrical cardioversion—synchronized DC shock.
- Rate control—if onset unclear, no major urgency for cardioversion or unlikely to remain in SR, then rate should be controlled with drugs which slow conduction at the AV node.

Long-term management

Patients with AF in association with valvular heart disease should be anticoagulated with warfarin. In non-valvular AF there is a 5–7-fold increase in the risk of stroke compared with controls without AF. Warfarin reduces that risk by 68%, and aspirin reduces it by 22%. Those at the highest risk benefit most from anticoagulation, so the

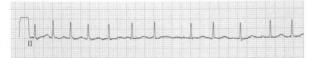

**Fig. 3.19** Atrial fibrillation with a rapid ventricular response. The baseline is chaotic with no organized atrial activity and the ventricular rhythm is irregularly irregular

---

| Box 3.21  Causes of atrial fibrillation |
|---|
| • Hypertension |
| • Ischaemic heart disease |
| • Mitral valve disease |
| • Thyrotoxicosis |
| • Alcohol |
| • Sepsis |
| • Pericarditis |
| • Pulmonary embolus |
| • Bronchial carcinoma |
| • Pneumonia |
| • Cardiac surgery |
| • Cardiomyopathy |

decision to anticoagulate is based on the individual's risk of thromboembolic events. There are a number of risk scoring systems, with the $CHA_2DS_2VASc$ score recently being recommended by the European Society of Cardiology.

Novel anticoagulants

Rivaroxaban and pixaban (oral factor Xa inhibitors) and dabigatran (oral direct thrombin inhibitor) have recently been shown to have similar efficacy and safety profiles to warfarin with the advantage that they are given in a fixed dose and anticoagulant monitoring is not required. They are an alternative to warfarin in patients with non-valvular AF and risk factors for thromboembolic complications.

Further management depends if AF is persistent or paroxysmal.

Paroxysmal AF

- The same indications for anticoagulation with warfarin apply.
- Antiarrhythmic therapy—β-blockers, class IC or class III antiarrhythmics.
- Amiodarone is the most effective antiarrhythmic drug, but the side effect profile is a major limiting factor (also interacts with warfarin).
- Potential cure can be offered with the catheter-based procedure of pulmonary vein isolation.

Persistent AF

- Rate control or rhythm control strategies are equivalent in well-tolerated AF.
- Rhythm control—cardioversion to SR with or without anti-arrhythmic therapy to maintain SR. For patients with significant symptoms attributable to AF.
- Rate control—first line therapies are β-blockers or rate-limiting calcium channel blockers (verapamil, diltiazem), adding digoxin if required, and anticoagulation as appropriate.

*Atrial flutter*

A regular, usually narrow complex tachycardia with ventricular rate ~150 bpm (Fig. 3.20). 'Typical' flutter, with a saw-toothed baseline in the inferior leads is due to a counter-clockwise macro-re-entrant circuit in the right atrium involving the cavo-tricuspid isthmus. The atrial rate is usually ~300 bpm, with the ventricular rate a multiple of this, although it may be irregular if there is variable block.

Treatment strategies are similar to AF, as are indications for anticoagulation, though very high cure rates of atrial flutter can be achieved with radiofrequency ablation of the cavo-tricuspid isthmus.

*Atrial tachycardia*

Caused by an ectopic atrial focus discharging at a rate of 150–200bpm. There may be one-to-one conduction, or varying degrees of block. Atrial tachycardia with AV block is associated with digoxin toxicity.

Treatment strategies similar to AF, but again cure with catheter ablation is possible.

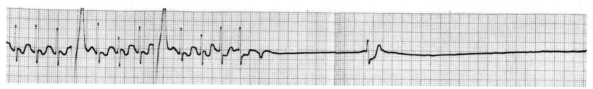

**Fig. 3.20** Atrial flutter with 2:1 ventricular response. Note the characteristic saw-toothed baseline in the inferior leads. The ventricular rate is 150bpm and regular. This could be mistaken for sinus tachycardia (lead V1), but intravenous adenosine is a very useful diagnostic test as it would slow the ventricular rate and unmask the flutter waves. © EKG World Encyclopedia http://cme.med.mcgill.ca/php/index.php , courtesy of Michael Rosengarten BEng, MD.McGill. This file is licensed under the Creative Commons Attribution-Share Alike 3.0 Unported (//creativecommons.org/licenses/by-sa/3.0/deed.en) license.

### Supraventricular tachycardia (SVT)

All the tachyarrhythmias discussed so far are supraventricular in origin but the term SVT is used specifically to describe atrioventricular re-entry tachycardias of which there are two main types:

- Atrioventricular nodal re-entry tachycardia (AVNRT).
- Atrioventricular re-entry tachycardia (AVRT).

In both cases there are two pathways for atrioventricular conduction. In AVNRT these are both within the AV node (dual AV nodal physiology) and in AVRT there is an accessory pathway (a bundle of myocytes connecting the atria and ventricles) remote from the AV node. In certain circumstances, such as with an atrial premature beat, conduction may occur down one pathway whilst the other is refractory. If this is conducted retrogradely back to the atria via the other pathway which is no longer refractory a re-entry circuit is created leading to a regular, narrow complex (usually) tachycardia (rate 140–250bpm) which will persist until the circuit is interrupted.

### Treatment of an acute episode

- Vagal manoeuvres:
  - Valsalva.
  - Carotid sinus massage.

- Adenosine (Fig. 3.21—3mg, 6mg, then 12mg given as IV bolus) into an antecubital vein and flushed through with saline as the half-life in plasma is <10 seconds.

If these measures fail or are only temporarily effective then try:

- 5mg verapamil as an intravenous bolus, or
- 2mg/kg flecainide, up to 150mg, as an intravenous infusion.

### Long-term treatment options

- No treatment other than for infrequent acute episodes.
- Regular therapy with β-blocker, verapamil, or flecainide.
- 'Pill in the pocket' approach—patient has a supply of tablets, e.g. flecainide 150mg, and only takes one if an episode occurs.
- Radiofrequency ablation (RFA)—this is an excellent option for a long-term cure with a 90–95% procedural success rate, and a risk of <1% for serious complications.

### Wolff–Parkinson–White syndrome

This is the finding of 'pre-excitation' on the 12-lead ECG in association with tachyarrhythmias (Fig. 3.21). There is a short PR interval and a delta wave (slurred upstroke in QRS complex) causing QRS prolongation. This is due to ventricular activation via an accessory pathway

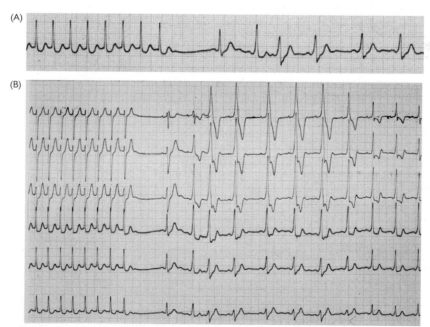

**Fig. 3.21** Cardioversion from SVT to sinus rhythm with adenosine. This patient has Wolff–Parkinson–White syndrome with a short PR interval and delta wave in sinus rhythm. Note how the wide QRS complex narrows as the AV node-blocking effect of the adenosine wears off and the contribution of AV nodal conduction to the QRS complex increases.

Reproduced from *Heart*, Rankin AC et al., 'Value and limitations of adenosine in the diagnosis and treatment of narrow and broad complex tachycardias.', 62, 3, pp. 195–203, 1989, with permission from BMJ Publishing Group Ltd.

*Favours VT*
- AV dissociation.
- Capture beats (a normal sinus beat within the tachycardia due to successful AV conduction).
- Fusion beats (a hybrid of a normal sinus beat and the ventricular complex.
- QRS >140ms.
- Extreme axis deviation/change in axis.
- Concordance across the limb leads.
- Specific QRS morphologies (e.g. Rsr′ in V1).
- VA relationship—atrial rate is a fraction of the ventricular rate, e.g. 2:1 VA block.

*Favours SVT*
- Slowing/termination with vagal manoeuvres or adenosine.
- Precipitated by atrial premature beat.
- Ventricular rate is a fraction of atrial rate, e.g. 2:1 AV block.
- Short VA time (RP interval <100ms).
- rSR′ in V1.

Box 3.23 Idiopathic forms of VT

- Catecholaminergic polymorphic VT:
  - Treat with β-blockers.
- Right ventricular outflow tract tachycardia:
  - LBBB morphology with inferior axis.
  - Treat with β-blockers, verapamil, or RFA.
- Left septal VT:
  - Fascicular tachycardia.
  - First-line treatment is verapamil.
  Other conditions associated with ventricular arrhythmias:
- Brugada syndrome:
  - Sodium channel abnormality.
  - ST elevation right precordial leads.
  - Associated with SCD.
  - Can be unmasked by flecainide challenge.
- Hypertrophic cardiomyopathy:
  - Risk stratification for sudden death allows targeted ICD therapy.
- Repaired tetralogy of Fallot:
  - VT secondary to re-entry at the site of repair in RVOT.
- Arrhythmogenic RV cardiomyopathy:
  - VT will have LBBB morphology.
- Long QT syndrome:
  - Causes torsades de pointes which can degenerate into VF. β-blockers first-line prevention.
  - ICD for primary prevention in high-risk cases, or for secondary prevention.

as well as the normal conduction system. Patients with AVRT can be cured by radiofrequency ablation of the accessory pathway.

### Broad complex tachycardias

The majority of these will be ventricular tachycardias with the remainder supraventricular arrhythmias with pre-existing bundle branch block, aberrant conduction, or antegrade conduction over an accessory pathway (Box 3.22).

#### Ventricular tachycardia (VT)

This is a regular, broad complex (QRS >120ms) tachycardia originating from the ventricles with a rate of 110–250bpm (Fig. 3.22). VT is said to be sustained if it lasts >30 seconds. It can be described as monomorphic if the QRS complexes are all of similar morphology, or polymorphic if the complexes continually change morphology.

Ventricular tachycardia most often occurs in the context of acute myocardial infarction, coronary artery disease, or impaired left ventricular function, although there are notable exceptions (Box 3.23).

The majority of ventricular tachycardias will have a RBBB morphology because the arrhythmia most frequently originates from the left ventricle.

*Treatment of an acute episode*

If there are signs of haemodynamic compromise, decompensated heart failure, chest pain, or impaired conscious level immediate DC cardioversion is indicated. Attempted pharmacological cardioversion with negatively inotropic agents may be harmful in this circumstance.

If haemodynamically stable, initial treatment with intravenous amiodarone may be appropriate. If this fails then DC cardioversion or overdrive pacing via a temporary pacing wire should be attempted.

*Long-term management*

In patients with sustained VT and haemodynamic compromise and/or left ventricular dysfunction implantable cardioverter defibrillators (ICDs) reduce mortality by aborting sudden cardiac death.

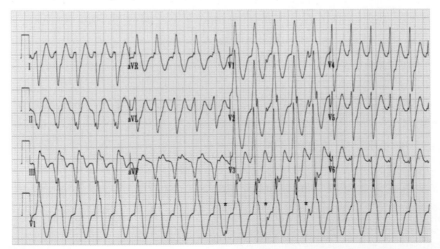

**Fig. 3.22** Ventricular tachycardia. A left ventricular origin is indicated by the right bundle branch block morphology. Close examination reveals the presence of independent atrial activity (asterisks) demonstrating atrioventricular dissociation. Note also the extreme axis deviation and the Rsr′ pattern in V1.

Courtesy of Professor AC Rankin.

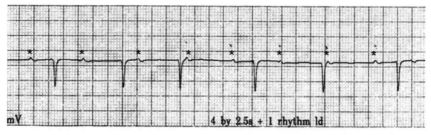

**Fig. 3.23** Mobitz type I second-degree AV block. P waves are identified by asterisks. Some P waves are followed by a QRS but with lengthening PR interval until a P wave is not conducted. This is the Wenckebach phenomenon which is usually a property of the AV node.

Amiodarone and sotalol are useful in preventing recurrent VT. In certain circumstances β-blockers or verapamil can suppress recurrent arrhythmias.

### Torsades de pointes

This is a form of polymorphic VT with the characteristic 'twisting' of the QRS amplitude around the isoelectric line. It occurs in the context of acquired or congenital QT interval prolongation. In congenital long QT syndrome, β-blockers prevent torsades de pointes and an ICD may be appropriate.

### Ventricular fibrillation

This most often occurs in the context of coronary artery disease and impaired LV function, although can rarely be idiopathic. Treat as per resuscitation guidelines.

## Bradyarrhythmias

Defined as a heart rate <60bpm.

### Sinus bradycardia

Often normal for that individual, or drug-induced. Other causes should be considered.

### Sick sinus syndrome

Inappropriate sinus bradycardia or episodes of sinus arrest due to sinus node dysfunction. Often associated with paroxysmal AF. Permanent pacing indicated for symptomatic bradycardia or sinus pauses and symptomatic chronotropic incompetence. May also be required to allow use of anti-arrhythmic drugs for AF.

### Atrioventricular node disease

#### First-degree heart block

Prolonged PR interval (>200ms) but every P wave followed by a QRS. No specific treatment required.

#### Second-degree heart block

The key feature is that some, but not all, P waves are conducted to the ventricles.

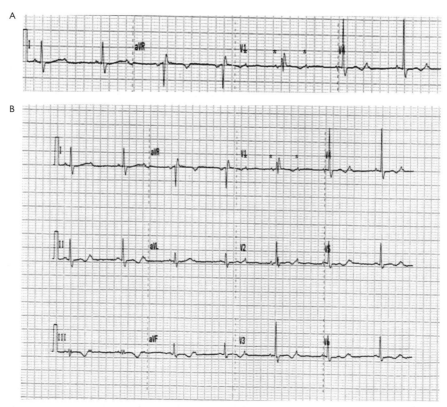

**Fig. 3.24** Mobitz type II second-degree AV block. Only every second P wave (asterisks) is conducted. This can be a subtle finding and may be overlooked unless every lead is examined for evidence of atrial activity. In this example the P waves are only clearly seen in V1, which is often the best lead for identifying atrial activity.

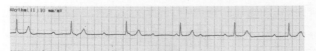

**Fig. 3.25** Complete heart block. There is no relationship between the P waves and the QRS complexes (AV dissociation).

*Mobitz type I second-degree AV block*

Also known as the Wenckebach phenomenon. P waves are conducted to the ventricles but with increasing AV delay until one P wave is blocked. The site of block is usually the AV node, and permanent pacing is not required unless there are symptoms clearly associated with the bradycardia or the site of block is below the bundle of His. See Fig. 3.23.

*Mobitz type II second-degree AV block*

This is characterized by non-conducted P waves without a preceding lengthening of the PR interval. It can be intermittent or persistent, e.g. with 2:1 conduction. The level of block is usually in the His–Purkinje system. This is an indication for permanent pacing even if asymptomatic if heart rate <40bpm, or pauses >3 seconds. See Fig. 3.24.

*Complete heart block (third-degree AV block)*

No P waves are conducted to the ventricles, and ventricular activation occurs from an automatic focus within the ventricles themselves, so there is no relationship between the P waves and the QRS complexes. Permanent pacing is generally indicated unless there is a reversible cause. See Fig. 3.25.

# 3.5 Pacemakers and devices

## Pacemakers

### Pacemaker systems

The basic concept of cardiac pacing is delivery of an electrical impulse of sufficient magnitude to cause depolarization of atrial or ventricular myocardium if there is no intrinsic electrical activity detected within a specified time interval. This requires all the components of the pacemaker system to be functioning appropriately:

- **Pulse generator:** contains power source, output, sensing and timing circuits, memory and rate adaptive elements.
- **Leads:** conductors which carry electrical impulses surrounded by insulation material. Connect to pulse generator headers.
- **Electrodes:** distal end of conductors which are in direct contact with myocardium. Deliver electrical impulse/conduct intrinsic electrical activity which is sensed by the pulse generator.

### Major indications for pacing

*Acquired atrioventricular block*

- Third-degree AV block.
- Mobitz type II second-degree AV block.
- Mobitz type I second-degree AV block with symptoms definitely correlated with bradycardia.
- AV block associated with atrial fibrillation or flutter if bradycardia associated with heart failure, pauses >5 seconds or escape rate <40bpm, especially if rate-limiting drugs are required to control tachycardia.
- Chronic bi-or trifascicular block with intermittent high-degree AV block or syncope not attributable to other causes.

*Sinus node dysfunction*

- Symptomatic bradycardia or sinus pauses.
- Asymptomatic bradycardia/sinus pauses when rate-limiting drugs are required to control tachyarrhythmias.

### Pacing mode

Internationally standardized nomenclature exists to describe the main functions of an antibradycardia pacemaker (Table 3.3).

*Mode selection*

Sequential atrioventricular activation optimizes cardiac haemo-dynamics although this has translated into only a minor benefit in clinical trials comparing pacing modes. Recent clinical studies have suggested that continuous RV pacing can be deleterious to left ventricular function, as a result of abnormal electrical activation. On this basis pacing mode is generally selected with the aim of maintaining sequential AV activation, and minimizing RV pacing, if possible.

VVI—Single chamber ventricular pacing. For AV block/symptomatic bradycardia in patients in atrial fibrillation.

VVIR—single-chamber ventricular pacing with rate response. Randomized trial data suggests this is as good as DDD(R) in elderly patients with AV block.

AAI(R)—single chamber atrial pacing—for symptomatic sinus node dysfunction with intact AV conduction. Superior to VVI pacing in sinoatrial disease.

DDD(R)—dual chamber pacing is appropriate for AV block, and also used commonly in sinus node dysfunction, especially if there is evidence of AV block. In this circumstance pacemaker algorithms designed at minimizing RV pacing should be employed.

## Implantable cardioverter defibrillators

ICDS are designed to detect and treat life-threatening ventricular arrhythmias.

### Detection

The device is programmed with heart rate zones for identifying VT or VF. If the intrinsic heart rate falls into one of these heart rate zones the device will deliver the programmed therapy (Fig. 3.26). Certain algorithms, and in fact an atrial lead, can help to discriminate ventricular and supraventricular tachycardias.

### Therapy

The pulse generator houses the power source and capacitors for generating a high-energy electrical impulse. This is delivered via the device itself and shocking coils in the ICD lead.

Internal defibrillation is painful and distressing for patients. Less aggressive therapies can be programmed for VT at a rate below the VF detection zone:

- **Antitachycardia pacing:** the device paces the RV at a rate above the VT rate to try and terminate the tachycardia.
- **Cardioversion:** the device attempts to terminate the tachycardia with a low energy (e.g. 11J) biphasic shock.
- **Defibrillation:** the device attempts defibrillation with a full energy biphasic shock (e.g. 35J).

### Indications

See Box 3.24.

- **Primary prevention:** for patients deemed to be at high risk of life-threatening ventricular arrhythmias.
- **Secondary prevention:** for survivors of a VF arrest or haemo-dynamically compromising VT.

## Cardiac resynchronization therapy (CRT)

Patients with left ventricular dysfunction often have abnormal electrical activation manifest by conduction abnormalities and a wide QRS complex on the surface ECG. Abnormal electrical activation can lead to atrioventricular and ventricular dyssynchrony which contributes to left ventricular dysfunction.

| Table 3.3 NASPE/BPEG Generic code for antibradycardia pacing | | | |
|---|---|---|---|
| **Chamber(s) paced** | **Chamber(s) sensed** | **Response to sensing** | **Rate response** |
| O = None | O = None | O = None | O = None |
| A = Atrium | A = Atrium | T = Triggered | R = Rate modulation |
| V = Ventricle | V = Ventricle | I = Inhibited | |
| D = Dual (A + V) | D = Dual (A + V) | D = Dual (T + I) | |

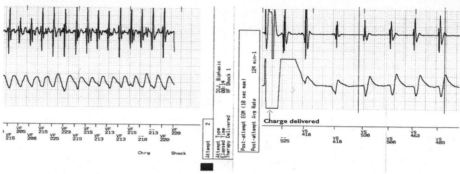

**Fig. 3.26** Printout from an ICD programmer. The top line is the intracardiac electrogram recorded from the tip of the ICD lead in the right ventricle. The bottom line is more analogous to a surface ECG recording, but is in fact the electrogram recorded between the tip of the ICD lead and a shocking coil in a more proximal portion of the lead. Each sensed ventricular event is labelled according to the preceding RR interval. On the left side of the trace the RR intervals are very short, and the device detects this as VF, which certainly looks appropriate from the lower electrogram. Once this is detected by the device, the capacitors are charged, and a 31J shock is delivered. This successfully defibrillates the VF as seen on the right side. VF: RR intervals falls within VF detection zone; VS: sensed ventricular event not falling within any tachycardia zone. The numbers below are the actual RR intervals in milliseconds.

---

**Box 3.24 NICE guidelines for implantable cardioverter defibrillators (indications for use in non-ischaemic cardiomyopathy not considered in this guidance)**

*Primary prevention*

A history of previous MI (>4 weeks) and:

Either

Left ventricular dysfunction with LVEF < 35% (NYHA ≤III)

and

NSVT on 24-hour Holter monitoring

and

Inducible VT on electrophysiological testing

or

Left ventricular dysfunction with LVEF < 30% (NYHA ≤III)

and

QRS duration ≥120ms

A familial cardiac condition with a high risk of sudden death including long QT syndrome, hypertrophic cardiomyopathy, Brugada syndrome, or arrhythmogenic right ventricular dysplasia.

*Secondary prevention*

- Survivors of cardiac arrest due to VT or VF.
- Sustained VT causing syncope or haemodynamic compromise.
- Sustained VT without syncope or haemodynamic compromise, but with LVEF less than 35% (NYHA ≤III).

National Institute for Health and Clinical Excellence (2006). Adapted from *TA 95 Arrhythmia – implantable cardioverter defibrillators*. London: NICE. Available from http://guidance.nice.org.uk/TA95 Reproduced with permission.

CRT restores atrioventricular and ventricular synchrony. The system comprises a pulse generator, standard atrial and right ventricular leads, and a left ventricular pacing lead (implanted via the coronary sinus) which allow optimization of the AV delay and synchronous activation of both ventricles. Clinical trials have demonstrated a reduction in mortality, improvement in symptoms, and a reduction in heart failure hospitalizations in selected patients with chronic heart failure symptoms, a wide QRS, and moderate to severe LV dysfunction.

- CRT-P—a standard biventricular pacing device.
- CRT-D—biventricular pacemaker with ICD incorporated.

# 3.6 Heart failure

## Background

Heart failure is the clinical syndrome that results from any cardiac disorder that impairs the ability of the heart to generate a cardiac output sufficient to meet the demands of the tissues. It can be acute or chronic. Acute heart failure (AHF) is reserved for either *de novo* heart failure or acute decompensations of chronic heart failure (CHF); cardiogenic shock is discussed in Section 1.2. This chapter will focus on CHF.

Note: asymptomatic left ventricular systolic dysfunction (LVSD) is considered a precursor to symptomatic CHF; some authors include it in the definition of CHF. CHF and LVSD should not be used interchangeably, as heart failure can arise from systolic dysfunction, diastolic dysfunction, valvular, endocardial, and pericardial diseases also.

## Epidemiology

- Population prevalence 1–2% (UK).
- Incidence increases with age (~0.2% in 45–54-year-olds vs. ~4% in 85–94-year-olds).
- The mean age at diagnosis of CHF is 74 years in the UK.
- ~50% of patients with LVSD are asymptomatic, and 50% with CHF have preserved LV ejection fractions (LVEF).

## Aetiology

The most common causes of CHF in the developed world are ischaemic heart disease (IHD) and hypertension. Clinically it is useful to consider underlying causes (i.e. conditions that can lead to CHF developing in previously-well patients) and precipitating causes (i.e. conditions that can cause deterioration in compensated CHF)—see Boxes 3.25 and 3.26.

## Pathophysiology

Irrespective of the cause of CHF, the syndrome involves haemodynamic dysfunction and neurohormonal activation. These changes are initially compensatory (Fig. 3.27) but ultimately pathophysiological.

Neurohormonal activation is a key component of the condition, and provides important targets for treatment:

---

**Box 3.25 Underlying causes of CHF**

- IHD.
- Hypertension.
- Valvular heart disease.
- Cardiomyopathy:
  - Idiopathic: drug-related (including alcohol); infiltrative disease (amyloid, haemochromatosis).
  - Infective, e.g. Chagas disease.
- Myocarditis.
- Pericardial disease:
  - Constrictive pericarditis.
  - Restrictive cardiomyopathy.
  - Pericardial effusion/tamponade.
- Endocardial disease, e.g. endomyocardial fibrosis.
- Arrhythmia, e.g. tachycardiomyopathy, heart block.
- High-output states:
  - Anaemia.
  - Hyperthyroidism.
- Pregnancy-related heart failure.
- Iatrogenic fluid overload (rare in normal heart).

---

**Box 3.26 Factors that precipitate decompensations of stable CHF**

- Acute coronary syndrome/silent myocardial ischaemia.
- Arrhythmia (tachy-, brady-), conduction disturbance (AV block).
- Drugs (verapamil, diltiazem, excessive beta-blockade, NSAIDs, glitazones, multiple antiarrhythmics, alcohol, toxins).
- Systemic infection.
- Inappropriate reduction of CHF therapy (fluid restriction, drug therapy (especially diuretics)); includes poor adherence.
- Anaemia.
- Renal dysfunction.
- Thyroid disease.
- Pulmonary embolism.
- Rapid progression of known valvular disease, e.g. precipitated by endocarditis.

---

- Sympathetic activation (probably in response to hypotension and reduced organ perfusion) promotes compensatory tachycardia and positive inotropy (maintains cardiac output initially).
- Sympathetic activation also increases pulmonary and vascular resistance (increasing afterload) and promotes energy expenditure.
- Direct effect of sympathetic nervous system on β1 adrenoceptors in juxtaglomerular apparatus in kidney promotes renin release, as does reduced renal perfusion (note: diuretics also increase renin secretion).
- Renin–angiotensin activation results in excessive amounts of angiotensin II (potent vasoconstrictor, enhances sodium-retention) and aldosterone release.
- Aldosterone promotes renal sodium and water retention and has direct fibrotic effects on myocardium and vasculature (reducing relaxation/compliance).

In response to progressive fluid retention, the heart and vasculature release compensatory peptides: ANP from the atria, BNP from the ventricles, and both promote natriuresis and vasodilatation. Despite an increase in whole body fluid, release of AVP from the hypothalamus in CHF may not be suppressed. CHF may also stimulate release of endothelins from the vasculature, which have potent cardiac, renal and vascular actions that may compound the syndrome of heart failure.

## Symptoms

- Dyspnoea.
- Orthopnoea, paroxysmal nocturnal dyspnoea (PND).
- Fatigue, reduced exercise capacity.
- Anorexia, nausea.
- Peripheral oedema (ankle or sacral swelling, anasarca).

## Clinical signs

Some, all, or none of the following may be elicited:
- General: malnourished ('cardiac cachexia'), pallor (anaemia).
- Pulse: alternans if severe heart failure, AF not uncommon.
- JVP elevated.
- Cardiac: displaced apex, gallop rhythm (S3 present), prominent P2 component of S2 (see Section 3.1).
- Pulmonary: bibasal crepitations, pleural effusions.
- Abdomen: hepatomegaly (could be pulsatile), ascites.
- Peripheral (dependent) pitting oedema.

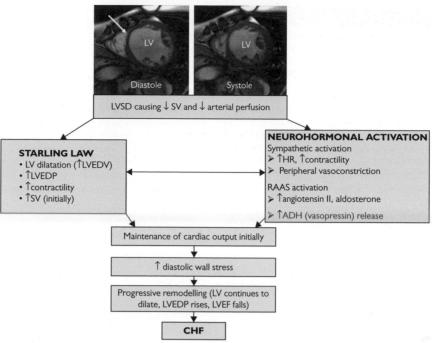

**Fig. 3.27** Pathophysiology of CHF. The cardiac MRI images show short axis biventricular views at end-diastole and end-systole, demonstrating reduced stroke volume due to a prior anteroseptal infarct; a thinned akinetic segment is seen (arrowed). This patient has CHF in the context of LVSD.
Key: ADH: antidiuretic hormone; HR: heart rate; LVEDV: LV end-diastolic volume; LVEDP: LV end-diastolic pressure; RAAS: renin–angiotensin–aldosterone system; SV: stroke volume.

## Diagnosis

Fatigue, dyspnoea, and oedema are by no means specific to CHF. Four basic tests can confirm or refute the diagnosis:

1. **ECG:** a normal ECG suggests that CHF is very unlikely; significant tachy- or bradycardia may precipitate CHF; the detection of LBBB has implications for certain management decisions (see later in section).

2. **CXR:** not only might the classical features of pulmonary oedema be seen (Fig. 3.28), but also alternative pulmonary diagnoses causing dyspnoea.

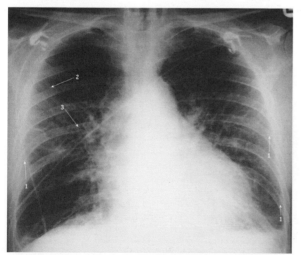

**Fig. 3.28** CXR of patient with pulmonary oedema. Note the following features: cardiomegaly, perihilar haziness, and small pleural effusions (better seen at the left base). Additionally: 1. Kerley 'B' lines; 2. Kerley 'A' lines; 3. Peribronchial cuffing.
Courtesy of Dr. C. Adams, RAH.

3. **Bloods:** FBC (anaemia), UEs (renal impairment; decisions concerning medication); TFTs (dysthyroidism); LFTs (congestion); glucose (diabetes). Cardiac biomarkers (e.g. troponin) should be checked in acute deteriorations of CHF.

4. **Echocardiography:** measurement of LVEF, wall thickness, regional wall-motion abnormalities; assessment of valves, pericardium, diastolic function (controversial), and dyssynchrony.

Some centres provide assays for serum natriuretic peptide quantification. Low–normal concentrations of BNP and its precursor NTproBNP in an untreated patient with possible CHF make the diagnosis very unlikely. Some centres utilize these assays in tailoring CHF treatment.
Other tests may be indicated after the four basic tests:

- Ferritin (exclude haemochromatosis), viral titres (possible myopericarditis), other bloods as in dilated cardiomyopathy (see Section 3.8).

- Additional non-invasive tests: stress echo, nuclear myocardial perfusion scintigraphy, cardiac MRI (see Section 3.2).

- Cardiac catheterization: coronary angiography (diagnostic and/or if planning revascularization in patients with ischaemic symptoms and CHF); invasive haemodynamic monitoring via Swan–Ganz catheter occasionally useful; valve assessment.

- Endomyocardial biopsy in unexplained CHF or else if significant diagnostic uncertainty (e.g. myopericarditis).

- Holter/event recorders if arrhythmia suspected (syncope).

## Treatment of chronic heart failure

Specific European guidelines exist (ESC Task Force, 2012) for the management of CHF. Patients can be classified as having CHF with reduced LVEF (HF-REF) and CHF with preserved LVEF (HF-PEF). Management is summarized as follows:

### Non-pharmacological management

- Patient and carer education: advice on fluid intake, diet, regular weighing to detect rapid gains, smoking cessation.

- Drug counselling: importance of adherence.

- Up to 50% of patients with CHF have preserved LV ejection fractions (Fig. 3.29).
- Compared to HF-REF, these patients are more often older, ♀, less likely to have IHD, and more likely to have hypertension (and LVH).
- AF is common—these patients may rely more on atrial contraction to improve diastolic filling of the LV; if this is lost, dyspnoea may rapidly worsen.
- No single drug treatment has been convincingly shown to reduce morbidity or mortality in HF-PEF. Recommendations from current guidelines are as follows:
  - Avoid precipitating factors (Box 3.26).
  - Treat any concomitant hypertension, arrhythmia, and/or myocardial ischaemia.
  - Diuretics if fluid overload present (but be cautious as can reduce preload excessively).

- Regular aerobic exercise if stable (as part of a structured programme).
- Vaccinations offered (influenza, pneumococcal).
- Avoidance of precipitating factors (Box 3.26).

## Pharmacological management

HF-PEF is common but less extensively investigated in clinical trials than HF-REF (Box 3.27). Medical treatment of HF-REF involves:

### ACE inhibitors

- Recommended for all patients with LVEF ≤40% (in addition to a beta-blocker) to reduce the risk of hospitalisation and premature death, if no contraindication.
- If fluid overload present, should be co-administered with diuretic as first-line treatment.
- Should be commenced at low dose and cautiously up-titrated to evidence-based dose (Table 3.4) or maximum tolerated dose.
- ACE inhibitors reduce all-cause mortality and reduce admission for worsening HF.

### Beta-blockers

- Recommended for all patients with LVEF ≤40% (in addition to an ACE inhibitor—or ARB) to reduce the risk of hospitalisation and premature death, if no contraindication.
- Only evidence-based β-blockers for use in CHF are: bisoprolol, carvedilol, metoprolol succinate, nebivolol.

- Initiation must be cautious (can cause initial myocardial depression): attain euvolaemia first, then start at low dose and cautiously up-titrate (Table 3.4).
- Even if only a low dose is tolerated, this may still provide morbidity and mortality benefit.
- Beta-blockers reduce all-cause mortality and reduce admission for worsening HF.

### Mineralocorticoid receptor antagonists

- Addition of spironolactone is recommended if the patient remains in NYHA class III–IV despite β-blocker and ACE inhibitor (Table 3.5).
- Addition of eplerenone is recommended if the patient is still in NYHA class II despite β-blocker and ACE inhibitor.
- Close electrolyte monitoring required (hyperkalaemia).
- Mineralocorticoid receptor antagonists reduce all-cause mortality and reduce admission for worsening HF.

### Angiotensin II receptor blockers (ARBs)

- Candesartan can be used as an alternative in patients intolerant of ACE inhibitors.
- Candesartan reduces cardiovascular mortality and hospitalization due to CHF when added to ACE inhibitor in patients with NYHA II–IV CHF with LVSD; valsartan reduces symptoms and CHF hospitalizations when added to ACE inhibitor therapy in symptomatic CHF.

### Ivabradine

- Ivabradine *should* be considered to reduce risk of CHF hospitalization in those in sinus rhythm, NYHA class II–IV, LVEF ≤35% with heart rate ≥70bpm despite evidence-based or maximal tolerated dose of beta-blocker.
- Ivabradine *may* be considered to reduce CHF hospitalization in those in sinus rhythm, NYHA class II–IV, LVEF ≤35% with heart rate ≥70bpm who are intolerant of a β-blocker.

### Diuretics

- Essential for symptomatic treatment if fluid overload is present (surprisingly there are no RCTs assessing their effect on survival).
- Loop diuretics used as first-line; higher doses required in more advanced CHF, and can lead to renal impairment. Malabsorption due to gut oedema can be an issue—if so, torasemide and bumetanide absorbed better than furosemide (or use IV initially).
- Thiazides (bendrofluazide, metolazone) have synergistic effect with loop diuretics but caution required—risk of rapid deterioration in renal function and hypokalaemia.

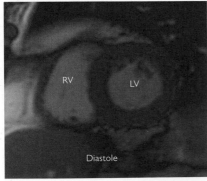
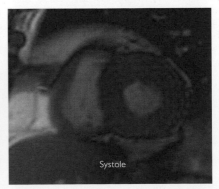

**Fig. 3.29** CHF with preserved LVEF (HF-PEF). Short axis cardiac MRI bi-ventricular views at end-diastole and end-systole of a patient with CHF with preserved LV ejection fraction. Note the thickened LV myocardium (compared to Fig. 3.27), and the narrow LV cavity at end-systole. Systolic function is normal.

**Table 3.4** (A) Recommended starting doses, up-titration regimens and evidence-based target doses of the approved β-blockers for CHF. (B) Recommended starting doses and maintenance doses for a selection of ACE inhibitors approved for use in CHF in Europe

**(a)**

| Beta-blocker | Starting dose | Increments | Target dose (mg) |
|---|---|---|---|
| Carvedilol | 3.125mg bd | 6.25, 12.5, 25, 50mg bd | 25-50mg bd |
| Bisoprolol | 1.25mg od | 2.5, 3.75, 5, 7.5, 10mg od | 10mg od |
| Metoprolol CR/XL | 12.5–25mg od | 25, 50, 100, 200mg od | 200mg od |
| Nebivolol | 1.25mg od | 2.5, 5, 7.5, 10mg od | 10mg od |

**(b)**

| ACE inhibitor | Starting dose | Maintenance dose |
|---|---|---|
| Ramipril | 1.25-2.5mg od | 2.5-5mg bd |
| Captopril | 6.25mg tds | 25-50mg tds |
| Enalapril | 2.5mg od | 10mg bd |
| Lisinopril | 2.5mg od | 5-20mg od |
| Trandolapril | 1mg od | 4mg od |

### *Others*

- Digoxin used to control ventricular rate in patients with AF and CHF, and may be considered to reduce symptoms and CHF hospitalizations in those with CHF in sinus rhythm, but does not improve survival.
- Hydralazine and isosorbide dinitrate combination can be used if ACE inhibitor and ARB intolerant. Shown to be efficacious in reducing mortality in African Americans already on an ACE inhibitor.

### Devices

Conventional single-lead RV pacing can worsen LV function and should be avoided in CHF. Patients with HF-REF who have a conventional indication for brady-pacing should be considered for CRT.

About 20% of severe CHF patients will have a prolonged QRS interval on ECG (≥120ms), many of whom will have ventricular dyssynchrony. CHF patients in sinus rhythm, with LVEF ≤35%, LBBB morphology, and QRS ≥120ms, who remain in NYHA class III/IV despite optimal medical therapy, and who are expected to survive at least 1 year, are recommended for CRT to improve symptoms, hospitalizations, and survival. Recent studies have demonstrated a beneficial effect on outcomes of CRT in patients with milder CHF symptoms, such that CRT is now also recommended in patients in NYHA class II with LVEF ≤30%, LBBB morphology, QRS ≥130ms, on optimal medical therapy and expected to survive at least 1 year, to reduce CHF hospitalizations and improve survival. CRT may be combined with an ICD ('CRT-D'); there are no data that conclusively demonstrate superior survival with CRT-D over CRT-pacemakers ('CRT-P').

ICD insertion is recommended to improve survival in patients who have survived cardiac arrest, and those with sustained VT (either poorly-tolerated, or in the context of LVSD). It is also recommended in patients with LVEF ≤35%, on optimal medical therapy for at least 3 months and expected to survive at least a year, to reduce the risk of sudden death.

**Table 3.5** New York Heart Association (NYHA) classification for heart failure

| Class | Exercise tolerance | Symptoms |
|---|---|---|
| I | No limitation | No symptoms during normal activity |
| II | Mild limitation | Comfortable at rest; ordinary activity causes symptoms |
| III | Moderate limitation | Comfortable only at rest; less than normal activity causes symptoms |
| IV | Severe limitation | Symptomatic at rest; any physical activity brings on discomfort |

Adapted with permission of Heart Failure Society of America.

**Box 3.28 Left ventricular assist devices (LVAD)**

*The standard LVAD consists of:*

- Pump, implanted in abdomen (Fig. 3.30).
- Inflow tube, attached to LV apex.
- Outflow tube, attached to aorta.
- Internal (one-way) valves.
- Power leads (pass through skin to external battery).
- Battery unit/controller (often on a belt worn by patient).

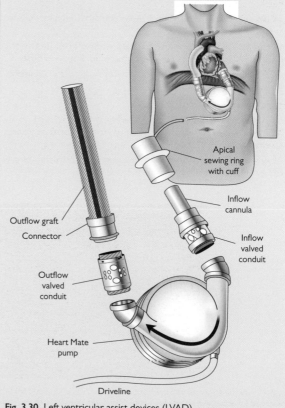

Apical sewing ring with cuff

Inflow cannula

Outflow graft
Connector

Inflow valved conduit

Outflow valved conduit

Heart Mate pump

Driveline

**Fig. 3.30** Left ventricular assist devices (LVAD).
Reprinted with the permission of the Cleveland Clinic Foundation.

| Box 3.28 Continued |
| --- |

*How it works:*

- Assists LV (does not 'replace' it).
- Blood flows into pump during ventricular systole.
- Some devices employ a suction effect, drawing more blood from the LV into the pump, during systole.
- During ventricular diastole, as LV fills with blood, pump forces blood into aorta and improves arterial perfusion.

*Indications:*

- Bridge to cardiac transplant.
- Acute severe myocarditis ('bridge to recovery').
- Long-term destination therapy for patients with severe refractory CHF deemed unsuitable for transplantation.

*Complications:*

- Infection.
- Mechanical failure of device.
- Thromboembolism.
- Complications of surgical insertion.

## Surgery

Surgical (or percutaneous) revascularization is recommended for CHF patients with angina and either significant left main stem disease or else two- or three-vessel coronary artery disease including the LAD, as long as the patient is suitable for revascularization and expected to survive at least 1 year with good functional status. There is no indication for revascularization in the absence of angina. Valve repair/replacement and LV aneurysmectomy may be indicated in selected patients (although operative mortality is high).

Advances in medical and device therapy have led to fewer patients undergoing cardiac transplantation. This should be considered in severe heart failure with no alternative treatment options. Conventional contraindications to organ transplantation apply.

Left ventricular assist devices are discussed in Box 3.28.

## Reference

The Task Force for the diagnosis and treatment of CHF of the European Society of Cardiology. Guidelines for the diagnosis and treatment of acute and chronic heart failure. 2012. *Eur Heart J* 2012; *14*: 803–69.

## Mitral valve disease

### Mitral stenosis

#### Aetiology
Almost always a result of rheumatic fever. ♀ preponderance.

#### Pathophysiology
As the mitral valve orifice reduces in size, a small pressure gradient at rest is required to maintain blood flow from left atrium to left ventricle. This results in an increase in left atrial pressure and in turn pulmonary venous and pulmonary capillary pressures. The long-term consequence of this is pulmonary arterial hypertension. Symptoms of dyspnoea first develop in the context of tachycardia which reduces the diastolic left ventricular filling time causing a further increase in left atrial pressure.

#### Clinical features
##### Symptoms
- Exertional dyspnoea.
- Orthopnoea.
- Haemoptysis.
- Chest pain.

##### Signs
- Malar flush.
- Atrial fibrillation.
- Tapping apex.
- Loud S1.
- Opening snap.
- Low-pitched, rumbling diastolic murmur with presystolic accentuation in sinus rhythm (best heard with the bell of the stethoscope in left lateral position and can be accentuated by exertion).
- Signs of pulmonary hypertension (see Box 3.29).

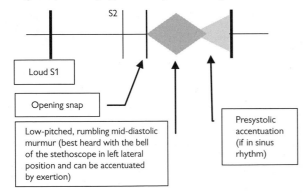

#### Investigations
- ECG—P mitrale in sinus rhythm, atrial fibrillation.
- CXR (see Fig. 3.31)—left atrial enlargement, pulmonary arterial enlargement, right heart enlargement, and interstitial oedema (depending on severity).

---

**Box 3.29 Signs of pulmonary hypertension**

- Right ventricular heave.
- Loud pulmonary component of S2.
- Elevated JVP.
- Pansystolic murmur of tricuspid regurgitation.
- Right ventricular S4.

---

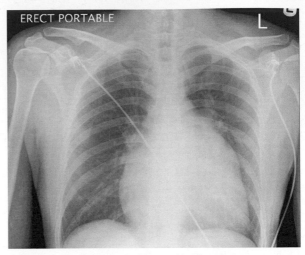

**Fig. 3.31** Chest radiograph of a 32-year-old male with severe mitral stenosis. There is cardiomegaly with a dilated left atrium (left atrial 'bulge' on left heart border and splaying of the carina) and pulmonary venous congestion. The left atrium measured 10cm on echocardiography (normal <3.8cm).

- Echocardiography—thickening and calcification of leaflets and subvalvular apparatus with stenotic mitral valve orifice. Characteristic 'doming' of anterior mitral valve leaflet in diastole (Fig. 3.32). Mitral valve area can be measured directly or calculated on the basis of pulsed-wave Doppler pressure half-time.

#### Natural history
In developed countries there is a delay of 15–20 years between an episode of acute rheumatic fever and symptoms of mitral stenosis (MS) developing. There is slow progression over 5–10 years from mild symptoms (NYHA II) to severe limitation (NYHA III–IV). In tropical and subtropical countries the progression to severe mitral stenosis is much more rapid.

#### Medical therapy
Oral diuretics can improve symptoms.

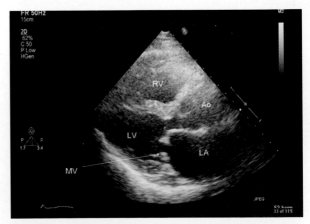

**Fig. 3.32.** There is evidence of rheumatic mitral stenosis with thickening of the valve and characteristic 'bowing' of the anterior mitral valve leaflet in diastole (*). Ao: aorta; LA: left atrium; LV: left ventricle; MV: mitral valve; RV: right ventricle.
Image courtesy of Dr NER Goodfield.

The onset of atrial fibrillation often precipitates symptoms, which can improve with rate control with digoxin and β-blockers/rate-limiting calcium channel blockers.

### Anticoagulation
Patients with atrial fibrillation in association with mitral stenosis should be anticoagulated with warfarin. This is also indicated in sinus rhythm with previous embolism or LA thrombus, and should be considered if spontaneous echo contrast (indicating low-velocity blood flow) or severe LA dilatation.

### Interventional treatment options
- Percutaneous balloon mitral valvuloplasty.
- Open surgical valvotomy.
- Mitral valve replacement (MVR).

The indications for intervention are moderate to severe mitral stenosis (mitral valve area <1.5cm$^2$) and significant symptoms (NYHA ≥II), although usually there is a higher threshold for surgical intervention (NYHA III or IV). See Table 3.6.

## Mitral regurgitation

### Aetiology
- MV annular calcification (age-related degeneration).
- Mitral valve prolapse.
- Rheumatic fever.
- Ischaemic heart disease—papillary muscle dysfunction or rupture.
- Infective endocarditis.
- LV dilation of any cause.
- Rupture of chordae tendinae (spontaneous, infarction, infective endocarditis, trauma).
- Others—HCM (hypertrophic cardiomyopathy), collagen abnormalities, connective tissue disorders.

### Pathophysiology
Significant mitral regurgitation (MR) results in a chronic volume overload state causing left ventricular and left atrial enlargement. Although there is an increase in left ventricular end-diastolic dimensions, the reduction in afterload associated with severe MR results in increased contractility and a reduction in end-systolic dimensions. Left atrial pressure is not normally dramatically increased in severe MR as the regurgitant jet is accommodated by an enlarging LA. Decompensation is often the result of a failing left ventricle due to chronic volume overload, often with prominent features of reduced cardiac output.

In acute severe MR there is reduced atrial compliance leading to a marked increase in left atrial pressure and resultant pulmonary venous hypertension and pulmonary oedema.

### Clinical features
#### Symptoms
- Exertional dyspnoea.
- Weakness and fatigue may be prominent due to diminished cardiac output.

#### Signs
- Normal or diminished volume pulse.
- Sharp upstroke of arterial pulse.
- Hyperdynamic apex displaced laterally.
- Diminished S1.
- Widely split S2 (early A2).
- S3 ± brief diastolic rumble (rapid early filling of LV).
- Pansystolic murmur—high-pitched, blowing, loudest at apex and radiating to axilla.

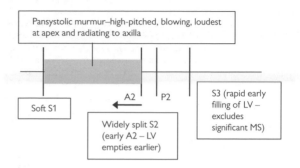

#### Investigations
- ECG—p mitrale or AF. May reflect LV enlargement or RV hypertrophy.
- CXR—most prominent feature is cardiomegaly with LA enlargement. Lung changes less prominent than in mitral stenosis.

#### Transthoracic echocardiography
- Cause—MV and subvalvular apparatus anatomy (Fig. 3.33).
- Severity—colour flow Doppler, transmitral flow velocities (Fig. 3.34).
- Consequences—LA and LV dimensions (particularly LVEF and end-systolic volume), TR, and estimated PASP (pulmonary artery systolic pressure), right heart function and dimensions.

#### Transoesophageal echocardiography
More detailed images of valvular anatomy and helps establish the severity of MR. Of particular importance when considering MV repair.

| Table 3.6 Therapeutic options for symptomatic mitral stenosis | |
| --- | --- |
| **Therapeutic option** | **Considerations** |
| Balloon mitral valvuloplasty (BMV) | Least invasive<br>Excellent long term outcome with restenosis in <20% at 10 years<br>Only applicable if suitable valvular anatomy on echo<br>Contra-indicated if significant MR or LA thrombus |
| Open mitral valvotomy | Requires cardiopulmonary bypass<br>Similar results to BMV<br>Can be applied to more distorted valves |
| Mitral valve replacement | Higher threshold due to higher operative mortality<br>Indicated for extensively calcified and distorted valves not amenable to valvotomy<br>First choice if significant MR |

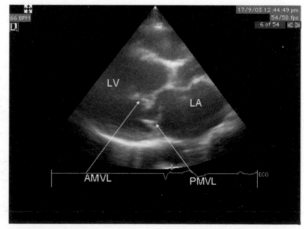

**Fig. 3.33** Parasternal long axis view of a transthoracic echocardiogram showing prolapse of the posterior mitral valve leaflet (PMVL). The leaflet tips fail to coapt and the posterior mitral valve leaflet clearly prolapses beyond the plane of the mitral valve annulus. AMVL: anterior mitral valve leaflet.

Image courtesy of Dr NER Goodfield.

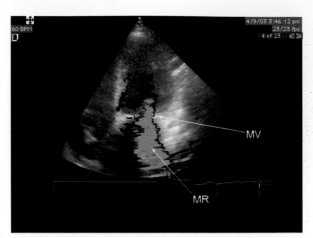

**Fig. 3.34** Apical four-chamber view with colour flow Doppler of a transthoracic echocardiogram demonstrating severe mitral regurgitation in the same patient as shown in Fig. 3.33. Turbulent flow is indicated by the yellow colour. There is a broad jet of mitral regurgitation filling virtually the entire left atrium (MR). MV: mitral valve.

Image courtesy of Dr NER Goodfield.

### Natural history

In chronic severe MR progression is usually indolent, but even if initially asymptomatic, surgery within 10 years is almost inevitable. The key is to operate before irreversible LV dysfunction occurs as this has a major adverse effect on postoperative survival.

### Medical therapy

Although reduction in afterload is effective, and in fact essential, in acute severe MR, there is little evidence of a benefit of long-term ACE inhibitor therapy in chronic asymptomatic severe MR. In patients with heart failure as a result of MR who are not candidates for surgery, aggressive heart failure therapy with diuretics, ACE inhibitors, and β-blockers is warranted.

### Surgical therapy

If technically feasible, MV repair rather than replacement is desirable due to reduced perioperative mortality (2% vs. 6%) and improved preservation of left ventricular geometry and function.

### Indications for surgery

The major issue is balancing the operative risk, and the risk of delaying surgery too long. By the time signs of reduced cardiac output and pulmonary congestion occur, irreversible left ventricular damage may have occurred leading to a poor outcome in spite of surgery. An increase in left ventricular end-systolic diameter (LVESD), and a reduction in left ventricular ejection fraction (LVEF) predict adverse surgical outcomes. Another factor to consider is whether repair is feasible; a lower threshold for surgery is appropriate due to reduced operative risk (Box 3.30).

## Aortic valve disease

### Aortic stenosis

#### Aetiology
Left ventricular outflow tract obstruction may result from a supravalvular or subvalvular membrane, or hypertrophic obstructive

---

**Box 3.30 Indications for surgery for mitral regurgitation**

Asymptomatic severe mitral regurgitation:
- Truly asymptomatic?—careful history/ETT.
- Surgery if evidence of **progressive** LV dysfunction (LVEF <0.60 or LVESD >45mm) on echocardiographic follow-up (6–12-monthly).
  Symptomatic severe MR (NYHA II–IV):
- Surgery is indicated (unless LVEF <0.30 and valve not suitable for repair).

---

**Box 3.31 Symptoms of severe aortic stenosis**

| | |
|---|---|
| Angina | May occur with normal coronary arteries due to increased myocardial oxygen demand (increased LV mass and increased systolic pressure) and also decreased supply (increased LV diastolic pressure impairs coronary perfusion, and diastolic duration is also diminished). |
| Exertional syncope | Is the result of systemic vasodilation in response to exercise in the presence of fixed LV outflow obstruction. |
| Exertional dyspnoea | Ultimately heart failure develops when pulmonary venous hypertension occurs. |

cardiomyopathy, but this section will concentrate on valvular aortic stenosis of which there are three main causes:
- Degenerative.
- Rheumatic—diminishing in frequency.
- Bicuspid—a congenitally bicuspid valve is subject to turbulent flow leading eventually to fibrosis and calcification of the valve leaflets and outflow obstruction.

### Pathophysiology
Progressive left ventricular outflow obstruction causes an increase in afterload and left ventricular pressures. Left ventricular hypertrophy develops to maintain cardiac output. The left atrium hypertrophies which helps maintain LVEDP due to vigorous left atrial contraction, and so protects from pulmonary venous hypertension. However, when aortic stenosis becomes severe (effective aortic valve orifice <1.0cm$^2$) though the stroke volume is maintained at rest, it cannot adequately increase with exertion.

### Clinical features

#### Symptoms
The three cardinal symptoms are angina, exertional dyspnoea, and exertional syncope (Box 3.31).

#### Signs
- Slow rising pulse.
- Low systolic BP and narrow pulse pressure.
- Sustained, undisplaced apical impulse unless left ventricular failure develops.
- Ejection systolic murmur loudest at the base of the heart and radiating to the carotids ± thrill.
- S2—aortic component diminishes as severity increases.
- S4.

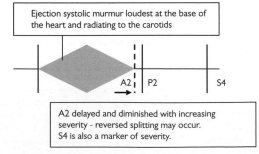

### Investigations
See Box 3.32 and Fig. 3.35.

### Natural history
There is very gradual left ventricular outflow obstruction and there is a long latent period where patients are asymptomatic in some cases in spite of severe stenosis. The onset of symptoms is an ominous sign and the average time from symptom onset to death without operative treatment is 2 years with heart failure, 3 years with syncope, and 5 years with angina. A major concern in asymptomatic severe aortic stenosis is the risk of sudden death (thought to be due to cerebral

| Box 3.32 Investigations in severe aortic stenosis | |
|---|---|
| ECG | LVH in 85% of severe aortic stenosis. Biphasic p wave in V1 suggestive of LA hypertrophy rather than LA dilation. |
| CXR | Heart size often normal. There may be calcification of aortic valve, and post-stenotic dilation of the ascending aorta. |
| Cardiac catheterization | Most haemodynamic data are now gathered from echocardiography, so this is mainly indicated to assess coronary artery anatomy prior to cardiac surgery. |
| Transthoracic echocardiography | Provides accurate information on aortic valve structure, pressure gradient across the valve (Doppler-derived) and associated abnormalities such as LVH, left ventricular dysfunction, and concomitant valvular pathology. |

| Box 3.33 Causes of aortic regurgitation | |
|---|---|
| *Valvular AR*<br>Rheumatic fever<br>Infective endocarditis<br>Calcific aortic valve disease<br>Bicuspid aortic valve disease<br>Deterioration of bioprosthetic aortic valve replacement<br>Inflammatory conditions such as SLE, rheumatoid arthritis | *Aortic root disease*<br>Age-related aortic dilation<br>Cystic medial necrosis (isolated or classical Marfan)<br>Aortic dissection<br>Syphilitic aortitis<br>Systemic hypertension<br>Osteogenesis imperfecta<br>Ankylosing spondylitis<br>Psoriatic arthritis<br>Arthritis associated with ulcerative colitis |

hypoperfusion followed by arrhythmia), but in fact this is very rare without prior symptoms (risk <1% in a large series).

### Medical therapy

Medical therapy has little to offer in aortic stenosis. Diuretics can treat fluid overload, and ACE inhibitors can be used if there is LV dysfunction, and operative intervention is not being considered. However ACE inhibitors, or any vasodilators, must be used with extreme caution in severe aortic stenosis as there is potential for causing profound hypotension.

### Surgical therapy

Symptomatic severe aortic stenosis—mortality 2–5%.

Asymptomatic severe aortic stenosis—consider if:
- Progressive left ventricular dysfunction.
- Abnormal BP response to exercise.

Transcutaneous aortic valve implantation (TAVI) is an alternative for some patients who are not operative candidates.

## Aortic regurgitation

### Aetiology

This can result from primary valvular disease, or aortic root dilation (Box 3.33).

### Pathophysiology

In significant aortic regurgitation the left ventricle is subject to chronic volume overload leading to left ventricular dilation, and increased afterload due to systolic hypertension. Normal wall tension is initially preserved by eccentric LV hypertrophy and LVEDP initially remains normal. The chronic LV strain does however lead to interstitial fibrosis in the LV wall, and decompensation in LV function will eventually occur with progressive LV dilation, rising LVEDP, LA pressure, PCWP, PA, RV, and RA pressures resulting in congestive heart failure.

### Clinical features
#### Symptoms
- Dyspnoea—initially exertional, progressing to orthopnoea and paroxysmal nocturnal dyspnoea.
- Angina—can occur with normal coronary arteries due to a mismatch in myocardial oxygen demand and supply (increased LV mass and wall tension, decreased diastolic BP, and increased LVEDP).
- Thoracic pain—dilated heart hitting the thoracic wall.
- Palpitations—the increased ejection of a severely dilated ventricle after a post-ectopic pause.

#### Signs
See Box 3.34.

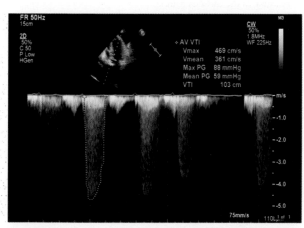

**Fig. 3.35** A continuous wave Doppler tracing in a patient with severe aortic stenosis. The Doppler signal is positioned in the left ventricular outflow tract. From the velocity of blood flow, the pressure gradient across the stenosed aortic valve can be calculated from the Bernoulli equation $P = 4V^2$, where P is the pressure gradient in mmHg and V is the velocity of blood flow. The peak and mean gradients can be calculated. This patient has atrial fibrillation resulting in some variability of the Doppler velocity.

Image courtesy of Dr NER Goodfield.

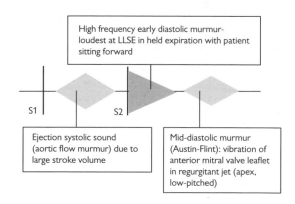

### Investigations
- ECG—left axis deviation.
- LV diastolic volume overload—prominent Q waves I, aVL, and V3–V6.
- LV hypertrophy and 'strain' pattern.
- CXR—cardiomegaly and aortic root dilation.

### Transthoracic echocardiography
- Cause—aortic valve and root anatomy.
- Severity—regurgitant jet on colour flow Doppler, pressure half-time of regurgitant jet from continuous wave Doppler.

- Collapsing pulse.
- Wide pulse pressure.
- Quincke sign—capillary pulsations in nailbeds (fingers).
- De Musset sign—head nodding with systole.
- Visible carotid pulsations.
- Pistol-shot femorals (loud 'crack' in systole and diastole over femoral arteries).
- Duroziez sign—systolic murmur over femoral artery when depressed proximally, and diastolic murmur when compressed distally.
- Apical impulse—diffuse, hyperdynamic and displaced inferiorly and laterally.
- Auscultation—ejection systolic sound due to large stroke volume, S3 if significant LV dilation, high frequency EDM loudest at LLSE in held expiration with patient sitting forward.

- Effect—left ventricular parameters, in particular LVEDD, LVESD, and LVEF. LVESD can be used to predict which asymptomatic patients are likely to progress to need surgery.

*Natural history*

In asymptomatic severe AR with normal LV function there is a 4–6% annual incidence of the endpoint of symptoms, asymptomatic LVD, and death. However 45% will remain asymptomatic with normal LV function at 10 years. Once symptomatic there is a rapid decline without surgical intervention. In the presurgical era death would occur on average 2 years after the onset of heart failure. Surgical outcome is worse if there is LVD, and this may be irreversible.

*Medical therapy*

There is unconvincing evidence that vasodilator treatment with dihydropyridine calcium channel blockers, ACE inhibitors, or hydralazine will delay the need for surgery in asymptomatic severe AR with normal LV function.

*Surgery*

*Indications*

- Symptomatic severe AR.
- Asymptomatic severe AR with signs of progressive LV dysfunction—LVEF <0.50, LVEDD >75mm, LVESD >55mm.
- The aim is to operate before irreversible LV dysfunction develops.

# Right heart valvular disease

## Tricuspid stenosis

*Aetiology*

Rheumatic fever (almost always associated with mitral stenosis).

*Clinical signs*

- Systemic venous congestion (raised JVP, hepatomegaly, ascites and peripheral oedema).
- Giant a waves on the jugular venous waveform in sinus rhythm.
- Opening snap and diastolic murmur loudest at the LLSE on inspiration, but often overlooked if mitral stenosis also present.

*Medical treatment*

Sodium restriction and diuretics.

*Surgery*

Rarely requires treatment in isolation. Open valvotomy should be performed at the time of mitral valve surgery if significant tricuspid stenosis.

## Tricuspid regurgitation

*Aetiology*

- Functional—secondary to RV dilation of any cause (most common—see Fig. 3.36).

- Valvular disease—rheumatic fever, carcinoid syndrome, infective endocarditis, and congenital heart disease.

*Symptoms*

TR is often well-tolerated unless there is pulmonary hypertension.

*Signs*

- Pulmonary hypertension.
- Atrial fibrillation.
- Prominent cv wave on the jugular venous waveform with a rapid y descent.
- Pansystolic murmur at the LLSE loudest on inspiration.
- Pulsatile hepatomegaly.
- Peripheral oedema.

*Surgery*

- Rarely indicated for TR alone.
- TR secondary to mitral valve disease should be repaired at the time of mitral valve surgery.
- Mechanical tricuspid valve replacement should be avoided if at all possible due to the risk of valve thrombosis.
- Infective endocarditis—often due to intravenous drug use, the valve may be completely excised if bacteriological control is not achieved and a bioprosthesis inserted at a later stage if appropriate.

## Pulmonary stenosis

Most commonly congenital, may also be caused by rheumatic fever or carcinoid syndrome. Significant pulmonary outflow obstruction causes RV hypertrophy. Signs include a harsh ESM in the pulmonary area loudest on inspiration, a RV heave, and signs of systemic venous congestion. Severe cases require valvotomy or pulmonary valve replacement.

## Pulmonary regurgitation

More common than pulmonary stenosis. Usually caused by dilation of the valve ring as a result of pulmonary hypertension. Rarer causes include infective endocarditis, carcinoid syndrome and iatrogenic, e.g. after treatment of tetralogy of Fallot. The RV volume overload is usually well tolerated unless there is pulmonary hypertension in which case right heart failure develops. Signs of pulmonary hypertension may predominate. There is often wide splitting of S2 due to prolonged RV ejection time. A diastolic murmur is heard in the third and fourth left intercostals spaces. PR itself does not usually require treatment unless it causes intractable right heart

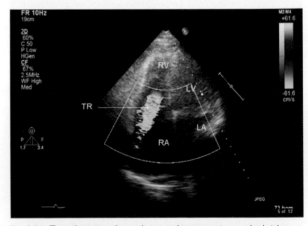

Fig. 3.36 Transthoracic echocardiogram demonstrating marked right atrial (RA) and right ventricular (RV) dilation. The right ventricle should be smaller than the left ventricle (LV) in this apical four-chamber view. The turbulent colour flow demonstrates a broad-based jet of severe tricuspid regurgitation (TR) secondary to tricuspid annular dilatation as a result of the right ventricular dilatation.

Image courtesy of Dr NER Goodfield.

failure, which really only occurs in PR secondary to repaired tetralogy of Fallot.

## Prosthetic heart valves

### Mechanical valve prostheses
There are three main types of mechanical valves in use:
- Caged-ball (e.g. Starr–Edwards)—excellent longevity though slight increase in incidence of thromboembolism compared with other mechanical valves.
- Tilting disc (e.g. Medtronic-Hall valve).
- Bileaflet—St Jude bileaflet is the most commonly used prosthetic valve worldwide.

These valves have excellent durability, but because of the increased risk of thromboembolism anticoagulation with warfarin is mandatory (Box 3.35).

The main complications are endocarditis, complications related to anticoagulation and valve thrombosis.

Valve thrombosis is a medical emergency. It should be suspected if there is acute dyspnoea and muffled valve clicks or a new murmur. Diagnosis is made by echocardiography. Treatment is with aspirin, heparin and thrombolysis or surgery (especially if they fail to respond or there are mobile thrombi visible on echo).

### Bioprosthetic heart valves
The most commonly used is the porcine heterograft (e.g. Carpentier–Edwards) but other options include a stentless porcine valve, bovine pericardial valves, homograft aortic valves (from cadavers), pericardial autografts and pulmonary autografts.

Anticoagulation—Box 3.35.

Bioprosthetic valves have limited durability compared to mechanical valves. There is a 30% rate of primary valve failure at 10 years, and freedom from valve failure is only 30–60% at 15 years. Deterioration is more likely in the mitral than the aortic position.

### Choice of valve prosthesis
This should be tailored to the individual needs of the patient. The major issues are the need for anticoagulation with the mechanical valves, and the limited durability of the bioprostheses (bearing in mind mortality from a redo valve surgery is double the initial surgery). Several studies have shown no difference in outcomes in the first 5 years after valve replacement. One long-term study demonstrated a survival benefit with a mechanical valve in the aortic position, but no difference in the mitral position. Another long-term study demonstrated survival with the original valve and without adverse valve related effects was greater for mechanical valves, though there was no clear mortality difference.

---

**Box 3.35 Indications for anticoagulation for prosthetic heart valves**

*Mechanical valves*
- Anticoagulation mandatory.
- Thromboembolic risk higher in mitral than aortic position.
- Moderate thromboembolic risk (bileaflet or tilting disc valves in the aortic position): target INR 2.0–3.0.
- High thromboembolic risk (AF, previous thromboembolism, all other mechanical aortic valve replacements, and all mechanical valves in the mitral position: target INR 2.5–3.5.

*Bioprosthetic valves*
- AVR—desirable for first 3 months only to allow endothelialization of valve ring unless another indication for warfarin.
- MVR—first 3 months only unless AF, heart failure, previous thromboembolism, or left atrial thrombus.
- If there is any other indication for anticoagulation, there is no benefit of bioprosthetic over mechanical valves.

---

## Infective endocarditis

This is a microbial infection affecting the endothelial surface of the heart, most commonly on the heart valves. Vegetations develop adherent to the valve. These are a heterogeneous mass of fibrin, platelets, micro-organisms and inflammatory cells. This condition can be caused by a wide variety of organisms. It most commonly occurs in patients with pre-existing valve disease or prosthetic heart valves, but no predisposing factors are found in 25% of cases. The incidence in the UK is 6–7/100,000 population.

### Causative organisms

| | |
|---|---|
| Streptococci | 30–65% |
| *Staphylococcus aureus* | 25–40% |
| Enterococci | 5–15% |
| Coagulase-negative staphylococci | 3–8% |
| Gram-negative bacilli | 5% |
| Culture negative | 5% |

This distribution of causative organisms applies to native valve endocarditis. There are special circumstances where the pattern is different:

*Intravenous drug users*
*Staphylococcus aureus* predominates (40–70%). There is also an increased incidence of Gram-negative bacilli and fungal endocarditis. Infection occurs mainly on right heart valves.

*Prosthetic valve endocarditis*
Accounts for 10–30% of all cases of endocarditis. Incidence 1.4–3.1% of valve replacements in the first year.

Classified as early (0–60 days post-surgery) and late (60 days+). Early infection is presumed to be secondary to the surgery. *S. aureus* and coagulase-negative staphylococci are the main causative organisms, and there is an increased frequency of Gram-negative bacilli and fungi. In reality this pattern of causative organisms persists to approximately 1 year post-surgery, after which a similar distribution to native valve endocarditis is found.

### Symptoms
These can be quite non-specific and include fever, lethargy, anorexia, and weight loss. There may be symptoms related to valve destruction (dyspnoea) or to embolic complications such as stroke.

### Signs
Fever and heart murmur are the most common. As the aetiology of IE has changed, and successful antibiotic regimes have been introduced, the classical peripheral signs of endocarditis (splinter haemorrhages, conjunctival petechiae, finger clubbing, Osler nodes, Janeway lesions, Roth spots) are increasingly rare.

### Diagnosis
Modified Duke Criteria (Box 3.36).

### Investigations
Full blood count—normocytic normochromic anaemia and normal white cell count in subacute illness, no anaemia and leucocytosis in acute illness.

ESR—elevated except possibly in heart failure, chronic renal failure, or disseminated intravascular coagulopathy.

Blood cultures—three separate sets of blood cultures should be taken from separate venepunctures over 24 hours prior to initiation of antibiotic therapy.

Echocardiography this can identify underlying cardiac lesions, vegetations (Fig. 3.37), and evidence of valve destruction. In native valve endocarditis transthoracic echocardiography (TTE) has a sensitivity of 65% for vegetations, and transoesophageal echocardiography (TOE) has a sensitivity of 85–95%. In prosthetic valve endocarditis the sensitivity of TTE is 15–35% compared with 82–96% for TOE.

Box 3.36 Modified Duke criteria for the diagnosis of infective endocarditis

| Major criteria | Positive blood culture |
| --- | --- |
| | Typical microorganism from two separate blood cultures |
| | Persistently positive blood cultures with typical microorganism |
| | Single positive blood culture for *Coxiella burnetii* |
| | Evidence of endocardial involvement |
| | Positive echocardiogram |
| | Oscillating intracardiac mass |
| | Abscess (Fig. 3.38) |
| | New partial dehiscence of prosthetic valve |
| | New valvular regurgitation |
| Minor criteria | Predisposition (predisposing heart condition or IV drug use) |
| | Fever ≥38.0°C |
| | Vascular phenomena—e.g. major arterial emboli |
| | Immunological phenomena—e.g. glomerulonephritis |
| | Microbiological evidence—positive blood culture not meeting the major criteria |

Definite endocarditis: two major criteria **or** one major and three minor criteria **or** five minor criteria.

Possible endocarditis: one major and one minor criterion or three minor criteria.

Reproduced from Li JS *et al.*, 'Proposed modifications to the Duke Criteria for the diagnosis of infective endocarditis', *Clinical Infectious Diseases*, 2000, by permission of Oxford University Press and Infectious Diseases Society of America.

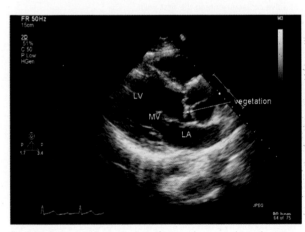

**Fig. 3.37** Parasternal long axis view of a transthoracic echocardiogram demonstrating a vegetation on the aortic valve.

Image courtesy of Dr NER Goodfield.

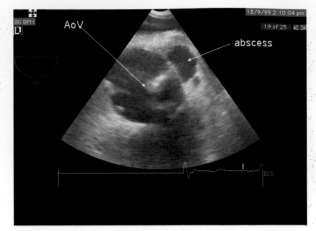

**Fig. 3.38** A short axis view of the aortic valve (AoV) on transoesophageal echocardiography. This patient was known to have aortic valve endocarditis, but this image clearly demonstrates that they have developed the complication of an aortic root abscess. This requires surgical treatment, but pending surgery the patient should have daily electrocardiograms to detect developing atrioventricular block. This is an acknowledged complication of an aortic root abscess (and aortic valve surgery) due to the proximity of the atrioventricular node.

Image courtesy of Dr NER Goodfield.

### Treatment

- Should be bactericidal rather than bacteriostatic.
- Combination treatment often required.
- Treatment must be prolonged with high tissue concentrations of antibiotics required (therefore intravenous therapy essential). It should be guided by microbiology advice based on blood culture results where possible.

### Indications for surgery

- Moderate to severe heart failure due to valve dysfunction.
- Uncontrolled infection in spite of optimal antimicrobial therapy.
- Intracardiac complication such as an abscess.
- Embolic complications.

## Antibiotic prophylaxis

The indications for antibiotic prophylaxis for patients with valvular heart disease undergoing dental and invasive procedures has been extensively revised. This is only recommended for high-risk patients undergoing high-risk procedures. The conditions for which antibiotic prophylaxis should be considered are prosthetic valves, previous endocarditis, and certain forms of congenital heart disease.

# 3.8 Structural heart disease

## Introduction

Advances in cardiac imaging have led to increased detection of structural abnormalities, frequently at a subclinical (or, perhaps more correctly, preclinical) stage. Such structural abnormalities may be congenital or acquired.

## Adult congenital heart disease: atrial septal defect

There are four main types of atrial septal defect (ASD):
1. Ostium secundum (most common type: defect in central fossa ovalis).
2. Ostium primum (often associated with mitral or tricuspid valvular defects, VSDs).
3. Sinus venosus defect (usually near superior vena cava opening in RA).
4. Coronary sinus defect (rare).

See Box 3.37 for conditions associated with ASD.

### Clinical presentation

*Paediatric*
- Most children asymptomatic—diagnosis made after discovery of a murmur.
- Primum ASDs often detected earlier due to associated AV valvular regurgitation/VSD if present.

*Adult*
- Progressive exercise intolerance (occurs by 3rd decade in 30%, 5th decade in >75%).
- Palpitations (due to supraventricular arrhythmias).
- Paradoxical embolism.

### Clinical signs
(If in PACES, usually a secundum ASD.)
- Low volume pulse; may be in AF.
- Left parasternal (RV) heave and loud P2 if pulmonary hypertension.
- Systolic pulmonary thrill with large L-to-R shunts.

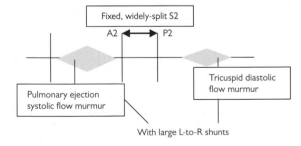

With large L-to-R shunts

### Investigations
- ECG: axis deviation to right (secundum) or left (primum); RBBB; first-degree heart block common in primum ASD, AF.
- CXR: cardiomegaly (due to dilated right heart), pulmonary plethora, small aortic knuckle.
- Echo: see Fig. 3.39. TOE may be needed to assess suitability for device closure; also good for delineating pulmonary venous drainage.
- Cardiac catheterization: often unnecessary; can confirm step-up in oxygen saturations allowing shunt identification.

---

### Box 3.37 Conditions associated with ASD

*Down syndrome*
- Ostium primum ASD.

*Noonan syndrome*
- ASD.
- Congenital pulmonary stenosis.
- Phenotype similar to Turner syndrome, but this has left-sided cardiac lesions; and Noonan right (PS).
- Autosomal dominant—chromosome 12.

*Lutembacher syndrome*
- Combined ASD and mitral stenosis, the latter either congenital or acquired (rheumatic).

*Holt–Oram syndrome*
- Autosomal dominant, but 50% are sporadic mutations.
- *TBX5* gene on chromosome 12 implicated.
- Abnormalities of upper limb and congenital heart defects (usually secundum ASD).
- Upper limb abnormalities include absent or triphalangeal thumb, syndactyly, clinodactyly, missing/malformed carpal bones or forearm bones.

*Eisenmenger syndrome*
Pulmonary hypertension caused by a congenital L-to-R shunt may reach systemic levels and result in reversal of the shunt, leading to cyanosis and heart failure. This is Eisenmenger syndrome and is irreversible.

**Common causes** include VSD ('Eisenmenger complex'), ASD, and patent ductus arteriosus (PDA).

**Clinical course:** may have healthy childhood but cyanosis develops by 2nd or 3rd decade; exercise intolerance develops by the 3rd decade. Most survive to adulthood, but die in their 30s.

**Complications:** AF/flutter (35%), VT (10%), pulmonary and cerebral embolism, endocarditis, (massive) haemoptysis (pulmonary infarction), respiratory infections.

**Clinical signs:** central cyanosis, clubbing, JVP 'a' waves or systolic cv waves visible if TR present, left parasternal heave, loud P2, Graham Steell murmur. Pansystolic murmur is TR, as VSD murmur disappears as R and L pressures equalize.

**Treatment** is based on prevention and symptoms: annual influenza vaccinations; endocarditis prophylaxis; antiarrhythmics, diuretics if necessary. Pregnancy strongly contraindicated—maternal mortality approaches 50%. The high pulmonary vascular resistance precludes closure of the primary defect, but heart-lung transplantation is an option.

---

### Management
- Spontaneous closure of ASD may occur in 1st year of life.
- Percutaneous device closure for secundum ASDs if suitable size of defect with enough surrounding septum (and away from AV valves).
- Open surgical closure if any of above points present, and for primum ASD (patch repair; AV valve may also need intervention).

Children with closed primum ASD need prolonged follow-up—risk of mitral regurgitation, subaortic stenosis, and AV block.

Other features that can be seen on transthoracic echo:
- Paradoxical septal motion (due to RV pressure overload).
- Direction of flow through ASD (reversed in Eisenmenger syndrome).
- Calculation of pulmonary-to-systolic flow ratio.

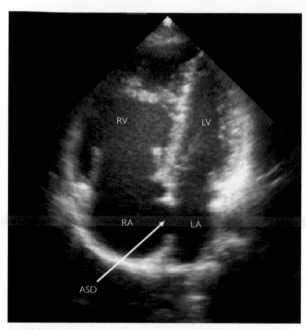

**Fig. 3.39** Transthoracic echo showing secundum ASD.

Note the anatomical features apparent from the still image in Fig. 3.39: not only is the ASD clearly seen, the right heart (both RV and RA) is significantly dilated, and indeed the right-sided chambers are larger than the left-sided chambers. The tricuspid valve annulus is stretched, and there will be significant tricuspid regurgitation. Pulmonary arterial pressure is likely to be elevated.

- Agitated saline ('bubble test')—rapid injection of 5–10mL agitated saline through a peripheral vein during real-time imaging will show direct transit of bubbles through ASD. Useful for smaller defects.

# Ventricular septal defect

Ventricular septal defects (VSDs) are among the most common congenital heart defects, occurring in 0.1–0.4% of live births, and constituting 20–30% of congenital heart lesions.

They can be classified by location within the interventricular septum: muscular, membranous, infundibular, AV canal defect, Gerbode defect (VSD connects LV and RA).

Can also be classified by pathophysiology:

- Restrictive: maintains large pressure gradient between LV and RV (pulmonary:aortic (P:A) systolic ratio <0.3); small shunt only and tend to be asymptomatic. May close spontaneously during childhood or even adulthood.
- Moderately restrictive: moderate shunt; P:A systolic ratio <0.66; may present with dyspnoea, progressive left atrial/ventricular dysfunction and pulmonary hypertension.
- Non-restrictive: large shunt; P:A systolic ratio >0.66; symptomatic, and if ratio reaches 1:1, Eisenmenger syndrome develops.

See Box 3.38 for associated conditions. VSDs can be single or multiple. Risk of SBE is reasonably high so antibiotic prophylaxis required.

## Clinical signs

- Thrill at lower left sternal edge.

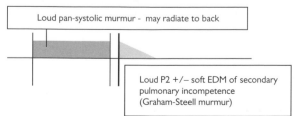

Loud pan-systolic murmur - may radiate to back

Loud P2 +/− soft EDM of secondary pulmonary incompetence (Graham-Steell murmur)

---

**Box 3.38 Associations of VSD**

- Patent ductus arteriosus (5–10%).
- ASD.
- Valvular lesions: pulmonary stenosis, aortic incompetence.
- Fallot tetralogy.
- Coarctation.

---

- No correlation between size and murmur intensity (Maladie de Roger: very small defect with very loud murmur).
- PSM lessens as shunt reverses and Eisenmenger develops.

### Investigations

Echo is gold-standard diagnostic test (Fig. 3.40).

The apical four-chamber view is shown (Fig. 3.40; see Section 3.2). Colour flow Doppler shows an obvious jet travelling from the left ventricle (LV) to the RV through the interventricular septum. This jet passes through the VSD, which lies in the membranous part of the septum.

### Indications for closure

- Haemodynamically significant VSD in absence of irreversible pulmonary hypertension.
- Recurrent SBE.

### Management

Surgical patch closure; percutaneous device closure possible with certain VSDs.

# Patent ductus arteriosus (PDA)

- The ductus arteriosus connects the proximal left pulmonary artery to the descending aorta, just distal to the left subclavian artery, allowing the fetal circulation to bypass the lungs *in utero*—it closes after birth, (becoming the ligamentum arteriosum).
- PDA more likely if born at high altitude, and ♀ sex.
- Associated with any congenital defect that causes hypoxia, e.g. coarctation, hypoplastic left heart syndrome.
- Small PDAs may be asymptomatic and of no clinical consequence, but larger ones can cause pulmonary hypertension and ultimately Eisenmenger syndrome (5% of cases).

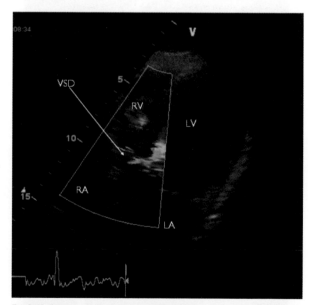

**Fig. 3.40** Echocardiogram of patient with VSD.

Image courtesy of Mrs C. Kemp, Cardiology Department, Royal Alexandra Hospital, Paisley.

- Signs: continuous murmur ('machinery') best heard in 2nd left intercostal space (often with associated thrill), wide pulse pressure with collapsing pulse, displaced apex, S3, differential cyanosis (feet > hands).
- Treatment:
  - **Infants:** indomethacin closes PDAs in >90% of cases; (prostaglandin E1 can prevent closure). Transcatheter device closure now recommended ahead of surgical closure, ideally within the first few years of life
  - **Adults:** transcatheter closure first-line, surgical closure second-line, unless irreversible pulmonary hypertension present (contraindication to closure).

## Aortic coarctation

- Narrowing of aorta most commonly found just distal to the origin of the left subclavian artery:
  - The coarctation (block arrow in Fig. 3.41) is seen within the aortic arch just beyond the origin of the left subclavian artery.
- 2–5× more common in ♂.
- Cardiac associations: bicuspid aortic valve, VSD, PDA, mitral valve disease.
- Non-cardiac associations: Turner syndrome (35% have coarctations), berry aneurysms of circle of Willis.
- Often asymptomatic, otherwise symptoms include headache, epistaxis, exertional leg weakness.
- Complications: intracranial haemorrhage, aortic dissection, premature coronary artery disease.
- Signs:
  - Upper limb systolic hypertension.
  - Radiofemoral delay.
  - Interscapular systolic murmur.
  - Crescendo-decrescendo systolic murmur.
  - Tortuosity of retinal vessels.
- Treatment: surgical excision with end-to-end repair.
- Re-stenosis in 5–10%—potentially amenable to angioplasty.
- Follow-up every 1–3 years (echo and/or cardiac MRI).

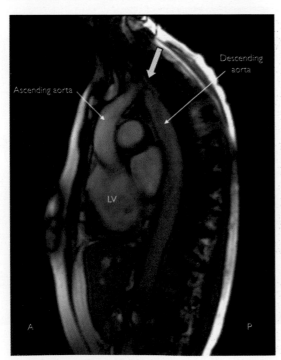

**Fig. 3.41** Coarctation of aorta (cardiac MRI, sagittal view).

### CXR abnormalities in aortic coarctation

- Enlargement of the aortic knuckle.
- Poststenotic aortic dilatation.
- Cardiomegaly.
- Pulmonary congestion.
- Rib-notching (undersurface of the ribs).

## Tetralogy of Fallot

Narrowing at the infundibulum of the pulmonary valve forces deoxygenated blood from the RV (arrow in Fig. 3.42) to pass through the VSD and into the aorta. The RV free wall hypertrophies, resulting in RVH (LV and RV walls are of comparable thickness).

- Commonest cause of cyanotic congenital heart disease.
- Symptoms tend to occur after first 6 months of life: cyanotic attacks, failure to thrive, squatting (adaptive response to increase systemic vasoconstriction and reduce R-to-L shunt), progressive exertional dyspnoea.
- Signs:

| | |
|---|---|
| Central cyanosis | RV heave |
| Left parasternal systolic thrill | Clubbing |
| Ejection systolic murmur (varies inversely with severity of RV outflow obstruction) | Single S2 |

- Treatment:
  - Definitive surgical repair now performed in early life, but occasionally a temporizing Blalock–Taussig shunt is required (diverts blood from subclavian to pulmonary arteries) until child suitable for surgical correction.
  - Surgery involves: (1) patch repair of VSD, (2) removal of RV outflow obstruction (may require pulmonary valve repair or replacement). Occasionally a conduit is created between RV and pulmonary artery—a Rastelli repair.

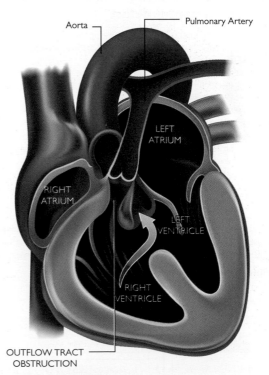

**Fig. 3.42** Tetralogy of Fallot.

# Pericardial disease

## Acute pericarditis

- Acute inflammation of the pericardium.
- Most commonly viral (*Coxsackie B* most commonly identified) but can be idiopathic, bacterial, fungal, traumatic, autoimmune (e.g. Dressler syndrome, SLE), post-MI, uraemic, paraneoplastic, radiotherapy-induced or drug-induced (e.g. tetracyclines, isoniazid, ciclosporin).
- Presents with sharp retrosternal chest pain classically altered by position (relieved by sitting forward). Pericardial friction rub may be heard, but examination most commonly normal.
- ECG: saddle-shaped (concave upwards) ST elevation either globally or, less common, regionally, with depressed P-Q segments and lack of reciprocal ischaemic changes.
- Echocardiography may show brightened pericardium (often non-specific) and should be performed to exclude pericardial effusion (tends to be small and of no haemodynamic significance if present).
- Management: treatment of underlying cause; symptomatic treatment with NSAIDs; steroids may be necessary in resistant (or autoimmune) cases.

## Constrictive pericarditis

- Increasingly rare condition in the Western world.
- Causes of constrictive pericarditis:

| Idiopathic (most common) | Radiotherapy |
|---|---|
| TB | Neoplastic |
| Bacterial pericarditis | Post-cardiac surgery |
| Uraemia | Drugs, e.g. methysergide |

- As entire pericardium involved, there is restricted filling of all cardiac chambers.
- Symptoms are of insidious onset: peripheral oedema and abdominal discomfort (due to hepatic congestion) may progress to exertional dyspnoea, jaundice, and ascites.

*Cardiovascular signs*
- Elevated JVP, rising on inspiration (Kussmaul sign).
- Pulsus paradoxus may be present.
- Pericardial knock: loud S3 in early diastole.

*Investigations*
- Echo: thickened, bright pericardium.
- CXR: calcified pericardium (suspect TB).
- Cardiac CT/MRI: thickened pericardium.
- Cardiac catheterization (differentiate from RCM).
Surgical pericardiectomy is the only definitive treatment. It carries a perioperative mortality of 5–15%.

## Pericardial effusion

- Fluid can accumulate in the pericardial space acutely or chronically.
- Cause: any cause of constrictive pericarditis, plus bleeding into pericardial space: aortic dissection, ventricular rupture post-MI, or iatrogenic during cardiac catheterization.
- Large effusions may cause:
  - Pulsus alternans; paradoxus if impending tamponade.
  - Impalpable apex and muffled heart sounds.
  - Elevated JVP.
  - Small complexes on ECG, and electrical alternans.
  - Cardiomegaly on CXR.
- Drainage via pericardiocentesis is indicated urgently if tamponade present, and in symptomatic large effusions.
- Smaller effusions may be managed conservatively, with regular echo follow-up.

## Cardiac tamponade

- Collection of fluid within the pericardial space sufficient to prevent cardiac filling.
- Speed of development of the effusion is the key factor: <250mL may cause tamponade if develops rapidly, while chronic effusions of >>1L may be very well-tolerated.
- Signs: hypotension, quiet heart sounds, elevated JVP (= Beck triad), pulsus paradoxus, tachycardia.
- Echo urgently required; features:
  - Diastolic collapse of right atrium/ventricle.
  - Variable mitral valve Doppler signal with respiration.
- Treatment is by urgent pericardiocentesis (if direct bleeding is the cause, contact cardiothoracic surgical team).
- Once the initial tamponade is relieved, it is usual practice to leave a pericardial drain *in situ* until no longer draining.
- Pericardiodesis (with sclerosant) or a pericardial window may be needed in recurrent (malignant) effusions.

# Myocarditis

- Acute inflammation of the myocardium.
- Pathophysiology poorly understood; often presumed to be viral, or part of a post-viral autoimmune syndrome. *Coxsackie* virus traditionally associated, but a large number of viruses—especially parvovirus B19—have been implicated.
- Non-viral (presumptive) causes include bacteria, fungi, rickettsiae, spirochaetes, protozoa, and drugs (e.g. methyldopa, sulphonamides, doxorubicin).
- Clinical features:
  - Patients usually younger.
  - Viral illness (concurrent or recent).
  - Fatigue, dyspnoea, chest pain, palpitations.
  - May present in heart failure.
  - White cell count usually mildly elevated.
  - Can develop (refractory) ventricular arrhythmias; risk of sudden cardiac death.
- Investigations:
  - ECG usually abnormal, with non-specific ST–T changes.
  - Cardiac enzymes often elevated in acute phase.
  - Autoantibodies/viral titres frequently measured but rarely helpful.
  - MRI may help differentiate from acute MI.
- Treatment:
  - Limitation of physical activities.
  - Supportive therapy; may need CHF treatment.
  - If severe, may need LVAD or transplant assessment.
  - Full recovery is possible (even if fulminant myocarditis).

# Cardiac tumours

These are rare (lifetime incidence <0.02%) and about 75% are benign, mostly myxomata. Malignant tumours are usually sarcomata.

## Cardiac myxoma:

- ♀:♂ incidence is 2:1; 75% occur in left atrium.
- Can cause mechanical obstruction (intracavitary or valvular), systemic emboli (in 30%), constitutional symptoms.
- Clinical signs include clubbing, transient mitral stenosis, tumour 'plop' (early diastole, shortly after S2).
- Atrial arrhythmias surprisingly uncommon.
- Bloods may reveal inflammatory response (elevated white cell count, ESR), haemolysis, raised immunoglobulins.
- Diagnosed on echo; TOE indicated prior to surgery.
- Treatment is surgical resection; recurs in at least 5% thus annual echo and/or TOE indicated for first 3 years, then periodically.

# 3.9 The cardiomyopathies

## Background

A group of conditions in which the predominant feature is direct involvement of the heart muscle. Detection rates are increasing as a consequence of the introduction of enhanced non-invasive cardiac imaging. There are three major pathophysiological types of cardiomyopathy: dilated, hypertrophic, and restrictive.

## Dilated cardiomyopathy (DCM)

### Epidemiology
- Incidence 5–8 per 100,000 per year.
- Three times more common in ♂ and Afro-Caribbeans.

### Pathology
- Cardiac enlargement and impaired systolic function of one or both ventricles; ventricles dilated more than atria.

### Aetiology
- > 50% cases are idiopathic.
- Inherited in 25–30% of cases; tends to be AD.
- ACE DD genotype more frequent in DCM.
- Otherwise results from a wide variety of pathologies:
  - Alcohol.
  - Autoimmune disease.
  - Arrhythmia (e.g. tachycardiomyopathy).
  - Viral infection (including HIV).
  - Nutritional deficiency (e.g. thiamine—beri beri).
  - Infiltrative diseases (e.g. sarcoid, haemochromatosis).
  - Dystrophia myotonica.
  - Muscular dystrophies.

### Symptoms/signs
- Can be asymptomatic for many years; symptoms develop gradually (usually in middle age but can occur at any age).
- Symptoms and signs are those of CHF.

### Investigations
- Bloods to exclude specific conditions that might contribute to DCM: iron studies, thyroid function tests, viral titres (if history suggests possible myocarditis), thiamine, selenium, serum ACE, calcium. Consider HIV screening.
- ECG: LBBB common.
- Echo: hallmark features of DCM; ventricular thrombi not uncommon.
- Cardiac MRI often indicated.
- Holter/event recorders if history suggestive of arrhythmia.

### Treatment
Standard CHF treatment, centred on ACE inhibitors, β-blockers, and diuretics.

Obstructive sleep apnoea is a common comorbidity and may require nocturnal CPAP.

## Hypertrophic cardiomyopathy (HCM)

### Epidemiology
- Population prevalence 1:500 to 1:1000.
- ♂=♀.
- Most often diagnosed in 4th or 5th decade.

### Pathology
See Fig. 3.43.
- Myocardial mass markedly increased, small LV/RV cavities.
- Often asymmetrical septal hypertrophy.
- Abnormal intramural coronary arteries may be seen (reduced luminal diameter—angina can occur).

### Aetiology
- AD inheritance in 50–70%; remainder are sporadic.
- >10 different genes and >150 mutations identified to date.
- Most familial HCM caused by one of three mutations (Table 3.7).
- Some mutations deemed 'high-risk' due to increased risk of sudden cardiac death.

### Pathophysiology
- Systolic anterior motion of the AMVL (Fig. 3.43); mechanism unclear. LV outflow tract obstruction results.
- Systolic LV function normal or even hyperdynamic.
- LV cavity narrow in systole ('sword-shaped' at catheterization).
- Abnormal myocardial relaxation results in increased LVEDP; dyspnoea, pulmonary congestion may result.
- Abnormal coronary arteries contribute to ischaemia, arrhythmia, and sudden death risk.

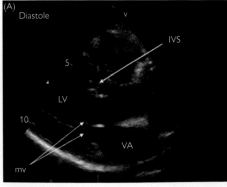
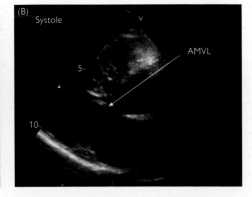

**Fig. 3.43** Echocardiograms of a patient with HCM.
(A) depicts the anatomy in end-diastole, with the mitral valve (mv) leaflets having just closed: the disproportionately thickened interventricular septum (IVS) is very apparent.
(B) taken during ventricular systole shows the anterior motion of the anterior mitral valve leaflet (AMVL), which contributes to obstruction of the LV outflow tract.
Image courtesy of Mrs C. Kemp, Cardiology Department, Royal Alexandra Hospital, Paisley.

| Table 3.7 Prevalence of HCM gene mutations | | |
|---|---|---|
| Gene | Chromosome | Prevalence |
| β myosin heavy chain | 14 | 35–50% |
| Myosin-binding protein C | 11 | 15–25% |
| Cardiac troponin T | 1 | 20% |

## Symptoms
- Most patients asymptomatic (HCM picked up on echo).
- If symptomatic, dyspnoea, angina, fatigue, presyncope and syncope may occur; palpitations, paroxysmal nocturnal dyspnoea and CHF rarer.
- First presentation may be sudden cardiac death.

## Signs
(For differentiation from aortic stenosis see Box 3.39.)
- Clinical examination may be normal.
- Large 'a' waves on JVP.
- Jerky carotid pulsation (bifid).
- Double apical impulse (forceful atrial contraction against stiff LV).
- Systolic thrill at left sternal edge.
- Harsh ejection systolic murmur.
- S4 frequent.
- Mitral regurgitation often coexistent.

## Investigations
- Echo is standard diagnostic test (Fig. 3.43).
- ECG usually abnormal:
    ST–T changes and LVH most common abnormalities.
    Prominent Q waves (inferior, anterior) in 20–50%.
    15–25% have normal ECG; these patients tend to have only minimal, localized hypertrophy.
- Cardiac MRI in selected cases.
- Cardiac catheterization rarely necessary—reserved for cases where angiography and septal ablation planned.
- Exercise testing, Holter monitoring for risk stratification.
- Family screening essential.

## Treatment
- Great variability in disease progression; patients classified as high-risk if ≥1 high-risk feature present (see Box 3.40).
- Avoid strenuous exercise, contact sports.
- Medical therapy:
    - β-blockers first-line.
    - Calcium antagonists (verapamil has most evidence).

| Box 3.39 Clinical differentiation of HCM from valvular aortic stenosis (AS) | | |
|---|---|---|
| | AS | HCM |
| **Carotid pulse** | Slow-rising | Jerky |
| **Thrill** | 2nd right interspace | Lower left sternum |
| **Ejection click** | May be present | Absent |
| **Early diastolic murmur** | Often present | Rare (post-surgery) |
| **Response to manoeuvres** | Fixed | Variable |

The systolic murmur in HCM is increased in intensity by Valsalva manoeuvre, and by standing from a squatting position. It is decreased during squatting, passive leg elevation and hand-grip.

| Box 3.40 High-risk features for HCM |
|---|
| • Onset of symptoms (especially syncope) in childhood. |
| • Exercise-induced hypotension. |
| • Marked outflow tract obstruction. |
| • High-risk genetic mutation. |
| • Family history of sudden cardiac death. |

### Cardiac amyloidosis
- Cardiac involvement common in primary amyloid (although clinically apparent in only 30%) but rare in secondary amyloid; occurs in 25% of familial amyloid patients.
- ♂>♀, rare <40 years.
- Clinical manifestations:
    - Restrictive cardiomyopathy
    - CHF
    - Orthostatic hypotension
    - Arrhythmia, AV block, sudden cardiac death
- Investigations:
    - **ECG**—low voltage; BBB and left axis deviation common; (inferior) Q waves. AF not infrequent.
    - **Echo**—undilated, stiff LV and RV; thickened valve leaflets (although not usually impairing valve function); 'speckling' appearance of interventricular septum (or other affected area). MRI is a useful adjunct.
    - **Tissue diagnosis**—endomyocardial biopsy may be required in cardiac amyloid; general investigations in amyloid covered in Chapter 16.
- Management:
    1. Treat cause of amyloidosis.
    2. CHF may be relatively refractory to diuretics; risk of hypotension with nitrates and other vasodilators.
    3. Sensitive to digoxin—avoid if possible.
    4. Pacemaker insertion may be indicated if evidence of conduction block.
- Prognosis dire: <5% alive at 5 years from diagnosis.

- Amiodarone if documented arrhythmia.
- Diuretics can be used cautiously if CHF present.
- (Avoid digoxin (if in sinus rhythm), nitrates, and inotropes.)
- ICD insertion (high-risk patients, evidence of sustained ventricular arrhythmia, aborted sudden cardiac death).
- Alcohol septal ablation.
- Surgical myomectomy.
- DDD pacing.

## Prognosis
Annual mortality 3% in adults, 6% in children.

# Restrictive cardiomyopathy (RCM)

RCM is much less common than DCM or HCM in the Western world. Causes include:

| | |
|---|---|
| Idiopathic (rare) | Endomyocardial fibrosis |
| Amyloidosis (see box above) | Hypereosinophilic syndrome |
| Systemic sclerosis | Carcinoid syndrome |
| Sarcoidosis | Metastatic cancers |
| Haemochromatosis | Cardiotoxic agents (e.g. anthracycline) |
| Radiotherapy | Drugs (serotonin, methysergide) |
| Fabry disease | Glycogen storage disorders |

Systolic LV (and RV) function is usually normal, but diastolic function is significantly impaired: the ventricular walls are very stiff and thus impede diastolic filling.

## Symptoms

- Exercise intolerance, fatigue, dyspnoea, and palpitations frequent. Symptoms tend to be inexorably progressive.

## Signs

- Elevated JVP, Kussmaul sign.
- Palpable apical impulse.
- S3 and S4 frequently present.
- Hepatomegaly.
- Peripheral oedema (may be marked).

## Investigations

RCM and pericardial constriction share several similar features, but can be differentiated on basis of the findings of echocardiography and cardiac catheterization. Other:

- ECG: AF frequent.
- Cardiac MRI: may show infiltration of myocardium.

## Treatment

No specific treatments exist, and surgery is usually unhelpful.

Certain causes may be managed medically to an extent: venesection/chelating agents if haemochromatosis, enzyme replacement if Fabry disease. These tend to delay progression rather than reverse existing pathology.

# 3.10 Hypertension

## What is hypertension?

British Hypertension Society (BHS) definitions are shown in Table 3.8.

## Epidemiology

- Prevalence of hypertension rises progressively with age in both sexes.
- Grade 1 hypertension detected in 22% of Europeans and 23% white Americans aged 35–44 years, and in 79% and 80% respectively >75 years of age.
- Afro-Caribbean and African American people have higher prevalence of hypertension at every age after adolescence.
- Population studies show that each 20mmHg rise in systolic BP, or 10mmHg rise in diastolic BP, causes at least a twofold increase in mortality due to stroke and coronary heart disease.

## Causes of hypertension

Hypertension can be primary (essential) or secondary.

### Essential hypertension

- ~95% of all hypertension is essential.
- Multifactorial aetiology presumed: age, genetic predisposition, (presumably polygenic), environmental factors, diet, smoking, stress; low foetal birthweight controversial.

### Secondary hypertension

- ~5% of cases of hypertension (or less).
- Renal disease is 10× more common than all other secondary causes put together (Box 3.41).
- Renal parenchymal disease is the commonest secondary cause, followed by renovascular disease.

## Symptoms/signs

- In secondary hypertension, disease-specific symptoms and signs may point towards diagnosis.
- Uncomplicated hypertension tends to be asymptomatic.
- If symptoms present, they tend to be non-specific: headache, dizziness, tinnitus, epistaxis (frequently anecdotal).
- Fundoscopy is mandatory in newly-diagnosed hypertensive, to assess presence of retinopathy (Fig. 3.44).

| Box 3.41 Secondary causes of hypertension |
|---|

*Renal disease*
- Renal parenchymal disease:
  - Glomerulonephritis (acute or chronic)
  - Diabetic nephropathy
  - Chronic pyelonephritis
  - Analgesic nephropathy
  - Adult polycystic kidney disease
- Renovascular disease:
  - Renal artery stenosis (atheromatous or fibromuscular hyperplasia)
  - Polyarteritis nodosa
- Any cause of chronic renal failure

*Adrenal disease*
- Cushing syndrome
- Phaeochromocytoma
- Conn syndrome
- Congenital adrenal hyperplasia

*Other endocrine causes*
- Diabetes
- Acromegaly
- Hyper- and hypo-thyroidism
- Hyperparathyroidism
- Renin-secreting tumours:
  - Pregnancy
  - Alcohol excess
  - Drugs
  - Glucocorticoids, contraceptive pill, monoamine oxidase inhibitors

## Investigation

It must be borne in mind that secondary hypertension is rare. Over-investigation of all patients with hypertension is time-consuming, costly, and inappropriately worrisome for the patient!

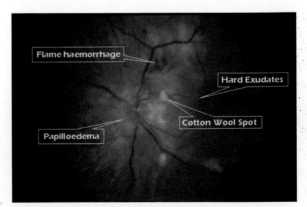

**Fig. 3.44** Hypertensive retinopathy. Retinal photograph displaying grade 4 hypertensive retinopathy.

Reproduced with permission from Dr KM O'Shaughnessy, Clinical Pharmacology Unit, Addenbrooke's Hospital, Cambridge University

| Table 3.8 BHS definitions of blood pressure and hypertension | Systolic (mmHg) | Diastolic (mmHg) |
|---|---|---|
| **Blood pressure** | | |
| Optimal | <120 | <80 |
| Normal | <130 | <85 |
| High-normal | 130–139 | 85–89 |
| **Hypertension** | | |
| Grade 1 (mild) | 140–159 | 90–99 |
| Grade 2 (moderate) | 160–179 | 100–109 |
| Grade 3 (severe) | ≥180 | ≥110 |

In most newly-diagnosed hypertensives, the following are sufficient screening tests:

1. Bloods: FBC with haematocrit; electrolytes and creatinine; fasting glucose and lipids; serum calcium; serum urate and thyroid function tests.

2. Urinalysis: presence of blood, protein, or glucose should prompt further investigation; microscopy for casts.

3. ECG: assess for LVH.

If these tests are abnormal, and suggest a secondary cause, appropriate further tests may be required. Likewise young patients, or those with refractory hypertension, warrant further investigation. This includes:

- Echocardiography.
- Renal ultrasound examination.
- Magnetic resonance angiography of renal vessels; occasionally invasive renal angiography required.
- Renal biopsy in selected cases.
- CT abdomen (with high-resolution adrenal slices).
- Urinary catecholamine analysis.
- Serum cortisol, renin, angiotensin, and aldosterone levels.

## Who should be treated (primary prevention)?

The treatment of hypertension and the primary prevention of cardiovascular disease should be based on total cardiovascular risk. Various calculators are available (see <http://www.bhsoc.org>) which provide a cumulative 10-year risk. The following are recommended by the BHS:

- General lifestyle measures apply to all levels of hypertension (and prevention thereof): smoking cessation, dietary advice (low salt), weight loss, exercise, etc.
- Sustained grade 2 hypertension (≥160/100mmHg) should be treated with medication.
- Grade 1 hypertension (140–159/90–99mmHg) should be treated medically if:
  - Any complication of hypertension present (see Box 3.42).
  - Evidence of end-organ damage.
  - 10-year cardiovascular risk ≥20% despite lifestyle advice.
- Grade 1 hypertension *not* treated medically, and those with high-normal blood pressure, require annual review.

Blood pressure treatment thresholds in secondary prevention (and in diabetes) vary and are covered in individual sections.

### Box 3.42 Complications of hypertension

- Cerebrovascular disease
- Left ventricular hypertrophy
- CHF
- Ischaemic heart disease
- Peripheral arterial disease
- Retinopathy (Box 3.43 and Fig. 3.44)
- Proteinuria
- Renal impairment

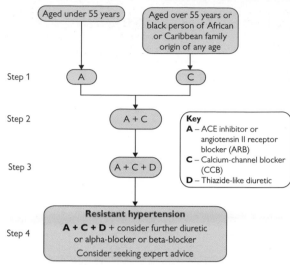

**Fig. 3.45** BHS/NICE treatment algorithm for hypertension.

National Institute for Health and Clinical Excellence (2011) CG 127 Hypertension: Clinical management of primary hypertension in adults. London: NICE.

Available from http://guidance.nice.org.uk/CG127. Reproduced with permission.

### Box 3.43 Grades of hypertensive retinopathy

1. Increased tortuousity + reflectiveness ('silver-wiring') of retinal arteries.
2. Arteriovenous nipping.
3. Flame-shaped haemorrhages, soft 'cotton wool' exudates; hard exudates may appear.
4. Papilloedema.

## Medical treatment

The BHS/NICE algorithm (2011 version) should be followed (Fig. 3.45). Notable points include:

- Hypertensive patients aged ≥55 years, or black patients of any age, should receive a calcium blocker or thiazide diuretic as first-line treatment.
- Hypertensive patients <55 years old should receive an ACE inhibitor as first-line.
- β-blockers are no longer considered first-line treatment for hypertension, but may still be used as such in younger patients, particularly if: ACE inhibitor/ARB intolerant or contraindicated; ♀ of child-bearing potential; evidence of enhanced sympathetic drive. In these patients, calcium blockers should be the second-line drug due to risk of diabetes on thiazide + β-blocker.

## Treatment targets (primary prevention)

- Optimal target (non-diabetic) <140/<85mmHg.
- Acceptable target (non-diabetic) <150/<90mmHg.

# 3.11 Aortic dissection

## Background

This is an uncommon but lethal condition with an incidence of ~3/100,000 per year and an untreated mortality of 25% in the 1st 24 hours, 50% in the 1st week, and 90% in the 1st year.

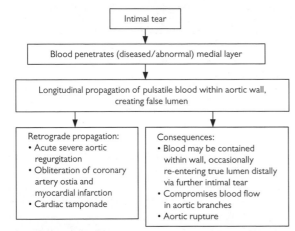

## Pathophysiology

Usually an intimal tear allows blood to penetrate a diseased medial layer with longitudinal propagation of pulsatile blood within the aortic wall and creation of a false lumen (Fig. 3.46). Propagation tends to be in an antegrade direction, but retrograde propagation occurs frequently. Retrograde propagation may lead to acute severe aortic regurgitation (AR), myocardial infarction due to obliteration of the coronary artery ostium by the dissection, or cardiac tamponade. The blood may re-enter the true lumen via a further intimal tear distally. It may be initially contained, may compromise blood flow in aortic branches, or lead to aortic rupture.

## Aetiology

Advanced age and hypertension are the major risk factors with a peak incidence in the 6th and 7th decades. In these cases there

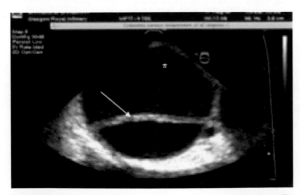

**Fig. 3.46** Transoesophageal echocardiogram of an aortic dissection. This shows a cross-sectional view of the thoracic aorta. The arrow points to the intimal flap. The false lumen (asterisk) is often the larger of the two.

is usually a degree of medial degeneration but not the classical cystic medial degeneration found in Marfan syndrome: elastin and vascular smooth muscle in the media are replaced by cystic spaces filled with mucoid material. This weakens the media and predisposes to aortic dissection. Patients with Marfan syndrome account for 5% of aortic dissections, but this tends to occur at a younger age. Other conditions associated with aortic dissection are Ehlers–Danlos syndrome, bicuspid aortic valve disease (5–7%), coarctation of the aorta and rarely pregnancy, cocaine abuse, and blunt trauma.

## Symptoms

The dominant symptom is pain—classically a sharp tearing anterior chest pain radiating between the shoulder blades. Tends to be as severe at onset as it ever becomes, rather than the crescendo-type pain in acute myocardial infarction. Other symptoms may be present depending on branch vessel involvement.

## Signs

### Hypertension
- 36% Type A (see Box 3.44).
- 70% Type B.

### Hypotension
- Falsely low due to dissection involving brachiocephalic vessel.
- Genuine hypotension—suspect tamponade, acute severe AR or aortic rupture.
- **Pulse deficits**—more common in type A dissection.
- **Aortic regurgitation**—murmur detected in 1/3 of proximal dissections.
- **CVA**—involvement of innominate or left carotid artery; 3–6%.
- **MI**—1–2%. Most commonly inferior STEMI due to dissection into right coronary ostium.

### Rare signs
- Hoarseness due to compression left recurrent laryngeal nerve.
- Upper airways obstruction.
- Horner syndrome.

---

**Box 3.44 Anatomical classifications of aortic dissection**

The Stanford classification is now more commonly used due to simplicity with types A and B corresponding to the definitive management strategies.

*Stanford*
- Type A—aortic dissection originating from intimal tear in ascending aorta (2/3 of cases).
- Type B—aortic dissection originating from intimal tear in the descending aorta (1/3 of cases).

*De Bakey*
- I—intimal tear in ascending aorta with propagation into descending.
- II—intimal tear in ascending aorta with dissection limited to ascending.
- III—Intimal tear and dissection in descending aorta only.

> **Box 3.45** Definitive management of aortic dissection
>
> *Surgical/endovascular repair*
> - Acute type A (proximal) dissection.
> - Acute type B (distal) dissection complicated by:
>   - Progression with vital organ compromise.
>   - Rupture or impending rupture (saccular aneurysm formation).
>   - Retrograde extension into ascending aorta.
> - Dissection in Marfan syndrome.
>
> *Medical management*
> - Uncomplicated Type B dissection.
> - Stable, isolated arch dissection.
> - Stable chronic dissection.
>
>   **Surgical treatment** involves resection of the diseased portion of the aortic root and reanastomosis, usually with an aortic root graft. Aortic valve replacement may be necessary, depending on the extent of aortic regurgitation.
>
>   **Medical management** consists of long-term tight BP control with β-blockers, and whichever other agents are necessary.

> **Box 3.46** Prognosis in aortic dissection
>
> If patients survive to hospital discharge, long-term outcomes are excellent regardless of the site of dissection, whether it was surgically or medically-managed, or whether it was acute or chronic.
>
> The main long-term concern is aneurysm formation. This is most common in the first 2 years, and CT surveillance is recommended—3 months, 6 months, then 6-monthly for 2 years, and annually thereafter.

## Routine investigations

- ECG—LVH in 1/3, normal in 1/3.
- CXR—widening of aortic silhouette (81–90%). Left pleural effusion is not uncommon. A small effusion may result from an inflammatory reaction around the aorta. A large effusion is more likely to represent a haemothorax due to transient rupture.

## Differential diagnosis

- Myocardial infarction/ischaemia.
- Pericarditis.
- Pulmonary embolus.
- Acute AR without dissection.
- Non-dissecting thoracic or abdominal aortic aneurysm.
- Mediastinal tumour.

In order to make the diagnosis, the possibility must be considered, and definitive investigations undertaken quickly and appropriately if there is sufficient clinical suspicion.

## Definitive investigations

### Contrast-enhanced CT

The first-line investigation of choice if it is readily available. Two distinct lumen separated by an intimal flap can be identified. Sensitivity and specificity are 96–100%. Advantages are that it is generally readily available, is non-invasive, and can identify branch vessel involvement and pericardial effusion. Disadvantages are that the site of the intimal tear is rarely visualized, and AR cannot be detected.

### Transoesophageal echocardiography

First-line investigation if CT not readily available, or patient unstable, but major role should be in assessing type A dissections pre-/perioperatively to determine aortic root anatomy, site of intimal tear, and aortic valve. Sensitivity is 98–99%, specificity 94–97%. Safe, non-invasive, can be done at the bedside and can detect AR and pericardial effusion. See Fig. 3.46.

### MRI

Excellent modality in this circumstance, but major limitation is the inability to safely monitor patient whilst in the scanner.

### Aortography

Previous gold standard, but now rarely performed due to improvements in non-invasive imaging.

## Management

With a mortality rate of 1% per hour in the first 24 hours timely diagnosis and management is essential.

### Initial management

Monitor in high dependency area.

Invasive BP monitoring.

Treat hypertension—it is crucial to reduce the force of left ventricular ejection, therefore reducing the change in aortic pressure with time (dP/dt) to try to prevent aortic rupture.

Intravenous labetalol is first-line therapy with intravenous sodium nitroprusside and additional antihypertensives as required. Labetalol will reduce BP and aortic dP/dt whereas vasodilators alone may actually increase dP/dt. Rate-limiting calcium channel blockers (verapamil or diltiazem) should be used if β-blockers are contraindicated. BP target is 100–120mmHg systolic.

### Definitive management

See Box 3.45.

### Prognosis

See Box 3.46.

# 3.12 Case history

## Background

A 55-year-old male self-presents to the accident and emergency department of a district general hospital. He gives a 6-hour history of severe central chest pain radiating to his neck and arms.

He is a smoker of 20 cigarettes per day. He has no other identified cardiovascular risk factors.

On examination he is pale and clammy, and in obvious distress. Heart rate is 90 beats per minute and blood pressure 130/80mmHg in both arms. Heart sounds are normal, JVP is not elevated, and his chest is clear to auscultation.

His 12-lead ECG is shown in Fig. 3.47.

## Diagnosis

Acute anterior ST-segment elevation myocardial infarction (STEMI).

## Immediate management

- Intravenous access and bloods.
- Opiate analgesia, eg 2.5mg diamorphine and 10mg metoclopramide.
- Aspirin 300mg (to be chewed to allow more rapid absorption via the buccal mucosa).
- Ticagrelor 180mg.
- Urgent reperfusion therapy:
  - The preferred option is primary PCI. There may be an argument for thrombolysis if he presented <3 hours after symptom onset and the door to balloon time would be >90 minutes, but at this relatively late-stage primary is clearly the best option.

He is transferred by blue light ambulance to the regional PCI centre.

## Further management

On arrival at the interventional centre he undergoes immediate coronary angiography. A view of his left coronary artery is shown in Fig. 3.48.

As anticipated from the anterior location of the infarct, the left anterior descending (LAD) artery is the culprit for the STEMI.

Primary PCI is undertaken and the artery is opened and stented with a good angiographic result in the epicardial vessel, though distal flow is a little sluggish. This phenomenon is not uncommon in primary or rescue PCI when there is often a large thrombus burden in the artery. Distal embolization can occur with balloon inflation or stent deployment resulting in impaired blood flow through the microcirculation.

He returns to CCU in a stable condition and his chest pain has settled, though there is no significant ST-segment resolution post-procedure.

## Day 1

He feels well.

HR 90/min; BP 115/70.

Heart sounds are normal and there are no signs of heart failure.

He remains on bed rest and a cardiac monitor.

Medications are aspirin 75mg and ticagrelor 90mg twice daily.

Ramipril is added at a dose of 2.5mg twice daily (AIRE study).

Atorvastatin 80mg is also introduced. The role of statins in secondary prevention was firmly established by the 4S study. In the PROVE-IT trial there was a 3.9% reduction in the primary end point in patients treated with high-dose statin (atorvastatin 80mg) compared to standard dose statin (pravastatin 40mg) in the context of an acute coronary.syndrome, although this was principally driven by a reduction in admission for unstable angina or repeat revascularization (Cannon et al., 2004).

## Day 2

Complaining of breathlessness.

HR 110/mm; BP 140/90.

Heart sounds normal, but there are fine inspiratory crepitations on auscultation of his chest.

A CXR confirms the diagnosis of pulmonary oedema.

He is treated with intravenous nitrate and diuretics.

An echocardiogram is undertaken. This shows a large anteroapical wall motion abnormality with severe left ventricular dysfunction and a left ventricular ejection fraction (LVEF) of 28%. There are no mechanical complications.

His symptoms improve.

116

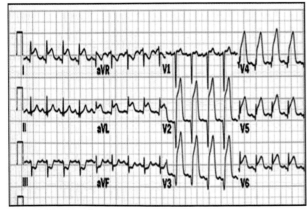

**Fig. 3.47** 12-lead ECG of a patient.

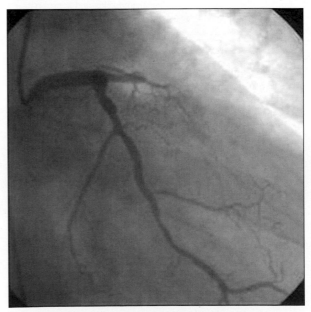

**Fig. 3.48** Coronary angiography of left coronary artery.

## Day 3

He feels better and his chest is clear.

Renal function is stable.

Heart rate is 90 with BP 110/70.

His dose of ramipril is increased to 5mg twice daily.

Eplerenone 25mg once daily is added on the basis of the EPHESUS study. This demonstrated that the addition of eplerenone 25–50mg once daily to standard therapy in patients with signs of heart failure and LVEF <40% (or diabetics with LV dysfunction alone) on day 3–14 after an acute MI resulted in a 2.3% absolute reduction in all-cause mortality (Pitt et al., 2003).

Mobile around his room and manages to shower.

## Day 4

Tolerating his increased medication and making steady progress.

Heart rate 85 and BP 105/70.

Begins to mobilize around the ward with no adverse effects.

## Day 5

Clinical condition is stable.

Decision to optimize his medication with the addition of a β-blocker. This is in the context of severe left ventricular dysfunction, so should be done with some caution.

Carvedilol 6.25mg twice daily is commenced based on the CAPRICORN study which demonstrated a 3% absolute mortality reduction with carvedilol in patients with left ventricular dysfunction post-myocardial infarction (Dargie, 2001).

## Day 6

Stable on all his medication and having been seen by the cardiac rehabilitation team he is fit for discharge.

It is planned that his eplerenone is up-titrated to 50mg once daily, and that his carvedilol is gradually up-titrated to 25mg twice daily over 4–6 weeks.

In view of the combination of an ACE inhibitor and an aldosterone antagonist his urea and electrolytes will be checked by his general practitioner at 1 and 4 weeks. He was also advised to discontinue this combination if he has any concurrent illness, particularly causing dehydration.

## Post-MI clinic

He is reviewed in the clinic 6 weeks after his admission. He is doing well and is established on all his therapy at appropriate doses. His echocardiogram is repeated and his LV function remains severely impaired. He is therefore considered for an implantable cardioverter defibrillator (ICD). On the basis of the MADIT I trial (Moss et al., 1996) he would be eligible for an ICD on the basis of his LV dysfunction if he had NSVT on Holter monitoring and inducible VT on electrophysiology study. However, a 24-hour Holter monitor was normal. On the basis of the MADIT II trial (Moss et al., 2002), which showed a 5.6% mortality reduction with the use of ICD in patients with a past history of MI, and LVEF <30% without any electrophysiological testing, he is eligible for ICD therapy. However, NICE has recommended that this evidence should only be applied if the QRS duration on a resting ECG is >120ms. His QRS duration is 96ms only, so an ICD is not implanted. He continues under clinic review.

## References

Cannon CP, Braunwald E, McCabe CH, *et al.*; Pravastatin or Atorvastatin Evaluation and Infection Therapy-Thrombolysis in Myocardial Infarction 22 Investigators. Intensive versus moderate lipid lowering with statins after acute coronary syndromes. *N Engl J Med* 2004; 350(15): 1495–504.

Dargie HJ. Effect of carvedilol on outcome after myocardial infarction in patients with left-ventricular dysfunction: the CAPRICORN randomised trial. *Lancet* 2001; 357: 1385–90.

Effect of ramipril on mortality and morbidity of survivors of acute myocardial infarction with clinical evidence of heart failure. The Acute Infarction Ramipril Efficacy (AIRE) *Study Investigators. Lancet* 1993; *342*: 821–8.

Moss AJ, Hall WJ, Cannom DS, *et al.* Improved survival with an implanted defibrillator in patients with coronary disease at high risk for ventricular arrhythmia. Multicenter Automatic Defibrillator Implantation Trial Investigators. *N Engl J Med* 1996; 335: 1933–40.

Moss AJ, Zareba W, Hall WJ, *et al.*; Multicenter Automatic Defibrillator Implantation Trial II Investigators. Prophylactic implantation of a defibrillator in patients with myocardial infarction and reduced ejection fraction. *N Engl J Med* 2002; *346*(12): 877–83.

Pitt B, Remme W, Zannad F, *et al.*; Eplerenone Post-Acute Myocardial Infarction Heart Failure Efficacy and Survival Study Investigators. Eplerenone, a selective aldosterone blocker, in patients with left ventricular dysfunction after myocardial infarction. *N Engl J Med* 2003; 348: 1309–21.

Randomised trial of cholesterol lowering in 4 444 patients with coronary heart disease: the Scandinavian Simvastatin Survival Study (4S). *Lancet* 1994; 344: 1383–9.

# Chapter 4

# Care of the elderly medicine

# 4.1 Science and physiological changes of ageing

## What is geriatric medicine?

Unlike other medical specialities which tend to be geared towards a particular system or group of diseases, geriatric medicine focuses on a subset of the population. Historically this has been determined solely by age, but a 'geriatric' patient is better defined as an elderly patient with multiple medical pathologies and resultant complicated social and discharge planning needs. Hence a fit and well 85-year-old need not necessarily be considered 'geriatric', whereas a 70-year-old with diabetes, ischaemic heart disease, peripheral vascular disease, and MS who needs a high level of care might be best managed by a geriatrician.

## Ageing population

Western populations are growing older (Fig. 4.1). Life expectancy is increasing as a result of improved living standards and medical care. The result of this is that the number of centenarians in the UK (9000 in 2004) is expected to more than double by 2020. In addition, declining fertility rates mean that the proportion of the population that is elderly is increasing as well. In 1991, 1.5% of the population were over 85 years old. This is projected to be 2.8% by 2020.

The increase in the numbers of elderly and very elderly people has a major impact on health care services. In 2002, the average number of GP consultations per year for those over 75 was eight, versus five for adults under 75. Similarly there was an average of 23 inpatient stays each year per 100 people aged over 75 versus 14 stays each year per 100 people for adults under 75. The average length of an inpatient stay in 2003 was 8 nights, but the average in those over 75 years old was 14. A similar weighting is also seen in prescribing as the oldest 15% of the population receive 40% of all drug prescriptions.

The demographic changes are not unique to the West. Many rapidly-developing countries, e.g. China will see dramatic increases in their elderly population over the next few decades.

## Ageing physiology

Differentiated tissues have a limited capacity for regeneration; the rate and efficiency with which they do so declines with age. The mechanism is poorly understood but popular theories include impaired cell division secondary to telomere shortening and cumulative damage to cellular structures by oxygen species released as a by-product of oxidative metabolism. 'Ageing' therefore results from a combination of as yet poorly understood genetic factors, damage to cells from the environment, and increasingly less effective regeneration.

The effect of this process is understandably more pronounced in those tissues with more limited ability to regenerate, such as neurons, renal tubules, and myocytes, and it is here where the deterioration with age is most marked.

Differentiating 'normal ageing' from 'pathological ageing' is difficult. Organ systems that would deteriorate gradually with time may have this process accelerated by environmental stresses, e.g. respiratory decline exacerbated by smoking. On the other hand, environmental factors may appear to slow the ageing process, e.g. bone mineral density and cardiovascular fitness will be better preserved in more active people. The result is more disparity between physical and biological age in a group of elderly people than in a group of younger people.

## Different presentation

The spectrum of presentations is much broader in the elderly and cardinal features may be more subtle or even absent. Presentations are likely to be more non-specific and may include several different problems. For instance, myocardial ischaemia may not present with chest pain but rather breathlessness, light-headedness, and lethargy; pneumonia may present with confusion and collapse rather than cough and shortness of breath; a fall may be precipitated by the combined effects of sepsis, hypovolaemia, sedation, and peripheral neuropathy and not merely be mechanical.

## Multiple pathologies

Elderly patients often have multiple pathologies. This results from:

- Increased prevalence of disease with ageing, e.g. hypertension, atrial fibrillation, Alzheimer disease, and cancer.
- An initial condition or risk factor predisposing to multiple future diseases, e.g.:
  - Renal failure, visual impairment, and neuropathy resulting from a 40-year history of diabetes.
  - Emphysema, lung cancer, peripheral vascular disease, and stroke as a consequence of a 60-pack-year smoking history.
- Increased risk as a result of ageing physiology, e.g. bed sores and DVT resulting from immobility.

## Ageing organ systems

### Cardiovascular

Cardiac performance decreases with age. Maximum heart rate decreases. Force of contraction reduces as does rate of relaxation and systolic or diastolic dysfunction can result. Furthermore, the prevalence of myocardial ischaemia, hypertension, and valvular disease increase and can further impact upon cardiac performance.

The vasculature is also affected, becoming less compliant with increasing age. This results in elevated blood pressure (particularly systolic) and increasing levels of atheroma which, although considered pathological, is seen almost universally as people age in economically developed countries.

### Renal

Kidney size decreases with age. The number of glomeruli reduces, the basement membrane becomes less permeable, and the result is a decrease in glomerular filtration rate (Fig. 4.2). Tubular function also decreases and the ability of the kidney to deal with a salt and water load or alternatively with water deprivation is impaired. As a result, elderly kidneys are more sensitive to changes in fluid balance and drugs.

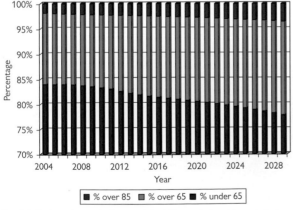

**Fig. 4.1** Projected spread of ages of the UK population. Not only is the population expected to increase, but the number of elderly people is also expected to increase as a proportion of the total.

Data from Office of National Statistics, 2007. Contains public sector information licensed under the Open Government Licence v2.0. http://www.nationalarchives.gov.uk/doc/open-government-licence/version/2/

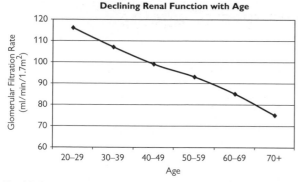

**Fig. 4.2** Demonstration of declining organ function with age. Chronic kidney disease is classified by GFR:

Stage 1—GFR 90+

Stage 2—GFR 60–89

Stage 3—GFR 50–59

Stage 4—GFR 15–29

Stage 5—GFR 14 or less

Thus most elderly people have a GFR at a level commensurate with mild renal impairment and many would be classed as stage 3, although this may be 'physiological' for their age.

Douville *et al.*, 'Impact of age on glomerular filtration estimates', *Nephrology Dialysis Transplantation*, 2009, 24, 1, by permission of Oxford University Press. Copyright European Renal Association, and European Dialysis and Transplant Association.

Impaired renal function is especially important to consider when prescribing, as decreased filtration may cause accumulation of drugs at lower doses than might be expected.

## Brain

Cerebrovascular disease is common in Western society. Imaging of elderly brains often shows cortical atrophy and evidence of small vessel ischaemia which may be associated with cognitive or functional impairment.

Stroke can be divided into haemorrhage (about 15%) and infarcts. The commonest causes for haemorrhage in the elderly are hypertension and amyloid angiopathy. Infarcts occur as a result of ischaemia and hypoperfusion. This can result from large vessel disease, small vessel disease, emboli, hypotension (watershed infarct), or venous thrombosis.

The effects of cerebrovascular disease include the widely-recognized motor dysfunction, visual field loss, and dysphasia. The cognitive and psychosocial effects are less well-acknowledged but equally disabling. These include visuospatial neglect, impaired memory and cognition, personality changes, and depression.

## Musculoskeletal

The two most common musculoskeletal disorders in the elderly are osteoarthritis and osteoporosis.

### Osteoarthritis

A degenerative condition as a result of wear of the cartilage covering joint surfaces. Weight-bearing joints are most commonly-affected. The result is decreased range of movement, pain, and ultimately decreased joint function and mobility.

### Osteoporosis

A condition of decreased bone mineral density and disrupted bone microarchitecture. Many factors affect peak bone mineral density and its rate of loss; however, the most common candidate is oestrogen/testosterone deficiency later in life. Osteoporosis is defined as a bone mineral density 2.5 or more standard deviations below peak bone mass. Osteoporotic patients are at increased risk of fractures and the associated complications.

## Respiratory

Alveoli are made until about age 20, after which the number starts to decrease. Increasing age is also associated with decreased elasticity and the result is a declining $FEV_1$ and FVC. This is not usually sufficient to compromise respiratory function and significant impairment usually only occurs following other lung insults such as smoking or environmental pollution.

# 4.2 Assessment of the elderly

## Introduction

Assessment of an elderly patient is not always as straightforward as assessment of a younger patient. The approach needs to be tailored towards the individual. In some instances the patient will be able to provide a coherent history and cooperate with the examination; in others they may be disorientated and unaware of why they are in hospital (making a witness history essential), and may be unable to cooperate with the clinical examination.

Consider if anything can be done to help with the clinical encounter. For instance, if the patient is hard of hearing, an amplification device will greatly facilitate communication. Written information regarding diagnoses and medication changes will help patients remember what has been said and also in communicating this to their relatives and carers.

## History

As with any patient it is important to establish the presenting complaint and past medical history. If relatives or carers are present, also record their account. In the case of a confused patient, a collateral history is essential in deciding whether this is acute or chronic, and determining any precipitating events. Additional information sources include the GP letter, ambulance transfer sheet, and any documentation from the nursing home. If a witness is not present, a phone call can help to clarify things.

Current medication, dosing regimens, and allergies should be clearly documented. Details of critical (e.g. Parkinson) medication should be brought to the attention of the nursing staff. Alternative routes of administration (nasogastric, rectal, or intravenous) may need to be considered if essential medication cannot be taken orally.

A detailed social history is very important, and if possible should be taken on initial clerking. Opinions of patient and relatives may differ about how well they feel they are coping.

### Points to address in a social history

- Where does the patient live?
- Do they live in a house, bungalow, flat, residential or nursing home?
- Do they need to negotiate stairs?
- Do they own their accommodation?
- Who else is living there with them?
- Do they have family/friends nearby?
- Is there a warden?
- Have they had additional social services support?
- What is their mobility like—at home and out and about?
- How do they transfer?
- Are they continent?
- Are they able to wash/bathe/shower?
- Do they use mobility aids?
- Do they feel they are coping?
- Do they feel they need increased help or support?
- Do family members agree with the patient's own assessment?

## Examination

Conventional systems examination is essential in a proper assessment of any patient and the elderly are no exception. Additionally several specific points should be considered.

## General appearance

- Is the patient well-nourished or is there evidence of recent weight loss (baggy clothing, muscle wasting)?
- What is their hydration like?
- Are they well looked after and groomed or is there evidence of neglect, either by themselves or from others?
- What is their mood like, are they making eye contact? Could they be depressed?
- What is their current cognitive function like? What is their Abbreviated Mental Test score?

## Joints and mobility

- Is the patient able to mobilize independently?
- What is their gait like? Are they unstable and at risk of falling?
- Have they got problems with any of their joints?
- Remember: 'look, feel, move' approach to examining.
- Functional examination—e.g. combing hair or reaching to put socks on—is more important than formal examination.

### Get-Up and Go Test

A useful screening test for identifying those at risk of falling who would benefit from further physiotherapy assessment.
Ask the patient to:
- Stand from a sitting position without using their arms for support
- Walk several paces (about 10 feet)
- Turn and walk back
- Sit back down, again without using their arms.
Can comment on:
- Sitting balance
- Transfer from sitting to standing
- Balance while walking and turning.

Data from Nordin et al., 'Prognostic validity of the Timed Up-and-Go test, a modified Get-Up-and-Go test, staff's global judgement and fall history in evaluating fall risk in residential care facilities', Age and Ageing, 2008, 37, 4, pp. 442–448.

## Miscellaneous

- Be aware of possible incidental diagnoses; does the patient look hypothyroid or have the expressionless facies of Parkinson?
- Look at the legs. Are there areas of ulceration? Are the legs well-perfused—is it safe to use thromboembolic prevention stockings?

Good communication skills are essential in dealing with elderly patients. Time should be taken to try and overcome barriers to successful communication such as visual or hearing impairments.

- Speak slowly and clearly
- Face the patient
- Amplification devices
- Use everyday language
- Pause frequently
- Present information in a variety of ways
- Take time for questions or requests for clarification.

Patients (e.g. dysphasic following CVA) may have difficulty communicating with you. Picture charts may enable simple ideas to be communicated and are easily used by all those involved in patient care.

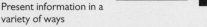

Shaded eye: Reproduced with permission of The Partially Sighted Society.
Ear: This image is in the public domain under the following licence: CC0 1.0 Universal (CC0 1.0) Public Domain Dedication http://creativecommons.org/publicdomain/zero/1.0/deed.en

- Can the patient swallow? An acute illness can exacerbate problems with swallowing and put the patient at risk of aspiration. If concerned, a ward swallow test or referral to a speech and language therapist is appropriate.

# Psychosocial factors

Individuals have their own beliefs, concerns, issues, and agendas. The elderly are no different and it is important to bear this in mind. Attitudes clearly vary from individual to individual but there are several 'themes' that are often seen:

### Embarrassment

Society was historically more reserved and this can be reflected in reluctance to admit to symptoms or problems of a more 'personal' nature. It is not uncommon to find elderly ladies with fungating breast tumours presenting late as a result of embarrassment, plus fear of the diagnosis.

### Burden

Patients can feel that they are burdening their friends, relatives, or society by being unwell and needing help, exacerbated by a reluctance to admit to declining independence. The result can be refusal of help even when it is there.

### Institutionalization

At the other extreme, individuals may relish the care and attention that comes along with hospitalization. Requiring help with tasks brings with it social contact and this may be enjoyed and encouraged by otherwise isolated and lonely individuals. The downside is that encouraging reliance on others results in increasing difficulty in managing tasks for oneself and loss of independence.

# End of life issues

Nobody lives for ever. There comes a time when, in spite of medical care, a patient dies. As well as addressing the acute medical problem, it is important for medical staff to be aware of palliative issues.

Every procedure or medical intervention carries side effects. There comes a point at which the likelihood of benefit is so small it ceases to outweigh the negative impact of treatment on quality of life. At this stage it may be more appropriate to focus on symptom control.

Similarly, it may be inappropriate to attempt cardiopulmonary resuscitation if it is unlikely to be successful, result in a quality of life that would be unacceptable to the patient, or if it is not what the patient wants. In such instances a 'do not attempt resuscitation' or DNAR order may be indicated.

End of life issues are understandably emotive. The best approach is to be open and honest in discussion with patients and their next of kin (where appropriate). It is important to emphasize that a DNAR order is just that and not a 'do not treat' order. When possible, issues are best discussed early and in advance of an acute deterioration as this allows for more discussion and acceptance of any decision amongst family members. Ultimately, however, decisions regarding treatments offered and resuscitation rest with the clinician in charge of a patient's care.

# National service framework

In 2001, the Department of Health published a national service framework (NSF) for older people, aiming to optimize the quality of care services available. The report was divided into eight 'standards' that those working with the elderly should follow, and these are still relevant today.

### Standard 1: Rooting out age discrimination

NHS services should be provided on the basis of clinical need and ability to benefit and patients should not be denied access to services as a result of their age alone. Aggressive investigation or treatment may be inappropriate, not because of age, but rather a result of medical comorbidities.

### Standard 2: Person-centred care

Treat patients with respect and dignity as individuals, and involve them in decisions about their care where possible. Efforts should be taken to ensure that diagnoses, treatments, and discharge plans are explained in a manner that patients understand so that, where possible, they can make an informed choice themselves rather than having such decisions (sometimes illegally) made on their behalf.

### Standard 3: Intermediate care

A new tier of care bridging the gap between home and hospital care was introduced. This aims to:

- Intervene to respond to a 'crisis' and where possible prevent the need for hospital admission. This may involve extra help coming into a patient's home in the short-term, or respite care in a residential setting.
- Facilitate earlier discharge from hospital by providing rehabilitation following a hospital stay, either in an interim residential placement, or at the patient's home, allowing more effective integration back into their environment.
- Support patients while long-term care is being considered. Interim care teams can provide a stop-gap to support the patient at home while plans for longer-term care can be made, avoiding 'social' hospital admissions.

### Standard 4: General hospital care

Older people should have access to specialist care with staff with the appropriate skills to meet their needs. This does not only include the medical staff, but all groups involved in patient care such as rehabilitation therapists and dieticians.

### Standard 5: Stroke

Emphasis is placed on primary prevention of stroke and targeting modifiable risk factors, and following a stroke of early access to diagnostic services, involvement of a stroke specialist and multidisciplinary rehabilitation team, plus appropriate secondary prevention. Clear evidence exists to show the outcome benefit of early admission to a dedicated stroke unit, with staff experienced in the management of acute stroke and its complications.

### Standard 6: Falls

Steps should be taken to identify those at high risk both of falls and the complications from falls. Frequent/unexplained fallers are ideally assessed in an integrated falls service.

### Standard 7: Mental health in older people

Increased awareness is required to improve detection rates of mental illness in the elderly. There should be support from integrated mental health teams and specialist care. There is an increased focus on dementia (National Dementia Strategy 2009).

### Standard 8: The promotion of health and active life in older age

Prevention of disease and illness is preferable to treating its complications. Evidence exists for some areas of primary prevention, e.g. control of hypertension, even in the very elderly. The NSF emphasizes a healthy lifestyle and targeting of risk factors to promote continued health and well-being.

### Appendix: Medicines management

A guide to prescribing in the elderly aiming to maximize therapeutic benefit whilst minimizing illness caused by excessive, inappropriate, or inadequate consumption of medicines.

# 4.3 Activities of daily living, disability, and rehabilitation

## Introduction

Older patients tend not to bounce back from acute illness as quickly as younger patients. This is likely to result from increased comorbidities, declining reserve, and ageing physiology. It is important to consider this in the care of elderly patients, as a substantial component of their treatment will involve rehabilitation to optimize their physical, mental, and social function.

## Types of rehabilitation

Rehabilitation can occur in any setting and any one patient is likely to receive therapy in several of these:

- Acute hospital setting: while medically unwell.
- Slow stream: this can either be on a rehabilitation ward in an acute hospital, or at a community hospital.
- At home: therapists visit an individual to provide rehabilitation in their own environment. This can follow an acute admission, or be an attempt to try and avert one.
- Specialist rehabilitation: dedicated centre used for certain types of rehabilitation, e.g. a stroke unit.

## The rehabilitation team

Rehabilitation is carried out by a multidisciplinary team. This should ideally include not only the medical and therapy staff formally looking after a patient, but also the patient's family. Typical members usually include the following:

### Medical staff

Involved in managing acute medical problem. Often chair multidisciplinary meetings and help coordinate inpatient stay.

### Nursing staff

More involved in day-to-day care of patients. Initially may provide majority of care, but should aim to encourage increasing patient independence as acute illness resolves.

### Physiotherapists

Work on joint function and mobility. This can range from passive to resistive exercise. Functional work involves transfers, stairs, and balance.

### Occupational therapists

Help to rehabilitate patients with their activities of daily living such as washing, dressing, and feeding as well as helping provide equipment to make such tasks easier.

### Speech and language therapists

As well has helping patients overcome communication and language problems, speech and language therapists are also skilled at assessing swallowing and advising on appropriate consistency of diet.

### Dietician

Reviews dietary needs of patients and advises on high-calorie supplements, alternative feeding regimens, and special diets (Fig. 4.3).

### Psychologist

Helps address cognitive issues or behavioural disturbance.

### Social worker

Is involved in helping plan for future social care of the patient. This involves assessment for care packages, residential or nursing homes, as well as advising on any benefits the patient may be entitled to.

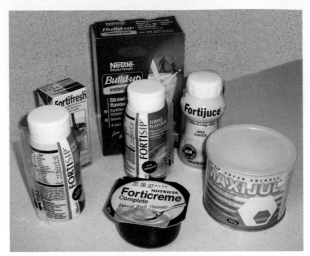

Fig. 4.3 Example of the various dietary supplements and build-up drinks available. Good nutrition is essential in supporting an active rehabilitation programme.

## Assessment tools

### Activities of daily living

Activities of daily living are used in the functional assessment of patients. Categories considered include:

- Continence of bowels
- Bladder control
- Personal care/hygiene
- Toilet use
- Eating
- Transferring
- Mobility
- Dressing and undressing
- Stairs
- Bathing

### Barthel Index

This is a standardized assessment used to score people in the ten listed categories of activities of daily living to give a result out of 20. Independence is suggested by a score of 20, 10–19 suggests moderate dependency, and 0–9 high dependence.

### Access visit

An occupational therapist may arrange to visit a patient's house to determine if it requires any modifications to facilitate the patient returning.

### Home visit

Therapists may take a patient on a 'visit' back to their home. This offers the same benefits as an access visit, but enables the therapists to specifically assess the patient in their own environment.

### Kitchen assessment

Verifies an individual's ability to prepare hot drinks and light meals.

### Stairs assessment

Ensures people are able to cope with stairs and highlights if they need supervision.

# Discharge destinations

## Home

Usually the preferred choice. Patients may manage at home independently, but may also require further support. This can come in the form of:

- Home modifications: can range from rails and ramps to hospital beds and hoists.
- 'Lifeline': a call button, usually worn around the neck, that contacts a call-centre who can then call neighbours/relatives should the patient need help.
- 'Meals-on-wheels': either delivering hot food or supplying frozen meals for microwaving.
- Carers: either individually or pairs. Can come up to four times a day to help patient with activities of daily living.
- 24-hour care: on-site carer.

## Sheltered accommodation

Essentially the patient has their own accommodation, but this is often purpose-built to enable easy access and assistance. There is usually a warden on site who is able to check on patients daily and can be called if needed via panic-alarms. The warden is, however, unable to provide significant levels of care.

## Day centres

Provide some structured activity as well as respite for carers.

## Residential homes

Live-in accommodation, usually with individual rooms and often en-suite bathrooms. Carers are on site to help with washing, dressing, feeding, etc. There are no formally trained nursing staff and patients usually need to be able to transfer independently or with the assistance of one person.

## Nursing homes

Are able to provide a higher level of care than residential homes and have at least one trained nurse present. Are equipped to look after individuals with higher nursing needs such as hoisting. Some nursing homes are able to provide subcutaneous fluids.

## DeE (dementia elderly) beds formerly elderly mentally infirm (EMI) placements

These can provide either residential or nursing level support but specialize in the care of patients with behavioural difficulties, usually as a result of cognitive impairment and dementia.

# Benefits and funding

## Winter Fuel Payment

Tax-free payment to people aged 63 years and over that is not means-tested to help with winter fuel bills. Additional cold weather payments are available to some people on income-related benefits during very cold spells.

## Personal Independence Payments

Since 2013, Personal Independence Payments (PIP) have replaced 'Disability Living Allowance' for people aged 16–64. This payment may help with the costs caused by long-term health or disability. The rate depends on how the condition affects you, not the condition itself.

## Attendance Allowance

This is a non-means-tested benefit for people aged over 65 years, with care—but not mobility—needs. Individuals are not eligible if living permanently in hospital or a local authority-funded home. They must have had care needs for at least 6 months, or be terminally ill. It is not necessary to actually be receiving help to address the care needs, only to have the needs. Two rates exist depending on the level of need.

## Carer's Allowance

This is a taxable allowance for people aged 16 or over who spend at least 35 hours a week caring for a disabled person in their own home. Eligibility is means-tested.

## Care funding

Social care is means-tested. Individuals can either be:

- Self-funded—the individual is responsible for meeting the full costs of carers or placement because they have assets (including property) above a set level. If a relative aged over 60, an incapacitated relative, or a relative aged under 16 lives at the property, this is not counted in the assessment of assets.
- Local authority funded—assets are below the limit for self-funding and the local authority pays for carers/placement up to a set limit. They only pay for care that they feel matches the individual's care needs. Depending on the assets, individuals may be required to make a contribution towards the costs.
- NHS funding—if care assessments determine that input is needed from a registered nurse in a nursing home, the NHS pays the cost of this (Registered Nurse Care Contribution) to the home. The remainder of the cost must be met through local authority or self-funding.
- NHS continuing care—if an individual has ongoing healthcare needs and meets certain criteria (relating to complexity, intensity, and unpredictability of the needs) such that they require regular medical supervision, they may be eligible for continuing care, in case which the NHS covers the entire cost of all care on a non-means-tested basis. Funding is usually approved through a panel and decisions are frequently contested, especially in the area of mental health.

# 4.4 Dementia and mental state examination

## What is dementia?

Dementia is not a diagnosis in its own right, but rather describes a cluster of symptoms of acquired global cognitive and memory impairment attributable to an underlying neurological pathology.

## Epidemiology

- A leading cause of morbidity and mortality.
- >750,000 people in the UK currently affected. 2.5% of those are under 65.
- The prevalence of dementia increases with age. One person in 20 over the age of 65 is affected and one person in 5 is over age 80.
- With an ageing population there is likely to be an increasing economic and social need for society to meet.

## Aetiology

Dementia can be the result of several separate disease processes. The most common three causes (discussed later) are:
- Alzheimer disease
- Vascular dementia
- Dementia with Lewy bodies

## Differential diagnosis

### Delirium

This is an acute deterioration in cognitive function commonly due to infection or electrolyte disturbance. It lacks the chronicity of dementia and collateral history is essential in differentiating the two. Delirium can also occur in the presence of dementia—acute-on-chronic confusion.

### Depression

This is common in the elderly owing to factors such as social isolation, bereavement, and concurrent illness. Up to 15% of the population aged over 65 may be affected by depression at any one time.

Presentation in the elderly may be atypical and is easily missed. It is important to consider, as treatment may bring significant improvement. The Geriatric Depression Scale is a useful tool for highlighting possible depression.

### Normal pressure hydrocephalus

Urinary incontinence          Abnormal broad-based gait (presents before dementia)

Dementia

(See Fig. 4.4B.)
Characterized by the triad:
- Disability is in excess of formal neurological signs.
- Potentially reversible cause of cognitive impairment.
- Treated by ventriculo-peritoneal shunting.

## Presentation and history

Presentation usually involves progressive memory loss, generally over several years, followed by impairment of other cognitive functions such as language, orientation, and worsening executive function. There are usually associated behavioural changes.

Collateral history is desirable in establishing a diagnosis; speed of onset, changes in personality, and ability to cope at home are often better described by a witness. It is only a collateral history of chronic symptoms that can differentiate a dementia from a delirium. Similarly a witness may be more able to provide an accurate family history.

History should include exploring the possibility of reversible causes of dementia or alternative diagnoses, e.g.:
- History of falls—consider subdural haemorrhage.
- Chronic high alcohol intake/malnutrition—could there be vitamin deficiency?
- Possibility of depression.

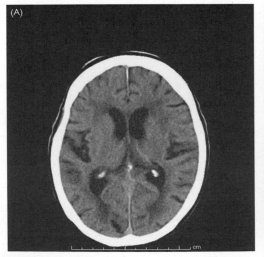

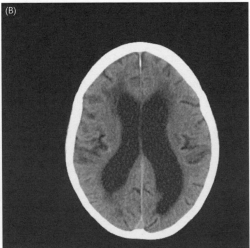

**Fig. 4.4** (A) CT image of moderate small vessel disease.
This image illustrates the typical appearance seen in the brain of a patient with vascular dementia with evidence of small vessel ischaemia. There is prominence of the cortical sulci with periventricular loss of white matter. There is also a more focal right parietal infarct.
(B) CT image of normal pressure hydrocephalus.
This demonstrates very prominent ventricles with disproportionately 'normal' cortical sulci and is suggestive of normal pressure hydrocephalus.

## Examination

Targeted towards excluding other possible causes of cognitive dysfunction, e.g. chest or urosepsis and/or constipation. Presence of cardiovascular disease or evidence of previous strokes supports the possibility of vascular dementia. Parkinsonian features should raise the question of dementia with Lewy bodies.

It is important to conduct a screening cognitive assessment. While limited time often precludes detailed assessment, an Abbreviated Mental Test Score can confirm cognitive impairment, indicate that further testing may be required, and provides an objective record for future comparison. More detailed assessment tools include the Mini-Mental State Examination (MMSE)—30 questions, or Addenbrooke Cognitive Assessment (ACE)—100 questions. These are able to explore orientation, language and comprehension, short-term memory, and visuospatial skills in more detail.

## Investigation

Should be geared towards excluding other causes of cognitive impairment and identifying modifiable risk factors:
- Septic screen
- U&Es
- Calcium
- Vitamin B$_{12}$
- Thyroid function tests
- Glucose
- Cholesterol
- Syphilis serology
- ECG, e.g. to identify AF
- CT head

## Management

Once again the importance of treating any possible reversible cause cannot be over-emphasized.

Patients should be nursed in a well-lit, non-cluttered environment. There should be clues to help orientate them to time and place, e.g. newspapers and signs. Their day should be based around a structured routine and unnecessary relocation should be avoided. Early medical intervention at home, with a view to admission avoidance, is particularly beneficial. This may be undertaken by the patient's GP or by a community geriatrician. Patients with an established diagnosis of dementia also benefit from the input of a community psychiatric nurse. If there is diagnostic uncertainty, marked behavioural problems, or coexisting depression, old age psychiatry teams may be involved.

Sometimes in spite of the simple approaches described, patients with dementia may become increasingly agitated and confused. In this instance, it is important to exclude a superimposed delirium. Management of patients in this situation can be difficult. It may be that patients respond better to familiar faces such as friends and family who may be willing to help. Similarly, a dedicated one-on-one nurse may be able to provide a greater degree of reassurance.

There will be times where agitation/aggression is such that the acutely confused patient is a risk to themselves. Pharmacotherapy may be required in these instances. If possible, patients should be encouraged to take oral medication but parenteral dosing may be required. Care must be taken not to overmedicate, as such patients are usually elderly and respond more readily to smaller doses. Local policies should be followed, but a usual starting dose is lorazepam 0.5–1mg orally and/or haloperidol 0.5mg PO/IM. The latter should not be used in patients with parkinsonism or where dementia with Lewy bodies is a possibility, owing to worsening of extrapyramidal symptoms.

An emerging field in dementia management involves the use of smart or assistive technologies. Equipment is installed in the patient's home which is able to monitor what they are doing and provide appropriate verbal prompting if needed.

Possible uses include:
- Prompting patients not to go out if they are noted to be opening the front door at an inappropriate time.
- Automatically turning off taps that are left running.
- Automatically turning on the lights if the patient starts wandering at night.
- Regularly orientating patients to time and place.
- Alerting care staff if the patient is noted not to be moving around as expected, which could indicate a fall.

An essential part of the management of dementia is the explanation—where applicable—to the patient and family of the disease process and its likely course. Providing such support and information may allow some prediction of future problems, particularly care and/or housing needs.

### Abbreviated Mental Test Score

| Question | Score |
|---|---|
| What is your age? | |
| What is the time to the nearest hour? | |
| Give the patient an address, and ask them to repeat it at the end of the test | |
| What is the year? | |
| What is the name of this place? | |
| Recognition of 2 people | |
| What is your date of birth? | |
| What are the dates (year of beginning or end) of the First World War? | |
| What is the name of the present monarch? | |
| Count backwards from 20 to 1 | |

Reproduced from Hodkinson HM, 'Evaluation of a Mental Test Score for Assessment of Mental Impairment in the Elderly', *Age & Ageing*, 1972, 1, pp. 233–238, by permission of Oxford University Press and British Geriatrics Society.

- Each question scores 1 point. There are no half marks.
- A score of fewer than 7 is suggestive of cognitive impairment and indicates that further assessment is warranted.
- Confounding factors include conditions that provoke an acute confusional state.
- An acute change from a baseline score when 'well' can indicate a delirium.

## Prognosis

Progressive deterioration in cognitive function means patients in the later stages of dementia have increasing difficulty in communication, continence, and appropriate social behaviour. They may experience hallucinations and delusions. Management becomes increasingly difficult and individuals may require more care than can be provided at home.

A common ethical dilemma concerns nutrition. Individuals with advanced dementia tend to become less interested in eating and may not manage to meet their nutritional needs. How such patients should be managed is controversial. One view is that decreased oral intake is part of the terminal phase of the disease process and the emphasis should be on palliation. The other view is that if the individual is not meeting their needs orally, other methods should be attempted, for instance, with a percutaneous endoscopic gastroscopy (PEG) placed feeding tube. There is no clear evidence that such interventions produce improvements in mortality, morbidity or quality of life. It is important in these situations to discuss the situation fully with the multidisciplinary team and patient's next of kin/representatives.

> ▶ Rarer causes of dementia

- Chronic alcoholism: cerebral atrophy, Korsakoff syndrome (vitamin $B_1$ deficiency)
- Frontotemporal dementia
- Frontal lobe dementia (Pick disease)
- Chronic subdural haematoma
- Multiple sclerosis
- Hypothyroidism
- Nutritional deficiencies: nicotinic acid (pellagra), vitamin $B_{12}$
- Infection: HIV dementia, neurosyphilis
- Inherited conditions, e.g. Huntington disease
- Prion diseases, e.g. Creutzfeldt–Jacob disease
- Motor neurone disease
- Non-progressive sequel to intracranial catastrophe, e.g. severe head injury, meningitis, cerebral anoxia

# Types of dementia

## Alzheimer dementia (AD)

- The most common cause of dementia (accounts for approximately half of all cases—see Figs 4.5 and 4.6).
- Prevalence increases with age and is higher in women.
- Onset is usually insidious with slow progression.
- Marked short-term memory impairment with early language and visuospatial deficits. Motor, sensory, and gait abnormalities only appear late.

### Pathogenesis

The exact pathophysiology remains poorly understood. On the macroscopic level there is cerebral atrophy. At the microscopic level AD is characterized by the formation of:

1. Senile plaques containing a central amyloid core. Amyloid also deposits in the cerebral vasculature.

2. Neurofibrillary tangles, composed of Tau protein (normally part of the axonal cytoskeleton).

The formation of amyloid β (Aβ), a cleavage product of the amyloid precursor protein (APP), appears central to the development of the cerebral pathology (Fig. 4.7). Increased production of Aβ may occur in a number of inherited conditions with early-onset familial AD. Aβ is resistant to proteolysis and forms insoluble plaques, which are infiltrated by microglial cells secreting cytokines. Aβ plaques are toxic to neurons and cell death results.

Chromosome 19 carries the apolipoprotein E gene (*ApoE*) with three alleles ε2/3/4; 2% of the global population are *ApoE* ε4 homozygotes (the majority are ε3/ε3). Increased allelic frequency of *ApoE* ε4 is found in the late-onset forms of sporadic and familial AD. It is thought that ε4 promotes plaque formation from otherwise soluble β-amyloid. Other genetic or environmental factors must be involved, however, as *ApoE* ε4 by itself does not guarantee the development of AD. A fault in the Tau phosphorylation pathway with the resultant formation of neurofibrillary tangles (which promote neuronal loss) is also implicated.

### Pharmacological management

Loss of cholinergic innervation has been observed in AD. Therapeutic intervention has targeted this by inhibiting cholinesterase to increase the levels of acetylcholine in the synaptic space. Randomized controlled trials have shown that the rate of deterioration in the treated population is less than that in the placebo group. Some studies even suggest a modest improvement in MMSE scores.

The three acetylcholinesterase inhibitors (donepezil, galantamine, and rivastigmine) have been recommended by the UK National Institute for Health and Care Excellence (NICE) as options in the treatment of mild to moderately-severe AD. Memantine (an NMDA receptor blocker) is recommended in moderate disease where acetylcholinesterase inhibitors are not tolerated or in severe disease. Treatment should only be initiated by specialists in the care of dementia (psychiatrists, neurologists, and care of the elderly physicians). Patients should only continue the drug while there is ongoing benefit. This and previous NICE guidance provoked some debate as they publicly highlighted the difficulty of balancing cost and benefit in a rationed healthcare system.

## Vascular dementia

- The second most prevalent cause of dementia.
- ♂ > ♀.
- Cognitive decline results from neuronal loss. This can either be focal, e.g. following an ischaemic stroke, or diffuse, such as occurs with multi-infarct dementia (see Fig. 4.4A).
- Associated with a higher mortality rate than AD—probably because of associated cardiovascular morbidity.

Vascular dementia tends to progress in a stepwise fashion with further cognitive decline occurring with further vascular events. It differs from other dementias which tend to have a more gradual deterioration.

Progression of vascular dementia can be slowed by targeting cardiovascular risk factors. Steps include:

- Stopping smoking
- Antiplatelet treatment—usually aspirin
- Anticoagulation in AF (taking into account the risks/benefits for the individual patient)
- Blood pressure control
- Cholesterol control
- Tight glycaemic control

## Dementia with Lewy bodies

Lewy bodies are cytoplasmic inclusions originally identified in the substantia nigra in patients with Parkinson disease. Lewy body

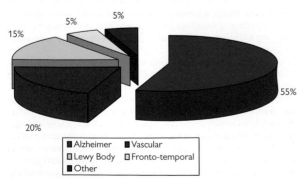

**Fig. 4.5** Frequencies of different types of dementia in the UK. Adapted with permission from Alzheimer's Society.

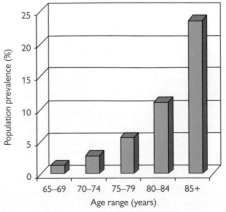

**Fig. 4.6** Prevalence of dementia in Western societies. Adapted with permission from Alzheimer's Society.

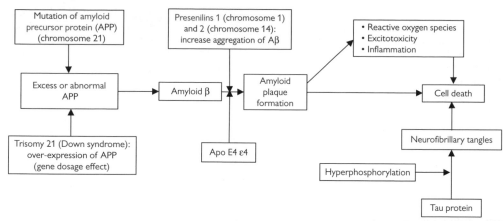

**Fig. 4.7** Postulated pathogenesis of Alzheimer disease (genes associated with *early-onset* familial AD in **red**). Mutations result in excess/abnormal amyloid precursor protein. This is then abnormally processed to amyloid β. This aggregates to form amyloid plaques (influenced by the presenilins and apolipoprotein E ε4). These result in cell damage and death, hence neuronal loss.

dementia is a smoothly progressing dementia, like AD, but progression may be more rapid.

Features suggesting Lewy-Body dementia over AD include:
• Fluctuating levels of consciousness
• Visual hallucinations
• Presence of parkinsonian features

As mentioned previously, dementia with Lewy bodies causes patients to become very sensitive to antidopaminergic drugs. This is most likely because of concomitant loss of dopaminergic innervation. This sensitivity means that antipsychotic drugs, e.g. haloperidol, should generally be avoided. The blurring between dementia with Lewy bodies and Parkinson disease means that individuals may develop parkinsonian motor disorders that respond to anti-Parkinson treatments. The difficulty is, however, that such treatments tend to exacerbate the hallucinations and confusion.

### Mixed dementia

Dementias often coexist and cognitive impairment in an individual may well be the cumulative result of several different disease processes. In particular, AD and vascular dementia often coexist.

The CT findings need to be correlated with the clinical picture in order to reach a diagnosis.

## Caring for someone with dementia

Caring for someone with dementia is not easy. Care is frequently provided by family members who are often faced with increased dependency and higher need for assistance in activities of daily living such as dressing, feeding, and toileting. In addition to this they have to face the emotional burden of witnessing the decline of a loved one with the associated behavioural problems and personality changes.

The challenge is in combining a dignified quality of life with appropriate care and at the same time not ignoring the needs of the carer. Ongoing deterioration frequently means carers are ultimately unable to cope at home and residential or nursing care may be needed. Behavioural problems may require placement in DeE (dementia elderly, formerly EMI) settings.

The Alzheimer's society (<http://www.alzheimers.org.uk/>) provides a wealth of information about all types of dementia and can provide advice and support to patients and their carers.

## Mental capacity

Historically, assessment of mental capacity in the UK has been covered by common law. In 2007, however, the 2005 Mental Capacity Act came into force.

Capacity describes the ability of an individual to make a decision. Lack of capacity implies an inability to make a decision on a specific topic at a given time. Any assessment of capacity is relevant only to a given decision at a given time and an individual may therefore not have capacity even if the impairment is only temporary.

An individual lacks capacity if:
• They are unable to understand information relevant to a decision.
• They are unable to retain the information for long enough to weigh the decision up.
• They are unable to use the information to make a decision.
• They are unable to communicate the decision by any means.

Of note, the information needs to be provided in a way appropriate to the individual's circumstances (e.g. avoiding excessive jargon and using his or her language!). Also, retention of the information only need be long enough to reach a decision and need not be indefinite. This is of particular relevance in patients with dementia who may be able to retain the information for long enough to decide, but be unable to recall it the next day.

### Mental Capacity Act 2005

The Mental Capacity Act 2005 presumes that individuals have capacity and guarantees their right to be supported to make their own decisions, even if these are apparently eccentric. Any assessment of capacity is relevant to a given decision, and does not result automatically from a given diagnosis, the person's age, or their behaviour.

For those who lack capacity, decisions need to be made in their best interests and in the least restrictive way. If the lack of capacity is temporary, decisions should only be made if absolutely necessary; otherwise they should be deferred until capacity is regained.

Assessment of best interest involves taking what is known about a person's feelings and beliefs into account; and consulting with relevant parties such as relatives, carers, and friends. If an individual lacking capacity has no representative to speak for them there is a statutory obligation to involve an independent mental capacity advocate (IMCA). Similarly, advance statements the person has made about their wishes need to be considered. Safeguards exist to ensure that advance decisions to refuse treatment are only valid to refuse life-saving treatment if they are in writing and specify 'even if life is at risk'.

The Act provides for an individual to plan for a period when they may lack capacity by granting a Lasting Power of Attorney. This allows for decisions concerning health and welfare as well as property and affairs. If appropriate, a deputy can also be appointed by the Court of Protection. Similarly the court may be required to decide in instances when there is a dispute between medical staff and the deputy. No decision can be made about marriage, sexual relationships, adoption, or voting on behalf of another individual.

### Capacity or not?

A 72-year-old lady with mild dementia is in hospital following recurrent falls. She wants to leave and go back home, where she lives in a period cottage on her own. Her mobility has deteriorated and the multidisciplinary team do not feel she will be safe at home.

**Scenario 1:** the lady is adamant that she will cope and feels that she will not have a problem at home. She does not agree that her mobility is unsafe and becomes aggressive, stating that she is being held against her will.

**Scenario 2:** the lady acknowledges that her mobility has deteriorated and she is at risk of falling and subsequent injury. Regardless of this risk she still wants to go home without further intervention.

---

**Consent to treatment**
- Need to have capacity.
- Be making the decision voluntarily and free from distress.
- Be provided with enough information to make the decision.

---

The lady in scenario 1 does not appear to be receptive to, or retaining, the fact that her mobility has deteriorated and she is at risk as a result. Her decision is therefore not being made in light of the available facts and she lacks capacity. The lady in scenario 2 is choosing to put herself at increased risk, but is showing insight into her condition and understands that risk. She has capacity.

# 4.5 Incontinence

## Introduction

Incontinence describes the situation in which an individual is unable to control voiding of urine or faeces. This is not only unhygienic and demoralizing, but has implications for social and nursing care. Inability to cope at home with incontinence is frequently a precipitating factor for residential care.

## Urinary incontinence

Urinary continence is maintained by urethral pressure exceeding detrusor muscle pressure. Voiding occurs when bladder pressure exceeds urethral pressure. Various causes for have been identified and may coexist.

### Causes

*Stress incontinence*

High urethral pressure is maintained through the action of the pelvic floor muscles. Weakening of these muscles means that transient increases in abdominal pressure, such as sneezing or coughing, cause bladder pressure to exceed urethral pressure resulting in voiding small amounts of urine. The most common cause for weak pelvic floor muscles is a result of pregnancy and childbirth. Tone does also decrease with age and can be affected by surgical procedures.

*Urge incontinence*

Occurs when a person has very little warning of needing to micturate and voids before reaching the toilet. Causes include:

- Local detrusor instability, e.g. increased irritability as a result of urinary or pelvic infection.
- Impaired neurological suppression of detrusor autonomy, e.g. MS, cord injury, dementia.

*Overflow incontinence*

Result of a full bladder which leaks urine even when an individual is not trying to void. Occurs when there is obstruction to full bladder emptying (benign prostatic hyperplasia), neurological impairment (MS, diabetes, spinal cord injury) or impaired contractility secondary to drugs, e.g. anticholinergics.

*Non-specific causes*

- Debilitation, impaired cognition, or acute illness may prevent an individual recognizing the need to pass urine. Eventually the bladder reflexes initiate voiding resulting in incontinence.
- Decreased mobility may mean individuals are unable to toilet themselves and without assistance will be incontinent. This may be exacerbated by drugs such as diuretics, or conditions such as poorly-controlled diabetes which will cause more urine to be produced.
- Constipation can cause bladder outflow obstruction, urinary retention, and overflow incontinence.

### Investigation

The mainstay of investigation is a detailed history of the circumstances in which incontinence occurs. Examination may suggest a urinary tract infection, constipation, urinary retention, prostate enlargement, or neurological condition.

Nitrites and leucocytes on urinalysis may suggest urinary infection—confirm with formal laboratory testing.

If no cause is evident, referral to a urologist or urogynaecologist should be considered. Urodynamic studies may be undertaken to look at bladder versus pelvic pressure, response to filling, flow rates, and residual volumes.

### Management

*Treatment strategies*

These obviously depend on the cause of incontinence:

- Exacerbating factors such as infection, constipation, diuretics, and uncontrolled hyperglycaemia should be addressed where possible. Caffeine should be avoided.
- Pelvic floor exercises can help to maintain urethral tone (> bladder tone) and minimize or prevent stress incontinence. Colposuspension repositions the bladder into a more physiological position and can also help.
- Alpha-blockers (e.g. tamsulosin) or antiandrogens (e.g. finasteride) can increase the size of the prostatic urethra, preventing outflow obstruction and thereby reducing residual volumes and overflow incontinence.
- Anticholinergics (e.g. tolterodine) or beta-3 adrenergic receptor agonists (e.g. mirabegron) can reduce bladder excitability and treat urge incontinence.
- Surgical treatment in some cases, e.g. intramural urethral bulking agents in stress incontinence.
- Bladder training/regular toileting: awareness of the need to void and toileting to pre-empt this is useful in cases of reduced mobility or awareness of a full bladder.

*Coping strategies*

These essentially all involve containment of urine. The simplest approach is to use absorbent continence pads to soak up urine. In male patients, a convene sheath placed over the penis can carry urine to a catheter bag. Urethral catheterization is effective at achieving continence, but increases the risk of infection as well as being more invasive. It can be intermittent or permanent. The benefits clearly need to be weighed against the risk. Longer-term, suprapubic catheterization may be preferable.

## Faecal incontinence

While rarer than urinary incontinence, this has greater hygiene and social implications. Causes include:

- Diarrhoea: more liquid stool requires greater sphincter tone to control and may precipitate incontinence in a usually unaffected individual.
- Decreased sphincter tone: secondary to muscle damage or neurological impairment (stroke, cord compression).
- Immobility/decreased awareness (e.g. dementia).

### History and investigation

Exclude reversible causes such as infective diarrhoea and constipation with overflow. Per rectum examination is mandatory (unless impossible to gain compliance) to exclude constipation, assess anal tone, and exclude inflammation or tumours (sigmoidoscopy may also be necessary).

### Management

- Address reversible causes.
- Regular toileting.
- Antidiarrhoeal medication (e.g. loperamide) may produce more formed and manageable stools. Rarely, a combination of antidiarrhoeals and enemas may be used to produce 'controlled' bowel motions.
- Surgery: sphincter repair may be possible. Colostomy may allow controlled collection of faeces, and although extreme may increase confidence and allow an individual to return to a normal lifestyle.
- Always consider **cord compression** or **cauda equina syndrome** in a patient with new-onset bladder and/or bowel incontinence. Delayed recognition can result in permanent loss of sphincter function and paraparesis. Check both rectal tone and perianal sensation to pinprick.

# 4.6 Falls

## Introduction

A fall is defined as when a patient moves from one position to a lower position unintentionally. This is opposed to syncope, which describes an episode of loss of consciousness as a result of transient cerebral hypoperfusion. As many people can not recall falling, both need to be considered as part of a falls assessment.

A fall may result in injury itself, but may also herald significant underlying pathology. Falls are a leading cause of morbidity and mortality with over 400,000 older people attending A&E a year as a result of a fall. Falls in the elderly are usually multifactorial and only rarely purely mechanical. Their successful diagnosis, investigation, and treatment require a multidisciplinary approach. The PROFET (Prevention of Falls in the Elderly Trial) study showed that medical and occupational therapist assessment of elderly people with falls can significantly reduce the number of subsequent falls.

## Clinical evaluation

A comprehensive history and assessment are essential to an accurate diagnosis both as to cause of the fall and in identifying injury (see Section 4.2). In particular:

### History

*This fall*

- Can patient recall falling?
- What were they doing and where were they when they fell?
- How did they feel before the fall? Were they light-headed, did they have palpitations?
- Did they lose consciousness? If so, for how long and when did they regain it? How were they afterwards?
- Have they fallen before? Was it under similar circumstances?
- Why do they think they fell?
- Any symptoms of infection?
- Was it witnessed?

*Falls risk*

- Pre-existing balance or gait disorder (e.g Parkinson).
- Polypharmacy (especially antihypertensives and sedatives).
- Poor vision.
- Dementia.
- Home hazards.
- Alcohol and drugs.

*Injury risk*

- Anticoagulation.
- Established osteoporosis (see Fig. 4.8).
- Osteoporosis risk factors:
  - Previous fragility fracture.
  - Long-term steroids.
  - Smoker.
  - Premenopausal hysterectomy.
  - High alcohol intake.
  - Low BMI.
  - Family history.

### Examination

*Baseline obervations*

- Temperature—infective focus, hypothermia?
- Heart rate—tachy/bradyarrhythmia (see Fig. 4.9)?

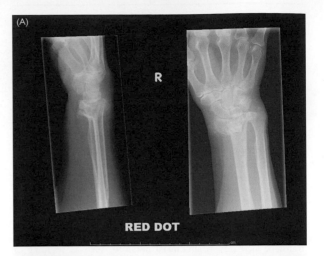

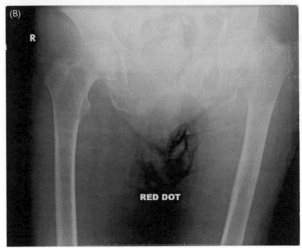

**Fig. 4.8** A fragility fracture (e.g. Colles in (A)) should initiate an osteoporosis risk assessment as treatment may be indicated to minimize further bone loss and prevent more debilitating injuries (e.g. fractured neck of femur in (B)) in the future.

- BP—hypotension, postural drop (see Box 4.1 and Fig. 4.10)?
- Oxygen saturations—hypoxia?

*Cardiovascular*

- Exclude significant valvular disease.

*Respiratory*

- Evidence of infection or failure?

*Neurological*

- Vision?
- Weakness?
- Impaired coordination?
- Impaired proprioception?
- Underlying diagnosis, e.g. Parkinson?

*Balance/gait*

- Is it normal or a factor in the fall? Watch the patient walk if possible.

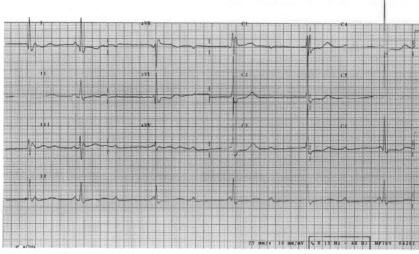

**Fig. 4.9** Mobitz type 2 heart block.

*Cognition*
- Any evidence of confusion:
  - Is it acute, a possible delirium?
  - Is it longstanding: possible dementia?

An ECG should be performed in all falls where syncope is a possibility. Any dysrhythmia (see Fig. 4.9) may be discovered.

| Common causes of 'falls' |
| --- |
| Environmental: |
| • Obstacles/loose carpets/ice/pets |
| • Poor lighting |
| • Unfamiliar surroundings |
| • Inappropriate footwear |
| Mobility: |
| • Degenerative joint disease |
| • Movement disorders (e.g. Parkinson). |
| Infective: |
| • Urosepsis |
| • Lower respiratory tract infection |
| Neurological: |
| • Seizure |
| • Stroke (NB: TIAs are **not** a cause of falls in the absence of focal neurology) |
| • Visual impairment |
| • Dementia/delirium |
| Metabolic/biochemical: |
| • Electrolyte disturbance |
| • Hypoglycaemia |
| • Alcohol and drugs |

| Causes of syncope |
| --- |
| • Cardiogenic: |
| • Hypotension (including postural) |
| • Dysrhythmia (tachy- or bradycardia) |
| • Carotid body hypersensitivity |
| • Valvular dysfunction |
| • Ischaemia |
| • Neurological: vertebrobasilar insufficiency |
| • Vasovagal |

| Consequences of a fall |
| --- |
| • Injury: |
| • Superficial (e.g. abrasion, bruising) |
| • Moderate (e.g. rib, pelvic, or vertebral fractures) |
| • Major (e.g. fractured neck of femur) |
| • Death (e.g. intracranial bleed) |
| • Inability to get up: |
| • Hypothermia |
| • Pressure sores |
| • Dehydration/renal failure |
| • Rhabdomyolysis |
| • Loss of confidence |
| • Social isolation |
| • Institutionalization |

**Investigation**

Unless there is good clinical reason not to, all falls patients should have a postural BP check and bedside ECG performed. Other investigations should be tailored to the case in hand. A balance needs to be struck between appropriate and over-investigation.

*Blood tests*
- Electrolytes (low sodium is common).
- Inflammatory markers.
- Full blood count.
- Vitamin $B_{12}$ (deficiency can contribute to dementia and peripheral neuropathy).
- Thyroid function tests.
- Corrected calcium (can cause confusion if elevated).
- Vitamin-D (deficiency associated with osteoporosis and proximal myopathy).
- INR (essential if on warfarin).
- Syphilis serology (although rare nowadays).

## Box 4.1 Orthostatic hypotension

Orthostatic (postural) hypotension is a common cause of falls as a result of syncope, or near-syncope. Such falls usually occur a short while after standing. Patients may describe feeling light-headed when they stand up.

Blood pressure (BP) should be taken with the patient lying down. They should then be stood up. The BP should ideally be repeated immediately and again at 2 minutes. A normal response is for no change, or a slight increase in BP. A fall of more than 20/10mmHg is significant.

Causes include hypovolaemia, antihypertensives, autonomic dysfunction and Addison disease.

Management involves reviewing any offending medication (antihypertensives, diuretics), fluids to correct hypovolaemia, and graded compression stockings to minimize venous pooling. Pharmacotherapy includes fludrocortisone (watch for possible cardiac failure). Midodrine (an alpha sympathomimetic) can increase peripheral tone and also helps reduce the fall in BP.

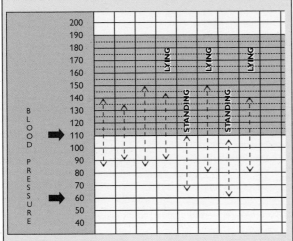

**Fig. 4.10** Orthostatic hypotension.

### Septic screen if suspicion of infective precipitant
- Urine dipstick and culture.
- Blood cultures.
- CXR.

### Imaging
- Bone radiographs if clinical concern.
- CT head if new focal neurology, loss of consciousness after head trauma, or fluctuating GCS.

### Cardiac investigations
- ECG.
- Carotid sinus massage.
- 24-hour tape.
- Echocardiogram.
- Tilt table.

### Other
- Dual-energy X-ray absorptiometry DEXA scan (identify possible osteoporosis—if aged over 75, female, and have had an osteoporosis-related fracture, guidance from NICE suggests a DEXA scan is not needed before treatment).

## Treatment

### Address ongoing pathology
- Infection.
- Electrolyte disturbance.
- Tachyarrhythmia.

- Haemodynamically-significant bradycardia—if no response to atropine may need temporary pacing.

### Address future risk
- Environment.
- Occupational therapy review may suggest home modifications such as rails, elevated toilet seats, ramps instead of steps, removal of loose rugs etc.
- Physiotherapist to advise on appropriate walking aids.
- Reduce alcohol intake.
- Drugs: stop unnecessary medications, especially antihypertensives/sedatives.

### Minimize risk of complications from falls
- Build bone mass:
  - Weight-bearing exercise.
  - Good nutrition.
  - Consider bisphosphonates and/or calcium and vitamin D supplementation.
- Stop smoking.
- Review anticoagulation: risks vs. benefits assessment.

### Rehabilitation
- Physiotherapy.
- Balance and strength training.
- Appropriate equipment.
- Coping strategies (e.g. getting up after fall).
- Aids to call for help (e.g. pendant alarm).

### Referral to specialist clinic
- Previous fragility fractures.
- Unexplained falls.
- Afraid of falling.
- Multiple risk factors.

## Performing carotid sinus massage

Contraindicated in carotid atherosclerosis—exclude history of recent TIA and stroke. First, auscultate to ensure absence of bruit. A history of VT or VF are relative contraindications. Atropine and resuscitation equipment should be to hand.
- Lay the patient down so they are comfortable.
- Connect them to cardiac monitor with printer.
- Locate the carotid artery at the midpoint of the medial border of sternocleidomastoid.
- Massage for 5 seconds looking for variation in heart rate. Ideally non-invasive, beat-to-beat BP monitoring is performed, but this is often not practical.
- If there is no response, try the other side.
A result is positive if there is:
- Asystole exceeding 3 seconds (cardioinhibitory hypersensitivity).
- A drop in BP of 50mmHg systolic (vasopressor hypersensitivity).
- A combination of the two (mixed hypersensitivity).

## Key points
- Falls are frequently multifactorial.
- Personal history may be unreliable and witness history may be required to identify cause.
- Syncope in the elderly is rarely benign.
- Frequent or unexplained falls should be investigated in specialist falls clinics.

# Hypothermia

Hypothermia is low core body temperature. Hypothermia develops when there is a mismatch between heat generation and loss. Falls commonly precipitate hypothermia in the elderly. After falling, an individual may be unable to get up again and may be left on the floor for some time. Ageing physiology and autonomic decline result in impaired homeostasis and heat production. In addition a cool environment (heating costs are rising) may mean the heat gradient is larger, accelerating heat loss.

Other causes include:

*Decreased heat production*

- Hypothyroidism.
- Hypoadrenalism.
- Malnutrition.
- Hypoglycaemia.

*Increased heat loss*

- Vasodilatation secondary to drugs.
- Wet clothing (spills or incontinence).
- Immersion (e.g. unable to get out of bath).

*Impaired thermoregulation*

- Damage to the skin (e.g. burns).
- Hypothalamic dysfunction.

*Hypothermia is categorized by severity.*

- Mild (32–35°C).
- Moderate (28–32°C).
- Severe (<28°C).

Mild hypothermia may be associated with confusion and shivering, moderate with delirium and slowed reflexes, and severe with coma, respiratory difficulties, and cardiac arrhythmias.

Management involves stabilizing the patient and monitoring closely for cardiac dysrhythmia. Wet clothing should be removed. Gently warm the patient with humidified oxygen, warmed IV saline, blanket/ Bair Hugger™ (warm air blanket).

# Rhabdomyolysis

Rhabdomyolysis describes the pathological breakdown of muscle fibres with leakage of toxic cellular contents. Rhabdomyolysis was initially described in crush injuries but can be caused by various factors including trauma, ischaemia, drugs, and exertion.

The commonest cause in the elderly is prolonged immobilization following a fall from which they are unable to get up. Symptoms include muscle ache, but are non-specific and a high index of suspicion should be maintained. Diagnosis can be confirmed biochemically with a CK that is elevated 5–10-fold. Myoglobinuria may be suggested by the presence of a urine dipstick positive for blood in the absence of red blood cells.

The most immediate threat from rhabdomyolysis is of hyperkalaemia owing to release of intracellular potassium from damaged cells. Potassium levels need to be monitored closely. The treatment of hyperkalaemia is detailed in Section 11.1. There is a risk of compartment syndrome as inflamed tissue swells and a fasciotomy may be necessary. The most serious medium- to long-term complication is acute kidney injury, which may develop over the first few days.

The mainstay of treatment is good hydration. IV fluids should be given to maintain a good urine output (ideally 100–200mL/hour). Limited evidence exists to support urinary alkalinization and this should be considered in severe cases.

Haemodialysis/filtration may be required in resistant hyperkalaemia, fluid overload, progressive renal failure or severe acidosis.

# 4.7 Prescribing in the elderly

## Background

The oldest 15% of the population receive 40% of drug prescriptions. It is rare to find someone in their 8th or 9th decade who is not on a multitude of medications. Drug interactions and side effects are therefore common, affecting the balance between benefit and harm.

## Evidence base

The vast majority of drug trials recruit fit, healthy people (often only male) between the ages of 18 and 65. Strictly speaking, conclusions drawn from such studies are only extendable to the population the subjects represented. Prescribing in the elderly is therefore less evidence-based, rather extrapolated and this should be borne in mind—especially in the very elderly whose life expectancy may be less than the time it takes treatment and non-treatment curves to diverge!

## Factors affecting prescription

Prescribing in the elderly is influenced by patient factors, pharmacokinetic and pharmacodynamic factors, as well as increased susceptibility to side effects and complications.

### Patient factors

A prescription is pointless if the patient is unable or unwilling to take the medication.

Compliance is a well-recognized problem in patients of all ages and the elderly are no exception. It is important to:

- Explain why medication is needed.
- Explain how and when to take it.
- Emphasize that for any medication it is important not to stop abruptly.

If a patient does not appear to be responding to a medication, always consider whether they are actually taking it. People may have cupboards full of collected prescriptions they never take.

The style of medication and its method of administration also need to be considered:

- Patients may have difficulty swallowing large tablets, whereas a soluble preparation would pose no problem.
- A diabetic patient with retinopathy may have poor glycaemic control simply because he is unable to read the dial on the insulin pen and has no one who can help him.
- Some inhalers may be too mechanically difficult for someone with marked rheumatoid arthritis to operate, whereas alternative devices would present no problem.
- Medication aids should be considered, e.g. dosette box.

### Pharmacodynamic and pharmacokinetic factors

Any part of a drug's progress through the body and its effect on its receptors may be influenced by the ageing process, for instance:

- Gastric emptying may be slower or bowel transit longer.
- Bioavailability may be affected by a hypoalbuminaemic state or increased fat to muscle ratio.
- Metabolism of drugs may be accelerated or reduced by other enzyme inducing or inhibiting drugs.
- Receptor sensitivity and/or number may vary.
- Elimination may be impaired owing to declining renal function causing toxicity.

---

### Key points

Is the drug needed?
- Would non-drug treatments be effective?

Can the patient manage to take it?
- Would alternative forms or delivery routes/mechanisms be more appropriate?

Is the dosing regimen suitable?
- A once-a-day drug may be preferable to a complicated regimen.

Start low and go slow.

Well-established drugs are preferred.

Review regularly:
- Is medication still needed?
- Are side effects occurring?
- May new drugs be interacting? Bear in mind enzyme-inducing or -inhibiting drugs.

---

## Side effects and complications

As a result of ageing physiology and altered pharmacodynamics and kinetics, the elderly are more prone to side effects, interactions, and complications. While these can be varied, a few merit special consideration.

### Acute kidney injury

Many elderly patients take diuretics and angiotensin system-modifying drugs. While beneficial in helping with heart failure and/or hypertension, they may increase the risk of pre-renal failure when further stresses such as gastrointestinal upset and volume depletion are present. Moreover, it is not uncommon for patients to report how, in spite of struggling to keep fluids down, they have forced themselves to take their tablets. It may be worth giving patients 'sick-day' rules to avoid diuretics, ACE inhibitors, ARBs, NSAIDs, etc. if they have diarrhoea and vomiting.

### Gastrointestinal haemorrhage

Older patients have increased susceptibility to drugs such as non-steroidal anti-inflammatories and steroids. These are known to increase the risk of upper gastrointestinal haemorrhage. It is prudent to consider whether such medications are truly needed, and if so is some form of acid suppression treatment also warranted? For example, when starting a frail elderly patient on aspirin and clopidogrel following an NSTEMI, consider a proton pump inhibitor.

### Falls

It is well-recognized that falls are more common in patients on four or more medications. This may in part be due to the fact that more medications imply more medical problems which could contribute to falls, but side effects are also a factor. Drugs particularly implicated include antihypertensives and sedatives.

### Confusion and CNS effects

Most drugs that cross the blood–brain barrier can cause confusion or sedation. Opiate analgesics often cause confusion (as well as nausea and constipation).

Smaller doses of sedatives and antipsychotics are usually needed for the same effect in the elderly. Treatment is best initiated at a low dose and only titrated slowly. Antidopaminergic side effects may cause extrapyramidal sequelae and drug-induced parkinsonism.

Confusion may limit dosing regimens in the elderly, e.g. in the middle-aged with Parkinson disease, dyskinesias usually limit the maximum dose of levodopa or dopamine agonists. In the elderly, confusion and/or hallucinations are often the dose-limiting factors.

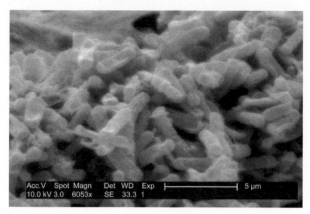

**Fig. 4.11** An electron micrograph of *Clostridium difficile* from a stool sample.

Courtesy of CDC/Louis S. Wiggs. This image is in the public domain. http://phil.cdc.gov/phil/details.asp (ID# 6256)

### Diarrhoea

Many drugs can cause diarrhoea as a side effect. Antibiotics are perhaps the greatest culprit, either as a direct side effect or through favouring *Clostridium difficile* infection (Fig. 4.11).

The *C. difficile* bacterium is an anaerobic, spore-forming Gram-positive rod. It occurs as a commensal organism in up to 30% of the population. As such it is not pathogenic because other bowel flora keep it in check. When patients are treated with antibiotics, the other flora are killed off, but the resistant spores enable *C. difficile* to survive. It then flourishes and causes a toxin-mediated diarrhoea.

Severity of infection may range from mild diarrhoea to life-threatening pseudomembranous colitis. Usual treatment is metronidazole (or oral vancomycin in cases that fail to respond). In extreme cases, intravenous immunoglobulins have been used.

### Anorexia

Any drug that can cause nausea and vomiting (e.g. SSRIs, donepezil, and codeine) may only cause anorexia instead and result in unexplained weight loss.

## Anticoagulation

Warfarin is notorious for interacting with other drugs and care always needs to be taken that medication changes do not result in over- or under-anticoagulation.

Frequent fallers are at increased risk of bleeding. Of greatest concern is the risk of intracranial bleeding following head trauma. The benefits of warfarin need to be weighed closely against the possible risks. If a patient has atrial fibrillation or paroxysmal atrial fibrillation and they are not given warfarin to decrease the chances of stroke, a reason must be documented.

▶▶ **Key point**

Check the drug list matches the list of problems the patient has. This is particularly useful in admission clerkings and discharge summaries.

# Chapter 5

# Clinical pharmacology and therapeutics

# 5.1 Pharmacodynamics

## Definitions

The study of the physiological and biochemical effects of drugs is termed pharmacodynamics. This discipline aims to understand the mechanism of drug action, paying attention to correlations between drug effects and chemical structure.

In its widest sense, a drug is a chemical entity (with the exclusion of food substances) which affects living processes. If the effect is beneficial, the drug is a medicine, whereas a poison is a drug with a detrimental effect. This distinction is often blurred in that a particular drug can be either a medicine or poison depending on the person using it and the conditions of use.

A drug may alternatively be defined as an agent used to diagnose, prevent, alleviate or cure disease. All definitions have limitations, however, as the latter would exclude contraceptives (pregnancy is not considered to be a disease).

## Drug classification and nomenclature

Various criteria are used to classify drugs, including chemical structure or pharmacological action; the preferred classification being the latter one.

Drugs have three or more names including:

- Chemical name—obeys the rules of nomenclature of chemical compounds.
- Brand (or trade) name—selected by manufacturer and always capitalized.
- Generic (or common) name—common established name which is not dictated by manufacturer.

Usually a drug bearing a particular generic name is equivalent to the same drug with a brand name. There are circumstances, however, when this equivalency does not hold true. For example, chemically identical drugs manufactured in different ways may differ in pharmacological action because of differences in isomerization, crystal structure (size, form, and hydration), purity (number and type of impurities), binders, coatings, vehicles, dissolution rate, and storage stability.

## Molecular aspects of drug action

Drugs produce effects in the body mainly in the following ways:

- By acting on receptors.
- By inhibiting carriers.
- By modulating or blocking ion channels.
- By inhibiting enzymes.
- Non-specifically.

### Receptors

Receptors are usually cellular proteins (membrane-bound or intracellular) which are stimulated by endogenous chemical mediators, such as hormones or neurotransmitters, to initiate a cellular response. Receptors allow the responses of individual cells to be co-ordinated. Drugs utilize receptors by causing either stimulation (so-called agonists) or by preventing receptor stimulation by endogenous agonists (so-called antagonists).

Receptors can be broadly grouped into four types:

1. G-protein coupled receptors (GPCRs); or metabotropic receptors—these have a basic structure consisting of a single polypeptide chain with seven transmembrane spanning domains. Signal transduction is mediated by activation of guanine nucleotide-binding proteins (G-proteins) that modulate the activity of ion channels and enzymes.

2. Ion channel-linked receptors; or inotropic receptors—these are ligand-gated ion channels located in cell membranes. The receptor and channel proteins may be a single entity. Signal transduction occurs in milliseconds. An example is the nicotinic acetylcholine receptor.

3. Receptors modulating gene transcription; or nuclear receptors—an example is the glucocorticoid receptor. This is located in the cytosol and migrates to the nucleus upon ligand binding.

4. Enzyme-linked receptors—these are transmembrane proteins with an extracellular binding site for ligands such as cytokines and growth factors. This is coupled to an intracellular enzymatic domain, usually having intrinsic tyrosine kinase activity. Upon receptor activation an intracellular signalling cascade is activated leading eventually to changes in gene transcription.

### Carriers

These are membrane transport proteins and their classification varies between authorities. In essence two main types exist:

1. Ion pumps with intrinsic ATPase activity—these include the sodium pump ($Na^+/K^+$-ATPase), the calcium pump, and the proton pump ($K^+/H^+$-ATPase). The latter is abundant in gastric parietal cells and is the target for proton pump inhibitors such as omeprazole.

2. Transporters or exchangers—including symporters and antiporters. Symporters utilize the transmembrane electrochemical gradient of one ion (often $Na^+$) to transport another ion (or several ions or molecules, e.g. glucose) across a cell membrane. Drugs can modify the action of symporters by binding site occupation (e.g. the action of furosemide on the $Na^+/K^+/2Cl^-$ symport in the nephron). Antiporters use the electrochemical gradient of one ion (usually $Na^+$) to drive another ion (or molecule) across the membrane in the opposite direction. An important example is the $Ca^{2+}$ exchanger (different from the $Ca^{2+}$ pump) which exchanges three $Na^+$ ions for one $Ca^{2+}$ ion. This is the target of the cardiac glycoside, digoxin.

### Ion channels

Drugs which act by direct interaction with ion channels include: local anaesthetics (which block voltage-gated $Na^+$ channels, e.g. lignocaine or lidocaine) and dihydropyridine $Ca^{2+}$ channel antagonists (which block voltage-gated L-type $Ca^{2+}$ channels). These ion channels should be distinguished from ion channels that function as inotropic receptors and open in response to ligand binding.

### Enzymes

Drugs affect enzymatic reactions by enzyme modification (reversible or irreversible) or through substrate competition. Some examples are shown in Table 5.1.

### Non-specific interactions

This refers to the physical effect of drugs on cells. For example, sucralfate is an ulcer-healing drug which forms a protective barrier by adhering to gastric mucosa. Drugs can also act outside of cells by chemical interactions. Neutralization of stomach acid by antacids is a good example.

## Mode of drug action

The action of drugs should be distinguished from their effects. Drug action refers to the physiological and biochemical mechanisms by which the drug leads to a response. The effect is the observable consequence

**Table 5.1** Drugs acting through alteration of enzyme reactions

| Substrate | Enzyme | Products | Inhibitor | Uses |
|---|---|---|---|---|
| HMG-CoA | HMG-CoA reductase | Mevalonic acid | Atorvastatin | Hypercholesterolaemia |
| Angiotensin I | Angiotensin converting enzyme (ACE) | Angiotensin II | Ramipril | Hypertension, myocardial infarction |
| Arachidonic acid | Cyclooxygenase | Prostanoids | Ibuprofen | Pain, inflammation |
| Hypoxanthine | Xanthine oxidase | Uric acid | Allopurinol | Gout |
| Folate | Dihydrofolate reductase | Tetrahydrofolate | Trimethoprim | Antibacterial |

of drug action. An example is the action of penicillin to inhibit bacterial cell wall synthesis and the effect is bacterial lysis and death.

A major problem in pharmacology is that drugs usually produce multiple effects. The desired therapeutic effect may be considered the primary effect with secondary effects listed as all other effects,

either beneficial or harmful. Drugs are often chosen to exploit differences between normal metabolic processes and the abnormalities associated with disease. It is because these differences may not be great that drugs are non-specific in their action, often altering normal functions leading to side effects.

# 5.2 Pharmacokinetics

## Background

Pharmacokinetics is defined as the pharmacological discipline that studies quantitatively the fate of administered substances, such as drugs. This includes the means and extent of drug absorption, the distribution of the drug throughout the compartments of the body, the successive metabolic transformations of the drug and its metabolites, and finally, the elimination of the drug and its metabolites or, in rare cases, their irreversible accumulation in the body. So in contrast to pharmacodynamics which explores what a drug does to the body, pharmacokinetics studies what the body does with the drug.

## Routes of drug administration

The main routes of administration are:
- Intravenous
- Oral
- Buccal
- Sublingual
- Rectal
- Intramuscular
- Transdermal
- Subcutaneous
- Inhalational
- Topical

The bioavailability of a drug is the fraction of an administered dose that reaches the systemic circulation, which by definition equals 100% for an intravenous injection. For other routes of administration it is dependent on absorption, local metabolic degradation, and first-pass metabolism. The latter is defined as drug removal from the portal circulation by hepatic enzymatic degradation such that the amount of drug reaching the systemic circulation is considerably less than the amount absorbed into the portal vein.

## Routes of drug elimination

The main routes by which drugs are removed from the body are:
- Hepatic metabolism.
- Renal excretion.
- Lungs (e.g. for volatile/gaseous anaesthetics).

### Hepatic metabolism

Metabolic alteration of drug molecules involves two kinds of biochemical reaction, which often (though not invariably) occur sequentially, known as phase I and phase II reactions.

Phase I reactions typically consist of oxidation, reduction, or hydrolysis. The products are usually more reactive and occasionally more toxic than the parent drug. The reactions are catalysed by a complex system of enzymes known as the mixed function oxygenases residing on smooth endoplasmic reticulum. Several enzymes are involved, with the most important being the cytochrome P450 system (consisting of 30–100 isoenzymes, each with differing substrate specificities and differing mechanisms controlling their expression).

Phase II reactions involve conjugation by addition of glucuronyl, sulphate, methyl, acetyl, glycyl, and glutamyl groups. This usually makes compounds less reactive and more water-soluble (and hence more easily excreted in urine or bile).

### Renal excretion

Drugs are handled by the kidney in very different ways with three basic processes accounting for these differences:

- Glomerular filtration.
- Active tubular secretion or reabsorption.
- Passive diffusion across tubular epithelium.

Glomerular capillaries will allow drug molecules with a molecular weight <20,000 to pass through into the glomerular filtrate. However, if a drug binds to plasma albumin (molecular weight 68,000), e.g. warfarin, its concentration in the filtrate will be less than the total plasma concentration.

Drugs can enter the tubular lumen from adjacent peritubular capillaries by two independent and non-selective carrier systems. One transports acidic drugs (and also acidic endogenous substances such as uric acid) whilst the other handles basic chemical moieties. The carriers transport drugs against their electrochemical gradients and can decrease the plasma concentration to nearly zero.

If the tubular epithelium is freely permeable to a drug, the drug concentration in the filtrate will closely resemble that of the plasma. Drugs with high lipid solubility have high tubular permeability and are therefore excreted slowly. Drugs will accumulate in the tubular fluid (and have greater renal excretion) if they are highly polar and of low tubular permeability.

## First-order kinetics

Most drugs are eliminated with first-order kinetics, i.e. a constant fraction of the drug in the body is eliminated per unit time. The rate of elimination is proportional to the amount of drug in the body and the plasma concentration–time curve shows an exponential decay (Fig. 5.1A).

For drugs which follow first-order kinetics a number of useful pharmacokinetic constants can be applied:

- Clearance (CL)—the volume of plasma from which the drug is completely removed per unit time.
- Elimination rate constant ($k_{el}$)—the fraction of the drug in the body eliminated per unit time. This is represented by the slope of the line of the $\log_e$ plasma concentration versus time.
- Volume of distribution ($V_d$)—is the theoretical volume of fluid a drug would require to be diluted in to achieve the plasma concentration. Drugs that are highly lipid-soluble, such as digoxin, have a very high $V_d$ (500 litres). Drugs which are lipid-insoluble, such as neuromuscular blockers, remain in the blood, and have a low $V_d$. The $V_d$ gives an indication of the expected plasma concentration for a given dose of drug.
- Half-life ($t_{1/2}$)—the time taken for plasma concentration to reduce by 50%. After 4 half-lives, elimination is 94% complete.

The following equations derive from these definitions:

$$\text{Rate of elimination} = \text{CL} \times \text{plasma concentration}$$
$$\text{Rate of elimination} = k_{el} \times \text{amount of drug in body}$$
$$\text{Amount of drug in body} = V_d \times \text{plasma concentration}$$
$$\text{CL} = k_{el} \times V_d$$
$$\text{Natural logarithm of 2 (ln 2)} = k_{el} \times t_{1/2}$$

An example may help to clarify: you have a container with 10mL of orange squash. You make this up to a litre by adding 990mL of water. The $V_d$ of the diluted orange squash is 1000mL. If each minute you discard 10mL of the diluted squash and replace this with water, the clearance is 10mL/min. The $k_{el}$ is 0.01min$^{-1}$ (10/1000) and the elimination $t_{1/2}$ is 70 minutes.

If the volume of the container is increased to 2000mL and the clearance remains the same the $t_{1/2}$ increases to 140 minutes.

The example describes a single compartment model, i.e. if the bloodstream is the only compartment in the body (or if $V_d$ = the blood volume). The human body is obviously more complex with many compartments (muscle, fat, brain, etc.). In order to describe this we use multi-compartment models.

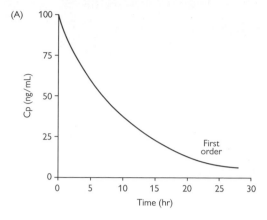

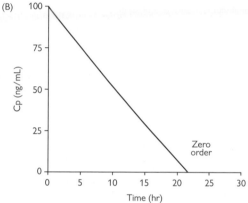

**Fig. 5.1** Plasma concentration (Cp)–time curves for drugs eliminated with (A) first-order and (B) zero-order kinetics.

## Multi-compartment models

When a patient is administered an intravenous injection of thio-pentone (a general anaesthetic) they wake up after 5 minutes, even though it takes several hours to eliminate this drug from the body. Initially the drug is completely contained in the blood. Organs with a rich vascular supply, such as the brain, accumulate drug rapidly. After several minutes the drug begins to re-distribute into other tissues such as fat, the concentration in the brain decreases and the patient wakes up. The explanation for the observed effect is, therefore, redistribution into other compartments.

Graphical representation of elimination from two compartments shows a bi-exponential pattern. A rapid fall in blood concentration is followed by a plateau phase and then a slower gradual fall. The first part (or alpha phase) is the rapid redistribution phase, the plateau is the equilibrium phase (when blood concentration = tissue concentration), and the slower elimination phase (or beta phase) is when blood and tissue concentrations fall in tandem. This is a simple two-compartment model. A mathematical description of multi-compartment models is beyond the scope of this chapter.

## Zero-order elimination

In a small number of cases where drugs are inactivated by enzymatic mechanisms, for example, ethanol, phenytoin, and salicylate, the time-course of drug elimination from plasma does not follow an exponential or bi-exponential pattern, but is initially linear (Fig. 5.1B). Drug is eliminated at a constant rate that is independent of its plasma concentration. This is termed zero-order (or saturation) kinetics. In the case of ethanol, the rate of disappearance from the plasma is constant at approximately 4mM per hour, irrespective of plasma concentration. The explanation is that the rate of oxidation by alcohol dehydrogenase enzymes reaches a maximum at low ethanol concentrations due to limited availability of the cofactor $NAD^+$.

Saturation kinetics has several important consequences. Firstly, the duration of action is more strongly dependent on dose than with drugs that do not show metabolic saturation. Another consequence is a steep and unpredictable relationship between dose and steady-state plasma concentration. This is particularly problematic if the drug has a low therapeutic index. It is for this reason that changes to the dose of phenytoin are made in very small increments, e.g. 300mg to 325mg.

## Dosage regimens

The strategy in calculating a dosing regimen is to give a dose rate sufficient to produce the desired therapeutic effect whilst minimizing the risk of toxic effects.

The maintenance dosing rate (given by dose/dose interval) is equal to the rate of elimination at steady-state (i.e. at steady-state, rate of elimination = rate of administration). It follows that:

Dosing rate = clearance × desired plasma concentration

Drugs accumulate in the body if the drug has not been fully eliminated before the next dose. As a general rule, it takes about five half-lives for the steady-state concentration to be achieved. It follows that to achieve a target plasma concentration rapidly, a loading dose must be administered, particularly if the drug has a long half-life. The loading dose can be derived from the volume of distribution:

Loading dose = volume of distribution × desired plasma concentration

# 5.3 Drug metabolism and prescribing in special circumstances

## Renal failure

Drugs can give rise to problems when used in patients with reduced renal function for one of the following reasons:

- Toxicity resulting from failure to excrete a drug and its metabolites.
- Sensitivity to a drug can be increased despite no change to its elimination.
- Patients in renal failure tend to tolerate drug side effects poorly.
- Drugs may be less effective in patients with renal failure.

One solution to some of these problems is to reduce the dose of drug or to use alternative drugs in renal failure.

### Dose adjustment in renal failure

Depends on:

- Drug toxicity.
- The extent of renal vs. hepatic elimination.

For drugs with minimal dose-related side effects, precise modification of the dosing regimen is unnecessary. More toxic drugs should be dosed according to glomerular filtration rate (GFR). Where there is evidence that efficacy and toxicity are closely-related to the plasma concentration, therapeutic drug monitoring may be recommended.

In patients with renal disease, nephrotoxic drugs should be avoided completely because reduced renal reserve means that the consequences of nephrotoxicity are exaggerated. In severe renal disease drug prescribing should be kept to a minimum.

A reduction in the dosing rate can be achieved by increasing the dose interval or by reducing the size of individual doses. One implication of a reduction in the maintenance dose is that a loading dose may be required to achieve a rapid response. This is because it takes about five times the drug half-life to reach a steady-state plasma concentration and drug half-life is often prolonged in renal failure, increasing the time taken to achieve a therapeutic plasma concentration. Usually the loading dose equates to the initial dose for a patient with normal renal function.

### Dosage tables

These tables are used to guide dose, based on the severity of renal impairment. Various measurements of renal function exist, e.g. GFR and creatinine clearance (CrCl). GFR is estimated from a formula derived from the Modification of Diet in Renal Disease study using serum creatinine, age, sex, and race. CrCl is best derived from a 24-hour urine collection but can also be calculated from a formula using serum creatinine, age, sex, and weight.

For dosing purposes, renal impairment is often graded according to the measured or estimated GFR which places patients into different stages of chronic kidney disease (CKD) as indicated in Table 5.2.

Renal function declines with age and many elderly patients have a GFR <50mL/min. This may not, however, be accompanied by a raised serum creatinine because of reduced muscle mass. A safe measure is to assume a mild degree of renal impairment when prescribing for the elderly.

Renal function should be checked before prescribing any drug which requires dose adjustment, if renal impairment is considered likely on clinical grounds.

## Liver failure

There are a number of mechanisms by which liver disease can alter drug responses. In severe liver disease drug prescribing should be kept to a minimum. This is particularly the case in patients with encephalopathy, jaundice, and ascites.

Although the liver is responsible for metabolizing a large array of drugs, the significant hepatic reserve means that hepatic failure has to be severe before significant effects on drug metabolism are seen. Liver function tests have poor predictive power in determining the extent to which hepatic drug metabolism is impaired. In cholestatic liver disease the biliary excretion of drugs is significantly impaired (e.g. fusidic acid and rifampicin).

Severe liver disease is often associated with hypoalbuminaemia. The effect of reduced protein binding capacity is to increase the toxicity of drugs which avidly bind plasma proteins, such as phenytoin and prednisolone. Clotting factor production is also reduced in liver disease. This leads to increased sensitivity to anticoagulants such as warfarin and phenindione.

Drugs can also precipitate and exacerbate encephalopathy. Those drugs which may impair cerebral function in severe liver disease include sedatives, opiates, drugs causing constipation, and diuretics (particularly those that cause hypokalaemia).

Liver disease is often associated with a state of secondary hyper-aldosteronism, accompanied by oedema and ascites. This is exacerbated by drugs that cause fluid retention such as non-steroidal anti-inflammatory drugs (NSAIDs) and corticosteroids.

Patients with liver disease are more prone to the side effects of hepatotoxic drugs (see Table 5.3). Both dose-related toxicity and idiosyncratic reactions are more likely in liver failure.

Table 5.3 Drugs causing a predominant hepatocellular, cholestatic, or mixed injury pattern.

| Category | Hepatocellular | Cholestatic | Mixed |
|---|---|---|---|
| Cardiac drugs | Amiodarone | Clopidogrel | Verapamil |
| | Statins* | Fosinopril | Enalapril |
| | Lisinopril | Irbesartan | Captopril |
| Antibiotics | Isoniazid | Flucloxacillin | Clindamycin |
| | Tetracycline | Erythromycin | Sulphonamides |
| | Ketoconazole | Terbinafine | Trimethoprim-sulphamethoxazole |
| CNS drugs | Valproic acid | Chlorpromazine | Trazodone |
| | Fluoxetine | Tricyclics | Carbamazepine |
| | Bupropion | Phenothiazines | Phenytoin |
| Miscellaneous drugs | Allopurinol | Azathioprine | Flutamide |
| | Diclofenac | Anabolic steroids | Cyproheptadine |
| | Troglitazone | Oral contraceptives | Ibuprofen |

*HMG-coA-reductase inhibitors.

Reproduced from 'Human Drug Hepatotoxicity: A Contemporary Clinical Perspective', Assis DN et al., Expert Opinion in Drug Metabolism & Toxicology, 2009, 5, 5, pp. 463–473, Taylor & Francis, reprinted by permission of the publisher (Taylor & Francis Group, http://www.informaworld.com).

Table 5.2 Grading of renal impairment by GFR

| Grade | GFR (mL/min) | CKD Stage |
|---|---|---|
| Mild | 30–60 | 3 |
| Moderate | 15–30 | 4 |
| Severe/dialysis-dependent | <15 | 5 |

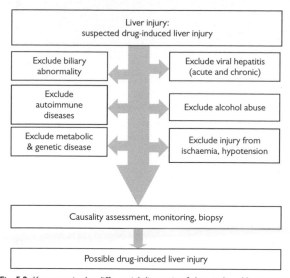

**Fig. 5.2** Key steps in the differential diagnosis of drug-induced liver injury. 'Human Drug Hepatotoxicity: A Contemporary Clinical Perspective', Assis DN *et al.*, *Expert Opinion in Drug Metabolism & Toxicology*, 2009, 5, pp. 463–473, Taylor & Francis, reprinted by permission of the publisher (Taylor & Francis Group, http://www.informaworld.com).

Hepatotoxic drugs should generally be avoided, or used only with extreme caution, in patients with severe liver disease.

Drug-induced liver disease can be difficult to diagnose. An algorithm to aid in the differential diagnosis of drug-induced liver injury is provided in Fig. 5.2.

## Pregnancy

The fetus is at risk of deleterious drug effects at all stages of its development, and this should be remembered when prescribing during pregnancy, and also in men and women trying to conceive.

The major concern in the first trimester is teratogenesis, or the risk of drug-induced congenital malformations. The period of greatest risk is the 3rd–11th week of fetal development.

In the second and third trimesters, the growth and functional development of the fetus may be affected by drug action. Drugs given shortly before term and during labour may adversely affect the physiology of labour and early neonatal development.

When considering whether to prescribe in pregnancy, the severity of the condition being treated should be weighed against the potential for adverse drug reactions. As a general rule, drugs should be prescribed when the expected benefit to the mother is perceived to be greater than the risk to the fetus and, if possible, all drugs should be avoided during the first trimester. Drugs of choice are those which have been extensively used in pregnancy and appear to be safe. The lowest effective dose should be prescribed. New or untried drugs should be avoided.

Few drugs are known conclusively to be teratogenic, but no drug is safe beyond all doubt in early pregnancy. As it is not ethical to test the safety of a new compound in pregnancy, we may never know the true teratogenicity of most drugs.

Drugs given to breastfeeding mothers may cause toxicity to the infant if they enter the milk in pharmacologically-significant quantities. Iodides, for example, can reach concentrations in breast milk that exceed the maternal plasma concentration, thereby posing a toxicity risk to the infant. Very low drug concentrations, which have minimal pharmacological effects, still pose the theoretical risk of hypersensitivity reactions in the infant. Drugs may also inhibit lactation (e.g. bromocriptine) and the infant's sucking reflex (e.g. phenobarbital).

# 5.4 Drug interactions

## Background

Two or more drugs given at the same time may interact. Such an interaction may be one of potentiation, of antagonism, or occasionally something else. Suspected adverse drug interactions should be reported to the Committee on Safety of Medicines (CSM).

Drug interactions may be classified as pharmacodynamic or pharmacokinetic.

## Pharmacodynamic interactions

These occur when drugs have either similar or antagonistic pharmacological effects. Drugs may compete for the same receptor site or modulate the same physiological system. Such interactions are predictable from the pharmacology of the interacting drugs and usually occur with all drugs of a particular class. To a greater or lesser extent, the interaction occurs in most patients receiving the interacting drugs.

## Pharmacokinetic interactions

Interactions of this type occur when the absorption, metabolism, excretion, or distribution of one drug is modulated by a second drug. In comparison to pharmacodynamic interactions, they affect only a small proportion of patients taking the combination of drugs and are not easily predictable. They show significant variation within any drug class.

They can be grouped as follows:

### Changes in absorption

Both the total amount of drug absorbed and the rate of absorption can be altered by drug interactions. Delayed absorption is only of clinical importance if a high peak plasma concentration is required for therapeutic efficacy (e.g. analgesics). A reduction in the total amount of drug absorbed is more likely to affect clinical efficacy. A good example is the reduction in antibiotic efficacy when tetracyclines are co-administered with divalent cations (e.g. milk, antacids, and calcium, magnesium, and iron salts).

### Changes in protein binding

Most drugs, to a variable extent, are loosely-bound to plasma proteins. As these binding sites are relatively non-specific, one drug can easily displace another drug in a dynamic equilibrium dependent on the concentration of each drug. As it is usually the concentration of unbound drug that determines pharmacological action, displacement from plasma proteins can result in a clinically-significant drug interaction. The effect is most dramatic with drugs which are >90% bound and have a low volume of distribution (i.e. are not widely distributed throughout the body). It is, however, rare for drug displacement interactions to produce significant potentiation since the increased concentration of free drug results in increased elimination.

An example is the potentiation of warfarin by sulphonamides and tolbutamide. This interaction is, however, more complex as warfarin metabolism is also inhibited by these agents.

### Altered metabolism

The metabolism of drugs in the liver can be increased by induction of the hepatic microsomal enzyme system leading to a reduction in drug concentration and reduced efficacy. The most important enzyme inducers are rifampicin, barbiturates, many anti-epileptics, and antifungals (such as griseofulvin). On withdrawal of the inducer, plasma concentrations increase with the risk of toxicity. Drugs whose metabolism is affected by enzyme induction include warfarin and oral contraceptives.

Conversely, some drugs may inhibit hepatic microsomal enzymes leading to higher plasma concentrations of other drugs. Known enzyme inhibitors include the antimicrobials isoniazid, erythromycin, ketoconazole, and sulphonamides.

The hepatic cytochrome P450 system consists of many isoenzymes which interact with a wide range of drugs. The interactions are complex with drugs acting as substrates, inducers, or inhibitors of different isoenzymes. Although much *in vitro* information is available on drug–enzyme interactions, the clinical effects of such interactions are difficult to predict. This is likely to be because drugs are usually eliminated by several metabolic routes as well as by renal excretion.

### Altered renal excretion

Drug elimination by the kidney involves glomerular filtration and active tubular secretion. Competition occurs between drugs sharing active transport systems in the proximal tubule. An example is the delayed excretion of methotrexate by salicylates with the risk of serious methotrexate toxicity.

## Relative importance of interactions

Drug interactions are usually harmless. Those which are potentially harmful occur in only a small proportion of patients and the severity of interaction varies from one patient to another.

Those at increased risk from drug interactions are the elderly and patients with renal or hepatic impairment.

Drug interactions are of greater significance when the therapeutic ratio is low and careful control of dosage is required. Examples include:

- Warfarin.
- Phenytoin.
- Oral contraceptives.
- Oral hypoglycaemics.
- Antihypertensives.
- Drugs acting on the brain.

# 5.5 Adverse drug reactions

## Background

The early reports of adverse reactions to drugs are of historical significance in that they led to regulatory changes. For example, the toxic effects of sulphanilamide led to the formation of the Food and Drug Administration (FDA) in the USA. In the UK, the debilitating side effects of thalidomide resulted in similar regulatory changes.

More recent examples, such as the side effects of benoxaprofen (Opren®), highlighted the need for caution in particular patient groups, such as the elderly.

## Statistics

Adverse drug reactions:
- Occur in 10–20% of hospital inpatients.
- Are implicated in up to 3% of inpatient deaths.
- Are responsible for up to 5% of hospital admissions.
- Are evident in 18% of patients taking one to five drugs and 80% of patients taking six or more.
- Drug interactions account for 7% of drug reactions but account for 1/3 of the deaths.

## Classification

Adverse drug reactions can be classified as follows:
- Dose-related—type A, augmented.
- Non-dose-related—type B, bizarre, or idiosyncratic.
- Long-term.
- Delayed.

### Dose-related

These account for the majority of adverse drug reactions. In theory they are avoidable if the dose is correct and providing the dose–response curves for therapeutic and side effects are disparate. These types of side effect account for between 75% and 90% of adverse drug reactions. They have three main causes:

1. **Pharmaceutical variation:** e.g. lithium, nifedipine, diltiazem. A good example occurred in Australia when the manufacturer of phenytoin changed the excipient from $CaSO_4$ to lactose. The result was a massive increase in the plasma phenytoin concentration and this led to some deaths.
2. **Pharmacokinetic variation:**
   - Pharmacogenetic differences—e.g. hepatic microsomal isoenzymes.
   - Liver disease—see Section 5.3.
   - Renal impairment—see Section 5.3.
   - Cardiac disease.
   - Thyroid disease—resistance caused by hyperthyroidism.
3. **Pharmacodynamic variation:**
   - Liver failure—drug effects on CNS are enhanced (e.g. risk of encephalopathy when patients with cirrhosis are given opiates).
   - Electrolyte and fluid abnormalities (e.g. hypokalaemia exacerbating digoxin action).

### Non-dose-related

These side effects are less predictable and more difficult to avoid. A history of allergy can be a useful guide.
They include:
- Immunological reactions—e.g. penicillin allergy. Prevalence is ~10 % and there is some overlap with cephalosporin allergy.
- Pharmacogenetic variations—extremely difficult to predict unless there is a positive family history. Examples include carbimazole-induced agranulocytosis and hydralazine-induced systemic lupus erythematosus.

### Long-term
These include:
- Adaptive changes—e.g. up-regulation of beta adrenoceptors during beta-blocker therapy, dopamine antagonists causing tardive dyskinesia.
- Rebound phenomena—occur upon sudden withdrawal of drug. Problematic with beta-blockers and corticosteroids (can be avoided by weaning drug slowly).
- Others: chloroquine effects on the retina, amiodarone resulting in tissue deposition of phospholipids.

### Delayed
Delayed drug side effects include:
- Teratogenicity.
- Impaired fertility.
- Carcinogenesis.

## Detection

Detection of adverse drug reactions can be very difficult. The rarer the side effect, the more difficult it is to detect. This difficulty is compounded if the background incidence of the adverse effect is high. To illustrate, a pre-market trial of 3000 patients will detect only one adverse effect if there is an incidence of 1 in 1000 and providing there is no background incidence.

Surveillance methods include:
- Anecdotal reporting.
- Voluntary reporting—e.g. Yellow cards in the British National Formulary (BNF).
- Other methods—intensive event recording, prospective cohort and case–control studies, population statistics, record linkage.

## Avoiding side effects

Methods to prevent adverse drug reactions include:
- Use low doses initially.
- Care in patients with renal or hepatic disease.
- Care in the elderly.
- Take a history about previous adverse effects.
- Warn patients about what to expect.
- Clear hand-writing (e.g. micrograms).
- Vigilance to drug interactions.

# 5.6 Drug development

## Background

- Can be classified into four phases (Fig. 5.3).
- The time taken to proceed through all four stages usually ranges around 8–12 years.
- For every 5000 compounds that enter preclinical testing, only one is approved for market use.
- The cost of getting a new drug to market averages £550 million.

## Phase 0 (preclinical studies)

- Non-clinical studies involving *in vitro* techniques.
- Use animal populations (e.g. rodents, dogs).
- Wide range of drug dosages are introduced to the animal subjects or to an *in vitro* substrate in order to obtain preliminary pharmacokinetic and toxicokinetic information.
- Various approaches are used to determine the dose range for first time in human studies, e.g. the no observed adverse effect level (NOAEL) and the minimum anticipated biological effect level (MABEL).

## Phase I

- First stage of testing in human subjects.
- A small group (20–100) of healthy volunteers (usually male) are selected.
- Trials assess the safety (pharmacovigilance), pharmacokinetics, pharmacodynamics, and side effect profile of a therapy.
- Patients are usually observed as in-patients until several half-lives of the drug have passed.

- A variety of dose-ranging studies are used, e.g. single ascending dose (or SAD) studies and multiple ascending dose (MAD) studies.
- Phase I trials occasionally use patients rather than healthy volunteers, such as with oncology and HIV drug trials.

## Phase II

- Designed to assess clinical efficacy and also continue safety assessments in a larger group of volunteers (100–300).
- The development process is often abandoned during phase II trials due to the discovery of poor efficacy or toxic effects.
- Often divided into phase IIA (dosing requirements) and phase IIB (study efficacy).

## Phase III

- Randomized controlled trials on large patient groups (1000–3000).
- Form the definitive assessment of efficacy of the new therapy relative to current 'Gold Standard' treatment.
- Expensive and time-consuming.
- A positive outcome in phase III is often known as a landmark study for a drug. A comprehensive documentation of the trial methodology and results, together with animal study data, manufacturing procedures, and formulation details make up the 'regulatory submission'. This is reviewed by various regulatory authorities in different countries, such as the European Medicines Agency (EMA) or the FDA in the USA prior to marketing approval.

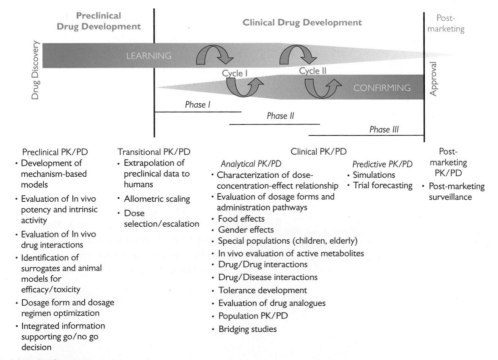

**Fig. 5.3** Clinical drug development.

*The AAPS Journal*, 10 (4), 2008, 552–9, 'Concepts and Challenges in Quantitative Pharmacology and Model-Based Drug Development', Zhang L, with kind permission from Springer Science and Business Media.

## Phase IV

- Involve the post-launch safety surveillance and ongoing technical support of a drug.
- May be mandated by regulatory authorities or may be undertaken by the sponsoring company for competitive or other reasons.
- Designed to detect any rare or long-term adverse effects over a much larger patient population and timescale than was possible during the initial clinical trials.
- May result in the withdrawal or restriction of a drug—recent examples include cerivastatin and rofecoxib.

# 5.7 Paracetamol poisoning

## Epidemiology and pathogenesis

Paracetamol poisoning is a common cause of admission to emergency departments. It is the most commonly abused substance in deliberate self-poisoning. Surveys have revealed the following facts:

- >50% obtained paracetamol with the specific intent of poisoning.
- ~60% overdosed on paracetamol because of its easy availability.
- ~40% overdosed on paracetamol because of its known dangers.
- Nearly 80% appreciated that overdose could cause death.
- Only 23% realized that the harmful effects could take >24 hours to appear.

Paracetamol is often overdosed alone, or in combination with other drugs (e.g. combination preparations such as co-codamol), or alcohol. Severe toxicity in adults occurs upon ingestion of doses of >250mg/kg of paracetamol, liver damage being the main complication. The risk of death is increased when paracetamol is taken in combination with other drugs, particularly opiates.

Following paracetamol overdose, 10% of patients develop liver damage and 2% would die of hepatic failure without treatment. In normal clinical doses, however, paracetamol has virtually no hepatotoxicity.

Paracetamol is metabolized in the liver by oxidation reactions requiring the cytochrome P450 system. These reactions generate a reactive quinone derivative which is removed by further reaction with glutathione and other sulphydryl-containing compounds. If glutathione stores are depleted, the quinone acts as an alkylating agent binding in a covalent fashion to other cellular proteins. The result is hepatocyte death leading to centrilobular necrosis. Protection against paracetamol poisoning is afforded by administration of the sulphydryl-containing compounds N-acetyl cysteine and methionine. These act to replenish hepatocyte glutathione levels. Liver enzyme induction, which occurs following barbiturate or alcohol ingestion, potentiates toxicity through increased production of intermediate quinine.

## Clinical features

Following a suspected overdose it is important to obtain a history of the drugs taken, how many were taken (number and dosage of tablets), and when.

Features are non-specific initially (often some nausea and vomiting); however, patients may have no symptoms in the first 24-hour period following ingestion.

After an apparent recovery, worrying examination findings include tender hepatomegaly with signs of hepatic failure and encephalopathy. In fulminant cases, hypotension, hypoglycaemia, and acute tubular necrosis ensue.

Emergency blood levels should be taken at least 4 hours after ingestion if paracetamol poisoning is suspected. One of the earliest signs of hepatic necrosis is a prolongation of the prothrombin time (PT), with a value >45 seconds indicating severe liver damage. Normal clotting 72 hours after ingestion offers reassurance.

## Management

Gastric lavage has a role if the patient presents within an hour of overdose. Activated charcoal (50g dose) should also be given.

If a significant overdose is suspected, a paracetamol antidote (N-acetylcysteine or methionine) should be administered immediately in advance of the 4-hour plasma level. When the 4-hour plasma concentration is known, this should act as a guide for further treatment. The plasma paracetamol concentration peaks at about 4 hours and therefore measurements before this time-point are of little value. Fig. 5.4 shows a treatment nomogram to guide whether antidote is required. Levels requiring antidote include 200mg/L at 4 hours, 70mg/L at 10 hours, and 50mg/L at 12 hours. The threshold for treatment should be halved in patients at risk of hepatic enzyme induction, e.g. alcoholics and those taking anticonvulsants.

Little harm is done if treatment has been initiated and the subsequent plasma concentration deems it unnecessary. In fact no fatalities have been associated with N-acetylcysteine use and it is therefore reasonable to administer it in doubtful cases. Patients who are discharged should be advised to return in the event of abdominal pain or vomiting.

The protocol for N-acetylcysteine infusion is as follows:

- 150mg/kg in 200mL of 5% dextrose over 15 minutes; then
- 50mg/kg in 500mL of dextrose over 4 hours; then
- 100mg/kg in 1 litre of dextrose over 16 hours

The effect is greatest in the first 8 hours and diminishes by 24 hours.

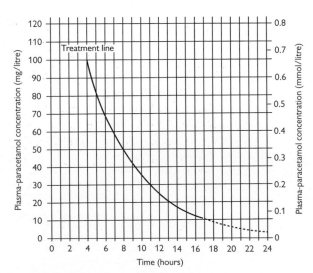

**Fig. 5.4** Treatment nomogram after paracetamol overdose.

This data is Crown Copyright and has been reproduced with the permission of the Medicines and Healthcare Products Regulatory Agency. You should contact this agency if you wish to reproduce or reuse this material.

Allergic (or anaphylactoid) reactions are common with N-acetylcysteine. They are managed by stopping the infusion, giving intravenous steroids and antihistamines, and then continuing N-acetylcysteine at a slower rate.

Methionine is an alternative antidote given orally at a dose of 2.5g. Repeated dosing at 4-hourly intervals to a maximum of 10g. If the patient is vomiting, absorption is unreliable.

It is of utmost importance to remember that if this management fails to prevent fulminant hepatic necrosis, the only life-saving treatment is liver transplantation. It is better to contact a liver transplant centre early. Indications for liver transplantation include:

- Acidosis (pH <7.3), or
- A combination of raised PT, renal failure, and encephalopathy.

# 5.8 Salicylate poisoning

## Background

Salicylate poisoning most commonly results from the ingestion of aspirin. The condition is common, with moderate to severe toxicity in adults occurring after ingestion of 15g (or 50 tablets).

Salicylates are also to be found in:

- Oil of wintergreen (contains methylsalicylate). This is particularly toxic when ingested orally due to rapid absorption. One teaspoonful is equivalent to 3.6g of aspirin.
- Keratolytic agents such as salicylic acid.

Aspirin is absorbed rapidly from the gastrointestinal tract when taken at low doses. Tablets can, however, adhere to form a bolus, which slows absorption. The result is that blood salicylate levels may continue to rise for up to 24 hours following a significant overdose. Features of toxicity occur when the blood salicylate level exceeds 250mg/L.

## Clinical features

The most important factors are patient age and the quantity of tablets taken. In adults, a characteristic sequence of events occurs with a respiratory alkalosis (due to stimulation of the respiratory centre) followed later by a metabolic acidosis. In children, the development of a metabolic acidosis is more rapid and, in the under-fives, a preceding respiratory alkalosis is rare.

Presenting features include restlessness, confusion, pyrexia, hyperventilation, and sweats. This progresses to severe vomiting with epigastric pain, tinnitus, and deafness. Fulminant toxicity manifests with coma (due to cerebral oedema), seizures, and adult respiratory distress syndrome (ARDS), and eventually leads to death.

Metabolic effects that accompany these symptoms include:

- Hypokalaemia and hyper- or hyponatraemia.
- Respiratory alkalosis (in adults) followed by metabolic acidosis.
- Dehydration.
- Deranged blood sugars (high or low).
- Hypoprothrombinaemia.
- Renal failure.

## Pathogenesis

Respiratory alkalosis results from direct stimulation of the respiratory centre. This is compensated for by the urinary excretion of bicarbonate together with sodium, potassium, and water. Eventually a metabolic acidosis ensues associated with dehydration and electrolyte depletion.

Salicylates result in the uncoupling of oxidative phosphorylation and inhibition of Kreb cycle enzymes. As lactate and pyruvate levels rise, so does the severity of acidosis. Changes in fat and protein metabolism lead to the production of ketones and the urinary excretion of amino acids.

## Investigations

- U&E and glucose.
- FBC.
- Clotting—prolonged PT.
- Arterial blood gases (ABGs)—to show the extent of acidosis (respiratory/metabolic) or hypoxia (lung damage).
- Plasma salicylate levels—samples should be taken early and repeated at 4-hourly intervals up to 24 hours post-ingestion. Plasma levels in the adult (in mg/L) can be interpreted as follows:
  - Therapeutic range: 150–250.
  - Mild poisoning: 250–500.
  - Moderate poisoning: 500–750.
  - Severe poisoning: >750.
- CXR: ARDS and pulmonary oedema.

## Management

- Gastric lavage is declining in popularity and lacks an evidence base but should be considered up to 24 hours after ingestion.
- 50g of activated charcoal.
- Replace fluid and electrolyte losses.
- Correct hypoglycaemia.
- Correct clotting abnormalities with vitamin K.
- Monitor fluid balance (input/output charts, urinary catheter).
- Monitor CVP due to risk of pulmonary oedema.

Further management is dependent on the degree of poisoning:

- Mild poisoning: the initial management should be sufficient.
- Moderate poisoning: administration of sodium bicarbonate to produce an alkaline diuresis. This promotes the ionization of salicylates in the urine and increases their rate of elimination. Carbonic anhydrase inhibitors should not be used and may increase mortality by exacerbating the pre-existing metabolic acidosis.
- Severe poisoning: requires haemodialysis and intermittent positive pressure ventilation (IPPV) in an ICU setting.

# 5.9 Lithium toxicity

## Background

Adverse effects are seen relatively frequently, even if blood levels are closely monitored, owing to the low therapeutic index of lithium.

Side effects occurring within the therapeutic range include weakness, a fine tremor (common), nausea, polydipsia, and polyuria. Usually these are not dangerous, but occasionally can indicate the onset of acute lithium toxicity.

Lithium levels in the desired therapeutic range can also produce hypothyroidism (sometimes with thyroid enlargement), ECG abnormalities, skin rashes, a diabetes insipidus-like state, and osteoporotic changes in bone. Some patients report a metallic taste in the mouth.

Acute lithium toxicity occurs when levels exceed 1.4mmol/L. The toxic syndrome is characterized by anorexia, vomiting, diarrhoea, cerebellar signs, confusion, and seizures. This may progress to a state of hyper-reflexia and increased tone and eventually to coma and irreversible neurological damage.

Long-term lithium use can also lead to interstitial nephritis and renal failure (Fig. 5.5).

Circumstances where the patient is particularly at risk of developing a toxic reaction include:

- Dehydration—exacerbated by hot weather, diarrhoeal illness, or excessive physical activity. Lithium treatment should be stopped if dehydration is severe.
- Renal failure.
- Elderly.
- Natriuretic drugs (e.g. diuretics).
- Drugs reducing lithium excretion (e.g. ACE inhibitors and NSAIDs).

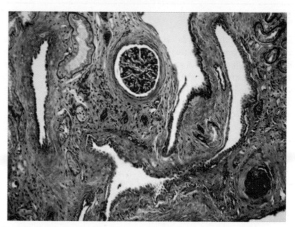

**Fig. 5.5** A renal biopsy from a 60-year-old patient treated with lithium for many years. This demonstrates tubular atrophy, interstitial fibrosis, and chronic inflammation (haematoxylin & eosin stain × 200).

Reprinted by permission from Macmillan Publishers Ltd: *Kidney International*, Alexander MP et al., 'Lithium toxicity: A double-edged sword', 73, 2 © 2007.

## Management

- Withhold lithium.
- Fluid resuscitation and correction of electrolyte abnormalities.
- Dialysis in severe toxicity.
- General supportive measures (e.g. treat seizures).

# 5.10 Digoxin toxicity

## Background

Digoxin (a cardiac glycoside) is a naturally occurring compound found in leaves of plants of the foxglove family. Acute overdose with digoxin is uncommon, despite its widespread use in the treatment of cardiac arrhythmias and heart failure. Nevertheless, digoxin toxicity is common due to its low therapeutic index. Toxicity can occur within the 'therapeutic range' —elderly patients being particularly at risk. Above concentrations of 2µg/L, toxicity is common and almost invariable > 3µg/L.

Factors that increase the risk of toxicity include:

- Hypokalaemia (digoxin competes with extracellular potassium when binding to its target, the $Na^+/K^+$-ATPase; Fig. 5.6).
- Hypomagnesaemia.
- Hypercalcaemia—digoxin increase intracellular calcium levels.
- Hyperkalaemia—exacerbates AV block.
- Renal impairment.

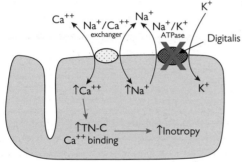

**Fig. 5.6** Mechanism of digoxin action in cardiac myocytes. Digoxin inhibits the $Na^+/K^+$-ATPase leading to a rise in intracellular $Na^+$ and a secondary rise in intracellular $Ca^{2+}$ (due to impaired $Na^+/Ca^{2+}$ exchange). Intracellular $Ca^{2+}$ binds to troponin C (TN-C) activating myocyte contraction (increased inotropy).
Reproduced with permission from Richard E. Klabunde, PhD (www.cvphysiology.com).

- Elderly.
- Hypoxia and acidosis (in combination).
- Hypothyroidism.

## Clinical features

- Arrhythmia (Box 5.1).
- Reduced appetite, nausea, and vomiting.
- Confusion (in the elderly).
- Yellow vision (xanthopsia), blurred vision, and photophobia.

## Management

Mild toxicity (e.g. nausea, ectopics) is managed conservatively:

- Withhold digoxin for several days.
- Oral potassium supplements if necessary.

Serious toxicity (e.g. persistent nausea with vomiting, significant arrhythmia, or heart failure) is managed initially with:

- Intravenous potassium (with cardiac monitoring).
- Intravenous magnesium (myocardial protection).
- Activated oral charcoal (consider).

If first-line treatment for digoxin toxicity fails, the treatment of choice is digoxin-specific Fab (DSFab) therapy:

- These are biologically active fragments of antibodies that inactivate digoxin.
- The response can be rapid with initial effects seen within 30 minutes.
- The dose of DSFab is calculated according to dose ingested or plasma concentration of digoxin.

Other treatments:

- Atropine—for bradyarrhythmias.
- Temporary pacing for persistent heart block.
- DC cardioversion—indicated in cases of life-threatening arrhythmia.

---

### Box 5.1 ECG changes associated with digoxin use

ST depression and T-wave inversion in V5–V6 in a reversed tick pattern (Fig. 5.7)—seen with plasma levels within the therapeutic range. Changes are more extensive in digoxin toxicity and include:

- Bradycardia.
- Prolonged PR.
- Shortened QT.
- Arrhythmias—the most common arrhythmias are ventricular extrasystoles, ventricular bigeminy/trigeminy, and atrial tachycardia with complete heart block.

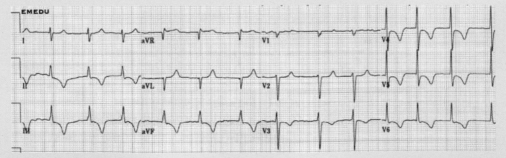

**Fig. 5.7** ECG showing reversed tick pattern due to digoxin effect.
© EMEDU. Reproduced with permission.

# 5.11 Carbon monoxide poisoning

## Background

Carbon monoxide (CO) is a colourless, odourless gas produced when carbon or organic fuels are burnt in a limited supply of oxygen. Cases of CO toxicity are mostly due to:

- Car exhaust fumes.
- Fuel combustion in an inadequate flue such as a blocked domestic boiler.

## Clinical features

- Headache is the most common complaint seen in 90% of cases.
- Vertigo in 50%.
- Nausea and vomiting in ~1/2 cases, which may mimic a viral gastroenteritis.
- Altered consciousness in ~1/3 cases.
- Subjective 'flu-like' weakness in ~1/5.

The absence of cyanosis is explained by the fact that carboxyhae-moglobin (COHb) has a deceptive pink colouration in the skin and mucous membranes.

Exposure to high concentrations of CO can result in:

- Acute confusional state.
- Cardiac toxicity with tachyarrhythmias and myocardial ischaemia.
- Neurological impairment with cerebellar ataxia, hemiplegia, parkinsonism, mutism, unconsciousness, and coma.
- Cherry red skin colouration is rarely seen and occurs when COHb concentrations exceed 20%.

CO is produced when the oxidation of carbon is incomplete. Following inspiration it diffuses rapidly into the bloodstream where its affinity for haemoglobin is 240 times greater than that of oxygen. COHb is, there-fore, formed preferentially and dissociates much less readily than oxy-haemoglobin. As a consequence, the oxygen-carrying capacity of the blood is reduced. The rate of dissociation of COHb can be increased sixfold if 100% oxygen is administered. An additional feature of CO toxicity is a leftward shift in the oxyhaemoglobin dissociation curve, i.e. interference with the unloading of oxygen (Fig. 5.8). CO binds avidly to other compounds containing the haem moiety. Interference with the intracellular cytochrome electron chain results in 'sick cell syndrome'. When bound CO dissociates from the chain, usually some 24 hours after exposure, a post-intoxication encephalopathy can ensue.

Clues to the diagnosis include:

- Several people in the same house affected.
- Improvement in symptoms when away from the house, e.g. when on holiday.
- Symptoms exacerbated in winter when boiler use increases.
- Symptoms related to use of gas cooker.
- Soot marks around fires, boilers, and stoves.
- Gas appliances burning with sooty yellow flames.
- Smoke accumulation due to faulty flues (although CO is odour-less, other combustion products have a smell).

## Investigations

- It is possible to measure CO levels in expired air although levels quickly subside as the subject is removed from the source.

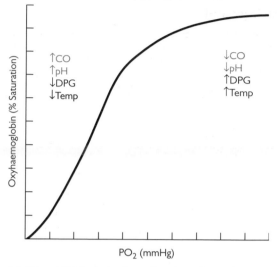

**Fig. 5.8** Effect of CO (and other factors) on the oxyhaemoglobin dissociation curve.

- Measure blood levels of CO—a level >5% suggests inhalation, but levels do not accurately predict poisoning severity.
- Pulse oximetry is not recommended because falsely high oxygen saturations occur due to the similar light absorbance of oxyhae-moglobin and COHb.

## Management

- Remove patient from CO source.
- Fit a tight mask and deliver 100% oxygen.
- Monitor COHb levels with serial ABGs. As a guide, COHb levels of:
  - 20% cause headache.
  - 40% cause lethargy and confusion.
  - 60% cause death.
- Give mannitol and dexamethasone in cases of cerebral oedema.
- Correct acid–base disturbances and provide other general sup-portive measures.
- Exclude cyanide poisoning in those exposed to house fires.
- Hyperbaric oxygen should be considered if COHb levels exceed 20%. Base this decision on:
  - Conscious level.
  - Neurological signs.
  - ECG changes indicating ischaemia or arrhythmia.
  - Pregnancy.

Hyperbaric oxygen decreases the half-life of COHb and there is some evidence that in severe CO poisoning it can reduce neurologi-cal and cognitive impairment.

# 5.12 Ethylene glycol poisoning

## Background

Ethylene glycol is a solvent found in products ranging from anti-freeze fluid and de-icing solutions to carpet and fabric cleaners. As little as 30mL of ethylene glycol can be fatal in adults. However, when treated appropriately, patients have survived much larger ingestions.

The primary pathology is metabolic acidosis (with an increased anion gap; Fig. 5.9) leading to acute renal failure. Death is uncommon in persons who receive prompt diagnosis and treatment.

Ingestion may be deliberate but usually it is taken accidentally as an ethanol 'substitute'. Ethylene glycol exerts its effects by the accumulation of toxic metabolites (aldehydes, glycolates, oxalates, and lactates) which can be prevented by blocking the initial degradative step catalysed by alcohol dehydrogenase.

## Clinical features

- Initially, vomiting, polyuria, and decreased level of consciousness ('inebriation' but without alcohol on the breath).
- Fits and focal neurological signs (e.g. ophthalmoplegias) are seen in the first 24 hours.

Anion gap: $Na - (Cl + HCO_3) = 12mM$

| Cations | Anions |
|---|---|
| Na = 140mM | Cl (104mM) |
| | Albumin, $SO_4$, $PO_4$ |
| K, Ca, Mg | $HCO_3$ (24mM) |

**Fig. 5.9** Calculation and normal constituents of the plasma anion gap. Some authorities calculate the anion gap as $(Na + K) - (Cl + HCO_3)$. Ethylene glycol poisoning increases the anion gap due to the generation of organic acid metabolites.

- Loin pain, haematuria, and acute tubular necrosis appear over the next 48 hours.

Late complications include oliguric renal failure (due to calcium oxalate crystal nephropathy; Fig. 5.10), cerebral oedema, and cardiovascular collapse. Non-cardiogenic pulmonary oedema and myocarditis have occasionally been described.

## Prognostic features

- Ethylene glycol is often taken with ethanol. This is actually protective, as it blocks the metabolism of ethylene glycol to its toxic metabolites.
- Renal failure may be averted if specific treatment is instituted early enough. Plasma levels of ethylene glycol (if available) may be useful in indicating severe overdose (>500mg/L = 8mM).
- Degree of acidosis is probably the best indicator of likely outcome.

## Management

- Gastric lavage is declining in popularity and is not routinely indicated. Nevertheless, it enables confirmation that ethylene glycol has been taken (commercial 'antifreeze' often contains fluorescein which is easily detected with a UV light source; also detectable in urine).
- Monitor plasma $Na^+$, $K^+$, $Cl^-$, $HCO_3^-$ allowing calculation of the anion gap (Fig. 5.9).
- Examine by microscopy a fresh urine sample looking for the needle-shaped crystals of calcium oxalate monohydrate (a pathognomonic sign).
- The half-life of ethylene glycol is short (3 hours) so, to prevent significant metabolism, an ethanol infusion should be started as soon as possible. The infusion should be continued until plasma ethylene glycol is undetectable.
- An alternative to ethanol infusion is the alcohol dehydrogenase inhibitor **fomepizole**.
- Haemodialysis is indicated for severe acidosis, declining vital signs, concentration >500mg/L, or oliguria. Haemo- or peritoneal dialysis may be used (the former is two- to threefold more effective). Normal renal function is generally restored in 7–10 days although permanent impairment has been reported.

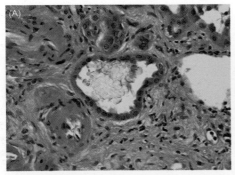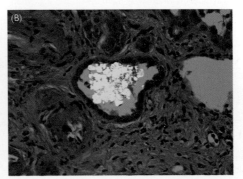

**Fig. 5.10** Oxalate crystals within a dilated renal tubule under normal light microscopy (A) demonstrate birefringence under polarized light (B) (both haematoxylin & eosin stain × 400).

'Calcium oxalate crystals in acute ethylene glycol: A confocal laser scanning microscope study in a fatal case', Pomara C, Fiore C, D'Errico S, *et al. Journal of Toxicology-Clinical Toxicology*, 2008, Taylor & Francis, reprinted by the permission of the publisher (Taylor & Francis Group, http://www.informaworld.com)

# 5.13 Tricyclic antidepressant poisoning

## Background

The ingestion of around 10mg/kg of tricyclic antidepressant (TCA) leads to mild–moderate poisoning, with severe poisoning occurring when ingestion exceeds 15–20mg/kg.

Ingestion of <1g rarely results in death.

Symptoms appear within 30–60 minutes of ingestion, reaching their peak intensity within 4–12 hours.

## Clinical features

These partly resemble those of cholinergic inhibition due to the interaction of TCAs with muscarinic receptors:

- Dilated pupils
- Sinus tachycardia
- Drowsiness
- Urinary retention
- Dry mouth
- Increased tendon reflexes
- Extensor plantar responses

In fulminant cases, death ensues from cardiac arrhythmias, seizures, or coma.

## Management

- Gastric lavage is theoretically useful up to 12 hours post-ingestion as TCAs delay gastric emptying.
- Activated charcoal—useful to reduce absorption in patients who present within 24 hours.
- ECG monitoring—cardiac monitoring is essential because of the risk of broad complex arrhythmias (Table 5.4). In general, anti-arrhythmic drugs should be avoided.
- Fluid resuscitation—required to correct hypotension. If insufficient to normalize blood pressure then inotropic support is indicated.

| Table 5.4 ECG changes associated with tricyclic antidepressant poisoning |
| --- |
| Non-specific ST or T wave changes |
| Prolongation of QT interval |
| Prolongation of PR interval |
| Prolongation of QRS interval |
| Right bundle branch block |
| Right axis deviation |
| AV block |
| Brugada wave (ST elevation in V1–V3 and right bundle branch block) |

Source: Thanacoody HK, Thomas SH. Tricyclic antidepressant poisoning: cardiovascular toxicity. *Toxicol Rev* 2005; 24: 205–14.

- Correction of hypoxia and acidosis.
- Check levels of paracetamol and salicylate to exclude combination overdose.

Factors associated with increased likelihood of major toxicity following tricyclic overdose are:

- ingestion of amitriptyline
- age ≥ 30 years
- heart rate ≥ 120bpm
- serum tricyclic antidepressant level ≥ 800ng/mL (highest odds ratio of 5.2)
- QRS interval ≥ 100ms
- QRS axis > 90 degrees
- QTc interval > 480ms
- A small number of trials support the use of TCA antibody fragments (TCA Fab).

As only a small fraction of drug is sequestered in the vascular compartment, haemoperfusion and haemodialysis are ineffective.

# Chapter 6

# Dermatology

# 6.1 Eczema/dermatitis

## Background

The terms eczema and dermatitis are used interchangeably to describe a chronic inflammatory disease affecting the skin. Several subsets of eczema are described:

- Atopic eczema
- Discoid eczema
- Seborrhoeic eczema
- Pompholyx eczema
- Varicose eczema
- Asteatotic eczema
- Contact dermatitis

## Atopic eczema

### Epidemiology

- Prevalence—20% of children are affected in the UK. It becomes less common in adulthood
- Age of onset—50% of patients are affected by 6 months and 90% by 1 year of age

### Aetiology

The pathophysiology of atopic eczema (AE) is not fully understood

- Genetic factors—there is a strong genetic component as 70% of patients have a family history of atopic disease. Twin studies show concordance rates of 77% in monozygotic twins and 15% in dizygotic twins. Inheritance is polygenic, with several genes relating to skin barrier function and inflammatory cytokines implicated. Recently, loss-of-function mutations in the *Filaggrin* gene have been shown to be a major risk factor for AE, particularly in northern European populations
- Immune dysfunction—Th2 CD4+ lymphocytes are involved in atopic responses through the release of IL-4, -5, and -13 which signal B cells to produce IgE
- Environmental factors—lack of exposure to infections during childhood may result in a shift of immune responses that follow a Th2-mediated pathway and thus favour atopy (the 'hygiene hypothesis'). Animal dander, food allergens, stress, and woollen clothing may precipitate or exacerbate AE

### Clinical features

*History*

- Itchy erythematous patches
- Distribution is characteristic and varies with age. Predominantly on flexural sites at most ages
- Remitting and relapsing course

*Examination*

- Poorly defined erythematous patches with fine scale
- Symmetrically distributed in flexures but can occur anywhere (Fig. 6.1)
- Excoriations from scratching
- In the acute state, the skin may be oedematous and lesions may be moist and crusted
- In the chronic state, repeated rubbing produces skin thickening with exaggerated skin markings—lichenification
- Post-inflammatory hypo- or hyperpigmentation particularly in pigmented skin
- Nail pitting may be seen
- Skin is generally dry and xerotic

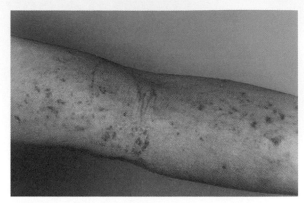

Fig. 6.1 Classical eczema affecting flexoral aspect of arm.

### Complications

- Bacterial sepsis produces crusting and pustules. The skin is said to be impetiginized. Antibiotics should cover *Staphylococcus*, *Streptococcus*, and occasionally *Pseudomonus* (all known to be causative agents)
- Eczema herpeticum (Kaposi varicelliform eruption; Fig. 6.2) secondary to infection with herpes simplex virus is a serious complication and requires prompt treatment with aciclovir
- Molluscum contagiosum is more common
- Conjunctival irritation, keratoconjunctivitis, and cataracts
- Retarded growth may be seen in patients with poorly controlled chronic disease

### Treatment

AE can have a huge impact on the quality of life of both the patient and their family. Parents need education and support about how to manage the disease.

*Conservative measures*

- Avoid known irritants
- Dietary manipulation with the assistance of a dietician

*Topical treatments*

- Bath oils and soap substitutes
- Emollients
- Corticosteroids (Box 6.1)

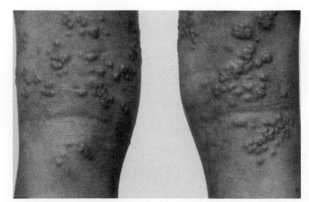

Fig. 6.2 Eczema herpeticum.

| Box 6.1  Classification of topical steroids | |
|---|---|
| Mild | 1% hydrocortisone |
| Moderately potent | 0.05% clobetasone butyrate |
| Potent | 0.1% betamethasone valerate |
| Very potent | 0.05% clobetasol propionate |

- Immunomodulators—tacrolimus and pimecrolimus are second-line alternatives to potent steroids. Unlike topical steroids they do not cause atrophy and hypopigmentation, but may cause localized irritation when first used
- Zinc and paste bandages

*Second-line agents*

- Ultraviolet light phototherapy
- Severe flares may require short courses of prednisolone
- Systemic immunosuppression with azathioprine or ciclosporin is used for resistant disease
- Sedating antihistamines help with poor sleep

**Prognosis**

90% of children are clear of disease by their teenage years.

# Discoid eczema

Well-demarcated, crusted, coin-shaped patches which show similar morphology to AE. Discoid eczema is more common in adults. Lesions frequently occur on the limbs and are prone to infection. The differential diagnosis includes psoriasis and early-stage mycosis fungoides. Emollients and topical steroids form the mainstay of treatment.

# Seborrhoeic eczema

This is caused by an abnormal immune response to the yeast *Pityrosporum ovale*, also called *Malassezia furfur*. It is characterized by redness and scaling in areas with active sebaceous glands such as the scalp and face, presternal area, axillae, groin, and glans penis. In babies it presents as cradle cap. Seborrhoeic dermatitis is more common in adults with Parkinson disease and HIV infection. Treatment is with a mild topical steroid combined with a topical antifungal such as miconazole. Topical tacrolimus is also effective and ketoconazole shampoo is used for scalp disease.

# Pompholyx eczema

Pompholyx eczema is confined to the hands and feet. Pruritic small vesicles or bullae develop on the palms, soles, and sides of the fingers. The fingertips may become scaly and fissured. An irritant or allergic contact dermatitis should be excluded. Occasionally a fungal infection at a distant site causes a similar vesicular eruption, the 'id reaction' and this too should be excluded. Treatment is with emollients and topical steroids. Resistant cases may need PUVA phototherapy.

# Varicose eczema

Varicose (or gravitational) eczema is associated with chronic venous disease and occurs on the legs. Other signs of venous disease may be present such as varicose veins, ulceration, haemosiderin deposition, venous flare, and atrophy blanche. In addition to treating the eczema with emollients and topical steroids, compression bandaging and hosiery will help the underlying venous disease.

# Asteatotic eczema

Asteatotic eczema is seen in the elderly and is related to frequent use of soaps and the low relative humidity in heated homes. Cracked and fissured skin is seen predominantly on the dorsum of the hands and lower legs. Patients should avoid soap, use liberal emollients for the xerosis, and topical steroids for the eczematous component.

# Contact dermatitis

Irritant and allergic contact dermatitis are exogenous forms of eczema. Diagnosis relies on a detailed history, focusing on occupation, hobbies, and exposure to chemicals and metals.

- Allergic contact dermatitis is a type IV delayed hypersensitivity reaction. With repeated exposure, susceptible individuals become sensitized and a dermatitis results after each exposure to the allergen. Common allergens include nickel, chromate in cement, perfumes, and plants. Allergens can be identified by patch testing
- Irritant contact dermatitis is caused by direct irritation. It can affect anyone at any site. Detergents and soaps are common culprits

In both cases the causative agent needs to be excluded. Emollients and topical steroids are used to treat the eczematous component.

# 6.2 Psoriasis

## Epidemiology

- Prevalence 1–2%
- ♂ = ♀
- Affects all races
- Common onset in young adults (although second peak between years of 50–60 reported)

## Aetiology/pathogenesis

- Polygenic, multifactorial disease
- A number of susceptibility genes (e.g. *PSORS1* gene on chromosome 6p21)
- 73% concordance in monozygotic twins compared with 27% in dizygotic twins
- Trigger factors include:
  - Physical trauma (Koebner phenomenon)
  - Infection (streptococcal)
  - Stress
  - Drugs (β-blockers, lithium, antimalarials)
  - Alcohol
  - Smoking
- More severe/atypical in HIV-infected individuals
- T-cell mediated disease with upregulation of Th1 cytokines such as IL-2, IFN-α, and TNF-α
- Characterized by epidermal hyperproliferation and increased angiogenesis

## Clinical evaluation

### History
- Plaques are usually asymptomatic though they may be itchy

### Examination
- Symmetrical, well-demarcated, red plaques with a thick, silvery-white scale, most common on the scalp and extensor surfaces (in psoriasis vulgaris), although they may appear anywhere on the body (Fig. 6.3)
- Auspitz sign—tiny bleeding points when scratched

- Nail signs include pitting (Fig. 6.4), onycholysis, oil-drop sign (yellow-brown spot under nail plate), subungual hyperkeratosis
- Associated arthropathy:
  - Symmetrical polyarthritis
  - Asymmetric oligoarthritis
  - Distal interphalangeal joint arthritis
  - Ankylosing spondylitis-like
  - Arthritis mutilans

### Investigations
- None usually required as diagnosis is clinical
- Skin biopsy shows regular acanthosis with parakeratosis, suprapapillary thinning, dilated capillaries in papillary dermis, and neutrophil microabscesses in epidermis
- Baseline blood tests if planning systemic treatment

## Classification

### Psoriasis vulgaris
- Chronic plaque type
- Subacute/acute—bright-red, tender, inflamed plaques
- Erythrodermic—>90% body surface area coverage

### Pustular psoriasis
1. Localized:
   - Palmoplantar:
     - More common in ♀.
     - Associated with smoking.
     - Characterized by sterile yellow-brown pustules on an erythematous background.
   - Acrodermatitis continua of Hallopeau:
     - Rare.
     - Sterile pustules on a digit associated with involvement of the nail.
     - Can slowly extend proximally.
2. Generalized (Fig. 6.5):
   - Pustular psoriasis of Von Zumbusch:
     - Sheets of sterile pustules on a background of painful erythema.
     - Occur in waves, exfoliating as they dry.
     - Unwell patient, generally with fever.

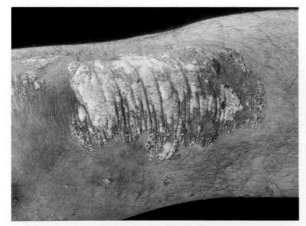

**Fig. 6.3** Classical chronic plaque psoriasis on extensor aspect of knee.

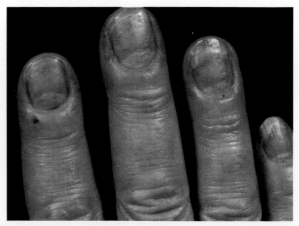

**Fig. 6.4** Nail pitting associated with psoriasis.

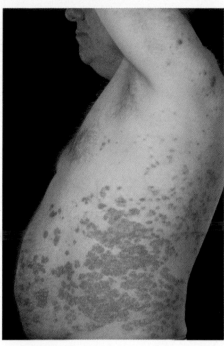

**Fig. 6.5** Generalized pustular psoriasis.
Reproduced with permission from Cambridge University Hospitals NHS Foundation Trust.

### Guttate psoriasis
- Small plaques affecting trunk and limbs, usually following a streptococcal sore throat

## Management

Factors to consider in choosing therapeutic option include type and severity of psoriasis, previous treatments, patient expectations, practicality of treatment, and comorbidity.

### Therapeutic options
- Topical:
  - Emollients.
  - Vitamin D analogues (e.g. calcipotriol)—avoid face and flexures.
  - Topical corticosteroids (for face and flexures).
  - Dithranol (but causes staining of skin and clothes).
  - Coal tar preparations (but messy and cause staining).
  - Topical retinoids (e.g. tazarotene).
- Phototherapy:
  - PUVA.
  - UVB/TLO-1 (narrowband UVB).
- Systemic agents: options include: methotrexate, acitretin, ciclosporin, hydroxycarbamide, and fumarates
- Combination therapy as well as rotation may be tried
- Palmoplantar variant may be treated with superpotent topical steroids ± coal tar, localized PUVA, or systemic agents (severe cases)
- Biological agents: in severe, unresponsive cases, options include etanercept, infliximab, ustekinumab, and adalimumab

## Outcome/prognosis

- Chronic plaque psoriasis is a lifelong condition but the majority of patients get intermittent remissions
- Guttate psoriasis usually clears up within 6–8 weeks but may recur or progress to chronic plaque psoriasis

## Erythroderma

This is characterized by >90% involvement of body surface area, and can be life-threatening.

### Causes of erythroderma
- Idiopathic
- Psoriasis
- Eczema
- Drugs
- Cutaneous lymphoma
- Pityriasis rubra pilaris
- Others (including paraneoplastic, HIV, immunobullous, e.g. pemphigus foliaceus)

### Complications
- Loss of thermoregulation
- Fluid loss leading to hypovolaemia
- Protein loss, iron deficiency
- Sepsis (skin, chest)
- High-output cardiac failure
- Thromboembolic disease

### Management
- Usually requires hospital admission and close monitoring
- Prevention and treatment of hypothermia, fluid and electrolyte imbalance, sepsis, and other complications
- Skin biopsy may be required to confirm underlying diagnosis
- Regular, topical, greasy emollients
- Treatment of underlying disorder (e.g. systemic agents: methotrexate for psoriasis, avoid phototherapy)

# 6.3 Blistering skin disorders

## Pemphigus

The term is derived from the Greek word pemphix meaning blister. It refers to a group of autoimmune blistering conditions affecting the skin and mucous membranes, characterized by acantholysis (loss of intracellular connections causing disruption to tissue integrity) and intraepidermal blistering. The main subtypes are:

- Pemphigus vulgaris
- Pemphigus foliaceus
- Paraneoplastic pemphigus
- IgA pemphigus

Drug-induced cases have also been reported (Box 6.2)

## Pemphigus vulgaris

### Epidemiology

- Accounts for 75% of all cases of pemphigus
- Annual incidence: 0.5–3.2/100,000 population
- Peak incidence: 40–60 years old (although all ages, including children and adolescents, may be affected)
- ♂ and ♀ equally affected

---

**Box 6.2  Causes of blistering skin disorders**

Inherited
- Epidermolysis bullosa (simplex, junctional, dystrophic)
- Incontinentia pigmenti
- Hailey–Hailey disease

Acquired
1. Autoimmune:
   - Intra-epidermal:
     - Pemphigus
   - Subepidermal:
     - Bullous pemphigoid
     - Mucous membrane pemphigoid
     - Pemphigoid gestationis
     - Dermatitis herpetiformis
     - Linear IgA disease
     - Epidermolysis bullosa acquisita
2. Infections:
   - Viral:
     - Herpes simplex
     - Varicella zoster
   - Bacterial:
     - Staphylococcal (cellulitis, impetigo, scalded skin syndrome)
3. Physical causes:
   - Friction, radiation, burns, chemical burns, electrical injury
4. Metabolic:
   - Diabetes
   - Porphyria
   - Amyloid
5. Others:
   - Acute contact dermatitis
   - Erythema multiforme/Stevens–Johnson syndrome/toxic epidermal necrolysis/drug reactions
   - Insect bite reaction

---

- Affects all races although more frequent in Ashkenazi Jews and Mediterranean races. There is a younger age of onset in patients from the Indian subcontinent

### Aetiology/pathogenesis

- Autoimmune disorder with antibodies against desmosomal proteins: desmoglein 3 ± desmoglein 1, leading to acantholysis
- Genetic background—increased frequency in certain races
- Association with other autoimmune conditions such as rheumatoid arthritis and pernicious anaemia
- HLA association: HLA-DR4, HLA-DR14

### Clinical evaluation

*History*
- Often starts with mucosal involvement only. Painful erosions affecting oral mucosa in up to 70% of cases. Epistaxis, hoarseness, dysphagia, and weight loss (due to reduced oral intake) may occur
- Cutaneous lesions are usually painful rather than pruritic

*Examination*
- Mucosal blisters which rapidly **rupture** leading to painful erosions
- May affect oral mucosa, pharynx, larynx, oesophagus, eyes, nasal mucosa, and anogenital mucosa
- Flaccid skin blisters that rupture easily leaving erosions. May be localized or generalized (Fig. 6.6)
- Most commonly involved sites include the scalp, face, flexures, trunk, and any pressure points
- **Nikolsky** sign positive (firm lateral pressure with a finger to areas of normal-looking skin produces a blister/erosion)
- Rarely, nails may be involved, with onycholysis, dystrophy and periungual bullae

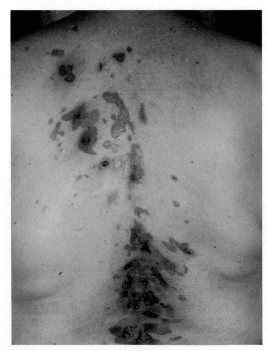

**Fig. 6.6** Pemphigus Vulgaris.

*Investigations*
- Skin biopsy (H&E staining) shows:
  - Suprabasal blistering with acantholysis.
  - Inflammatory infiltrate with eosinophils.

*Definitive diagnosis*

Direct immunofluorescence demonstrating intercellular staining with IgG (anti-desmoglein autoantobodies) and C3 in the epidermis on perilesional skin biopsy
- Serum: circulating autoantibodies (anti-desmoglein 3 ± anti-desmoglein 1 on ELISA, ANCA)

**Management**
- **Corticosteroids**: high-dose oral corticosteroids (60–100mg/day prednisolone) are the mainstay of treatment. Pulsed IV methylprednisolone may be required
- Adjuvant **immunosuppressive** therapy: including azathioprine, methotrexate, cyclophosphamide, mycophenolate mofetil, IVIG, and rituximab

**Outcome/prognosis**
- Prior to the introduction of corticosteroids, this was a progressive and almost invariably fatal condition
- Current mortality is ~5–10%, usually due to sepsis (cutaneous, respiratory), thromboembolism, or complications of treatment
- Treatment may need to be life-long, although ~75% may be able to stop treatment after 10 years

# Pemphigus foliaceus

- Characterized by more superficial blistering in the epidermis and associated with predominance of antibodies against desmoglein 1
- Least severe type of pemphigus
- Often starts on the scalp and does not involve the oral mucosa

# Paraneoplastic pemphigus

- Commonly-associated malignancies include: lymphoma (non-Hodgkin and CLL), thymoma and Castleman disease (tumours in lymph node tissue)
- Mucosal involvement is often severe and resistant to treatment

# Drug-induced pemphigus

- Clinically, most closely resembles pemphigus foliaceus
- Penicillamine and captopril are the most common causes

# Bullous pemphigoid

Bullous pemphigoid (BP) is a chronic, autoimmune, subepidermal, blistering skin disease that rarely involves mucous membranes.

**Epidemiology**
- Relatively common condition
- Peak age of onset 60–80 years although cases have been reported even in children
- ♂ and ♀ equally affected
- No racial predilection reported

**Aetiology/pathogenesis**

Autoantibodies against a 230kDa and 180kDa (BP antigens 1 and 2) protein in the hemidesmosomes at the basement membrane probably play an aetiological role in this condition.

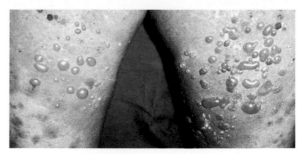

Fig. 6.7 Bullous pemphigoid.

**Clinical evaluation**

*History*
- Often a prodromal urticarial eruption that subsequently blisters
- May be extremely pruritic

*Examination*
- Tense **intact** blisters usually arising on an urticated erythematous background (Fig. 6.7). Straw-coloured or haemorrhagic
- May be localized or generalized
- Erosions and crusting may develop
- A rare variant called mucous membrane pemphigoid affects mucosae and causes scarring

*Investigations*
- Skin biopsy (H&E): subepidermal blister, chronic inflammatory infiltrate with prominent eosinophils
- Direct IF: basement membrane zone staining with IgG and C3
- Serum: circulating autoantibodies (IgG) to basement membrane zone in 70% of cases

*Management*
- Oral prednisolone (30–60mg/day)
- Adjuvant immunosuppressive therapy (e.g. azathioprine, methotrexate, or mycophenolate mofetil) sometimes necessary
- Tetracyclines plus nicotinamide may be helpful (anti-inflammatory properties) for control of milder cases
- Topical highly-potent corticosteroids have been reported to control less severe cases

*Outcome /prognosis*
- Patients often go into permanent remission and treatment may be withdrawn after 2–3 years
- Local recurrences may be controlled with topical corticosteroids

# Dermatitis herpetiformis

Dermatitis herpetiformis (DH) is a chronic, recurrent, intensely pruritic eruption occurring symmetrically in an extensor distribution, associated with a gluten-sensitive enteropathy.

**Epidemiology**
- Most common age of onset: 30–40 years (although can occur at any age)
- ♂:♀ = 2:1

**Aetiology /pathogenesis**

IgA-mediated disease, occurring in association with a gluten-sensitive enteropathy.

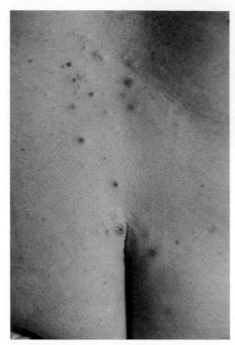

**Fig. 6.8** Dermatitis herpetiformis.
Reproduced with permission from Cambridge University Hospitals NHS Foundation Trust.

### Clinical evaluation

*History*

- Intense, episodic pruritus
- May have associated bowel symptoms although enteropathy is frequently asymptomatic

*Examination*

- Erythematous papules or vesicles in groups symmetrically distributed on extensor surfaces: elbows, knees, buttocks, scapular, and sacral areas most frequently affected (Fig. 6.8)
- Mostly excoriated so rare to see intact vesicles

*Investigations*

- Skin biopsy (H&E): subepidermal blisters with neutrophils and papillary tip microabscesses
- Direct IF: dermal staining with granular deposits of IgA
- Serum: anti-reticulin, endomysial or tissue transglutaminase antibodies may be present
- Anaemia (secondary to iron or folate deficiency)
- GI investigations for evidence of coeliac disease

*Management*

- Dapsone (associated with rapid, dramatic relief of symptoms)
- Gluten-free diet may allow withdrawal of dapsone, but can take several years to be effective for the skin lesions

*Outcome/prognosis*

Course is prolonged although some patients may have a spontaneous remission.

# 6.4 Bacterial and viral infections of the skin

## Erysipelas and cellulitis

These are acute bacterial infections of the dermis and subcutaneous tissues respectively, and may be associated with profound systemic disturbance.

### Aetiology

- Erysipelas is almost always caused by group A β-haemolytic *Streptococcus*, while cellulitis may be caused by *Streptococcus* or *Staphylococcus aureus*
- It may occur at any age, but elderly, alcoholics, and malnourished are particularly prone
- The point of entry of the infection may be a minor abrasion, surgery or fungal infection (e.g. tinea pedis)

### Clinical evaluation

- Abrupt onset of fever ± rigors associated with usually a unilateral erythema and oedema mostly affecting the face or leg (Fig. 6.9). Blistering and erosions may follow
- Patients can become unwell and complications include septicaemia and nephritis
- Inflammatory markers such as neutrophils, CRP, and ESR are elevated
- Skin swabs for microscopy and culture may help though they are often negative. Blood cultures should be taken if systemic upset is present

### Management

- Treatment with IV (or oral if mild infection) penicillin and flucloxacillin is usually very effective. Erythromycin is a suitable alternative (e.g. penicillin-allergic)
- Recurrent attacks can be prevented by using prophylactic low-dose penicillin
- If the portal of entry of the organism can be identified it may be worth treating (e.g. antifungal agents if tinea pedis present)

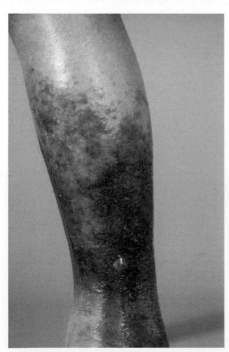

Fig. 6.9 Cellulitis.

## Necrotizing fasciitis

This is a rapidly advancing soft tissue infection with systemic toxicity and high mortality (also known in the popular press as 'flesh-eating bug').

### Aetiology

- It can be caused by a number of organisms, most often group A *Streptococci* and *Staphylococcus aureus*, but also anaerobic bacteria
- Predisposing factors include diabetes mellitus, immunosuppression, increasing age, underlying malignancy, and alcohol excess

### Clinical evaluation

- There is localized painful erythema progressing rapidly over a matter of hours to haemodynamic collapse with high fever
- Associated blistering and necrosis of the skin may occur, and these findings can affect any part of the body. In the early stages, there is an apparent disproportionate level of pain
- The diagnosis is clinical, although microbiology may help
- Aspiration of blister fluid may reveal streptococci on microscopy and tissue biopsy should be sent for culture
- CRP and ESR usually very elevated (CK may also be)

### Management

- Urgent aggressive surgical treatment with debridement of affected areas is indicated
- IV antibiotics such as penicillin, flucloxacillin, and metronidazole are required
- Supportive care possibly on an ICU or HDU required
- The mortality rate is quite high, but can be reduced by prompt diagnosis and intervention

## Viral warts

### Aetiology/epidemiology

- Very common, particularly in children and young adults
- Caused by human papilloma virus (HPV) infection, a DNA virus that causes squamous epithelial cell proliferation. There are >70 subtypes of HPV:
  - Palmar and plantar (common) warts are usually caused by HPV-1.
  - Mosaic warts: HPV-2.
  - Flat/plane warts: HPV-3.
  - Genital warts: HPV-6, -10, -11, -16, -18 (Fig. 6.10).
- HPV-16 and -18 have been implicated in malignant transformation in the cervix, vulva, and penis
- HPV-5 is associated with epidermodysplasia verruciformis, a rare autosomal recessive disorder characterized by widespread HPV infection and a predisposition to cutaneous squamous cell carcinoma
- Warts are contagious and spread through contact (especially if local trauma)

### Clinical evaluation

- **Common** warts: asymptomatic, discrete, flesh-coloured papules with a rough surface occurring anywhere (but particularly on the hands and feet)
- **Flat** warts: flesh-coloured, very slightly raised, well-defined, flat-topped lesions and can occur anywhere (but particularly the face and limbs). They exhibit Koebner phenomenon

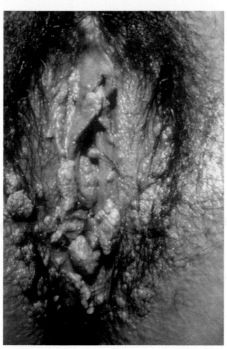

Fig. 6.10 Genital warts.

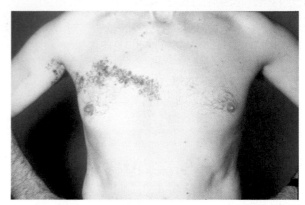

Fig. 6.11 Shingles.

- **Verrucae**: discrete lesions with a roughened surface on the feet. Can be painful. Paring with a scalpel usually reveals minute bleeding points and helps differentiate them from callosities
- **Mosaic** warts: plaques of roughened skin within which delineated individual warts are seen (usually on the soles)
- **Anogenital** warts: usually seen in adults and are sexually transmitted. They can be filiform, keratotic, or cauliflower-like (condylomata acuminata)

### Management

- Most resolve spontaneously after months to years
- Therapeutic options include:
  - Topical salicylic acid preparations daily (after paring down), for at least 3 months.
  - Cryotherapy, cautery, surgery (curettage).
  - Anogenital warts: podophyllin and topical imiquimod. Referral to GUM clinic should be made to exclude other coexisting STDs.

## Herpes zoster

Also known as shingles, this is a painful dermatomal eruption usually seen in older individuals although any age group can be affected (Fig. 6.11). Both sexes are affected.

### Aetiology

- Caused by human herpesvirus 3 (also known as varicella zoster virus: VZV), which also causes chickenpox
- Shingles is due to a reactivation of the virus that remains dormant in dorsal root ganglia
- Healthy individuals may be affected (particularly during periods of stress)
- More common in the setting of immunosuppression (e.g. lymphoma, leukaemia, iatrogenic, diabetes mellitus, HIV infection)

### Clinical evaluation

*History and examination*

- Prodrome: abrupt onset of pain usually in a dermatomal distribution

- Usually in a unilateral dermatomal distribution
- Thoracic nerves most commonly affected followed by the trigeminal nerves
- Lesions are clustered on an erythematous base and progress over 2–3 weeks from papules to vesicles to pustules which may become haemorrhagic, and then scab over
- Lesions at different stages of evolution may be seen
- More than one dermatome sometimes involved, and lesions may cross the midline or become disseminated particularly in the context of immunosuppression

### Investigation

- Clinical features usually diagnostic, but blister fluid samples for virology (electron microscopy looking for viral particles or PCR for VZV DNA) are sometimes useful

### Complications

- Secondary bacterial infection
- Ocular involvement in cases involving the ophthalmic division of the trigeminal nerve. A useful clue is involvement of the side and tip of the nose (nasociliary branch)
- Ramsay–Hunt syndrome: vesicles involving the external auditory canal, associated with an ipsilateral facial nerve palsy
- Sacral nerve involvement: retention of urine and difficulty with defaecation may result
- Post-herpetic neuralgia persists long after the cutaneous eruption has healed and responds poorly to analgesics
- Disseminated herpes zoster can occur in the setting of immunosuppression. Visceral organ involvement may occur, with a significant mortality rate

### Management and prognosis

- Resolves spontaneously in the majority of cases, although occasional complications as described earlier
- Early treatment with antiviral therapy (oral aciclovir, valacyclovir) has been reported to reduce the incidence of post-herpetic neuralgia
- Treatment may be indicated in the setting of immunosuppression and may have to be delivered intravenously in disseminated cases

## Pityriasis rosea

### Epidemiology/aetiology

- Common in autumn and winter
- Most frequent in adolescents and young adults
- Small outbreaks have been reported
- Human herpesvirus 7 has been implicated

## Clinical evaluation

*History*

- Usually asymptomatic but may be itchy in up to 50% of cases
- Patients may recall an initial herald patch followed a few days later by a widespread truncal rash

*Examination*

- **Herald patch**: an oval pink patch 3–6cm in diameter with a peripheral collarette of scale
- Multiple oval macules 1–3cm with a collarette of scale usually in a 'Christmas tree' distribution on the trunk and proximal limbs symmetrically
- Atypical forms may occur without a herald patch, in an inverse distribution affecting face and neck or in a localized pattern

## Investigations

- None usually required

## Differential diagnosis

- Herald patch: tinea corporis
- Truncal eruption:
  - Pityriasis versicolor

- Guttate psoriasis
- Seborrhoeic dermatitis
- Drug eruption
- Secondary syphilis
- Lichen planus

## Management

- This is usually symptomatic:
  - Oral sedative antihistamines for pruritus
  - Emollients
  - Topical corticosteroids
  - Phototherapy may be helpful in severe cases

## Outcome/prognosis

- Resolves spontaneously over 1–2 months
- Second attacks are unusual

Superficial cutaneous infections are caused by three groups of fungi:

- *Pityrosporum*
- *Candida*
- Dermatophytes

# 6.5 Fungal infections and infestations

Subcutaneous and systemic fungal infections will not be discussed in this section.

---

## Pityriasis versicolor

### Epidemiology/aetiology
- Relatively common, usually affects young adults
- Caused by the yeast *Pityrosporum ovale*, previously called malassezia furfur. This is a normal commensal on the skin but has been implicated in pityriasis versicolor, seborrhoeic dermatitis, and pityrosporum folliculitis

### Clinical evaluation
- Usually presents on the trunk with asymptomatic slightly scaly erythematous macules which, after sun exposure, tend to appear hypopigmented due to tanning of the surrounding skin
- Scrapings for mycology help to confirm the diagnosis

### Management
- Options include:
  - Selenium sulphide shampoo applied daily for 1 week to the body (20 minutes then washed off)
  - Ketoconazole shampoo alternate days for 1 week
  - Topical imidazoles twice daily for 2 weeks
  - Oral itraconazole 200mg once daily for 1 week
- The hypopigmentation may take months to return to normal

---

## Candidal infections

### Epidemiology/aetiology
- *Candida albicans* is the most common pathogen and is found as a commensal in the GI tract in most individuals. It is an opportunistic infection.
- Predisposing factors include extremes of age, pregnancy, menses, immunosuppression (e.g. HIV, diabetes, underlying malignancy), uraemia, oral antibiotics, and oral steroids as well as occlusion and damage to the stratum corneum.

### Clinical evaluation
- **Mucosal**: oral candidiasis may present with a sore mouth and white patches on the mucosal surfaces that can be scraped away leaving a red surface (thrush). Angular cheilitis is a red, scaly, often raw condition affecting the angles of the mouth. Candidal vulvovaginitis and balanitis may occur.
- **Skin**: candidal intertrigo affecting the flexures is common particularly in overweight individuals. It is characterized by raw, erythematous skin in the flexures with satellite pustules. It can affect toe web spaces and mimic tinea pedis.
- **Nail**: frequent immersion of the hands in water can lead to candidal paronychia. It can also mimic tinea unguium.
- Swabs may help confirm the diagnosis.

### Management
- Oral candidiasis:
  - Nystatin oral suspension
  - Amphotericin lozenges
  - Oral fluconazole in the immunosuppressed
  - + Oral hygiene
- Genital:
  - Imidazole creams or pessaries in women
  - Oral fluconazole sometimes required

- Intertrigo:
  - Topical imidazole (e.g. clotrimazole)
  - Oral imidazoles (severe cases)

---

## Dermatophyte infections

### Epidemiology/aetiology
- Any age, although usually more common in children
- ♂ >♀
- Three types of dermatophyte are relevant:
  - Trichophyton
  - Epidermophyton
  - *Microsporum* species

  These can only be differentiated on culture
- They may be geophilic, zoophilic, or anthropophilic
- Host factors play a role, and impaired cell-mediated immunity predisposes to these infections

### Clinical evaluation
The clinical appearance depends on the part of the body affected and the host response:
- **Tinea corporis**: erythematous, scaly, asymmetrical patches with an advancing raised edge and central clearing. May be itchy. As a rule, any asymmetrical scaly patches should be scraped for mycology
- **Tinea cruris**: well-demarcated, erythematous, scaly plaques in the groin. Satellite pustules are usually absent
- **Tinea pedis**:
  - Interdigital (athlete's foot) with web space maceration
  - Chronic with scaling on the soles (moccasin type)
  - Bullous (can be confused with pompholyx eczema)
- **Tinea manuum**: asymmetrical, erythematous scaling of the palms
- **Tinea capitis**: usually in children (Fig. 6.12). Subtypes include grey patch, black dot, favus, and kerion. Usually associated with alopecia
- **Onychomycosis** or **tinea unguium:** more common with increasing age. Usually starts at the distal or lateral edge of nail and spreads. Asymmetrical discoloration and thickening of nails with subungual debris
- **Tinea incognito**: misdiagnosis and treatment with topical steroids tends to modify the appearance of tinea, hence the name

### Investigations
- Skin scrapings, nail clippings and hair pluckings are sent for mycology to confirm the diagnosis

### Management
- Localized skin infections can be treated with topical antifungals (e.g. terbinafine, clotrimazole)
- Systemic options include oral terbinafine (not licensed in children), oral itraconazole and oral griseofulvin. Indications for systemic treatment include:
  - Scalp infections (8 weeks of oral griseofulvin in children)
  - Nail infections (oral terbinafine: 6 weeks for fingernails, 12 weeks for toe nails, may need longer)
  - Tinea incognito infections (oral terbinafine for 2–4 weeks)

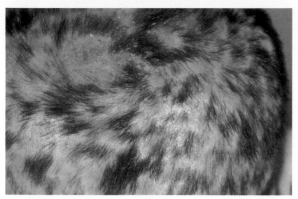

Fig. 6.12 Tinea capitis.

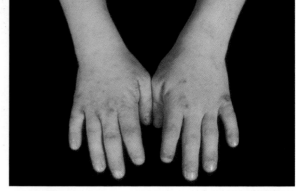

Fig. 6.14 Scabies—hands.

## Scabies

This is an intensely pruritic, contagious eruption caused by infestation with the scabies mite.

### Epidemiology/aetiology

- The causative mite, *Sarcoptes scabiei* (Fig. 6.13) is transmitted from one individual to another by prolonged physical contact
- Can occur at all ages, though most frequently affects children and young adults
- Affects both sexes and all races

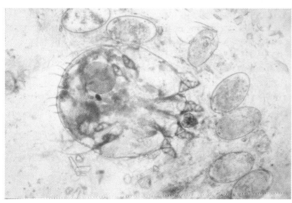

Fig. 6.13 Scabies mite.

### Clinical evaluation

- Extremely itchy (itch is typically worse at night). There is often a history of itchy contacts
- Burrows (typically on the sides of fingers and on the wrists) are diagnostic but not always present (Fig. 6.14). These are usually found early in disease course, followed a few weeks later by an erythematous eruption predominantly on the trunk. This is believed to be an immunological reaction to the mite
- Penile papules and nodules on the breasts and buttock regions point to a diagnosis of scabies. Widespread excoriations may be seen
- Diagnosis confirmed by finding scabies mites on microscopy of a scraping of a lesion/ burrow in potassium hydroxide
- Norwegian or crusted scabies occurs in elderly or immunosuppressed individuals and is extremely infectious. It presents as a scaly rash with hyperkeratotic, crusted lesions on the hands and feet. It is particularly difficult to treat

### Management

- Can be very difficult and requires a lot of explanation and attention to instructions
- Topical application of a scabicide such as **permethrin** or **malathion** from the neck downwards, washed off after 12 hours and repeated after 1 week
- All close contacts need to be treated even if asymptomatic
- The preparation must be reapplied after washing hands
- Pruritus may persist for a few weeks and a mild topical steroid with an emollient may be helpful. Antihistamines can also be given
- Oral **ivermectin** (unlicensed) may be used in resistant cases and in cases of Norwegian scabies

# 6.6 Erythema multiforme

## Background

Erythema multiforme (EM) is a common skin disorder of unknown aetiology.

It usually follows infection or drug exposure.

The clinical condition may range from a mild self-limiting rash (common) to a severe life-threatening mucosal disorder (Steven–Johnson syndrome, rare).

## Epidemiology

- Usually young adults (peak incidence 2nd/3rd decades)
- ♂ >♀

## Aetiology

- Idiopathic
- Infection (especially HSV or mycoplasma)
- Drugs (e.g. penicillins, sulphonamides, anticonvulsants, allopurinol)
- Some recurrent cases are associated with SLE

## Clinical evaluation

### History

- Lesions evolve over a few days and may be pruritic or painful (especially if affecting mucous membranes)
- May be associated with constitutional symptoms such as fever, malaise, or weakness
- Preceding history of cold sores (HSV) or specific medication
- Previous episodes of EM

### Examination

- Typical lesions are targetoid (but may be vesicular or bullous) (Fig. 6.15)
- Lesions may be localized or generalized. Typical sites include: dorsa of hands, palms, and soles; face and forearms
- Mucosal involvement: erosions may affect lips, oropharynx, nasal/conjunctival/vulvar/anal/penile mucosae. In EM minor, there is little or no mucosal involvement, whilst in EM major there is extensive mucosal involvement (see Stevens–Johnson syndrome, Section 6.6)

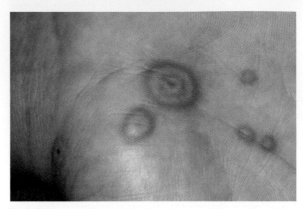

**Fig. 6.15** Close-up of target lesion in erythema multiforme. Reproduced from Sue Lewis-Jones, *Oxford Specialist Handbook: Paediatric Dermatology*, 2010, Figure 4.12, with permission from Oxford University Press.

## Investigation

- Diagnosis is usually clinical although in some cases a skin biopsy may be helpful, and shows lichenoid histology with marked inflammation and necrotic keratinocytes
- If the history is suggestive, look for underlying causes: viral swabs for HSV and mycoplasma serology

## Management

- **Steroids**: short-term use of oral prednisolone may be helpful in severe cases although clinical trial evidence for this is lacking
- **Aciclovir** may be used at the first sign of a cold sore in HSV-triggered cases, or prophylactically in cases of recurrent EM

## Outcome/prognosis

- Usually self-limiting, provided offending agent removed/treated
- In recurrent cases, underlying recurrent HSV or SLE should be excluded

# 6.7 Stevens–Johnson syndrome/toxic epidermal necrolysis

## Background

These conditions are not clearly-defined or classified.

Most authors regard **Stevens–Johnson syndrome** (SJS) as an extreme variant of EM major with severe mucosal involvement (<10% epidermal detachment).

**Toxic epidermal necrolysis** (TEN), however, involves epidermal detachment (cell death causes the epidermis to separate from the dermis) affecting >30% body surface area.

## Epidemiology

- Any age but most frequent in adults >40 years
- ♂ = ♀

## Aetiology

- >50% SJS cases and the majority of TEN are drug-associated. The most commonly implicated drugs are: sulphonamides, anticonvulsants, penicillins, allopurinol, NSAIDs
- Other causes of SJS include HSV and mycoplasma infections
- Some cases may be associated with malignancy (carcinomas, lymphoma) whilst in up to 50% no cause is identified (idiopathic)

## Clinical evaluation

### History

- Usually appears 1–3 weeks after first drug exposure, although may be faster on re-challenge
- Often a prodromal flu-like illness with fever for several days followed by painful mucocutaneous lesions

### Examination

- **Skin**: commences with EM-like lesions. These may be purpuric or tender. Small macules then coalesce to form larger areas and the epidermis may detach in sheets leaving denuded red dermis. Nikolsky sign may be positive
- **Mucosa**: involvement of mucosal surfaces may be severe, with erythema and erosions affecting lips, buccal mucosa, and conjunctivae, genital and anal mucosae (Fig. 6.16). Keratitis and corneal erosions may develop
- **Systemic**: patients are generally unwell with high fever. There may be systemic involvement with respiratory and GI erosions and renal failure

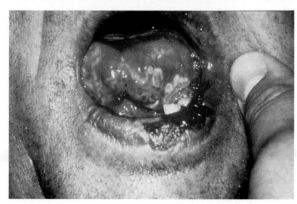

Fig. 6.16 Oral involvement in Stevens–Johnson syndrome.

## Investigations

- The diagnosis is usually clinical and can be confirmed by skin biopsy
- Comprehensive blood screening is required to ascertain potential cause and detect any complications

## Management

- Early diagnosis and withdrawal of the offending drug (as appropriate) are critical
- Fluid and electrolyte replacement are essential to avoid renal complications
- The patient may need to be cared for in a burns unit or ICU
- Reverse barrier nurse to avoid infection
- Emollients topically, eye care, and ophthalmology advice as necessary
- Systemic corticosteroids are controversial and not usually recommended (increase incidence of secondary infections)
- High-dose IVIG if administered early may halt progression in severe cases
- The management of complications such as infection/systemic sepsis/renal failure is essential

## Outcome/prognosis

- Advise against re-challenge with the offending drug
- Mortality rates: ~5% (SJS), ~30% (TEN)

# 6.8 Erythema nodosum

## Background

This condition is characterized by painful nodules on the lower legs, and may be due to one of a number of causes.

## Epidemiology

- Most common in young adults
- ♀ > ♂
- Affects all races

## Aetiology

May be due to any of the following:
- Idiopathic
- Drugs (e.g. sulphonamides, barbiturates, oral contraceptives)
- Infections:
  - Bacterial (e.g. streptococcal, TB, leprosy, *Yersinia, Salmonella*, cat scratch disease).
  - Fungal (e.g. coccidioidomycosis, histoplasmosis, blastomycosis).
  - Viral (e.g. EBV) and chlamydial (e.g. psittacosis).
- Systemic disorders:
  - Sarcoidosis.
  - Ulcerative colitis/Crohn disease.
  - Hodgkin lymphoma.
  - Behçet disease.

## Clinical evaluation

### History
- Acute onset of painful, red nodules usually on the legs (Fig. 6.17)
- May be associated with a mild fever, arthralgia, and malaise

### Examination
- Bilateral tender, red, indurated/deep-seated nodules 3–4cm in diameter usually on the anterior shins
- Ulceration is **not** usually a feature and if present should raise the possibility of erythema induratum (a tuberculid) or nodular vasculitis

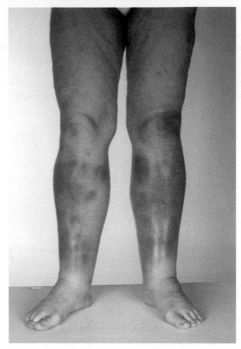

Fig. 6.17 Erythema nodosum.

### Investigations
- Elevated WBC, ESR, CRP
- Skin biopsy shows a septal panniculitis on H&E stain
- Investigate to exclude known associations (e.g. throat swab, anti-streptolysin O titre, stool culture, Mantoux, CXR)

### Management
- Identify and treat underlying cause (if found)
- Bed rest, light compression, NSAIDs
- Systemic steroids are sometimes used if the aetiology is known and infections have been adequately excluded

### Outcome/prognosis
- Depends on underlying aetiology, but usually resolves spontaneously over 6–8 weeks without scarring

# 6.9 Drug eruptions

## Background

Drugs are notorious for causing rashes.

Almost any type of cutaneous reaction (eczematous, psoriasiform, lichenoid, acneiform) can be brought on by a drug, and this must be borne in mind when considering the differential diagnosis for most rashes.

The most frequent type of drug rash is a maculopapular rash or a 'toxic erythema' (Fig. 6.18). Withdrawal of the offending agent usually results in resolution of the rash over 8–10 days.

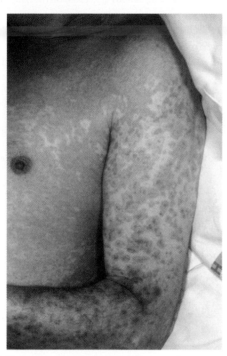

**Fig. 6.18** Maculopapular rash caused by a drug reaction.

The most common causes of drug rashes are listed in Box 6.3.

The most serious drug reactions are erythroderma, toxic epidermal necrolysis, and drug hypersensitivity syndrome. The first two of these are discussed elsewhere.

## Drug hypersensitivity syndrome

### Aetiology

- Typically caused by anticonvulsants: carbamazepine, phenytoin, phenobarbitone, clonazepam

### Clinical evaluation

- Usually comes on after a few weeks of taking the relevant drug
- Generalized rash ± mucosal involvement, high fever, lymphadenopathy, arthralgia or hepatosplenomegaly. Occasionally the skin may pustulate
- There may be peripheral eosinophilia and hepatitis. Severe cases can lead to multi-organ failure

### Management

- Stop the offending agent. The listed anticonvulsants cross-react (as do the newer ones, vigabatrin and lamotrigine), and so they must all be avoided. Sodium valproate may be a suitable alternative
- Oral corticosteroids may be indicated

# 6.10 Benign skin tumours

## Non-melanocytic lesions

### Seborrhoeic keratosis (SK)

- Very common benign skin tumours, often seen in older people
- Can occur in isolation but usually appear as multiple brown papules or plaques with a warty surface and 'stuck-on' appearance (Fig. 6.19). Some lesions may be pruritic
- Can vary in colour from light–dark brown and may sometimes be confused with melanoma
- The sudden appearance of multiple SKs in association with an internal malignancy is known as Lesser–Trelat sign
- Dermatosis papulosa nigra is a benign inherited condition affecting black skin, characterized by multiple hyperpigmented sessile and pedunculated papules appearing on the face. Histologically these lesions look similar to SKs
- Treatment options include cryotherapy, shave excision, and curettage and cautery

### Epidermoid cyst

- These lesions are derived from the cystic enclosure of stratified squamous epithelium with a well-formed granular layer within the dermis. They are thin-walled and rupture easily, releasing a malodorous cream-coloured, paste-like discharge
- Commonly occur on the face, neck, trunk, and scrotum, where they may calcify
- Usually solitary nodules with a central punctum (but may be multiple)
- Inflamed or troublesome lesions can be surgically excised

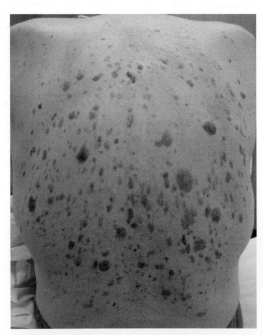

**Fig. 6.19** Multiple seborrhoeic keratoses on the back.
Author: James Heilman MD. This file is licensed under the Creative Commons Attribution-Share Alike 3.0 Unported (//creativecommons.org/licenses/by-sa/3.0/deed.en) license.

### Pilar cyst

- Also known as a trichilemmal cysts, these lesions occur on the scalp as smooth, firm, dome-shaped nodules that are often multiple
- There is often a family history of cysts with autosomal dominant inheritance pattern
- There is no central punctum and inflammation is not usually a feature
- The cyst wall is thick and can usually be excised intact. It is also lined by stratified squamous epithelium but without the granular layer
- Troublesome lesions can be surgically excised

### Dermatofibroma

- This is a common dermal tumour that is often found on the limbs (legs > arms). There may be a history of insect bite
- Lesions are typically solitary, dome-shaped papules or nodules that can be skin-coloured, red/brown, or more darkly pigmented, mimicking a melanoma
- Lateral compression between the thumb and index finger produces the characteristic 'dimple sign'
- They may involute spontaneously but can otherwise be surgically excised

## Melanocytic lesions

### Solar lentigo

- Tan-coloured, even-outlined macules or patches that occur at sites of sun exposure, usually the face, upper trunk, arms, and hands
- Multiple lesions may occur. No treatment is required

### Acquired melanocytic naevi (moles)

- Benign tumours due to proliferation of melanocytes. They first appear in childhood, reach their final number in early adulthood, and then tend to disappear. New lesions are rare >40 years
- The density of naevi is partly proportional to sun exposure and can act as a marker for an individual's risk of melanoma
- Multiple lesions may occur. No treatment is required

### Classification and clinical features

This is determined by the site of the naevus cells:

- **Junctional** naevi—found at the dermo-epidermal junction, above the basement membrane. The lesions appear in childhood and are flat, uniformly-pigmented macules with regular borders
- **Compound** naevi—found in the dermis and at the dermo-epidermal junction. The lesions appear in adolescence and are slightly raised or more elevated papules or nodules. The surface can be smooth or papillomatous and there may be more than one pigment present, which may not be distributed evenly. Hairs may project from the surface
- **Intradermal** naevi—found exclusively in the dermis. The lesions appear after adolescence and are typically skin-coloured papules or nodules which commonly occur on the face and scalp. They are occasionally hairy. There is no malignant potential
- These naevi frequently evolve from junctional to compound to intradermal in the first four decades of life
- **Halo** naevi—a benign melanocytic naevus becomes encircled by a halo of depigmentation. With time, the naevus disappears and the halo re-pigments. The naevus within the halo should be evaluated

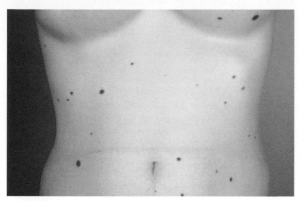

Fig. 6.20 Dysplastic naevus syndrome.

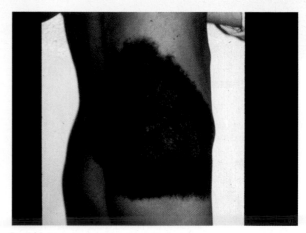

Fig. 6.21 Large congenital melanocytic naevus.

for signs of malignancy (e.g. variable pigmentation and irregular outline) as a halo can occasionally develop around a malignant melanoma

### Treatment

Any naevus with junctional activity has the potential for malignant change. However, this is an infrequent event in comparison with the prevalence of these lesions and therefore prophylactic excision is not recommended. If a diagnosis of melanoma cannot be excluded, the naevus should be excised.

## Atypical mole syndrome

This diagnosis should be suspected in anyone with >100 moles, or moles >5mm in diameter. If two or more moles have dysplastic histology, the diagnosis is made.

Dysplastic naevi tend to be larger than benign melanocytic naevi, have slightly irregular, less distinct margins and more variable pigmentation (Fig. 6.20). They may occur in unusual sites such as the scalp, buttocks, soles, and iris. Affected individuals are at higher risk of malignant melanoma. It is prudent they avoid excessive sun exposure and must regularly examine their moles.

## Congenital melanocytic naevi

Congenital melanocytic naevi (CMN) arise from nests of melanocytes that are found deep in the dermis and are present at birth. They are seen in 1–2% of newborns.

### Aetiology

The aetiology is unclear. One explanation is that there is a mutation in the embryonic neuroectoderm precursor cells as they migrate to the skin to form melanocytes.

### Classification

CMN are classified according to their size:
- Small CMN are <1.5cm
- Medium CMN are <20cm
- Large CMN are ≥20cm (Fig. 6.21)

### Clinical features
- Brown patches or plaques that are present at birth
- Smooth or verrucous surface
- Pigmentation and nodularity may increase with age

## Neurocutaneous melanosis

Large CMN are associated with neurocutaneous melanosis. This is a rare congenital syndrome where melanocytic cells are found in both the skin and meninges. Melanoma can develop at both these sites. Patients can also develop symptoms of raised intracranial pressure. MRI scanning will reveal leptomeningeal involvement.

### Treatment
- Small and medium-sized CMN can be monitored by regular surveillance
- Patients with a large CMN have a 5–7% lifetime risk of developing a malignant melanoma. Therefore, if possible, the lesion should be partially or completely excised. This may involve the use of skin grafts, flaps and tissue expanders to close large defects. Curettage and laser treatment have also been used with limited success

# 6.11 Malignant skin tumours

## Premalignant lesions

### Actinic keratosis

- Premalignant lesions that arise on sun-damaged skin. They are also known as solar keratoses
- Lesions consist of ill-defined erythematous, keratotic plaques with very adherent scale which is painful to remove
- Common on sun-exposed skin
- Histologically there is dysplasia of the basal keratinocytes
- The risk of transformation to squamous cell carcinoma is small
- Lesions occasionally involute spontaneously but can require treatment. Options include cryotherapy, topical treatment with diclofenac, 5-fluorouracil or imiquimod, curettage, and cautery

### Bowen disease

- Bowen disease is *in situ* squamous cell carcinoma
- Lesions consist of solitary erythematous scaly plaques that may be mistaken for eczema or psoriasis
- They are most common on sun-exposed sites
- Malignant change should be suspected if the lesion becomes nodular, indurated, or eroded
- Histologically there is full-thickness dysplasia of the epidermis
- Treatment includes cryotherapy, topical 5-fluorouracil or imiquimod, photodynamic therapy, curettage, and surgical excision

## Malignant lesions

### Squamous cell carcinoma

Squamous cell carcinoma (SCC) is the second most common type of skin cancer. It is a malignant tumour of keratinocytes arising in the epidermis and stratified squamous mucosa. It may develop from pre-cancerous lesions (see Premalignant lesions, above) and has the potential to metastasize. The incidence of SCC is rising and men are affected two to three times more than women, probably because of their higher UV exposure.

### Aetiology

- UV radiation—cumulative lifetime sun exposure is a major risk factor for SCC. Patients with Fitzpatrick skin types I and II (very fair/fair skin) are most at risk, as are those with oculo-cutaneous albinism who have lost their protective melanin pigment
- UV exposure leads to the production of pyrimidine dimers in keratinocyte DNA resulting in defective DNA replication and transcription
- Inactivation of the tumour suppressor gene $p53$ is seen in 90% of SCCs. Mutations in $p16^{INK4A}$ and $p14^{ARF}$ have also been documented
- Human papilloma virus (HPV)—HPV-16 and 18 have been associated with the development of anogenital and periungual SCC. Their oncogenic activity is thought to be mediated by the HPV E6 protein which functionally inactivates the $p53$ tumour suppressor gene
- HPV-5 and 8 have also been implicated in the development of cutaneous SCC
- Immunosuppression—solid-organ transplant recipients, individuals receiving long-term systemic immunosuppressive treatments and those infected with HIV are at increased risk of UV light and HPV-induced SCC
- Old scars—SCC can develop within a chronic ulcer and is referred to as Marjolin ulcer in this context. However, any scarred area is susceptible such as old burn sites or disease processes that result in scarring such as epidermolysis bullosa (a group of inherited blistering diseases)
- Chronic inflammation—lesions resulting from discoid lupus erythematosus, erosive lichen planus, or lichen sclerosus et atrophicus are also at increased risk of developing SCC
- Chemicals—arsenic and polycyclic hydrocarbons found in tar, pitch, and soot
- Genetic diseases—oculo-cutaneous albinism, xeroderma pigmentosum and epidermodysplasia verruciformis

### Clinical features

- The lesion is commonly on the head and neck or another sun-exposed site
- There may be a slowly-enlarging keratotic papule or plaque, arising *de novo*, or within a patch of Bowen disease. The surface can be crusted, scaly, eroded, or ulcerated (Fig. 6.22)
- Nodular lesions may develop at the margin of a chronic ulcer or on the vermillion border of the lip
- Anogenital SCC presents with pruritus or tenderness and a nodule or erosion may be found on examination
- Regional lymph nodes should be examined for metastases. Lesions on the ear, vermillion border, and in the anogenital region are more likely to metastasize, as are lesions in chronically immunosuppressed patients

### Diagnosis

An incisional biopsy can be taken to confirm the diagnosis.

### Treatment

- Surgical excision—simple excision with a 4mm margin of surrounding skin is required for low-risk tumours. A wider margin of 6mm should be taken for high-risk tumours (those >2cm in diameter or high-risk sites—eye, ear, nose, lip, and scalp; poorly-differentiated

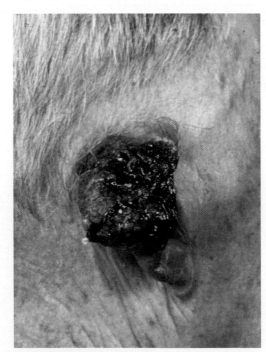

**Fig. 6.22** Squamous cell carcinoma.

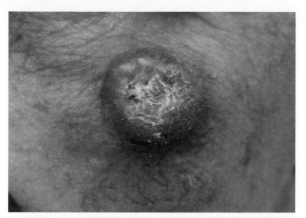

Fig. 6.23 Keratoacanthoma.

tumours and when there is perineural invasion or extension into subcutaneous tissue). These cases are best managed with Mohs micrographic surgery (see Basal cell carcinoma, below)

- Radiotherapy—useful if surgery is not feasible
- Curettage and cautery or cryotherapy—can be used for some small low-risk tumours

## Keratoacanthoma

This is a rapidly-enlarging nodule with a central keratin-filled crater that grows over several weeks, reaches a plateau, and then spontaneously involutes, leaving behind a pitted scar (Fig. 6.23). Histologically it is difficult to distinguish from a well-differentiated SCC but there is minimal epithelial dysplasia and few mitoses. The lesion should be removed by curettage and cautery or completely excised to rule out the possibility of SCC. Multiple keratoacanthomas are found in Ferguson–Smith syndrome.

## Basal cell carcinoma

Basal cell carcinoma (BCC) is the most common form of skin cancer. It is a locally destructive tumour derived from the basal cells of the epidermis and rarely metastasizes. It is more common in men and has a peak incidence between the ages of 55–75 years.

### Aetiology

- UV radiation—both cumulative lifetime exposure and intense intermittent exposure predispose to BCCs. Fair skinned people who burn easily and tan poorly (Fitzpatrick skin types I and II) are most at risk
- Loss of function mutations in the *PTCH* (patched) gene and activating mutations in the *SMO* (smoothened) gene have been found in both sporadic and familial BCCs and UVB-induced mutations in the *p53* tumour suppressor gene are found in 40–50% of sporadic cases
- X-ray treatment and ionizing radiation
- Arsenic ingestion
- Immunosuppression (e.g. post-organ transplantation)
- Genetic syndromes (e.g. Gorlin syndrome, xeroderma pigmentosa, and epidermodysplasia verruciformis)

### Clinical features

- Most commonly found on the head and neck, but can affect skin at any site
- Lesions are usually painless but they may bleed and form crusts that do not heal
- BCCs near the eyes, ears, and nose can be locally destructive as they enlarge (Fig. 6.24)

### Subtypes

- Nodular BCC ('rodent ulcer')—the most common type of BCC. It presents as a papule or nodule that has a rolled pearly edge with surface telangiectasia. As the lesion enlarges, it may ulcerate centrally. Represents 60% of BCCs
- Cystic BCC—a well-defined papule or nodule that does not ulcerate, with a translucent telangiectatic surface
- Morphoeic BCC—indurated plaque that often resembles a scar. The margins of the tumour can be difficult to define clinically
- Superficial BCC—appears as a thin, red, scaly plaque with fine telangiectasia and a thin rolled edge. More common on the trunk and limbs and multiple lesions may be present
- Pigmented BCC—similar to nodular variant but with pigmented margins

### Diagnosis

- An incisional or punch biopsy from the lesion may be taken to confirm the diagnosis of BCC and the histological subtype
- The diagnosis of BCC can also be made from skin scrapings taken for cytology

(A)

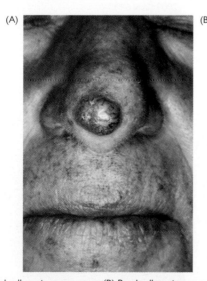

(B)

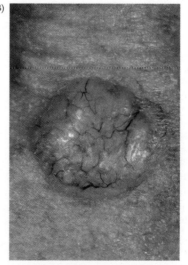

Fig. 6.24 (A) Nodular basal cell carcinoma on nose (B) Basal cell carcinoma on nose (right: magnified view)

(A) M. Sand, D. Sand, C. Thrandorf, V. Paech, P. Altmeyer, F. G. Bechara: *Cutaneous lesions of the nose*. In: *Head & face medicine* Band 6, 2010, S. 7, ISSN 1746-160X. doi:10.1186/1746-160X-6-7. PMID 20525327. (Review). Open Access. © 2010 Sand *et al*. This file is licensed under the Creative Commons Attribution 2.0 Generic (//creativecommons.org/licenses/by/2.0/deed.en) license. (B) Reproduced with permission from Cambridge University Hospitals NHS Foundation Trust

## Treatment

This is influenced by the nature of the tumour (site, size, and subtype), the patient (age and comorbidities), and what facilities are locally available.

- Topical 5-fluorouracil and imiquimod cream and cryotherapy can be used to treat superficial BCCs
- Curettage and cautery can be used for small (<1cm) BCCs that are not deeply ulcerated at low-risk sites
- Surgical excision with primary closure, secondary intention healing, skin flaps or grafts can be used to treat most lesions
- Radiotherapy—useful in elderly patients if surgery is not feasible. Should be avoided on the ear, calf, and dorsum of the hand as radionecrosis is more likely at these sites
- Photodynamic therapy—can be used to treat superficial BCCs
- Mohs micrographic surgery is a specialist treatment that is becoming increasingly available. It is a staged procedure that involves serial frozen section examination and resection. Indications include tumours at high-risk sites (around the eyes, ears, nose, and on the scalp) when tissue preservation is important, morphoeic BCCs, recurrence after surgery or radiotherapy and if there is perineural invasion

## Prognosis

With adequate treatment cure rates of 95% can be expected.

## Gorlin syndrome (basal cell naevus syndrome)

- Gorlin syndrome is an autosomal dominant condition caused by mutations in the *PTCH* gene located on chromosome 9q21–31. This is the human equivalent of the *Drosophila patched* gene and it is involved in the hedgehog signalling pathway
- Patients develop BCCs from childhood onwards
- Other associated abnormalities include palmar and plantar pits, odontogenic keratocysts, bilamellar calcification of the falx cerebri, and bifid or splayed ribs
- The BCCs can be treated by any of the previously mentioned modalities except radiotherapy which should be avoided as these individuals are particularly sensitive to the effects of ionizing radiation. The development of multiple BCCs within irradiated fields in affected patients is well-described

## Malignant melanoma

This is the most serious form of skin cancer with a rising incidence and a relatively high mortality. Early diagnosis is of paramount importance in reducing this mortality. All age groups can be affected although it is rare in childhood.

### Aetiology/pathogenesis

Predisposing factors include:
- Genetic:
  - Family history of melanoma in first-degree relative.
  - Familial atypical mole/melanoma syndrome (FAMM).
  - Susceptibility genes include *CDKN2A* on chromosome 9 (encoding p16); *CDK4* on chromosome 12.
- Fair skin, red hair, multiple freckles, Fitzpatrick skin types 1 and 2
- Atypical mole syndrome, giant congenital melanocytic naevus
- Severe intermittent sun exposure (sunburns) particularly in childhood as well as chronic sun exposure, PUVA, use of tanning salons
- Xeroderma pigmentosa

### Molecular pathology

- Advances in molecular biology have helped identify numerous chromosomal gains/losses (e.g. 6p25, 6q23, 11q13), activation of oncogenes (*BRAF, NRAS*), and deletion of tumour suppressor genes (p16—*CDKN2A*), with potential diagnostic and prognostic utility
- Melanomas on acral and mucosal sites have been associated with *KIT* oncogene mutations, and anecdotal reports of the use of kinase inhibitors (imatinib) to treat these lesions are emerging
- In addition there are differences in these findings related to site and degree of sun exposure, i.e. chronic sun exposure (face), intermittent sun exposure (trunk, arms, legs), minimal sun exposure (palms and soles), and no sun exposure (mucosal)

### Clinical features—subtypes

- Superficial spreading melanoma. Enlarging irregularly pigmented lesion that enlarges radially before entering vertical growth phase
- Nodular melanoma (Fig. 6.25). Rapidly growing nodule, usually pigmented, occasionally amelanotic
- Lentigo maligna melanoma. Usually on the face of older individuals. Enlarging irregularly pigmented lesion (lentigo maligna), which may become invasive (lentigo maligna melanoma)
- Acral lentiginous melanoma. Palmar, plantar, or subungual lesions. Usually present late. Most common subtypes in dark-skinned individuals
- Other subtypes are quite rare

### Checklist for diagnosis

Superficial spreading melanoma, if diagnosed early and excised, has a relatively good prognosis. The ABCD criteria and Glasgow 7-point checklist (Box 6.4) may be useful in differentiating these lesions from benign or atypical naevi.

### Diagnosis

- Clinical evaluation as previously described
- Excision biopsy with 2mm margin. Histopathology remains the 'gold standard' in diagnosis of melanoma. Important prognostic factors include:
  - Breslow thickness (vertical distance in mm from the granular cell layer to the deepest melanoma cell).
  - mitotic rate (per mm$^2$).
  - presence of ulceration.

### Staging/prognosis

- The new AJCC criteria for staging of melanoma were published in 2009 (Box 6.5)
- Investigation (LDH, CXR, CT, PET) may be indicated in melanomas with Breslow thickness >1mm
- 5-year survival rates range from >95% in stage 1 disease to <15% in stage 4 disease

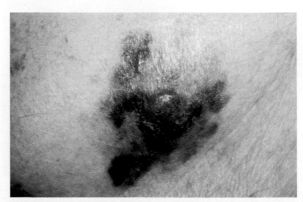

Fig. 6.25 Nodular malignant melanoma.

**ABCD criteria**
- A Asymmetry of lesion.
- B Irregular border.
- C Variegated colour.
- D Diameter >6mm.
- E Enlargement.

**Glasgow 7-point checklist**
- Change in size.
- Change in shape.
- Change in colour.
- Diameter >7mm.
- Inflammation.
- Oozing.
- Change in sensation.

## Management

Melanomas should be managed by teams that are experienced in the management of these tumours, and as part of a skin cancer multidisciplinary team.
- Surgery:
  - Wide local excision is the treatment of choice (1cm margins for melanomas with Breslow thickness <1mm, 2cm margins if Breslow >1mm).
  - Sentinel lymph node biopsy for lesions with Breslow thickness >1mm. This has definite prognostic importance in the management of melanoma, and recent evidence suggests that it may improve disease-free survival, although data on improved overall survival is lacking.
  - Elective lymph node dissection, in cases where there is lymph node involvement.
- Chemotherapy/immunotherapy for advanced disease
- Radiotherapy may have a role in palliation and in the treatment of lentigo maligna (*in situ* component)

Box 6.5 Simplified staging—malignant melanoma

- Stage 1: no nodal or distant metastasis; <1mm thick or ≤2mm without ulceration.
- Stage II: no nodal or distant metastasis; >1mm thick with ulceration or >2mm thick.
- Stage III: regional metastases.
- Stage IV: distant metastases.

Source: American Joint Committee on Cancer (AJCC) melanoma staging and classification. *J Clin Oncol* 2009; 27(38): 6199–206.

# Xeroderma pigmentosum

- Xeroderma pigmentosum (XP) is a rare autosomal recessive disorder that affects all races and both sexes
- It is characterized by defective enzymatic repair of UV light-induced damage to epithelial DNA
- Seven XP repair genes (*XPA–G*) have been identified and seven complementation groups are described, corresponding to the defective gene products. Prenatal diagnosis is available
- Affected patients show an exaggerated sunburn response and early onset of chronic photo-damage and premalignant and malignant skin lesions (BCC, SCC, and melanoma) from childhood onwards
- Ocular involvement is common with photophobia, conjunctivitis, ectropion, and ulceration as well as progressive neurological disease including deafness, microcephaly, and poor intellectual function
- ~25% of cases are termed XP variant. They exhibit a similar but milder phenotype to classical XP
- Sun avoidance is paramount and patients need regular skin and ophthalmological surveillance. Oral retinoids may be helpful in slowing down the onset of tumours

# Skin manifestations of malignancy

- Malignant acanthosis nigricans—adenocarcinoma
- Tripe palms—bronchial and gastrointestinal carcinoma
- Generalized pruritus—lymphoma
- Pyoderma gangrenosum—myeloproliferative disorders
- Acquired ichthyosis—lymphoma
- Acquired palmoplantar keratoderma—ovarian, breast, and lung carcinoma
- Dermatomyositis
- Erythema gyratum repens—bronchial carcinoma
- Necrolytic migratory erythema—glucagonoma
- Erythroderma—lymphoma and leukaemia
- Hypertrichosis lanuginose acquisita—colorectal and bronchial carcinoma
- Sister Joseph nodule—umbilical metastatic deposit of gastric carcinoma
- Leukaemia cutis—cutaneous metastases of leukaemia
- The sign of Lesser–Trelat—multiple seborrhoeic keratoses with gastric carcinoma
- Migratory superficial thrombophlebitis—pancreatic carcinoma
- Paraneoplastic pemphigus
- Bazex syndrome—upper respiratory/GI carcinoma

# 6.12 The skin and systemic disease

## Diabetes and the skin

Skin disease is a common complication in diabetes.

### Infection

- Candida—mucosal and cutaneous
- Dermatophytoses—tinea pedis and onychomycosis
- Erythrasma—pink/brown patches in intertriginous sites caused by *Corynebacterium minutissimum* infection. Porphyrins released by the bacteria produce coral-pink fluorescence when Wood's light is shone on involved sites. Treatment is with antiseptic washes, topical clindamycin, and topical or oral erythromycin
- Furuncles, carbuncles, paronychia, and cellulitis are more common

### Necrobiosis lipoidica (NL)

*Epidemiology*

- Average age of onset is 30 years
- ♀: ♂ = 3:1
- Affects 0.3% of diabetics but a large proportion of patients with NL have diabetes, impaired glucose tolerance, or a family history of diabetes. NL precedes the onset of diabetes in 15% of patients

*Aetiology*

- The cause is unknown but may be related to diabetic microangiopathy
- The course of NL is unrelated to diabetic control

*Clinical features*

- History—a slowly enlarging lesion on the shin, lateral calf, or dorsum of the foot. Less commonly found on the face, upper limbs, and abdomen
- Examination—a well-defined slightly raised plaque with a red-brown border and a waxy yellow atrophic centre with prominent telangiectasia. Ulceration may occur. Lesions heal to leave depressed scars

*Pathology*

- Histologically there is distortion of the collagen bundles, (necrobiosis) with a granulomatous reaction in the deep dermis. Foam cells are often present and dermal blood vessels show endothelial thickening
- Direct IF demonstrates C3 deposition in blood vessel walls

*Differential diagnosis*

- Granuloma annulare
- Sarcoidosis

*Treatment*

- Corticosteroids—potent topical steroids under occlusion or intralesional triamcinolone
- Ciclosporin
- PUVA photochemotherapy
- Antiplatelet aggregation therapy with aspirin and dipyridamole or pentoxifylline
- Ulcerated areas may need to be excised and grafted

### Granuloma annulare

Granuloma annulare (GA) is a common inflammatory dermatosis of unknown aetiology. It has been associated with diabetes and thyroid disease.

*Epidemiology*

- Affects children and young adults
- ♀: ♂ = 2:1

*Clinical features*

There are several subtypes:

- Localized GA—red or flesh-coloured papules, 2–3mm in diameter, arranged in an annular fashion or annular plaques. The dorsum of the hand is the most common site but lesions can occur anywhere
- Generalized GA—multiple red, brown, or flesh-coloured papules and nodules that may coalesce into plaques. Several sites are symmetrically affected
- Subcutaneous GA—firm, non-tender, red or flesh-coloured nodules on the extremities
- Perforating GA—umbilicated papules that are usually on the extremities. More common in children

*Differential diagnosis*

- Localized GA—necrobiosis lipoidica, tinea corporis, annular lichen planus
- Generalized GA—lichen planus, sarcoidosis
- Subcutaneous GA—rheumatoid nodules
- Perforating GA—molluscum contagiosum, perforating collagenosis

*Pathology*

- Palisading histiocytes around foci of necrobiosis

*Treatment*

- Spontaneous resolution may occur
- Potent topical steroids with or without occlusion
- Intralesional triamcinolone
- Generalized GA—PUVA phototherapy, isotretinoin, and hydroxychloroquine

### Diabetic dermopathy

- Red-brown oval or round macules on the shins that arise in crops and resemble scars. Lesions may blister
- The cause is unknown but may be related to microvascular disease or an exaggerated response to trauma
- Usually seen in older diabetics with chronic disease and poor diabetic control

### Acanthosis nigricans (AN)

- AN is the velvety hyperpigmentation of the skin that is principally seen in the axillae and neck but may be found in other intertriginous areas (Fig. 6.26)
- **Benign** AN: associated with several endocrine diseases where insulin resistance is a feature including: diabetes, acromegaly, Cushing and Addison diseases and hypothyroidism
- **Pseudo** AN: a complication of obesity and more common in darker-skinned patients. Multiple skin tags may also be seen. It improves with weight loss
- **Malignant** AN: a paraneoplastic phenomenon associated with adenocarcinoma, commonly of the GI tract. In contrast to the benign variant, it appears suddenly, is rapidly progressive, and there may be associated hyperkeratosis of the palms and soles. Malignant AN may precede the appearance of malignancy by 5 years
- Other causes of AN include drugs such as nicotinic acid and the oral contraceptive pill and, in some cases, hereditary factors

### Adverse drug reactions

- Insulin-induced—lipoatrophy and lipohypertrophy at injection sites. Urticaria and serum sickness-like illness
- Oral hypoglycaemic agents—urticaria, eczematous reactions, erythema multiforme, and photosensitivity

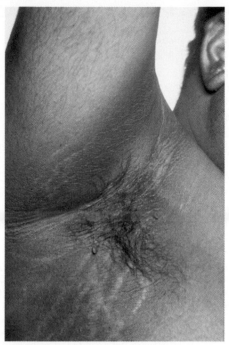

Fig. 6.26 Acanthosis nigricans.

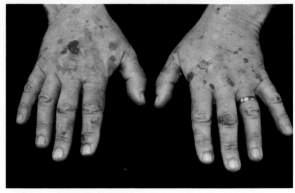

Fig. 6.27 Porphyria cutanea tarda.

### Other problems seen in diabetic skin

- Ulceration—the combination of peripheral vascular disease, atherosclerosis, and peripheral neuropathy commonly leads to foot ulcers. These are common over bony prominences, particularly on the sole. There is increased risk of gangrene
- Autonomic neuropathy leads to anhidrosis, xerosis, and fissuring on the skin of the legs and feet
- Diabetic bullae—spontaneous blistering on the extremities
- Eruptive xanthomas resulting from hypertriglyceridaemia related to poor diabetic control
- Sclerodema of Buschke—waxy thickening and hardening of the skin secondary to mucin deposition between collagen bundles
- Kyrle disease—an acquired reactive perforating dermatosis that is associated with diabetes, chronic kidney disease, and hepatic dysfunction. Numerous papules and nodules with central keratin-filled plugs appear on the legs and forearms. There is no specific treatment
- Localized GA—red or flesh-coloured papules, 2–3mm in diameter, arranged in an annular fashion or annular plaques. The dorsum of the hand is the most common site but lesions can occur anywhere
- Generalized GA—multiple red, brown, or flesh-coloured papules and nodules that may coalesce into plaques. Several sites are symmetrically affected
- Subcutaneous GA—firm, non-tender, red or flesh-coloured nodules on the extremities
- Perforating GA—umbilicated papules that are usually on the extremities. More common in children

## The porphyrias

This is a group of disorders caused by abnormal metabolism in the synthetic pathway for haem (usually a partial enzyme deficiency which may have a genetic basis).

As a result, there is an accumulation of porphyrins which may be **phototoxic** leading to skin photosensitivity.

Involvement of other organs can occur. Not all types of porphyria have skin manifestations.

### Subtypes

Affecting skin only:
- Porphyria cutanea tarda (PCT)
- Congenital erythropoietic porphyria
- Erythropoietic protoporphyria

Affecting skin and causing acute attacks with systemic manifestations:
- Hereditary coproporphyria
- Variegate porphyria

Acute attacks with systemic manifestations only:
- Acute intermittent porphyria

### Porphyria cutanea tarda (PCT)

- Commonest porphyria involving a genetic predisposition in 25% (the remainder are acquired and usually result from liver damage, e.g. alcohol or hepatitis C-related)
- Presentation in middle-age with trauma-induced blisters in light-exposed areas of skin (usually dorsal aspect of hands, sometimes face or upper chest; Fig. 6.27)
- Blisters heal with scarring, and milia formation is common. Hypertrichosis on the face may develop

### Congenital erythropoietic porphyria

- Very rare, autosomal recessive disorder presenting in childhood with severe photosensitivity and haematological disease
- Infants present with severe blistering on light-exposed areas (even during winter months). Scarring with thickening of the skin and deformities develop over time
- Cataracts, brown teeth, and haemolysis (with splenomegaly) are also features

### Variegate porphyria

- Rare, autosomal dominant inheritance
- Skin involvement usually starts in adolescence and features are similar to PCT
- ~17% of patients will suffer an acute attack

### Acute intermittent porphyria (AIP)

- Second most common form of porphyria
- Autosomal dominant inheritance
- Attacks occur more commonly in women than men
- Features include: abdominal pain, constipation, vomiting, dehydration, tachycardia, motor neuropathy with weakness and confusion. Respiratory paralysis may be fatal
- Dietary factors (including alcohol), infection, menstruation and pregnancy, drugs and hormones which are metabolized by liver cytochrome P450 may all precipitate acute attacks

### Diagnosis

- Usually suspected on clinical grounds and confirmed by biochemical analysis of blood, urine, and stool to detect raised levels of porphyrins

### Management

- Photoprotection is paramount for skin manifestations
- Avoidance of precipitating drugs
- Aggressive treatment of coexisting infection
- Dietary changes may be advised (high carbohydrate diet)
- Genetic counselling

## Pyoderma gangrenosum

- Observed as an extraintestinal feature of IBD (both Crohn disease and ulcerative colitis) in ~5% of patients
- Single or multiple erythematous macules develop, most commonly on the lower limbs, and often in association with local trauma
- Necrosis of the dermis leads to deep ulceration and often a sterile, purulent exudate (Fig. 6.28)
- Lesions may be correlated with disease activity in some individuals, where management of the underlying bowel disease with immunosuppression leads to resolution of the skin manifestations. Anti-TNF therapies may have a particular role
- Always exclude/treat superimposed infection

## Dermatomyositis

### Background

Dermatomyositis is an inflammatory disorder of striated muscle that is associated with characteristic cutaneous findings. The lungs (interstitial pneumonitis), heart, GI tract, blood vessels, and joints can also be affected.

### Subtypes

- Dermatomyositis
- Polymyositis (myopathy without skin involvement)
- Malignancy-associated dermatomyositis or polymyositis
- Juvenile dermatomyositis/polymyositis
- Connective tissue disease associated with dermatomyositis/polymyositis
- Amyopathic dermatomyositis: skin disease without myopathy
- Postmyopathic dermatomyositis: persistent severe skin disease after myopathy controlled

### Epidemiology

- ♀: ♂ = 2:1
- All ages can be affected: peak age of onset in children is 5–10 years and in adults 50 years

### History

- Pruritus
- Scaly scalp or diffuse hair loss
- Photosensitivity (50%)
- Fatigue
- Proximal muscle weakness causing difficulty rising from sitting, climbing stairs, and brushing hair
- Dysphagia and dysphonia
- Symptoms related to an underlying malignancy

### Examination

- Heliotrope rash: violaceous oedema of the upper eyelids and periorbital skin. The mauve/erythematous discoloration may extend to the scalp, cheeks, neck, upper chest, and extensor surfaces of the limbs
- Gottron papules: violaceous papules, nodules or plaques usually overlying the knuckles and interphalangeal joints, sometimes the elbows, knees and feet (Fig. 6.29)
- Poikiloderma: variegated erythema with hypo- or hyperpigmentation, atrophy, and telangiectasia. This is seen in sun-exposed sites especially over the extensor surface of the arms, the 'V' of the neck, upper chest and back (shawl sign)
- Nailfold changes: periungual erythema with telangiectasia. The cuticles look overgrown, thickened, and unkempt
- Cutaneous vasculitis and calcinosis are seen in juvenile disease
- Other cutaneous findings include panniculitis, hyperkeratosis of the lateral/palmar aspects of the fingers (mechanic's hands), cutaneous mucinosis, and acquired ichthyosis
- Muscle findings: symmetrical proximal muscle weakness ± atrophy and tenderness. Occasionally the facial, bulbar, pharyngeal, and oesophageal muscles become involved
- Joint swelling is sometimes seen. The associated arthritis is not erosive or deforming
- Patients with interstitial pneumonitis may have crepitations on pulmonary auscultation

### Differential diagnosis

- Lupus erythematosus, lichen planus, and psoriasis
- Exclude other causes of myopathy, e.g. corticosteroids and thyroid disease
- Mixed connective tissue disease

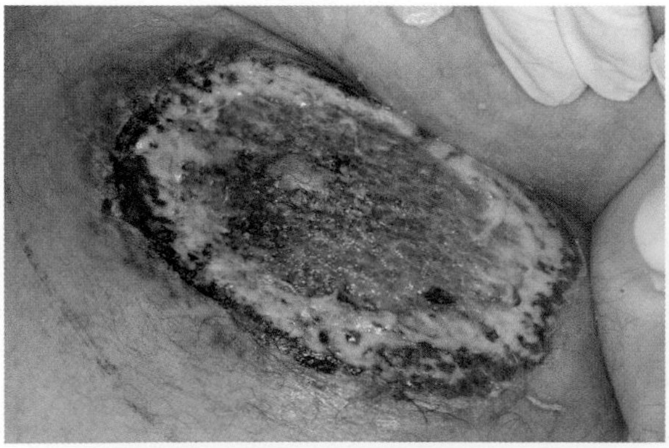

**Fig. 6.28** Pyoderma gangrenosum.
Reproduced with permission from Cambridge University Hospitals NHS Foundation Trust.

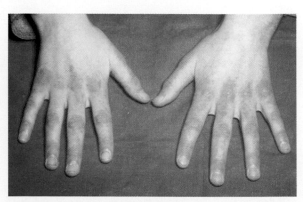

**Fig. 6.29** Dermatomyositis—Gottron papules.

## Investigations

- Raised muscle enzymes: CK is the most sensitive (but LDH, aspartate aminotransferase, and aldolase can also be used)
- Electromyography
- Muscle biopsy

The diagnosis of dermatomyositis is confirmed when proximal muscle weakness is found in association with at least two of the listed criteria. Polymyositis does not require the presence of cutaneous findings.
Additional tests that can be helpful include:

- MRI—affected muscles show increased signal intensity. MRI can be used to select a site for muscle biopsy
- Skin biopsy (interface dermatitis)
- CXR and PFTs (interstitial pneumonitis)
- Barium swallow ± oesophageal manometry
- ECG
- Autoantibodies—these are not routinely used in diagnosis. A positive ANA at a low titre is a common finding in dermatomyositis. Myositis-specific antibodies occur in 30% of patients with dermatomyositis or polymyositis. Anti-Jo1 is more commonly associated with polymyositis and pulmonary involvement. Anti-PM/Scl autoantibodies are found in patients with polymyositis overlapping with scleroderma. Anti-Ku antibodies are found in patients with myositis overlapping with other connective tissue diseases
- An underlying malignancy should be excluded in adult patients

## Treatment

Once malignancy has been excluded, immunosuppression is required to treat the myopathy:

- Prednisolone: starting at 40–60mg daily is used as initial therapy
- Azathioprine: 2–3mg/kg/day is used as a steroid-sparing agent
- Methotrexate, mycophenolate mofetil, and IVIG have also been used
- Topical steroids and hydroxychloroquine can be useful with widespread cutaneous involvement
- Protective clothing, sun avoidance, and regular use of high-factor sunscreen help in photosensitive skin disease

## Prognosis

Patients with an underlying malignancy, cardiac, or pulmonary involvement, severe muscle weakness and older age have a worse prognosis. Remission is seen in about 20% but relapse is common. The 8-year survival rate is 70–80%.

# 6.13 Cutaneous lupus erythematosus

## Background

Systemic lupus erythematosus (SLE) is a multisystem autoimmune disease associated with polyclonal B-cell activation. The clinical manifestations range from limited cutaneous disease to a severe life-threatening systemic illness (Box 6.6). There are three categories of lupus-specific skin disease:

1. **Chronic discoid**
2. **Subacute**
3. **Acute**

## Chronic discoid cutaneous lupus erythematosus

Discoid lupus erythematosus (DLE) is a chronic, scarring, photosensitive dermatosis. DLE lesions may occur in up to 25% of patients with SLE and 5% of patients with DLE may progress to SLE.

### Epidemiology
- Age of onset: 20–45 years
- ♀: ♂ = 2:1
- Race: Afro-Caribbean more commonly affected

### History
- Lesions precipitated by sunlight to exposed sites, particularly the face, ears, and scalp. The disease is localized to these areas in 90% of patients
- In generalized disease, lesions typically involve the upper chest, back, and arms. These patients are more likely to progress to full SLE
- Lesions are occasionally pruritic
- Features of SLE may be present

### Examination
- Well-defined red papules that evolve into plaques which can be annular or polycyclic with irregular borders (Fig. 6.30)
- Surface changes include scale, hyperkeratosis, and follicular plugging (dilatation of the follicular openings with a keratin plug)
- The lesions expand peripherally and regress centrally with atrophy and scarring
- Active lesions are bright red whilst burned out lesions appear pink or white. Squamous cell carcinomas occasionally develop within chronic lesions
- Scarring alopecia is seen if the scalp is affected
- Lips, tongue and oral mucosa can also be affected
- Lesions may also become hypertrophic or verrucous

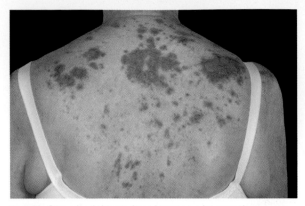

Fig. 6.30 Generalized chronic discoid cutaneous lupus erythematosus. Reproduced with permission from Cambridge University Hospitals NHS Foundation Trust.

### Investigations
- **Skin histology:** liquefactive degeneration of the basal layer, follicular plugging, hyperkeratosis and epidermal atrophy, dermal oedema, and a perivascular and peri-appendiceal lymphocytic inflammatory infiltrate
- **Direct immunofluorescence:** granular deposition of immunoglobulin and complement at the dermo-epidermal junction is characteristic of cutaneous lupus. The presence of immunoreactants in the basal layer is not specific for lupus
- **Autoantibodies**: antinuclear antibody (ANA) is positive in 20% of patients with DLE
- **Other tests:** ± raised ESR, low complement (C3/C4) levels and cytopenias

### Treatment
- UV light protection: high-factor sunscreen, protective clothing, and sun avoidance
- Cosmetic measures: wigs (alopecia)
- Corticosteroids: moderate or potent topical steroids and intralesional triamcinolone for mild or localized disease
- Calcineurin inhibitors: topical tacrolimus
- Antimalarials: hydroxychloroquine
- Others: dapsone, mepacrine, thalidomide, methotrexate, mycophenolate mofetil, and azathioprine

## Subacute cutaneous lupus erythematosus

Subacute cutaneous lupus erythematosus (SCLE) is a non-scarring photosensitive dermatosis that accounts for 10% of cases of cutaneous lupus. Patients with SCLE frequently have a few of the criteria used to define SLE and serological abnormalities.

### Epidemiology
- Mean age of onset: 43 years
- ♀: ♂ = 4:1
- More common in Caucasians

### History
- Photosensitive rash on exposed sites (upper trunk, arms, and hands) that is mostly asymptomatic. The face may be spared
- Arthralgia is common
- Fatigue
- Features of SLE may be present

---

**Box 6.6 Cutaneous features of SLE**

- Malar rash
- Photosensitivity
- Oral lesions: painful ulcers, gingivitis and chelitis
- Non-scarring, diffuse alopecia
- Nail changes: periungual erythema, dilated nailfold capillaries
- Raynaud phenomenon
- Palmar erythema
- Livedo reticularis
- Perniosis/chilblains
- Vasculitis including urticarial vasculitis

### Examination

Two distinct types of lesion are seen:

1. Papulosquamous—erythematosus papules and small plaques with fine scale.
2. Annular—red polycyclic lesions with central clearing:
   - Non-scarring
   - No follicular plugging

### Investigations

- Skin histology: vacuolar degeneration of the basal layer with a patchy perivascular and peri-appendiceal lymphocytic inflammatory infiltrate. There is slight hyperkeratosis but follicular plugging is less common than in DLE
- Direct IF: 60% have immune deposits at the dermo-epidermal junction
- Autoantibodies: 60–80% ANA positive. Anti-Ro antibodies are present in up to 90% and anti-La antibodies in up to 50% of cases
- Other: cytopenias, low complement levels, and raised ESR may also be present

### Treatment

- UV light protection
- Topical and intralesional steroids
- Antimalarials: hydroxychloroquine
- Others: thalidomide
- Women with anti-Ro antibodies may give birth to babies with neonatal lupus and congenital heart block and should be counselled about this

## Acute cutaneous lupus erythematosus

Acute cutaneous lupus erythematosus (ACLE) has a strong association with SLE. ACLE lesions have been noted in 20% of SCLE patients but are uncommon in DLE.

### Clinical features

- Butterfly rash: erythematous macular eruption in a malar distribution that can extend to the forehead, periorbital area, and neck (Fig. 6.31). The lesions are well-defined with fine scale
- Generalized ACLE: generalized photosensitive eruption that can blister and mimic toxic epidermolysis bullosa
- The lesions typically last a few weeks and are exacerbated by sunlight
- Post-inflammatory pigmentation may result but scarring is not usually a feature
- Superficial ulceration of the oral and nasal mucosae

### Investigations

As ACLE and SLE are often closely related, the laboratory findings are similar:

- Skin histology: upper dermal oedema, liquefactive degeneration of the basal layer, and a sparse lymphocytic infiltrate. Direct IF positive

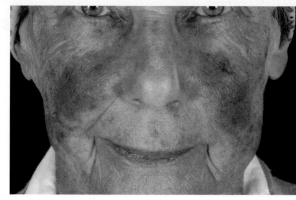

**Fig. 6.31** Classic butterfly rash of acute cutaneous lupus erythematosus. Reproduced with permission from Cambridge University Hospitals NHS Foundation Trust.

- Autoantibodies: positive ANA in most patients. Double-stranded DNA (dsDNA) antibodies and anti-Sm antibodies are specific for SLE
- Low complement levels
- Cytopenias, renal dysfunction, and a raised ESR may be seen in patients with systemic involvement

### Treatment

- Systemic corticosteroids in systemic disease
- Antimalarials: hydroxychloroquine
- Others: azathioprine, cyclophosphamide, and thalidomide

### Lupus profundus

- A rare panniculitis that can occur with SLE, DLE, or independently
- Involvement of the deep dermis and subcutaneous fat resulting in tender nodules which appear on the buttocks and limbs
- Overlying skin can be normal, or show changes of DLE, scarring, or hyperpigmentation. Ulceration is common

### Drug-induced lupus

- Can be precipitated by hydralazine, procainamide, isoniazid, methyldopa, D-penicillamine, and minocycline. These drugs do not seem to affect existing SLE
- Multiple organs may be affected but nephritis and central nervous system involvement are uncommon. Cutaneous disease affects 25–50% of patients. Purpura, erythema nodosum, and erythematous papules are seen
- ANA is usually positive
- Antihistone antibodies are seen in most cases
- The offending drug should be stopped

# 6.14 Systemic sclerosis (scleroderma)

## Background

Systemic sclerosis (SS) is a connective tissue disease characterized by hardening of the skin with involvement of the internal organs, particularly the lungs, kidneys, GI tract, and heart.

## Epidemiology

- Age of onset: 30–50 years
- ♀: ♂ = 4:1
- Affects all races
- Rare (prevalence ~65–265 per million population)

## Classification

Limited cutaneous SS (lcSS):
- Skin involvement limited to distal limbs and face
- Prolonged time to visceral disease
- Anticentromere antibodies found in many patients
- Include CREST syndrome (**C**alcinosis, **R**aynaud phenomenon, o**E**sophageal dysfunction, **S**clerodactyly and **T**elangiectasia)

Diffuse cutaneous SS (dcSS):
- Widespread skin involvement including trunk and proximal limbs
- Early internal organ involvement
- Antitopoisomerase I (Scl-70) antibodies found in 1/3 of patients

Scleroderma sine scleroderma:
- Internal organ involvement without skin disease
- Usually diagnosed postmortem

## Clinical evaluation

### History
- Raynaud phenomenon—digital pain and tingling with triphasic colour change: white, blue, red
- Migratory polyarthritis
- Shortness of breath, dry cough
- Dysphagia, constipation, diarrhoea, malabsorption, and weight loss
- History of renal failure

### Examination
- Hands:
  - Non-pitting oedema of hands and feet.
  - Sclerodactyly—tapered fingers with bound down hardened skin.
  - Nail-fold capillaries (periungual telangiectasia).
  - Loss of distal phalanges due to bony resorption and fingertip ulceration.
  - Beaked nails and nail dystrophy.
  - Subcutaneous calcification over fingertips and bony prominence.
- Face:
  - Small sharp beaked nose.
  - Microstomia with thin lips and radial perioral furrowing.
  - Loss of facial lines due to oedema and fibrosis.
  - Mat telangiectasia.

Box 6.7  American College of Rheumatology diagnostic criteria for systemic sclerosis

One major or two or more minor criteria are required
- **Major criteria:** proximal sclerosis affecting the face, arms, and/or neck.
- **Minor criteria:** sclerodactyly, bibasal pulmonary fibrosis, erosions or atrophy of the fingertips.

Source: Preliminary criteria for the classification of systemic sclerosis (scleroderma). Subcommittee for scleroderma criteria of the American Rheumatism Association Diagnostic and Therapeutic Criteria Committee. *Arthritis Rheum* 1980; 23: 581–90).

- Other:
  - Thickened indurated skin on distal extremities in lcSS and on trunk and proximal extremities in dcSS.
  - Areas of hypo- and hyperpigmentation.
  - Hypertension.
  - Hepatomegaly (association with primary biliary cirrhosis).

The diagnosis is clinical, based on the American College of Rheumatology guidelines (Box 6.7).

## Investigations

- Skin biopsy
- Autoantibodies: positive ANA with anticentromere and antitopoisomerase I antibodies
- Capillaroscopy—dilated capillary loops

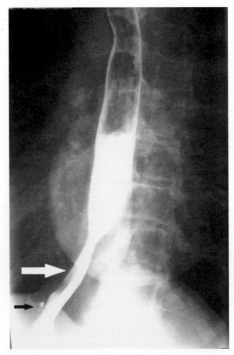

**Fig. 6.32** Barium swallow examination in patient with scleroderma, showing long distal oesophageal peptic stricture (large arrow) and mucosal ulceration (small arrow).

Reproduced with permission of Dr. Hany Elmadbouh.

190

- Bloods:
  - Anaemia (iron deficiency from chronic oesophagitis, $B_{12}$ and folate deficiency from malabsorption, normocytic normochromic due to chronic disease, microangiopathic haemolytic anaemia).
  - Raised urea and creatinine with renal involvement.
  - Raised CK with muscle involvement.
- CXR, PFTs, and HRCT
- Echocardiogram
- Barium swallow (Fig. 6.32)

## Differential diagnosis

Eosinophilic fasciitis, scleromyxoedema, chronic graft versus host disease, lichen sclerosus et atrophicus.

## Management

- Education and psychological support
- Treat Raynaud phenomenon:
  - Avoid cold, wear protective clothing, stop smoking.
  - Calcium channel blockers (e.g. nifedipine).
  - IV prostaglandins/prostacyclin analogues (e.g. epoprostenol).
- Proton-pump inhibitors for reflux symptoms
- Renal disease—ACE inhibitors for renal crisis
- Pulmonary disease—prostacyclin analogues and vasodilators (e.g. sildenafil)
- Systemic treatment—methotrexate, ciclosporin, cyclophosphamide, chlorambucil, and interferon alpha

None proven to be consistently beneficial.

## Prognosis

Patients with limited cutaneous disease have the most favourable prognosis. Death is usually due to internal organ involvement (renal, pulmonary, or cardiac):

- GIT: dysphagia, oesophageal reflux, abdominal bloating, constipation, diarrhoea, malabsorption
- Kidney: glomerulonephritis, hypertension
- Lungs: fibrosis, pulmonary hypertension
- Heart: myocardial fibrosis

# 6.15 Vasculitis

## Background

Vasculitis refers to a heterogeneous group of disorders characterized by inflammation of the blood vessels.

Any size vessel can be affected within any organ. The size of the affected vessels can be used to classify the different types of vasculitis.

## Classification

### Large vessel vasculitis
- Giant cell (temporal) vasculitis
- Takayasu arteritis

### Medium vessel vasculitis
- Polyarteritis nodosa (PAN)
- Kawasaki disease

### Small vessel vasculitis
- Cutaneous leucocytoclastic vasculitis
- Henoch–Schönlein purpura
- Granulomatosis with polyangiitis (GPA, formerly known as Wegener granulomatosis)
- Eosinophilic granulomatosis with polyangiitis (EGPA, formerly known as Churg–Strauss syndrome)
- Microscopic polyangiitis (MPA)

## Leucocytoclastic vasculitis

Leucocytoclastic vasculitis (LCV) is the most common form of cutaneous vasculitis. LCV refers to the histological change that occurs in the skin. The vessels of the papillary and reticular dermis are dilated and show fibrinoid necrosis with fragmentation of neutrophil nuclei which is associated with the extravasation of red blood cells into the connective tissue.

### Cause

LCV can be localized to the skin or it may be part of a systemic disease in any of the primary small vessel vasculitides. In addition, there are several secondary causes that are more common and should also be considered (Box 6.8).

---

| Box 6.8 Secondary causes of a leucocytoclastic vasculitis |
|---|
| **Idiopathic**: |
|   Drugs: β-lactam antibiotics, thiazide diuretics, NSAIDs |
| **Infection**: |
|   β-haemolytic streptococci |
|   Hepatitis B and C |
|   HIV |
|   Neisseria |
|   Rickettsia |
|   Meningococcal disease |
| **Connective tissue disease**: |
|   Rheumatoid arthritis |
|   SLE |
|   Sjögren syndrome |
|   Sarcoidosis |
| **Inflammatory bowel disease**: |
|   Crohn disease |
|   Ulcerative colitis |
|   Malignancy |

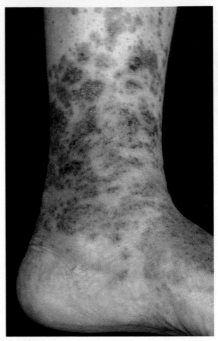

Fig. 6.33 Vasculitic rash.

## Clinical features
- Palpable purpura (non-blanching red papules) on the lower extremities or dependent areas (Fig. 6.33)
- Livedo reticularis
- Blistering, ulceration, or necrosis of purpura
- Lesions typically last 1–4 weeks
- Pruritus, burning, and pain can occur
- Symptoms and signs of any underlying disease

## Investigations
Investigations are directed at determining the presence of internal organ involvement and identifying an underlying disorder:
- FBC
- ESR
- Renal function tests and urine dipstick
- LFTs
- CRP, blood cultures
- Hepatitis B and C serology
- HIV test
- Antistreptolysin O titre (ASOT)
- ANA, dsDNA, ENA, ANCA, complement, and ACE levels
- Cryoglobulins
- Serum electrophoresis
- CXR
- Skin biopsy for histology and direct IF

## Differential diagnosis
Thrombocytopenia, coagulopathy, scurvy, or septic/atherosclerotic plaque emboli.

**Treatment**

- Treat any underlying disease
- Elevate legs
- Compression stockings
- If the disease is confined to the skin, systemic steroids, colchicine and dapsone can be used to control symptoms until the disease goes into remission

## Henoch–Schönlein purpura

Henoch–Schönlein purpura (HSP) is an IgA-mediated leucocytoclastic vasculitis that affects the skin, joints, kidneys, and GI tract.

### Epidemiology

- Children and young adults
- ♂ : ♀ = 1.5:1

### Clinical features

- History: recent URTI, colicky abdominal pain or bloody diarrhoea
- Skin: palpable purpura on legs, buttocks, and forearms
- Joints: arthralgia
- Kidneys: microscopic/macroscopic haematuria and proteinuria. Renal involvement may occur late and has a worse prognosis
- Neurological: headache, seizures, and coma (rare)
- Fever, malaise, myalgia, lymphadenopathy

### Investigations

- Throat swab and ASOT
- Skin biopsy with immunofluorescence
- Abdominal and renal investigations if indicated
- Exclude other causes of a LCV

### Treatment

- HSP is usually a self-limiting disease
- Corticosteroids and additional immunosuppression can be used in renal disease

## Background

The skin is the largest organ in the body and is composed of several layers containing specialized cells and appendages (sweat glands, sebaceous glands and hair follicles). It serves multiple functions. Functions of the skin:

- Barrier against injury, infection, excess water loss or gain
- Protection against UV radiation
- Thermoregulation
- UV light-induced vitamin D synthesis
- Antigen presentation
- Sensory function (pain, temperature, and touch)

## The epidermis

The epidermis is derived from the ectoderm and is composed of stratified squamous epithelium. It consists of four layers:

- Basal cell layer
- Prickle cell layer
- Granular cell layer
- Cornified layer (stratum corneum)

## Keratinocytes

Keratinocytes are the main cell type found in the epidermis. They originate in the basal cell layer and advance up the epidermis by the process of maturation. The cells are initially columnar and aligned at right angles to each other in the basal cell layer. As they mature, they become polygonal in the prickle cell layer and acquire keratohyaline granules in the granular cell layer. In the cornified layer keratinocytes have lost their nuclei, are flattened in shape, and lie in parallel to each other, forming a waterproof barrier.

## Melanocytes

Melanocytes are derived from the neural crest. In healthy skin, they are only found in the basal cell layer. They secrete the pigment melanin and protect against UV radiation. Skin colour is determined by the amount and type of melanin that is produced, not the number of melanocytes.

## Langerhans cells

Langerhans cells are dendritic cells that are found in the suprabasal layer of the skin. They act as antigen-presenting cells.

## Merkel cells

Merkel cells arise from the neural crest. They are often associated with sensory nerve endings and may have a neuroendocrine function.

## Basement membrane zone

The basement membrane zone is a complex structure that anchors the epidermis to the dermis. It consists of four major structural components:

- Basal cell plasma membrane
- Lamina lucida
- Lamina densa
- Sublamina densa zone

Pathology in this region may give rise to blistering diseases.

## The dermis

The dermis is derived from the mesoderm and lies beneath the epidermis. It is divided into the superficial papillary layer, and the deeper reticular layer. It is composed of collagen, elastin, and ground substance and this provides strength and elasticity to the skin. In addition to containing blood and lymphatic vessels, nerves, and muscles, the dermis supports the skin appendages.

## Sebaceous glands

- Produce sebum, a complex lipid mixture
- Become active during puberty
- Most concentrated on the face and scalp

## Apocrine sweat glands

- Found in the anogenital region and axillae
- Become active during puberty

## Eccrine sweat glands

- Found on all skin surfaces except mucous membranes
- Most concentrated on the palms and soles, forehead, and axillae

## The subcutaneous layer

The subcutaneous layer is mostly composed of adipose tissue which contains blood vessels and nerves. Its physiological function is to provide insulation and act as a lipid store.

## Hair

- Hair covers all the body except the palms and soles and the mucous membranes of the genitalia. **Lanugo** hair is present at birth. It is non-medulated (see later), soft and fine. **Terminal** hairs are medullated and are the thick, coarse hairs found on the scalp, beard, and pubic regions. **Vellus** hair is non-medullated, short, and fine and can be found all over the body

- The hair follicle is made up of several layers. The external layer is the outer root sheath and is continuous with the epidermis. The inner root sheath is keratinized. The hair shaft has an inner medulla (may be absent) and an outer cortex and cuticle. Hair growth occurs at the distal end of the follicle in the bulb which surrounds the richly innervated and vascularized dermal papilla

- Hair growth is cyclical, consisting of a growth phase (**anagen**), arrest phase (**catagen**), and the resting/shedding phase (**telogen**). Hair length is related to the length of the anagen phase which is from 2–6 years on the human scalp. Catagen is about 2 weeks and telogen 1–3 months

## Nails

The nail is a keratinized plate that arises from the nail matrix. The visible portion of the nail matrix is the lunula. The nail bed lies between the lunula and the hyponychium. The nailfold is the cutaneous soft tissue that encases the nail. Adult fingernails grow at an average rate of 3mm per month.

## Psoriasis

- Nail changes are seen in 50% of cases
- Pitting (Box 6.9)
- Transverse ridges
- Brittle nail plate
- Onycholysis—detachment of the nail plate from the nail bed (Box 6.10 and Fig. 6.34)
- Oil spots
- Subungual hyperkeratosis

| Box 6.9  Causes of nail pitting |
| --- |
| • Psoriasis |
| • Eczema |
| • Alopecia areata |
| • Normal variant |

| Box 6.10  Causes of onycholysis |
| --- |
| • Psoriasis |
| • Lichen planus |
| • Trauma |
| • Thyrotoxicosis |
| • Infection—onychomycosis |
| • Hereditary |
| • Drugs |

## Lichen planus

- Nail plate becomes thin and brittle
- Longitudinal ridges

- Onycholysis
- Subungual hyperkeratosis, and pterygium formation
- Permanent anonychia
- All 20 nails can be affected without involvement of the skin—20-nail dystrophy

## Acrolentiginous malignant melanoma

- Subungual or periungual brown-black discoloration of the nail with or without nail dystrophy (Fig. 6.35)
- Hutchinson sign: periungual extension of pigmentation onto proximal and lateral nailfold
- More common on thumb and great toe nails
- Afro-Caribbean >Caucasian
- Poorer prognosis than cutaneous melanoma as often presents late

## Nail changes in systemic disease

- Leuconychia—hypoalbuminaemia in chronic liver disease
- Koilonychia—physiological, iron deficiency anaemia
- Splinter haemorrhages—physiological, traumatic, psoriasis, vasculitis, embolic (e.g. in bacterial endocarditis)
- Beau lines—transverse band like depressions in the nail plate—acute severe febrile illness, systemic disease, cytotoxic drugs, trauma
- Clubbing—congenital cyanotic heart disease, bronchial carcinoma and other malignancies, bronchiectasis, acromegaly, thyroid acropachy, hypertrophic osteoarthropathy
- Dilated nailfold capillaries and erythema—systemic sclerosis, dermatomyositis, systemic lupus erythematosus, rheumatoid arthritis

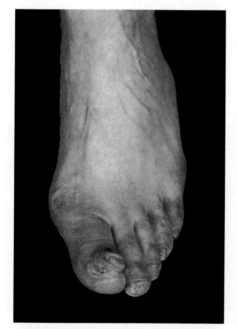

Fig. 6.34 Onycholysis.

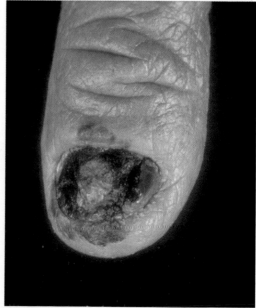

Fig. 6.35 Subungual malignant melanoma.

# 6.18 Alopecia

## Background

Alopecia can be due to a number of causes and these are generally divided into scarring (Box 6.11) and non-scarring (Box 6.12), differentiated clinically by the destruction or preservation of hair follicles respectively.

Initial blood tests are used to exclude metabolic, nutritional, or endocrine causes of alopecia, and a biopsy for H&E and direct IF may be helpful in determining the cause, particularly in scarring alopecia.

## Alopecia areata

### Epidemiology
- Onset usually in children and young adults
- ♂ = ♀
- Common condition affecting up to 1% of the population at some stage

### Aetiology/pathogenesis
- Cause is unknown though it is thought to be an autoimmune condition, and has an association with other autoimmune conditions such as vitiligo, thyroid abnormalities, and pernicious anaemia. Some patients may have a family history of autoimmune conditions

### Clinical evaluation
*History*
- Gradual loss of hair over weeks. Usually asymptomatic. May be progressive or stable and may spontaneously regrow. There may be a history of recurrent episodes

*Examination*
- Well-demarcated patches of non-scarring alopecia with 'exclamation-mark' hairs at the periphery (Fig. 6.36)
- May become confluent and cause alopecia totalis (loss of all scalp hair) or alopecia universalis (loss of all body hair)
- Regrowth may initially be with white hairs
- There may be evidence of nail pitting

### Investigations
- The diagnosis is usually clinical, but if there is evidence of inflammation or scarring a biopsy may be indicated
- Blood tests to exclude other autoimmune conditions

### Management
- No curative treatment available, and treatment may not affect course or outcome

---

**Box 6.11  Non-scarring alopecia**
- Alopecia areata.
- Androgenic alopecia.
- Telogen effluvium.
- Trichotillomania.
- Endocrine disorders: hypo-/hyper-thyroidism.
- Infections: tinea, syphilis.
- SLE.
- Drugs (e.g. chemotherapy).
- Metabolic or nutritional: iron/zinc deficiency.
- Traction alopecia.

---

**Box 6.12  Scarring alopecia**
- Discoid lupus erythematosus.
- Lichen planus.
- Idiopathic (pseudopelade).
- Folliculitis decalvans.
- Dissecting cellulitis.
- Infections: kerion/VZV.
- Tumours (e.g. BCC, SCC, metastases).
- Physical (e.g. burns, radiation).
- Dermal infiltrate (e.g. scleroderma, sarcoidosis).

---

- Options include:
  - Topical or intralesional steroids.
  - Oral corticosteroids (although hair loss decreases only during therapy and significant side effects).
  - Contact sensitization with diphencyprone.
  - Phototherapy with PUVA.
  - Hair pieces may be useful in severe cases.

### Outcome/prognosis
- Most patients' hair regrows, although recurrent episodes are common
- In some cases the course may be progressive, and poor prognostic factors include:
  - Recurrent episodes.
  - Widespread involvement.
  - Positive family history of alopecia areata.
  - Personal history of atopy.
  - Nail pitting.
  - Ophiasis pattern (alopecia affecting the scalp margins, usually occipital margin).

---

## Androgenic alopecia

Most common type of non-scarring alopecia.

### Epidemiology
- ♂ >> ♀
- Onset after puberty in ♂, being fully expressed in their 40s. Later onset in ♀
- Affects all races

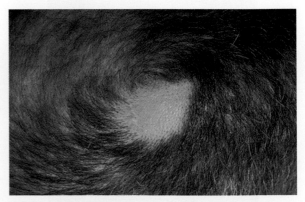

**Fig. 6.36** Alopecia areata.

### Aetiology/pathogenesis

- Inherited component (may be polygenic or autosomal dominant)
- Locally increased androgen receptors and changes in androgen metabolism of the scalp hair follicles are thought to play a part
- In women, polycystic ovarian syndrome (PCOS) may need to be excluded as an underlying cause

### Clinical evaluation

*History*

- Gradual thinning of hair over months to years
- There may be a family history of androgenic alopecia
- In women, need to inquire about acne, hirsutism, irregular menses, or virilization

*Examination*

- Miniaturization of hair at sites of hair loss
- Men usually start with fronto-temporal recession progressing to loss over the vertex
- Women usually have more diffuse hair loss over the vertex

### Investigations

- Blood tests to exclude other treatable causes of non-scarring alopecia such as ferritin, zinc, and thyroid function
- In women, may need to check LH, FSH, testosterone, free androgen index, DHEAS, sex hormone binding globulin, ± ovarian USS

### Management

- Difficult, and active treatment may not be necessary
- Therapeutic options include topical minoxidil, oral finasteride (5-alpha reductase inhibitor), in men and oral anti-androgens in women. Hair transplantation and hair pieces may be helpful

### Outcome/prognosis

- Alopecia usually gradually progresses over many years

# Telogen effluvium

An acute diffuse hair loss that occurs usually a few months after a major event.

### Epidemiology

- Can occur at any age
- ♀ >♂

### Aetiology/pathogenesis

- Precipitating factors include significant medical illness (especially with high fever), profound emotional stress, crash dieting, surgical shock, postpartum haemorrhage, major trauma; usually 3–4 months prior to hair shedding
- Thought to be due to a premature shift of anagen hairs into the telogen phase

### Clinical evaluation

*History*

- Increased hair loss, anxieties about going bald
- History of preceding precipitating event

*Examination*

- Positive hair pull test (several hairs may be shed on passing fingers through patient's hair)
- Diffuse non-scarring thinning of scalp hair
- Nails: Beau lines as a response to the precipitating event

### Investigations

- Diagnosis is usually made clinically, but blood tests are carried out to exclude iron and zinc deficiency, thyroid abnormalities, and SLE
- Trichogram shows increased telogen hairs

### Management

- Reassurance. No intervention is required

### Outcome/prognosis

- Complete regrowth of hair is the rule, though it may go on for a year after the precipitating event

# 6.19 Hirsutism and hypertrichosis

## Background

Hirsutism refers to male pattern hair growth in females (Fig. 6.37), while hypertrichosis refers to excess hair growth at sites which are not usually hairy and can affect males and females.

## Hirsutism

### Causes of hirsutism

1. **Increased androgen production**:
   - Ovarian (PCOS, ovarian tumours)
   - Adrenal (adrenal tumour/hyperplasia, hyperpituitarism).
2. **Ovarian failure:** postmenopausal, post-oophorectomy.
3. **Androgens:** steroids, danazol.
4. **Constitutional/racial:** Middle Eastern, Indian, African races.

### Investigations

- FBC, early morning cortisol, testosterone, DHEAS, prolactin, LH/FSH, ovarian USS, radiography of the pituitary fossa (as indicated)

### Management

- If virilizing features are present, full endocrine investigations should be carried out
- Once underlying causes are excluded, it is labelled as constitutional hirsutism
- Therapeutic options include:
  - Physical methods (e.g. plucking, shaving, waxing, electrolysis, bleaching, laser therapy).
  - Medical therapy (anti-androgens).

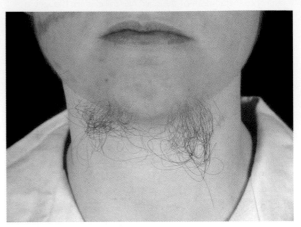

Fig. 6.37 Hirsutism.

## Hypertrichosis

Generalized hypertrichosis occurs in:
- Anorexia nervosa
- Porphyria
- Underlying malignancy
- Drugs (e.g. ciclosporin and corticosteroids)

# 6.20 Acne vulgaris

## Background

Acne is a common inflammatory condition of the pilosebaceous units affecting the face and sometimes the trunk, often causing significant psychosocial morbidity.

## Epidemiology

- Most common skin disease in adolescence (>80% teenagers aged 13–18 years affected at some point)
- Increasing incidence of adult acne (cause unknown)
- ♂ and ♀ equally affected
- All races

## Aetiology and pathogenesis

- Genetic susceptibility
- Increased androgens during puberty
- Increased sebum production
- Ductal hyperkeratosis and blockage of pilosebaceous unit
- Proliferation of *Propionibacterium* acnes (anaerobic bacterium)

## Clinical evaluation

### History

- Appearance of 'spots'
- Pain
- Perimenstrual flares in women

### Examination

- Open (blackheads) or closed (whiteheads) comedones (Fig. 6.38)
- Papules, pustules
- Nodules, cysts
- Scarring
- Post-inflammatory pigmentation
- Distribution on face, chest, upper back

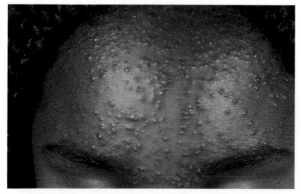

Fig. 6.38 Acne affecting the forehead in a young female.

## Investigations

- Usually none required
- In older women, consider excluding hyperandrogenaemia and PCOS

## Differential diagnosis

- Rosacea, perioral dermatitis
- Steroid folliculitis, drug-induced acne (contraceptives, androgens)
- Bacterial or *Pityrosporum* folliculitis

## Therapeutic options

### Topical

- Antibiotics: erythromycin, clindamycin
- Keratolytics: benzoyl peroxide, azelaic acid
- Retinoids: tretinoin, adapalene

### Systemic

- Antibiotics: tetracyclines, erythromycin, trimethoprim
- Antiandrogens (in women): cyproterone acetate (Dianette®)
- Isotretinoin (Roaccutane®)
  - Indications: severe nodulocystic or scarring acne, unresponsive to other therapies.
  - Contraindications: pregnancy.
  - Adverse effects: teratogenic, dry skin and mucosae, raised lipids, hepatotoxicity, mood swings, possibly depression.
  - Monitoring: baseline liver function and lipids, regular pregnancy testing (see Box 6.13).

## Complications

- Acne fulminans:
  - Mostly young ♂.
  - Severe crusted and necrotic lesions.
  - Systemic features include fever, arthralgia, fatigue.
  - Treated with oral prednisolone, followed by oral isotretinoin.
- Multiple miliary osteoma cutis (rare complication, may require surgical intervention)
- Psychosocial effects

## Prognosis

Facial acne persists over the age of 25 years in only ~3% men and 12% women.

---

**Box 6.13 Precautions when prescribing isotretinoin to women of child-bearing age**

- Effective contraception for 1 month before, during, and 1 month after treatment (usually two forms of contraception).
- Consent form showing understanding of teratogenicity and agreement to effective contraception measures.
- Baseline and monthly pregnancy tests.

# 6.21 Rosacea

## Background

Rosacea is a common condition, characterized by a range of clinical signs, including erythema, telangiectasia, papules, and pustules. Facial flushing may also be a feature.

## Epidemiology

- Peak incidence between 40–50 years
- ♀ >♂ (although rhinophyma occurs more often in ♂)
- More common in fair skin types

## Aetiology/pathogenesis

- Cause is unknown
- Problem with vasomotor stability of blood vessels a possibility
- Potential role of *Demodex* mites
- Spicy foods, alcohol, and hot beverages may trigger flushing but unlikely to have a role in basic pathogenesis

## Clinical evaluation

### History

- May be a long history of episodic flushing (especially in response to triggers)
- Concern regarding cosmetic appearance

### Examination

- Symmetrical localization on the face (cheeks, chin, forehead, glabella, and nose). Rarely neck, chest, and back may be involved
- Persistent erythema with telangiectasia (Fig. 6.39)
- Tiny papules and pustules (no comedones)
- Marked sebaceous hyperplasia and lymphoedema in late stages causing disfigurement of the nose (rhinophyma), forehead, eye-lids, ears, and chin
- Eye involvement may occur, with blepharitis, conjunctivitis, or episcleritis. Rosacea keratitis can be a serious problem with development of corneal ulcers

## Management

- Avoid topical corticosteroids (which may exacerbate or even precipitate the condition)

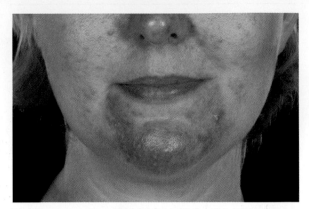

Fig. 6.39 Rosacea affecting the chin.
Reproduced with permission from Cambridge University Hospitals NHS Foundation Trust.

- **Prevention:** avoidance of alcohol and hot beverages may help some patients
- **Topical:**
  Metronidazole gel or cream may be helpful.
  Topical azelaic acid.
- **Systemic:**
  - Oral tetracyclines for 6 weeks usually helpful (but more prolonged courses/maintenance treatment may be required).
  - Oral isotretinoin (often in low doses) may help, but is reserved for severe cases.
- **Physical:** intense pulse light or pulsed-dye laser may help with erythema and telangiectasia

| Causes of facial rashes |
| --- |
| • Acne vulgaris |
| • Rosacea |
| • Perioral dermatitis |
| • Seborrhoeic dermatitis |
| • Atopic dermatitis |
| • Contact dermatitis |
| • Dermatomyositis |
| • Lupus erythematosus |
| • Photosensitive eruptions |

# 6.22 Hidradenitis suppurativa

## Background

This is a chronic, suppurative, often scarring condition affecting mainly the flexures.

## Epidemiology

- Onset usually after puberty
- ♀ >♂
- Can affect all races

## Aetiology/pathogenesis

- Thought to be a disorder of apocrine glands but the cause is unknown
- Predisposing factors:
  - Obesity.
  - Genetic predisposition in some families to acneiform or follicular occlusive disorders.

## Clinical evaluation

- History: painful lesions in the axillae and/or groins with intermittent discharge
- Examination: papules, nodules, cysts, abscesses or sinuses leading to scarring in flexures: axillae, groins and natal cleft most frequent sites
- Investigations: swabs for microscopy and culture

## Management

- Generally very difficult
- Weight loss
- Prolonged courses of antibiotics
- Oral retinoids
- Anti-androgen therapy (in ♀ patients)
- In severe cases, infliximab has recently been shown to be of benefit
- Surgery may be an option in severe, localized disease

## Outcome/prognosis

- Spontaneous resolution in some cases
- Often relapsing/remitting/progressive course
- May remit after the menopause

## Background

Pigment of the skin is produced by melanocytes of the epidermis and is called melanin. Pigmentary disorders may be classified into generalized/localized and increased/decreased pigmentation.

## Classivfication

### Generalized increase in pigmentation
- Addison disease
- Acanthosis nigricans (initially more pronounced in flexures)
- Primary haemochromatosis
- Drugs: minocycline, amiodarone

### Localized increase in pigmentation
- Melasma
- Café au lait macules (neurofibromatoses)
- Post-inflammatory

### Generalized decrease in pigmentation
- Albinism

### Localized decrease in pigmentation
- Piebaldism
- Vitiligo
- Leprosy
- Post-inflammatory

The more common conditions are described in the following sections.

## Melasma

This is more common in women and associated with increased levels of oestrogen during pregnancy, lactation, and with the combined oral contraceptive pill. It affects the sun-exposed parts of the face with a diffuse, usually well-defined increase in pigmentation. It fades in the winter with lack of sun exposure, but will darken rapidly with minimal sun exposure in the spring. Treatment should be with careful, broad-spectrum sun protection.

## Post-inflammatory pigmentary changes

Both increased and decreased pigmentation can occur after an inflammatory condition of the skin. Eczema, for example, can lead to both. Lichen planus is particularly prone to causing marked post-inflammatory hyperpigmentation. Once the inflammation is treated

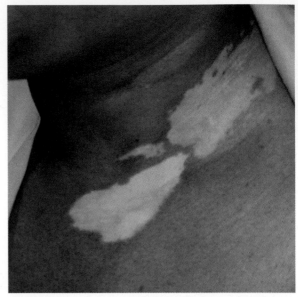

Fig. 6.40 Vitiligo.

(whatever the cause), the pigmentary change will usually improve, although this may take 6–12 months.

## Vitiligo

Focal destruction of melanocytes caused by autoimmune mechanisms is thought to be the cause of this condition. It is often associated with other autoimmune disorders. Well-defined patches of depigmentation occur (Fig. 6.40), usually symmetrically and starting acrally and in a peri-orofacial distribution. In fair-skinned people the condition may not be noticeable until sun exposure leads to tanning of the surrounding normal skin. It is a significant cosmetic problem in darker-skinned individuals. The usual clinical course is for gradual extension of depigmentation over many years, although repigmentation is also known to occur without treatment.

Treatment consists of counselling regarding the diagnosis, as in some races depigmentation carries the stigma of possible leprosy. Sun protection is important, especially in fair-skinned individuals. Cosmetic camouflage can be very helpful. Repigmentation is difficult to achieve, but topical corticosteroids and calcineurin inhibitors may have a role. Phototherapy (narrow-band UVB treatment) can produce a 50% improvement in ~50% of patients.

# 6.24 Urticaria and angio-oedema

## Background

These conditions result from histamine, bradykinin, leukotriene C4, prostaglandin D2, and other vasoactive substances released from mast cells and basophils in the skin.

In **urticaria,** the swelling is dermal and individual lesions usually resolve within 24 hours.

In **angio-oedema,** the resulting swelling is deeper in the subcutaneous tissues and often more prolonged in duration.

## Urticaria

The majority of cases have no identifiable cause. In some cases, intermittent urticaria can be caused by type 1 hypersensitivity to specific foods such as prawns or strawberries. In these cases, the cause is usually obvious to the patient.

In ~50% of chronic ordinary urticaria, autoantibodies against the high-affinity IgE receptor are believed to be pathogenic.

### Subtypes

- Chronic ordinary urticaria: lasts >6 weeks
- Physical urticaria:
  - Dermatographism
  - Pressure urticaria
  - Cold urticaria
  - Solar urticaria

### Clinical features

*History*
- Pruritus
- Red wheals or hives which come and go within 24 hours
- May occur daily or intermittently
- Exacerbation with certain drugs (aspirin, NSAIDs, codeine, alcohol)

*Examination*
- May be normal at the time of examination
- Wheals of various sizes and forms (Fig. 6.41)

### Investigations

Laboratory investigations may not be required at all. Tests should be selected based on clinical suspicion:
- FBC and differential
- TFT
- Autoantibody screen
- Stool sample for ova, cysts, and parasites

### Treatment

- Identify and stop any drugs which may be exacerbating the condition
- Antihistamines (H1 antagonists) are the mainstay of treatment. In severe cases, higher than usual doses and combinations of different antihistamines may be required

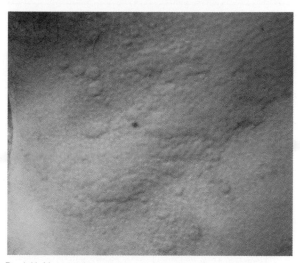

**Fig. 6.41** Urticaria demonstrating pink erythema with raised, slightly swollen, well defined plaques which come and go within 24 hours.
Author: James Heilman MD. This file is licensed under the Creative Commons Attribution-Share Alike 3.0 Unported (//creativecommons. org/licenses/by-sa/3.0/deed.en) license.

- Addition of H2 antagonists can help in some patients
- Oral steroids will work, but due to the chronicity of some patients' disease, long-term use of oral corticosteroids is likely to do more harm than good
- In severe, chronic cases, immunosuppression with non-steroid agents may be tried. Oral ciclosporin has been shown to be effective

### Prognosis

The majority of cases of urticaria resolve within a few weeks, although they may periodically recur.

Prolonged urticaria is less common, but can continue for months or years.

It is difficult to predict which cases are likely to be chronic.

## Angio-oedema

Angio-oedema may occur alone or in conjunction with urticaria. Any skin or mucosal surface may be involved, but mouth, eyelids, hands, and genitals are common sites. The tongue and pharynx may be involved and this may lead to life-threatening difficulties in breathing (anaphylactic reaction).

When occurring without urticaria, angio-oedema may be caused by a rare hereditary deficiency of C1 esterase inhibitor.

The ACE-inhibitor class of antihypertensive drugs may be a cause of acquired angioedema.

# 6.25 Photosensitivity

## Classification

See Box 6.14.

## Diagnosis of photosensitivity

Diagnosis of a photosensitive eruption may, in many cases, rely on history alone.

Careful elucidation of the details of onset, resolution, and distribution of the rash in relation to sun exposure and season is vital.

Examination of a photosensitive rash may reveal a sharp demarcation in sun-protected sites such as the top of the arms (Fig. 6.42), the V of the neck, or around the wrists, depending on the type of clothing that is customarily worn. It is also important to look for sparing of sun-protected sites (e.g. behind ears, under chin, and between fingers).

The two more important idiopathic photosensitive disorders are described in more detail as follows.

## Polymorphic light eruption

This is a recurrent, abnormal reaction to sunlight that occurs after a delay following exposure and heals without scarring.

### Epidemiology
- Common, prevalence 10–20% in Europe and USA
- Increasing prevalence further from the equator
- Most common in young ♀

### Aetiology/pathogenesis
- Cause is unknown
- Probable inherited predisposition
- Possibly a delayed-type hypersensitivity to an unidentified endogenous antigen

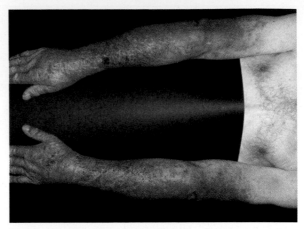

Fig. 6.42 Photosensitivity rash affecting arms.

### Clinical evaluation
*History*
- Pruritus or tingling sensation
- Appears in spring/early summer, tends to get better towards the end of summer
- Onset several hours after exposure to sunlight, lasting a few days to 2 weeks after sun avoidance

*Examination*
- Papules and/or vesicles, although urticated plaques/wheals may be seen
- Affects forearms, V of the neck and occasionally the trunk
- Often spares the face

### Investigations
- Autoantibody screen (ANA, ENA) usually negative (excluding lupus)
- Porphyrin screen negative
- Provocation with a monochromator may reproduce the eruption (phototesting)

### Management
- Sun avoidance and protective measures
- Prophylactic phototherapy/photochemotherapy in the spring may reduce the frequency or severity of subsequent eruptions
- Short courses of oral prednisolone (20–30mg/day) as soon as eruption appears may help in the acute setting or on sunny holidays

## Chronic actinic dermatitis

This is a rare, chronic eczematous photosensitive eruption affecting face, neck, and hands.

### Epidemiology
- Uncommon
- Most common age of onset 60–70 years
- Predominantly affects ♂
- All races can be affected

### Aetiology/pathogenesis
- Cause is unknown, but is thought to be a delayed hypersensitivity disorder

- Initially, may be a contact dermatitis or a photodermatitis, but progresses to a persistent photosensitivity

## Clinical evaluation

*History*

- Gradual onset of rash (which may be itchy) affecting the face and hands

*Examination*

- Erythema and scaling, with thickening
- May have leonine appearance
- Affects face, back of hands, and back of neck. May extend to affect covered areas, and can lead to erythroderma

## Investigations

- Phototesting reveals severe sensitivity to UVA, UVB, ± visible light

- Patch testing reveals multiple contact allergies in up to 2/3 of patients
- Histology is eczematous, although may appear pseudolymphomatous

## Management

- Strict sun avoidance (UV and visible light in some cases): clothing, strong sunscreens, screens in house, and car windows
- Avoid contact allergens
- Topical steroids and emollients
- Oral steroids
- Immunosuppression with azathioprine may be required

## Outcome/prognosis

- Usually a chronic course
- Anecdotal reports of progression to cutaneous lymphoma

# 6.26 Lichen planus

## Background

Lichen planus (LP) is a common pruritic inflammatory dermatosis affecting the skin and mucous membranes, and there may be associated nail dystrophy and/or hair loss.

## Epidemiology

- Affects up to 1% of the population
- ♂ = ♀
- All races are affected
- Can occur at any age but most frequent between the ages of 30–60 years

## Aetiology/pathogenesis

- Cause is unknown
- Most cases are idiopathic
- Drugs such as gold, penicillamine, and antimalarials can cause a similar eruption
- In Italy, an association with hepatitis C infection has been reported

## Clinical evaluation

### History

- Acute onset of a very itchy eruption

### Examination

- Characterized by shiny, violaceous, flat-topped, polygonal papules 1–10mm in diameter with a fine white scale on the surface (Wickham striae). See Fig. 6.43
- Symmetrical distribution
- Sites of predilection include flexor aspects of wrists, hands, forearms, ankles, shins, lumbosacral region, and genitalia, although it can occur anywhere and may be generalized
- Post-inflammatory hyperpigmentation common
- Variants include:
  - Hypertrophic LP (thick plaques usually on the shins/feet).
  - Lichen planopilaris (follicular form leading to scarring alopecia).
  - Bullous LP (rare variant, vesicles/bullae within skin lesions).
  - Annular LP (papules develop in a ring distribution, sometimes with central sparing).
  - Actinic LP (photosensitive eruption, seasonal, more common in Middle Eastern countries).
- ~ 50% have mucosal involvement (usually lacy white hyperkeratosis on the buccal mucosa, although erosive or ulcerative lesions occur) (Fig. 6.44). Genital involvement is also relatively common
- Scalp involvement with a scarring alopecia may occur
- Nails may be affected with longitudinal ridges, destruction of the nail fold/nail bed and pterygium formation

## Investigation

- Skin biopsy for H&E shows saw-tooth acanthosis, hypergranulosis, basal vacuolar degeneration, a lymphohistiocytic infiltrate

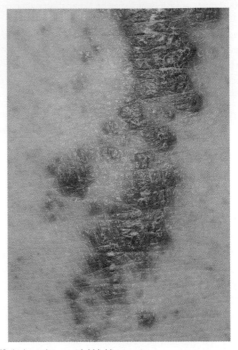

**Fig. 6.43** Lichen planus with Wickham striae.
Reproduced with permission from Cambridge University Hospitals NHS Foundation Trust.

at the dermo-epidermal junction (lichenoid infiltrate), pigment incontinence (loss of melanin from epidermis), and apoptotic keratinocytes

## Differential diagnosis

- Includes lichenoid eczema, lichenoid drug eruptions, scabies, and graft versus host disease

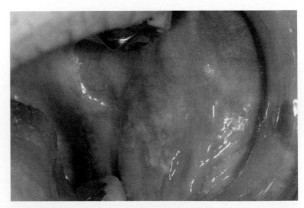

**Fig. 6.44** Mucosal involvement with lacy white hyperkeratosis on buccal mucosa.
Reproduced with permission from Cambridge University Hospitals NHS Foundation Trust.

## Management

Therapeutic options include:

- Topical: super-potent topical steroids
- Phototherapy with narrow-band UVB or PUVA
- Systemic: oral prednisolone 30mg daily reduced over 3–4 weeks. This is required for extensive or unresponsive symptomatic disease, scalp involvement, or nail involvement. The aim is to arrest disease progression and prevent scarring. Oral acitretin (retinoid) or ciclosporin may be helpful

## Outcome/prognosis

- The majority of cases clear within 9–18 months and rarely recur. There may be an increased risk of squamous cell carcinoma with oral and genital LP

# Chapter 7

# Endocrine

# 7.1 Endocrine physiology

## Hormones

- A hormone is any compound produced by a gland or cell which, acting locally or at a distance, facilitates communication between different cells/tissues/organs, thereby coordinating their activities.
- The physiological roles of the major hormones can be broadly classified into three areas:
  - Control of growth and differentiation.
  - Maintenance of homeostasis.
  - Regulation of reproduction.
- Many hormones have multiple functions, while biological effects often reflect the combined activation of several different endocrine pathways.
- Although classical endocrinology has viewed hormones as the products of specialized glands/cells (e.g. thyroid, parathyroid, pituitary, adrenals), it is now recognized that hormones are also produced by a diverse array of tissues/organs that have not been traditionally viewed as endocrine glands (e.g. the numerous hormone-secreting cells of the gastrointestinal tract—releasing gastrin, secretin, vasoactive intestinal peptide, etc.—and adipose tissue, the source of leptin (a key appetite regulator) and many other so-called 'adipo-cytokines').

### Hormone classification

In general, hormones can be classified in to:
- Peptides/proteins and their derivatives—e.g. hypothalamic-releasing factors (typically small peptides), insulin and growth hormone (larger polypeptides), and biogenic amines (e.g. catecholamines and serotonin, which are derived from amino acids). The majority of peptide/protein hormones interact with cell surface (membrane-bound) receptors, which activate one or more intracellular signalling pathway(s) that in turn leads to a change in cellular function. Many hormones are secreted as larger polypeptides (prohormones, e.g. proinsulin), which are subsequently cleaved to generate smaller functional peptides. Some also undergo post-translational modification (e.g. addition of carbohydrate side chains to generate the glycoprotein hormones thyroid-stimulating hormone (TSH), luteinizing hormone (LH), follicle-stimulating hormone (FSH))
- Steroids and other lipophilic substances—e.g. cortisol, oestrogen, testosterone (which are derived from cholesterol), vitamin D and retinoic acid (synthesized from dietary substrates), and thyroid hormones (produced by modification of tyrosine residues in thyroglobulin). In general, these hormones cross the plasma membrane to interact directly with intracellular receptors.

### Control of hormone production/release

Classical endocrine axes feature hormone production by one gland, which is secreted into the circulation and then travels to a distant tissue/organ to bring about a change in function. Perhaps the best known examples of this involve the hypothalamus and pituitary gland and a variety of target tissues (e.g. gonads, thyroid and adrenal glands) (Fig. 7.1). Endocrine homeostasis is carefully maintained through a 'feedback loop', in which hormones released by the target tissue (e.g. cortisol, testosterone, inhibin) repress hypothalamic/pituitary function to ensure hormone production does not continue in an unregulated manner.

However, in addition to these classical endocrine systems, other types of local regulatory pathway exist:
- **Paracrine:** in which factors released by one cell type in a given tissue act on an adjacent cell in the same tissue (e.g. testosterone from Leydig cells of the testes exerts effects on nearby Sertoli cells to enhance spermatogenesis).
- **Autocrine:** in which a factor acts upon the same cell from which it is produced (e.g. interleukin-2 and T-lymphocytes).

Coordinated hormone release may occur in response to certain stimuli—for example, stress activates various hypothalamic–pituitary pathways (adrenocorticotrophic hormone (ACTH), growth hormone (GH), prolactin) and causes catecholamine release from the adrenal medulla. In contrast, intercurrent/chronic illness or nutritional deficiency may impair hormone synthesis/release.

Several hormones are also released in a rhythmic (e.g. ACTH/cortisol) and/or pulsatile (e.g. GH, LH, FSH) manner.

*Clinical relevance*
- Measurement of hormone levels during periods of intercurrent illness/stress is generally not advised unless there is a strong clinical suspicion that endocrine dysfunction is the primary problem. For example, non-thyroidal illness (so-called 'sick euthyroid syndrome') is typically associated with subnormal TSH and free triiodothyronine (FT3) levels, and low normal free thyroxine (FT4), which may be erroneously interpreted as suggestive of hypopituitarism.
- Nutritional imbalances and weight fluctuations (e.g. obesity, anorexia) may result in suppression of hypothalamic–pituitary–gonadal function.
- Interpretation of LH, FSH, and oestradiol levels is dependent on the stage of the menstrual cycle. Ideally, samples should be taken in the follicular (first half of the cycle) phase.
- Random measurements of hormones that are released in a rhythmic (e.g. ACTH/cortisol) or pulsatile (e.g. GH) manner are only occasionally of use in diagnosing states of hormone excess or deficiency.

### Hormone binding proteins

Many lipid soluble hormones are transported in the circulation bound to proteins produced by the liver, e.g. cortisol binding globulin (CBG), thyroid binding globulin (TBG), sex hormone binding globulin (SHBG). The bound form is in equilibrium with the free form and readily dissociates if free hormone levels fall, thus acting as a 'reservoir'.

*Clinical relevance*

Production of hormone binding proteins by the liver can be increased (e.g. CBG levels rise in pregnancy and with oestrogen therapy), or decreased (e.g. SHBG levels are lower in obese subjects), and thus affect measurements of total, but not free, hormone levels. As it is the free form of the hormone that mediates receptor activation, then endocrine function is generally unaffected by changes in binding protein levels. However, if only total hormone levels are measured, hyper- or hypo-function may be erroneously suspected. Therefore, where possible, most laboratories offer free hormone assays (e.g. FT4, FT3), but this is not universally the case (e.g. the majority of currently available serum cortisol and testosterone assays measure total, not free, hormone levels).

### Hormone action

Hormones mediate biological responses through interactions with receptors located either on the cell membrane or intracellularly in the cytoplasm or nucleus. Examples of different cell surface and nuclear receptors are shown in Tables 7.1 and 7.2.

In the majority of cases, ligand (hormone) interaction with a given receptor is highly specific, conferring selectivity for activation of the relevant signalling pathway; there are some notable exceptions, for example both cortisol and aldosterone can activate the mineralocorticoid receptor (MR) (however, inactivation of cortisol, through its conversion to cortisone by the renal enzyme 11β-hydroxysteroid dehydrogenase type 2 (11β-HSD 2) serves to prevent inappropriate activation of MR in the kidney).

*Clinical relevance*

Supraphysiological cortisol levels (e.g. in Cushing syndrome) may overwhelm the renal 11β-HSD 2 enzyme, leading to activation of MR by cortisol, and yielding clinical features of mineralocorticoid excess.

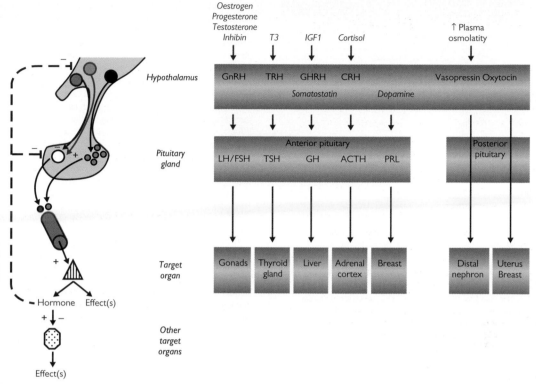

**Fig. 7.1** Hypothalamic–pituitary–target organ axes.

- Hypothalamic releasing factors (GnRH, TRH, GHRH, CRH) are released into the portal venous system and travel to the anterior pituitary gland (adenohypophysis) to promote hormone synthesis and release.
- Somatostatin and dopamine negatively regulate somatotroph (GH) and lactotroph (prolactin) function respectively; somatostatin and dopamine receptor expression on other cell types (e.g. somatotroph, corticotroph, thyrotroph) may facilitate medical treatment with somatostatin analogues and/or dopamine agonists in some cases of acromegaly, Cushing disease, or thyrotropinoma.
- Hormones released by the anterior pituitary then travel to a variety of target organs.
- The posterior pituitary gland (neurohypophysis) serves as a store for the hypothalamic hormones vasopressin (antidiuretic hormone (ADH)) and oxytocin.
- Hormones released by target organs, together with other factors, feedback to control hypothalamic–pituitary function in a series of tightly regulated feedback loops.
- *Italics* have been used to denote factors mediating negative regulation.
Reproduced from Warrell et al., *Oxford Textbook of Medicine*, 2010, Figure 13.1.1, with permission from Oxford University Press.

Hormones that bind to membrane receptors utilize effector proteins (e.g. G-proteins, adenylate cyclase, phospholipase C) to activate second messenger pathways which, in turn, trigger a cascade of intracellular kinases that ultimately change gene transcription or modulate a biochemical pathway to bring about a physiological response. In contrast, hormones that act through nuclear receptors (NRs) are either actively or passively transported across the cell membrane, and then bind to their respective receptors in the cytoplasm (prior to transport in to the nucleus) or in the nucleus itself. NRs bind specific recognition sequences in the promoter regions of target genes to alter gene transcription (up- or down-regulation), and hence protein synthesis.

# The posterior pituitary gland

- The neurohypophysis secretes two nine-amino-acid peptides, arginine vasopressin (also known as antidiuretic hormone, ADH) and oxytocin.
- Both are synthesized in nerve cell bodies in the supraoptic and paraventricular nuclei of the hypothalamus as precursor

| Table 7.1 | Membrane receptor families | |
|---|---|---|
| **Type** | **Subtypes** | **Examples** |
| G-protein-coupled | Glycoprotein hormones | TSH, LH, FSH, hCG |
| | Biogenic amines | Adrenaline, noradrenaline, dopamine, serotonin |
| | Peptides | TRH, CRH, PTH, calcitonin, angiotensin, vasopressin, gastrin, glucagon |
| | Small molecules | Calcium, GABA |
| Tyrosine kinase | | Insulin, IGF-1 |
| Cytokine | | GH, prolactin, leptin, EPO |
| Serine/threonine kinase | | Activin, inhibin |

TSH: thyroid stimulating hormone; LH: luteinizing hormone; FSH: follicle stimulating hormone; hCG: human chorionic gonadotropin; TRH: thyrotropin releasing hormone; CRH: corticotropin-releasing hormone; PTH: parathyroid hormone; GABA: γ-aminobutyric acid; IGF-1: insulin-like growth factor 1; GH: growth hormone; EPO: erythropoietin.

**Table 7.2 Nuclear receptors**

| Type | Receptor | Hormone/ligand |
|---|---|---|
| Homodimeric | GR | Cortisol |
| | MR | Aldosterone |
| | ERα/β | Oestradiol |
| | PR | Progesterone |
| | AR | Testosterone, di-hydrotestosterone |
| Heterodimeric | TRα/β | T3 |
| | RARα/β/γ | All-trans retinoic acid |
| | RXRα/β/γ | 9-cis retinoic acid |
| | VDR | 1,25-dihydroxy vitamin D3 |
| | PPARα/β/γ | Unsaturated fatty acids, eicosanoids |

GR: glucocorticoid receptor; MR: mineralocorticoid receptor; ER: oestrogen receptor α or β subtypes; PR: progesterone receptor; AR: androgen receptor; TR: thyroid hormone receptor α or β subtypes; RAR: retinoic acid receptor α, β, or γ subtypes; RXR: retinoid X receptor α, β, or γ subtypes; VDR: vitamin D receptor; PPAR: peroxisome proliferator-activated receptor α, β, or γ subtypes; T3: triiodothyronine.

molecules comprising a signal peptide, the active nonapeptide and a specific neurophysin (carrier protein).

- They are processed as they pass along the nerve axons to be secreted—separate from their neurophysins—into the systemic circulation from the posterior pituitary.

### Antidiuretic hormone

- ADH has a short half-life in the circulation (5–15 minutes).
- Under physiological conditions it is a key player in the control of blood osmolality, water excretion, and extracellular fluid volume.
- ADH release is stimulated by:
  - Increase in blood osmolality.
  - Hypotension/intravascular volume depletion.
  - Nausea/vomiting/pain.
  - Smoking.
- The principal action of ADH is to reduce the renal excretion of water. It has pressor actions at very high serum concentrations, e.g. when stimulated by hypotension/intravascular volume depletion.

*Clinical relevance*

- Deficiency of ADH leads to cranial diabetes insipidus.
- In the syndrome of inappropriate antidiuretic hormone secretion (SIADH), unregulated ADH release occurs.
- Cortisol has a permissive effect on free water excretion by the kidney and in hypocortisolaemic states coexistent diabetes insipidus may be masked. Subsequent cortisol replacement can result in a profound aquaresis.

### Oxytocin

The effects of oxytocin are mainly confined to pregnancy and the postpartum period:

- Stimulation of the nipple leads to oxytocin secretion and milk ejection from the lactating breast (the suckling reflex).
- Release of oxytocin following distension of the cervix of the pregnant uterus is part of the initiation of parturition.

*Clinical relevance*

- Infusion of oxytocin may be used to induce and augment labour.

## The anterior pituitary gland

### Growth hormone–insulin-like growth factor 1 axis

- Pituitary growth hormone (GH) secretion occurs in a pulsatile manner (most secretion at night). During puberty, activation of the hypothalamic–pituitary–gonadal axis increases GH secretion and leads to the growth spurt.

- GH secretion is subject to both positive (via growth hormone releasing hormone (GHRH)) and negative (via somatostatin) hypothalamic regulation, with a variety of factors (fasting, sleep, catabolic states) stimulating GHRH release (Fig. 17.1). In addition, ghrelin, a potent endogenous growth hormone secretagogue (GHS) is released by the stomach and promotes GH secretion, probably acting at both the hypothalamic and pituitary levels.
- GH has anabolic and catabolic effects. The majority of its actions are mediated through insulin-like growth factor 1 (IGF-1), produced mainly in the liver, and which mediates important anabolic effects, e.g. through actions on protein metabolism. IGF-1 circulates bound to a number of high-affinity binding proteins (e.g. IGFBP3). Proteolytic cleavage of IGFBP3 results in IGF-1 release, thus allowing it to bind and activate its cell surface receptors. The IGFs have endocrine, paracrine and autocrine effects, regulating metabolism, cell survival, differentiation, and cell death.
- GH itself has direct 'anti-insulin' actions, stimulating lipolysis and raising free fatty acid concentrations, which leads to a rise in plasma glucose levels.

*Clinical relevance*

- Due to the pulsatile nature of its release, measurement of random GH levels is not a reliable means of excluding GH excess or deficiency. Although IGF-1 has a longer half-life in the circulation, it still has significant limitations in diagnosing disorders of GH secretion (especially GH deficiency). Accordingly, dynamic tests (e.g. the insulin tolerance test (ITT) for diagnosing GH deficiency and the oral glucose tolerance test (OGTT) for diagnosing GH excess) are used.

### Hypothalamic–pituitary–adrenal axis

See Figs 7.1–7.3.

- The adrenal cortex is subdivided into two major functional regions—an outer cortex and inner medulla. The latter is the source of catecholamines (e.g. adrenaline and noradrenaline). The cortex is subdivided into three zones—an outer zona glomerulosa (ZG—the source of aldosterone), middle zona fasciculata (ZF—site of cortisol synthesis), and inner zona reticularis

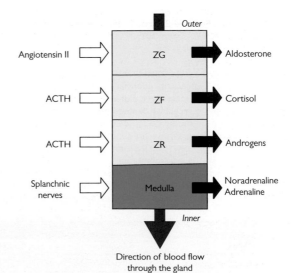

**Fig. 7.2** Schematic representation of the anatomical structure and function of the adrenal gland showing the outer cortex and inner medulla. Steroid biosynthesis occurs in three separate regions of the cortex, but with overlap between the ZF and ZR. The direction of blood flow through the gland ensures that cortical steroids are delivered to the medulla—in particular cortisol which has a permissive effect on the enzyme phenylethanolamine N-methyltransferase (PNMT) that facilitates conversion of noradrenaline to adrenaline. ACTH: adrenocorticotrophic hormone; ZF: zona fasciculata; ZG: zona glomerulosa; ZR: zona reticularis.

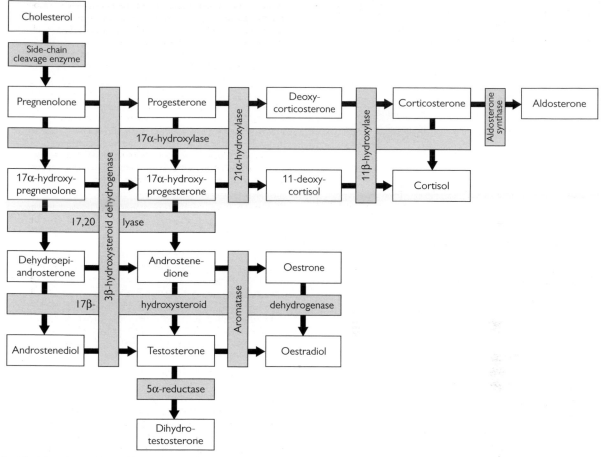

**Fig. 7.3** Adrenal cortical steroid biosynthetic pathways.

(ZR—where adrenal androgens, e.g. dehydroepiandrosterone, are synthesized). Both the ZF and ZR are under hypothalamic (corticotropin-releasing hormone (CRH))—pituitary (ACTH) control. In contrast, aldosterone production is regulated by the renin–angiotensin system.

- Basal CRH and ACTH secretion occurs in a diurnal fashion; cortisol levels tend to be highest just before waking, then fall progressively throughout the day to reach a nadir late at night. Various factors including 'stress' (physical or emotional) may cause additional 'spikes' in cortisol secretion, which are superimposed on the background rhythm.

- ~80% of the total circulating cortisol is bound to CBG, 10% is bound to albumin, and 10% is free (metabolically active).

- Cortisol has multiple metabolic effects, regulating protein degradation, hepatic glucose output and lipolysis. It has key immunomodulatory effects, and is important in the maintenance of normal circulatory function.

*Clinical relevance*

- In primary hypoadrenalism (i.e. primary adrenal failure), cortisol, aldosterone and androgen insufficiency are all present, and ACTH levels are elevated.

- In secondary hypoadrenalism, cortisol and androgen levels are low, but aldosterone production is preserved. ACTH levels are inappropriately low/normal.

- Random cortisol measurements rarely confirm or exclude hypocortisolism. Timed measurements are more useful (e.g. a 9am cortisol of <100nmol/L is highly suggestive of adrenocortical insufficiency, while an elevated sleeping midnight cortisol is consistent with Cushing syndrome).

- Where possible, cortisol replacement should be given in a regimen that 'mimics' endogenous cortisol production, i.e. with a larger dose in the morning and smaller doses later in the day (e.g. 10mg hydrocortisone on waking, with 5mg at midday and a further 2.5–5mg at 4–5pm).

- Increased oestrogen levels (e.g. in pregnancy or with oral contraceptive pill usage) induce hepatic CBG production, thereby raising total, but not free, serum cortisol levels. Accordingly, where possible, it is desirable to discontinue exogenous oral oestrogen therapy for 6 weeks before assessing cortisol levels. However, further investigation should not be delayed in a patient presenting acutely, but results should be interpreted with caution.

- Cushing syndrome, resulting from prolonged exposure to supraphysiological cortisol levels, is associated with marked metabolic derangements and immunosuppression.

**Hypothalamic–pituitary–thyroid axis**

- Hypothalamic thyrotropin-releasing hormone (TRH) stimulates pituitary TSH secretion, in turn directing thyroid hormone synthesis and release from the thyroid gland (Fig. 7.1).

- The thyroid gland secretes T4 and T3 in a ratio of approximately 14:1 (Fig. 7.4).

- T3 and T4 are transported around the circulation bound to thyroid-binding globulin (TBG), albumin and pre-albumin (>99% bound). As with cortisol, only free hormone is available for tissue uptake (via specific transporters) and subsequent action.

- T3 is the biologically active hormone (signalling via the thyroid hormone receptor), and conversion of T4 to T3 is mediated by a family of deiodinase enzymes, which can also convert T4 and T3 to inactive metabolites (e.g. reverse T3 (rT3) and T2).

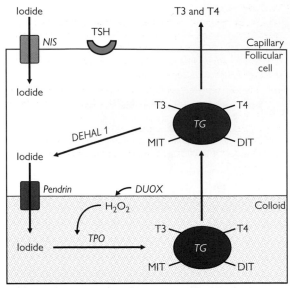

**Fig. 7.4** Thyroid hormone synthesis in a thyroid follicular cell. DEHAL1: dehalogenase 1; DIT: diiodotyrosine; DUOX: dual oxidase; MIT: monoiodotyrosine; NIS: sodium-iodide symporter; T3: triiodothyronine; T4: thyroxine; TPO: thyroid peroxidase; TG: thyroglobulin; TSH: thyrotropin.

- Thyroid hormones regulate a diverse array of biological processes, ranging from development and functioning of the nervous system to metabolism and reproduction.

*Clinical relevance*

- TSH is a very sensitive indicator of primary thyroid dysfunction, and changes rapidly in response to minor changes in FT4/FT3 levels—it is an ideal screening test for primary hypo- or hyperthyroidism. However, it is not a reliable indicator of thyroid status in the presence of pituitary disease, and measuring TSH alone may fail to identify central hypothyroidism or a TSH-secreting pituitary adenoma.
- Most laboratories offer free thyroid hormone assays, thereby negating potential confounding effects of changes in binding protein concentrations.
- Autoantibodies against TPO are detectable in the serum of many patients with autoimmune thyroid disease, especially hypothyroidism.
- Autoantibodies capable of binding to, and activating the TSH receptor on thyroid follicular cells are found in patients with Graves disease.
- A small amount of thyroglobulin (TG) 'escapes' into the circulation and can be measured in serum. In patients with differentiated forms of thyroid cancer, in whom total thyroidectomy has been undertaken, TG can serve as a useful tumour marker.
- Iodide is taken up into thyroid follicular cells by the sodium-iodide symporter (NIS).
- Once inside the cell, it is then transferred to the colloid (via a second transporter—Pendrin) where it is oxidized by thyroid peroxidase (TPO).
- Organification of tyrosine residues in TG (a process involving iodination of phenolic rings) generates mono- and di-iodotyrosine, which are then coupled to form T3 or T4.

**Hypothalamic–pituitary–gonadal axis**

See Fig. 7.1.

*Testis*

- LH promotes testosterone production by Leydig cells.

- FSH is important in the initiation of spermatogenesis, possibly through increasing intratubular concentrations of dihydrotestosterone (the active form) via an effect on Sertoli cells.
- ~2% of total circulating testosterone is unbound, with the remainder bound to albumin (~55%) and SHBG (~43%).
- Testosterone, oestradiol, and inhibin provide negative feedback regulation of the axis.

*Clinical relevance*

- Most laboratory assays measure total, and not free, serum testosterone. Accordingly, changes in the levels of binding proteins such as SHBG may confound interpretation of blood levels, e.g. obesity is associated with low SHBG resulting in borderline low total testosterone levels, but with normal LH (because free testosterone levels are normal).
- Testosterone secretion is diurnal, and ideally levels should be measured in the early morning.

*Ovary*

- A schematic representation of the changes in LH, FSH, oestradiol and progesterone levels during a 'classical' 28 day menstrual cycle are shown in Fig. 7.5.
- LH induces ovulation of the mature follicle and stimulates oestrogen production by promoting the synthesis of androgen precursors in theca cells (the pathways of steroidogenesis are similar to those of the adrenal gland). Diffusion of these androgens into adjacent granulosa cells is followed by aromatization into oestrogens under the influence of FSH. LH also helps to sustain the corpus luteum during the second half of the cycle by stimulating progesterone synthesis.
- In addition to its role in promoting oestrogen synthesis, FSH is responsible for the development of the mature follicle which ovulates in response to the LH surge in mid-cycle.
- ~2% of the total circulating oestradiol is unbound, with the remainder bound to albumin (~60%) and SHBG (~38%).
- Progesterone is produced by the corpus luteum, and has 'progestational' effects, inducing secretory activity in the endometrium.
- Oestradiol and progesterone, together with inhibin, provide negative feedback regulation of the axis.

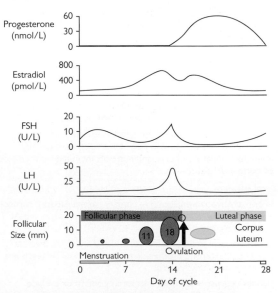

**Fig. 7.5** Hormonal changes during the normal menstrual cycle.
Reproduced from Royal College of Physicians. *Medical Masterclass: Endocrinology*, 2nd edition. London: RCP, 2013. Copyright © 2013 Royal College of Physicians. Reproduced with permission.

- Non-steroidal hormones and growth factors (including insulin and the IGFs) also have autocrine and paracrine effects in the regulation of ovarian function, follicular maturation, and steroidogenesis.

*Clinical relevance*

- During the ovulatory surge, concentrations of LH and FSH may reach 'postmenopausal' levels, and thus repeat measurements, together with a paired oestradiol sample, must be checked before making a diagnosis of premature ovarian failure.
- A high mid-luteal phase progesterone concentration indicates that the cycle was ovulatory.

*The breast*

- A number of different hormones and growth factors (including prolactin, oestradiol, progesterone, GH/IGF-1) act synergistically to promote ductal and alveolar development of the mammary gland.
- High levels of placentally derived oestradiol and progesterone during pregnancy prime the breast for milk production, but inhibit lactation.
- After parturition, the sudden fall in oestradiol and progesterone levels releases the inhibition of lactation. Both the anticipation of nursing (including the sight and sound of the baby) and nipple stimulation promote oxytocin release from the posterior pituitary, resulting in myoepithelial contraction and milk expulsion. The 'milk ejection reflex' can be inhibited by stress.
- Prolactin is released from the anterior pituitary in response to nipple stimulation and maintains lactogenesis (Fig. 7.1). It also inhibits hypothalamic secretion of gonadotropin-releasing hormone (GnRH) and gonadal steroid production, thus inhibiting ovulation; however, women should still be advised to use appropriate contraceptive precautions while breastfeeding.
- Physiological involution of the mammary gland occurs when lactation is complete, and after the menopause.

*Clinical relevance*

- Suckling by the infant is essential to the maintenance of milk production. Hence, early support to establish successful breast-feeding is critical to avoid failure of lactation.
- Continued nipple stimulation after weaning may result in unwanted postpartum galactorrhoea.
- Pathological hyperprolactinaemia often manifests with hypogonadotrophic hypogonadism due to the inhibitory effect of prolactin on GnRH secretion.
- Dopaminergic agonists such as bromocriptine and cabergoline inhibit prolactin production and may be used in the treatment of pathological hyperprolactinaemia and after a still birth.

# Parathyroid hormone and calcium homeostasis

- Most of the calcium in the body is found in bone and teeth, with only ~1% in extracellular fluid and cells.
- Extracellular calcium is bound to albumin (45%), complexed to citrate, phosphate, or bicarbonate (5%), or in a free ionized (active) form.
- Both PTH and vitamin D are key regulators of calcium homeostasis (Fig. 7.6).
- 1,25-dihydroxycholecalciferol ($1,25(OH)_2D_3$), the active form of vitamin D, is synthesized from precursors generated in the skin in response to ultraviolet light, and to a lesser extent from dietary sources. 25-hydroxylation of cholecalciferol occurs in the liver and 1-hydroxylation in the kidneys (Fig. 7.7).
- Calcitonin, produced by the parafollicular C cells of the thyroid gland, has uncertain significance in calcium metabolism in humans.

| Organ | PTH | | | Vitamin D | | |
|---|---|---|---|---|---|---|
| | Action | Serum calcium | Serum phosphate | Action | Serum calcium | Serum phosphate |
| 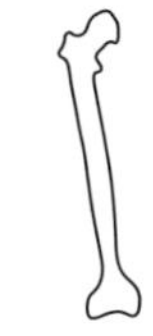 *(bone)* | ↑ osteoclastic bone resorption | ↑ | | Enhancement of action of PTH, with ↑ osteoclastic bone resorption<br><br>↑ bone mineralisation | ↑ | |
| 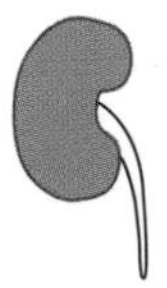 *(kidney)* | ↑ tubular calcium reabsorption | ↑ | | ↑ tubular calcium reabsorption | ↑ | |
| | ↓ tubular phosphate reabsorption | | ↓ | ↑ tubular phosphate reabsorption | | ↑ |
| | ↑ 1α-hydroxylase activity leading to ↑ production of 1,25 dihydroxy-cholecalciferol | ↑ | ↑ | | | |
| 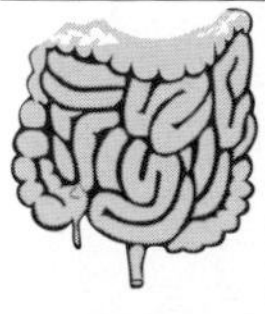 *(intestine)* | | | | ↑ gut calcium absorption | ↑ | |
| | | | | ↑ gut phosphate absorption | | ↑ |

Fig. 7.6 Roles of parathyroid hormone (PTH) and vitamin D in calcium and phosphate homeostasis.

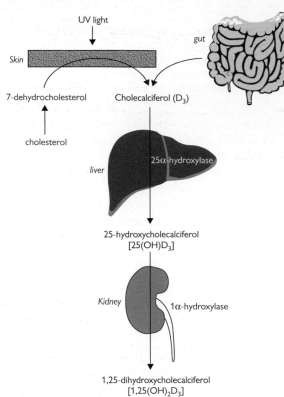

**Fig. 7.7** Schematic representation of the key steps in vitamin D synthesis/metabolism.

## Clinical relevance

- $25(OH)D_3$ is the main storage form of vitamin D, and most laboratories offer measurement of this rather than $1,25(OH)_2D_3$ as an index of vitamin D status.

- Measurement of $1,25(OH)_2D_3$ is generally reserved for certain clinical settings, e.g. sarcoidosis where extra-renal synthesis of the active form may lead to hypercalcaemia.

- In moderate to severe renal failure abnormalities of vitamin D metabolism (reduced $1\alpha$-hydroxylation) and PTH secretion (secondary hyperparathyroidism) can occur and, if untreated, may lead to severe bone disease (renal osteodystrophy). Treatment with active metabolites (most commonly alfacalcidol ($1\alpha$-hydroxycholecalciferol); less commonly calcitriol ($1,25$-dihydroxycholecalciferol)) is used to prevent this, although total parathyroidectomy is required in some cases.

- In contrast, in the majority of patients with simple vitamin D deficiency (due to inadequate sunlight exposure $\pm$ dietary insufficiency), and in whom hepatic and renal function are normal,

replacement with non-activated forms is generally preferred, e.g. ergocalciferol (vitamin $D_2$) or c(h)olecalciferol (vitamin $D_3$).

- There is no role for calcitonin measurement in the routine management of calcium and bone disorders.

## The endocrine pancreas

The pancreas comprises two distinct functional organs:
- Exocrine pancreas—a major source of digestive enzymes.
- Endocrine pancreas—comprising four major cell types within the Islets of Langerhans:
  1. A ($\alpha$) cells that secrete glucagon.
  2. B ($\beta$) cells that secrete insulin.
  3. D ($\delta$) cells that secrete somatostatin.
  4. F (PP) cells that secrete pancreatic polypeptide.
These hormones regulate the rate of absorption of various dietary constituents, their cellular storage and metabolism.

### Insulin

*Insulin synthesis and secretion*
- The human insulin gene is located on chromosome 11.
- The initial gene product, a precursor molecule, preproinsulin, is cleaved almost immediately after synthesis to proinsulin, which is stored in secretory granules.
- Subsequent processing of proinsulin releases insulin and a smaller connecting peptide (C-peptide) through cleavage at two sites within proinsulin (Fig. 7.8).
- The insulin molecule comprises two peptide chains (A and B), connected by two disulphide bridges (Fig. 7.8).

*Clinical relevance*
- C-peptide levels in plasma can be measured to provide an index of endogenous insulin production. This may be helpful in distinguishing between type 1 (insulinopenic) and type 2 (insulin resistant) diabetes mellitus.

- Measurement of C-peptide is also helpful in distinguishing hypoglycaemia due to endogenous insulin hypersecretion (e.g. insulinoma—C-peptide levels detectable/elevated) from exogenously administered insulin (e.g. insulin overdose—C-peptide levels are low/suppressed). Note that hypoglycaemia due to sulfonylurea therapy is associated with elevated C-peptide levels, as sulfonylureas promote endogenous insulin secretion from pancreatic $\beta$ cells.

Glucose is a potent stimulus to insulin release, entering the pancreatic $\beta$ cell by diffusion and via a glucose transporter (GLUT2). Insulin secretion in response to glucose is biphasic: an early phase response, which is relatively short-lived, occurs almost immediately with rising glucose levels, but if glucose levels are maintained, a late phase response is seen that is more gradual in onset but sustained.

A number of other factors have been shown to regulate insulin release in humans including:
- Dietary components, e.g. amino acids.
- Hormones, e.g. incretins such as glucagon-like peptide-1 (GLP-1).
- Drugs, e.g. diazoxide, somatostatin analogues.

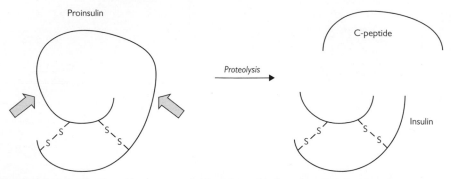

**Fig. 7.8** Schematic representation of proinsulin and its cleavage to insulin and c-peptide through proteolysis at two sites.

*Clinical relevance*

- GLP-1 agonists/analogues (e.g. exenatide, liraglutide) are licensed for use in type 2 diabetes mellitus, promoting insulin secretion, suppressing glucagon secretion, and preventing weight gain (and in some cases promoting weight loss).

- Diazoxide inhibits insulin release and may be used in the treatment of insulinoma prior to surgery or when surgery is not curative. Somatostatin also inhibits insulin secretion and somatostatin analogue therapy is an alternative for patients intolerant of/inadequately controlled by diazoxide, but also has suppressive effects on other counter-regulatory hormones, e.g. glucagon, and may therefore worsen hypoglycaemia in some patients.

## Insulin action

- Insulin exerts its effects through binding to specific receptors (Table 7.1) on the surface membranes of target cells. The receptors are membrane glycoproteins composed of α (extracellular, containing the hormone binding domain) and β (predominantly transmembrane and cytoplasmic, and containing the tyrosine kinase function) subunits.

- Binding of insulin triggers a cascade of intracellular signalling pathways, which ultimately facilitate transport of nutrients into insulin target tissues, an important mechanism being the migration of the GLUT-4 glucose transporter to the cell surface, promoting glucose uptake.

- Activation of the insulin signalling cascade also promotes glycogen, lipid, and protein synthesis, and, through alternative pathways, insulin is able to influence mitogenesis and cellular differentiation.

*Clinical relevance*

- Lack of insulin leads to increased glycogenolysis, lipolysis, and gluconeogenesis, with resultant hyperglycaemia and hyperketonaemia, e.g. diabetic ketoacidosis.

## Insulin metabolism

First-pass metabolism in the liver removes half of the insulin in the portal vein. Within the plasma it circulates in unbound form, is freely filtered by the glomeruli, and then rapidly reabsorbed and metabolized by the renal tubules. The plasma half-life of insulin is ~5 minutes.

*Clinical relevance*

- Metabolism of insulin by the kidneys is impaired in renal failure: diabetics may be at risk of hypoglycaemia if they remain on their 'normal treatment' regimen in the face of deteriorating renal function.

### Glucagon

Glucagon release from pancreatic α cells occurs in response to falling blood glucose levels; its predominant action is within the liver, where it promotes mobilization of glycogen and gluconeogenesis.

*Clinical relevance*

- IM glucagon can be given to treat hypoglycaemia when it is not safe/possible to give sugar by mouth. Once the patient is conscious, carbohydrates should be given to help restore liver glycogen supplies (depleted by glucagon).

- Glucagon is not recommended for the treatment of chronic/recurrent hypoglycaemia, or in patients with significant hepatic impairment, because its efficacy is limited by absence of liver glycogen stores.

# Glucose and energy homeostasis

- The key steps involved in the maintenance of normal blood glucose levels are depicted in Figs 7.9 and 7.10.

- Energy homeostasis involves regulation of food intake and energy expenditure.

- Leptin, an adipose tissue-derived hormone, acts via hypothalamic pathways (e.g. melanocortin 4) to reduce food intake; conversely, rising gastrointestinal production of ghrelin preprandially stimulates food intake.

- Thyroid hormone is an important determinant of resting energy expenditure or basal metabolic rate.

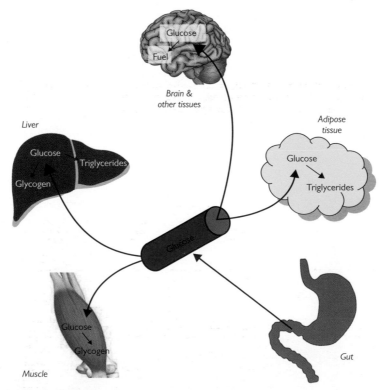

**Fig. 7.9** Glucose homeostasis during the fed state.

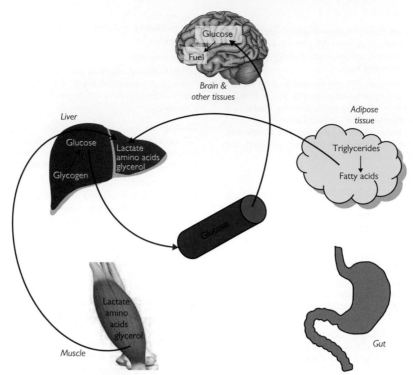

**Fig. 7.10** Glucose homeostasis during the fasting state.

- Metabolic effects are mediated by several hormones: insulin lowers blood glucose by enhancing its cellular uptake and promoting glycogen synthesis; conversely, GH, cortisol, glucagon and adrenaline act as counter-regulatory hormones to raise blood glucose.

- Glucagon and adrenaline stimulate glycogenolysis and, together with cortisol, promote gluconeogenesis.

- Other metabolic pathways are also influenced by these hormones: GH and cortisol are lipolytic whereas insulin mediates lipogenesis; insulin and GH are also anabolic by promoting protein biosynthesis, whereas cortisol increases protein breakdown. Adiponectin, another adipose tissue-derived hormone, enhances tissue insulin sensitivity.

# 7.2 Acid–base balance

## Background

- Control of acid–base (pH) balance within a narrow range is essential for the normal functioning of cellular processes.
- The amount of acid generated from cellular metabolism (mainly catabolism of dietary protein) corresponds to 40–80**milli**mol/day (~1mmol/kg/day) of $H^+$, yet the extracellular pH is maintained at the **nano**molar level (45–35nmol/L or pH 7.35–7.45).
- This is achieved by buffers that minimize the change in pH: bicarbonate within tissues, and bicarbonate plus haemoglobin in the bloodstream (Fig. 7.11).
- Bicarbonate is the key buffer, reacting with protons thus:

$$H^+ + HCO_3^- \leftrightarrow H_2CO_3 \leftrightarrow H_2O + CO_2$$

- Complete metabolism of carbohydrate and fat also generates $CO_2$.
- $CO_2$ tension is regulated by respiration, $HCO_3^-$ concentration by the kidneys, and pH is thus determined by the activity of both:

$$pH \propto \frac{[HCO_3^-]}{PaCO_2} \begin{matrix}\text{(kidneys—normally ~25mmol/L)} \\ \text{(lungs—normally ~5.3kPa)}\end{matrix}$$

(simplified Henderson–Hasselbach equation)

- Renal or pulmonary disease can lead to disturbance of body pH.
- Respiratory acidosis results from decreased $CO_2$ removal.
- Respiratory alkalosis results from increased $CO_2$ removal.
- Metabolic acidosis or alkalosis can result from renal disease or as a consequence of other systemic upset, e.g. lactic acidosis in shock, gastrointestinal $HCO_3^-$ losses in severe diarrhoea.
- An increase in acid production and reduction in $[HCO_3^-]$ will reduce the pH, stimulating the respiratory centre to increase ventilation and hence reduce $pCO_2$, returning the pH **towards** normal. This is the basis of 'compensation', by which the lungs or

kidneys can minimize the change in pH induced by an abnormality in the other's function.

- If the respiratory system maintains $pCO_2$ around a set point, the role of the kidneys is to replenish $HCO_3^-$ and excrete excess acid (Fig. 7.12). Two separate processes occur:
  1. $HCO_3^-$ is freely filtered at the glomerulus and must be reclaimed to prevent catastrophic bicarbonate wasting. This is largely a function of the proximal tubule.
  2. The additional acid produced by metabolism must also be secreted into the urine, a function of specialized cells within the distal nephron.

## Sodium homeostasis

- Sodium is the most abundant extracellular cation and is thus the major determinant of extracellular volume.
- Sodium concentration is tightly regulated (range 135–145mmol/L).
- Sodium is freely filtered at the glomerulus, at a rate of ~1000mmol per hour. Rather than eat 2kg of sodium chloride per day, the kidneys reabsorb 99% of filtered sodium.
- Different proportions of the filtered load of NaCl are reabsorbed in each nephron segment (see Fig. 7.12). However, the driving

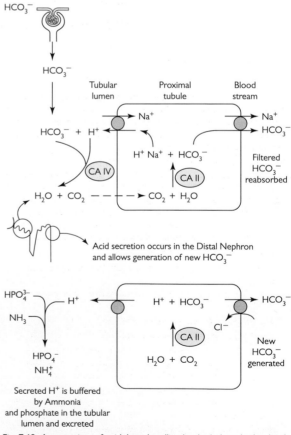

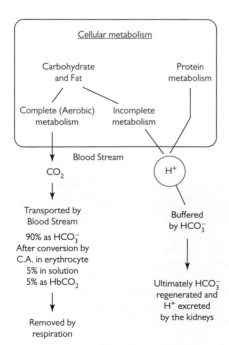

**Fig. 7.11** Acid–base: the basics. CA: carbonic anhydrase.

**Fig. 7.12** An overview of acid–base handling by the kidney. In the distal nephron acid excretion is performed by type A (α-) intercalated cells. CA II/IV: carbonic anhydrase types II and IV.

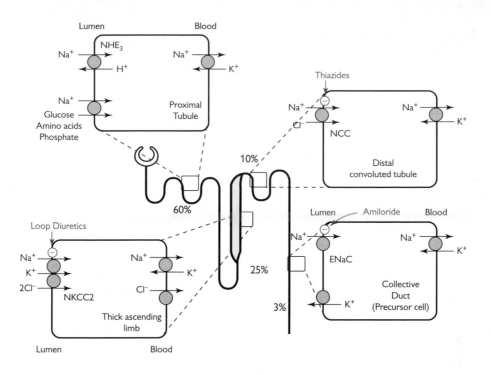

In blue = Proportion of Na+ reabsorbed in Nephron Segment.

$NHE_3$ = $Na^+/H^+$ – exchanger 3

$NKCC_2$ = $Na^+/K^+/2Cl^-$ co-transportor

NCC = $Na^+/Cl^-$ co-transportor

ENac = Epithelial $Na^+$ Channel

Fig. 7.13 Mechanisms of renal sodium handling.

force behind this process is the same throughout the nephron—the basolateral membrane $Na^+/K^+$-ATPase which returns filtered NaCl to the bloodstream. This generates an inward gradient for $Na^+$ uptake from the tubular lumen via a variety of channels (specific to nephron segments).

Renal reabsorption of $Na^+$ (Fig. 7.13) is controlled by:

1. Glomerulotubular balance. An intrinsic property of the kidney to maintain reabsorption of a constant **proportion** of filtered $Na^+$ by the proximal tubule (and not a constant **amount**): fractional excretion of $Na^+$ remains constant. ↑ GFR → ↑ oncotic pressure in the peritubular capillaries (arising from glomerular efferent arteriole), and ↑reabsorption, dampening the effect of ↑GFR.

2. Renin–angiotensin–aldosterone system.
   - Renin is released by cells of the juxtaglomerular apparatus (JGA) in response to:
     - NaCl concentration at the macula densa: ↓ $[Na^+]$ → ↑ renin release.
     - ↓ afferent arteriole perfusion pressure.
     - Activity of renal sympathetic nerves.
   - Renin cleaves angiotensin I to active angiotensin II:
     - Preferentially vasoconstricts efferent arteriole, maintains GFR and ↑ proximal tubular $Na^+$ and $H_2O$ reabsorption.
     - Directly ↑ proximal tubule $Na^+$ reabsorption.
     - Stimulates aldosterone release and $Na^+$ reabsorption by the distal tubule.

3. Other hormones also play a role: ADH, atrial natriuretic peptide, prostaglandins. and catecholamines.

## Potassium homeostasis

- Potassium is the major intracellular cation, with an intracellular concentration of ~150mmol/L, compared to an extracellular fluid concentration of ~4mmol/L.

- This distribution of $K^+$ determines the membrane potential of cells—especially important in excitable tissues (e.g. nerve and muscle)—and is maintained by the $Na^+/K^+$-ATPase, present in virtually all cells. Various channels exist to control potassium 'leak' out of cells.

- Multiple factors can modify cellular uptake or leak of $K^+$ (Fig. 7.14):

| ↑ cell $K^+$ uptake → ↓ serum $K^+$ | ↑ cell $K^+$ leak → ↑ serum $K^+$ |
| --- | --- |
| Insulin | Hyperglycaemia |
| $\beta_2$-adrenoceptor agonists | β-blockers |
| Alkalosis | Acidosis |
| α-adrenoceptor antagonists | α-adrenoceptor agonists |

### Potassium handling by the kidney

- Potassium reabsorption and site:
  - 65–70%: proximal convoluted tubule.
  - 30%: loop of Henle (thick ascending limb).
- **Excess** $K^+$ is **secreted** by cells of the collecting duct (unlike $Na^+$, where any excess is lost by not being absorbed).

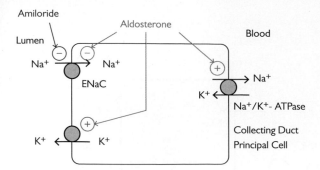

Potassium Secretion Influenced by:

- Distal Na⁺ Delivery (↑Luminal Na⁺ → ↓ Electro-
  Chemical Gradient for K⁺ Secretion)
- Luminal Flow (↑Flow: (A)↑Gradient for K⁺ Secretion
  And (B) Directly Stimulates some K+ Channels)
- Aldosterone (Hence ↑K⁺ Effect of Sprinolactone).

Fig. 7.14 Mechanisms of renal potassium handling.

# 7.3 Thyrotoxicosis

## Background

The term thyrotoxicosis refers to the clinical disorder resulting from exposure to supraphysiological thyroid hormone levels. The term hyperthyroidism is more specific and implies hyperfunction of the thyroid gland.

## Aetiology

See Table 7.3.

## Clinical evaluation

### Signs and symptoms

See Fig. 7.15. Many of the clinical manifestations of thyrotoxicosis reflect increased sensitivity to circulating catecholamines. Included

### Table 7.3 Aetiology of thyrotoxicosis

| Cause | Frequency | Condition |
| --- | --- | --- |
| Primary | Common | Graves disease |
| | | Toxic multinodular goitre |
| | Less common | Toxic adenoma |
| | | Thyroiditis |
| | | Drug induced, e.g. amiodarone |
| | | L-T4 therapy—iatrogenic or factitious |
| | Rare | Follicular thyroid carcinoma |
| | | Struma ovarii |
| Secondary | Rare | hCG-mediated (e.g. gestational) |
| | | Thyrotropinoma (TSHoma) |
| | | Resistance to thyroid hormone (RTH) |

amongst these are the eye signs 'lid retraction' and 'lid lag'; other eye signs are specific to Graves disease (see later in section).

### Complications
- Atrial fibrillation (AF), cardiac failure.
- Hepatic dysfunction (deranged LFT, hypoproteinaemia).
- Osteopenia/osteoporosis.
- Hypercalcaemia.

### Investigations
*Laboratory findings*
Typically:
- Thyroid hormones (thyroxine/T4; triiodothyronine/T3) are elevated.
- TSH (thyroid-stimulating hormone) is fully suppressed (i.e. <0.1mU/L and often <0.01mU/L in more modern sensitive assays).

Most laboratories routinely measure free thyroid hormone levels (i.e. FT4 and FT3), thereby negating the effects of changes in binding protein levels (e.g. oestrogen therapy can increase thyroid binding globulin (TBG) levels, and therefore raise total T4 and T3, but FT4 and FT3 are unchanged).

The finding of elevated FT4 and/or FT3 levels with non-suppressed TSH is unusual and may indicate laboratory assay interference, drug effects (e.g. amiodarone, heparin), thyrotropinoma (TSHoma), or the genetic disorder resistance to thyroid hormone (RTH).

Subclinical hyperthyroidism:
- TSH suppressed but FT4 and FT3 within reference ranges.
- Associated with AF and reduced bone mineral density.
- Decision to treat and choice of therapy made per individual.

## Graves disease (GD)

### Epidemiology
- Most common thyroid disease in areas of iodine abundance.
- Prevalence = 2.7% in ♀; ♀:♂=10:1.

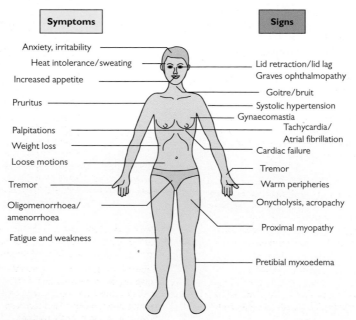

**Fig. 7.15** Clinical features of thyrotoxicosis.

Symptoms: Anxiety, irritability; Heat intolerance/sweating; Increased appetite; Pruritus; Palpitations; Weight loss; Loose motions; Tremor; Oligomenorrhoea/amenorrhoea; Fatigue and weakness

Signs: Lid retraction/lid lag; Graves ophthalmopathy; Goitre/bruit; Systolic hypertension; Gynaecomastia; Tachycardia/Atrial fibrillation; Cardiac failure; Tremor; Warm peripheries; Onycholysis, acropachy; Proximal myopathy; Pretibial myxoedema

- Incidence 1:1000 over 20 years.
- Most common in 3rd–4th decade of life.

### Pathogenesis
- Autoimmunity against thyroid peroxidase ('microsomal' Ag), thyroglobulin, and TSH receptor.
- Environmental 'triggers' (possibly infections, stress, pregnancy, drugs) combine with genetic susceptibility (e.g. HLA-DR3 and CTLA4 variants).

### Symptoms and signs (specific for GD)
- Infiltrative orbitopathy: irritation, dryness, periorbital oedema, chemosis, exophthalmos and proptosis (may be unilateral), ophthalmoplegia with diplopia (Figs 7.16A and B).
- Beware the patient with apparently mild eye disease but in whom visual acuity and colour vision are impaired; in these patients raised pressure within the orbit is compressing the optic nerve. Immediate referral to an ophthalmologist is mandatory.
- Dermopathy (classically 'pretibial myxoedema'—hyperpigmented, non-pitting induration, sometimes plaque like; Fig. 7.16C).
- Thyroid bruit—signifying a highly vascular gland.
- Thyroid acropachy (looks like clubbing).

### Investigations
- Typically markedly elevated FT4 and FT3 (FT3 rise may be relatively >FT4 rise).
- TSH receptor antibody (TRAb) detectable.
- Diffusely increased radioactive iodine/technetium uptake (not required if clinical signs of Graves disease and detectable TRAb) (Fig. 7.18A).
- TRAb titres should be measured in pregnancy (especially if the mother has developed prior hypothyroidism and is therefore unable to mount a thyrotoxic response herself to circulating TRAb) as it facilitates estimation of risk of intrauterine/neonatal thyrotoxicosis.
- Antithyroid peroxidase (TPO) antibodies are not positive in all patients with Graves disease.
- Thyroid USS is not indicated in the majority of cases.

### Treatment
- β-blockers (preferably non-selective e.g. propranolol 20–40mg three times daily) for rapid relief of symptoms.
- Antithyroid drug (ATD) therapy (e.g. carbimazole (CBZ) or propylthiouracil (PTU)—Box 7.1) results in long-term remission in ~40–50% of cases. Regimens include:
  - 'Titration' according to FT4/FT3 levels—typically given for 12–18 months.
  - 'Block and replace': higher doses of CBZ/PTU, combined with thyroxine (L-T4) replacement, for 6–12 months
- TSH may stay suppressed for several months despite normalization of FT4/FT3. L-T4 should therefore be commenced once FT4 has fallen to just above, or into the upper part of the reference range. This is particularly important in those with active Graves eye disease, which can be markedly exacerbated by the development of hypothyroidism.
- Radioiodine (RAI $^{131}$I) (300–800MBq) may be used as first–line therapy or for ATD failure; using higher doses reduces rates of relapse, but increases risk of hypothyroidism; ATDs must be discontinued prior to RAI to allow adequate uptake of the isotope, but can be restarted 5–7 days later and continued for 2–3 months, at which point residual thyroid status should be assessed.
- RAI is **not** recommended in patients with moderate–severe active Graves ophthalmopathy. Prednisolone (30–40mg/day) may be used to prevent worsening of ophthalmopathy in those with milder eye disease who wish to undergo RAI therapy.

(A1)

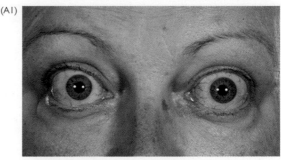

(A2)

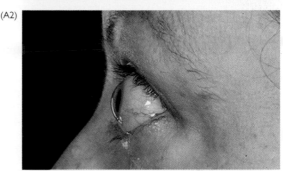

(B)

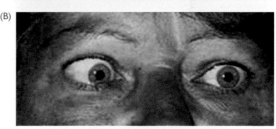

(C)

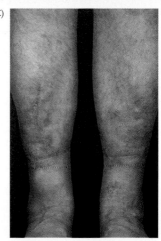

**Fig. 7.16** Specific clinical features of Graves disease. (A) Exophthalmos and mild periorbital oedema. (B) Ophthalmoplegia—note the patient's inability to look to the left. (C) Pretibial myxoedema.

- RAI is contraindicated in pregnancy, which should be avoided for 6 months after treatment. Men are normally advised not to attempt to father a child for 4 months after RAI therapy.
- Subtotal thyroidectomy is generally reserved for those with relapsing thyrotoxicosis who decline or are not suitable for RAI, or if there are significant compressive symptoms; potential complications include haemorrhage, vocal cord paresis, hypoparathyroidism and hypothyroidism.

- Rashes are the most common side effect of ATD therapy (~5%)—the use of an antihistamine for milder cases, or switching from carbimazole to propylthiouracil may resolve the problem.
- A small number (~0.5%) of patients may experience life-threatening agranulocytosis and/or thrombocytopenia, which requires immediate cessation of therapy. All patients on ATDs must be warned of this possibility, and given instructions (including in written format) advising them to immediately stop treatment and attend their GP or accident and emergency department for a full blood count if they develop a sore throat, mouth ulceration (Fig. 7.17) or fever. Once confirmed, the patient should **not** be restarted on/switched to an alternative ATD as the risk of recurrence is high.

Patients should be rendered euthyroid prior to thyroidectomy, or surgery covered with a β-blocker, to minimize the risks of precipitating dysrhythmias/thyroid storm.

## Toxic multinodular goitre

- More common in patients >50 years of age; ♀ >♂.
- Autonomy evolves over time; iodine exposure (food, drugs) may influence risk of development.
- Biochemical thyrotoxicosis generally milder, but cardiovascular manifestations common (AF, tachycardia with heart failure).
- Retrosternal extension and obstructive symptoms more common (consider CT neck/thoracic inlet, flow volume loop).
- Increased patchy radioactive iodine/technetium uptake (Fig. 7.18B)
- TRAb and TPO negative.
- ATDs control, but do not cure, thyrotoxicosis; RAI is the treatment of choice; surgery if significant compressive symptoms.

## Toxic adenoma

- Typically in patients 30–40 years of age.
- Follicular adenoma.
- Symptoms usually less marked than in Graves disease.
- May present with palpable thyroid nodule.
- Isolated 'hot spot' on radioactive iodine/technetium scan, with suppression of remainder of the gland (Fig. 7.18C).

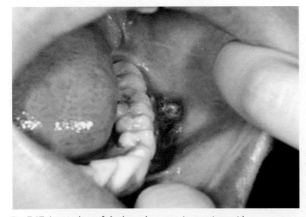

Fig. 7.17 Large ulcer of the buccal mucosa in a patient with carbimazole-induced neutropaenia.

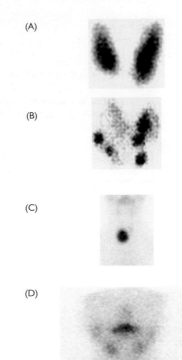

Fig. 7.18 Thyroid ⁹⁹ᵐtechnetium isotope scans. (A) Uniform high uptake in Graves disease. (B) Patchy uptake in toxic multinodular goitre. (C) Solitary right-sided toxic adenoma. (D) Absent thyroidal uptake in a patient with thyroiditis—note normal salivary gland uptake bilaterally.

- RAI is preferred, as the suppressed normal gland usually recovers function in due course.

## Thyroiditis

- Several different forms are recognized, many of which produce only transient thyrotoxicosis:
  - Autoimmune: 'hashitoxicosis' preceding development of hypothyroidism; high anti-TPO Ab titre; firm thyroid due to lymphocytic fibrosis; painless.
  - Subacute (De Quervain): classically following viral upper respiratory tract infection (URTI); relatively sudden onset of pain, worse with neck movement; tender thyroid++; ESR increased++, but WBC normal.
  - Postpartum: typically <6 months postpartum; painless.
  - Other: pyogenic, radiation, amiodarone-induced, Riedel (extensive fibrosis, 'rock hard' thyroid, often obstructive symptoms).
- Very low/absent radioactive iodine/technetium uptake (Fig. 7.18D).
- TRAb negative, but may be TPO positive.
- ATDs ineffective; β-blockers control symptoms.
- A hypothyroid phase often follows initial thyrotoxicosis; may be permanent in a small number of cases (more likely if TPO Ab titre raised).

# Thyroid storm/crisis

- Rare, but potentially life-threatening.
- Typically arises in patients with poorly controlled disease; precipitants include intercurrent illness, surgery, or RAI therapy.
- Manifestations include: hyperpyrexia, profuse sweating, restlessness, psychosis, cardiac failure, coma.

## Management

- **Obtain specialist endocrine advice and do *not* wait for thyroid function results.**
- **Stop synthesis of new hormone**: ATD—CBZ 20mg or PTU 200mg immediately and continued 4–6-hourly thereafter.
- **Impair release of stored hormone**: sodium iodide 0.5–1g IV 12-hourly or saturated solution of potassium iodide 6–8 drops orally every 6 hours
- Iodide must **not** be started before ATD therapy—risk of providing further substrate for hormone synthesis.
- The radiographic contrast agents ipodate and iopanoate may also be used to reduce thyroid hormone release and have the added benefit of markedly impairing T4 to T3 conversion.
- **Block peripheral manifestations of excess thyroid hormones:** propranolol 0.5–2mg IV slowly, followed by 40–80mg orally every 6–8 hours; the short-acting agent esmolol is preferred in those with pre-existing cardiac disease where impairing remaining sympathetic drive to the myocardium may result in sudden decompensation. Verapamil is a suitable alternative for those with a history of asthma
- **Dexamethasone:** 2mg orally or IV every 6–8 hours reduces peripheral conversion of T4 to T3
- **Supportive measures:** O$_2$ therapy, intravenous fluids, active cooling, diuretics, chlorpromazine—as indicated. Involve critical care teams as appropriate.

# 7.4 Hypothyroidism

## Background

The term hypothyroidism describes the clinical syndrome resulting from a lack of thyroid hormone.

## Aetiology

See Table 7.4.

- Hashimoto thyroiditis and atrophic thyroiditis account for >90% of cases.
- Hashimoto thyroiditis is 7× more common in ♀ than in ♂.
- Congenital hypothyroidism occurs in 1 in 3000–4000 live births in the UK.

| Table 7.4 Aetiology of hypothyroidism | | |
|---|---|---|
| **Cause** | **Type** | **Clinical condition** |
| Primary | Autoimmune | Hashimoto thyroiditis |
| | | Atrophic thyroiditis |
| | Iatrogenic | Thyroidectomy |
| | | Radioiodine therapy |
| | | Neck irradiation |
| | | Drugs, e.g. antithyroid agents, lithium |
| | Transient | Thyroiditis (e.g. subacute, postpartum) |
| | Defects of hormone synthesis | Iodine deficiency (or excess) |
| | | Inborn errors |
| | Infiltration | Tumour, amyloidosis |
| | Thyroid hypoplasia/agenesis | |
| Secondary | Hypothalamic or pituitary disease | |

## Classifications

- Primary vs. secondary (pituitary) vs. tertiary (hypothalamic).
- Congenital vs. acquired.
- Clinical vs. subclinical.

## Clinical evaluation

### History and examination

- The majority of symptoms and signs of hypothyroidism are independent of the underlying cause, of insidious onset, and often vague or absent in mild disease (Figs 7.19 and 7.20).
- Features of associated conditions (e.g. primary adrenal failure and type 1 diabetes mellitus in patients with primary hypothyroidism, or hypopituitarism in subjects with central disorders), may also be present.
- Thyroid examination may point to a specific diagnosis (e.g. non-palpable thyroid in cases of agenesis/hypoplasia; diffuse goitre in Hashimoto) (Fig. 7.21).

### Myxoedema

- Symptom complex arising from severe thyroid hormone deficiency.
- Characterized by cardiac failure + neuropsychiatric manifestations (cerebellar ataxia, psychosis, encephalopathy).
- Left untreated, coma ensues with hypothermia, bradycardia, hypotension, hypoglycaemia, hyponatraemia, hypoxia, and hypercapnia.
- Precipitated by intercurrent infection, myocardial infarction, sedative drugs, or cold exposure.

### Cretinism

- Syndrome of mental retardation, deafness, and short stature; characteristic puffy appearance of face and hands.
- Consequence of untreated congenital hypothyroidism.

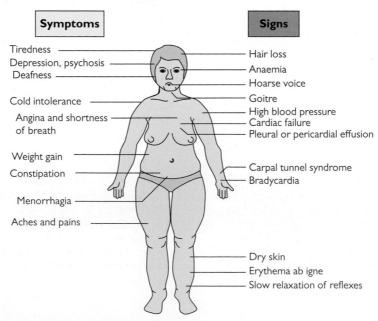

**Symptoms**
- Tiredness
- Depression, psychosis
- Deafness
- Cold intolerance
- Angina and shortness of breath
- Weight gain
- Constipation
- Menorrhagia
- Aches and pains

**Signs**
- Hair loss
- Anaemia
- Hoarse voice
- Goitre
- High blood pressure
- Cardiac failure
- Pleural or pericardial effusion
- Carpal tunnel syndrome
- Bradycardia
- Dry skin
- Erythema ab igne
- Slow relaxation of reflexes

**Fig. 7.19** Schematic representation of the clinical features of hypothyroidism.

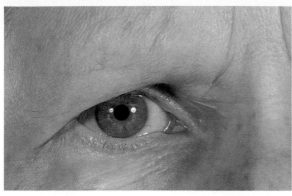

**Fig. 7.20** Classical thinning of the eyebrows (with particular loss of the outer 1/3) in a patient with longstanding hypothyroidism.

## Investigations

- The diagnosis is traditionally based on clinical findings and biochemical confirmation of hypothyroidism. Thyroid imaging or biopsies are only warranted in exceptional cases (e.g. concomitant thyroid nodule).

*Laboratory findings*
Typically:

- Thyroid hormones (T4, T3) are low (routine measurement of FT3 is not required in most cases).
- Thyrotropin (TSH) is raised (usually markedly so).
- ▶ The finding of low FT4 and FT3 levels with a normal or low TSH is suggestive of central hypothyroidism and an underlying pituitary disorder must be excluded.

Subclinical hypothyroidism:

- TSH mildly raised but FT4 and FT3 within respective reference ranges.
- Estimated to affect up to 10% of ♀ >50 years of age.
- Associated with hypercholesterolaemia.
- Decision to treat made on individual basis.

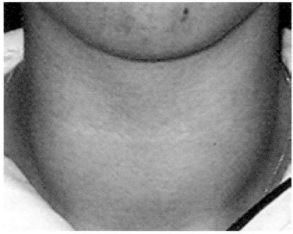

**Fig. 7.21** Diffuse goitre in a patient with Hashimoto thyroiditis.

- Anti-TPO antibodies are typically found in the early stages of autoimmune hypothyroidism (especially Hashimoto), but may wane and become undetectable in 'burnt out' disease.
- Anaemia is common in hypothyroidism and multifactorial (microcytic if menorrhagia, macrocytic if coexisting pernicious anaemia, or normocytic).
- Hypercholesterolaemia and raised creatine kinase denote hepatic and muscle hypothyroidism respectively.

## Management

### Levo-thyroxine (L-T4)

Standard treatment is with thyroxine supplementation/replacement—usually beginning with a dose of 50mcg/day, and increasing up to 1.6mcg per kg per day in those requiring full replacement; however, elderly subjects typically need lower doses, while requirements may be greater in younger subjects or in those taking confounding medications (e.g. exogenous oral oestrogen or enzyme-inducing agents).

- Reassess clinically and check TSH and FT4 at 4–6-weekly intervals until stabilized on treatment.
- In primary hypothyroidism titrate L-T4 to achieve a TSH in the lower half of the reference range (i.e. 0.4–2mU/L); this may be associated with a FT4 level which is in the upper half or even just above the upper limit of the respective reference range.
- In secondary hypothyroidism titrate L-T4 therapy against symptoms and the FT4 level—remember TSH is unreliable in this setting.
- ▶ In elderly patients or those with known/suspected ischaemic heart disease cautious titration of L-T4 (e.g. beginning with 25mcg/day or on an alternate day basis) is necessary. Consider admission to hospital with ECG monitoring if appropriate.
- ▶ In subjects with suspected coexistent hypoadrenalism do not start L-T4 until the diagnosis has been excluded or confirmed and hydrocortisone replacement commenced.

Treatment of subclinical hypothyroidism is controversial, but should be considered if the patient is symptomatic, has hypercholesterolaemia, or if there is a high likelihood of progression to overt hypothyroidism (e.g. TSH >10mU/L; positive TPO titre).

### Pregnancy

- Untreated maternal hypothyroidism is associated with higher rates of miscarriage, stillbirth, and congenital abnormalities. It has been reported that even mild maternal hypothyroidism may have consequences for the subsequent intellectual development of the unborn child.
- L-T4 requirements may increase by 50–100% during pregnancy, especially in the later stages.
- Thyroid function tests should ideally be checked prior to conception and at regular intervals during pregnancy with early/prompt dose titration.

### Myxoedema coma

Myxoedema coma is a medical emergency (see Section 1.12); treatment includes:

- Ventilatory and circulatory support.
- Correction of hypothermia and hypoglycaemia.
- Treatment of precipitating event(s).
- Hydrocortisone replacement until normal adrenal reserve demonstrated.
- L-T4 or L-T3 therapy—dose and regimen should be decided in conjunction with an endocrinologist.

# 7.5 Goitre and thyroid nodule

## Background

The term 'goitre' is used to describe a swelling in the neck due to enlargement of the thyroid gland (see Fig. 7.21, Section 7.4). Subjects with a goitre may be hyper- (e.g. 'toxic goitre'), hypo- (e.g. due to iodine deficiency), or euthyroid.

## Epidemiology

- In unselected American men and women thyroid nodules were palpable in 1.5% and 6.4% respectively.
- In autopsy series nodules are reported in 1/3 to 1/2 of all subjects, and prevalence rises with increasing age.
- Iodine deficiency is a predisposing factor.
- Histologically 1/20 thyroid nodules are malignant (no difference between solitary and multiple nodules). Clinically relevant malignancy is rare (<1% of all cancers and <0.5% of cancer-related mortality).

## Causes

(See Table 7.5.) Given the high prevalence, and the fact that the vast majority of goitres/thyroid nodules are benign and do not progress to malignancy, the decision whether a thyroid lesion warrants further investigation is difficult. Remember:

- Diffuse goitres can be physiological.
- Diffuse goitres, cysts without solid components, and 'toxic' nodules are usually benign.
- A family history for simple goitre, Hashimoto thyroiditis, or hyper-/hypothyroidism favour benign disease.
- A sudden increase in the size of a nodule, with pain or tenderness, is suggestive of an expanding cyst (e.g. haemorrhage into cyst) or subacute thyroiditis.

Patients at higher risk for thyroid cancer:

- History of head and neck irradiation (especially at young age— e.g. Chernobyl nuclear accident).
- Positive family history for thyroid cancer or multiple endocrine neoplasia.
- Clinical features suspicious of malignancy such as fixation to skin, voice changes, palpable neck lymph nodes, and hoarseness (recurrent laryngeal nerve compression).

| Table 7.5 Causes of goitre and thyroid nodules | | |
|---|---|---|
| | **Type** | **Examples** |
| Diffuse goitre | Physiological | Puberty, pregnancy |
| | Autoimmune | Graves disease, Hashimoto thyroiditis |
| | Thyroiditis | Subacute (de Quervain), Riedel |
| | Endemic | Iodine deficiency |
| | Goitrogens | Antithyroid drugs, lithium, iodine excess |
| | Dyshormonogenesis | |
| Nodular goitre | Multi-nodular goitre | Toxic/non-toxic |
| | Solitary nodule | Follicular adenoma, benign nodule/cyst, thyroid malignancy, lymphoma, metastasis |
| | Infiltration (rare) | Tuberculosis, sarcoidosis |

- Enlarging nodule on a background of Hashimoto (may signify thyroid lymphoma).

## Signs and symptoms

- Thyroid enlargement is often asymptomatic, but neck discomfort and globus sensation are not uncommon.
- Large goitres can displace or compress anatomical structures in the thoracic inlet resulting in inspiratory stridor, dysphagia, and a choking sensation (often positional).
- Features of hyper- or hypothyroidism may be present.

## Investigations

### Biochemistry

- Establish thyroid status: TSH, FT4.

### Radiology

- If clinically suspected, exclude significant retrosternal extension or tracheal compression (neck CT or MRI, flow-volume loops) (Fig. 7.22).
- Thyroid ultrasound can be used to evaluate the morphology of nodules (e.g. presence of cysts, microcalcifications, multiple or solitary, vascularity, etc.).
- $^{99m}$Technetium scintigraphy assesses functional status (cold, hot or warm) of nodules, but is generally reserved for those with evidence of biochemical thyrotoxicosis.

### Biopsy

Non-toxic solitary or dominant nodules within a multinodular goitre (commonly a cut off of >1cm diameter is used) require histological assessment by fine needle aspiration biopsy (±ultrasound guidance) (sensitivity and specificity >90%). In the UK, the THY grading system is used to classify appearances on FNA biopsy and ranges from 1 (non-diagnostic) to 5 (diagnostic of malignancy).

Malignancy can not always be completely excluded and surveillance (+/− repeat biopsy or further investigation) may be required in some patients.

## Management

Monitoring by periodic clinical examination and thyroid function testing is often sufficient, for example, in an asymptomatic patient with a simple goitre. Treat the underlying cause if possible. Suppressive therapy with T4 (i.e. at a dosage that lowers TSH to the low-normal range) may result in goitre shrinkage in the context of Hashimoto thyroiditis. Indications for surgery may include:

- Cosmetic reasons.
- Local pressure symptoms.
- Suspicion of malignancy.

$^{131}$Iodine therapy of non-toxic nodular goitres may result in some reduction in gland volume and is therefore a possible treatment option, especially when surgery is deemed high-risk.

## Thyroid cancer

- The commonest endocrine cancer.
- Molecular pathogenesis has been elucidated for some subtypes, e.g. BRAF (V600E) mutation or RET-PTC rearrangements in papillary carcinoma; p53 mutations in anaplastic carcinoma; RET germline mutations in MEN-2.

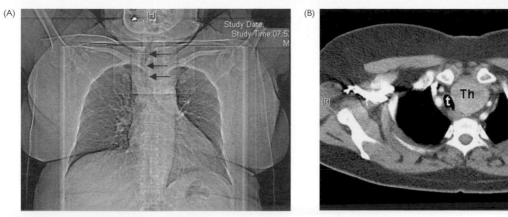

**Fig. 7.22** Goitre and thyroid nodules. (A) Planning coronal CT scan demonstrating tracheal deviation (arrows) to the right as a consequence of an enlarged left lobe of thyroid (see B) in a patient with local compressive symptoms. (B) CT scan showing deviation and compression of the trachea (t) by an enlarged left thyroid lobe (Th).

- A WHO histological classification (as follows) is widely used; the TNM-system is used for staging. Together papillary and follicular cancers account for ~90–95% of cases.

**Papillary**
- Peak incidence during the 4th and 5th decades of life, although smaller peak also seen in 2nd and 3rd decades.
- Slowest growing of thyroid cancers. Local spread to cervical lymph nodes common at presentation, but distant metastases rare.
- Total thyroidectomy followed by an ablative dose of radioactive iodine is recommended for all, except very small tumours. Treatment may include lifelong T4 therapy to fully suppress TSH.
- Targeted therapies (e.g. Kinase Inhibitors) are attracting increasing interest and may be used in patients with disease refractory to conventional treatment.
- Thyroglobulin is useful as tumour marker following total thyroidectomy.
- Cancer-related death in <5% during 10-years of follow-up.

**Follicular**
- Peak incidence during the 5th decade of life.
- More aggressive than papillary carcinoma. Spread into local lymph nodes or into blood vessels with distant lung and bone metastases.
- Treatment as per papillary carcinoma.
- Cancer-related death in 5–10% during 10 years of follow-up.

**Anaplastic**
- <5% of all cases.

- Peak incidence 60–75 years of age.
- Aggressive form of thyroid cancer. Typically presents with painful, rapidly expanding thyroid mass.
- Despite combined treatment (surgery, radiotherapy ± chemotherapy), few patients survive long-term.

**Medullary (MTC)**
- <5% of all cases.
- Peak incidence during 4th–5th decades for sporadic MTC, much earlier age for hereditary.
- Associated with MEN-2 syndromes. Both (i.e. sporadic and hereditary) MTC linked to RET mutations.
- More aggressive than papillary or follicular, but less so than anaplastic cancer. Locally invasive with distant spread via lymphatics and blood.
- Calcitonin virtually always raised.
- Total thyroidectomy may be curative in early stages, hence rationale for genetic screening of relatives. Radiotherapy and chemotherapy are usually of little benefit.
- Long-term survival is variable.

**Lymphoma**
- <1% of all cases.
- May arise as a primary thyroid or as part of generalized lymphoma.
- Variable prognosis and response to radiotherapy.

Beware an enlarging nodule on a background of Hashimoto goitre—the diagnosis of thyroid lymphoma should be assumed until proven otherwise.

# 7.6 Cushing syndrome

## Background

- **Cushing syndrome** (CS; Harvey Cushing, 1869–1939, American neurosurgeon) describes the clinical manifestations of chronic exposure to excessive levels of glucocorticoids.
- **Cushing disease** (CD) refers exclusively to CS due to an adrenocorticotrophic hormone (ACTH)-secreting pituitary adenoma.
- Endogenous (intrinsic) CS is rare, but often queried because typical manifestations include common and non-specific symptoms, e.g. weight gain, weakness, low mood.

## Epidemiology

Incidence ~1–2 per million population per year, although in cohorts of obese individuals with hypertension and type 2 diabetes mellitus prevalence rates of 2–5% have been reported.

## Pathophysiology

- Hypothalamic corticotropin-releasing hormone (CRH) stimulates pituitary corticotrophs to secrete ACTH, which in turn stimulates adrenocortical fasciculata cells to produce glucocorticoids. Autonomous overproduction of hormones at any level → CS (Table 7.6).
- By far the commonest cause of CS is treatment with supraphysiological **exogenous** glucocorticoids (>5–7.5mg prednisolone or >20–30mg hydrocortisone/day), i.e. iatrogenic CS.
- **Cyclical/periodic CD:** some autonomous ACTH-producing tumours exhibit cyclical and intermittent secretion resulting in cyclical symptoms and signs. Such cyclicity can extend over months to years and delay the diagnosis.
- **Pseudo-cushingoid states:** high alcohol intake, depression, and extremes of body weight can lead to clinical and biochemical features of CS, which improve when the underlying disorder has resolved.

## Clinical evaluation

### History and examination

Obesity and weight gain (95%), facial plethora (90%), 'moon' face (90%), reduced libido (90%), thin skin (85%), menstrual irregularity (80%), hypertension (75%), hirsutism (75%), depression/emotional lability (70%), easy bruising (65%), glucose intolerance (60%), weakness, especially proximal myopathy (60%), osteopenia or fracture

**Table 7.6** Aetiology of endogenous Cushing syndrome

| Type | Example |
|---|---|
| ACTH-dependent | Pituitary adenoma (70%) |
| | Ectopic ACTH syndrome (EAS, 10%) |
| | Ectopic CRH secretion (very rare) |
| ACTH-independent | Adrenal adenoma (10%) |
| | Adrenal carcinoma (5%) |
| | AIMAH |
| | PPNAD (Carney complex or sporadic, very rare) McCune–Albright syndrome (very rare) |

ACTH: adrenocorticotrophic hormone (corticotropin); AIMAH: ACTH-independent (bilateral) macronodular adrenal hyperplasia; CRH: corticotropin-releasing hormone; PPNAD: primary pigmented nodular adrenal disease.

(50%), nephrolithiasis (50%), striae (50%), oedema (50%), 'buffalo hump' (50%).

Signs of protein wasting most reliably differentiate CS from pseudo-cushingoid states, e.g. proximal myopathy, easy bruising, and thin skin (Fig. 7.23).

### Investigation

Because many of the features of CS are non-specific and prevalent in the general population, appropriate and cost-effective screening is important. No single test excludes or confirms CS. Investigation involves two phases:

*1. Confirm clinical suspicion.*

This typically involves two or more of the following:

*24-hour urinary free cortisol (UFC) measurement*

Three consecutive collections: excess cortisol is excreted in urine when it exceeds the binding capacity of cortisol binding globulin (CBG). 1 in 4 UFC results are in the normal range in up to 15% of patients with subsequently confirmed CS.

*Low-dose dexamethasone suppression test (LDDST)*

0.5mg 6-hourly for 48 hours: in CS serum cortisol fails to suppress to <50nmol/L. May yield false positive result in the presence of (1) enzyme inducing drugs (e.g. phenytoin, rifampicin), which increase dexamethasone clearance and (2) agents that raise CBG levels (e.g. oestrogen)—most serum assays measure total and not free cortisol. Many centres use the more convenient overnight DST as a screening test for CS (1mg at 11pm followed by measurement of 9am serum cortisol the next day). False positive rates of 15–30% have been reported with both tests.

*Cortisol day curve and late night/midnight cortisol*

Physiologically, cortisol levels are highest on rising and lowest around midnight. Midnight sleeping cortisol <50nmol/L excludes CS. Conditions (e.g. hyperthyroidism) or substances (e.g. oestrogen), which increase CBG elevate serum total cortisol and may yield false positive results. In contrast, salivary cortisol can be collected at home and the assay measures free hormone levels.

*Combined LDDST-CRH stimulation test*

May help to distinguish true CS (in particular CD) from pseudo-cushingoid states.

*2. Identify the underlying cause*

*ACTH*

'Undetectable' or low in CS due to adrenal pathology. ACTH is normal or elevated in CD and in ectopic ACTH syndrome (EAS).

*Plasma potassium*

Often low in EAS even in the absence of confounding drug treatments, but may also be low in some cases of CD.

*Imaging*

Pituitary MRI (in CD) (Fig. 7.24), adrenal CT (in adrenal adenoma or carcinoma) (Fig. 7.25A and B), and chest/abdominal CT ± whole body scintigraphy (e.g. octreotide) or positron emission tomography (e.g. FDG-PET) studies (in EAS) can visualize the source of ACTH/ cortisol excess, but should only be requested once the diagnosis of CS has been confirmed biochemically (in view of the high rate of 'incidentalomas', which may lead to erroneous interpretation of equivocal test results).

*Bilateral inferior petrosal sinus sampling (BIPSS)*

Best test to distinguish CD from EAS (sensitivity + specificity ~95%): in CD the ratio of ACTH sampled in the inferior petrosal sinuses (drain venous blood from the pituitary gland—Fig. 7.26) to that in peripheral veins is >2:1 before and >3:1 after administration of CRH; also aids lateralization of pituitary adenoma in ~2/3 of cases.

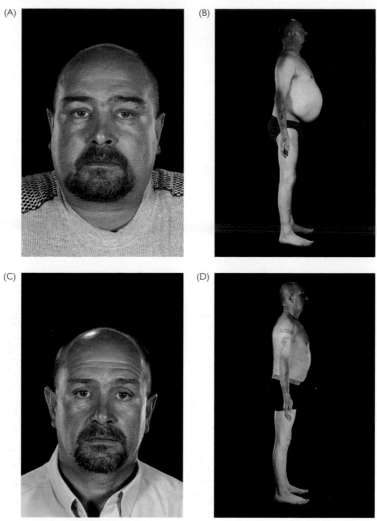

Fig. 7.23 Clinical features of a patient with Cushing syndrome before (A and B) and after (C and D) treatment.

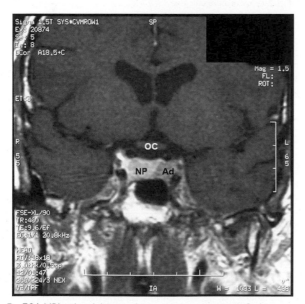

Fig. 7.24 MRI with gadolinium enhancement in a patient with Cushing disease. Note the bright appearance of the normal pituitary gland (NP), which contrasts with the relative lack of enhancement of the left-sided microadenoma (Ad). The position of the optic chiasm (OC) is also shown.

Dynamic non-invasive investigations can also be used to help differentiate CD from EAS, but their performance is considerably less than that of IPSS such that some centres no longer routinely recommend their use:

*High-dose dexamethasone suppression test (HDDST)*
2mg 6-hourly for 48 hours or 8mg overnight test: in ~80% of cases of CD some negative feedback remains (cortisol at 9am after test ≤50% of basal level, i.e. level before commencing dexamethasone suppression) vs. ≤10% of EAS.

*CRH stimulation test*
100mcg IV: ACTH (and cortisol) rise is exaggerated in 80–90% of CD. EAS only rarely responds.

## Management

Prolonged exposure to hypercortisolaemia is associated with increased mortality and significant comorbidities. Management of patients with CS in tertiary centres with surgical teams specializing in adrenal and pituitary surgery results in the best outcome.

### Treatment of the underlying cause
*Transsphenoidal surgery (TSS)*
The therapy of choice for CD. 80–90% cure rates for micro- and 50% for macroadenomas with experienced surgeon.

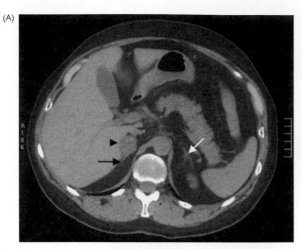

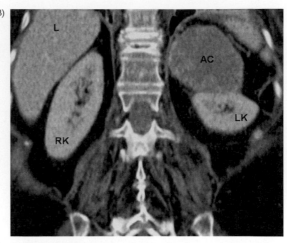

Fig. 7.25 Adrenal causes of Cushing syndrome. (A) CT scan showing a right adrenal adenoma (black arrowhead). Note that the morphology of the postero-medial limb of the right adrenal has been preserved (black arrow). The normal left adrenal gland is clearly seen (white arrow). (B) Coronally reconstructed CT scan demonstrating large left adrenal carcinoma (AC), compressing the adjacent kidney (LK). L: liver; RK: right kidney.

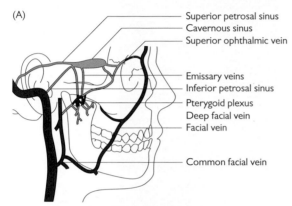

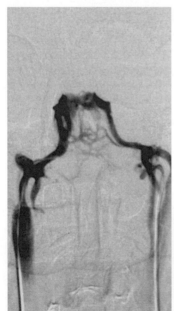

Fig. 7.26 (A) Inferior petrosal sinus anatomy. (B) Plain radiograph showing bilateral symmetrical catheter placement in the inferior petrosal sinuses in a patient undergoing IPSS for investigation of ACTH-dependent Cushing syndrome.

Reproduced from Royal College of Physicians. *Medical Masterclass: Endocrinology*, 2nd edition. London: RCP, 2013. Copyright © 2013 Royal College of Physicians. Reproduced with permission.

### Pituitary irradiation
Indicated in some patients who have undergone unsuccessful pituitary surgery or who have undergone bilateral adrenalectomy (in the latter group to prevent pituitary proliferation (Nelson syndrome) due to loss of negative feedback).

### Adrenal surgery
Adrenal adenomas should be removed, ideally by laparoscopic adrenalectomy. Survival of non-metastatic adrenal cancer is prolonged with surgery. Bilateral adrenalectomy is an option in CD when therapies targeting the pituitary have failed, and in EAS when the primary tumour evades detection or is unresectable.

### Excision of ectopic ACTH-secreting tumours
May occasionally be curative, but prognosis with such tumours is generally guarded.

### Medical treatments to lower cortisol levels
If curative procedures fail, or in preparation for surgery, hypercortisolism can be controlled with metyrapone (dose range: 250mg 12-hourly, up to 1g 6-hourly) and ketoconazole (400–1200mg daily), which block steroidogenic enzymes. Mifepristone, which antagonizes cortisol signalling via the glucocorticoid receptor, may also be tried. Cabergoline and other dopamine agonists have found use in some cases of CD.

Recently, the novel multireceptor somatostatin analogue pasireotide has been licensed for use in the treatment of CD. There is considerable interest in the potential roles of this agent in primary medical therapy and as an adjunct to surgery. However, its use is frequently complicated by the development of glycaemic disturbance.

The adrenolytic agent mitotane is an important adjunct in the treatment of adrenal cancer.

### Other considerations
Sequelae of CS such as osteoporosis, insulin resistance, and hypertension improve once cortisol levels fall, but may require independent treatment.

## Prognosis

Patients with incompletely controlled CS have a 5× excess mortality. Following curative TSS long-term mortality of patients with CD is marginally increased. Adrenal and other cancers (e.g. small cell lung disease) associated with CS still carry a poor prognosis. Comorbidities may persist even after curative treatment.

Labels in Fig 7.26(A):
- Superior petrosal sinus
- Cavernous sinus
- Superior ophthalmic vein
- Emissary veins
- Inferior petrosal sinus
- Pterygoid plexus
- Deep facial vein
- Facial vein
- Common facial vein

# 7.7 Acromegaly

## Background

**Acromegaly** is the clinical syndrome resulting from growth hormone (GH) excess.

**Pituitary gigantism** refers to pre-pubertal GH excess, i.e. arising prior to the fusion of the epiphyseal growth plates, leading to excessive linear growth, which does not occur in acromegaly.

## Epidemiology

- Rare with 3–5 reported cases per 1 million persons per year and a prevalence of 40–70 per million.
- Mean age at diagnosis is 40–45 years.
- Onset of symptoms commonly predates the diagnosis by 5–15 years.
- Mortality is increased 1.5–4-fold (increased cardiovascular and respiratory disease).

## Pathophysiology

- At diagnosis ~75% of patients with acromegaly have a GH secreting pituitary macroadenoma (>1cm in diameter) and ~25% a microadenoma (<1cm in diameter).
- Very rarely acromegaly results from ectopic growth hormone-releasing hormone (GHRH) secretion (e.g. peripheral neuroendocrine tumours).

- The clinical features of acromegaly are attributable to high levels of GH and insulin-like growth factor (IGF)-1. IGF-1 is produced by the liver in response to GH.
- Excess GH and IGF-I have both somatic, i.e. tissue growth, and adverse metabolic effects (see later in section).
- Mass effects of the enlarging pituitary adenoma can lead to central nervous system symptoms/signs (see 'History and examination').
- Acromegaly may arise as part of the MEN-1 syndrome (parathyroid, pancreatic, and pituitary tumours) or Carney complex (cardiac and cutaneous myxomas, primary pigmented nodular adrenal disease causing CS, benign testicular tumours, and acromegaly) (see Section 7.18). Germline mutations in the *AIP* gene are an increasingly recognized cause of acromegaly in patients presenting at a younger age, and may be associated with relative resistance to somatostatin analogue therapy (see 'Medical therapy').

## Clinical evaluation

### History and examination

The onset of acromegaly is often insidious and its progression slow (Figs 7.27 and 7.28). Commonly patients first attend other specialists, e.g. rheumatologists, dentists, or optometrists, for specific manifestations or complications of acromegaly, triggering a referral to an endocrinologist.

(A)

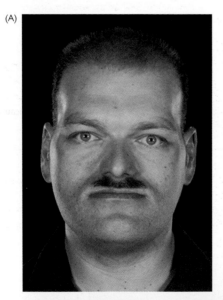

(B)

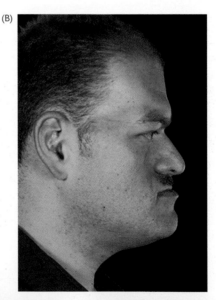

(C)

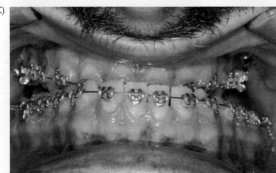

(D)

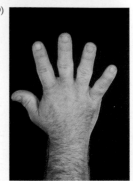

**Fig. 7.27** Clinical features of a patient with acromegaly. Note the typical coarse appearance, prominence of the supraorbital ridges, prognathism, dental separation, and 'spade-like' hands.

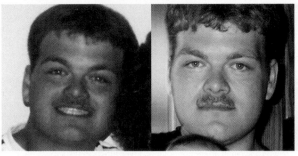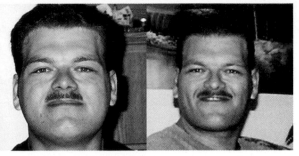

**Fig. 7.28** Serial photographs over a 16-year period showing progressive development of acromegalic features.

Typical signs and symptoms include:

*Somatic effects of GH/IGF-1 hypersecretion*

- Increase in the size of the hands and feet (changes in ring and shoe size, 'spade-like hands') (Fig. 7.27D).
- Coarsened facial features (deep skin folds, frontal bossing) (Fig. 7.27A,B); ask to see old photographs (Fig. 7.28).
- Crowding of the tongue, gapped teeth, over-bite, and prominence of the lower jaw (prognathism) (Fig. 7.27B,C).
- Carpal tunnel syndrome.
- Sweating and oily skin.
- Snoring (indicating sleep apnoea, see 'Complications').
- Arthralgia (bone and cartilage overgrowth).
- Cardiac failure (combination of hypertension—see 'Complications'—and a disease-specific cardiomyopathy).

*Metabolic effects of GH/IGF-1 hypersecretion*

- Insulin resistance and diabetes mellitus (glycosuria, osmotic symptoms).
- Dyslipidaemia (high triglycerides).
- Hypertension.

*Mass effects of the pituitary adenoma*

- Headaches.
- Visual disturbances (typically bitemporal hemianopia—Fig. 7.29).
- Pituitary dysfunction (amenorrhoea, loss of libido or erectile dysfunction, lack of stress hormone response, secondary hypothyroidism).

### Investigations

*GH/IGF-1*

- Single GH measurements are generally considered insufficient to diagnose acromegaly because of the pulsatile nature of GH secretion.

- Biochemical confirmation utilizes a 75g OGTT. Normally GH is suppressed to <1mcg/L (although many endocrinologists recommend a lower cut-off of <0.4mcg/L for modern GH assays). In acromegaly, GH levels show a paradoxical rise or a failure to suppress.
- The IGF-1 concentration is typically elevated above the age- and sex-matched reference range.

*Pituitary function*

- A detailed assessment of pituitary function must be carried out (see Section 7.4).
- 20–25% of GH-producing tumours co-secrete prolactin.

*Radiology/ophthalmology*

- MRI (or CT) of the pituitary fossa should be undertaken once the diagnosis has been established biochemically.
- If the pituitary adenoma is situated close to the optic chiasm, formal assessment of visual acuity and visual fields is mandatory (Fig. 7.29).

*Other*

- Cardiovascular: ECG, echocardiography, lipid profile.
- Metabolic: fasting and 120-minute glucose in OGTT, HbA1c.
- Respiratory: sleep assessment (e.g. polysomnography).
- Gastrointestinal: colonoscopy (see 'Complications').

### Management

Aims:

- To normalize GH and IGF-1 secretion (thereby reversing excess morbidity and mortality).
- To preserve/improve existing pituitary function.
- To contain mass effects of the pituitary tumour.

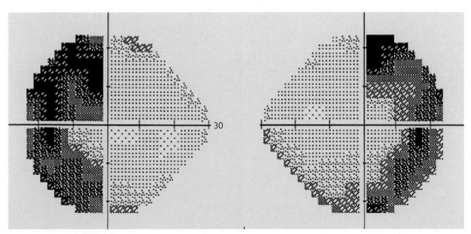

**Fig. 7.29** Visual perimetry demonstrating a bitemporal field defect due to pituitary macroadenoma.

Ideally, complete resection of an adenoma should be associated with normalization of GH secretion (and appropriate suppression during the OGTT). However, in those cases where cure is not achieved/possible, then the aim is to 'control' GH hypersecretion. In this context, the biochemical 'minimum acceptable target' has been the subject of considerable debate—recent consensus guidelines utilize a combination of nadir GH during OGTT, 9am GH and IGF-1 to differentiate 'active' from 'controlled' disease. At its simplest level, if 9am GH is <1 mcg/L and IGF-1 normal, then more detailed testing is generally considered unnecessary.

### Surgery

Transsphenoidal adenomectomy is the treatment of first choice for acromegaly. Experienced neurosurgeons report cure rates of >80% for microadenomas, but only 40–70% for macroadenomas.

### Radiotherapy

Useful for residual tumours and persistent GH elevation postoperatively or if the patient is deemed unfit for surgery. On average, 2 years after conventional fractionated radiotherapy GH levels decrease by ~50% and by ~75% after 5 years. A significant proportion of patients only achieve 'safe' GH suppression after 10 years. Radiosurgery (in which the total dose is given in a single fraction, unlike the multiple fractions over many weeks of conventional radiotherapy), may provide an alternative in selected patients, and allow more rapid control of residual disease activity.

### Medical therapy

The role of medical therapy in the management of acromegaly is evolving, but is still considered interim or second-line therapy, i.e. if pituitary surgery fails or is not appropriate.

**Dopamine agonists (e.g. bromocriptine, cabergoline):** suppress GH levels sufficiently in ~15–25% of cases, and often need to be given at high doses, but are useful for prolactin co-secreting tumours or in combination with somatostatin analogues.

**Somatostatin analogues (octreotide, lanreotide):** control symptoms reducing GH to 'safe' levels in ≤80%, and constrain growth or induce tumour shrinkage in a significant number of cases. They are only available as injections, and may cause GI side effects (transient nausea, diarrhoea, gallstone formation). Pasireotide is a novel SSA with potentially greater efficacy than octreotide and lanreotide, although its use is likely to be limited due to relatively high rates of glycaemic disturbance.

**Growth hormone receptor antagonist (pegvisomant):** normalizes IGF-1 levels in >90% of cases improving many of the clinical features of acromegaly. However, it does not reduce pituitary tumour size and GH levels rise during treatment. Pegvisomant is expensive and is administered by subcutaneous injection. Currently, its use is limited to patients for whom all other treatment options have failed to achieve adequate control. Liver function tests must be monitored and pituitary MRI repeated at regular intervals during treatment.

## Complications

**Treatment of cardiovascular risk factors:** important to improve the prognosis of acromegaly. Particular attention should be paid to hypertension, diabetes mellitus, dyslipidaemia and sleep apnoea.

**Screening colonoscopy:** should be offered once the patient is of an appropriate age, as the risk of colonic neoplasia in acromegalic subjects is increased.

Other **comorbidities** should be addressed, often requiring a multidisciplinary approach (rheumatology, orthopaedics, dentists, maxillofacial surgeons, psychologists).

## Follow-up

Lifelong follow-up with periodic pituitary MRI, visual fields, and pituitary function assessment is required. IGF-I and 9am GH measurement should be undertaken at regular intervals. Repeat OGTT (off treatment) may be required in cases where there is uncertainty regarding possible low level relapse.

# 7.8 Hyperprolactinaemia

## Background

Prolactin is produced solely by lactotroph cells in the anterior pituitary gland. Dopamine, a hypothalamic neurotransmitter which reaches the pituitary gland via the pituitary stalk, acts on D2 receptors of lactotroph cells and inhibits prolactin secretion.

## Causes

Hyperprolactinaemia can be physiological (e.g. pregnancy) or pathological if lactotroph cells become autonomous (e.g. prolactinoma), or if the inhibitory effect of dopamine is disrupted (e.g. by pituitary stalk compression or dopamine antagonist therapy). See Table 7.7.

## Clinical evaluation

### Symptoms and signs

*Hormone **hyper**secretion*

*Galactorrhoea*
- Non-bloody, usually milky nipple discharge.
- 30–80% of cases.
- Occasionally seen in ♂ and normoprolactinaemic individuals.

*Hormone **hypo**secretion*

*Hypogonadism*
May arise even in the absence of significant mass effect because of the inhibitory action of hyperprolactinaemia on hypothalamic gonadotropin-releasing hormone (GnRH) secretion. Manifestations include:
- ♀: oligo/amenorrhoea and infertility.

- ♂: low libido, impotence, infertility, and gynaecomastia (the latter is predominantly a consequence of low testosterone levels rather than hyperprolactinaemia per se).
- Longstanding hypogonadism is associated with osteopenia/osteoporosis.

*Hypopituitarism*
Compression of the pituitary stalk and/or the remaining normal pituitary gland may lead to varying degrees of hypopituitarism (see Section 7.4).

*Local mass effects*
- Hypopituitarism (see Section 7.4).
- Reduced visual acuity/impaired visual fields—due to chiasmal/optic nerve compression.
- Diplopia—due to cavernous sinus extension and compression of cranial nerves III, IV, and VI.

### Investigations

Unless there is a clear explanation for hyperprolactinaemia (e.g. a mild rise in serum prolactin temporally related to commencing medication (Table 7.7)), then consistently elevated prolactin levels require further investigation including:
- U&E, LFT.
- FT4, TSH:
- Pituitary function tests (see Section 7.4).
- Visual acuity and field assessments (Fig. 7.30).
- Pituitary MRI (Fig. 7.31).
- The extent to which the prolactin level is elevated may provide a clue as to the aetiology.
- **Hook effect:** very high circulating levels of prolactin 'overwhelm' the antibodies used in the immunoassay, thus yielding a falsely low reading. Dilution of the serum usually helps to reveal the true level.

| Table 7.7 Causes of hyperprolactinaemia | | |
|---|---|---|
| **Type** | **Conditions** | **Examples** |
| Physiological | Pregnancy | |
| | Lactation | |
| | Stress | |
| | Sexual intercourse, physical activity | |
| | (Following seizure) | Epilepsy—may help to distinguish genuine from pseudo-seizure |
| Pathological | 'Idiopathic' | May actually be due in some cases to tiny microprolactinomas that are not readily visualized on MRI |
| | Hypothalamic-pituitary stalk dysfunction | Suprasellar (e.g. craniopharyngioma, meningioma) or intrasellar (e.g. non-functioning adenoma) tumour causing stalk compression; empty sella; granuloma; infiltration (e.g. sarcoidosis); trauma; surgery; cranial irradiation |
| | Prolactinoma | Micro- or macroadenoma |
| | Other endocrine disorders | Primary hypothyroidism (TRH is trophic for prolactin secretion); PCOS |
| | Systemic disorders | Chronic renal failure (reduced prolactin clearance), hepatic cirrhosis, chest wall pathology (e.g. zoster) |
| Pharmacological | Neuroleptics* | Haloperidol, chlorpromazine, risperidone, sulpiride |
| | Antidepressants | Tricyclics (e.g. amitriptyline), SSRIs (e.g. fluoxetine) |
| | Antiemetics | Metoclopramide, domperidone |
| | Antihypertensives | Verapamil, methyldopa |
| | H2 antagonists | Cimetidine |
| | Opiates | Morphine |

PCOS: polycystic ovarian syndrome; SSRI: selective serotonin reuptake inhibitor; TRH: thyrotropin-releasing hormone.

*Quetiapine, olanzapine, and clozapine are antipsychotics with no or minimal effect on prolactin.

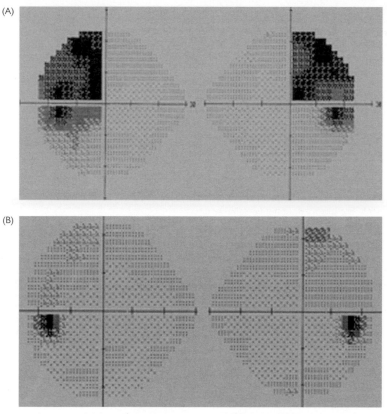

**Fig. 7.30** Visual fields in a patient with a macroprolactinoma (presenting prolactin 45,000mu/L). (A) Prior to treatment there is evidence of a dense bilateral upper temporal quadrantanopia due to compression of the optic chiasm from below. (B) Shortly after starting cabergoline, the field defect has resolved. Note the position of the normal blind spot just below the horizontal meridian in each eye.

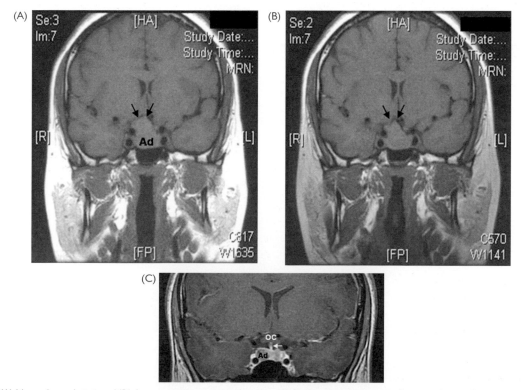

**Fig. 7.31** (A) Non-enhanced pituitary MRI demonstrating a macroprolactinoma (Ad) with asymmetric suprasellar extension causing compression of the optic chiasm against the adjacent brain (arrows) (same patient as in Fig. 7.30). (B) Shortly after commencing cabergoline therapy there is a small but definite reduction in the size of the suprasellar component (arrows), which was sufficient to decompress the chiasm (Fig. 7.30B). (C) MRI with gadolinium showing a non-enhancing microprolactinoma (Ad). The position of the optic chiasm (OC) and pituitary stalk (arrow) are also shown.

- **Macroprolactinaemia:** prolactin complexed to an immuno-globulin; it is biologically inactive but may remain immunoreactive depending on the laboratory assay used to measure serum prolactin. Impaired renal clearance of prolactin in the complex leads to elevated serum levels.

## Management

Hyperprolactinaemia may be entirely asymptomatic and not require treatment (e.g. in postmenopausal women) unless there is existing or impending mass effect (e.g. due to a pituitary macroadenoma). Addressing secondary causes where possible often results in normalization of the prolactin level.

*Dopamine receptor agonist (DA) therapy*

- Almost always the treatment of choice for macro- and microprolactinomas.
- Visual impairment due to macroprolactinoma can improve within hours of starting DA therapy, but surgery must not be deferred if improvement is not rapid and sustained.
- Commonly used DAs include bromocriptine (side effects: hypotension, nausea, sleepiness, depression) and cabergoline and quinagolide (side effects: generally fewer and milder than with bromocriptine). DA should be up-titrated slowly until serum prolactin normalizes.
- Ergot-derived DAs (e.g. bromocriptine, cabergoline) may predispose to fibrotic disorders (pulmonary, cardiac, retroperitoneal). Although the doses used to treat hyperprolactinaemia are generally much lower than those used in other clinical settings (e.g. Parkinson disease, where high rates of cardiac valvular incompetence have been noted in patients on cabergoline), patients should be carefully monitored for symptoms and signs, and baseline echocardiography, pulmonary function tests, and assessment of renal function considered for those likely to need relatively high-dose long-term therapy.

*Subsequent management*

May include:

- Pituitary surgery—if intolerant/resistant to DA treatment.
- Correction of pituitary hormone deficits.
- Osteoporosis prophylaxis/treatment.

The decision to discontinue DA therapy in the longer term is based on the extent to which treatment lowers circulating prolactin levels and promotes tumour involution. Regular endocrine clinic follow-up is advised. Periodic MRI follow-up is generally recommended for macroprolactinomas, but microadenomas can often be managed through a combination of clinical and biochemical surveillance.

*Pregnancy*

- Some patients experience rapid normalization of gonadal function shortly after commencing DA therapy, and accordingly all patients must be warned that pregnancy is possible even before menstruation is re-established.
- 1/3 of macroadenomas enlarge in pregnancy (microadenomas generally not) and require careful pregnancy planning and occasionally pre-emptive surgery. Bromocriptine and cabergoline appear to be safe for use in pregnancy. For most microprolactinomas, and for macrorolactinomas which have significantly involuted, treatment can often be discontinued once pregnancy is confirmed. In other patients DA therapy is continued throughout pregnancy. In all cases, close surveillance is recommended.

## Extra

Occasionally prolactinomas are a manifestation of multiple endocrine neoplasia type 1 (*MEN1*—see Section 7.18).

# 7.9 Hypopituitarism

## Background

- The clinical condition arising as a consequence of impaired synthesis and/or secretion of one or more pituitary hormones.
- Estimated adult incidence of ~10 per million per year.

## Anterior pituitary hormones

Produced within specialized cells in well-defined locations within the pituitary gland:

- **Growth hormone** (GH) regulates growth and metabolism.
- **Gonadotrophins** (Gn), **luteinizing**, and **follicle stimulating hormones** (LH and FSH) regulate testicular/ovarian function.
- **Prolactin** induces lactation.
- **Adrenocorticotrophic hormone** (ACTH) regulates adrenal cortisol and androgen, but **not** aldosterone, production.
- **Thyroid stimulating hormone** (TSH) regulates thyroid hormone (thyroxine/T4 and triiodothyronine/T3) production.

## Posterior pituitary hormones

Produced in the hypothalamus, transported along the pituitary stalk and secreted from the posterior pituitary gland:

- **Antidiuretic hormone (ADH—vasopressin)** regulates water excretion in the kidneys.
- **Oxytocin** facilitates parturition and initiation of lactation.

## Aetiology and pathophysiology

Destruction/compression of normal pituitary tissue or reduction in the blood supply (including the hypothalamo–hypophyseal portal circulation) accounts for most cases. See Table 7.8.

## Clinical evaluation

### History and examination

Clinical presentation depends on multiple factors:

| Table 7.8 Aetiology of hypopituitarism | |
|---|---|
| **Common** | Pituitary/peri-pituitary tumours (e.g. pituitary adenoma, craniopharyngioma, suprasellar meningioma) or as a complication of treatment (e.g. surgery, radiotherapy) |
| **Less common** | Vascular (e.g. pituitary apoplexy, Sheehan syndrome, intrasellar carotid artery aneurysm) |
| | Pituitary infiltration (e.g. metastasis, haemochromatosis, sarcoidosis, histiocytosis, granulomatosis with polyangiitis (Wegener)) |
| | Infection (e.g. tuberculosis, pituitary abscess) |
| | Autoimmune (lymphocytic) hypophysitis |
| | Traumatic (e.g. post-head injury) |
| | Low body weight (e.g. anorexia nervosa, excessive exercise, malnutrition) |
| | Drug-induced (e.g. exogenous glucocorticoids, sex steroids) |
| | Congenital (e.g. isolated or combined pituitary hormone deficiencies) |
| | Idiopathic |

*Gender*

- Hypopituitarism is typically diagnosed earlier in pre-menopausal women due to menstrual disturbance.

*Extent of pituitary hormone loss*

- Resilience of pituitary cells to damage differs: with local compression (e.g. due to a pituitary macroadenoma) GH secretion is typically compromised first, followed by LH and FSH, then ACTH, and finally TSH.
- Following cranial irradiation GH deficiency and hyperprolactinaemia are often the earliest manifestations, but TRH(/TSH) deficiency may develop at a relatively early stage and in the absence of LH/FSH and ACTH deficiency.
- Prolactin deficiency is rare (typically only occurs with complete pituitary destruction e.g. apoplexy), and the only symptom is failure of lactation; in contrast, hyperprolactinaemia is common (pituitary stalk compression leads to loss of dopaminergic inhibition of lactotrophs—see Section 7.8).
- ACTH deficiency may mask diabetes insipidus (cortisol is required for renal free water excretion).
- Patients with panhypopituitarism are typically pale (absence of melanocorticotrophic effects of ACTH), lethargic (↓ ACTH and TSH), and hypogonadal (↓ LH and FSH).
- Symptoms of GH deficiency vary; may include tiredness/lethargy and generally impaired quality of life. ↓ bone mineral density, altered body composition (↑ fat mass, ↓ lean mass) and metabolic dysfunction may be evident.
- ADH deficiency presents with diabetes insipidus (DI; see Section 7.10).

*Speed of onset*

Sudden development of hypopituitarism can be dramatic (i.e. hypovolaemic shock, vomiting) pointing to a vascular cause (e.g. pituitary apoplexy). Gradual progressive impairment leads to more subtle signs and suggests a slow-growing pituitary or hypothalamic tumour.

*Age of onset*

In congenital forms the severity of the phenotype often depends on the age of onset (e.g. dwarfism, cretinism).

*Aetiology*

- Some causes of hypopituitarism have classical presentations: e.g. craniopharyngioma often results in diabetes insipidus; autoimmune hypophysitis is most commonly seen in late pregnancy/early postpartum.
- Hypothalamic–pituitary irradiation typically produces hypopituitarism (consistency issue) which evolves over years.
- In autoimmune hypophysitis hormonal deficits may be transient (1/3 of cases).

### Investigations

Hypopituitarism may develop insidiously, and signs and symptoms are often subtle and non-specific. Therefore, a high index of suspicion is required. In circumstances where there is a significant risk of hypopituitarism developing, e.g. post-cranial irradiation, lifelong periodic screening is indicated.

*Basal pituitary profile*

A simple screen of pituitary status should include:

| | |
|---|---|
| • Cortisol. | • FT4 and TSH. |
| • Prolactin. | • LH/FSH and testosterone or oestradiol. |
| • IGF-1. | • Paired plasma and urine osmolalities and electrolytes, urea and creatinine if DI suspected. |

- The sample should ideally be taken at 9am to allow for the diurnal variations in cortisol and testosterone secretion.

- ACTH measurement is rarely helpful unless a paired serum cortisol at 9am is very low (<100nmol/L).
- IGF-1 levels may lie within the normal range even in the presence of severe GH deficiency.

Accordingly, if ACTH and/or GH deficiency are suspected, dynamic testing is required:

### Insulin tolerance test (ITT)

Insulin-induced hypoglycaemia (laboratory blood glucose <2.2mmol/L) provides a strong stimulus to the hypothalamic–pituitary–adrenal axis (serum cortisol rises to >500nmol/L), and to growth hormone secretion (serum GH ↑ to > 10mcg/L and often >20mcg/L).

| ITT contra-indicated if: | • Epilepsy.<br>• IHD/dysrhythmias.<br>• 9am cortisol <100nmol/L. |
|---|---|

- Ideally, FT4 should also be normal, but see later in this section regarding correction of hypocortisolism before starting thyroxine therapy.

### Arginine and glucagon stimulation tests

Alternative means for assessing GH reserve.

### Short Synacthen® test

- 250mcg Synacthen® IM/IV. Measure cortisol at 0 and 30 minutes. May be used to assess adrenal reserve. Ideally perform at 9am so the basal cortisol level can also be compared to the population reference range.
- A normal post-Synacthen® peak cortisol response does not exclude partial pituitary ACTH deficiency (i.e. decreased pituitary reserve) in patients whose basal ACTH production is sufficient to prevent adrenal atrophy, but in whom the CRH-ACTH response to stress is impaired.

### Assessment of posterior pituitary function

See Section 7.10.

### Pituitary imaging & ophthalmic assessment

- Request pituitary MRI (or CT) once hypopituitarism has been confirmed biochemically. May be required periodically as surveillance for a known structural lesion (Fig. 7.32).
- Visual acuities and visual fields (perimetry).

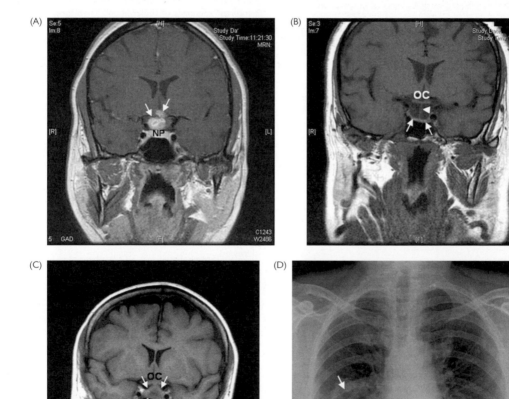

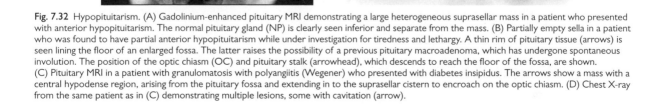

**Fig. 7.32** Hypopituitarism. (A) Gadolinium-enhanced pituitary MRI demonstrating a large heterogeneous suprasellar mass in a patient who presented with anterior hypopituitarism. The normal pituitary gland (NP) is clearly seen inferior and separate from the mass. (B) Partially empty sella in a patient who was found to have partial anterior hypopituitarism while under investigation for tiredness and lethargy. A thin rim of pituitary tissue (arrows) is seen lining the floor of an enlarged fossa. The latter raises the possibility of a previous pituitary macroadenoma, which has undergone spontaneous involution. The position of the optic chiasm (OC) and pituitary stalk (arrowhead), which descends to reach the floor of the fossa, are shown. (C) Pituitary MRI in a patient with granulomatosis with polyangiitis (Wegener) who presented with diabetes insipidus. The arrows show a mass with a central hypodense region, arising from the pituitary fossa and extending in to the suprasellar cistern to encroach on the optic chiasm. (D) Chest X-ray from the same patient as in (C) demonstrating multiple lesions, some with cavitation (arrow).

# Management

| Includes: | • Correction of hormone deficiencies.<br>• Identification and treatment of underlying condition.<br>• Cardiovascular risk modification.<br>• Patient education. |
|---|---|

## Hormone replacement
*Sex-hormones*

| Required for: | • Normal sexual function.<br>• Prevention of osteoporosis.<br>• Maintenance of body composition. |
|---|---|

• Women may be prescribed either the combined oral contraceptive pill (COCP) or hormone replacement therapy (HRT) until review at the menopause (typically ~50 years).

► Check personal/family history of breast disorders and thromboembolic disease before starting oestrogen therapy.

• Testosterone can be replaced using a variety of preparations (see Section 7.15).

• Check personal/family history of prostate disease and, if appropriate, discuss surveillance with digital rectal examination and PSA measurement.

• LFT and haematocrit should also be checked prior to, and periodically after starting, testosterone replacement. Secondary polycythaemia is a relatively common side effect, especially with injectable testosterone, and may require periodic venesection if treatment is to be continued safely.

• Fertility treatment usually requires spermatogenesis/ovulation induction with gonadotropins.

*Growth hormone*

In adults, replacement may:

• Increase lean body mass.
• Prevent/reverse low bone mineral density.
• Improve exercise capacity and quality of life.
• Correct/attenuate metabolic dysfunction, e.g. dyslipidaemia.

Recombinant human GH is given by self-administered daily SC injection. Side effects occasionally include oedema and arthralgia.

*Cortisol*

Usually replaced using hydrocortisone, typically given thrice daily to mimic normal circadian rhythm (e.g. 10mg on waking, 5mg lunchtime, and 5mg teatime). A long-acting slow-release oral preparation has recently been licensed and may find use in those who find it difficult to adhere to a thrice daily regimen.

• It is important to avoid over-replacement, which in the longer-term may have detrimental effects on metabolic parameters and bone mineral density.

► Patients should receive written advice re: 'sick day rules' (e.g. doubling normal hydrocortisone dose during intercurrent illness, seeking early medical attention if vomiting), be advised to carry a steroid card or alert bracelet, and provided with an emergency injection pack.

Fludrocortisone replacement is not required for secondary hypoadrenalism.

*Thyroid hormones*

• Thyroxine (L-T4) is given once daily.

• TSH is generally considered unreliable and cannot be used to monitor adequacy of replacement. Therefore, titrate L-T4 therapy against FT4 level.

► Always correct hypocortisolism before starting L-T4 (risk of hypoadrenal crisis).

*ADH*

See section 7.10.

Individual pituitary hormone axes may recover in cases where the underlying cause of the hypopituitarism can be treated effectively (e.g. transsphenoidal surgery of a pituitary tumour), and therefore re-testing after temporary withdrawal of hormone replacement is occasionally indicated. See Section 7.10.

## Associated conditions

• Prolonged sex steroid and GH deficiency predisposes to osteoporosis, which should be assessed and monitored with periodic bone densitometry (see Section 7.26).

• Cardiovascular risk is increased in patients with hypopituitarism. Other risk factors such as dyslipidaemia and smoking should be addressed.

# 7.10 Diabetes insipidus

## Background

- Defined as the excretion of excessive or 'copious' volumes of urine (traditionally >3L per 24 hours).
- Plasma osmolality is normally tightly regulated by hypothalamic antidiuretic hormone (ADH—also called vasopressin), which is transported along axonal projections in the pituitary stalk to the posterior pituitary gland. Here it is stored and subsequently secreted in order to regulate aquaresis (excretion of free water) via activation of renal vasopressin type 2 (V2) receptors.

## Aetiology/pathophysiology

Classically three types of diabetes insipidus (DI) are recognized (Table 7.9):

- **Primary polydipsia** (PPD) or **dipsogenic DI** (DDI): caused by excessive water intake. Sometimes referred to as psychogenic DI, although this term is not appropriate in all cases and is therefore best avoided.
- **Nephrogenic DI** (NDI): normal ADH secretion, but renal ADH resistance.

### Table 7.9  Causes of diabetes insipidus

| Cranial (hypothalamic) diabetes insipidus | | |
|---|---|---|
| Primary | Genetic | AD, AR, DIDMOAD (Wolfram) syndrome |
| | Developmental syndromes | Laurence–Moon–Biedl syndrome, septo-optic dysplasia |
| | Idiopathic | |
| Secondary | Trauma | Head injury, post-neurosurgery (e.g. pituitary surgery) |
| | Tumour | Craniopharyngioma, metastasis (especially breast, bronchial), germinoma, (only very rarely a presenting feature of pituitary adenomas) |
| | Inflammatory | Sarcoidosis, histiocytosis, infection, autoimmune hypophysitis |
| | Vascular | Aneurysm, infarction, Sheehan syndrome |
| **Nephrogenic diabetes insipidus** | | |
| Primary | Genetic | XR, AR, AD |
| | Idiopathic | |
| Secondary | Chronic renal disease | Obstructive uropathy, polycystic kidney disease |
| | Metabolic disorders | Hypercalcaemia, hypokalaemia |
| | Osmotic diuretics | Glucose, mannitol |
| | Drug induced | Lithium, demeclocyclin |
| | Systemic disorders | Amyloidosis |
| | Pregnancy | |
| **Primary polydipsia (dipsogenic diabetes insipidus)** | | |
| Habitual or compulsive water drinking | | |
| Affective disorders | | |
| Response to a dry mouth | Therapy with anticholinergic agents, Sjögren syndrome | |
| Structural hypothalamic damage | Sarcoidosis, tumours, head injury, tuberculous meningitis | |

AD: autosomal dominant; AR: autosomal recessive; XR: X-linked recessive.

- **Central or cranial DI** (CDI), or hypothalamic DI (HDI): absolute or relative lack of ADH secretion from the hypothalamic–posterior pituitary axis.

## Clinical evaluation

### History

- Polydipsia—often associated with a preference for ice-cold water and a need to carry fluids at all times.
- Polyuria and nocturia (on several occasions); many patients refuse to visit places where ease of access to toilets is not guaranteed!
- Features of anterior pituitary dysfunction and the underlying disorder may also be present.

### Examination

- Reduced visual acuity and visual field defects may be evident in those with HDI due to a structural lesion.
- Check carefully for evidence of anterior pituitary hormone insufficiency.
- Clinical signs of the underlying disorder may be evident.

### Investigations

*1. Confirm polyuria*

Collect all urine output for 24 hours; ask patient to record fluid intake for the same period.

*2. Exclude common causes of polyuria*

E.g. diabetes mellitus, hypercalcaemia, hypokalaemia, drug-induced.

*3. Confirm diagnosis of DI*

*Plasma and urine osmolalities*

Measurement of paired early morning plasma and urine osmolalities, together with U&E, following limitation of fluid intake overnight may help to exclude cases in which the clinical index of suspicion is low. In this setting, the demonstration of a concentrated early morning urine sample (>750mosmol/kg), with normal electrolytes and plasma osmolality, excludes DI.

⚠ Note that this 'unsupervised' form of water deprivation should not be used in cases where genuine DI is suspected.

*Water deprivation test*

- Fluid restriction prior to the test is not required, but the patient should be advised to avoid excessive drinking where possible, and to record fluid intake for the 12 hours before the test.
- Allow a light breakfast, but no tea or coffee.
- Under direct supervision the patient is required to abstain from any fluid or food intake for 8 hours. Do not allow him/her to smoke.
- At baseline (time zero), ask patient to empty bladder, record body weight, measure serum electrolytes, urea and glucose, and plasma and urine osmolalities.
- Record hourly urine output.
- Measure plasma and urine osmolalities at 0, 2, 4, 6, and 8 hours
- Weigh patient at 0, 2, 4, 6, 7, and 8 hours.
- At conclusion of test give desmopressin 2mcg IM and continue collecting hourly urine samples and measuring urine osmolalities for a further 4 hours. Allow access to fluids and food during this time, but avoid excessive fluid intake.
- ▶ If at any point during the test the patient loses ≥3% body weight compared to baseline, check plasma osmolality urgently: if this has risen to >295mosmol/kg give desmopressin 2g IM, allow the patient to drink and continue monitoring urine output/osmolality as indicated earlier; otherwise consider continuing the test under close supervision. Abandon if patient loses ≥5% body weight.

*Interpretation of water deprivation test results*

- In PPD urine volume decreases as the urine concentrates, and plasma osmolality remains within the reference range.
- Excessive fluid intake in the 12 hours prior to the test may result in an apparent continued 'diuresis', especially during the early stages of the test. However, plasma osmolality remains <295mosmol/kg.
- In CDI the urine does not adequately concentrate, a 'diuresis' is maintained and plasma osmolality increases. Desmopressin reverses these abnormalities.
- In NDI the findings are similar to CDI, but there is no or only slight improvement with desmopressin.
- In practice the interpretation of the water deprivation test can be challenging with equivocal results. In these circumstances a hypertonic saline infusion test, with direct measurement of plasma ADH levels, may be required. This should only be undertaken in a specialist endocrine unit.

*4. Determine cause and associated complications in CDI*

*Assess anterior pituitary functional status*

- See Section 7.9.
- NB: cortisol is permissive for free water excretion. Therefore, DI may be masked in the presence of cortisol deficiency, and may only become apparent once glucocorticoid replacement has been commenced.

*MRI (or CT) scan*

Imaging the hypothalamus and pituitary fossa is mandatory to:

- Exclude a structural lesion.
- Check for the presence of the posterior pituitary bright spot (Fig. 7.33)—reflecting stored ADH.

*Ophthalmic assessment*

- Visual acuity.
- Visual fields (e.g. perimetry).

## Management

- Wherever possible, the underlying cause should be addressed, e.g. correction of metabolic disturbances.
- The treatment of PPD is challenging, and often focuses on reduction of fluid intake through behavioural approaches.
- ADH replacement in the form of the analogue desmopressin, nasally (typically 10–40mcg/day), parenterally (0.5–4mcg/day), or orally (100–1200mcg/day) is the mainstay of therapy for CDI.
- NDI can sometimes be alleviated by ADH used at higher doses (e.g. ≥5mcg/day SC). Thiazide diuretics may reduce glomerular filtration rate and ease polyuria.

249

(A)

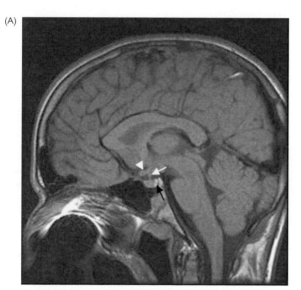

(B)

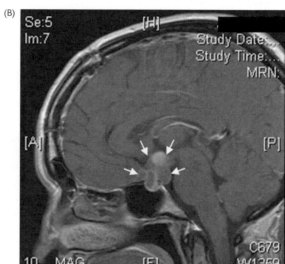

**Fig. 7.33** (A) Unenhanced sagittal MRI showing the normal posterior pituitary bright spot (black arrow). The position of the pituitary stalk (white arrow) and optic chiasm (white arrowhead) are also shown. (B) Loss of the high signal from the posterior pituitary gland in a patient with a multicystic craniopharyngioma extending anterior, posterior and superior to the fossa (arrows). The patient presented with DI.

# 7.11 Adrenal incidentaloma

## Background

Any adrenal mass (>1cm diameter) detected incidentally—typically during radiological imaging—when no adrenal disease is suspected by the clinical presentation.

## Epidemiology

- The prevalence of adrenal incidentaloma (AI) is not known with accuracy.
- Autopsy series report rates of 1–9% depending on the criteria used to define AI.
- Consistent with this, imaging studies identify AI in ~4–7% of all patients undergoing abdominal CT/MRI, with lesions increasingly common with advancing age.

## Aetiology

See Table 7.10.

## Clinical evaluation

### History and examination

- Although by definition an AI is an incidental finding (the majority of which are non-secretory benign adenomas), on closer questioning some patients will report features consistent with adrenal cortical (hypercortisolism, hyperaldosteronism or very rarely hyperandrogenism) or medullary (phaeochromocytoma) hyperfunction.
- Most AI that secrete glucocorticoids do not manifest with overt Cushing syndrome, reflecting relatively low-grade autonomous cortisol production—hence the terms subclinical hypercortisolism (SH), subclinical Cushing syndrome, or subclinical autonomous glucocorticoid hypersecretion (SAGH). However, the effects of long-term, low-grade hypercortisolism should not be underestimated, and an increased rate of cardiovascular risk factors (hypertension, diabetes mellitus, central obesity) and osteoporosis have been observed. Several recent studies have also reported increased mortality in this group of patients.
- Hypertension and hypokalaemia occurring in a patient with an AI should raise suspicion of hyperaldosteronism.
- Adrenocortical carcinoma can be functioning or non-functioning with respect to hormone hypersecretion. Co-secretion of cortisol and androgens should alert the clinician to the possibility of malignancy. Excess androgen secretion is usually clinically obvious.

| Table 7.10 Aetiology of adrenal incidentalomas/enlargement | |
| --- | --- |
| Aetiology | Approximate % of cases* |
| Adrenal adenoma (benign) | 40–50 |
| Metastases | 5–20 |
| Adrenocortical carcinoma | 5–10 |
| Myelolipoma | 5–10 |
| Phaeochromocytoma | 5–10 |
| Others e.g. cysts, infection (tuberculosis, histoplasmosis), haemorrhage, adrenal hyperplasia, infiltration | 10–15 |

*Varies according to case series and local reporting criteria. Although bilateral adrenal enlargement/masses may be seen with most of these conditions, if bilateral masses are present specific consideration should be given to excluding metastases, phaeochromocytoma (especially if arising in the setting of a genetic syndrome, e.g. multiple endocrine neoplasia type 2), infection, haemorrhage, hyperplasia.

- Normotension in a patient with an adrenal mass does not exclude the possibility of a phaeochromocytoma.
- Metastases to the adrenal glands are frequently bilateral and the primary tumour is usually obvious (e.g. lung, breast, kidney, colon, pancreas, liver, stomach, melanoma, lymphoma). Impairment of adrenal function is rare except when there is gross destruction/replacement of both adrenals.

## Investigations

The diagnostic work up of AI revolves around two questions:

1. Is the lesion hormonally inactive or active?
2. Is the lesion benign or malignant?

In addition to the clinical clues described, biochemical and radiological findings are important in answering these key questions.

### Biochemical screening

*To exclude subclinical hypercortisolism*

The overnight (1mg) dexamethasone suppression test provides a useful means of excluding autonomous cortisol secretion. Further investigations (see Section 7.6) are required in those with positive results or in whom there is a high index of clinical suspicion.

*To exclude hyperaldosteronism*

Measurement of renin and aldosterone levels is usually recommended to exclude hyperaldosteronism (see Section 7.12).

*To exclude hyperandrogenism/sex-hormone hypersecretion*

Screening to exclude hypersecretion of adrenal androgens (e.g. dehydroepiandrosterone sulphate—DHEAS) or oestrogens is generally unproductive in the absence of overt clinical features.

*To exclude phaeochromocytoma*

Plasma or urinary fractionated metanephrines afford the most sensitive means of excluding a phaeochromocytoma (see Section 7.14).

### Radiological findings
#### CT/MRI

Increasingly, CT and MRI provide valuable information regarding the likely nature of adrenal lesions (Fig. 7.34). Clues from the imaging that a lesion is likely to be a benign adenoma include:

- Round/smooth contour, sharp margination, homogeneous appearance.
- Diameter <3cm.
- Low attenuation value (<10 Hounsfield units (HU)) on unenhanced CT—reflecting the high lipid content of adrenal adenomas (Fig. 7.34B).
- Rapid washout of contrast on enhanced CT.
- 'Chemical shift' evidence on MRI (loss of signal on the out-of-phase images as compared with in-phase images is typical of an adrenal adenoma).

Adrenal carcinomas are usually larger and heterogeneous in appearance (often containing mixed solid and cystic components) (Fig. 7.34C). A 'cut-off' of 4cm in diameter has been proposed as a trigger for recommending surgical removal, as the prevalence of malignancy increases significantly in lesions greater than this size. However, if the radiological appearances are strongly suggestive of a benign lesion, some centres consider it reasonable to offer continued surveillance rather than surgery even in this group.

Although phaeochromocytomas may exhibit characteristic findings on CT and MRI, they can also present as large heterogeneous masses with necrotic/cystic degeneration. Hence biochemical screening is mandatory before invasive procedures/surgery is contemplated for such an adrenal mass.

#### Nuclear medicine

Although not typically required, nuclear medicine imaging may help to delineate the nature of AI, e.g. [123]I-MIBG scanning in phaeochromocytoma.

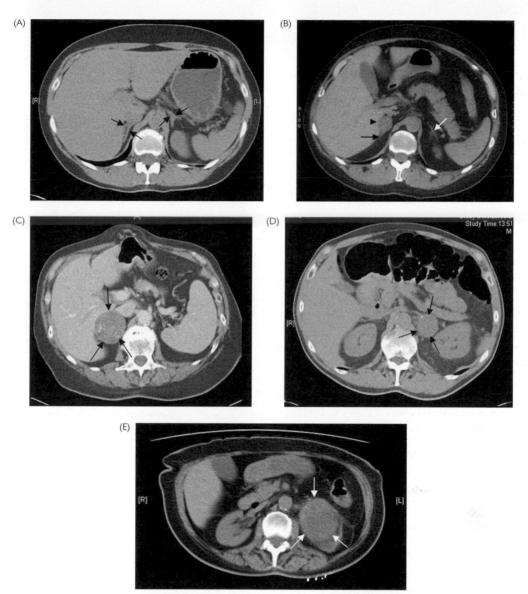

**Fig. 7.34** Adrenal incidentalomas identified on CT scans in individuals undergoing imaging for non-endocrine purposes. (A) CT scan showing normal right and left adrenal glands for reference. (B) Right adrenal adenoma (black arrowhead). Note the low attenuation on this pre-contrast scan, in keeping with a high lipid content. The morphology of the postero-medial limb of the right adrenal has been preserved (black arrow). The normal left adrenal gland is clearly seen (white arrow). (C) Right adrenal carcinoma. Note the heterogeneous appearance with flecks of calcification. (D) Left adrenal phaeochromocytoma. (E) Large left adrenal mass in a patient with known malignant melanoma. Adrenalectomy confirmed haemorrhage in to a metastatic deposit.

*Fine needle aspiration (FNA)*
Only occasionally indicated and should not be undertaken if there is concern regarding the possibility of phaeochromocytoma unless adequate α-blockade established. Currently, it is not possible to reliably distinguish a benign from malignant adrenocortical lesion on FNA.

## Management

• When the morphological features and/or hormonal profile support surgical removal of an AI, then laparoscopic adrenalectomy is generally preferred, although some centres advise open adrenalectomy for suspected adrenocortical carcinoma.

• In cases where there is evidence of autonomous cortisol secretion, then peri-operative (and continued post-operative) hydrocortisone cover is mandatory until the hypothalamic–pituitary–(remaining) adrenal axis has been shown to have recovered.

• If the adrenal lesion is hormonally inactive and malignancy is deemed unlikely, then 'watchful observation' is reasonable. The frequency of follow-up (clinical, biochemical, and radiological) remains a matter of debate. One suggested approach is to repeat imaging at 6–12 months, and clinical/biochemical assessment annually for 4 years. Patients with lesions which remain stable on imaging, and in whom hormone hypersecretion is not evident, may not require further follow-up.

# 7.12 Primary hyperaldosteronism

## Background

- Excessive aldosterone production (i.e. autonomous from the renin–angiotensin control system) leads to excessive sodium reabsorption in the distal nephron and subsequent hypertension.
- Potassium ($K^+$) and hydrogen ion ($H^+$) exchange for sodium leads to urinary $K^+$ wastage and alkalosis.
- The term 'Conn syndrome' is classically reserved for primary hyperaldosteronism (PHA) due to a benign adrenal adenoma.

## Epidemiology

The prevalence of PHA varies depending on the population studied, but is now believed to account for 5–10% of all hypertension and for ~25% of patients with so-called refractory hypertension.

## Aetiology

See Table 7.11.

## Clinical evaluation

### History and examination

- The majority of cases come to light during investigation of hypertension or unexplained hypokalaemia.
- Features of potassium depletion include weakness, lassitude, and polyuria (nephrogenic diabetes insipidus).
- The degree of hypertension varies from mild to severe, and may be 'resistant' to treatment with more commonly used antihypertensive agents.
- Evidence of target-organ damage should be sought (e.g. hypertensive retinopathy, left ventricular hypertrophy).

### Investigations

All patients with hypertension should have serum electrolytes checked and urinalysis performed. Further investigations, i.e. measurement of plasma renin and aldosterone, are particularly indicated in patients with:

- Associated unprovoked or marked hypokalaemia.
- Refractory hypertension.
- Young age at onset of hypertension (e.g. <40 years).
- Strong family history of hypertension (and/or associated complications, e.g. cerebral haemorrhage).
- Adrenal incidentaloma.

Some clinicians reason that measurement of plasma renin (looking for low renin states) can be justified in virtually all patients with hypertension given the apparently high prevalence of PHA.

Table 7.11 Aetiology of primary hyperaldosteronism

| Aetiology | Comments |
|---|---|
| Aldosterone-secreting adrenal adenoma (benign) | = Conn syndrome |
| Idiopathic hyperaldosteronism/ bilateral adrenal hyperplasia | |
| Adrenocortical carcinoma | Rare |
| Familial hyperaldosteronism | E.g. glucocorticoid-remediable (suppressible) hyperaldosteronism* |

*Autosomal dominant disorder in which the 11β-hydroxylase gene promoter is fused to the aldosterone synthase gene, thereby permitting ACTH-sensitive aldosterone production in the zona fasciculata.

### Screening tests
*Urea and electrolytes*

- The classical pattern is one of hypokalaemic alkalosis, although many patients are normokalaemic at presentation. Serum sodium is typically high normal/borderline high.

*Plasma renin and aldosterone*

- Measurement of paired plasma renin and aldosterone distinguishes primary (suppressed renin) and secondary (hyper-reninaemic, e.g. due to renal artery stenosis, cardiac failure) hyperaldosteronism. Hence, the ratio of plasma aldosterone to plasma renin activity (or plasma renin mass) is a useful screening test (ARR, aldosterone renin ratio).

  - Various drugs can affect plasma renin and aldosterone levels, and hence the ratio. For example, renin secretion is suppressed when β-adrenergic input to the juxtaglomerular apparatus is attenuated (e.g. with β-blocker therapy—thus leading to a falsely elevated ratio), but increased during treatment with ACE inhibitors (thereby potentially masking true primary hyperaldosteronism). Calcium channel antagonists may partially suppress aldosterone secretion even in cases of PHA.
  - Hypokalaemia can impair aldosterone secretion. Ideally therefore, renin and aldosterone levels should be measured in the absence of interfering medications and following correction of hypokalaemia. However, this is not always feasible, and experienced clinicians will sometimes interpret levels taking into account the predicted effects of confounding medications (e.g. persistent renin suppression in the face of ACE inhibition is strongly suggestive of a true low renin state).

- Comparison of supine and ambulatory plasma renin levels is only occasionally helpful: in normal subjects renin secretion is stimulated by adopting an upright posture for 4 hours; in contrast in primary hyperaldosteronism plasma renin remains suppressed despite ambulation.

### Confirmation of diagnosis
*Salt-loading tests*

- In normal subjects volume expansion due to salt and water retention will suppress plasma renin and aldosterone, whereas in primary hyperaldosteronism this does not have the same suppressive effects on aldosterone secretion. Salt-loading can be achieved by increasing dietary sodium intake, infusing saline, administering exogenous mineralocorticoid (e.g. fludrocortisone), or a combination, but should only be undertaken under expert supervision, and not in subjects prone to fluid overload.
- Care should be taken to ensure hypokalaemia is corrected during salt-loading.

### Determining the cause
*Plasma aldosterone*

- It is said that adrenal adenomas classically exhibit sensitivity to ACTH (adrenocorticotrophic hormone) and hence aldosterone levels fall in parallel with the circadian cortisol rhythm in patients with Conn adenomas. In contrast, so-called idiopathic hyperaldosteronism (typified by bilateral adrenal hyperplasia) is not associated with ACTH sensitivity. However, many consider this to be an unreliable means of distinguishing the two entities.
- In familial cases of primary hyperaldosteronism, consider genetic screening for glucocorticoid remediable (hyper)aldosteronism (GRA).

*CT/MRI of adrenals*

- Many, although not all, adrenal adenomas are readily identified on cross-sectional imaging (Fig. 7.35).

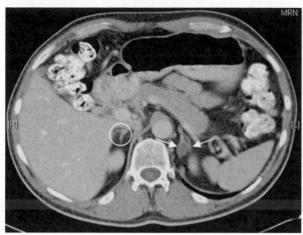

**Fig. 7.35** CT scan showing adrenal adenoma arising between the posteromedial and posterolateral limbs of the **left** adrenal gland (white arrows). The normal **right** adrenal gland is clearly seen (enclosed within white circle).

- However, the existence of a coincidental adrenal incidentaloma (see Section 7.11) may confound interpretation/localization.
- In bilateral adrenal hyperplasia both glands can appear enlarged or normal in size.

Cross-sectional imaging alone is therefore insufficient to reliably distinguish unilateral and bilateral disease in many patients.

*Adrenal venous sampling*

- Useful in confirming that a structural lesion seen on CT/MRI is the source of autonomous aldosterone secretion, and in distinguishing unilateral from bilateral disease (Fig. 7.37). Concomitant cortisol measurement confirms successful cannulation of the adrenal veins (which can be 'tricky' on the right side where the vein drains directly in to the inferior vena cava). An aldosterone/cortisol ratio between sides of >4:1 is suggestive of unilateral disease—providing satisfactory cannulation of both adrenal veins has been achieved (gauged by looking for a 'step up' in cortisol between samples taken from the IVC and those collected from the adrenal veins).

*Radionuclide/PET imaging*

- Radionuclide scanning with labelled cholesterol isotopes is an alternative means of confirming functionality in an adrenal lesion, but has reduced sensitivity and specificity compared with CT/MRI and venous sampling.
- PET-CT imaging with novel ligands (e.g. [11]C-metomidate), which are taken up by adrenocortical tissue, has recently been reported as an alternative to venous sampling, potentially offering greater sensitivity and specificity than conventional radionuclides.

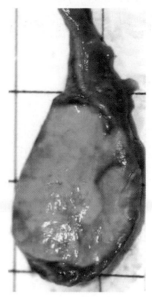

**Fig. 7.36** Typical appearance of a resected Conn adenoma.

# Management

- If an unequivocal diagnosis of a unilateral aldosterone-secreting adrenal adenoma is made, then laparoscopic adrenalectomy is widely regarded as the treatment of choice and will cure or improve hypertension in the majority of patients. Adrenal adenomas typically present a characteristic 'golden' appearance (reflecting the high lipid content of the adenoma) (Fig. 7.36).
- Where surgery is not an option, or if bilateral adrenal lesions/hyperplasia has been identified, medical therapy can be highly effective. It is based on two principles: (1) antagonism of aldosterone action at the mineralocorticoid receptor and/or (2) inhibition of sodium-potassium exchange in the renal tubule.
  - **Spironolactone** (12.5–200mg/day) is the most potent and cost-effective mineralocorticoid antagonist, but side effect prone e.g. gynaecomastia, reduced libido (due to antagonism of androgen receptor signaling), and menstrual irregularities.
  - **Eplerenone** (25–100mg/day) is a more specific mineralocorticoid-blocker with fewer side effects, but more expensive and less potent.
  - **Amiloride** (2.5–20mg/day) is an effective inhibitor of sodium–potassium exchange.
  - Regular monitoring of serum/plasma sodium, potassium, and renal function is mandatory in all cases.
- Calcium channel antagonists (e.g. amlodipine) may also help to control hypertension.

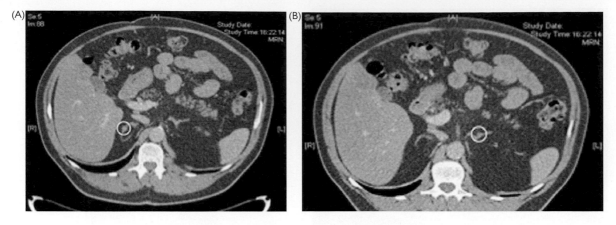

(C)

|  | Aldosterone (pmol/L) | Cortisol (nmol/L) | Aldosterone/ Cortisol |
|---|---|---|---|
| Left | 1250 | 560 | 2.23 |
| Right | 26540 | 522 | 50.84 |
| IVC | 750 | 250 | 3.0 |

**Fig. 7.37** Localization of source of hyperaldosteronism. (A and B) CT scan showing bilateral adrenal nodules (circled—(A) right; (B) left) in a patient with primary hyperaldosteronism. (C) Venous sampling revealed the right adrenal lesion to be the predominant source of excess aldosterone (aldosterone/cortisol = 50.84 on right vs. 2.23 on left). Note the step up in cortisol levels between the IVC (250) and right (522) and left (560) adrenal veins confirming successful bilateral cannulation.

# 7.13 Adrenal insufficiency

## Background

- Adrenocortical insufficiency may be primary or secondary in origin.
- The term 'Addison disease' (Thomas Addison, 1793–1860, physician at Guy's hospital, London) is reserved for cases of primary hypoadrenalism due to destruction or dysfunction of the adrenal cortex itself.
- Secondary hypoadrenalism occurs when central (hypothalamic CRH, and/or pituitary ACTH) drive to the adrenal cortex is impaired.

## Epidemiology

- Prevalence of Addison disease is estimated at 90–140/million adults, peaking in the 4th decade of life.
- Secondary adrenal insufficiency is more common (prevalence: 150–280/million, peaking in 6th decade of life).
- For both types ♀ are more commonly affected.

## Anatomy and physiology

- On CT/MRI scans the adrenals appear as distinct inverted Y-shaped structures situated above, but separate from, the kidneys (see Fig. 7.34A, Section 7.11).
- Anatomically they are divided into a medulla, which produces adrenaline (epinephrine) and noradrenaline (norepinephrine), and a cortex.
- The cortex is subdivided into three zones named (from inside out) 'zona reticularis' (source of androgens, e.g. dehydroepiandrosterone sulphate (DHEAS)), 'zona fasciculata' (source of glucocorticoids, e.g. cortisol), and 'zona glomerulosa' (source of mineralocorticoids, e.g. aldosterone).

## Aetiology and pathophysiology

See Table 7.12.

- The commonest cause of primary hypoadrenalism in the developed world is autoimmune adrenalitis (~70% of cases).
- Exogenous supraphysiological glucocorticoid therapy (see Box 7.2) accounts for a significant number of cases of secondary adrenal insufficiency.
- In primary hypoadrenalism typically all three layers of the cortex are affected, resulting in combined glucocorticoid, mineralocorticoid, and sex-steroid deficiency.
- In secondary hypoadrenalism, ACTH deficiency results in diminished glucocorticoid and sex-steroid synthesis/secretion, with associated atrophy of the corresponding layers of the adrenal cortex. However, in contrast, mineralocorticoid secretion is largely preserved, reflecting its control by the renin–angiotensin system.
- The rare disorder X-linked adrenoleucodystrophy must be considered in any young ♂ presenting with primary adrenal insufficency that is not autoimmune in origin.

## Clinical evaluation

### History and examination

The salient clinical features of both primary and secondary adrenal insufficiency are outlined in Table 7.13.

Cortisol insufficiency alone (i.e. in the absence of mineralocorticoid deficiency) may not manifest with significant haemodynamic compromise until the patient suffers an intercurrent illness/stress.

### Table 7.12 Causes of adrenal insufficiency

| | Cause | Examples |
|---|---|---|
| Primary adrenal insufficiency | Autoimmune adrenalitis | Isolated |
| | | Polyglandular syndromes (type 1 or 2) |
| | Infectious adrenalitis | Tuberculosis |
| | | Fungal, e.g. histoplasmosis |
| | | Opportunistic infections, e.g. in AIDS (*Cytomegalovirus*, *Cryptococcus*) |
| | Genetic disorders | Congenital adrenal hyperplasia |
| | | Adrenoleucodystrophy |
| | Bilateral adrenal haemorrhage | Anticoagulants |
| | | Meningococcal septicaemia, severe sepsis |
| | Bilateral adrenal infiltration | Metastases* |
| | | Lymphoma |
| | | Amyloidosis |
| | | Haemochromatosis |
| | Iatrogenic | Bilateral adrenalectomy |
| | | Drug-induced, e.g. metyrapone, ketoconazole, etomidate |
| Secondary adrenal insufficiency | Hypothalamic/pituitary tumours | Pituitary adenoma** (very rarely pituitary carcinoma) |
| | | Craniopharyngioma |
| | | Suprasellar meningioma |
| | | Metastases |
| | Pituitary infiltration | Sarcoidosis |
| | | Histiocytosis X |
| | | Granulomatosis with polyangiitis (Wegener) |
| | | Haemochromatosis |
| | Infection | Tuberculosis |
| | Pituitary inflammation | Autoimmune (lymphocytic) hypophysitis |
| | Pituitary apoplexy | Sheehan syndrome |
| | Iatrogenic | Surgery, cranial irradiation |
| | Post-traumatic | Head injury (especially with skull-base fractures) |
| | Isolated ACTH deficiency | |
| | Previous glucocorticoid therapy | |

AIDS: acquired immunodeficiency syndrome. * Although adrenal metastases are relatively common in certain malignancies (e.g. lung, breast, kidney), clinically-relevant hypoadrenalism is only occasionally seen; ** Patients with Cushing disease are particularly prone to postoperative secondary hypoadrenalism (even following selective adenomectomy) as a consequence of long-term suppression of normal pituitary corticotrophs.

- **Adrenal crisis**—most commonly seen in primary adrenal failure and may be a life-threatening first presentation. Characterized by: severe hypotension or shock, nausea and vomiting, abdominal pain, fever, hypoglycaemia. Responsiveness to treatment with vasopressors may be attenuated (lack of permissive effect of glucocorticoids on catecholamine action).

### Investigations

*Urea, electrolytes, glucose*

- Hyponatraemia is seen in both primary and secondary hypoadrenalism.

- Hyperkalaemia is typically only present in primary hypoadrenalism (mineralocorticoid insufficiency); blood urea levels are often raised in Addison disease.
- Hypoglycaemia may occasionally occur, especially during adrenal crisis.

### Random serum cortisol (±ACTH) measurement

- Of limited value except in the setting of suspected adrenal crisis, when samples should be taken and hydrocortisone administered without delay.

### 9am serum cortisol with paired ACTH

- Although these may be diagnostic of primary (high ACTH with low cortisol (<100nmol/L)) or secondary (low/inappropriately normal ACTH with low cortisol (<100nmol/L)) hypoadrenalism, in less severe cases cortisol and ACTH levels may fall within the normal range.

### Short Synacthen® test (SST)

- Plasma cortisol measured before and 30 minutes after 250mcg Synacthen® (tetracosactide = ACTH 1−24) IM (or IV).
- Ideally the test should be carried out at 9am, thereby allowing a reference comparison for the basal level, but this is not obligatory.
- A peak cortisol <500nmol/L (threshold varies according to laboratory) is suggestive of adrenal insufficiency.
- In primary hypoadrenalism the cortisol increment is typically small (<200nmol/L) or absent as the adrenals are already maximally stimulated by endogenous ACTH.

The SST may yield an apparently 'normal' result despite significant ACTH deficiency if testing is carried out in the early stage following

**Table 7.13** Clinical features of adrenal insufficiency

| | Features |
|---|---|
| Primary adrenal insufficiency | Tiredness, fatigue |
| | Weakness (typically generalized) |
| | Anorexia/weight loss/nausea/vomiting/gastrointestinal disturbance |
| | Pigmentation (generalized, but especially in sunlight-exposed areas; also check palmar creases, buccal mucosa and scars) (Figs 7.38 and 7.39) |
| | Dizziness/postural hypotension |
| | Generalized 'aches and pains' |
| | Reduced axillary and pubic hair; decreased libido (♀) |
| | 'Salt craving' |
| | Hypoglycaemia (typically with more severe cases) |
| Secondary adrenal insufficiency: as for primary adrenal insufficiency except: | Absence of pigmentation (lack of ACTH—skin is often pale) |
| | No features of mineralocorticoid deficiency |
| | Evidence of more global hypopituitarism may be present |
| | Local compressive symptoms and signs if pituitary/suprasellar mass |

Features of other associated endocrinopathies (e.g. primary hypothyroidism, type 1 diabetes mellitus, hypogonadism), and non-endocrine manifestations of autoimmune polyglandular syndromes (e.g. vitiligo, alopecia, vitamin $B_{12}$ deficiency) may also be evident in patients with primary adrenal insufficiency.

---

### Box 7.2 Adrenal insufficiency due to exogenous steroid therapy

An individual's susceptibility to suppression of the hypothalamic–pituitary–adrenal (HPA) axis, and rate and extent of recovery of adrenal function following withdrawal of exogenous corticosteroids (oral, inhaled, or topical 'steroids'), is extremely variable. Taking oral corticosteroid in the morning and alternate day therapy may lessen the likelihood of adrenal suppression.

Systemic corticosteroids may be stopped abruptly in those who have received treatment for 3 weeks or less and who are not included in the patient groups described here.

The possibility of axis suppression, and therefore gradual withdrawal of oral corticosteroids, should be considered in those who have:

- Recently received repeated courses (particularly if taken for >3 weeks).
- Taken a short course within 1 year of stopping long-term therapy.
- Received >40mg daily prednisolone or equivalent.
- Received >3 weeks of treatment.
- Been given repeat doses in the evening.
- Other possible causes of adrenocortical insufficiency.

During corticosteroid withdrawal, the dose can be reduced rapidly (primary disorder permitting) to a physiological replacement level (see later in box for steroid equivalents), and then tapered more slowly.

Dynamic testing (either in the form of an ITT or, more commonly, a SST) is generally not needed in the majority of corticosteroid-treated patients in whom axis suppression is unlikely or not suspected. It should only be undertaken when the corticosteroid dose has been tapered down to a physiological replacement level, to assess whether or not the axis is suppressed, with this helping to determine the rate at which replacement can be further reduced or even discontinued. In a patient whose axis is known to be suppressed (and who is on partial or full glucocorticoid replacement), dynamic testing may be used to assess whether the HPA axis is recovering, to guide the tempo of further withdrawal of glucocorticoid replacement. The HPA axis may remain chronically suppressed in patients who have been treated with corticosteroids long-term.

Patients with a slightly subnormal cortisol response during dynamic testing, but no symptoms, may require no regular glucocorticoid replacement, but should be advised to take supplementary glucocorticoid (e.g. hydrocortisone 5mg twice daily) during intercurrent illness (Sick day rules, see later in box).

Approximate equivalent physiological replacement doses of glucocorticoid are:

- 20mg hydrocortisone (given in divided doses, e.g. two or three times daily regimen; slight mineralocorticoid activity at this dosage, compared with higher dosages (e.g. >50 mg) when significant mineralocorticoid activity may be observed).
- ~5mg prednisolone (given once daily or in divided doses; minimal mineralocorticoid activity).
- ~0.5mg dexamethasone (given in divided doses, typically twice daily; no mineralocorticoid activity).

Adjunctive management of HPA axis suppression should include:

- 'Sick day rules.'*
- 'Steroid card' (see Fig. 7.40) and/or 'Alert' bracelet/necklace.
- Emergency pack.

*Patients with HPA axis suppression are unable to respond adequately to stresses such as intercurrent infection, trauma, or surgery. Accordingly, individuals on partial or full glucocorticoid replacement need to increase dosage of treatment; individuals who do not routinely require glucocorticoid replacement, but who demonstrate a suboptimal response to dynamic testing, should receive glucocorticoid supplementation during intercurrent illness.

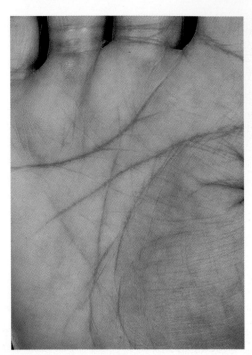

Fig. 7.38 Palmar crease pigmentation.

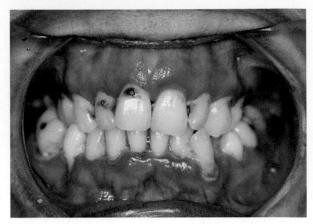

Fig. 7.39 Gingival pigmentation.

insult/injury to the hypothalamus/pituitary—when the adrenal cortex has not yet atrophied and responds to the supraphysiological ACTH challenge. In this setting there may be a discordance between the basal cortisol level (which is reflective of endogenous ACTH output) and the peak response (following exogenous Synacthen®)—hence the added value of undertaking the test at 9am.

*Insulin tolerance test (ITT)*
- Gold standard for diagnosing hypoadrenalism, especially secondary.
- Serum glucose and cortisol (and growth hormone if hypopituitarism suspected) are measured before and 15, 30, 45, 60, 90, and 120 minutes after a bolus of IV fast-acting insulin (typically 0.15U/kg, although higher doses may be required, especially in subjects with insulin resistance). Adequate hypoglycaemia = plasma glucose <2.2mmol/L; normal peak cortisol response >500nmol/L.

Most serum cortisol assays measure total cortisol (i.e. bound and free hormone). Therefore, conditions in which the major binding protein CBG (cortisol binding globulin) is raised (e.g. exogenous oral oestrogen therapy or pregnancy) may provide falsely reassuring results. Where possible, repeat testing in the absence of confounding factors (e.g. exogenous oral oestrogen therapy should be discontinued for 6 weeks prior to testing).

*Adrenal cortex autoantibodies, 21-hydroxylase autoantibodies*
Detectable in many, but not all, patients with autoimmune adrenalitis.

*Imaging*
Not routinely required in primary hypoadrenalism unless suspicion of non-autoimmune aetiology. In cases of secondary hypoadrenalism that are not attributable to exogenous steroid therapy, pituitary imaging is indicated.

*Other*
Measurement of very long chain fatty acids in suspected cases of adrenoleucodystrophy.

## Management

### Routine replacement
- **Hydrocortisone:** 5–10mg/m²/day, in two to three divided doses (e.g. 10mg/5mg/2.5mg per day).

- **Fludrocortisone:** 50–200mcg/day, taken either as a single dosage or in two divided dosages (morning and evening).
- **DHEA:** 25–50mg/day, as single dosage (morning); although studies have shown some benefits in both primary and secondary hypoadrenalism, the value of routine replacement remains a matter of debate.

### Adrenal crisis
- 100mg hydrocortisone IV (IM) stat, followed by 150–400mg/24 hours (see earlier). Samples for cortisol and ACTH should be drawn beforehand, but administration must not be delayed (see Section 1.15). Alternatively, following an initial intravenous bolus, a continuous hydrocortisone infusion may be used to provide a smoother profile of cortisol replacement.
- Fluid resuscitation (0.9% saline).
- Correct hypoglycaemia.
- Investigate for (and treat) precipitant(s).
- ► Care must be taken if the patient is significantly hyponatraemic at presentation, as too rapid correction may result in central pontine myelinolysis.
- Patients taking enzyme-inducing agents (e.g. phenytoin, carbamazepine, rifampicin) typically require a higher replacement dose to compensate for enhanced glucocorticoid metabolism.
- Mineralocorticoid replacement is only required in patients with primary hypoadrenalism.
- At higher dosages, hydrocortisone exerts mineralocorticoid activity and fludrocortisone replacement may be temporarily suspended until hydrocortisone dosage is returned to physiological levels (40–50mg hydrocortisone yields the equivalent of ~50–100mcg of fludrocortisone activity).

### Surveillance
The need for routine biochemical assessment of the adequacy of cortisol replacement (e.g. cortisol day curve) is controversial, with some clinicians arguing that symptoms and signs are sufficient to guide dose adjustments in the majority of patients. Fludrocortisone dose is titrated based on clinical (blood pressure (including postural), peripheral oedema) and biochemical (serum Na/K and plasma renin) parameters. DHEAS is typically restored to the middle of the age- and sex-matched reference range. In patients with autoimmune primary hypoadrenalism periodic screening for linked disorders (see Table 7.13) is recommended. Similarly, more global assessment of pituitary function is required in those with secondary hypoadrenalism.

### Education and follow up
Prevention of adrenal crisis (annual risk ~3%) is of paramount importance. Regular 'refresher training': reiterate 'sick day rules' (doubling

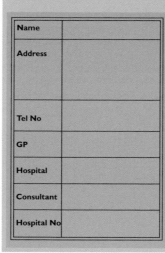

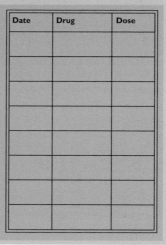

**STEROID
TREATMENT
CARD**

**I am a patient on STEROID
treatment which must
not be stopped suddenly**

- If you have been taking this
  medicine for more than three
  weeks, the dose should be
  reduced gradually when you
  stop taking steroids unless
  your doctor says otherwise.

- Read the patient information
  leaflet given with the medicine

- Always carry this card with you
  and show it to anyone who
  treats you (for example a doctor,
  nurse, pharmacist or dentist).
  For one year after you stop the
  treatment, you must mention
  that you have taken steroids.

- If you become ill, or if you come
  into contact with anyone who
  has an infectious disease, consult
  your doctor promptly. If you
  have never had chickenpox, you
  should avoid close contact with
  people who have chickenpox or
  shingles. If you do come into
  contact with chickenpox, see
  your doctor urgently.

- Make sure that the information
  on the card is kept up to date.

| Name | |
|------|--|
| Address | |
| Tel No | |
| GP | |
| Hospital | |
| Consultant | |
| Hospital No | |

| Date | Drug | Dose |
|------|------|------|
| | | |
| | | |
| | | |
| | | |
| | | |
| | | |
| | | |

**Fig. 7.40** Traditional steroid card. Although still in widespread use, this card is more suited to patients taking time-limited courses of supraphysiological corticosteroids (e.g. as anti-inflammatory agents). A new card is currently under development which is likely to be more relevant to those taking adrenal replacement dosages of corticosteroids.

of dose if unwell; seek medical attention if diarrhoea and/or vomiting), update steroid emergency card/bracelet, and renew parenteral hydrocortisone emergency kit. Patients should be aware to take an additional 5–10mg hydrocortisone prior to strenuous exercise, and that for most surgical procedures parenteral steroid cover is required (e.g. hydrocortisone 150–400mg/24 hours—depending on body weight/route of administration/concomitant drug usage/procedure etc.).

# 7.14 Phaeochromocytoma and paraganglioma

## Background

These tumours arise from the neuroectoderm and occur within the adrenal medulla ('**phaeochromocytoma**'; ~80%), or in extra-adrenal chromaffin cells, e.g. (sympathetic) ganglia of the spinal cord or (parasympathetic) carotid body ('**extra-adrenal phaeochromocytoma**', or '**paraganglioma**'; ~20%). Both may occur in isolation or as part of an inherited genetic syndrome. The abbreviation PPGL is now commonly used to denote disorders associated with phaeochromocytoma and/or paraganglioma.

## Epidemiology

- Rare, accounting for <0.5% of all cases of hypertension. Autopsy studies report prevalence rates of ~0.05%.
- Sporadic cases are typically diagnosed between the ages of 30–50 years: inherited forms present/diagnosed earlier. Even in patients without initial evidence of a wider syndrome or a positive family history, germline mutations in one or other of the recognized genes are subsequently identified in a significant proportion (currently approximately 40%) of patients.
- Paragangliomas are more likely to be malignant and recur.

## Aetiology and pathophysiology

See Table 7.14.
- Sporadic tumours are more commonly unilateral and <10cm in diameter.

### Table 7.14 Hereditary syndromes associated with phaeochromocytoma/paraganglioma

| **Von Hippel–Lindau syndrome (VHL) (type 2) (see Section 7.18)** |
| --- |
| VHL (tumour suppressor gene) mutations |
| Phaeochromocytomas in ~20%; higher percentage in some kindreds (type 2) |
| ~5% are malignant |
| **Multiple endocrine neoplasia (type 2) syndrome** |
| RET (proto-oncogene) mutations |
| Phaeochromocytomas occur in ~50% of cases |
| **Type 2A**—medullary thyroid carcinoma, phaeochromocytomas, hyperparathyroidism |
| **Type 2B**—medullary thyroid carcinoma, phaeochromocytomas, marfanoid habitus, mucosal neuromas |
| **Neurofibromatosis (type 1) (see Section 10.9)** |
| NF1 gene mutations |
| Phaeochromocytomas in <5% of cases (20% bilateral) |
| **Hereditary paragangliomas** |
| Mutations identified in succinate dehydrogenase complex subunits B, D, C, A, AF2 (i.e. SDHB, SDHD, SDHC, SDHA, SDHAF2) |
| Paraganglioma and/or phaeochromocytoma (PPGL), rare renal cancers, gastrointestinal stromal tumours (GIST); head and neck paragangliomas may occur in addition to, or independent of, abdominal/thoracic PPGL. |
| **Familial phaeochromocytomas** |
| TMEM127 mutations—phaeochromocytomas and rare renal cancers |
| MAX mutations—mainly PPGL |
| **Polycythaemia-paraganglioma syndrome** |
| EPAS mutations—polycythaemia, PPGL, somatostatinoma |
| **Leiomyomatosis and renal cell cancer** |
| Fumarate hydratase (FH) mutations—cutaneous and uterine leiomyomas, type 2 papillary renal carcinoma, rare PPGL |

- Adrenal phaeochromocytomas typically secrete both noradrenaline (NAd) and adrenaline (Ad), whereas paragangliomas secrete either NAd alone or are non-secretory.
- Phenylethanolamine-N-methyl-transferase (PNMT) is required for conversion of NAd to Ad; its action is dependent on local cortisol production by the adjacent adrenal cortex. Paragangliomas therefore lack PNMT activity.
- Occasional tumours secrete pure dopamine (DA), which may be associated with hypotension. These tumours are more likely to be malignant.

## Clinical evaluation

### History and examination

- Clinical features are variable and often non-specific (Table 7.15), leading to a delay in diagnosis.
- Most symptoms occur in a paroxysmal fashion (several times daily to once every few months), reflecting intermittent excess catecholamine secretion, and may be triggered by specific stimuli (exercise, anaesthesia, tumour manipulation, drugs, e.g. metoclopramide, opiates, glucocorticoids).
- Hypertensive paroxysms occur either on a background of sustained hypertension or normal BP.
- Unexplained orthostatic hypotension in a patient with hypertension is an important clue to the diagnosis.
- In cases associated with genetic syndromes (Table 7.14) other clinical features of the respective syndromes are commonly, but not necessarily, present (e.g. medullary thyroid carcinoma in MEN2; see Section 7.18).
- Complications are shown in Table 7.16.

### Table 7.15 Clinical features of phaeochromocytoma/paraganglioma

| System | Features |
| --- | --- |
| General | Sweating and heat intolerance<br>Pallor<br>Apprehension/anxiety ('sense of impending doom')<br>Fever |
| Cardiovascular | Sustained or episodic hypertension<br>Palpitations/tachycardia<br>Orthostatic hypotension<br>Chest pain, dyspnoea |
| Neurological | Headache<br>Visual disturbance/seizures |
| Gastrointestinal | Abdominal pain, nausea, constipation, weight loss |

### Table 7.16 Complications of phaeochromocytoma/paraganglioma

| System | Features |
| --- | --- |
| Cardiovascular | Hypotension/shock—often multifactorial, e.g. intravascular volume depletion + cardiovascular emergency (myocardial infarction, dysrhythmia, aortic dissection)<br>Left ventricular failure<br>Dysrhythmia<br>Dilated cardiomyopathy |
| Neurological | Cerebrovascular accident<br>Hypertensive encephalopathy |
| Metabolic | Hyperglycaemia<br>Hypercalcaemia |

### Screening

Should be considered in the following situations:

- Patients with the classic triad of headache, palpitations, and sweating, whether or not they have hypertension.

- Therapy-resistant hypertension.

- Young patients with hypertension.

- Paradoxical BP response during anaesthesia.

- Hereditary predisposition, or features suggestive of an associated genetic syndrome (Table 7.14).

- Patients with an adrenal 'incidentaloma' (see Section 7.11).

- Unexplained cardiomyopathy.

### Investigations

This is normally approached in two stages:

1. Biochemical confirmation of diagnosis.

2. Localization of tumour.

#### Biochemical testing

The potentially fatal consequences (Table 17.16) of a missed diagnosis necessitate a sensitive test for initial screening.

#### Catecholamines and metanephrines

Until recently, many centres offered measurement of catecholamines (Ad, NAd ± DA) in urine (24-hour collections) as their front-line screening test (sensitivity ~85%). However, most laboratories have now moved over to assays for urinary fractionated metanephrines (sensitivity ~97%) or plasma-free metanephrines (sensitivity ~99%).

▶ Increased sensitivity of metanephrines compared with catecholamines is due to **continuous** production of O-methylated metabolites in tumours (i.e. unlike the highly variable release of catecholamines).

One problem with using sensitive tests for screening is that false positive tests may occur, which divide into two groups:

- True catecholamine excess—physiological stimuli, drugs (e.g. tricyclic antidepressants, monoamine oxidase inhibitors) or clinical conditions (e.g. hypertension, heart failure, obstructive sleep apnoea) that increase circulating catecholamines ± their metabolites.

- Analytical interference: assay-dependent, may occur with coffee, β-blockers, paracetamol, sympathomimetics, L-dopa.

The magnitude of elevation of catecholamines and their metabolites may help to distinguish true from false positive results, but there is considerable overlap.

#### Other investigations

- Clonidine suppression test: clonidine suppresses NAd release from the sympathetic nervous system helping distinguish sympathetic activation from a phaeochromocytoma/paraganglioma. Measurement of plasma normetanephrine levels pre- and post-clonidine yields high positive (100%) and negative (96%) predictive values.

- Genetic testing: genetic screening in phaeochromocytoma/paraganglioma syndromes is currently generally limited to those with a positive family history for linked syndromes, or those aged <50 years, or with bilateral or extra-adrenal disease.

#### Tumour localization

- CT/MRI: imaging of the chest, abdomen, and pelvis is indicated in most cases (Fig. 7.41). Head and neck imaging may also be required in some cases of paraganglioma.

- [123]I-metaiodobenzylguanidine ([123]I-MIBG) scanning: [123]I-MIBG is taken up by chromaffin cells and localizes both adrenal and extra-adrenal tumours. Pre-treatment with potassium iodide prevents thyroidal uptake.

- PET: [18]F-fluorodopa and [18]F-fluorodopamine PET offer excellent sensitivity and specificity, especially in [123]I-MIBG negative cases. [18]F-fluorodeoxyglucose (FDG) PET is useful in malignant disease.

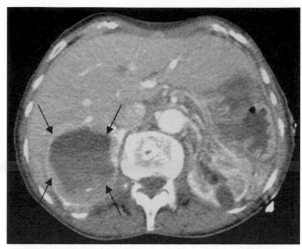

**Fig. 7.41** Contrast-enhanced abdominal CT scan. Large right adrenal phaeochromocytoma (arrows) indenting the liver.

## Management

### Medical therapy

To mitigate the vasoconstricting and arrhythmogenic effects of excessive circulating catecholamines, combined α- and β-adrenoceptor blockade is indicated in most patients.

▶ The sequence in which blockade is established is crucial—use of β-blockers before satisfactory α-blockade has been achieved may precipitate a hypertensive crisis due to unopposed α-adrenoceptor-mediated vasoconstriction.

#### α-blockade

- The non-competitive α-adrenoceptor antagonist phenoxybenzamine is generally preferred (begin with 10mg twice daily and titrate to normalize BP—most patients require 0.5–2mg/kg per day in divided doses). Orthostatic hypotension is a common early side effect of treatment (as vasoconstriction is relieved, the contracted circulating volume is insufficient to compensate), and the patient must therefore be rendered euvolaemic, with IV saline if necessary.

- Doxazosin can be used in patients intolerant of phenoxybenzamine, but blockade may be less effective due to the competitive nature of its α-adrenoceptor antagonism.

- Intravenous phentolamine provides an alternative when rapid control of BP is required, e.g. in theatre or in a patient with a hypertensive crisis.

#### β-blockade

- The non-selective agent propranolol is preferred (20–80mg 8-hourly), although other β-blockers may be used.

- Short-acting IV esmolol is an effective alternative when control of life-threatening arrhythmias is urgently required.

### Surgery

**Laparoscopic resection** is the treatment of choice for most phaeochromocytomas, but requires meticulous preoperative preparation (see earlier in this section). Open adrenalectomy is generally reserved for larger tumours in which there is suspicion of local invasion.

▶ Postoperative hypotension and hypoglycaemia are not uncommon, and patients should be monitored in a high-dependency area for 24–48 hours after surgery.

### Adjunctive therapy for malignant tumours

- High-dose (i.e. therapeutic) [131]I-MIBG may be useful in treating locally recurrent/metastatic disease.

- Long-term combined α- and β-blockade is usually required.

- α-methylparatyrosine (blocks tyrosine hydroxylase; rate-limiting step in catecholamine biosynthesis) may be useful.
- Chemotherapy has limited efficacy, but may help with symptom control in some patients; initial trials with tyrosine kinase inhibitors suggest a potential benefit in some patients.
- External beam radiotherapy for pain (bony metastases).

## Follow-up and prognosis

- Lifelong follow-up is required even in patients with a benign solitary tumour and no relevant family history.

- Clinical assessment and monitoring of catecholamine/metanephrine levels is generally sufficient, with imaging reserved for those with suspected recurrence or metastatic disease. Chromogranin A may be a useful tumour marker in malignant phaeo/paraganglioma.
- Although BP improves in most patients following surgery, some (~25%) will have persistent hypertension.
- Even patients with malignant tumours frequently survive for many years.

# 7.15 Male hypogonadism and gynaecomastia

## Male hypogonadism

Male hypogonadism is commonly used to denote clinical and/or biochemical evidence of testosterone deficiency, although it can also refer to impaired spermatogenesis irrespective of testosterone levels.

### Normal physiology

- Hypothalamic gonadotropin-releasing hormone (GnRH) stimulates pituitary gonadotrophs to secrete LH and FSH.
- LH then stimulates the Leydig cells of the testes to produce testosterone, while FSH stimulates Sertoli cells to produce sperm and secrete inhibin.
- Testosterone and inhibin impair GnRH, LH and FSH secretion in a negative feedback manner.

Only 1–2% of circulating testosterone is free (the remainder is bound to SHBG and albumin). Accordingly, conditions which lower or raise SHBG (Table 7.17) decrease or increase total testosterone levels respectively. As most laboratories measure total and not free serum testosterone, estimation of SHBG (and calculation of a free testosterone index) can be helpful in circumstances where binding protein levels are likely to be altered.

### Aetiology

#### Primary hypogonadism
See Table 7.18. Primary gonadal pathology → ↓ testosterone/inhibin ↓ negative feedback → ↑ LH and FSH levels.

#### Secondary hypogonadism
See Table 7.19. Hypothalamic and/or pituitary dysfunction ↓ LH/FSH, ↓ testosterone and impaired spermatogenesis.

### Signs and symptoms

#### Testosterone deficiency in utero/infancy
Ambiguous genitalia, micropenis, cryptorchidism.

#### Testosterone deficiency prior to/at puberty
Delayed onset of puberty, short stature, and all of the features as listed for adulthood if not corrected.

#### Table 7.17 Conditions associated with abnormal SHBG levels

| SHBG increased | Hyperthyroidism<br>Pregnancy<br>Oestrogen therapy |
| --- | --- |
| SHBG decreased | Cirrhosis<br>Obesity<br>Androgen therapy<br>Hypothyroidism<br>Acromegaly |

#### Table 7.18 Causes of primary hypogonadism in males

| Cause | Example(s) |
| --- | --- |
| Congenital | Klinefelter syndrome, disorders of androgen synthesis, myotonic dystrophy |
| Idiopathic | |
| Iatrogenic | Surgery, chemotherapy, radiotherapy |
| Environmental | Irradiation, environmental toxins |
| Local pathology | Varicocoele, testicular torsion, trauma |
| Infections | Viral orchitis (e.g. mumps) |
| Chronic disease | Liver cirrhosis, chronic renal failure |
| Autoimmune | |

#### Table 7.19 Causes of secondary hypogonadism in males

| Cause | Example(s) |
| --- | --- |
| Congenital | Kallmann and Prader–Willi syndromes, isolated hypogonadotrophic hypogonadism |
| Constitutional delay | |
| Hypothalamic/pituitary disorders | Hypothalamic/pituitary tumour/infiltration/surgery/radiotherapy |
| | Hyperprolactinaemia |
| | Pituitary trauma/apoplexy |
| Other endocrine | Cushing syndrome |
| Medication | Opiates, exogenous androgens, glucocorticoids |
| Chronic disease | Haemochromatosis, anorexia |
| Idiopathic | |

#### Testosterone deficiency in adulthood
Impaired general sense of well-being, reduced energy/stamina, decreased strength/muscle mass, reduced facial and body hair (Figs 7.42 and 7.43), loss of libido, erectile dysfunction, infertility, gynaecomastia, and osteoporosis.

### Investigations

- U&E, LFT.
- Testosterone (9am sample).
- LH, FSH (distinguishes between primary and secondary hypogonadism).
- SHBG if indicated (see 'Normal physiology').
- Semen analysis if indicated.

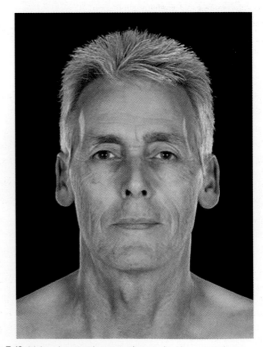

**Fig. 7.42** Male subject with acquired secondary hypogonadism as a consequence of a non-functioning pituitary macroadenoma. Note the smooth facial appearance.

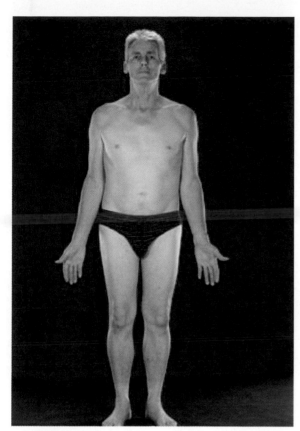

**Fig. 7.43** Male subject with acquired secondary hypogonadism as a consequence of a non-functioning pituitary macroadenoma. Note lack of male pattern body hair.

Also consider the following:
- Bone densitometry.
- Karyotyping (e.g. in Klinefelter syndrome).
- Pituitary screen in cases of secondary hypogonadism.
- Dexamethasone suppression test/circadian cortisol rhythm if Cushing syndrome suspected.
- Transferrin saturation (screen for haemochromatosis).
- USS to identify testes in cases of cryptorchidism.
- Genetic screening (e.g. Kallmann syndrome if absent sense of smell; *HFE* gene if suspect haemochromatosis).

## Management
- Explain diagnosis—many ♂ will find this a sensitive issue to discuss.
- Where possible (e.g. pituitary tumour, Cushing syndrome) treat the underlying cause.
- Where appropriate, institute gonadal replacement therapy.
- Refer for specialist fertility advice if indicated.

*Testosterone replacement therapy*
Although most hypogonadal ♂ should be offered testosterone replacement therapy, some may decline treatment (e.g. elderly ♂ with long-standing hypogonadism), preferring to adopt other measures for bone protection/treatment (e.g. bisphosphonate).

*Delivery*
- **Transdermal:** e.g. testosterone gel—generally effective and well-tolerated, although may cause local skin irritation, and younger ♂ may not achieve fully therapeutic levels with transdermal delivery.
- **Intramuscular:** short acting (every 3 weeks) or depot (every 3 months).
- **Implants:** pellets of crystallized testosterone implanted subcutaneously every 4–6 months.

*Contraindications*
Prostate cancer, breast cancer, history of primary liver tumours, hypercalcaemia, uncontrolled polycythaemia.

*Side effects*
Cholestatic jaundice, polycythaemia, acne, infertility, gynaecomastia, mood swings, sleep apnoea. May exacerbate pre-existing—or reveal latent—prostate disease.

*Monitoring*
- Clinical assessment.
- Biochemically (most (but not all) preparations require a trough measurement (i.e. just before the next administration), aiming for a level toward the lower end of the reference range.
- FBC (haemoglobin and haematocrit), LFT, and lipid profile should be checked prior to commencing treatment and periodically thereafter.
- ♂ of an appropriate age should be counselled regarding the pros/cons of prostate surveillance.

# Gynaecomastia
Benign proliferation of glandular tissue of the ♂ breast:
- Caused by an increase in the ratio of oestrogen to androgen acting on the breast, either as a consequence of ↓ androgen production/action, or ↑ oestrogen formation (including conversion of circulating androgens to oestrogens by aromatization).
- ~50% of cases due to drug therapy or idiopathic (Table 7.20).
- Gynaecomastia must be distinguished from lipomastia (excess breast fat), and the rare, but important condition of ♂ breast carcinoma.

## Clinical evaluation
*History*
- Age of onset—physiological gynaecomastia is commonly seen at the time of puberty and in elderly ♂.
- Uni- or bilateral? The former may be simple gynaecomastia, but warrants careful consideration of a sinister cause.
- Weight gain/loss, tenderness, discharge, discrete lumps; galactorrhoea suggests associated hyperprolactinaemia.
- Drug history (see Table 17.20).
- Symptoms of hypogonadism and hypopituitarism. Features of systemic disorders (e.g. thyrotoxicosis, chronic kidney disease, cirrhosis).
- The patient's main concern—e.g. appearance, or possibility of a sinister cause, etc.?

*Examination*
- Look for evidence of systemic disorders (e.g. renal or liver impairment, thyrotoxicosis).
- Confirm that the patient has genuine gynaecomastia (check for discrete lumps, axillary lymph nodes, and galactorrhoea).
- Look for evidence of hypogonadism or hypopituitarism.
- Examine both testes—volumes and masses.
- Consider Klinefelter syndrome.

*Investigations*
Some clinicians contend that gynaecomastia at puberty or in elderly subjects is so common that (in the absence of features of another underlying condition), it does not require further investigation; others however, argue that further investigation is merited in all patients. Screening tests include:
- Renal, liver, and thyroid function tests.
- Oestradiol, LH, FSH and testosterone (± SHBG); possibly DHEAS levels (a marker of adrenal androgen production).
- HCG and AFP tumour markers.

**Table 7.20** Causes of gynaecomastia

| Cause | Example(s) |
|---|---|
| Physiological | Neonatal, puberty, elderly, familial |
| Idiopathic | |
| Drugs | Antiandrogens (e.g. cyproterone acetate, spironolactone); GnRH analogues; oestrogens; digoxin; cimetidine; ketoconazole; metronidazole; anti-tuberculous therapy; alkylating agents; recreational use/abuse of anabolic steroids |
| Hypogonadism | Primary (e.g. Klinefelter syndrome, post-orchidectomy)<br>Secondary (e.g. hyperprolactinaemia, hypopituitarism, Kallmann syndrome) |
| Tumours | Oestrogen- or androgen-producing adrenal or testicular tumours (excess androgens are aromatized to oestrogens)<br>hCG producing tumours (e.g. testicular germ cell or bronchogenic carcinoma) |
| Other endocrine | Thyrotoxicosis (↑ hepatic SHBG production ↓ circulating free testosterone levels); androgen insensitivity syndromes; |
| Systemic | Cirrhosis; chronic renal impairment; HIV infection |
| Other | Obesity (increased aromatization in adipose tissue) |

Depending on clinical features and initial investigations, consider:
- Pituitary profile if suspicion of hypopituitarism.
- USS of testes if palpable mass or ↑ tumour markers.
- Karyotype analysis if Klinefelter syndrome suspected.
- Breast ultrasound ± biopsy if concern re: breast mass.

## Management

### Observation and treatment of underlying cause

Gynaecomastia may regress spontaneously (puberty related) or when the underlying cause (drug therapy, hypogonadism) is addressed. Social embarrassment and/or localized pain/tenderness may be indications for additional independent treatment.

### Medical therapy

Treatment to re-establish the balance between oestrogen and androgen action—aromatase inhibitors (e.g. anastrozole) or selective-oestrogen-receptor-modulators (e.g. tamoxifen).

However, results are often disappointing, although local discomfort may improve even without significant regression of the gynaecomastia.

### Surgery

Typically reserved for persistent gynaecomastia despite correction of any underlying disorder and/or in whom medical therapy has proved ineffective. May involve direct surgical excision of the glandular tissue and/or liposuction through a periareolar incision.

# 7.16 Menstrual disorders and anovulation

## Normal menstruation

- Hypothalamic gonadotropin-releasing hormone (GnRH) stimulates the pituitary to secrete follicle stimulating hormone (FSH) and luteinizing hormone (LH).
- Stimulated by FSH, ovarian follicles grow (follicular phase) and produce increasing amounts of oestrogen.
- Oocyte-expulsion (**ovulation**) triggered by mid-cycle LH surge.
- Ovulation initiates luteal phase during which the corpus luteum (comprising the remaining follicular granulosa cells) produces increasing amounts of progesterone; when levels of the latter decline (as corpus luteum involutes), menstruation occurs with shedding of the endometrium (see Section 7.1).
- Menstruation typically occurs for the first time (menarche) at the age of 10–14 years and continues until the menopause at the age of 46–55 years.
- The average cycle lasts 28 days (range 21–35 days), and recurs regularly. The first day of menstrual bleeding is taken as the first day of the cycle, and menstruation normally lasts for 3–5 days (range 2–7 days).
- Mean blood loss = 35–40mL; occasional small clots are normal.

## Abnormal menstruation

- Any bleeding pattern falling outside these parameters requires further investigation. The initial **history** and **examination** should help to exclude an extra-uterine source of bleeding (e.g. vulva, cervix, bladder).
- Consider the patient's **age**: it may indicate specific physiological causes of menstrual disturbance (pregnancy, menopause) or specific pathologies (ovulatory disturbances if age >20 years, when the hypothalamic–pituitary–ovarian axis is fully matured, are more likely pathological).
- **Categorizing** menstrual disturbances using the following criteria helps in establishing the underlying cause.

### Ovulatory menstrual disturbances

A regular cycle suggests ovulation is likely to be occurring normally and abnormal **menstrual** bleeding may therefore reflect local anatomical causes (polyps, fibroids, neoplasms, foreign bodies), coagulation disorders, infection, or trauma.

**Intermenstrual bleeding:** bleeding that occurs between menses, or between expected hormone withdrawal bleeds.

**Menorrhagia:** denotes excessive (>80mL) and/or prolonged (>7 days) menstrual bleeding.

**Premenstrual spotting:** light bleeding before regular menses.

### Anovulatory menstrual disturbances

Irregular, infrequent (>35 days between cycles) and absent menses are typically associated with anovulation.

**Oligomenorrhoea:** bleeding that occurs at an interval of >35 days. This is classically seen in the polycystic ovarian syndrome (PCOS) (see Section 7.17).

**Primary amenorrhoea:** failure of menarche by age 16 years. Commonest causes are anatomical (imperforate hymen, congenital uterine anomalies) or genetic (gonadal dysgenesis in Turner syndrome, androgen insensitivity syndrome).

**Secondary amenorrhoea:** absence of bleeding for >6 consecutive months in a woman who has previously menstruated.

**Breakthrough bleeding:** in the absence of the normal progesterone surge (second half of menstrual cycle), prolonged high oestrogen levels may cause endometrial hyperplasia, and thus erratic/excessive menstrual (breakthrough) bleeding.

## Causes of anovulation/oligomenorrhoea/secondary amenorrhoea

Any interference with the coordinated actions of the hypothalamus (GnRH), pituitary (LH, FSH), ovaries (oestrogen, progesterone), and uterus (functional endometrium) may disturb ovulation/menstrual function:

**Physiological:** pregnancy is a very common cause of secondary amenorrhoea—do not forget to consider this possibility—the patient may not have realized! Other physiological causes include lactation and postmenopausal status.

**Hypothalamic causes:** weight loss, nutritional deficiency, excessive exercise, and emotional/physical stress adversely affect the pulsatile secretion of GnRH, as do structural lesions in the vicinity of the hypothalamus (e.g. craniopharyngioma, hypothalamic glioma).

**Pituitary causes:** hormonal over- (e.g. hyperprolactinaemia, Cushing syndrome) or under-production (e.g. hypopituitarism) can affect LH/FSH secretion. Menstrual disturbance may be the first sign of evolving hypopituitarism in a woman.

**Ovarian causes:** ovarian failure with premature depletion of oocytes (chemotherapy, irradiation, autoimmune disease, idiopathic) and PCOS are commonly associated with menstrual disturbance/anovulation. Rarely androgen-secreting tumours (ovarian and adrenal) may present in this manner.

**Uterine causes:** scarring of the endometrium (Asherman syndrome) secondary to repeated uterine infections or excessive curettage can lead to light or absent menses.

## Investigations

Tailor to the history and examination, but may include:

- Pregnancy test—then you are unlikely to be surprised!
- TSH to exclude thyrotoxicosis.
- LH, FSH (distinguishes between primary and secondary hypogonadism), with paired oestradiol—timed to the follicular phase where possible.
- Prolactin to identify hyperprolactinaemic disorders (see Section 7.8).

Also consider the following:

- Testosterone ± DHEAS (dehydroepiandrosterone sulphate) if evidence of hyperandrogenism.
- Pituitary screen in secondary hypogonadism: prolactin, TSH and FT4, 9am cortisol, IGF-1, and pituitary MRI.
- Karyotyping (e.g. in Turner syndrome).
- Dexamethasone suppression test/circadian cortisol rhythm if Cushing syndrome suspected.
- Bone densitometry to identify those in need of bone-protective measures.
- USS to determine endometrial thickness (an indicator of oestrogen exposure) and to assess if ovaries polycystic.
- A 'progesterone challenge' can be used to assess the adequacy of oestrogenization: at the end of a short (5–10-day) course of progesterone, endometrial shedding and menstruation is expected if there has been sufficient preceding oestrogen exposure to allow endometrial proliferation.

## Management

Treat the underlying cause: behavioural therapy in anorexia, dopamine agonists in hyperprolactinaemia, insulin-sensitizing medication and weight loss in PCOS.

If regular ovulation cannot be achieved/restored, management focuses on prevention/treatment of complications (e.g. HRT to prevent osteoporosis due to oestrogen deficiency). Any infertility treatment offered depends on the underlying cause (ovulation induction in PCOS, egg donation in premature ovarian failure or gonadal dysgenesis).

# 7.17 Hirsutism and the polycystic ovarian syndrome

## Hirsutism

Excess of thick, pigmented, body hair in ♂ distribution (extent assessed using Ferriman–Gallwey score). Hirsutism, plus androgenic alopecia and acne, can occur with normal/only mildly increased serum levels of androgens. For causes see Table 7.21.

**Virilization:** increased muscle bulk, deepening of the voice, clitoromegaly. Usually due to a significant increase in circulating levels of androgenous hormones.

Opinions differ as to the extent to which women with hirsutism should be investigated—essentially the more severe and rapid the onset of hirsutism, the more detailed the investigation (especially if any evidence of virilization).

## Polycystic ovarian syndrome

Polycystic ovarian syndrome (PCOS) is very common among ♀ of reproductive age (prevalence: ~8% in ♀ overall; 75% in hirsute ♀; 75–90% in ♀ with irregular periods).

The cause remains a matter of debate, with environmental and genetic factors implicated in the pathogenesis involving:

- The ovaries (theca cells over-produce androgens and retain insulin sensitivity).
- The hypothalamic–pituitary axis (excessive LH secretion).
- Primary defects of insulin action, i.e. insulin resistance (leading to high insulin levels, which drive ovarian androgen production).

♀ usually seek medical advice for a specific manifestation of PCOS, e.g. hirsutism, oligo/amenorrhoea, infertility.

### Definition

Two out of three of the following:

- Oligomenorrhoea and/or anovulation.
- Clinical and/or biochemical features of hyperandrogenism.
- Polycystic ovaries.

► Ovarian USS is not essential to diagnose PCOS, but if performed the transvaginal route is preferred. USS evidence of polycystic ovaries in the absence of oligomenorrhea or hyperandrogenism is insufficient to diagnose PCOS.

Other causes of menstrual irregularity and/or hyperandrogenism (e.g. hyperprolactinaemia, congenital adrenal hyperplasia, androgen-secreting tumour, Cushing syndrome) must be excluded.

Table 7.21  Causes of hirsutism (idiopathic hirsutism and polycystic ovarian syndrome (PCOS) account for the majority of cases)

| Frequency | Condition |
|---|---|
| Common | Idiopathic |
| | Racial/familial |
| | PCOS |
| Less common | Congenital adrenal hyperplasia (non-classical) |
| | Adrenal/ovarian androgen-secreting tumours |
| | Ovarian hyperthecosis |
| | Cushing syndrome |
| | Hypothyroidism |
| | Drugs, e.g. anabolic steroids |
| | Severe insulin resistance states |

The metabolic disturbance and other features of PCOS would be predicted to increase CV risk, but the strength of any such link is still debated and the subject of ongoing research. Meanwhile, it seems sensible to treat/minimize individual risk factors (e.g. stop smoking).

## Insulin resistance (IR)

IR is key to the pathogenesis of PCOS, and reducing excess weight (present in >75% of cases) is central to management. The risk of impaired glucose tolerance (IGT) and overt diabetes is higher in obese subjects with than without PCOS.

## Management

### Weight/insulin resistance

*Lifestyle measures*

Even modest weight loss (diet and exercise) can restore ovulation, improve biochemical/clinical hyperandrogenism and lower the risk of IGT/diabetes mellitus.

*Insulin sensitizing therapy*

Metformin stabilizes (and may even reduce) weight, normalizes menses, and improves fertility.

### Hyperandrogenism

Serum androgen levels may be mild to moderately elevated in PCOS, but this is neither a universal finding nor a diagnostic requirement. However, late (>30 years, no excessive weight gain) or rapid onset of symptoms and/or signs of virilization should raise suspicion of an ovarian/adrenal neoplasm.

*Oestrogen/anti-androgen therapy*

The most effective treatment is a combined oral contraceptive preparation (COCP) containing ethinyl-oestradiol and a progestogen with minimal androgenicity (e.g. desogestrel). Risks and side effects of COCPs are similar to those for women without PCOS (e.g. increased risk of venous thromboembolism).

COCP effectiveness can be increased if combined with additional anti-androgen therapy, e.g. cyproterone acetate (side effects: reduced libido, LFT changes) or spironolactone (side effects: LFT changes, hyperkalaemia, hyponatraemia). The use of flutamide (more potent anti-androgen) and finasteride (5α-reductase inhibitor, blocks conversion of testosterone to dihydrotestosterone) is controversial and should only be undertaken by a specialist with experience in their use.

► Any unlicensed anti-androgen use requires appropriate consent and combination with effective contraception.

*Cosmetic measures*

Shaving, waxing, depilatories, electrolysis, or laser therapy may be most effective. Topical eflornithine cream retards hair growth but needs continuous use to be effective, while minoxidil solution (2–5%) can alleviate androgenic alopecia.

Metformin (in the absence of weight loss) does not generally improve hyperandrogenism.

### Anovulation

High prevalence in PCOS. For management of resulting menstrual disturbances and infertility see Section 7.16.

### Associated health problems

- Dyslipidaemia: low HDL-C with high triglycerides is typical in PCOS.
- IR/IGT/type 2 diabetes: given the high rate of IGT in obese PCOS patients, those with a BMI >27kg/m² should be offered an oral glucose tolerance test if fasting plasma glucose and HbA1c are normal.
- Non-alcoholic fatty liver disease (NAFLD) and steato-hepatitis (NASH): ALT frequently elevated in PCOS, especially if overweight.
- Sleep apnoea syndrome: relatively common in obese patients with PCOS (up to 30%).
- Increased cardiovascular (CV) risk.

# 7.18 Multiple endocrine neoplasia and other genetic endocrine tumour syndromes

- There are a variety of genetic syndromes characterized by neoplastic transformation in different tissues, including endocrine glands.
- Recognition of such disorders allows:
  - Avoidance of the complications of untreated endocrine dysfunction.
  - Pre-emptive treatment of potentially malignant endocrine tumours.
  - Effective family screening.

## Multiple endocrine neoplasia

### Multiple endocrine neoplasia type 1 (MEN1)

- Autosomal dominant disorder.
- Many, but not all, patients harbour a germline mutation in the coding region of the *MENIN* (tumour suppressor) gene (on chromosome 11q13).
- MEN1 is rare (estimated prevalence ~1 in 10,000).
- The clinical diagnosis requires two of the three main MEN tumours (Table 7.22) to be present.

There are several important differences when compared with sporadically occurring tumours:

- Hyperparathyroidism (HPT—also see Section 7.25) occurs at a younger age (typically <40 years vs. >60 years), and multigland involvement is the rule (vs. single adenomas)
- Gastro/entero/pancreatic neuroendocrine tumours (NET—also see Section 7.19) tend to be multifocal and more aggressive.

**Genetic screening** is generally recommended for:

- Patients with two or more MEN1 tumours.
- First- and second-degree relatives of patients with MEN1.

270

It should also be considered if:

- HPT occurs at young age (<40 years), especially if multiglandular involvement.
- NET with multifocal disease (e.g. gastrinoma).

**Biochemical screening** in MEN1 mutation carriers is typically undertaken on an annual basis (Table 7.23). Requirements for **radiological screening** (MRI pituitary and abdomen) are debated, but many endocrinologists advocate performing baseline scans, with, e.g. 3-yearly abdominal imaging thereafter, and pituitary imaging if there is clinical and/or biochemical suspicion of a pituitary adenoma at any stage.

*Treatment*

- Surgery remains the mainstay of treatment for primary HPT with either complete or 3½ gland removal. Some patients harbour an ectopically-sited gland (e.g. mediastinal). Life-long vitamin D replacement with either alfacalcidol (1α-hydroxylated) or calcitriol (1,25-dihydroxylated) is required.
- Calcimimetics (e.g. cinacalcet) have recently been tried with some success in patients with relapsing/refractory disease or those who are unfit for surgery.
- Pituitary adenomas are treated along conventional lines.
- Resection of NETs requires an experienced surgeon and should only be undertaken after careful discussion with the patient. Aggressive surgery with its attendant comorbidity (e.g. endocrine and exocrine pancreatic insufficiency) must be balanced against the risk of local and distant tumour recurrence if resection is incomplete.

### MEN type 2 (MEN2)

- MEN2 is a rare, autosomal dominant disorder associated with activating mutations in the *RET* proto-oncogene (on chromosome 10q11.2).
- The disorder has a high penetrance and, unlike MEN1, there is a strong correlation between genotype and clinical phenotype, thus helping with the planning/timing of treatment.
- Traditionally, MEN2 is divided in to three subtypes: MEN2A, MEN2B, and familial medullary thyroid carcinoma (FMTC) (Table 7.23).

*Clinical features*

- MTC is often the initial manifestation, and is typically multifocal. In MEN2b it may present at a very early stage and is frequently more aggressive. Treatment involves total thyroidectomy and central compartment lymph node ± radical neck dissection. Other treatment modalities are relatively ineffective.
- Genetic screening and prophylactic thyroidectomy (if affected) should be offered to all MEN2 kindreds.
- Plasma calcitonin is a useful tumour marker, especially following total thyroidectomy.
- Screening and treatment for HPT is as per MEN1.

▶ Phaeochromocytomas occur in up to 50% of cases and may be bilateral. Even in the absence of symptoms, screening (see Section 7.14) is advisable on an annual basis, and **must** be undertaken before any form of surgery or invasive procedure is contemplated.

## Von Hippel–Lindau disease

- Von Hippel–Lindau disease (VHL) is a highly penetrant autosomal dominant disorder (prevalence 1:30-40,000) that is characterized by the development of diverse tumours (retinal angiomas, central

| Table 7.22 Clinical features of multiple endocrine neoplasia syndromes | | |
|---|---|---|
| **Type 1** | Primary hyperparathyroidism | >90% |
| | Pituitary tumours (prolactinoma, acromegaly, rarely non-functioning or Cushing) | ~30% |
| | (Gastro-entero-) pancreatic tumours (gastrinoma, insulinoma, rarely glucagonoma, VIPoma, PPoma or non-functioning tumour) | ≤70% |
| | Cutaneous tumours (angiofibromas, collagenomas) | ~75% |
| | Others (adrenal cortical tumours, carcinoid tumour, phaeochromocytoma) | Variable |
| **Type 2A** | MTC | >90% |
| | Phaeochromocytoma | ~50% |
| | Parathyroid hyperplasia | ≤30% |
| **Type 2B** | MTC | ~100% |
| | Phaeochromocytoma | ~50% |
| | Marfanoid habitus | ~75% |
| | Mucosal neuromas | |
| | Intestinal ganglioneuromatosis | |
| **FMTC** | MTC only | ~100% |

Key: VIP, vasoactive intestinal peptide; PP, pancreatic polypeptide; MTC, medullary thyroid carcinoma; FMTC, familial MTC.

**Table 7.23** Biochemical screening in MEN1

| Condition | Biochemical tests |
|---|---|
| Hyperparathyroidism | Serum calcium and phosphate |
| | PTH |
| Pituitary adenoma | Prolactin and IGF-1 |
| | Other basal anterior pituitary function tests |
| Neuroendocrine tumours | Fasting gut hormones |
| | Chromogranin A |
| | ±24-hour urinary 5HIAA± fasting glucose* |

5HIAA: 5-hydroxyindole acetic acid; IGF-1: insulin-like growth factor-1; PTH: parathyroid hormone.

* Some centres do not routinely measure fasting glucose in the absence of symptoms, while others check paired fasting glucose and insulin levels (± HbA1c).

nervous system haemangioblastomas, renal cysts/carcinomas, phaeochromocytomas, pancreatic tumours/cysts).

- Affected subjects harbour mutations in the *VHL* gene (on chromosome 3p25).
- VHL may be subdivided into types 1 and 2, depending on the risk for developing phaeochromocytomas and renal cell carcinoma:

| Type 1 | • Low risk for phaeochromocytoma. |
|---|---|
| Type 2A | • Phaeochromocytomas (high risk). <br> • Renal cell carcinoma (low risk). |
| Type 2B | • Phaeochromocytomas (high risk). <br> • Renal cell carcinomas (high risk). |
| Type 2C | • Phaeochromocytomas only. |

- Annual biochemical screening combined with abdominal MRI (especially where also required for renal/pancreatic surveillance), is advised for all patients with type 2 disease.
- Treatment is with combined α- and β-adrenoceptor blockade followed by surgery (also see Section 7.14).
- More than 2/3 of patients with VHL will develop pancreatic tumours, of which ~10% are neuroendocrine in origin (see Section 7.19). Most of these are asymptomatic and slow growing, but secretory tumours can occur, and some lesions may metastasize. Accordingly, annual screening is indicated once a pancreatic lesion is identified.

# Carney complex

Carney complex (CNC) is a rare, autosomal dominant syndrome, characterized by cardiac, cutaneous, and neural myxomatous tumours, as well as a variety of pigmented skin and mucosal lesions. Endocrine complications include:

- Primary pigmented nodular adrenal disease (PPNAD)—manifesting with biochemical evidence of autonomous cortisol secretion or overt Cushing syndrome.
- GH/prolactin-secreting pituitary adenoma (somato-lactotroph hyperplasia may also occur)—causing acromegaly and/or hyperprolactinaemia.
- Large-cell calcifying Sertoli cell tumours (LCCSCT) of the testes (occasionally ovarian cysts in affected ♀).
- Thyroid adenoma.

Linkage with two different genetic loci on chromosomes 2p16 and 17q22–24 has been shown, and the latter has resulted in the identification of mutations in the protein kinase A regulatory subunit-1-alpha (*PRKAR1A*) gene (chromosome 17q) in several affected families.

# Neurofibromatosis type 1

- Neurofibromatosis type 1 (NF1; see Section 10.9) is a highly penetrant autosomal dominant disorder characterized by café-au-lait spots, axillary freckling, and multiple cutaneous and subcutaneous neurofibromas.
- Up to 5% of NF1 patients have phaeochromocytomas, which may be multifocal and occasionally extra-adrenal.
- In a small number of patients optic gliomas may impinge on adjacent tissues and disrupt hypothalamic–pituitary function.
- NF2 has no commonly associated primary endocrinopathies (secondary hypothalamic–pituitary dysfunction may complicate treatment for intracranial tumours).

# McCune–Albright syndrome

- A genetic—but not inherited—disorder arising as a consequence of postzygotic somatic mutations in the *GNAS* gene (on chromosome 20q13).
- These result in constitutive, agonist-independent, cAMP stimulation by disrupting the intrinsic GTPase activity that normally terminates G protein activation.

The condition is characterized by:

- Polyostotic fibrous dysplasia causing bone deformity, pathological fractures, pseudoarthrosis (especially in the pelvis and femora).
- Café-au-lait macules.
- Endocrine dysfunction, e.g. precocious puberty, thyroid nodules (± thyrotoxicosis), Cushing syndrome (due to adrenal hyperplasia or adenoma), growth hormone- or prolactin-secreting pituitary adenomas, and hypophosphataemic rickets.

# 7.19 Neuroendocrine tumours

## Background

The majority of neuroendocrine tumours (NETs) arise as a consequence of autonomous growth of neuroendocrine cells of the gastro-entero-pancreatic axis, which share a common embryological origin and the ability to secrete multiple polypeptides and biogenic amines. Occasionally carcinoid tumours arise in other sites (e.g. the lung).

NETs may initially secrete one particular peptide, recur secreting a different peptide, and metastasize to produce yet another peptide. They may occur sporadically or as part of a tumour syndrome such as MEN1 (see Section 7.18). They are often <1cm in size, slow growing, and metastasize prior to the patient developing clinical symptoms, which can be intermittent. The diagnosis and management of NETs is therefore challenging.

A variety of NETs are recognized and include:

- Carcinoid tumours.
- Insulinomas.
- Gastrinomas.
- PPomas (PP, pancreatic polypeptide).
- VIPomas (VIP, vasoactive intestinal peptide).
- Glucagonomas.
- Other (e.g. somatostatinomas).
- Non-functioning tumours.

## Carcinoid tumours

- Occur in 2–3/100,000 population, although this may be an underestimate.
- Classically divided in to those arising from the foregut, midgut, or hindgut, but may also develop in other sites, e.g. bronchial or thymic carcinoids.
- Multiple secretory products have been identified including serotonin, histamine, tachykinins, kallikrein, and prostaglandins.

Carcinoid tumours classically present with the carcinoid syndrome (CS), caused by elevated circulating serotonin levels. Features include:

- **Cutaneous flushing** (85%, spontaneous or induced, e.g. by certain food types, alcohol, or exercise).
- **Diarrhoea** (80%, watery, up to 30×/day, explosive).
- **Wheezing** due to bronchospasm (20%, often during flushing).
- **Pellagra-like skin lesions** (due to nicotinamide deficiency secondary to excessive tryptophan metabolism).

CS only develops if vasoactive secretory products escape metabolism by the liver. Therefore, gastrointestinal carcinoids only present with CS once liver metastases have occurred; in contrast, other carcinoid tumours (e.g. bronchial) may produce CS even in the absence of metastases.

- **Carcinoid heart disease:** high serotonin levels can be associated with plaque-like deposits of fibrous tissue on the endocardium of valvular cusps and leaflets. The tricuspid and pulmonary valves are most commonly affected.
- Some patients present with small bowel obstruction due to local adhesions.
- Ascites is also a recognized feature.

### Diagnosis

Screening tests include:

- 24-hour urinary 5-hydroxyindoleacetic acid (5-HIAA) excretion (the end-product of serotonin metabolism)
- Chromogranin A.

Following biochemical confirmation tumour localization may require a combination of cross-sectional imaging (CT and/or MRI), ultrasound (including endoscopic), somatostatin-receptor scintigraphy (e.g. with [111]indium-labelled octreotide) or PET-CT (e.g. [68]gallium-DOTATOC).

## Management of CS and NETs

- Surgical resection rarely affords cure as the majority of patients with CS present with liver metastases, and therefore treatment often focuses on symptom control using somatostatin analogues (e.g. octreotide, lanreotide), and palliative procedures (e.g. hepatic wedge resection, chemo-embolization of liver metastases).
- Recent evidence suggests that somatostatin analogue therapy can slow/halt tumour growth in some NET patients.
- Radioactive isotopes (e.g. [90]YDOTA octreotide and [177]Lu octreotate) have also shown promise in achieving partial remission and relief of symptoms.
- Conventional chemotherapy (e.g. 5-fluorouracil (or its prodrug capecitabine) and streptozotocin) may be tried, but responses are often short-lived.
- Tyrosine kinase inhibitors (e.g. sunitinib) may improve progression-free and overall survival in pancreatic NETs.

## Insulinoma

- Rare (incidence ~1–2 cases per million population/year).
- Usually present with neuroglycopenic (e.g. confusion, visual change, unusual behaviour) and autonomic (palpitations, diaphoresis, tremulousness) symptoms.

### Diagnosis

- Before embarking on investigation of possible hypoglycaemia it is important to ensure that the criteria for Whipple triad (symptoms/signs of hypoglycaemia, low plasma glucose concentration, resolution of symptoms/signs after plasma glucose concentration is raised) are met.
- When a spontaneous hypoglycaemic episode can not be observed, it may be possible to provoke hypoglycaemia during a formal supervised 72-hour fast.
- Although a cut-off of <2.2mmol/L has traditionally been used to define biochemical hypoglycaemia, recent guidelines suggest that a higher threshold (<3.0mmol/L) may be acceptable for triggering further investigation, provided that Whipple triad is present.
- In insulinoma, absolute insulin levels are not necessarily elevated, but are inappropriate for the ambient glucose concentration; C-peptide levels are also inappropriate, and the proinsulin:insulin ratio is typically elevated (insulin is derived from proinsulin after cleavage of C-peptide).
- ► C-peptide and sulfonylurea assays are helpful to exclude factitious insulin and sulfonylurea use.
- Preoperative localization often requires several modalities, e.g. CT/MRI abdomen (Fig. 7.44), endoscopic ultrasound, selective angiography (Fig. 7.45), octreotide scintigraphy (Fig. 7.46).

### Treatment

- Surgical resection is often curative.
- In cases where surgery is not feasible or is incomplete, treatment with diazoxide and octreotide may be effective in ameliorating hypoglycaemia, although the latter can exacerbate hypoglycaemia in some patients (through suppression of other counter-regulatory hormones, e.g. glucagon).

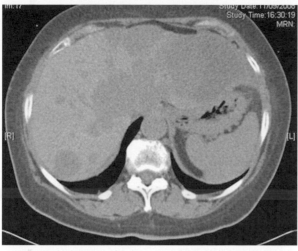

Fig. 7.44 Abdominal CT scan showing multiple hepatic metastases in a patient with malignant insulinoma.

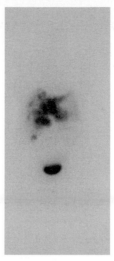

Fig. 7.46 $^{111}$In-labelled octreotide scintigraphy confirming avid uptake by metastatic insulinoma (same patient as in Fig. 7.44).

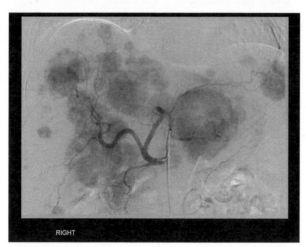

Fig. 7.45 Selective coeliac axis angiography demonstrating multiple tumour blushes, indicating multiple hepatic metastases (same patient as in Fig. 7.44).

## Gastrinoma

- Gastrinomas are rare (estimated prevalence of 1 per million population), but should be suspected if oesophageal/peptic ulcer disease is associated with breakthrough symptoms/frequent recurrence despite medical therapy, there are multiple ulcers, or if ulcers are located distal to the duodenum.
- ▶ Although ideally fasting plasma gastrin levels should be measured off PPI therapy, this may not be feasible due to symptoms, and in some patients can put them at risk of major/ life-threatening GI haemorrhage.
- A fasting gut hormone profile and chromogranin A levels should also be checked.
- Tumour localization is usually carried out using similar tests to those described for insulinoma. Endoscopic ultrasound can be particularly helpful in localizing small tumours in the head of the pancreas or wall of the duodenum.
- Medical treatment with high-dose PPI and H$_2$-blocker therapy is often required to control symptoms. Surgery is typically non-curative due to the multifocal nature of the disease.

# 7.20 Acid–base disorders

## Background

- Recall:
$$pH \propto \frac{[HCO_3^-]}{PaCO_2} \text{ or } \frac{kidneys}{lungs} \text{ (metabolic disorders)}$$
- The clinical approach to acid–base disturbances centres around correct evaluation of the type of abnormality, and then integrating this with the patient's history, examination findings and investigation results to get the correct differential diagnosis (Fig. 7.47).

## Alkalosis

### Metabolic alkalosis

- Gastrointestinal acid losses (vomiting).
- Hypokalaemia.
- Renal acid loss:
  - Mineralocorticoid excess
  - Diuretics
- Milk-alkali syndrome
- Post-hypercapnic alkalosis.
- $HCO_3^-$ administration.

NB: a very high serum $[HCO_3^-]$ (>45mmol/L) is only seen with repeated vomiting.

### Respiratory alkalosis

- Due to CNS stimulation:
  - Anxiety
  - Hypoxia
  - Salicylate poisoning (+ metabolic acidosis)
  - Encephalitis
  - Brainstem injury.
- Due to pulmonary disease:
  - Asthma
  - Pneumonia
  - Pulmonary embolism

| Normal values | |
| --- | --- |
| Arterial blood pH | 7.35–7.45 |
| $[HCO_3^-]$ | 24–30 mmol/L |
| $pCO_2$ | 4.7–6.0 kPa (35–45 mmHg) |
| Base excess | +/–2 mmol/L |
| Anion gap | 8–12 mmol/L |

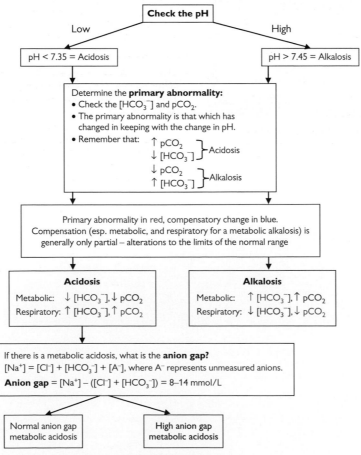

Fig. 7.47 Decision tree for acid–base analysis, based on arterial blood gas analysis.

- Pulmonary fibrosis
- Pulmonary oedema.

## Acidosis

### Metabolic acidosis

- Has deleterious effects on the function of many organ systems, although the clinical picture may also be due to the underlying cause.
- Reduces cardiac contractility, predisposes to arrhythmias, and vasodilates central vessels (but causes peripheral vasoconstriction).
- Causes impaired consciousness.
- Respiratory compensation = increased ventilation; deep, sighing, Kussmaul respiration. Check the $[HCO_3^-]$ in patients presenting with dyspnoea and no obvious cause! See Box 7.3.
- Acidosis also causes hyperkalaemia: $H^+$ entry into cells $\rightarrow \uparrow K^+$ exit (to maintain a normal membrane potential).
- The buffering action of bone in chronic acidosis results in $Ca^{2+}$ loss from the skeleton.

*Causes of a normal anion gap metabolic acidosis*
Loss of bicarbonate or failure of acid secretion. The fall in plasma $[HCO_3^-]$ is accompanied by an equal rise in chloride $[Cl^-]$.
- Diarrhoea.
- Urinary diversion procedures (ureterosigmoidostomy/ileal conduit)—the bowel exchanges $Cl^-$ in the urine for $HCO_3^-$.
- Renal tubular acidosis (see Section 17.17).
- Acetazolamide.

*Causes of a high anion gap metabolic acidosis*
Addition of a new acid to the body ($H^+A^-$).
- Ketoacidosis (diabetic or alcoholic).
- Lactic acidosis (tissue hypoxia or ischaemia (shock, bowel infarction), drugs (metformin)).
- Severe renal failure (uraemic acidosis).
- Ingested acid:
  - Ethylene glycol (antifreeze)
  - Methanol
  - Salicylates.

### Treatment of metabolic acidosis

- Should be guided by **diagnosis and treatment of the underlying cause**. Correction of circulatory disturbance, hypovolaemia, hyperkalaemia, and treatment of infection and hyperglycaemia are priorities.

- Administration of exogenous $HCO_3^-$ is generally of little benefit. At high concentrations (8.4%) it may actually worsen the intracellular acidosis ('paradoxical acidosis'), and the associated sodium load can exacerbate fluid overload.
- Isotonic (1.26%) $NaHCO_3$ may be useful as part of fluid replacement in the moderately unwell patient with acidosis and hyperkalaemia who is euvolaemic.
- Haemodialysis or continuous renal replacement therapy (haemofiltration) are of superior utility in the correction of acidosis in the unwell patient with renal impairment, especially when combined with care in an ICU/HDU environment.

### Respiratory acidosis

- Chronic obstructive pulmonary disease, neuromuscular disorders, opiate overdose—any cause of respiratory failure (see Section 18.4).
- This is type II respiratory failure: low $PaO_2$ (<8kPa) and elevated $PaCO_2$ (>6.5kPa).
- With chronic respiratory acidosis the respiratory centre loses its response to increases in $PaCO_2$ and respiratory drive becomes dependant on hypoxia—hence the caution required when administering high concentrations of inspired $O_2$ to such patients; their stimulus to respiration disappears as $PaO_2$ rises.

# 7.21 Sodium disorders

## Hyponatraemia

- Hyponatraemia results from an imbalance between body sodium and water content. It is relatively common in medical inpatients, and is associated with a poor prognosis. See Fig. 7.48.
- Diagnosing the cause depends on thorough history taking and accurate clinical assessment of volume status (Box 7.4).
- Hyponatraemia is almost invariably associated with hypo-osmolality (if plasma osmolality and sodium are discordant look for the presence of another osmotically active agent, e.g. glucose).

### Clinical presentation

- This depends on the rate of change in serum sodium as much as the absolute value.
- Elderly patients with chronic hyponatraemia may not exhibit any symptoms, whereas a young patient whose sodium has rapidly fallen from normal to 125mmol/L may be extremely symptomatic.
- Most patients with a serum $Na^+$ >125mmol/L are asymptomatic. Neuropsychiatric symptoms dominate once the serum $Na^+$ falls below 125mmol/L.
- In ↑ order of severity:
  - Anorexia
  - Headache
  - Nausea and vomiting
  - Lethargy
  - Personality change
  - Muscle cramps and weakness
  - Confusion
  - Ataxia
  - Drowsiness
  - Hyporeflexia
  - Convulsions
  - Coma
  - Death
- As serum $Na^+$ falls the extracellular fluid becomes increasingly hypotonic. This causes movement of water into the brain and hence cerebral oedema. However, if the change in serum $Na^+$

276

---

### Box 7.4 Clinical assessment of volume status

- History:
  - Diarrhoea/vomiting.
  - Diuretics.
  - Improving or worsening oedema.
- Examination:
  - Jugular venous pressure.
  - Postural blood pressure.
  - Presence or absence of oedema.

---

is not too abrupt, the brain can adapt to the reduced osmolality through loss of electrolytes (over hours), and later loss of organic solutes (hours–days).

### Treatment of hyponatraemia

- Correctly assess the patient for an underlying cause and find any recent/past U&E.
- The rate of change of serum sodium, and presence of symptoms, are the most important guides to therapy.

Acute, symptomatic, hyponatraemia (i.e. onset within 48 hours and with laboratory evidence to confirm this):

- Patients with neurological manifestations, especially seizures and coma, require correction of their serum $Na^+$ with hypertonic saline. Seek senior advice.
- Seizures should be treated as usual with IV benzodiazepine.
- Hypertonic saline (3% NaCl) should be infused at a rate of 1–2mL/hour per kg body weight, aiming to increase serum $Na^+$ by 1–2mmol/L per hour until symptoms resolve or serum $Na^+$ is >125mmol/L (also see next page).
- Regular re-assessment of the patient's clinical condition and serum electrolytes is absolutely essential. The patient should be managed in a HDU, or similar.
- Loop diuretics may be used to ↑ free water clearance.

**NB:** various equations exist to guide sodium replacement (Adrogué HJ & Madias, 2000a) and can be very useful, but most don't account for ongoing $Na^+$ losses. Repeated clinical and biochemical assessment is still mandatory.

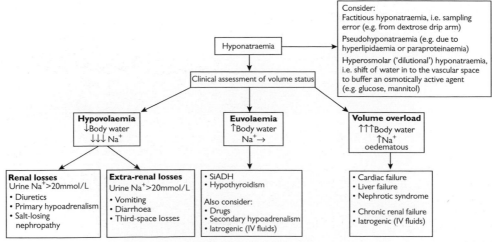

**Fig. 7.48** Algorithm for the assessment of the hyponatraemic patient.

## Box 7.5 Central pontine myelinolysis (CPM)

- The brain slowly adapts to hyponatraemia and hypotonicity by loss of organic solutes. This (partially) corrects the brain swelling that occurs with hypotonicity.
- After this process, the brain contains relatively less solute and rapid infusion of hypertonic fluids can lead to brain shrinkage and osmotic demyelination. Pontine neurones are particularly susceptible.

*Risk factors*
- Chronic alcoholism and/or liver failure.
- Malnutrition.
- Potassium depletion.
- Severe burns.
- Most importantly the **severity** (Na <120mmol/L) and **chronicity** (>48 hours) of hyponatraemia.

*The clinical picture is of a biphasic illness with:*
- Encephalopathy associated with rapid rise in serum Na$^+$.
- 2–3 days later:
  - Behavioural changes.
  - Cranial nerve palsies.
  - Progressive weakness → quadriplegia.
  - 'Locked-in' syndrome.

*Diagnosis*
- Pontine demyelination on T2-weighted MRI.
- Lesions may not be evident for 1-2 weeks after the event.

### Chronic, symptomatic, hyponatraemia

- If hyponatraemia is known to be chronic, or the rate of onset is unknown, then correction should be instituted much more cautiously—these are the patients at greatest risk of over-zealous correction and central pontine (CPM) or extrapontine myelinolysis (see Box 7.5).
- If neurological manifestations, then aim to raise the serum Na$^+$ by 1mmol/L per hour in the early stages of correction, but not more than 10–12mmol/L over 24 hours.
- Again, regular clinical and biochemical assessment is crucial and treatment should only be undertaken in a HDU or similar.

### Chronic, asymptomatic, hyponatraemia

- Gentle, gradual correction is the key for these patients
- Seek and treat the underlying condition where possible
- For SIADH (Box 7.6) consider fluid restriction, demeclocyline may help (blocks action of ADH on the kidney), vaptans (specific vasopressin V$_2$ receptor antagonists).

## Box 7.6 Syndrome of inappropriate ADH (SIADH)

- This is a diagnosis of exclusion.
- Inappropriately high levels of ADH secretion relative to the plasma osmolality → water reabsorption by the kidneys and formation of inappropriately concentrated urine.
- Said to be common in hospitals, but probably less so if the criteria are rigorously applied (Clayton et al., 2006).

*Causes*
See Table 7.24.

*Diagnostic criteria*
- True hyponatraemia (<135mmol/L).
- Plasma hypo-osmolality (<275mosmol/kg).
- Less than maximally dilute urine (osmolality >100mosmol/kg).
- Excessive urinary Na$^+$ excretion (>30mmol/L).
- Clinical euvolaemia.
- Normal renal, adrenal, and thyroid function.
- No recent diuretic therapy.

### Table 7.24 Causes of SIADH

| | | |
|---|---|---|
| Malignancy (ectopic ADH) | • Lung (especially small cell) | • Prostatic |
| | • Pancreatic | • Duodenal |
| CNS disorders (↑ release ADH) | • Meningoencephalitis | • Sub-arachnoid/ subdural haemorrhage |
| | • CNS tumours | • Head injury |
| | • Cerebral abscess | • Stroke |
| | • Guillain–Barré syndrome | |
| Chest disease | • Tuberculosis | • Abscess |
| | • Pneumonia (esp. *Legionella*) | • Aspergillosis |
| | • Positive pressure ventilation | |
| Drugs (lots of 'Cs') | • Chlorpromazine | • Cytotoxics |
| | • Carbamazepine | • Tricyclic antidepressants |
| | • Psychotropics | • Opiates |
| | • SSRIs | • Ecstasy |
| | • Desmopressin (DDAVP) | • Nicotine |
| Other | • Porphyria (acute intermittent) | • HIV |
| | • Postoperative: severe nausea, pain | |

# Hypernatraemia

- Represents a deficit of water relative to Na$^+$ (Fig. 7.49).
- Always associated with hyperosmolality.
- Requires either an inability to access sources of water, or an impairment of thirst.
- Thus most common in:
  - Infants.
  - Patients with an impaired mental status.
  - The elderly, where the cause is often multifactorial.
  - ITU patients.
- Na$^+$>160mmol/L in adults is associated with 75% mortality, although this is at least in part due to associated morbidity.

## Clinical features

- Reflect rate of change of serum Na$^+$ in addition to absolute value.
- Excessive thirst (but may disappear as Na$^+$ ↑↑).
- Confusion, convulsions, coma.
- Signs of dehydration (if present).

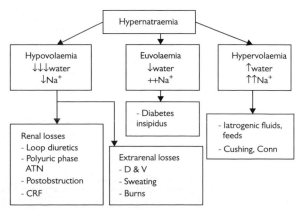

Fig. 7.49 Causes and assessment of hypernatraemia.

- Neurological features result from the increasing plasma osmolality causing water loss from the brain and brain shrinkage. Similar chronic adaptive measures occur as in hyponatraemia.

### Treatment

- Can correct rapidly if an acute change is obvious (generally iatrogenic infusions).
- Otherwise, gradual correction is the aim, ideally with oral/nasogastric water.
- Aim to reduce serum $Na^+$ by <10mmol/L/day.
- If IV fluids are needed, consider beginning with 0.9% sodium chloride (which is likely to be relatively hypotonic compared with the patient), but remember it contains 154mmol/L NaCl which may not be sufficiently hypotonic, and giving a sodium load may worsen some situations. Close monitoring is required (HDU or ITU). If serum sodium does not fall with 0.9% sodium chloride, then consider changing to 0.45% sodium chloride. 5% dextrose is another option, but presents the risk of inducing unduly rapid correction.
- Seek senior advice. Formulae exist to help calculate water deficits (Adrogué HJ & Madias, 2000b).

## References

Adrogué HJ, Madias NE. Hyponatraemia. *N Engl J Med* 2000a: *342*: 1581–9.

Adrogué HJ, Madias NE. Hypernatraemia. *N Engl J Med* 2000b: *342*: 1493–9.

Clayton JA, Le Jeune IR, Hall IP. Severe hyponatraemia in medical in-patients: aetiology, assessment and outcome. *QJM* 2006: *99*(8): 505–11.

## Hypokalaemia

- Results from increased renal or GI losses, or increased cellular uptake (Fig. 7.50).
- Rare in the absence of other disease or medications.
- Diuretics (and Conn syndrome) cause ↓ K⁺ by increasing Na⁺ delivery to the distal tubule where uptake of Na⁺ is accompanied by secretion of K⁺ to maintain electrochemical balance.
- Whilst vomiting directly causes some K⁺ loss, the majority of the hypokalaemia results from the metabolic alkalosis and volume contraction, both of which stimulate renal K⁺ excretion (the latter via activation of the renin–aldosterone axis).
- Hypokalaemia is associated with a metabolic alkalosis, except in the case of renal tubular acidosis (see Section 17.17).

### Clinical presentation

- Palpitations (arrhythmias).
- Muscle weakness and cramps.
- Incidental finding on U&E.
- Polyuria/nocturia (nephrogenic DI).

### The ECG in hypokalaemia

- Prolonged PR interval.
- Flattened T waves, followed by a prominent U wave.
- ST segment depression.
- Peaked P wave.

### Management

- Discontinuation of offending drugs.
- If serum K⁺ >2.5mmol/L and asymptomatic, then oral replacement is appropriate (e.g. Sando-K® tablets).
- If serum K⁺ <2.5mmol/L or evidence of cardiac arrhythmias, then IV therapy is necessary, aiming to replace at a rate <20mmol/hour (e.g. give 1L 0.9% saline containing 20–40mmol/L KCl over a few hours).
- Continuous ECG monitoring may be required until abnormalities resolve.
- Always remember to check serum Mg²⁺: hypomagnesaemia may make hypokalaemia refractory to treatment.
- ↓ Mg²⁺ promotes cellular K⁺ uptake and ↓ renal excretion.
- Causes of ↑ cellular uptake include insulin, β₂-agonists and alkalosis (see Potassium homeostasis).

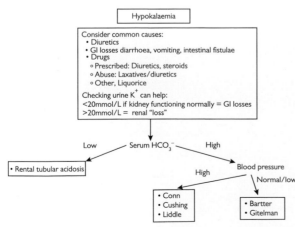

Fig. 7.50 Assessment algorithm for hypokalaemia.

## Bartter syndrome

- Autosomal recessive. Mutations in the genes encoding NKCC2 (see Fig. 7.13 in Section 7.2), K⁺ or Cl⁻ channels also in the same cell.
- Normal BP despite high renin levels because of volume contraction.
- See Section 17.17.

### Gitelman syndrome

- Autosomal recessive. Mutations inactivate NCCT, the thiazide-sensitive Na⁺/Cl⁻ co-transporter in the distal convoluted tubule.
- Present later than Bartter (often adulthood), with ↓ K⁺, muscle weakness, cramps, tetany (↓ Mg²⁺).
- See renal tubular acidosis (see Section 17.17).

### Liddle syndrome

- Autosomal dominant
- Activating mutations in the epithelial Na⁺ channel (ENaC) in the collecting duct (see Fig. 7.13 in Section 7.2).
- Salt-retention leads to volume expansion and early-onset hypertension; presents in teens and young adults.
- Hypokalaemic metabolic alkalosis.
- Appears similar to Conn syndrome, but low renin/aldosterone.

*Treatment*

- Amiloride/triamterene (block ENaC).
- Salt-restriction and potassium replacement.

### Hypokalaemic periodic paralysis

- Rare, often with autosomal dominant inheritance.
- Episodic paralysis, classically at night while patient asleep.
- Legs >arms; proximal >distal; rarely bulbar/respiratory.
- Precipitated by: alcohol, large carbohydrate meals, high salt diet, anxiety/stress, IV glucose + insulin.
- Treatment: K⁺ supplements, K⁺-sparing diuretics.
- Associated with thyrotoxicosis in Asian (Chinese, Japanese) men aged 20–50 years.
- May see hypokalaemia-associated arrhythmias.
- Correct K⁺, then treat thyroid disease which prevents paralysis.
- Propranolol effective.

## Hyperkalaemia

- ⚠ Severe hyperkalaemia is a medical emergency:
- Most of the body's K⁺ is intracellular where it determines the resting membrane potential of excitable cells (see Potassium homeostasis, Section 7.2).
- In the myocardium, increased excitability follows a rise in extracellular K⁺—demonstrated by ECG changes and the development of cardiac arrhythmias.

### Causes

- The kidney is responsible for K⁺ excretion and hyperkalaemia most commonly results from reduced renal excretory capacity.
- Hyperkalaemia may also be due to a shift in K⁺ out of cells, either due to reduced cellular uptake or cell death (Table 7.25).
- The hyperkalaemia of acute renal failure is thus often multifactorial: reduced renal excretory capacity (possibly compounded by

| Table 7.25 Causes of hyperkalaemia | | |
|---|---|---|
| Reduced renal K⁺ excretion | • Oligo-anuric renal failure<br>• ACE inhibitors, ARBs, K⁺-sparing diuretics<br>NSAIDs (via ↓ prostaglandins which mediate K⁺ excretion)<br>Trimethoprim & pentamidine (both block K⁺ excretion)<br>Calcineurin inhibitors<br>• Primary hypoadrenalism<br>• Hyperkalaemic distal renal tubular acidosis (type IV) | |
| K⁺ shift out of cells | Reduced cellular K⁺ uptake | • Metabolic acidosis (acute phase of diabetic ketoacidosis, uraemic)<br>• Digoxin |
| Others | Release from damaged cells | • Rhabdomyolysis<br>• Tumour lysis syndrome<br>• Burns |
| | Iatrogenic | • Excess IV K⁺ therapy |
| | Artefactual | • Haemolysed sample |

| Table 7.26 ECG changes in hyperkalemia | |
|---|---|
| Serum K⁺ (mmol/L) | ECG changes |
| 6–7 | Peaked or 'tented' T waves (present in all leads) |
| 7–8 | Flattening of p waves and prolongation of QRS |
| 8–9 | Sine wave pattern |
| > 9 | Ventricular fibrillation or asystole |

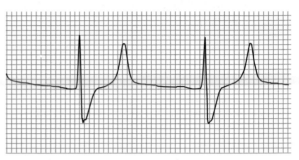

**Fig. 7.51** The ECG in hyperkalaemia.

concomitant drug therapy), uraemic acidosis driving K⁺ out of cells, and potentially K⁺ release (rhabdomyolysis).

### ECG changes in hyperkalaemia

- A typical pattern of ECG changes follows the progression of hyperkalaemia (Table 7.26).
- These changes may not always be present and patients with a normal baseline ECG may also develop arrhythmias.

Fig. 7.51 shows an ECG taken from a patient with a serum K⁺ of 8.0mmol/L demonstrating the classic changes of hyperkalaemia: tented T waves, flattening of P waves and prolongation of the QRS complex.

### Clinical presentation

- Most commonly an incidental finding on 'routine' U&E or ABGs.
- May present with weakness or palpitations.

### Management

- Urgent treatment of hyperkalaemia should be instituted if serum K⁺ >6.5mmol/L, or if any ECG changes are present.
- See Section 1.11.

# 7.23 Hypocalcaemia

## Aetiology/pathophysiology

Hypocalcaemia is mostly commonly related to abnormalities of parathyroid hormone (PTH) secretion/action, and vitamin D deficiency/resistance. The major causes of hypocalcaemia are shown in Table 7.27.

▶ As 40–45% of serum calcium is protein-bound, a fall in binding protein (e.g. albumin) levels will be associated with a decrease in measured total serum calcium but not free, bioavailable calcium—for this reason most laboratories also report a corrected calcium level, i.e. adjusted for variations in albumin:

cCa = serum Ca + 0.02 × (normal albumin—patient albumin)

The balance between total and free calcium is also affected by changes in acid–base status and occasionally by the presence of anions (e.g. citrate), such that clinical manifestations of hypocalcaemia may occur in alkalosis and following extensive blood transfusion, even though the measured total serum level lies within the normal range—in these cases the direct measurement of free (= ionized) calcium level can be helpful.

## Clinical evaluation

### Signs and symptoms

Clinical features depend on the duration and severity of the hypocalcaemia.

Acute/severe falls in serum calcium are associated with:

- Tetany: characterized by neuromuscular irritability with symptoms ranging from mild (e.g. perioral numbness, paraesthesia (especially hands and feet) and muscle cramps) to severe (e.g. carpopedal spasm, laryngeal spasm and seizures):
  - Carpopedal spasm is characterized by adduction of the thumb, flexion of the metacarpophalangeal joints, extension of the interphalangeal joints, and flexion of the wrist.
  - Trousseau sign—carpopedal spasm induced by inflation of a sphygmomanometer cuff above systolic blood pressure for 3 minutes.
  - Chvostek sign refers to contractions of the facial muscles elicited by tapping the facial nerve anterior to the ear (may occur in up to 10% of normocalcaemic subjects).
- Papilloedema.

Clinical manifestations of chronic and disease-specific hypocalcaemia include:

- Lethargy/malaise and, rarely, psychosis.
- Dry coarse skin, brittle sparse hair with patchy alopecia, brittle nails with characteristic transverse grooves.

- Dental abnormalities (e.g. enamel hypoplasia) if hypocalcaemia occurs during the development of permanent teeth; may be associated with skeletal (e.g. craniofacial) abnormalities.
- Candidiasis (resistant to antifungals) in polyglandular autoimmune hyoparathyroidism.
- Basal ganglia calcification with extrapyramidal features, cataracts and keratoconjunctivitis in chronic hypoparathyroidism.
- Cardiac arrhythmias and conduction abnormalities (e.g. prolongation of QT interval).

*Pseudohypoparathyroidism*

- Reflects resistance to the action of PTH, resulting in hypocalcaemia and hyperphosphataemia despite elevated PTH levels.
- May also be associated with resistance to TSH.
- Classical phenotypic features include short stature, rounded face, short 4th and 5th metacarpals, obesity (= Albright hereditary osteodystrophy); = type 1A.
- Some patients lack the skeletal manifestations; = type 1B or type 2.
- Other patients exhibit the classical skeletal features, but have normal calcium metabolism—traditionally referred to as pseudopseudohypoparathyroidism.

### Investigations

▶ As with hypercalcaemia, measurement of paired serum PTH and calcium levels is the key to determining the cause of hypocalcaemia in most patients:

- Serum PTH is reduced or inappropriately normal in patients with hypoparathyroidism.
- Serum PTH is elevated in acute or chronic kidney disease, vitamin D deficiency, and pseudohypoparathyroidism.
- Serum PTH is typically normal or low in patients with hypomagnesaemia (routine serum Mg measurement is advised).

Other investigations will be determined by the clinical presentation and may include:

- FBC, electrolytes, renal/liver/bone function tests, arterial blood gas, vitamin D metabolites (25-hydroxyvitamin $D_3$ and 1,25-dihydroxyvitamin $D_3$), amylase, urinary calcium and magnesium excretion.
- Modified Ellsworth–Howard test—to demonstrate a failure to increase urinary cAMP and phosphate excretion in response to infused PTH in pseudohypoparathyroidism.
- Targeted imaging ± isotope bone scintigraphy in suspected cases of malignancy.

| Table 7.27 Causes of hypocalcaemia | | |
|---|---|---|
| Low PTH (i.e. hypoparathyroidism) | High PTH/vitamin D related | Others |
| Destruction/failure of parathyroid glands:<br>  Idiopathic<br>  Post surgery<br>  Autoimmune polyglandular syndrome type 1<br>  Irradiation<br>  Infiltration (e.g. haemochromatosis, Wilson disease, granulomatous disorders, metastatic cancer)<br>Abnormal parathyroid development:<br>  Di George syndrome<br>Impaired PTH secretion:<br>  Hypomagnesaemia<br>  Activating mutations of the calcium sensing receptor<br>  Cinacalcet therapy (calcimimetic) | Resistance to PTH action:<br>  Drugs that impair osteoclastic bone resorption, e.g. bisphosphonates, calcitonin<br>  Renal failure<br>  Pseudohypoparathyroidism<br>Vitamin D deficiency/resistance:<br>  See Table 7.30, Section 7.27 | Calcium chelators, e.g. citrate<br>Osteoblastic metastases<br>Acute, necrotizing pancreatitis<br>Alkalosis (increased albumin binding), e.g. during hyperventilation<br>Severe hyperphosphataemia:<br>  Tumour lysis<br>  Rhabdomyolysis<br>  Acute renal failure |

*Inherited vitamin D disorders*
See Section 7.27.

# Management

### Severe symptomatic hypocalcaemia

- Severe symptomatic hypocalcaemia is treated with 10–20mL of 10% calcium gluconate IV (containing 90mg = 2.25mmol of elemental calcium per 10mL ampoule).
- ► Calcium-containing solutions **must** be infused slowly (e.g. 10mL of calcium gluconate given over a 10-minute period) to reduce the risk of precipitating arrhythmias—cardiac monitoring is advised.
- Thereafter, a continuous infusion is often required for the first 24 hours (e.g. 40mL of 10% calcium gluconate infused over 24 hours), with frequent monitoring of serum calcium.
- Oral calcium and vitamin D supplementation should be initiated concurrently (see management for chronic hypocalcaemia).
- ► Refractory hypocalcaemia occurs in patients with hypomagnesaemia, and hence magnesium levels should be checked and hypomagnesaemia corrected.

### Chronic hypocalcaemia

- Wherever possible, the underlying cause should be corrected. Mg levels should always be normalized.
- For hypoparathyroidism, PTH replacement is not routinely available, and therefore the more potent forms of vitamin $D_3$ (alfacalcidol or calcitriol) are used to maintain plasma calcium. For patients with adequate dietary calcium intake additional calcium supplements are often not required.
- The aim of treatment in hypoparathyroidism is to achieve a 'safe' serum calcium level—typically at, or just below, the lower limit of the reference range. Use of higher vitamin D doses in an attempt to fully normalize serum calcium levels results in hypercalciuria (due to the absence of PTH) increasing the risk of nephrolithiasis and nephrocalcinosis.
- Preliminary data suggests PTH replacement (administered as an s.c. infusion) may offer some benefits, but further studies (including of longer term renal outcomes) will be required before this can be considered for routine practice.
- For treatment of osteomalacia, see Section 7.27.

# 7.24 Hypercalcaemia

## Aetiology/pathophysiology

True hypercalcaemia occurs when the free (ionized) calcium level is elevated. In an outpatient setting the majority of cases are due to primary hyperparathyroidism (see Section 7.25), while in sick inpatients ~50% of cases are associated with malignancy. The major causes of hypercalcaemia are shown in Box 7.7, and mechanisms of malignant hypercalcaemia in Box 7.8.

▶ The degree of hypercalcaemia may provide a clue to the underlying diagnosis: in primary hyperparathyroidism serum calcium levels are commonly <3.0mmol/L, while values >3.25mmol/L are more suggestive of malignancy. However, there is considerable overlap, and for any cause calcium levels may rise further in the event of intercurrent illness with superadded dehydration.

▶ As 40–45% of serum calcium is protein-bound, a rise in binding protein (e.g. albumin) levels will be associated with an increase in measured total serum calcium but not free, bioavailable calcium—for this reason most laboratories also report a corrected calcium level, i.e. adjusted for variations in albumin:

cCa = serum ca + 0.02 × (normal albumin—patient albumin)

## Clinical evaluation

### Signs and symptoms

Mild hypercalcaemia (serum calcium <3.0mmol/L) is often asymptomatic and an incidental finding, although with the benefit of hindsight patients may report non-specific symptoms including constipation, fatigue, and depressive features. Even serum calcium levels of 3.0–3.5mmol/L may be remarkably well tolerated if the onset is gradual.

Other patients may present with clinical features perhaps best remembered according to the mnemonic 'stones, bones, abdominal groans, and psychic moans':

* 'Stones'—nephrolithiasis, renal colic, nephrocalcinosis.

### Box 7.8 Mechanisms of hypercalcaemia in malignancy

* Tumour secretion of parathyroid hormone-related peptide/protein (PTHrP) (e.g. squamous cell carcinoma of lung).
* Osteolytic metastases with local release of osteoclast activating cytokines (e.g. breast, bronchus, kidney or thyroid cancer).
* Production of cytokines that promote bone resorption (e.g. receptor activator of nuclear factor κB ligand (RANKL) in multiple myeloma).
* Production/activation of vitamin D within tumour tissue (e.g. rarely in lymphoma).

* 'Bones'—muscle weakness, bone pain, arthritis, reduced cortical bone mass, low-impact fractures.
* 'Abdominal groans'—nausea, vomiting, constipation, anorexia, peptic ulcer disease, pancreatitis.
* 'Psychic moans'—anxiety, depression, cognitive dysfunction. Lethargy, confusion, stupor, and coma may occur in severe cases.

Other typical presentations include polyuria (due to nephrogenic diabetes insipidus), polydipsia, acute or chronic renal failure, renal tubular acidosis, dehydration, anorexia, nausea, and changes in sensorium.

These signs and symptoms are either a direct consequence of the high calcium level itself (e.g. polyuria, polydipsia) or arise from complications secondary to a chronically elevated calcium level (e.g. renal stones, osteoporosis).

Band keratopathy, signifying subepithelial calcium phosphate deposits in the cornea, is a rare manifestation of chronic hypercalcaemia.

▶ Shortening of the QT interval on ECG may also be seen in hypercalcaemic states. Arrhythmias (e.g. bradycardia and first-degree atrioventricular block) and digitalis sensitivity can occur.

A careful drug history should be taken in all patients with hypercalcaemia (Box 7.7), and a family history sought for evidence of familial parathyroid disorders, including multiple endocrine neoplasia (MEN) (see Section 7.18), and familial hypocalciuric hypercalcaemia (FHH). The latter is a rare genetic disorder associated with loss-of-function mutations in the calcium-sensing receptor in the parathyroid glands and the kidney, leading to elevated PTH levels and hypercalcaemia. However, unlike primary hyperparathyroidism, complications are rare and treatment is generally not required.

### Investigations

▶ Measurement of paired serum PTH and calcium levels is the key to determining the cause of hypercalcaemia in most patients:

* Elevated or inappropriately normal PTH levels with hypercalcaemia signify hyperparathyroidism. The investigation and management of hyperparathyroidism is discussed in Section 7.25.
* Hypercalcaemia with suppressed PTH levels requires further investigations. An underlying malignant disorder must be excluded before ruling out other, rarer causes (Box 7.7).

Other investigations will be determined by the clinical presentation, but may include:

* FBC, ESR, electrolytes, renal/liver/bone function tests, serum ACE level.
* Chest radiograph—looking for changes of sarcoidosis (bilateral hilar lymphadenopathy, infiltrates) and primary or secondary malignancy.
* Abdominal radiograph or renal ultrasound to rule out nephrolithiasis/nephrocalcinosis.
* Targeted imaging ± isotope bone scintigraphy in suspected cases of malignancy.
* Serum electrophoresis, urinary testing for Bence Jones protein, and skeletal survey for possible myeloma.

### Box 7.7 Causes of hypercalcaemia

*Parathyroid dependent*
* Primary hyperparathyroidism.
* Tertiary hyperparathyroidism.
* Lithium therapy.
* Familial hypocalciuric hypercalcaemia (FHH).

*Parathyroid independent*
* Malignancy (see Box 7.8).
* Vitamin D related:
  * Excess ingestion.
  * Granulomatous disorders.
  * William syndrome.
* Endocrine disorders:
  * Thyrotoxicosis.
  * Adrenal failure.
  * Phaeochromocytoma.
* Other causes:
  * Drugs, e.g. thiazide diuretics.
  * Acute renal failure.
  * Milk-alkali syndrome (excess ingestion of calcium and absorbable alkali).
  * Prolonged immobilization.
  * Vitamin A intoxication.
  * Jansen metaphyseal chondrodysplasia.

- 1,25-dihydroxyvitamin D if extra-renal production (e.g. in sarcoidosis, certain malignant tumours) or vitamin D intoxication is suspected.
- PTH related peptide (PTHrp, see Box 7.7) measurement is possible, but not routinely undertaken.
- Thyroid function tests, Synacthen® test, urinary/plasma metanephrines/catecholamines.
- 24-hour urinary calcium: measurement of the calcium to creatinine clearance ratio (very low in FHH) can help to distinguish FHH from primary hyperparathyroidism.

## Management

### Mild asymptomatic hypercalcaemia

- No immediate treatment is required if the patient is asymptomatic with a corrected calcium of <3mmol/L.
- However, he/she should be advised to avoid factors that may aggravate hypercalcaemia, e.g. excess dietary calcium (including calcium-containing antacids) and/or vitamin D ingestion, offending drugs (e.g. thiazide diuretics, lithium), dehydration, prolonged bed rest or inactivity.
- Treatment can then by directed at the underlying cause once further investigations have been completed.

### Moderate–severe hypercalcaemia

- Although some patients with moderate hypercalcaemia (i.e. 3.0–3.5mmol/L) remain relatively asymptomatic, they are at significant risk of developing more marked hypercalcaemia, e.g. during intercurrent illness, and the majority of patients with serum calcium levels in excess of 3.0mmol/L require active treatment in addition to the lifestyle measures previously outlined.
- The extent and aggressiveness of intervention is dependent on symptoms, comorbidity, magnitude of hypercalcaemia, and underlying cause, but may include:

*Rehydration*

- Intravenous 0.9% saline: typically 3–6L over the first 24 hours, aiming to maintain a urine output of at least 100–150mL/hour. In most cases this alone will reduce calcium levels sufficiently.
- Caution should be exercised in those with renal impairment and/or cardiac failure (consider CVP monitoring).

*Active promotion of renal calcium excretion*

- Loop diuretics (e.g. furosemide) are generally reserved for those patients at risk of fluid overload—in all other patients the risk of exacerbating intravascular depletion probably outweighs any potential benefit of promoting renal calcium excretion.
- In those with severe hypercalcaemia and renal impairment, dialysis may help to stabilize fluid balance and reduce serum calcium levels.

*Bisphosphonates*

- Following adequate rehydration, an intravenous bisphosphonate (e.g. disodium pamidronate, typically 30–60mg in a single infusion or in divided doses—up to a maximum of 90mg) may be used to lower calcium levels over the next few days. The hypocalcaemic effect usually lasts for several weeks, but repeat courses may be required depending on the reversibility of the underlying cause. Oral bisphosphonates can be substituted once the acute phase has settled. Reduced doses are required in those with significant renal impairment.

*Other treatments*

- Glucocorticoids (e.g. prednisolone 40–60mg/day) may be effective in hypercalcaemia due to certain malignancies (e.g. lymphoma, myeloma), sarcoidosis or vitamin D toxicity.
- Calcitonin (initially 5–10 units/kg per day s.c. or i.m. in divided doses) lowers serum calcium levels rapidly in severe/refractory hypercalcaemia, but the effect is often short-lived and side effects (nausea, vomiting, diarrhoea, abdominal pain, flushing) are relatively common.

# 7.25 Hyperparathyroidism

## Background

In **primary hyperparathyroidism**, PTH is overproduced and secreted in an unphysiological manner that is not governed by circulating serum calcium levels. PTH may be raised or normal, but the levels are inappropriate for the ambient serum calcium level.

In **secondary hyperparathyroidism**, PTH secretion is increased as part of the homeostatic response to chronically low serum calcium, typically as a consequence of underlying renal disease and deficiency of activated vitamin D. 1α-hydroxylation of vitamin D occurs within normal kidneys, but this activity diminishes with increasing renal impairment. Thus, secondary hyperparathyroidism is a physiological attempt to restore serum calcium levels to normal, albeit at the expense of bone demineralization. If this process continues unchecked then parathyroid gland function may become autonomous and result in hypercalcaemia (so-called **tertiary hyperparathyroidism**).

## Epidemiology

- With greater automation of biochemical testing, elevated serum calcium levels are detected with increasing frequency in asymptomatic individuals.
- The overall prevalence is estimated at ~0.5% of the population in North America, with a ♀ preponderance (♀:♂ ~2:1).
- Occurs at any age, but is more common in those >45 years.

## Pathophysiology

- The cause of the vast majority of primary hyperparathyroidism cases is unknown.
- The incidence of primary hyperparathyroidism is increased by neck irradiation and lithium treatment.
- Rarely genetic and chromosomal abnormalities cause primary hyperparathyroidism, the most common being multiple endocrine neoplasia (MEN) type 1 (see Section 7.18).
- A single parathyroid adenoma is present in ~90%, whereas in genetic primary hyperparathyroidism all four glands are typically enlarged (parathyroid hyperplasia). The incidence of parathyroid carcinoma is ≤1%.

## Signs and symptoms

- Usually asymptomatic, but neuromuscular and psychiatric symptoms can be subtle. Patients labelled as 'asymptomatic' often 'feel better' following definitive therapy.
- Due to hypercalcaemia (see Section 7.24)
- Due to hyperparathyroidism, e.g. hyperparathyroid renal disease (nephrocalcinosis, nephrolithiasis) or hyperparathyroid bone disease with accompanying bone pain and osteoporosis.

## Differential diagnosis

- Hypercalcaemia due to other causes almost invariably leads to PTH suppression.
- Primary hyperparathyroidism is almost always benign. Parathyroid carcinoma (very high PTH, patients usually have symptoms, palpable neck mass) is very rare.
- Familial hypocalciuric hypercalcaemia (FHH—a genetic disorder caused by loss-of-function mutations in the calcium-sensing receptor, PTH is often normal) is a benign condition which does not require specific treatment and therefore needs to be excluded by demonstrating very low (vs. normal or high in primary hyperparathyroidism) urinary calcium excretion.

## Investigations

Investigations are necessary to:
- Confirm the diagnosis of hyperparathyroidism.
- Exclude alternative diagnoses (e.g. FHH).
- Screen for treatment-determining complications (e.g. reduced bone mineral density, renal complications).
- Localize the parathyroid adenoma preoperatively to facilitate minimally invasive parathyroidectomy.

### Routine biochemistry

- Serum calcium levels are elevated, while serum phosphate levels are low-normal or frankly low. Alkaline phosphatase levels are usually normal or mildly elevated. U&E and eGFR may reveal associated renal impairment.
- 24-hour urinary calcium excretion and/or the calcium:creatinine excretion ratio is typically high in primary hyperparathyroidism (but low in FHH, see earlier in section).
- Vitamin D (see Box 7.9).
- PTH—most laboratories use an assay which does not detect the smaller PTH–related peptide (PTHrP, see Section 7.24).

### Imaging

- Abdominal ultrasound or plain X-ray: useful for identifying/excluding nephrocalcinosis or nephrolithiasis (Fig. 7.52).
- Bone density scan (see Section 7.26): in addition to the hip and vertebral bones the distal radius should be scanned, which is particularly affected in primary hyperparathyroidism.
- Preoperative tumour localization: not necessary in all cases (e.g. for first conventional neck exploration for uncomplicated primary hyperparathyroidism), but very helpful in planning for minimally invasive parathyroidectomy (i.e. only one side of the neck is explored) and in cases requiring surgical re-exploration. Localization imaging/tests include:
  - Ultrasonography (Fig. 7.53).
  - $^{99m}$Tc–sestamibi (Fig. 7.54).
  - CT/MRI of neck and thorax.
  - Venous sampling.

---

**Box 7.9** Vitamin D deficiency in hyperparathyroidism

- Vitamin D deficiency in primary hyperparathyroidism is a relatively common finding. This is because vitamin D deficiency *per se* is common in the general population and because hydroxylation of 25-hydroxy-vitamin D to 1,25-dihydroxy-vitamin D is increased in the presence of elevated PTH levels; however, commonly used assays only measure 25-hydroxy-vitamin D.
- Vitamin D deficiency can lead to secondary and tertiary hyperparathyroidism or worsen primary hyperparathyroidism. Vitamin D should therefore be replaced to increase plasma levels to the season-adjusted, upper reference range under careful monitoring of plasma calcium levels (risk of hypercalcaemia). If PTH levels normalize, significant autonomous parathyroid dysfunction can be considered unlikely and parathyroidectomy avoided.

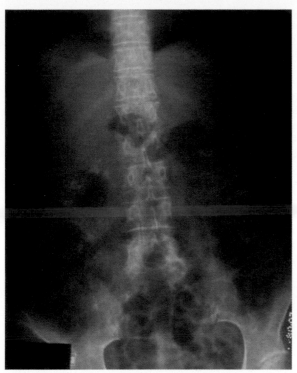

Fig. 7.52 Plain abdominal radiograph demonstrating bilateral nephrocalcinosis in a patient with primary hyperparathyroidism.

Reproduced from Royal College of Physicians. *Medical Masterclass: Endocrinology*, 2nd edition. London: RCP, 2013. Copyright © 2013 Royal College of Physicians. Reproduced with permission.

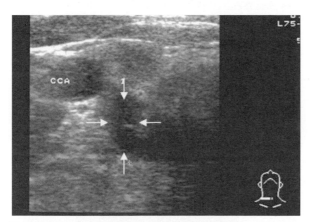

Fig. 7.53 Preoperative localization of parathyroid adenoma—ultrasonography.

Reproduced from Royal College of Physicians. *Medical Masterclass: Endocrinology*, 2nd edition. London: RCP, 2013. Copyright © 2013 Royal College of Physicians. Reproduced with permission.

## Management

### Emergency/short term

See Section 7.24.

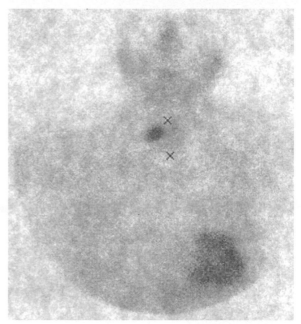

Fig. 7.54 Preoperative localization of parathyroid adenoma—$^{99m}$Tc–sestamibi scintigraphy.

Reproduced from Royal College of Physicians. *Medical Masterclass: Endocrinology*, 2nd edition. London: RCP, 2013. Copyright © 2013 Royal College of Physicians. Reproduced with permission.

### Long term

Long-term management pursues two aims: to normalize/optimize serum calcium levels and to prevent/ameliorate adverse effects on kidneys and bones. If or when to proceed to parathyroidectomy remains controversial.

- A widely accepted consensus is to favour surgery in all symptomatic patients, in asymptomatic patients if age <50 years, if serum calcium >0.25mmol/L above upper limit of normal, if urinary calcium excretion >10mmol/day, if creatinine clearance <30%, and when osteoporosis is present (T score <−2.5 in hip, lumbar spine, or distal radius), or if follow-up is judged to be difficult.

- Surgical treatment is improving (e.g. fast track, minimally invasive parathyroidectomy is performed as a day case) with success rates of >90%. There is prospective, long-term data demonstrating superiority above a conservative approach. For hyperparathyroidism arising in the context of MEN, full neck exploration is required, as all four glands are likely to be involved.

- Many patients with late onset, mild hyperparathyroidism remain asymptomatic without adverse effects on kidneys or bones and sometimes calcium levels normalize spontaneously. Therefore, observation with periodic calcium checks may be sufficient, ensuring good hydration and avoiding calcium raising drugs (e.g. thiazide diuretics).

- Oral biphosphonates are not generally deemed to be beneficial in the longer term treatment of hypercalcaemia, but may be used to treat/prevent concomitant osteoporosis.

- Calcimimetics (e.g. cinacalcet), which lower serum PTH and calcium levels, can be used for patients with recurrent disease or deemed unsuitable for surgery.

- Some patients require vitamin D replacement for concomitant insufficiency, but this must be undertaken with caution because of the risk of inducing marked hypercalcaemia (see Box 7.9).

# 7.26 Osteoporosis

## Background

- A disease characterized by low bone mass and microarchitectural deterioration of bone tissue, leading to enhanced bone fragility and an increase in fracture risk.
- In clinical practice the diagnosis can be made if the bone mineral density (BMD) derived by dual-energy X-ray absorptiometry (DXA) is >2.5 standard deviations (SDs) below peak bone mass or if susceptibility fractures have occurred, such as non-traumatic vertebral fractures, low-impact (fall from standing height or less) hip or Colles fracture.

## Epidemiology

- In the UK ~50% of ♀ and ~30% of ♂ will suffer an osteoporotic fracture in their lifetime; 22.5% of ♀ and 5.8% of ♂ aged >50 years have a BMD >2.5 SD below the sex-adjusted mean peak BMD.

## Pathophysiology

- Osteoporosis develops when there is a mismatch between bone resorption and formation. Assessment of the past medical history should focus on risk factors and conditions associated with bone loss, summarized in Table 7.28.
- ► Osteoporosis is **not** a disorder of calcium metabolism (serum calcium, phosphate, and alkaline phosphatase are usually normal, unless there has been a recent fracture).

## Clinical evaluation

### Signs and symptoms

- Often asymptomatic.
- Pain due to fractures (usually self-limiting within 3 months).

- Immobility and chronic pain due to secondary osteoarthritis.
- Loss of height (vertebral compression deformity).
- Kyphosis (vertebral wedge deformity).
- Abdominal protrusion (shortened spine).
- Superior iliac crest pain (ribs impinging on pelvic brim).
- Features of any predisposing condition may be present.

| Aims: | • To determine the overall risk of fracture. |
|---|---|
| | • To identify any treatable cause of secondary osteoporosis. |

## Investigations

### Radiology

- Bone loss >30% leads to detectable plain X-ray changes, (trabecular thinning, empty shell appearance of vertebral bodies, low density vs. soft tissue). These findings should be confirmed by DXA scan, as they are of low sensitivity and unreliable (e.g. overexposure of X-ray).
- More reliable radiological changes include: vertebral deformity (anterior wedge (Fig. 7.55), cod fish, compression) and obvious fragility fractures.
- ⚠ Posterior wedging is uncommon and may indicate an underlying destructive lesion.

### DXA

- Mainstay of—but not always required for—diagnosis (Fig. 7.56).
- Dependent on the difference in X-ray absorption by bone and soft tissue.

### Table 7.28 Factors influencing bone mass

| | Predisposing to bone loss | Protective against bone loss |
|---|---|---|
| Lifestyle | Increasing age<br>Salt-rich diet<br>High caffeine intake<br>Low body weight<br>Immobility<br>High alcohol intake<br>Smoking | Calcium-rich diet<br>Overweight<br>Physical activity<br>(especially weight bearing) |
| Genetic | ♀ gender<br>Family history<br>Caucasian | ♂ gender<br>Afro-Caribbean |
| Endocrine | Hypogonadism<br>Thyrotoxicosis<br>Hyperparathyroidism<br>Cushing syndrome<br>Growth hormone deficiency<br>or excess (osteoporosis occurs<br>in a subgroup of patients with<br>acromegaly) | |
| Drugs | Corticosteroids<br>Heparin<br>Cytotoxic therapy<br>Ciclosporin | Anabolic agents (e.g.<br>oestrogen therapy)<br>Agents that reduce<br>bone turnover (e.g.<br>bisphosphonates) |
| Chronic disease | Coeliac disease<br>Crohn disease<br>Malabsorption/poor nutrition<br>Rheumatoid arthritis<br>Chronic liver disease<br>Multiple myeloma | |

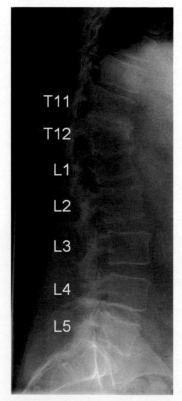

**Fig. 7.55** Osteoporotic vertebral fracture. Plain lateral X-ray of the spine showing an anterior wedge compression fracture of T12 vertebral body with 50% loss of height anteriorly in a patient with Cushing disease.

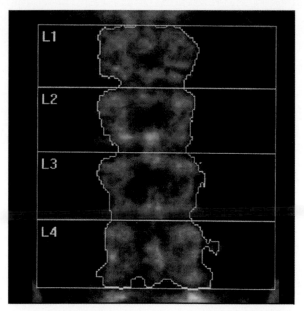

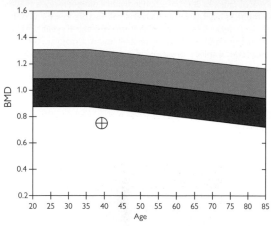

| Region | Area (cm²) | BMC (g) | BMD (g/cm²) | T-Score | PR (%) | Z-Score | AM (%) |
|--------|-----------|---------|-------------|---------|--------|---------|--------|
| L1 | 12.91 | 9.27 | 0.718 | −2.6 | 71 | −2.6 | 71 |
| L2 | 13.33 | 10.67 | 0.800 | −2.7 | 73 | −2.7 | 73 |
| L3 | 14.50 | 10.21 | 0.704 | −3.6 | 64 | −3.6 | 64 |
| L4 | 15.71 | 12.06 | 0.768 | −3.4 | 67 | −3.4 | 67 |
| Total | 56.45 | 42.21 | 0.748 | −3.1 | 69 | −3.0 | 69 |

**Fig. 7.56** Bone densitometry. DXA scan in a 39-year-old man with hypogonadism and associated osteoporosis. Both T-scores and Z-scores for the lumbar spine are shown.

- Low-dose X-ray
- Accurate, reproducible, well-validated for prediction of fracture risk.
- Results expressed in SD as gender-specific T- or Z-scores.
  - **T-score:** comparison with young adult (= peak bone mass) reference range. A drop in 1SD equates to a 12% spine density loss and doubles fracture risk.
  - **Z-score:** comparison with age-matched adult reference range.
  - Table 7.29 shows the World Health Organization classification for BMD based on T-scores.

*Other investigations*
- Quantitative CT/USS, bone biopsies rarely used.
- Biochemical markers of bone turnover, e.g. osteocalcin or procollagen type 1 N-terminal propeptide (P1NP) (osteoblastic) and

| Table 7.29 WHO classification of BMD (based on T-scores) | |
|---|---|
| BMD | Description |
| Above −1 SD | Normal |
| Below −1 SD but above −2.5 SD | Osteopenia |
| Below −2.5 SD | Osteoporosis |
| Below −2.5 SD with fragility fracture | Established osteoporosis |

C-terminal telopeptide of type 1 collagen (osteoclastic) can be used to monitor treatment efficacy: changes are faster and more closely linked with fracture risk reduction than changes in BMD.

*Screening for underlying cause*
- Dependent on clinical context, but may include: serum calcium, PTH, ALP, TSH, testosterone, oestradiol, FBC, ESR, protein electrophoresis, urinary Bence Jones protein, 24-hour urinary creatinine and calcium excretion.

**Differential diagnosis**
- Renal osteodystrophy; osteomalacia; multiple myeloma; osteogenesis imperfecta.

## Management

### Pain control
- Analgesia.
- Transcutaneous nerve stimulation.
- Physical measures (lumbar support, wrist splints).
- Calcitonin and balloon kyphoplasty in patients with treatment resistant pain due to vertebral fractures.

### Treatments to increase bone mass
Current NICE recommendations for treatment of established osteoporosis can be found at <http://www.nice.org.uk>.

    **Biphosphonates**—often considered first choice therapy, but strong oesophageal irritants:
- Alendronate (10mg/day or 70mg weekly), risedronate (5mg/day or 35mg weekly), ibandronate (150mg/month or 3mg IV 3-monthly)—reduce spine, hip, and wrist fractures
- Zoledronate—an extremely potent bisphosphonate, which is usually given as a once a year infusion, repeated on 2 occasions in the first instance.

▶ Oral bisphosphonates should be taken 30 minutes before breakfast on an empty stomach with a full glass of water, and the patient should remain upright for 30 minutes after taking the tablet. These measures ensure maximum efficacy and minimize the risk of oesophageal reactions.

    Osteonecrosis of the jaw is an extremely rare complication of bisphosphonate therapy (usually IV); typically in context of concomitant oral infections or dental procedures.

    Recent concerns have been raised regarding increased rates of atypical femoral fractures in those receiving long-term bisphosphonate therapy. Accordingly, a period off therapy is increasingly recommended.

*Other, second-line, treatments*
- Raloxifene—selective oestrogen receptor modulator (SERM); reserved for bisphosphonate failure or intolerance; increased risk of venous thromboembolism; only shown to reduce spine fractures
- Strontium ranelate—reduces spine, hip, and wrist fracture; DXA derived BMD artificially increased; however, concerns now exist regarding increased rates of cardiovascular and venous thromboembolic disease in those receiving treatment with strontium; its use is therefore now restricted for patients unable to tolerate other treatments, and should be prescribed only by a clinician experienced in its use and supervision.

- Teriparatide (recombinant PTH)—very effective, but very expensive; reserved for severe osteoporosis
- Sex hormone replacement therapy in hypogonadal ♂ and amenorrhoeic ♀ <50 years; HRT may also be considered in postmenopausal women in whom the risks of venous thromboembolic disease and breast cancer have been assessed and discussed.
- Calcium (500mg/day) and/or vitamin D supplementation (400–800IU/day) should be provided, if adequate calcium intake and/or vitamin D repletion is uncertain. However, if co-prescribed with a weekly bisphosphonate then calcium and vitamin D should only be taken on the other 6 days of the week.

## Prevention of fractures

- Fall prevention—walking frames; minimize drugs known to cause falls due to drowsiness, loss of balance, and postural hypotension; optimize living environment to minimize risk of falls (handle bars, stair lifts).
- Protection—hip protectors, carpets.
- Physiotherapy—improves balance and righting reflexes.

## Treatment of secondary causes

Wherever possible underlying conditions should be addressed, e.g. treat thyrotoxicosis, hyperparathyroidism.

## Monitoring treatment effects

Unpredictable response to drug therapy requires BMD monitoring (changes in BMD may not be evident for up to 2 years). Bone loss in untreated osteoporosis averages 2% per annum, while rate of bone gain with anti-resorptive treatments averages 3% per annum.

## Primary prevention

| Aims: | • Maximize peak bone mass.<br>• Reduce rate of bone loss. |
|---|---|
| Measures: | • Regular and weight-bearing exercise.<br>• Ensuring calcium and vitamin D replete diet.<br>• Avoidance of excessive alcohol intake.<br>• Non-smoking. |

- In general, prophylactic therapy is not required if bone mass is normal, but may be considered for osteopenia in postmenopausal ♀, in the presence of severe/multiple risk factors, or if accelerated bone loss demonstrated on serial DXA scans.

▶ In prolonged treatment with high doses of glucocorticoids (equivalent to ≥7.5mg of prednisolone/day) bisphosphonate therapy for at least the duration of the steroid therapy should be considered.

The WHO classification (and therefore the T-score) should ideally only be used in postmenopausal ♀ and ♂ >50 years of age. In pre-menopausal ♀, younger ♂, and children (who have not reached peak bone mass) the Z-score can be used for diagnostic purposes, but only in the clinical context (presence of fragility fractures, significant risk factors, etc.)—in these groups the relationships between BMD and fracture risk are not well established.

The FRAX® tool has been developed by WHO to evaluate fracture risk of patients. It is based on individual patient models that integrate the risks associated with clinical risk factors as well as BMD at the femoral neck. The FRAX® algorithms give the 10-year probability of hip fracture and the 10-year probability of a major osteoporotic fracture (clinical spine, forearm, hip, or shoulder fracture).

# 7.27 Osteomalacia

## Background

Impairment of mature bone matrix mineralization, resulting in weakness and increased propensity to fracture with subsequent deformity; termed 'rickets' if it occurs during childhood prior to fusion of epiphyseal growth plates, (i.e. a disorder of the growing skeleton).

## Epidemiology

Definitive diagnosis depends on bone histology making accurate estimation of prevalence problematic. However, biochemical features of osteomalacia are found in ~5–10% of the elderly and ~10–20% of patients with hip fractures.

## Pathophysiology

(See Table 7.30.) Defective bone mineralization due to:
- Altered vitamin D metabolism.
- Phosphate deficiency.
- Mineralization defects.

### Table 7.30 Aetiology of osteomalacia

| Disorder | Mechanism | Cause (examples) |
|---|---|---|
| Vitamin D deficiency/altered metabolism | ↓ substrate | Under-exposure to sunlight |
| | | Inadequate dietary intake |
| | | Small bowel malabsorption (coeliac, intestinal resection) |
| | | liver disease (primary biliary cirrhosis) |
| | ↑ clearance | Enzyme-inducing agents (phenytoin, carbamazepine) |
| | ↓ hydroxylation | Renal disease (↓ 1α hydroxylation) |
| | | Vitamin D-dependent rickets type I (AR)* |
| | | ↓ 25 hydroxylation—v. rare hereditary defects reported |
| | ↓ action | Vitamin D-dependent rickets type II (AR)** |
| Hypophosphataemia | ↓ intake | Phosphate binding medication (antacids) |
| | ↑ loss | X-linked hypophosphataemia (vitamin D resistant rickets, XLD) |
| | | Fanconi syndrome and/or Renal tubular acidosis |
| | | Oncogenic osteomalacia (mesenchymal tumours; occasionally adenocarcinomas, myeloma) |
| Defective mineralization | | High dose bisphosphonate therapy |
| | | Hypophosphatasia |
| Defective bone matrix | | Fibrogenesis imperfecta ossium |

*25-hydroxyvitamin D 1α-hydroxylase deficiency. **Defective vitamin D receptor signalling.

AR: autosomal recessive; XLD: X-linked dominant.

## Clinical evaluation

### History and examination
- Frequently asymptomatic.
- Generalized muscle aches and pains, worse with activity.
- Past history may include: gastric surgery, coeliac disease, long-term anticonvulsant use, immigration (reduced sun exposure ± dietary deficiency in certain ethnic groups).
- Proximal myopathy.
- Bone pain and fractures (including pathological).
- Deformities (spinal, thoracic, and pelvic) are rare nowadays and only seen in severe and longstanding cases.
- Occasionally features of hypocalcaemia are present.
- Rickets is characterized by growth retardation, bone pain and fracture, and skeletal deformity.

### Investigations
*Biochemistry*
- ► Much of the biochemistry is attributable to progressive secondary hyperparathyroidism. Other features vary with the underlying cause—see Table 7.31.
- In addition to ↓ serum calcium/phosphate and ↑ alkaline phosphatase, patients with oncogenic osteomalacia or Fanconi syndrome may exhibit aminoaciduria, while acidosis is a feature of Fanconi syndrome and renal tubular acidosis.
- In primary mineralization disorders all parameters may be normal, with bone biopsy required to confirm diagnosis.

*Radiology*
- 'Cod-fish' vertebrae secondary to ballooning of intervertebral disc.
- Looser's zones or 'pseudofractures' in pelvis, long bones, ribs (low density areas = unmineralized osteoid).
- Widened epiphyses + cupped metaphyses in rickets.
- Features of secondary hyperparathyroidism, e.g. subperiosteal resorption of phalanges, bone cysts, and resorption of distal ends of long bones.

## Management

Where possible, correct the underlying disorder.

### Vitamin D supplementation
Preparation, dose, and route of delivery depend upon the cause and severity of the deficiency, e.g.:
- 400–800IU/day of oral vitamin $D_2$ (ergocalciferol) may suffice in cases of limited sunlight exposure and/or dietary insufficiency (typically given with a calcium supplement).
- In contrast, deficiency caused by malabsorption usually requires pharmacological doses of vitamin D, e.g. ≥50,000IU of oral (or parenteral) ergocalciferol weekly.
- Vitamin D requires 1α-hydroxylation by the kidney to its active form and therefore the hydroxylated forms alfacalcidol (1α-hydroxycholecalciferol) or calcitriol (1,25-dihydroxycholecalciferol) are required in patients with moderate to severe renal impairment.
- ► All patients receiving pharmacological doses of vitamin D or the more potent preparations (alfacalcidol, calcitriol) should have their serum calcium level checked regularly.

Table 7.31 Osteomalacia and associated biochemical features

| Underlying cause | Biochemical features | | | | | |
|---|---|---|---|---|---|---|
| | Serum calcium | Serum phosphate | Serum 25-hydroxy vit D | Serum 1,25-dihydroxy vit D | Serum alkaline phosphatase | plasma PTH level |
| Vitamin D deficiency | ↓ | ↓ | ↓ | ↓ | ↑ | ↑ |
| Renal failure | ↓ | ↑ | ↔ | ↓ | ↑ | ↑ |
| Vitamin D-dependent rickets type I | ↓ | ↓ | ↔ | ↓ | ↑ | ↑ |
| Vitamin D-dependent rickets type II | ↓ | ↓ | ↔ | ↑ | ↑ | ↑ |
| X-linked hypophosphataemia | ↔ | ↓ | ↔ | ↔ | ↑ | ↔/↑ |
| Phosphate depletion | ↔ | ↓ | ↔ | | ↑ | |

- When the underlying cause of vitamin D deficiency is potentially reversible, care must be exercised to avoid over-treatment; pharmacological replacement should be substituted by physiological replacement once the deficit has been corrected.

**Phosphate replacement**

Required for phosphate deficiency/wasting disorders. Vitamin D therapy is often co-prescribed to maintain normal calcium homeostasis.

# 7.28 Paget disease

## Background

- Named after Sir James Paget (1814–1899, British surgeon).
- Osteitis deformans—**focal** skeletal disorder characterized by an accelerated rate of bone turnover with uncoupling of bone resorption and formation.
- Pathognomonic 'mosaic' pattern of lamellar bone.

## Epidemiology

- Marked geographic variation; common in USA (~3% of ♂ aged >45 years and ~10% of ♂ aged >80 years) and Europe, but rare in Asia. A disease of Anglo-Saxons.

## Pathophysiology

- Genetic (7–10-fold increased risk for family members).
- Association with viral infections described, but contentious.
- Increased bone resorption leads to increased, but abnormal, bone formation, and ultimately deformities and fractures. Spine, pelvis, skull, femur, and tibia are commonly involved sites.

## Clinical evaluation

### History and examination

- Often asymptomatic (<10% of patients with radiological features develop symptoms).
- Pain ('painful pagetic lesions', nerve impingements, fractures, secondary osteoarthritis).
- Deformities (bowing of long bones, skull invagination, increase in skull size).
- Nerve entrapment (hearing loss, blindness, facial palsy).
- Increased vascularity: warmth over affected bone, prominent temporal arteries, bounding pulse, very rarely high output heart failure, paralysis secondary to vascular steal syndromes.
- Increased incidence of bone tumours (benign giant cell tumour, rarely osteosarcoma).
- 🛈 In a patient with Paget disease, soft tissue swelling, increased pain, or a rapidly rising alkaline phosphatase level should alert the clinician to the possibility of osteosarcoma.

### Investigations

*Biochemistry*
- Typically isolated increase in alkaline phosphatase (bony origin). Serum calcium and phosphate usually normal, unless recent fracture or immobility.
- Primary (in up to 20%, reason unknown) and secondary hyperparathyroidism (if increased calcium demands not met) may be seen in Paget disease and can exacerbate the condition.

*X-ray*
- Evidence of chaotic new bone formation with expanded bones; localized areas of both sclerosis and osteolysis; osteoporosis circumscripta of skull ultimately leading to 'cotton wool' appearance (Fig. 7.57); bowing of long bones (Fig. 7.58).

*Isotope bone scan*
- Most sensitive test for determining the extent of disease, but low specificity.

## Management

### Bisphosphonates

- Mainstay of therapy in symptomatic patients.

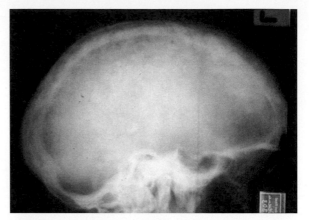

**Fig. 7.57** Plain lateral skull X-ray demonstrating thickening of the vault and typical 'cotton wool' appearance.

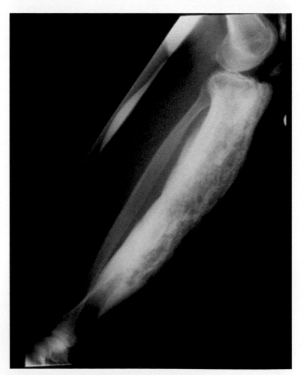

**Fig. 7.58** Plain X-ray of the tibia and fibula showing the classical 'sabre tibia' with anterior and lateral bowing.
Reproduced from Royal College of Physicians. *Medical Masterclass: Endocrinology*, 2nd edition. London: RCP, 2013. Copyright © 2013 Royal College of Physicians. Reproduced with permission.

- Reduce bone turnover by inhibiting osteoclast activity.
- Typically reduce alkaline phosphatase and bone scan uptake.
- May be analgesic.
- Role in asymptomatic patients is controversial, but should be considered if complications due to hypervascularity or disease progression are likely (e.g. imminent fractures, nerve compression).

### Other measures

- Simple analgesia.
- Treatment of associated osteoarthritis.
- Salmon calcitonin may be tried in those intolerant of bisphosphonates.

# 7.29 Dyslipidaemia

## Background

- For definitions and a brief overview of the essential steps in lipoprotein metabolism see Box 7.10.
- Dyslipidaemia can be defined as low-density lipoprotein (LDL) or triglycerides (TG) >90th or HDL <10th percentile, but the association with increased cardiovascular risk is linear without a threshold.
- In cohort studies 75–85% of patients with premature (<60 years) ischaemic heart disease have dyslipidaemia, which is familial in 85%.
- LDL has pathogenic importance for atherosclerosis: small, dense LDL penetrates endothelial barriers and accumulates in subendothelial macrophages where LDL is modified (e.g. oxidized) leading to the formation of 'foam cells'. These promote atheromatous plaque instability and platelet aggregation mainly through their pro-inflammatory properties.
- The link between high TG and atherosclerosis is weaker, but still of clinical relevance.

## Primary dyslipidaemia

- Genetic abnormalities in lipoproteins or in lipoprotein receptors result in overproduction and/or impaired removal of lipoproteins.

---

**Box 7.10 Definitions and overview of essential steps in lipoprotein metabolism**

**Lipoproteins** such as chylomicrons, VLDLs, LDLs, and HDLs transport insoluble lipids (cholesterol and triglycerides) in the plasma for energy utilization, lipid deposition, steroid hormone production, and bile acid formation.

Lipoproteins can be measured directly or indirectly in the plasma.

**Apoproteins** (e.g. Apo A-1, Apo B-100, Apo-E) are lipoprotein components, which determine the metabolism of lipoproteins as co-factors for enzymes and ligands for specific lipoprotein receptors.

Lipoprotein metabolism is best divided into three functional groups:

1. **Exogenous lipoprotein metabolism**: dietary cholesterol and triglycerides (= free fatty acids (FFA) and glycerol) are absorbed as *chylomicrons*, which release FFA by interacting with *endothelial lipoprotein lipase* (LPL) and ultimately undergo hepatic clearance through interaction of the Apo E ligand on *remnant chylomicrons* with *hepatic chylomicron remnant receptors*.

2. **Endogenous lipoprotein metabolism**: VLDL is excreted by the liver into the circulation and 'shrinks' to remnant VLDL (also referred to as intermediate density lipoprotein or IDL), releasing FFA through interaction with endothelial LPL. Most remnant VLDL is remodelled to LDL by *hepatic lipase* (HL). LDL contains Apo B-100, which interacts with the *LDL receptor* facilitating absorption into hepatic and extra-hepatic cells.

3. **Reverse lipoprotein metabolism**: the liver secretes '*lipid-poor Apo A-1 particles*' which interact with peripheral *ATP-binding cassette transporter* (ABCA1) to take up excess cellular cholesterol forming *pre-ß-HDL*, which is converted to 'mature' HDL by *lecithin-cholesterol acyltransferase* (LCAT). HDL cholesterol is then either taken up by the liver through interaction of HDL with *hepatic scavenger receptors* (SR-B1) or transferred to VLDL and LDL through the action of *cholesteryl ester transfer protein* (CETP).

---

- Primary dyslipidaemias are classified according to plasma electrophoresis patterns (Fredrickson system) or to their known or suspected causes as follows:

### Familial hypercholesterolaemia (FH)

- Various LDL receptor gene mutations (autosomal dominant) result in reduced LDL clearance. The severity of LDL elevation is milder in heterozygotes (1:500) vs. homozygotes (1:10$^6$) and varies with specific mutations (e.g. LDL receptor absent vs. partially functional).
- **Familial defective apolipoprotein B-100** (autosomal dominant) is identical to FH in its manifestations and treatment. However, the reduction in LDL clearance is due to a defective LDL receptor ligand Apo B-100 (LDL receptor normal).

*Clinical features*

- Excess LDL is deposited in the arteries (atheroma), tendons (xanthomata) and skin (xanthelasma, corneal arcus).
- Can lead to aortic stenosis in 50% of homozygotes.
- LDL deposits are visible in >75% of heterozygotes throughout their lifetime.

*Diagnosis*

- Without a family history in a 40-year-old, LDL >6.7mmol/L (and typically normal TG) is considered diagnostic for FH.
- Diagnostic LDL cut-offs are lower in the presence of a family history or in younger patients (e.g. >4mmol/L in 18-year-old with affected first-degree relative). Tendon xanthomata are pathognomic and can confirm a positive family history (for which premature heart disease is suggestive). LDL receptor defects can be confirmed biochemically.

*Management*

- Potent HMG (3-hydroxy-3-methyl-glutaryl)-CoA reductase inhibition (atorvastatin, rosuvastatin) is the treatment of choice.
- Ezetimibe (cholesterol absorption inhibitor) or cholestyramine (bile acid sequestrant) can be added.
- In treatment-resistant cases, cholesterol absorption and production can be treated with ileal bypass surgery portacaval anastomosis, liver transplantation, and LDL apheresis.

### Polygenic hypercholesterolaemia

A diagnosis of exclusion, characterized by moderate and isolated LDL elevations without clinical stigmata, but premature IHD within a family.

- Although probably polygenic, hypercholesterolaemia has been associated with Apo E4 alleles (10–20% of general population). The resulting Apo E4 ligand has a higher affinity for the LDL receptor leading to a down-regulation of LDL receptors driven by negative-feedback.
- Statins are the treatment of choice.

### Familial combined hyperlipidaemia (FCH)

- FCH occurs in up to 2% of the general population (autosomal dominant) and is characterized by an overproduction of liver-derived Apo B-100 (genetic cause unknown). The FCH clinical and biochemical phenotype varies between affected individuals, and may even vary over time within a given patient.

*Diagnosis*

- Triglycerides (VLDL) and/or LDL (especially small dense LDL) are raised.
- HDL is typically low.
- LDL/Apo B ratios of <1.2 (normally >1.4) is suggestive of FCH and **hyperapobetalipoproteinaemia**, probably a variant of FCH with population average LDL.

*Management*

- The phenotype dictates therapeutic strategies:
  - TG can be lowered with fibrates (bezofibrate, fenofibrate) or nicotinic acid and LDL with statins.
  - Combination therapy, which is associated with a higher risk of side effects (myositis, rhabdomyolysis, LFT changes), may be required.
  - Gemfibrozil should be used with caution (paradoxical increase in LDL; high side effect rate in combination therapy).

### Familial dysbetalipoproteinaemia

- Characterized by increased VLDL and chylomicron remnants due to expression of two Apo E2 alleles (autosomal recessive). The Apo E2 ligand has lower affinity for the Apo receptor and thus clearance of VLDL and chylomicrons is reduced. Consistently elevated VLDL leads to the formation of β-VLDL (denser than VLDL).
- Tuberoeruptive xanthomas and palmar crease xanthomas are pathognomonic.
- Beta-VLDL can be detected by gel electrophoresis. Apo E isoform analysis can be performed by isoelectric focusing.
- Therapy focuses on avoidance of causes of high TG and/or fibrates.

### Familial hypertriglyceridemia

- Characterized by moderate VLDL elevations (TG 2.3–5.6mmol/L) due to an over-production of VLDL-TG disproportionate to normal Apo-B production (autosomal dominant, genetic defect unknown).
- LDL is normal, HDL is typically low.
- The condition becomes clinically relevant in the presence of secondary causes of high TG. Avoidance of these is usually sufficient as therapy.

### LPL and Apo C II deficiencies

- Rare and characterized by TG >99th percentile.
- Very high chylomicron levels, not processed by LPL (Apo C II is a vital cofactor for LPL), lead to **eruptive xanthomata**,

hepatomegaly and acute symptoms (pancreatitis, memory disturbances, lipaemia retinalis) if chylomicrons are very high.

- A creamy plasma supernatant is typical.
- In LPL deficiency lipase activity does not rise after IV heparin (displaces LPL from the endothelium).
- Treatment entails a fat-free or low-fat diet. TG lowering medications (fibrates) are of limited benefit.

## Secondary dyslipidaemia

- Secondary causes of high TG and LDL levels are summarized in Table 7.32.
- TG elevations are amenable to lifestyle changes, in contrast to LDL levels, which are mainly determined genetically.
- Treatment focuses on the underlying cause, but may require specific LDL and TG lowering therapies.

| Table 7.32 Secondary causes of dyslipidaemia | | |
|---|---|---|
| **LDL increase** | **TG increase** | **HDL reduction** |
| Diet (high in saturated fats) | Diet (high in carbohydrates) | |
| Anorexia | Alcohol | Smoking |
| Drugs (corticosteroids, diuretics, ciclosporin) | Drugs (β-blockers, oestrogen, isotretinoin) | Drugs (anabolic steroids) |
| Nephrotic syndrome | Chronic renal failure | |
| Liver disease (chronic,cholestatic) | | |
| | Type 2 diabetes, insulin resistance, obesity | |
| Pregnancy | | |
| Hypothyroidism | | |

# 7.30 Porphyria

## Aetiology

- The porphyrias are a group of inherited or acquired metabolic disorders resulting from enzymatic defects in the haem biosynthetic pathway (Fig. 7.59).
- In the majority of cases inheritance occurs in an autosomal dominant fashion, although autosomal recessive and X-linked forms are also recognized.
- Porphyria cutanea tarda shows heritability in only a small percentage of cases.
- Various classifications have been proposed, including **acute** versus **non-acute** and **hepatic** versus **erythropoietic** (Table 7.33).

### Triggering factors
Attacks of porphyria may be triggered by:
- Drugs, e.g. barbiturates, sex steroids, enzyme inducers.
- Alcohol.
- Stress, including intercurrent infections.
- Electrolyte disturbances.
- Hormonal changes, e.g. during the menstrual cycle.

## Clinical evaluation

### Signs and symptoms
The clinical manifestations are diverse and depend on the subtype of porphyria (Table 7.33). However, in general the acute porphyrias predominantly exhibit neurovisceral symptoms and the non-acute porphyrias are characterized mainly by skin manifestations, although there is some overlap.

*Acute porphyrias*
Features may include:
- Abdominal pain, vomiting, and constipation.
- Sensorimotor neuropathy, seizures, coma, bulbar paralysis quadriplegia, respiratory muscle weakness.
- Psychiatric disorders including psychosis.
- Sinus tachycardia, hypertension, and rarely left ventricular failure.
- Hyponatraemia may occur in acute intermittent porphyria (AIP); due to the syndrome of inappropriate antidiuretic hormone (SIADH).

AIP, the most common type of porphyria, has no cutaneous features, whereas variegate porphyria (VP) and hereditary coproporphyria (HCP) often present with additional cutaneous manifestations (e.g. chronic blistering lesions on sun-exposed areas of the skin, particularly the back of the hands).

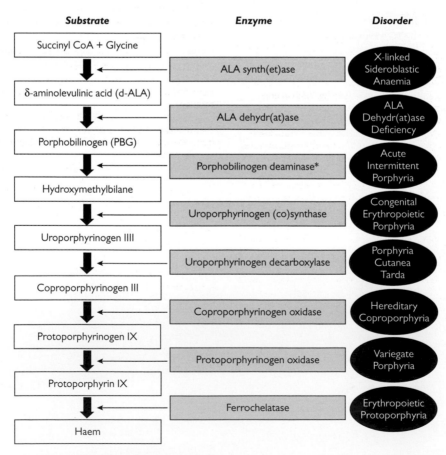

\* Also known as hydroxymethylbilane (HMB) synthase

**Fig. 7.59** Schematic representation of the major substrates, key enzymes, and associated inherited or acquired defects in porphyria.

**Table 7.33** Classification, enzyme defects, and core clinical features in porphyria

| Type of porphyria | Enzyme defect (inheritance) | Main clinical features |
|---|---|---|
| **Hepatic porphyria** | | |
| ● Acute intermittent porphyria | ● Porphobilinogen deaminase (AD)* | ● (Acute) Neurovisceral |
| ● Porphyria cutanea tarda | ● Uroporphyrinogen decarboxylase (AD) | ● (Non-acute) Cutaneous |
| ● Hereditary coproporphyria | ● Coproporphyrinogen oxidase (AD) | ● (Acute) Cutaneous and neurovisceral |
| ● Variegate porphyria | ● Protoporphyrinogen oxidase (AD) | ● (Acute) Cutaneous and neurovisceral |
| **Erythropoietic porphyria** | | |
| ● X-linked sideroblastic anaemia | ● ALA-synth(et)ase (XR) | ● Pallor, fatigue, hepato-splenomegaly |
| ● Congenital erythropoietic porphyria | ● Uroporphyrinogen (co) synthase (AR) | ● (Non-acute) Cutaneous |
| ● Erythropoietic protoporphyria | ● Ferrochelatase (AD) | ● (Non-acute) Cutaneous |

AD: autosomal dominant; AR: autosomal recessive; XR: X-linked recessive.

*Also known as hydroxymethylbilane synthase.

*Non-acute porphyrias*

The non-acute porphyrias are typically associated with photosensitivity due to activation of porphyrins in the skin by ultraviolet light:

- Porphyria cutanea tarda (PCT) presents as a bullous photosensitive rash that heals by scarring. Other features include hepatomegaly and an association with haemochromatosis.
- Erythropoietic protoporphyria (EPP) differs from other cutaneous porphyrias as the photosensitive rash is usually non-blistering. EPP may present in childhood. Additional features include paraesthesia and hepatic dysfunction.
- Congenital erythropoietic porphyria (CEP) presents with a bullous photo-sensitive rash, dystrophic nails, discolouration of teeth, anaemia, and splenomegaly.

**Investigations**

The diagnosis of acute porphyria is readily established during an acute episode by finding a substantial elevation of urinary porphyrins in a spot urine sample.

- Porphobilinogen (PBG) accumulation (PBG is one of the earliest substances in the porphyrin pathway—see Fig. 7.59) in urine during an acute attack yields a red/brown colour, due to a high concentration of porphobilin, a brownish auto-oxidation product of PBG, and porphyrins, which are reddish. PBG in fresh urine can be detected by the development of a characteristic pink/red colour on mixing with Ehrlich reagent, which is not absorbed out by chloroform or other organic solvents.
- AIP is confirmed by finding increased urinary excretion of both PBG and δ-aminolevulinic acid (ALA), along with decreased enzymatic activity of porphobilinogen deaminase (HMB synthase).
- AIP, HCP, and VP all cause increases in PBG and can be differentiated from each other by profiling blood, urinary and faecal porphyrins, together with assessment of enzymatic (e.g. PBG deaminase) activity.
  - ► Testing must be undertaken during an acute attack as results may be normal between episodes. Samples should be protected from light and sent immediately to the laboratory.

- Genetic screening for mutations in specific enzymes helps to confirm the diagnosis, and affords the opportunity for screening family members.
- Liver function tests are often abnormal during an acute episode.
- Nerve conduction studies may help to confirm the presence of neuropathy.

**Management**

Acute episodes are treated with supportive measures, including:

- Fluids and correction of electrolyte disturbances.
- Treatment of intercurrent infection/illness.
- Discontinuation of potential triggers, e.g. medications, alcohol.
- Ventilatory support.
- Analgesia (codeine, morphine, and diamorphine are thought to be safe—see following comments).

For all symptomatic patients, a high carbohydrate diet should be instituted without delay—often requiring intravenous dextrose (10% solution).

For patients with severe life-threatening disease, and in those not responding to the initial administration of carbohydrate, intravenous haem (e.g. haem arginate) at a dose of 3mg/kg per day (for 4 days) may be required.

► Once the acute episode has subsided, patient education regarding potential triggers is important.

► A list of drugs which are considered 'unsafe' in porphyria is available in the BNF, while an up-to-date list of treatments which are considered 'safe' is available at <http://www.wmic.wales.nhs.uk/porphyria_info.php>.

For the cutaneous porphyrias:

- Avoidance of sunlight is important.
- PCT may respond to venesection to reduce iron overload.
- Beta-carotene may improve sunlight tolerance in EPP.

# 7.31 Adult inborn errors of metabolism

## Background

- Huge range of inherited disorders too numerous and rare to be listed in any detail.
- The charity CLIMB (Children Living with Inherited Metabolic Diseases) recognizes >700 conditions that affect children. However, many of these significantly reduce longevity and affected patients often do not survive beyond childhood or early adulthood.
- A number of treatable and manageable conditions are screened for at birth: UK newborn screening programme (Guthrie heel prick test) for the most common mutations causing phenylketonuria (PKU) and medium-chain acyl-CoA dehydrogenase deficiency (MCADD) + others
- Can classify according to biochemistry (e.g. amino acid and urea cycle disorders—homocystinuria, PKU), affected organelle (e.g. mitochondrial disorders—MELAS); but simplest is **probably** by mode of inheritance—Table 7.34.

## Phenylketonuria

### Incidence

- ~1/10,000 live births in UK.

### Pathophysiology

- Absence of liver enzyme phenylalanine hydroxylase.

### Diagnosis

- Dried blood spot testing for phenylalanine levels.

### Presentation

- Normal at birth, ingestion of phenylalanine leads to mental retardation from build-up in cerebral tissues.
- Symptoms begin with failure to thrive, musty odour, an itchy rash, and progress to neurological symptoms such as hypertonicity, ataxia, and seizures.

### Treatment

- Phenylalanine-free diet, generally low protein with special formulas to provide all amino acids except phenylalanine.

### Effects in adults

- Almost impossible to stick to completely free diet, although with diet it is possible to limit effects.

- Women with PKU becoming pregnant must be especially careful to avoid elevated levels affecting fetal growth.

## Medium-chain acyl-CoA dehydrogenase deficiency

### Incidence

- ~1/10,000 live births in UK.

### Pathophysiology

- Lack of enzyme leads to difficulty breaking down medium-chain fatty acids to produce energy.

### Diagnosis

- Dried blood spot testing either for specific mutation K329E or levels of acylcarnitines

### Presentation

- Children generally well with symptoms appearing during metabolic crises, usually following infection and/or fasting.
- Presentation is with hypoglycaemia, lethargy, and seizures, progressing to respiratory, cardiac or neurological deterioration, coma, and death if untreated.
- Some individuals can present with fatty acid build-up in the liver, leading to hepatomegaly, hyperammonaemia, and cerebral oedema. This can lead to developmental delay.

### Treatment

- Frequent food intake with supplements during infection and careful monitoring can prevent crises.
- Diet can be helpful in reducing fatty acid accumulation.

### Effects in adults

- Vary depending on crises. If well treated, no significant effects.

## Gaucher disease

### Incidence

- Varies from ~1/50,000 (type I) to 1/100,000 (types II and III).

### Pathophysiology

- Lysosomal storage disorders resulting from various mutations in glucocerebrosidase, different mutations give rise

| Table 7.34 The commoner metabolic disorders divided according to their inheritance | | |
|---|---|---|
| **Autosomal dominant** | **Autosomal recessive** | **X-linked dominant** |
| Acute intermittent porphyria<br>Hyperlipidaemia type II*<br>Hypokalaemic periodic paralysis*<br>Pseudohypoparathyroidism (previously thought X-linked dominant) | Albinism<br>Ataxia telangiectasia<br>Congenital adrenal hyperplasia<br>Cysteinuria<br>Gilbert syndrome<br>Glycogen storage disorders<br>Homocysteinuria<br>Tay Sachs disease<br>Gaucher disease<br>Niemann–Pick disease<br>Mucopolysaccharidoses: except Hunter syndrome<br>Phenylketonuria<br>Wilson disease | Rett syndrome<br>Vitamin D-resistant rickets |
| **X-linked recessive** | **Mitochondrial** | **Chromosomal** |
| Fabry disease<br>Glucose-6-phosphate dehydrogenase deficiency<br>Hunter disease<br>Lesch–Nyhan syndrome<br>Wiscott–Aldrich syndrome | Leber optic atrophy<br>MELAS<br>MERRF<br>Kearns–Sayre syndrome | Turner syndrome |

to the differing phenotypes through accumulation of glucocerebroside.

### Diagnosis
- Bone marrow aspirate looking for Gaucher cells (swollen macrophages).
- Differentiation between forms of Gaucher involves specific enzyme deficiency analysis or mutation analysis.

### Presentation
- Typically with hepatosplenomegaly and bone marrow insufficiency leading to anaemia and/or thrombocytopenia.
- Bone pain from expansion of marrow cavities with accumulation of abnormal macrophages (Gaucher cells).
- Neurological involvement involves slowly progressive ataxia, dysarthria, and cognitive deterioration.

### Treatment
- Enzyme replacement therapy is now available and, although expensive, is very effective.

### Effects in adults
- Type III onset is in mid- to late childhood, but some individuals can present much later.
- Adults with Gaucher have an increased risk of Parkinson disease.

## Homocystinuria

### Incidence
- Worldwide ~1/350,000, Ireland 1/65,000.

### Pathophysiology
- Commonest enzyme deficiency is of cystathionine synthetase, but all causes lead to accumulation of homocysteine by preventing its breakdown into cysteine.

### Diagnosis
- Urinary cysteine levels.

### Presentation
- Initially well infants present with developmental delay; older individuals have a marfanoid body habitus, with moderate mental retardation, connective tissue abnormalities, especially downward dislocation of the lens (inferior ectopica lentis) and development of myopia with spontaneous retinal detachment.
- Seizures may occur though behavioural difficulties and psychiatric manifestations are more common.
- Patients are at increased risk of thromboembolism.
- Typically individuals have pale skin and fair hair due to inhibition of tyrosinase by homocysteine.

### Treatment
- High-dose pyridoxine (vitamin $B_6$) can be used to treat some patients by increasing conversion of homocysteine to cysteine, others require strict dietary restriction limiting methionine intake and cysteine supplementation.

### Effects in adults
- Thromboembolic events tend to present in adulthood, use of the oral contraceptive pill is therefore discouraged.

## Glycogen storage disease type I (Pompe disease)

### Incidence
- Ranges from 1/15,000 (black population) to 1/50,000 (most white populations).

### Pathophysiology
- Deficiency of lysosomal enzyme acid alpha-glucosidase leads to inability to break down glycogen, therefore accumulates in lysosomes of most tissues.

### Diagnosis
- Serum creatine kinase often raised but non-specific.
- Biopsy of skin, muscle or blood sampling (either leucocytes or dried blood spot) reveals low enzyme activity, <1% of normal in infantile forms, ranging up to 40% of normal in adult-onset forms. Histology can also demonstrate accumulation of glycogen within muscle lysosomes.

### Presentation
- Differs to other forms of glycogen storage disorder. The infantile form presents with cardiomyopathy and hypotonia. Juvenile- and adult-onset forms present with skeletal muscle weakness.

### Treatment
- Enzyme replacement therapy is available but is expensive and requires long-term use. Funding in the UK is difficult, particularly for adult-onset (and hence milder) forms.

### Effects in adults
- Adult-onset form presents between 2nd and 6th decade with gradually progressive muscle weakness, affecting skeletal muscles more than cardiac muscle.
- Respiratory insufficiency is the major cause of morbidity and mortality.

## Lesch–Nyhan syndrome

### Incidence
- ~1/350,000–400,000.

### Pathophysiology
- Deficiency of hypoxanthine-guanine phosphoribosyl transferase (HGPT) leads to overproduction of uric acid, therefore hyperuricaemia.
- It is unclear exactly what influence HGPT has on the neurological manifestations of Lesch–Nyhan syndrome.

### Diagnosis
- Raised plasma urate and urine urate/creatinine ratio.

### Presentation
- Infantile forms present at a few months of age with hypotonia and developmental delay, progressing to extrapyramidal spasticity and movement disorders such as choreoathetosis or ballismus.
- Progression of motor dysfunction continues until about 6 years of age but then remains static.
- Some patients present with symptoms related to hyperuricaemia such as recurrent UTIs or 'orange sand' in nappies from crystallization.
- Later recurrent renal stones, gouty arthritis, and tophi can develop.
- Behavioural problems are common, with aggressive and impulsive behaviours, classically severe self-injury, although severity of problems varies significantly.

### Treatment
- Allopurinol can be useful to reduce uric acid levels to within the normal range (titrate as low levels can also be harmful) and hydration is essential, particularly during intercurrent illness.
- Benzodiazepines and antispasmodics can be useful for the neurological syndromes.
- Behavioural problems are difficult to manage.

### Effects in adults
- Life expectancy for infant-onset forms is rarely beyond 40 years due to progressive renal impairment.
- Some forms can present later in life with choreiform movements, dysarthria, and renal impairment secondary to recurrent nephrolithiasis.

# 7.32 Obesity

## Background

Traditionally body mass index (BMI = weight in kg divided by height in m$^2$) has been used to categorize body weight. BMI overestimates the obesity in very muscular individuals and fails to discriminate between different distributions of excess adiposity, e.g. global vs. visceral vs. gluteal/limb (Fig. 7.60).

### WHO classification of obesity
- BMI <18.5 = underweight.
- BMI 18.5–24.9 = normal.
- BMI >25 = overweight (in Asian people >23).
- BMI >30 = class I obesity.
- BMI >35 = class II obesity.
- BMI >40 = class III ('severe', 'morbid') obesity.

## Epidemiology

- Obesity constitutes a worldwide epidemic, increasingly affecting both developed and developing countries.
- The prevalence of overweight/obesity has been estimated to be >50% in most Western societies.
- Obesity is associated with a significant increase in mortality and risk of many disorders, including diabetes mellitus, hypertension, dyslipidaemia, heart disease, stroke, sleep apnoea, dementia, and cancer.

## Aetiology

- The vast majority of cases of obesity are the result of a sedentary lifestyle coupled with overeating (Table 7.35).

- However, there is now clear evidence that genetic variation may mean that some individuals are more prone than others to gain weight.
- Medications are a common cause of weight gain (Table 7.36).
- Screening for rarer endocrine causes is usually only justified if there is a reasonable clinical index of suspicion.

## Clinical evaluation

Aim to identify underlying genetic, endocrine, or other specific causes of obesity (Tables 7.35 and 7.36).

### History
- Age at onset of weight gain.
- Previous attempts at weight loss and degree of success.
- Change in dietary patterns/alcohol consumption.
- Exercise level, medications, and smoking history (all current and past).
- Family history.
- Specific symptoms of endocrine disorders (e.g. hypothyroidism, Cushing syndrome).

### Examination
- In the majority of patients with simple obesity excess weight is distributed globally, although ♂ often display central/visceral adiposity (Fig. 7.60).
- Cutaneous markers of dyslipidaemia and insulin resistance (e.g. acanthosis nigricans (Fig. 7.61), multiple skin tags).
- Assess cardiovascular status, including blood pressure.
- Specific features of an underlying endocrine (e.g. hypothyroidism, Cushing syndrome) or genetic (e.g. Laurence–Moon–Biedl syndrome) cause of obesity should be sought.

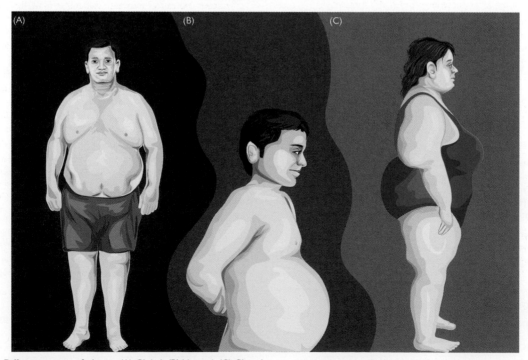

**Fig. 7.60** Differing patterns of obesity. (A) Global. (B) Visceral. (C) Gluteal.

| Table 7.35 Aetiology of weight gain/obesity | |
|---|---|
| **Type** | **Example** |
| Dietary obesity | Simple over-eating (high-fat, energy rich foods) |
| Limited exercise | Sedentary work/lifestyle |
| | Enforced inactivity (e.g. post-operative) |
| | Aging |
| Social and behavioural factors | Psychological, socioeconomic, ethnic (e.g. Binge- and night-eating syndromes) |
| Iatrogenic causes | Drugs (see Table 7.36) |
| Endocrine disorders | Hypothyroidism |
| | Hypogonadism |
| | Cushing syndrome |
| | Hypothalamic disorders |
| | Growth hormone deficiency |
| Genetic disorders | Leptin deficiency and leptin receptor defects |
| | Melanocortin 4 receptor (MC4R) defects |
| | Prader–Willi syndrome |
| | Laurence–Moon–Biedl syndrome |
| Other | Low birth weight |

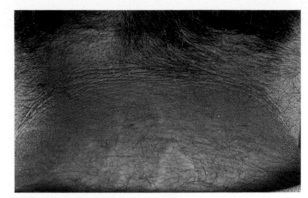

**Fig. 7.61** Acanthosis nigricans in the skin creases of the neck of a young obese man with severe insulin resistance. Note the pigmented, thickened, velvety appearance.

## Investigations

Investigations should assess the patient's cardiovascular (CV) risk profile and any suspected or confirmed obesity-related comorbidities. Occasionally screening for specific secondary causes of obesity is indicated (described earlier in this section).

## Management

### Cardiovascular risk

The threshold for preventative medication, such as aspirin and statin therapy, may need to be lowered if the CV risk profile cannot be improved sufficiently with other measures (e.g. weight loss and increased exercise).

Not all obese subjects exhibit features of the **metabolic syndrome**, but if present these increase CV risk substantially.

*Hypertension*
Common; treat aggressively. An inappropriately small cuff size spuriously elevates blood pressure readings.

*Smoking cessation*
A priority in all obese smokers.

### Glucose intolerance/diabetes mellitus

Given the high prevalence of type 2 diabetes, all obese individuals should have a fasting glucose (± HbA1c) checked annually. In the

| Table 7.36 Drugs that predispose to weight gain/obesity | |
|---|---|
| **Class** | **Example** |
| Anticonvulsants | Sodium valproate, gabapentin, phenytoin |
| Antidepressants | Tricyclics, SSRIs, mirtazapine, lithium |
| Antipsychotic agents | Especially atypicals, e.g. olanzapine, clozapine, |
| β–blockers | Propranolol, atenolol |
| Glucocorticoids | Prednisolone, dexamethasone |
| Oral contraceptives | Combined and progesterone-only preparations |
| Hypoglycaemic agents | Glitazones, sulphonylureas, insulin |

presence of osmotic symptoms (e.g. polyuria, nocturia), or signs of insulin resistance (Fig. 7.61), perform an oral glucose tolerance test if the fasting glucose level is normal and/or HbA1c equivocal.

*Dyslipidaemia*
Low HDL cholesterol and hypertriglyceridaemia are common findings in subjects with insulin resistance.

### Other comorbidities

Osteoarthritis and sleep apnoea are more common in obese subjects. Weight gain in women with PCOS often exacerbates hirsutism, menstrual disturbance, and may increase CV risk.

### Weight reduction

- Occasionally specific surgery or medication may facilitate dramatic weight loss, e.g. following treatment of Cushing disease or hypothyroidism.
- However, in the majority of overweight and obese subjects no specific underlying disorder is identified and long-term 'treatment' and support is required to achieve and maintain weight loss.
- 10% reduction in body weight significantly reduces all-cause cardiovascular and cancer mortality, diabetes mellitus, dyslipidaemia, and hypertension. Aiming for 5% weight loss by 6 months is a realistic target.
- Any given therapy can be deemed 'successful' if weight loss is maintained and associated with improved CV risk.

*Behavioural therapy*
The basis of any treatment regimen for obesity—maladaptive eating and exercise patterns contribute to weight gain and can be modified with techniques such as meal planning, self-monitoring, group therapy, stimulus control, and goal setting.

*Dietary therapy*
22–25kcal/kg/day is required to maintain 1kg of body weight in an average adult. Hence, calorie restriction to 800–1200kcal/day should result in weight loss in most adults if adhered to. 400kcal/day diets confer no extra benefits in terms of weight loss when compared to an 800kcal/day diet.

*Physical activity*
Resting in bed equates to an energy expenditure of around 0.8kcal/min (1150kcal/day) for a normal-weight adult. High levels of physical activity can increase this by a factor of 4–5. Loss of weight reduces energy expenditure making it even more difficult to maintain or reduce weight further.

303

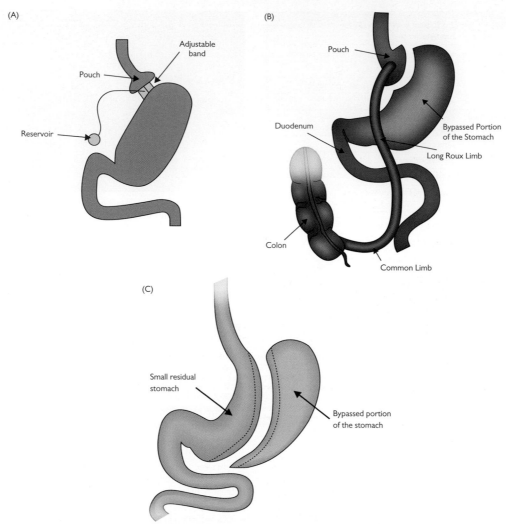

**Fig. 7.62** Types of bariatric surgery. (A) Adjustable gastric band—a small bracelet-like band is placed around the top of the stomach to create a small pouch thereby limiting food intake; the outlet size can be varied by injecting/removing saline from a small reservoir connected to the band. (B) Roux-en-Y—works by restricting food intake and by decreasing the absorption of food; a small pouch (similar in size to the adjustable gastric band) is created; in addition, absorption is reduced by 'excluding' most of the stomach, duodenum, and upper small intestine and routing food directly from the pouch into more distal small bowel. (C) Vertical sleeve gastrectomy—works by reducing the capacity of the stomach and altering gastric emptying.

*Medical therapy*
- Consider if dietary modifications and exercise alone fail.
- Orlistat (a gastric and pancreatic lipase inhibitor) facilitates mild–moderate weight loss; however, malabsorption of fat-soluble vitamins, and faecal urgency/soiling (if non-compliant with dietary restriction) may complicate treatment.
- In clinical trials glucagon-like peptide 1 (GLP-1) agonists/analogues (e.g. exenatide, liraglutide, lixisenatide—currently licensed for use in type 2 diabetes mellitus) can lead to significant weight loss in some individuals.

*Surgical therapy*
*Liposuction*
- Subcutaneous fat removal by aspiration; does not appear to improve insulin sensitivity or cardiovascular risk.

*Bariatric surgery*
- The most effective treatment for obesity (achieving on average a 60% reduction in excess weight).

- Surgical options are based on restrictive (gastric banding or stapling), malabsorptive (bypassing small bowel) or mixed (e.g. Roux-en-Y) strategies (Fig. 7.62).
- Indications for surgery vary among healthcare systems.

## Prognosis

In the absence of an underlying disorder (Cushing syndrome, hypothyroidism), the degree to which weight loss is achieved/maintained with lifestyle measures or medical therapy is dependent, to a large extent, on patient motivation.

Bariatric surgery is effective in promoting significant weight reduction but may be associated with other sequelae e.g. malabsorption.

# Chapter 8

# Diabetes

# 8.1 Diabetes mellitus

## Background

- Diabetes mellitus is a collective term for a group of metabolic diseases whose key feature is hyperglycaemia.
- The elevated glucose levels result either from a failure of insulin secretion or from resistance to the action of insulin, or both.
- The importance of this condition arises from the temporal association of chronically elevated glucose levels with damage to kidneys, nerves, eyes, heart, and vasculature.
- Diabetes affects infants, children, young people, and adults of all ages.
- In 2014 there were an estimated 3.3 million people with a diagnosis of diabetes in the UK (~6.2% of the population); prevalence and diagnosis data estimates that ~600,000 individuals with type 2 diabetes may be as yet undiagnosed.
- The prevalence is predicted to increase to ~5 million by 2025—the majority of which will be associated with the rise in the prevalence of obesity.
- Worldwide prevalence—see Fig. 8.1.

## Diagnosis

Diabetes may be diagnosed if any of the following three conditions are met (WHO, 2006):

- Symptoms of diabetes (polyuria, polydipsia, and unexplained weight loss) plus a random plasma glucose concentration ≥11.0mmol/L, or
- A fasting plasma glucose ≥7.0mmol/L on at least two occasions, or
- A 2-hour post load glucose ≥11.0mmol/L during a 75g oral glucose tolerance test.

An amendment by the WHO in 2011 now allows HbA1c to be used as a diagnostic test, providing it is adequately standardized. An HbA1c ≥48mmol/mol (6.5%) is diagnostic, however a value less than this, does not exclude diabetes if it has been diagnosed using glucose tests.

### Pre-diabetes

There are also intermediate conditions where individuals have higher glucose levels than normal but do not yet meet the criteria for the diagnosis of diabetes. These are:

- **Impaired fasting glucose**: fasting plasma glucose is ≥6.1mmol/L but <7.0mmol/L.
- **Impaired glucose tolerance**: 2-hour postload glucose ≥7.8mmol/L but <11.0mmol/L.

Individuals with either impaired fasting glucose or impaired glucose tolerance have a high risk of progression to overt diabetes and have an elevated risk of cardiovascular disease compared with individuals with normal glucose values (fasting plasma glucose ≤6.0mmol/L and 2-hour glucose <7.8mmol/L).

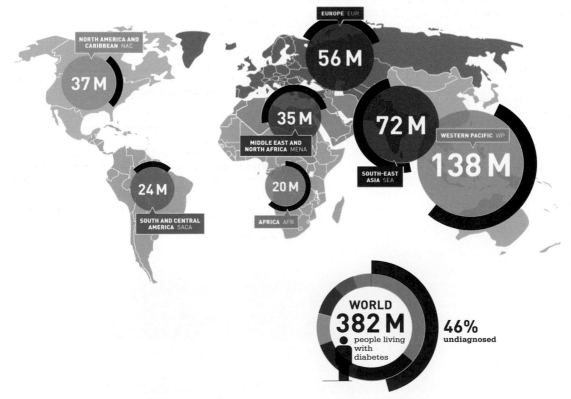

**Fig. 8.1** Worldwide prevalence of diabetes.
International Diabetes Federation. *IDF Diabetes Atlas, 6 ed.* Brussels, Belgium: International Diabetes Federation, 2015.

| Table 8.1 Differences between type 1 and type 2 diabetes | | |
|---|---|---|
| | Type 1 diabetes | Type 2 diabetes |
| Peak age at onset | 12 years | 60 years |
| Gender difference | ♂ > ♀, Europe ♀ > ♂, Africa, Asia | ♂ > ♀ |
| UK prevalence | 0.25% | 5–7% |
| Aetiology | Autoimmune mediated destruction of β cells | Defects in insulin action (insulin resistance) or insulin secretion |
| Phenotype | Usually lean | Frequently obese |
| Presentation | Acute; polyuria, polydipsia, and weight loss | Often incidentally discovered; complications often present at diagnosis |
| Ketoacidosis | Occurs | Rare |
| Treatment | Lifestyle change (diet and exercise) and insulin | Lifestyle change (weight loss), oral hypoglycaemic agents, and/or insulin |

# Classification

See Table 8.1.

## Type 1 diabetes

Pancreatic β-cell destruction leading to absolute insulin deficiency (5–25% of cases):

1. Immune-mediated—associated with anti-islet cell, anti-insulin, and anti-glutamic acid decarboxylase antibodies.
2. Idiopathic (no demonstrable autoimmunity).

## Type 2 diabetes

Insulin resistance or defects of insulin secretion or both (75–95% cases).

## Other types

1. Genetic defects of β-cell function:
   - Maturity onset diabetes of the young (MODY)
   - Mitochondrial DNA mutations.
2. Genetic defects of insulin action:
   - Type A insulin resistance
   - Leprechaunism/Donohue syndrome
   - Rabson–Mendenhall syndrome
   - Lipoatrophic diabetes.
3. Diseases of the exocrine pancreas:
   - Pancreatitis
   - Trauma/surgery (pancreatectomy)
   - Pancreatic infiltration, e.g. cystic fibrosis, haemochromatosis, neoplasia.
4. Endocrinopathies:
   - Cushing syndrome
   - Phaeochromocytoma
   - Hyperthyroidism
   - Acromegaly

   - Glucagonoma
   - Somatostatinoma.
5. Drug or chemical induced:
   - Glucocorticoids
   - Nicotinic acid
   - Thiazides
   - Diazoxide
   - α-Interferon.
6. Infections:
   - Congenital rubella
   - CMV.
7. Genetic syndromes associated with diabetes:
   - Down syndrome
   - Klinefelter syndrome
   - Turner syndrome
   - Prader–Willi syndrome
   - Lawrence–Moon–Biedl syndrome
   - Myotonic dystrophy
   - Friedreich ataxia
   - Wolfram syndrome/DIDMOAD (diabetes insipidus, diabetes mellitus, optic atrophy, and deafness).

## Gestational diabetes

Diabetes first diagnosed during pregnancy—irrespective of type.

- LADA—latent autoimmune diabetes of adulthood or type 1 1/2. Patients present with hyperglycaemia, but may lack signs of insulin resistance and are difficult to control with oral hypoglycaemic agents.
- They often rapidly progress to insulin therapy. They have auto-antibodies (antiGAD) and have a history of other autoimmune conditions.
- Prevalence estimated at 5–10% of diabetes.

# 8.2 Diabetic emergencies

## Diabetic ketoacidosis

### Diagnosis

- Diabetic ketoacidosis (DKA) is a disorder of absolute insulin deficiency and hence predominates in those with type 1 diabetes.
- It is rare but not impossible for those classified as type 2 to develop DKA.
- It is usually diagnosed based on a triad of biochemical abnormalities:
  - Ketonaemia (ketones (beta-hydroxybutyric acid and acetoacetic acid) positive in blood greater than or equal 3mmol/L)/on urinalysis (> 2+)).
  - Hyperglycaemia (glucose >11.0mmol/L).
  - Acidosis (venous pH <7.3, serum bicarbonate <15mmol/L).
- It has a mortality of 2–5% mainly due to delays in presentation and diagnosis.

### Epidemiology

- One in 11 subjects in the European IDDM (insulin-dependent diabetes mellitus) complications study reported hospitalization for DKA over a 12-month period.
- The incidence is 5–8/1000 diabetic patients per year.
- 25% of cases are new presentations of diabetes, but up to 50% of cases occur in known diabetics and are precipitated by infection.
- Poor compliance and/or manipulation of insulin doses (for a variety of reasons) is the next most common precipitant.
- For these reasons, DKA is more common in individuals <19 years of age, with a slight ♀ preponderance.

### Pathogenesis

- Insulin's main function with respect to blood glucose regulation is to increase peripheral glucose uptake and utilization, whilst stimulating hepatic glycogen synthesis and peripheral fat deposition to mop up any excess.
- DKA occurs as a result of absolute insulin deficiency. Although blood glucose levels are high, they cannot be utilized, and glucose is the primary energy substrate of the body. Hence the liver increases production of glucose by gluconeogenesis together with the breakdown of liver glycogen stores by glycogenolysis.
- Levels of the main counter-regulatory hormones (i.e. glucagon, cortisol, catecholamines, growth hormone) increase in response to the stress and alternative energy substrates are mobilized, including free fatty acids from adipose tissue. The by-product of fatty acid metabolism is ketone production, which results in a metabolic acidosis.
- Both glycosuria and ketonuria promote an osmotic diuresis with resultant hypovolaemia and hypotension.

### Clinical features

- When DKA occurs as a first presentation of diabetes, symptoms are usually present over a number of days with progressive dehydration, ketosis, and weight loss.
- However, DKA can develop very rapidly in a patient with established diabetes, particularly when insulin therapy has been forgotten, deliberately omitted, or disrupted. Children on continuous subcutaneous insulin infusions (CSII–'pump' therapy) seem susceptible.
- Other symptoms of dehydration such as muscle cramps may be present and deep regular rapid breathing (Kussmaul respiration) may occur as a result of acidosis, while the breath can smell of ketones.
- Vomiting, confusion, or abdominal pain may occur, as can symptoms of an underlying infection.
- Hypovolaemia—with accompanying losses of both sodium and potassium—can be profound (up to 6L or 10% of body weight) at presentation.

### Management

**Fluid resuscitation must be initiated as soon as the diagnosis is recognized**. Most hospitals will have their own written electronic protocol for management (Fig. 8.2). However, it was increasingly recognized that the management of DKA was suboptimal, even if local guidelines were present. To this extent the Joint British Diabetes Societies (JBDS-IP) Inpatient Care Group published 'national' guidance on the management of DKA in adults in 2010, revised in 2013 (https://www.diabetes.org.uk/About_us/What-we-say/Specialist-care-for-children-and-adults-and-complications/The-Management-of-Diabetic-Ketoacidosis-in-Adults/).

The National Inpatient Diabetes Audit of 2012 reported 170 out of 216 hospitals introduced new DKA guidance, the majority based upon the JBDS-IP.

- Fluid replacement, then treatment of hyperglycaemia, are the two first priorities.
- Complete a brief history and examination to assess the clinical condition of the patient and to establish the presence of precipitating factors/comorbidities. Remember to examine for signs of infection (don't forget the feet) and properly assess the patient's level of consciousness (GCS).
- The principles of JBDS-IP guidance move to make use of the rapid improvement in technology, particularly blood ketone measurement. They also utilize a fixed rate intravenous insulin infusion (FRIII) rather than the traditional sliding scale (variable rate intravenous insulin infusion (VRIII)).

*Treatment aims*

- Clear the blood of ketones and suppress ketogenesis.
- Achieve a fall of ketones of at least 0.5mmol/L/hour.
- In the absence of ketone measurement, bicarbonate should rise by 3mmol/L/hour and blood glucose fall by 3mmol/L/hour.
- Maintain serum potassium in normal range.

*Initial investigations*

- U&E.
- Urinalysis/venous/POC (Point of Care) sampling for ketones.
- Venous blood gases to evaluate the acid–base status of the patient.
- A FBC (leucocytosis does not always indicate concomitant infection).
- Cultures of blood and urine and a CXR (septic screen) as clinically indicated.
- ECG (arrhythmias due to potassium abnormalities/silent myocardial ischaemia).
- Other investigations depending on the presentation.

*Fluids*

- In the normotensive individual, i.e. SBP >90mmHg:
  - 1L IV 0.9% saline over 1 hour, continued according to national guidelines
  - 5% dextrose is usually commenced when the blood glucose is 10–15mmol/L. NICE (NG17) recommend no more than 2L in 24 hours. The aim is to allow continued infusion of insulin to suppress ketosis. It is not volume replacement.
  - Up to 7L of fluid may be required in the first 24 hours depending on the clinical condition of the patient
- If the patient is shocked (SBP <90mmHg), fluids may need to be given more rapidly.
- If the patient is elderly or has signs of cardiac/renal failure, more gradual fluid replacement is indicated.

| Guidelines for the management of diabetic ketoacidosis | | | |
|---|---|---|---|

**Diagnostic Criteria**
- Glucose >13mmol/L
- pH < 7.3
- Ketonaemia/Ketonuria
  (All three criteria essential)

**Fluids**

| Time | Primary Infusion | Rate |
|---|---|---|
| 1st hour | 1L 0.9% saline | 999mL/hr |
| next 2h | 1L 0.9% saline + KCl 20mmol | 500mL/hr |
| next 2h | 1L 0.9% saline + KCl 20mmol | 500mL/hr |
| next 4h | 1L 0.9% saline + KCl 20mmol | 250mL/hr |
| next 4h | 1L 0.9% saline + KCl 20mmol | 250mL/hr |
| next 6h | 1L 0.9% saline + KCl 20mmol | 170mL/hr |
| Reassess | | |

- Administer primary infusion via a volumetric pump
- If hypotensive give 500ml of 0.9% saline stat
- If hypokalaemic (K < 3.8mmol/L) use 0.9% saline with 40mmol/L of KCl
- Consider use 0.45% saline if $Na^+$ >155mmol/L
- Once BS <12mmol/L and patient still ketotic, add 10% glucose 12 hourly (83mL/hr) and modify saline infusion to avoid fluid overload
- When pH normal and non-ketotic use 0.18% saline/4% dextrose with 20mmol KCl if IV fluids are still required

**A continuous insulin infusion is essential to treat ketosis**

- Actrapid[R] Insulin (soluble insulin) 6 units IV bolus
- Actrapid[R] Insulin 50 units in 50mL 0.9% saline (1 unit/mL) via a syringe driver
- Use FRIII - Fixed rate intravenous insulin infusion as per JBDS guidelines
- Only stop insulin on senior medical review

**Other measures:**
**Continue long acting/intermediate insulin:**
**e.g. Determir (Levemir), Glargine (Lantus) Insulatard**
- NG tube if drowsy or vomiting.
- S/C LMWH as per NICE
- Antibiotics if evidence of bacterial infection
- CVP line if elderly, hypotensive, cvs or renal disease
- Consider critical care referral (blp 759) if severe acidosis (pH<7.1) or if invasive monitoring indicated

**Initial Investigations**
- Lab blood glucose
- U&E
- FBC
- Arterial/Venous blood gases
- Urine for Ketones and MSSU
- CXR & ECG
- Blood and other appropriate cultures

Monitoring

| Parameter | How often? | Comment |
|---|---|---|
| ECG | Once | Ideally in all patients with severe DKA (pH<7.1) in view of rapid changes in serum $K^+$. |
| Pulse/BP/T° | Hourly | If hypotensive give 500ml of colloid stat and consider urine output and CVP monitoring |
| Urine output | Hourly | Catheterize if oliguric (<30mL/h) in first 2h, or if indications for CVP monitoring exist |
| Capillary Bld sugar | Hourly | May be unreliable if > 20mmol/L |
| Venous (Lab) Glucose | 0, 2, 6, 12 & 24h | Especially if fingerprick blood glucose > 20mmol/L. Document results in notes. |
| U&E + venous $HCO_3$ | 0, 2, 6, 12 & 24h | Aim for $K^+$ of 4–5.5mmol/L |
| Arterial blood Gases | 0, 2h | Repeat if deteriorating. Omit if pH > 7.3 and $HCO_3$ > 17. Document results and time. |
| CVP (if needed) | Hourly | Infusion rates may need to be adjusted accordingly |
| Ketone assessment | 2 Hourly | Gives an indication of persistent ketosis |

| If emergency advice required at any time contact the diabetologists. |
|---|

Fig. 8.2 Example of a DKA management protocol.

- Central venous pressure monitoring and urinary catheterization may help guide rate of fluid replacement.

*Potassium*

Serial serum potassium measurements **need** to be made to guide the rate of replacement:

- Patients are profoundly potassium deplete, despite normal to high serum levels on initial electrolytes.
- Insulin is required to drive potassium into cells. In the insulin-deficient state potassium shifts from a predominantly intra- to an extracellular cation. The kidneys try to maintain homeo-stasis by increasing potassium excretion—resulting in a significant total body potassium deficit.
- Insulin initiation causes a massive shift of potassium back into the intracellular space—often resulting in significant extracellular hypokalaemia.
- Potassium replacement is usually required even if the initial levels are within normal limits.
- Regular reassessment of plasma potassium is essential (every 1–2 hours).
- Cardiac arrhythmia makes a significant contribution to the mortality of DKA. Consider continuous cardiac monitoring if the potassium concentration is abnormal.

*Insulin*

- The JBDS-IP guidelines have moved away from a sliding scale to a fixed rate insulin infusion.
- No initial bolus is required.
- Soluble insulin (e.g. 50 units. Actrapid® in 50mL 0.9% saline) is given by a fixed rate intravenous infusion at a rate calculated according to the patient's weight, i.e. 0.1 unit/kg/hour (e.g. 7mL/hour if weight is 70kg).
- Insulin is administered primarily to switch off the ketosis; normalization of blood sugars is a secondary endpoint. Insulin infusion is continued until after the ketoacidosis has cleared.

- If the patient normally uses a basal insulin (analogue or human) continue this at the usual dose and usual time.

**Additional therapies**

- Management in a HDU or ITU setting may be appropriate.
- Sodium bicarbonate is rarely indicated as it can paradoxically worsen intracellular acidosis and result in hypernatraemia and fluid overload. Use is usually restricted to severe acidosis pH <6.9mmol/L and only within the intensive care setting.
- In the absence of access to blood ketone measurement venous bicarbonate measurement should be used to assess improvement in acid–base status—this avoids repeated arterial punctures.
- Antibiotics are required for a confirmed or suspected infection; note C-reactive protein may increase modestly secondary to the ketosis, even in the absence of infection.
- Prophylactic anticoagulation (LMWH) may be necessary in an immobile patient.
- Nasogastric tube insertion should be considered in the confused/agitated individual. Acidosis profoundly delays gastric emptying, increasing the risk of aspiration.

**Complications**

Children are particularly prone to cerebral oedema as a complica-tion of DKA. They are highly sensitive to rapid changes in serum osmolality. It typically presents as a declining level of consciousness 8–24 hours after commencement of intravenous fluid replacement. Mortality can be up to 90%. Although mannitol and dexamethasone are frequently used in this situation, clear benefit has not been shown.

**Subsequent treatment**

Subcutaneous insulin can be commenced once the ketoacidosis has cleared, blood glucose levels are stable, and the patient is eating and drinking normally. There should be an overlap between subcutane-ous insulin administration and discontinuation of the intravenous insulin infusion to ensure that the patient does not become insulin deficient.

Education about the causes of DKA and their avoidance/early recognition must be given. In recognition of the complexity of management DKA attracts a best practice tariff.

# Hyperosmolar hyperglycaemic state (HHS)

## Diagnosis

- HHS (previously known as hyperosmolar, non-ketotic hyperglycaemia, HONK) affects patients with Type 2 diabetes.
- Although similar to DKA, patients usually have sufficient insulin to suppress ketoacidosis but not enough to prevent hyperglycaemia (typically the patient with type 2 diabetes who still produces some insulin).

The cardinal features of this condition are:

- Hyperglycaemia (frequently plasma glucose >30mmol/L).
- Elevated serum osmolality (may be in excess of 350mOsmol/kg).
- Absence of ketonaemia/ketonuria (ketones may be present if the patient has not eaten for a prolonged period or has been vomiting).
- Absence of acidosis.
- Hypovolaemia.

Hyperglycaemia and hyperosmolarity lead to signficant osmotic diuresis and an osmotic shift of fluid to the intravascular space, resulting in further intracellular dehydration.

## Epidemiology

- HHS typically affects an older population than DKA.
- The mortality can be as high as 50% often reflecting the impact of multiple comorbidities.
- High refined carbohydrate intake dehydration, infection, myocardial infarction, and drugs (e.g. glucocorticoids, thiazide and loop diuretics) are common precipitants of this condition.

## Pathogenesis

The presence of some insulin production is sufficient to inhibit hepatic ketogenesis and thus prevents the development of ketosis and acidosis in this condition; however, the amount of residual endogenous insulin secretion is usually insufficient to prevent the development of hyperglycaemia. The latter is also exacerbated by excess counter-regulatory hormone secretion.

## Clinical evaluation

- Presentation is often very non-specific but associated with severe dehydration and confusion.
- Coma may also occur particularly if serum osmolality is very high.
- Marked dehydration predisposes to hypercoagulability and patients are at significant risk of venous thromboembolic events.

## Management

- As per DKA, the JBDS-IP has produced national guidance, 2012 (https://www.diabetes.org.uk/About_us/What-we-say/Specialist-care-for-children-and-adults-and-complications/Management-of-the-hyperosmolar-hyperglycaemic-state-HHS-in-adults-with-diabetes/
- Fluid resuscitation.
- Electrolyte correction.
- Insulin infusion.
- Patients with HHS are at significant risk of developing cerebral oedema—particularly in response to rapid shifts in serum osmolality, this can be avoided by controlled lowering of the serum osmolality and glucose levels.
- Hourly review and adjustment of insulin doses is recommended. U&E should also be rechecked regularly.
- In elderly patients, especially those with significant comorbidities, fluid replacement often needs to be less vigorous than for DKA and central venous monitoring of fluid status may be required. Use measured or calculated osmolality to help guide treatment.
- Suggested sequential fluid regimen:

- The aim is to correct significant hypovolaemia in those who are often frail with multiple comorbidities.
  - A target would be to replace 50% of the deficit within the first 12 hours.
  - Choice of fluid is controversial, but JBDS-IP recommends fluid choice based upon initial osmolality and slow correction of abnormalities. They would recommend 0.9% saline.
  - 0.45% saline is recommended if osmolality fails to fall despite adequate rehydration and glycaemic control.
- Aim for a reduction in blood sugar of no more than 5mmol/L per hour—a target sugar of 10–15 is reasonable. JBDS-IP recommends FRIII, 0.05 units per kg per hour. Be aware that initial hydration often reduces blood sugar, accompanied by a fall in osmolality. JBDS-IP recommends, in a non-ketotic individual, to withhold insulin until the fall in glucose precipitated by hydration has stabilised.
- Treatment dose anticoagulation (LMWH) is usually advised even in the absence of signs of clinical thrombosis.
- Intravenous antibiotics need to be considered if an infection is suspected.
- A nasogastric tube should be placed in patients with reduced level of consciousness as there is an increased risk of aspiration (pneumonia).

## Complications

- Hypernatraemia often worsens as the glucose levels are lowered, which can occur with rehydration alone. As long as the osmolality continues to fall do not be concerned.
- Over-aggressive correction of glucose and sodium abnormalities carries a risk of precipitating cerebral oedema (mortality of up to 70%).
- Pancreatic stunning, extremely high levels of glucose are toxic to the pancreatic beta cells, and it is not uncommon for the patient to temporarily require insulin to prevent ketosis in the short term.

# Hypoglycaemia

## Definition

- Biochemical hypoglycaemia is defined as a blood sugar <3.5mmol/L, however in the context of adults with treated diabetes, less than 4mmol/L is the treatment threshold. 'Mild' hypoglycaemic episodes are self treated. 'Severe' hypoglycaemic episodes require third party intervention.
- Classical symptoms do not have to be present.
- Hypoglycaemia frequency and severity should be assessed at annual review, as should awareness of hypoglycaemia. NICE (NG 17) recommends the use of standardized scores. Remember to discuss driving (Section 8.3).

## Pathogenesis

- Glucose homeostasis in the normal individual is tightly regulated by a variety of counter-regulatory mechanisms (e.g. insulin, glucagon, cortisol, adrenaline).
- However, the use of exogenous insulin or insulin secretagogues perturbs normal homeostasis.
- Most people with diabetes learn how to regulate their blood sugar levels through a combination of medication, diet, and exercise. However, relatively subtle changes to daily routine can provoke hypoglycaemia, e.g.:
  - A missed or delayed meal.
  - Increased physical activity.
  - Excess alcohol.
  - Overdose (usually non-deliberate) of insulin or oral hypoglycaemic agent.
- Longer-acting, renally excreted sulphonylureas such as glibenclamide are particularly troublesome as they accumulate in patients with renal impairment and may cause severe prolonged hypoglycaemia.

## Clinical evaluation

*Symptoms and signs*

- Hunger, blurred vision, and weakness.
- Autonomic—sweating, tremor, palpitations, peripheral vasoconstriction.
- Neuroglycopenia—occur with plasma glucose <3.6mmol/L, e.g. headache, impaired concentration, drowsiness, coma (glucose <1.5mmol/L).

The autonomic symptoms usually provide early warning, sufficient for the individual to treat their blood glucose levels before they become unable to help themselves. However the autonomic response is often down-regulated after recurrent bouts of severe hypoglycaemia and they can be completely absent in autonomic neuropathy. Adrenergic blocking drugs (β-blockers) may also 'dampen' warning signs, however the majority of diabetologists would still prescribe β-blockers for their cardiovascular benefits, due to their established benefit rather than the 'theoretical' hypoglycaemia risk.

## Management

➔ Remember: Four is the Floor! Hypo treatment is required.
  Think Six! Do I need to to do something to prevent a Hypo?

The initial treatment of hypoglycaemia should be the administration of rapid-acting carbohydrate, followed by long-acting carbohydrate, be it the next meal or an additional carbohydrate.

It is best practice after the event to determine why it happened, particularly in the hospitalised patient. Is there anything further I should do to prevent a recurrent episode?

*If the individual is conscious, and able to swallow:*

- Advise 15–20g short-acting carbohydrate (CHO), e.g. 90–120mL Lucozade™, glucose tablets check manufacturers guidance, all vary, or 150–200mL pure orange juice.
- Recheck blood glucose in 10–15 minutes and repeat above a maximum of two times if still <4mmol/L—seek medical help.

- Follow-up with longer-acting CHO—1 slice toast, 2 biscuits, normal meal.

*Semi-conscious: i.e. confused, non cooperative but able to swallow*

- Apply glucose gel 1–2 tubes (GlucoGel™) to buccal mucosa or 1mg glucagon IM.
- Recheck blood glucose in 10–15 minutes and repeat above a maximum of two times if still <4mmol/L. Only administer glucagon once.
- Once recovered follow up with longer acting CHO.

*Unconscious:*

- 'ABC' and resuscitation if needed.
- 75–80mL of 20% dextrose (via large vein with generous flush) if in a medical setting.
- Follow-up with 10% glucose IV until stable with repeat glucose testing after 10 minutes, 60 minutes, and then 2-hourly.
- Or 1mg glucagon IM in the community. Once conscious, follow up with longer-acting CHO. Follow local policies for treatment of pre-op patients who are NBM.
▶ Individuals who do not have good glycaemic control may experience hypoglycaemic symptoms with blood sugars well within the normal range.
- Treatment will reverse their symptoms—their body has adapted to chronically high sugar levels!
▶ More than one episode of third-party hypoglycaemia within 12 months can lead to the loss of a group 1 driving license.

The Joint British Diabetes Societies Inpatient Care Group, has published guidance on the management of hypoglycaemia in adults in 2010 (revised 2013). (available at: https://www.diabetes.org.uk/About_us/What-we-say/Specialist-care-for-children-and-adults-and-complications/The-hospital-management-of-Hypoglycaemia-in-adults-with-Diabetes-Mellitus/).

# 8.3 Diabetes—long-term management

## Background

- Diabetes is a lifetime diagnosis.
- Hyperglycaemia, however mild, has now been definitively proven to be deleterious and associated with a significant increase in morbidity and mortality.
- Maintenance of normoglycaemia, along with aggressive cardiovascular risk management, has been shown in the landmark diabetes trials, UKPDS—type 2 diabetes, and DCCT—type 1 diabetes, to be beneficial in terms of reducing morbidity, increasing life expectancy, and increasing quality of life.

Despite these findings, general provision of diabetes services in primary care, where the majority of patients are cared for, was historically poor. This changed with the introduction of the QOF—Quality Outcome Framework structure—which required general practitioners to hold up-to-date diabetes registers including risk factor management. Reimbursement from the government was dependent upon reaching set population targets.

Secondary care is advised for all patients with type 1 diabetes and for those type 2 patients with significant comorbidities/complications. It is also recommended for paediatrics, adolescents, pregnancy, and those receiving insulin via continuous subcutaneous insulin infusion—CSII, i.e. pump therapy.

NICE recommends that any adult person with diabetes should be reviewed at least twice a year. One appointment should include screening for complications—the annual review. NICE also have specific clinical guidelines for the management of both type 1 and type 2 diabetes.

## Annual review

These following targets, based upon NICE and JBS (Joint British Societies) guidelines, are for the 'average' patient with diabetes—and should be individualized according to need:

- Glycaemic control—target HbA1c ≤6.5% (<53mmol/mol). This should also include hypo/hyperglycaemia assessment and education.
- Blood pressure—target ≤140/80mmHg; ↓ if complications.
- Cholesterol—target total <4.0mmol/L, LDL <2.0mmol/L. Other cardiovascular risk factors, smoking status, and antiplatelet therapy should be reviewed.
- Albumin:creatinine ratio—target ♀ <3.5, ♂ <2.5.
- Retinal review.
- Foot review—pulses, vibration sense, 10g monofilament.
- Erectile dysfunction/pregnancy/contraception.
- Depression screening.

## Lifestyle advice

- A diagnosis of diabetes is a life-changing event. Any chronic illness is a risk factor for depression, and after the diagnosis patients frequently evolve through a typical grief reaction. Psychological support is of proven benefit, and recommended in the national service framework (NSF); unfortunately very little support is generally available on the ground.
- Successful diabetes management is dependent upon full acceptance of the diagnosis with the willingness to undertake the lifestyle changes required. The impact of dietary modification and exercise is often under-rated, but is paramount to success.
- Patients should have immediate referral to a qualified dietician with an interest in diabetes. Written as well as verbal information should be given.

Those **diagnosed with type 1 diabetes** should be instructed in home blood glucose monitoring (HBGM) and prescribed insulin therapy. The latter should be initiated by a health professional—usually a diabetes specialist nurse—who is conversant with the latest devices and their suitability for an individual's needs. The first experiences of a person with diabetes, with their future healthcare services providers, significantly influences their acceptance of the disease.

For those **diagnosed with type 2 diabetes**, intensity of glucose monitoring (HBGM vs. urinalysis vs. periodic HbA1c) is dependent upon: the therapy initiated, age, and prognosis; e.g. a young 25-year-old female diagnosed with type 2 controlled with OHGA will usually undertake HBGM striving for normoglycaemia whilst an 80-year-old, diet-controlled, may simply require periodic HbA1c evaluation.

All should be offered structured education programmes: e.g. DESMOND™ and DAFNE™ which are recognized and validated for type 2 and type 1s respectively.

## Insulin therapy

- Insulin therapy + lifestyle advice (diet and exercise) is the required treatment for type 1 diabetes. It is also used for type 2 diabetes after other therapies have failed.
- Initiation of insulin therapy has several social implications.

## Driving

The Driver and Vehicle Licensing Agency (DVLA) needs to be informed once insulin is initiated, and these patients will need to renew their standard licences (Group 1) every 1–3 years. It is a legal requirement that blood sugar is tested within 2 hours of driving, and every 2 hours whilst on a long journey. "Blood glucose of 5 is safe to drive!" Do not drive if HBGM<4, treat as a hypo and then wait for 45 minutes before driving. Patients on oral hypoglycaemic therapies only need to inform the DVLA if they develop hypoglycaemia. The automatic ban to hold a group 2 license whilst on insulin (larger vehicles and some passenger carrying vehicles) has now been lifted—licenses are now issued after individual independent medical assessment providing strict criteria are met. Those on any oral hypoglycaemic therapies who hold a Group 2 license need to inform DVLA. (https://www.gov.uk/guidance/assessing-fitness-to-drive-a-guide-for-medical-professionals https://www.gov.uk/diabetes-driving https://www.diabetes.org.uk/Guide-to-diabetes/Living_with_ diabetes/Driving/).

## Insurance policy

All insurance policies held, e.g. life assurance, car insurance, need to be informed of the diagnosis of diabetes. By law, companies are not allowed to discriminate. The major UK diabetes charity (Diabetes UK) mediates with companies to offer competitive rates.

## Employment law

Various occupations used to be excluded to those on insulin—air traffic control, armed forces, etc. However many blanket bans have been fought in court using disability discrimination laws, and now employers are advised to act upon an individual basis.

## Insulin type and frequency

- In the UK the majority of patients administer insulin via subcutaneous injection. Those with type 2 diabetes are typically commenced on a basal insulin (intermediate/long acting) once or twice daily to work in conjunction with their oral hypoglycaemic agents (OHGAs).

- The insulin therapy of individuals with type 1 diabetes should mimic human physiology as closely as possible. Currently for the majority this is achieved by multiple injection therapy (MIT): the basal-bolus system. Individuals inject a once/twice-daily long-acting basal insulin, NICE (NG17) now recommends an insulin analogue, to mimic basal pancreatic secretion. When the individual eats, a short-acting, analogue, insulin is administered to cover the glycaemic peak of carbohydrate intake. The average person eats thrice daily, hence the average number of injections given is four/five per day.

- For this system to be effective, individuals have to tailor their short-acting analogue dose according to their pre-meal blood glucose, carbohydrate content of the meal, and planned activity.

- Some individuals, for a variety of reasons, cannot cope with this system and fare better on a twice-daily pre-mixed insulin, the twice-daily regimen. It suits sedentary predictable lifestyles and can achieve acceptable control.

- For newly-diagnosed type 1 patients in the UK, insulin analogues, i.e. insulins which have been modified to mimic endogenous insulin action, are now recommended. The short-acting analogues allow eating and injecting to occur simultaneously as they have a more rapid onset of action than the previously used soluble insulins (Actrapid®). The long-acting analogues, insulin glargine (Lantus®) and insulin detemir (Levemir®), were designed to be peakless to provide a more stable level of basal insulin with a reduced risk of hypoglycaemia, particularly nocturnal (Table 8.2). NICE (CG87) does not recommend basal analogues as first line for type 2 diabetes.

- The insulin delivery device, e.g. disposable or cartridge, should be determined by patient choice/acceptability and then according to acquisition cost.

- Animal insulins—bovine and porcine are still available. They should not be initiated in newly diagnosed individuals, but continued as a treatment of choice for those reluctant to change. A switch to animal insulin was often used in individuals who had lost all hypoglycaemic warning, but no evidence backs this up.

### Prescribing insulin

When insulin was first discovered in 1922, it was prepared in concentrations of 20 units/mL, and later 40 and 80 units/mL. However, the only standardized insulin syringe at that time was designed with 20 marks per mL. This led to many dosing areas with adverse patient outcomes. In the early 1980s the UK adopted U100 insulin (100 units per mL), following the US, Canada, Australia, and New Zealand, with the aim of improving patient safety.

However, in 2010 the then National Patient Safety Agency (NPSA) put out a Rapid Response Report following over 3000 wrong dose insulin reports over a 6-year period. Common themes included the use of non-insulin syringe to draw up insulin and the abbreviation of 'U' or 'IU' for units e.g. 10 U is read as 100. The writing of 'U' instead of units is now classified as a significant drug error.

With increasing type 2 diabetes and insulin resistance, many patients are requiring significant quantities of insulin at every injection. Hence the volume of insulin needed to be injected becomes impracticable. So in the more recent years U500 has become

available i.e. 500 units per mL. This has been prescribed in the UK for a minority of individuals because of safety concerns over incorrect dosing. Individuals have to be educated on calculating their dose safely using U100 insulin syringes. Lately, given the rise in obesity, insulin production companies have launched U200 and U300 versions of their insulins. Safety has been taken into consideration and the insulin administration devices have been designed such that the dose that is 'dialed up' is the dose (in units) that is delivered irrespective of the concentration of the insulin within the device.

### Continuous subcutaneous insulin infusion (CSII)—pump therapy

CSII is currently the most physiological method of insulin delivery available.

- Rapid-acting insulin is delivered continuously (24 hours) subcutaneously via a small pump—the basal rate. The basal rate is configured on an hourly basis and individualized to a patient's needs. The basal rate can also be adjusted 'instantaneously' upwards or downwards to account for exercise and intercurrent illness, for example. Similar to MIT, a bolus dose is programmed into the pump by the patient to be delivered at each carbohydrate intake. Advantages of CSII over MIT bolusing include the ability to give the calculated dose of insulin all at once or staggered over time to match the glycaemic index of the carbohydrate consumed. Dosing is much more accurate, down to 0.01 units, compared to 0.5 units with pen/syringes.

- NICE currently recommend pump therapy for adult type 1 patients who have failed to gain adequate glycaemic control on MIT, or whose control cannot be improved because of the risk of/or fear of significant hypoglycaemia.

- Pump therapy is expensive in terms of material costs, but with correct patient selection the benefits are enormous in terms of improved quality of life, ability to work, etc. as well as improved glycaemic control. Pumps can be used in tandem with continuous glucose monitoring systems (CGMS; Figs 8.3 and 8.4). CGMS continuously samples glucose levels in the subcutaneous tissues, feeding back the information to the pump. The new-generation pumps, according to individual pre-programmed targets will set off an alarm when glucose levels rise or fall out of target. Some will pump suspend, i.e. stop insulin, if you do not respond to a low alarm. Robust evidence to support the additional cost of CGMS is not yet available; hence NHS funding is on an individual patient basis, or self-funding.

- The artificial pancreas (closed loop system) combines insulin pump and sensor technology with a tablet/smart phone. The computer is programmed with a mathematical algorithm which in real time takes over control of basal insulin delivery by the pump. Individuals still have to bolus for meals. Trial results are very promising.

- AGP (ambulatory glucose profile) is a new form of glucose monitoring. Using sensor technology, companies have now developed commercially viable hand-held blood glucose meters that also download sensor data to provide individual glucose profiles. They can be a useful tool to improve glucose control.

▶ Note CGM and AGP glucose data is not blood data so is currently not accepted for driving or insulin dosing.

| Type of insulin | Examples | Peak activity (hours) | Duration of action (hours) |
|---|---|---|---|
| Rapid analogue | Lispro | 0.5–1.5 | <6 |
| | Aspart | | |
| | Apidra | | |
| Basal analogue | Detemir | Peakless | 24 |
| | Glargine | | |
| Short acting | Human Actrapid® | 1–3 | <8 |
| Intermediate | Human Insulatard® | 4–8 | <24 |
| Long acting | Human Ultratard® | 6–24 | <36 |

Table 8.2 Common insulins: name, peak activity, and duration

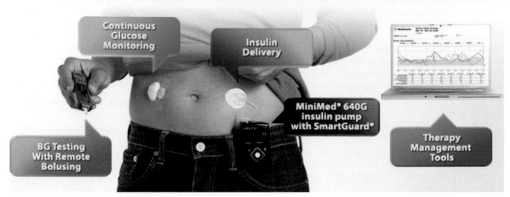

**Fig. 8.3** Combined CSII and CGMS.
Reproduced with permission of Medtronic.

Trend Graph
2 weeks up to 10.05.2011

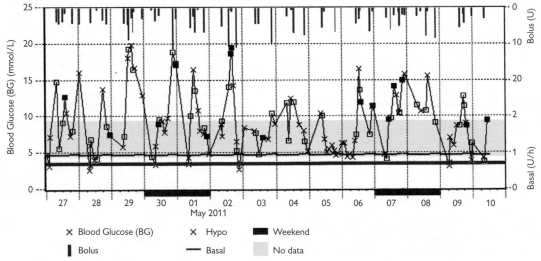

**Fig. 8.4** Example of downloaded pump data.

### Inhaled insulin

- The first to the UK market was Exubera® a rapid-acting insulin (delivered via an inhaler device)—hence a long-acting insulin injection was still required.
- In January 2008, it was withdrawn from the market as it did not meet customers' needs or financial expectations. Post-marketing surveillance has also highlighted a potential concern regarding increased lung cancer rates in treated individuals.

### Buccal insulin

- Buccal insulin is a short-acting form of recombinant insulin that is sprayed into the oral cavity, where it is absorbed into the blood stream.
- It is currently in clinical trials.

## Oral hypoglycaemic agents

- See Table 8.3.
- Most patients with type 2 diabetes should be given a 3-month trial of diet, exercise, and weight loss before initiation of drug therapy. In those patients with an acute presentation, drug therapy may

need to be initiated from diagnosis; however, lifestyle advice is also paramount.

- The choice of OHGA is becoming more diverse, although the majority of people with type 2 diabetes are initiated on metformin. Intensification of drug treatment should be in a stepwise logical manner taking into account the individual's glucose target, in accordance with NICE type 2 diabetes (NG28).
- Metformin remains the first-line agent, increased slowly to minimise GI side effects, Metformin modified release is reserved for those with GI intolerance.
- This is followed by a first intensification of treatment, dual therapy, i.e. two non-insulin blood glucose–lowering therapies—metformin plus. The second intensification would include triple therapy, three non-insulin therapies, or any treatment combination containing insulin. Quadruple therapy is four non-insulin-based therapies.
- Glitazones are contraindicated in those with heart failure and those at risk of osteoporosis. Rosiglitazone has been implicated in causing more ischaemic heart disease-related deaths and has been withdrawn by the European Medicines Agency (EMA). Pioglitazone has a Medicines and Healthcare products Regulatory

**Table 8.3** Oral hypoglycaemic agents

| Class | Mechanism of action | Major side effects | Expected HbA$_{1c}$ reduction |
|---|---|---|---|
| Biguanides, e.g. metformin | Decrease hepatic gluconeogenesis and increase muscle glucose uptake | Gastrointestinal disturbance. Lactic acidosis (rarely) | 0.8–2.0 |
| Sulphonylurea, e.g. glipizide, gliclazide | Stimulate insulin secretion from the pancreatic β cells | Hypoglycaemia, weight gain | 1.5–2.5 |
| Prandial glucose regulators, e.g. repaglanide | Stimulate insulin secretion from the pancreatic β cells | | 0.5–1.9 |
| α-Glucosidase inhibitors, e.g. acarbose | Inhibit breakdown of carbohydrates into monosaccharide components | Postprandial fullness, abdominal pain, flatulence | 0.4–0.7 |
| Thiazolidinediones/glitazones, e.g. rosiglitazone, pioglitazone | Increase insulin sensitivity of adipose tissue and muscle by activating the PPARγ receptor | Fluid retention, weight gain CVS risk (rosiglitazone), bladder cancer (pioglitazone) | 0.6–1.5 |
| Dipeptidyl peptidase-4 (DPP-4) inhibitors (the 'gliptins'), e.g. sitagliptin, vildagliptin | Inhibit the degradation of GLP-1 and GIP which results in ↑insulin secretion and suppression of glucagon release | Nasopharyngitis, headache | 0.6–1.0 |
| Sodium-glucose co-transporter 2 inhibitors, e.g. dapagliflozin | Inhibit reasorption of glucose in proximal tubule | Urinary tract infection, genital Infection | 0.32–0.84 |

Agency (MHRA) warning regarding a small increased risk of bladder cancer.

- Other drug classes include the prandial glucose regulators. Like sulfonylureas they stimulate pancreatic insulin secretion but have a much shorter half-life, hence are taken with each meal. The risk of hypoglycaemia is reduced.
- SGLT2 (sodium glucose transporter 2) inhibitors are the newest agents to be introduced in the market, e.g. dapagliflozin. Its action is glucose dependent, but independent of insulin, leading to a favourable profile with respect to hypoglycaemia. It prevents reabsorption of glucose from the proximal renal tubule. Post-marketing surveillance has led to an FDA warning regarding ketosis. Canaglifozin has an FDA warning regarding reduced bone density and fractures.

# Incretin mimetics

## DPP-4 inhibitors

- Oral agents, the gliptins, are inhibitors of the enzyme DPP-4 dipeptidyl peptidase-4, which degrades endogenous GLP (glucagon-like peptide). Endogenous GLP-1 levels are enhanced, promoting glucose-dependent insulin release.
- They have been proven to be as effective as all other OHGA in terms of lowering glucose levels, but as they are glucose dependent, the incidence of hypoglycaemia is low. Some agents in the class are metabolized hepatically, some renally. All are weight neutral. Further evidence is beginning to show beneficial class effects with respect to lowering of blood pressure and alterations in lipid profiles. The majority now have a license for use with insulin.

## GLP-1 agonists

- GLP-1 agonists are injectable non-insulin therapies e.g. exenatide, liraglutide, and lixisenatide. As mimetics of the incretin GLP-1, they increase insulin release in response to eating and suppress glucagon. They are licensed for use with oral hypoglycaemic agents, and insulin. They are injected subcutaneously once/twice daily/once weekly and typically achieve an ~1% reduction in HbA1c levels, without the risk of hypoglycaemia unless used concomitantly with a sulphonylurea/insulin.
- NICE (NG28) recommend them for use in the second intensification treatment stage, provided the individual has a BMI >35 kg/m$^2$ and specific psychological or other medical problems associated with obesity; or BMI <35kg/m$^2$ and for whom insulin therapy would have significant occupational implications or weight loss would benefit other significant obesity related comorbidities.

- The main advantage of these GLP-1 agonists is that they promote significant weight loss (insulin is associated with weight gain). This is as a consequence of delayed gastric emptying promoting early satiety and central effects promoting reduced appetite. They can delay the progression to insulin initiation for a few years if successful.
- Their predominant side effect is nausea and occasionally vomiting. Pancreatitis is emerging as a possible side effect in post-marketing surveillance.
- Combination therapies—2015 saw the license of the first medicine that combines insulin with another therapy, in this case a GLP-1 agonist. Xultophy combines insulin degludec with GLP-1 liraglutide. 1mL of Xultophy contains 100 units of insulin degludec and 3.6mg of liraglutide. Xultophy is administered once daily, subcutaneously. It is administered in 'dose steps'. One dose step is equivalent to 1 unit of degludec and 0.036mg liraglutide. The initial dose recommended is 10 dose steps if adding on to oral therapies, or 16 dose steps if transferring from a basal insulin.

# Islet cell transplantation

- Islet cell function is replaced by islet cells from a human donor. The donor islets are injected into the portal vein/liver or in the spleen. Most people require two transplants. Within two to six weeks they start producing insulin.
- Islet cells transplants are not a cure for diabetes. Although the donor islets produce insulin, few patients will become 'injection' free. The majority, however, will require significantly less insulin.
- Islet cell transplantation is reserved for those patients with type 1 diabetes who have recurrent severe hypoglycaemia (despite the best medical therapy, including pump therapy) or for those with a functioning kidney transplant on immunosurpressive therapy. Benefits include reduced frequency of hypoglycaemia, improved awareness of hypoglycaemia, reduced fear of hypoglycaemia, and increased quality of life. These need to be balanced against the risk of life long immunosuppression to prevent rejection of the transplanted islets. As of 2103, 95 transplants had been performed in 65 patients in the UK.
- Whole pancreas transplantation is an alternative option. The majority of patients will have normal glucose levels, but is generally only used in conjunction with renal transplantation in patients with end-stage renal failure secondary to diabetic nephropathy. It is a procedure associated with much more significant risk.
- Multivisceral transplantation is occasionally considered for those whose lives are disabled by severe gastroparesis and are dependent upon parenteral nutrition.

# 8.4 Diabetic retinopathy

## Background

As well as the retinopathies, ophthalmic complications of diabetes include:

- Corneal abnormalities
- Glaucoma
- Iris neovascularization
- Cataracts
- Neuropathies.

Although the most common ocular abnormalities in diabetes are cataracts, the most sight-threatening are the retinopathies. Retinopthies include background, proliferative, and maculopathy.

## Epidemiology

- Diabetic retinopathy remains the most common cause of blindness in individuals aged 20–74 years in the developed world.
- Proliferative retinopathy is more common in type 1 diabetes and maculopathy in type 2.

### Prevalence of retinopathy

*Type 1*
- <5 years (since diagnosis of diabetes): rare.
- 5–10 years: 30%.
- 10 years: 70–90%.

*Type 2*
- 10 years: 67% retinopathy, of which 10% will have proliferative diabetic retinopathy.

### Prevalence of macular oedema at 10 years
  - Type I patients: 20%.
  - Type 2 patients (non-insulin treated): 14%.
  - Type 2 patients (insulin treated): 25%.
- Diabetic retinopathy is more common in ethnic minorities than in Caucasians.

## Classification

Classification and severity grading were previously based on ophthalmoscopic examination findings. These did not necessarily reflect functional severity. Two different approaches to classification have emerged: those aimed at the ophthalmologist covering the full disease spectrum (e.g. the Early Treatment Diabetic Retinopathy Study (ETDRS)); and those used in population screening.

There is considerable overlap between the two. The following is one of the many classifications:

1. Retinopathy:
   - Background retinopathy:
     - Microaneurysms.
     - Haemorrhages (dot and blot/flame-shaped).
     - Hard exudates (lipid deposits).
   - Pre-proliferative retinopathy:
     - Soft exudates (cotton wool spots, nerve fibre infarcts).
     - Intra-retinal microvascular abnormalities (IRMAs).
     - Venous changes (e.g. beading).
   - Proliferative retinopathy (Fig. 8.5)
     - New vessels at the disc or within one disc diameter of it (NVD).
     - New vessels elsewhere (NVE).
     - Rubeosis iridis (iris neovascularization).
2. Maculopathy (Fig. 8.6):
   - Focal oedema.
   - Diffuse oedema.
   - Haemorrhages and hard exudates at the macula.
3. Advanced disease:
   - For example, retinal detachment.
4. Cataract.

## Pathophysiology

- Diabetic retinopathy is classically regarded as a microvascular complication (Fig. 8.7). However, as with all diabetic complications, a combination of vascular and metabolic factors is likely to contribute to its development. Increased erythrocyte and platelet aggregation and adhesion may predispose to a sluggish circulation. Endothelial damage and focal capillary occlusion result in retinal ischaemia.
- Sorbitol accumulation (aldose reductase pathway) as a result of hyperglycaemia leads to thickening of the capillary basement membranes and pericyte loss. This in turn results in weakness and eventual saccular outpouching (microaneurysms) of capillary walls.
- Increased permeability of these vessels results in leakage of fluid and proteinaceous material, which appears clinically as retinal thickening and exudates.

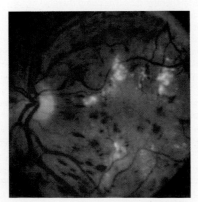

Fig. 8.5 Proliferative diabetic retinopathy with neovascularization.

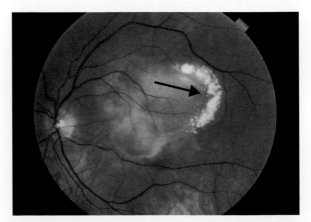

Fig. 8.6 Diabetic maculopathy: oedema and characteristic hard exudates around the macula (arrow).

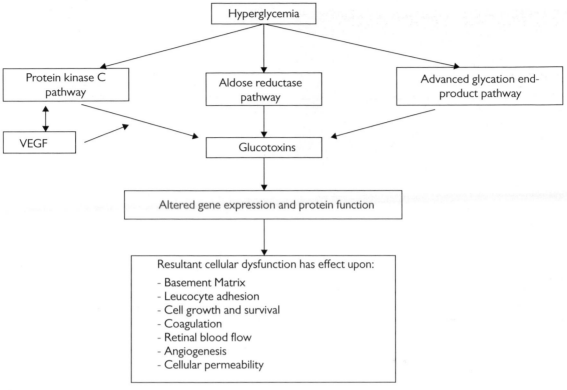

**Fig. 8.7** Pathophysiology of diabetic eye disease.

- As the disease progresses, closure of the retinal capillaries occurs leading to hypoxia. Infarction of the nerve fibre layer leads to the formation of cotton-wool spots.
- Further increases in retinal ischaemia trigger the production of vasoproliferative factors such as vascular endothelial growth factor (VEGF) and basic fibroblast growth factor (bFGF) that stimulate new vessel formation.

## Risk factors for development of diabetic retinopathy

### Duration of diabetes
There is a clear relationship between the duration of diabetes and development of retinopathy in both type 1 and 2 diabetes.

### Poor glycaemic control
Improved glycaemic control is the most important factor in reducing the development and progression of retinopathy, in both type 1 and 2 diabetes.

A 1% reduction in glycosylated haemoglobin reduces by ~1/3 the risk of requiring laser treatment.

### Hypertension
Observational studies have shown that hypertension is associated with retinopathy. Accordingly, treating hypertension reduces the risk of development and progression of diabetic retinopathy and maculopathy. ACE inhibitors are better at regulating retinal blood flow than β-blockers.

### Age
Older patients per se have an increased risk of visual impairment.

### Pregnancy
Pregnancy is associated with an unpredictable and sometimes rapid progression from background to proliferative retinopathy in a small number of individuals. They remain at risk until a year postpartum. Numerous factors have been implicated including poor pre-pregnancy glycaemic control, rapid improvement in glycaemic control during the pregnancy, and pregnancy-related hypertension. Patients should ideally be counselled prior to conception.

### Diabetic nephropathy
- All stages of diabetic renal impairment are associated with increased incidence of retinopathy.
- Transplantation, however, can be associated with an improvement in retinopathy.

### Miscellaneous risk factors
- Hypertriglyceridaemia
- Severe anaemia
- Puberty
- Intercurrent infection.

## Treatment

Untreated proliferative diabetic retinopathy leads to vitreous haemorrhage. Later in the disease, fibrotic tissue around the new vessels contracts with recurrent vitreous haemorrhage and tractional retinal detachment.

### Treatment of risk factors
- Both the United Kingdom Prospective Diabetes Study (UKPDS: type 2 diabetes) and the Diabetes Control and Complications Trial (DCCT: type 1 diabetes) showed a reduction in the risk of development and a slowing in the rate of progression of retinopathy with improved glycaemic control.
- The UKPDS also reported a 35% reduction in the need for laser therapy in patients with improved blood pressure control.
- Although some studies have shown a relationship with hyperlipidaemia, postulating deleterious effects of oxidized LDL-cholesterol in endothelial cells, no randomized controlled trial of treating hyperlipidaemia has shown a benefit.

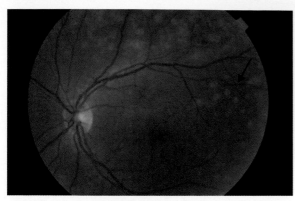

**Fig. 8.8** Panretinal photocoagulation (arrow).

### Treatment of established retinopathy

- For patients with severe proliferative retinopathy pan-retinal laser photocoagulation (PRP) reduces visual loss by >80%. PRP works in two ways:
  1. Multiple 'burns' to the peripheral retina reduces oxygen demand, reducing ischaemia-driven new vessel proliferation.
  2. New vessels can be 'lasered' to prevent leakage/haemorrhage (Fig. 8.8).

### Treatment of Maculopathy (DMO—Diabetic Macular Odema)

- Anti-VEGFA therapy, ranibizumab (NICE TA274, 2013) is approved in DMO if retinal thickness is >400mm. By inhibiting VEGFA, oedema and visual loss is reduced. It is administered monthly by intravitreous injection, until maximum visual acuity is achieved, which in practice is when vision has been stable for three consecutive months. It is gaining use in proliferative retinopathy.
- Aflibercept (NICE TA346, 2015) is an anti-VEGFA and B-inhibitor, as well as anti-placental growth factor. Again administered as an intravitreal injection.

- Intravitreal corticosteroid therapy: NICE TA349, 2015, recommended the use of dexamethasone intravitreal implant for the treatment of DMO, if there is an artificial lens, or if the patient's oedema has not improved with other treatments. It suppresses inflammation and prevents oedema. It contains 700mcg dexamthasone, and is degraded over time, approximately 6 months, when the treatment can be repeated.
- Laser therapy: it is possible to laser the macular, with effective results.
- Oral protein kinase C inhibitors (e.g. ruboxistaurin) are in development.

### Miscellaneous treatments

- For patients with vitreous haemorrhage or scarring, a vitrectomy may help to restore vision and reduce retinal traction.
- Cataract extraction is of benefit in affected patients.

## Prevention/screening

- Adequate control of blood glucose and blood pressure will help reduce the risk of developing of diabetic eye complications.
- Adult Patient with diabetes should undergo an annual eye examination from diagnosis. Children from age 12. NICE recommends screening with digital retinal photographs through dilated pupils. Visual acuity should be part of the review. There is now a National Diabetes Eye Screening Programme (DESP).
- Referral to ophthalmologists and recall are based upon screening classifications.
- Urgent referral to an ophthalmologist is indicated for patients with:
  - Sudden loss of vision
  - Rubeosis iridis
  - Pre-retinal or vitreous haemorrhage
  - Retinal detachment.

► Aspirin therapy does not reduce the risk of developing retinopathy, nor does it increase the risk of retinal haemorrhage.

Thrombolytic therapy in the treatment of myocardial infarction is **not** contraindicated.

# 8.5 Diabetic neuropathy

## Background

- One of the microvascular complications of diabetes.
- The exact pathogenesis is not fully understood, but metabolic (deposition of advanced glycation end-products) and vascular changes have been implicated in its aetiology. Other potential contributory factors include reduced levels of local nerve growth factor production, oxidative stress, and accumulation of sorbitol and fructose (aldose reductase pathway) with decreased levels of myo-inositol and glutathione.

## Epidemiology

- In a cohort of 4400 Belgian patients, 7.5% already had clinical evidence of neuropathy when diagnosed with type 2 diabetes. After 25 years, the number with neuropathy rose to 45%.
- Additional methods of detection, such as autonomic or quantitative sensory testing, may increase the prevalence.
- ♂ patients with diabetes usually have a higher incidence of diabetic neuropathy than ♀ patients, and symptomatic presentation is more common in individuals over the age of 50 years.

## Classification

### Sensory neuropathy

- The most common form of neuropathy.
- Early symptoms are often intermittent and affect the extremities—most commonly the feet. Patients report dysaesthesia (tingling and burning) often worse at night, affecting sleep quality. Symptoms gradually progress to chronic severe pain.
- Peripheral sensorimotor neuropathy is usually symmetrical and affects the longest fibres (feet) first with gradual progression proximally in a 'glove and stocking' manner.
- Symptoms often precede clinical detection. Absent ankle reflexes and decreased perception of vibration with a 128Hz tuning fork are commonly the first abnormalities found on examination. Loss of perception of a 10g monofilament also indicates a foot 'at risk' of ulceration (Fig. 8.9).

### Motor neuropathy

- Proximal motor neuropathy (diabetic amyotrophy) is relatively rare. Involvement of the lumbosacral plexus results in severe pain and paraesthesia of the proximal thighs with quadriceps wasting. Marked cachexia can also occur with this condition. Recovery is possible, with time, often in association with improved glycaemic control.
- Acute mononeuropathies are well recognized and may be the presenting symptom of diabetes, e.g. cranial nerve palsies III, IV, and VI, lateral common peroneal nerve palsy. Recovery is variable.

### Autonomic neuropathy

- Erectile dysfunction (ED) is the most common presentation of autonomic dysfunction, although the true aetiology of ED is both vascular and neurological.
- Otherwise autonomic dysfunction is generally a late consequence of long-term poor glycaemic control.
- Gastroparesis occurs if the vagus nerve is affected—stomach emptying is delayed resulting in nausea, vomiting, bloating, and weight loss.
- Cardiovascular symptoms include postural hypotension and painless ischaemia.
- Other causes of peripheral neuropathies need to be considered, particularly if symptoms occur early in a well-controlled patient with diabetes, e.g. alcohol-related neuropathy, vitamin B$_{12}$ deficiency.

## Treatment

- Improving glycaemic control is usually advocated as first line; however, it will only reverse symptomatology in those with relatively mild neuropathy of recent onset.
- Antihypertensive agents which act as vasodilators (ACE inhibitors, α-blockers) may be of benefit in some cases.

(A)
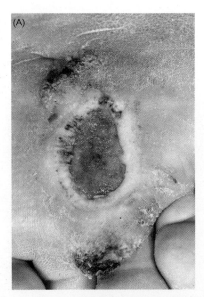

(B)
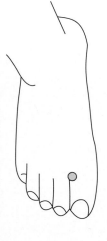
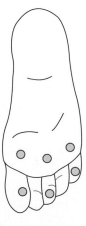

**Fig. 8.9** Neuropathic ulcer in a diabetic patient with sensory neuropathy (A) and recommended points for testing with 10g monofilament (B).

- Aldose reductase inhibitors have shown benefit in animal studies but their use in humans, to date, has been limited by toxicity; newer agents are currently undergoing trials.
- For painful (small fibre) neuropathies, topical agents such as 0.075% capsaicin are frequently commenced as first-line agents, often in conjunction with simple analgesia. However, NICE Clinical Guidance 173, *Neuropathic Pain* (November 2013), now advocates a choice of amitryptiline, duloxetine, gabapentin, or pregabalin, switching between drugs if one is not tolerated or effective. Emphasis is placed on non-pharmacological therapies, coping mechanisms, and managing expectations. Refer to specialist pain services if needed, with a potential trial of tramadol as a rescue agent only, whilst awaiting review.
- Antioxidants and exogenous nerve growth factor treatments are also currently under investigation.
- Gastroparesis may benefit from prokinetic drugs, e.g. metoclopramide, domperidone, erythromycin. Botulinum toxin therapy to the pyloric muscle and gastric neurostimulators have had some benefit in very resistant cases as has multivisceral organ transplantation.

- ED may respond to phosphodiesterase-5 (PDE5) inhibitors, but due to its mixed aetiology referral to speciality urological ED clinics is recommended if not successful. Hypogonadism, in those with type 2 diabetes, is now being increasingly recognized. Several studies have shown testosterone replacement to be beneficial in these individuals.

## Prevention

- Tight glycaemic control decreased the risk of neuropathy by 60% in 5 years in the Diabetes Control and Complications Trial.
- Neuropathic assessment is a key part of the diabetic annual review process.
- For those with 'at-risk' feet, education regarding daily foot care is essential with regular podiatry/chiropody support. The use of suitable footwear has been shown to prevent some problems from developing.

# 8.6 Diabetic nephropathy

## Background

- Diabetic nephropathy (DN) is a clinical syndrome characterized by persistent albuminuria, leading to proteinuria and a progressive decline in glomerular filtration rate, ultimately resulting in end-stage renal failure (ESRF).
- DN is the most common cause of ESRF in the Western world (and increasingly in developing nations), accounting for 20–40% of patients starting on renal replacement therapy.
- ~20–30% of patients with diabetes will develop DN.
- Diabetic patients developing nephropathy have a higher mortality than those without nephropathy: the majority die from cardiovascular complications.

## Epidemiology

- **Type 1 diabetes mellitus** (T1DM):
  - DN is rare in the first 5 years.
  - 10 years after onset, the annual incidence of nephropathy increases dramatically, to a peak of 3% per year at ~15 years.
  - The annual incidence than falls and those who have not developed nephropathy 35 years after disease onset are unlikely to do so.
  - Overall, about 30% of patients with T1DM develop DN.

- **Type 2 diabetes mellitus** (T2DM):
  - Nephropathy is present in 10% at presentation (reflecting previous undetected hyperglycaemia).
  - The 20-year cumulative risk of nephropathy is 25% in Caucasians, but is higher (up to 50%) in other ethnic groups (e.g. Afro-Caribbeans, Asian Indians, Japanese).
  - ~20% of people with T2DM with nephropathy develop ESRF.
  - The overall numbers of patients with T2DM and DN is much higher than T1DM and DN, given the greater population prevalence of the former.

## Aetiology

- **Chronic hyperglycaemia** and poor glycaemic control increases the risk of nephropathy in part due to the non-enzymatic glycation of proteins, resulting in higher levels of advanced glycosylation end products (AGEs). Cytokine production by macrophages and mesangial cells results in increased synthesis of type IV collagen. Hyperglycaemia also reduces the mesangial cells degradation of proteins accumulating in the extracellular matrix. Tubular cell TGF-ß also worsens this situation.
- **Hypertension** is a risk factor for nephropathy, and normalizing BP can slow disease progression. BP control by inhibition of the renin–angiotensin system seems to be most beneficial.
- **Genetic factors** play a role in susceptibility to both diabetes itself, and to the development of nephropathy. As with conditions such as SLE, genome-wide association studies in both type 1 and type 2 DM have identified several genetic mutations that are associated with an increased risk of developing the disease.

## Pathology

Renal pathology is characterized by increased deposition and/or decreased degradation of mesangial matrix, culminating in the obliteration of the glomerulus and sclerosis (Figs 8.10 and 8.11). The typical progression is:

- Increasing glomerular basement membrane thickness.
- Glomerular and tubular hypertrophy.
- Increasing deposition of extracellular matrix.
- Hyalinization of arterioles.
- Progressive mesangial sclerosis culminating in nodular glomerulosclerosis (Kimmelstiel–Wilson nodules).

## Clinical evaluation

From the time of diagnosis of diabetes, patients should be monitored closely for signs of nephropathy. The disease usually follows a well-characterized pattern, detailed here for T1DM:

- **Stage 1**: when a diagnosis of diabetes is made, the GFR is usually elevated, up to 120% of age matched controls. Urinary ACR is also often elevated. As glycaemic control is achieved with insulin (or other) therapy, both the GFR and the urinary ACR usually fall.
- **Stage 2**: during this stage, which may last 5–15 years, glomerular hyperfiltration with expansion of the mesangium may be seen. The ACR is not usually elevated.
- **Stage 3**: begins when microalbuminuria is detected (ACR 20–200mg/mmol). GFR may still be elevated or have

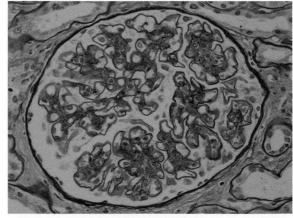

Fig. 8.10 Diabetic nephropathy.

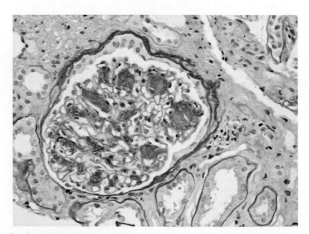

Fig. 8.11 Diabetic nephropathy.

normalized: significant renal damage has occurred before the serum creatinine rises. This stage usually lasts 10–15 years.
- **Stage 4**: 'established' nephropathy commences as the GFR declines. Proteinuria increases and is detectable on conventional urinalysis. Most patients are hypertensive and 30% become nephrotic. Renal biopsy shows diffuse glomerulosclerosis, with Kimmelstiel–Wilson lesions in 10%.
- T2DM is thought to progress in a similar fashion. Sometimes, these patients may present very late, and develop stage 4 nephropathy soon after diagnosis with diabetes.
- This may present diagnostic difficulties, and a renal biopsy may be required to exclude another cause for the renal impairment and heavy proteinuria.
- Generally, nephropathy is associated with retinopathy (common basement membrane pathology), and therefore rapid onset renal impairment in a diabetic without retinopathy may be an indication for renal biopsy. Non-diabetic renal pathology should also be considered if there is significant haematuria, very difficult-to-control hypertension, or other systemic illness.

## Management

- Good glycaemic control (both types of DM) can prevent development of DN.
- Screening allows early detection and treatment of microalbuminuria, and is highly cost effective as ESRF is expensive, as well as conferring an increase in morbidity and mortality:
  - Following diagnosis with DM, patients should be screened annually for albuminuria. Serum creatinine should be measured and used to estimate GFR.

### Clinical trials in diabetes mellitus

- The Diabetes Control and Complications Trial Research Group (DCCT)—1441 patients with T1DM were randomly assigned to either intensive therapy with three or more daily insulin injections guided by frequent blood glucose monitoring or to conventional therapy with one or two daily insulin injections. The patients were followed for a mean of 6.5 years. Intensive therapy delayed the onset and slowed progression of diabetic retinopathy, nephropathy, and neuropathy in patients with T1DM.
- In the United Kingdom Prospective Diabetes Study (UKPDS), 5102 patients with newly diagnosed type 2 diabetic patients were followed for an average of 10 years to determine whether intensive use of pharmacological therapy to lower blood glucose levels would result in clinical benefits. In addition, patients with T2DM who were also hypertensive were randomized to 'tight' or 'less tight' BP control. The study found that microvascular complications (retinopathy, nephropathy, and possibly neuropathy) benefited by lowering blood glucose levels with intensive therapy. Lowering BP to a mean of 144/82mmHg significantly reduced microvascular complications as well as stroke, diabetes-related deaths, heart failure, and visual loss. Epidemiological analysis showed a continuous relationship between the risk of all the above outcomes and SBP increasing above 130mmHg.

- Patients with persistently elevated albumin excretion rates require:
  - Good glycaemic control. This can slow the progression of the kidney lesion once microalbuminuria has developed. Worse glycaemic control is associated with a faster decline of the GFR in those with established DN.
  - Good BP control. Maintaining BP at <130/80mmHg can slow the decline in GFR in patients with stage 4 nephropathy.
  - ACE inhibitors and ARBs. These have been shown to slow the time to doubling of the serum creatinine and delay ESRF in patients with overt DN. This effect seems to be partly independent of their effect on BP. Combination therapy is not recommended.
  - Cardiovascular risk reduction. Cardiovascular risk is much higher in patients with DM and particular attention should be paid to standard cardiovascular risk factors: aspirin is advised for all patients with DN, statins for lipid management, and smokers should be encouraged to stop.
- Nephrological referral should be made according to local guidelines. In general, this is advised when the GFR falls below 50mL/min, i.e. during CKD stage 3, where sequelae such as anaemia and renal bone disease may occur. Preparation for renal replacement therapy can therefore be instituted as appropriate. Where possible, those with stage 4/5 CKD should receive a pre-emptive kidney transplant, which may be combined with a pancreas transplant. Late referral to nephrology services (within 6 months of requiring dialysis) is associated with a higher mortality.

## Outcome

- Patients with T1DM have a 20-fold greater mortality than the general population. This already increased risk is magnified 25-fold in those with proteinuria, and death is usually from cardiovascular disease.
- Diabetic patients with ESRF on dialysis have the highest mortality of all, at 30% in 2 years.
- Transplantation improves the mortality rate, such that the 5-year survival post transplant is 45–75%.

## Other renal/urinary tract-related complications

- Papillary necrosis—sloughing of the renal papilla due to impaired blood flow in the vasa recta. This can predispose to infection and the sloughed papillae may cause ureteric obstruction.
- Autonomic dysfunction affecting the bladder may lead to outflow obstruction, with or without ureteric reflux, and subsequent chronic kidney disease.
- ▶ Remember that insulin is renally excreted; an unexplained reduction in insulin requirements or new-onset recurrent/prolonged hypoglycaemia could indicate a decline in renal function.

# 8.7 The diabetic foot

## Background

- Diabetic foot problems are responsible for more hospital bed days than any other complication of diabetes. They also place a significant demand on community care services—district nurses, podiatrists, etc.
- Among patients with diabetes, 10% develop a foot ulcer, and 12–24% of individuals with a foot ulcer require amputation. Diabetes is the leading cause of non-traumatic limb amputation.
- Foot ulceration is a marker of disease severity, with 70% dying within 5 years of amputation.

## Pathophysiology

- Diabetic foot problems result from either neuropathy, ischaemia (Fig. 8.12), or more usually a combination of both.
- Sensory loss results in reduced sensation protection, leading to unnoticed foot injury. Impaired motor control to the small muscles of the foot may lead to deformity—e.g. claw toes, increasing the risk of injury. Autonomic dysfunction compromises blood flow to capillary beds. 1 in 3 people over the age of 50 with diabetes will have peripheral vascular disease.
- Healing is also impaired due to a variety of factors including impaired fibroblast function, growth factor deficiencies, and extracellular matrix abnormalities.
- The main features of both of these conditions are summarized in Table 8.4.

## Prevention and management

Increased prevalence of diabetes is likely to result in an increased prevalence of foot ulceration. Prevention through partnerships between patients and professionals based around annual structured foot surveillance is a key priority. A strong focus on patient education is also essential. NICE (CG19) currently classifies foot risk as:

- Low current risk. No risk factors present.
- Moderate risk. 1 risk factor present.
- High risk. >1 risk factor or previous ulceration/amputation and or on renal replacement therapy.
- Active foot problem: ulceration, spreading infection, etc.

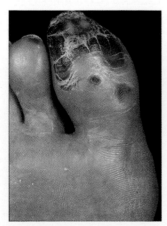

Fig. 8.12 Ischaemic great toe.

Risk factors include

- Neuropathy—use a 10g monofilament
- Limb ischaemia
- Ulceration
- Callus
- Infection and/or inflammation
- Deformity
- Gangrene
- Charcot arthropathy

### Management of infection

- Assess and document size, depth, and position of ulcer. Use one of the standardized severity scores.
- Ulcers are frequently infected. Wound swabs often show a combination of Gram-negative, Gram-positive, and anaerobic organisms.
- Osteomyelitis is very common, ulcers should be probed to see if bone is involved, and samples sent for sensitivities if at all possible. Prolonged antibiotic therapy is required.
- Plain x-rays will only demonstrate established osteomyelitis, but may reveal unsuspected foreign bodies or fractures.
- MRI is effective at demonstrating osteomyelitis and extent of infection.
- Wounds need regular dressing changes; negative pressure wound therapy can be useful. Debridement should only be undertaken by those with the training to do so.
- Offloading: offer non-removable casting to off-load plantar non-ischaemic non infected ulceration.
- Consider revascularization if appropriate. Systemic antibiotic therapy for non-healing/progressive ulcers is often required, resorting to surgery if progression despite treatment.

### Management of vascular insufficiency

- All patients with active ulceration require vascular assessment. Examine the femoral, popliteal, and foot pulses.
- Ankle–brachial pressure index (ABPI), of which manual measurements are preferable to automated systems may be falsely high due to arterial calcification; imaging is often required.
- First-line imaging is arterial duplex ultrasound, followed by contrast enhanced MRA (magnetic resonance angiography), or CT angiography in case of contraindications to MRI.
- Atheroma has a predilection for the medium-sized vessels, e.g. popliteal trifurcation in diabetes. The extent of disease is often widespread, as opposed to discreet lesions, making angioplasty less successful; femoro-distal bypass grafting is then required.

| Table 8.4 Features of ischaemic vs. neuropathic foot | |
|---|---|
| **Ischaemic foot** | **Neuropathic foot** |
| Cool | Warm |
| Absent or decreased foot pulses | Normal/bounding foot pulses |
| Trophic changes, e.g. hair loss | Dry skin |
| Pain associated with ulcers | Painless ulcers |
| Intermittent claudication or rest pain | Callus/Charcot changes of ankle may be present |
| On elevation, pallor of the skin increases; on dependency the foot reddens | |

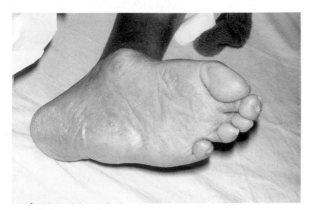

Fig. 8.13 Charcot ankle joint.

## Charcot arthropathy

- Joint destruction (Figs 8.13 and 8.14) secondary to neuropathy—a combination of motor (loss of motor control of muscles) and sensory (loss of proprioception) neuropathy usually affecting the large joints such as the knees or ankles. Charcot may develop post fracture.
- It characteristically presents as swelling and heat and is often mistaken in the early phase for cellulitis. Suspect if the skin is intact! Joint instability and trophic changes in the bone occur and if not recognized lead to major and severe deformities of the foot. This predisposes the foot to future ulceration.
- Diagnosis is usually clinical, but a weight bearing x-ray may be of benefit.
- If it is recognized early, the mainstay of treatment is to prevent foot deformity and destruction by offloading, using a non-removable device e.g. total contact cast.
- Bisphosphonates are no longer recommended, unless part of a clinical trial.

## Limb threatening or life-threatening diabetic foot

Each hospital should have a named consultant and a care pathway for the inpatient care of those with diabetic foot problems.

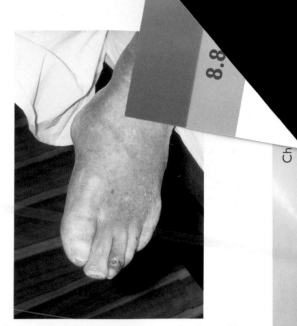

Fig. 8.14 Charcot joint (ankle). Note small ulceration (toes) caused by rubbing on ill-fitting shoes.

All patients admitted should be referred to the foot MDT (multi disciplinary team) within 24 hours of admission or detection of a foot problem.

If patients present with

- Ulceration with fever or any signs of sepsis
- Ulceration with limb ischaemia
- Gangrene

They should be referred immediately to acute services, who will then according to local protocols refer to the foot MDT for urgent individualized treatment and assessment. Often this involves urgent decompression surgery, with revascularisation and definitive surgery at a later stage.

# Diabetic skin

## Background

The most common skin conditions seen in diabetes are infections particularly genital candidiasis, often a presenting complaint in young males, and folliculitis caused by *Staphylococcus aureus*.

Other skin manifestations of diabetes include:

- **Scleroderma diabeticorum:** a thickening of the skin on the back of the neck and upper back which mainly affects people with T2DM.
- **Pretibial diabetic dermopathy:** shin spots, pigmented pretibial papules.
- **Bullosis diabeticorum:** painless blisters that usually occur on the fingers, hands, toes, feet, legs or forearms, particularly in patients with poor glycaemic control and diabetic neuropathy.
- **Necrobiosis lipoidica diabeticorum:** thought to be caused by changes in the collagen and fat content of the subcutaneous tissues leading to reddening and thinning of the overlying skin (Fig. 8.15).
- **Granuloma annulare:** sharply defined, ring or arc-shaped areas on the skin.
- **Vitiligo:** areas of depigmentation seen particularly in patients with type 1 diabetes. Of autoimmune aetiology.
- **Acanthosis nigricans:** darkening and thickening of the skin particularly in areas of skinfolds such as the axillae. This is usually seen in patients with insulin resistance.
- **Eruptive xanthomatosis:** firm, yellow, waxy bumps on the skin usually seen on the buttocks or face. This condition tends to occur in patients with hypertriglyceridaemia.

## Insulin-induced skin changes

### Atrophy

- Insulin-induced lipoatrophy—localized necrosis of subcutaneous fat tissue.

- Atrophy is now relatively rare and usually occurs at the site of multiple injections.
- The mechanism is not fully understood but involves both local autoimmunity and inflammation.

### Hypertrophy

- Insulin-induced lipohypertrophy—localized accumulation of subcutaneous fat tissue at the site of multiple injections (Figs 8.16 and 8.17).
- In its mildest form it is very common, a side effect caused by failure to adequately rotate insulin injections. Routine checking of injection sites should be part of the annual review.
- In the odd case it can be extreme, if the patient repeatedly injects at the same site.
- The advantage for the individual is that the hypertrophied site is relatively painless to inject into, however the hypertrophied tissue impedes the 'smooth' absorption of the injected insulin, resulting in either unexpected hyper- or hypoglycaemia.

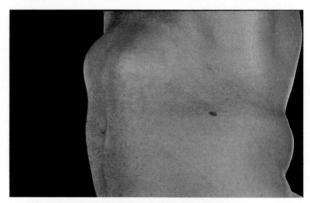

Fig. 8.16 Lipohypertrophy of the abdomen.

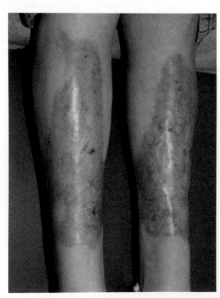

Fig. 8.15 Necrobiosis lipoidica

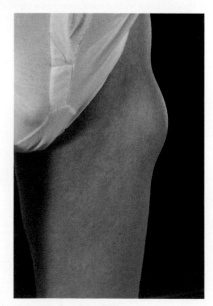

Fig. 8.17 Lipohypertrophy of the thigh.

# 8.9 The diabetic pregnancy

## Background

- There are ~700,000 deliveries per annum in England and Wales; 30,000 of them will be associated with diabetes (2–5%).
- Pre-gestational diabetes, i.e. diabetes that is recognized prior to conception, accounts for the minority percentage (7.5% T1DM, 5% T2DM), with gestational diabetes accounting for 87.5%.

## Pre-gestational diabetes

- It has long been recognized that the pregnancies in women with T1DM are high risk—with poor fetal and maternal outcomes.
- This risk was quantified by the CEMACH (Confidential Enquiry into Child and Maternal Health) report on women with diabetes (2007). The perinatal mortality rate was elevated 3–5× and the congenital malformation rate 4–10×, when compared with the general population. Of greater concern were the panel enquiries that highlighted suboptimal care in a substantial proportion of mothers with diabetes with adverse outcomes.
- The CEMACH report and other studies also published during this time also highlighted that the congenital anomaly rate and total adverse outcomes were as high in women with T2DM as in those with T1DM—dispelling the myth of 'mild' diabetes.

The congenital malformations included:

**Caudal regression syndrome:**

| Arises: | Between 3rd/4th embryonic week. |
|---|---|
| Features: | Sacral agenesis and hypoplasia of the femora. |
| Relative risk: | ↑200×. |

**Central nervous system anomalies:**

| Arises: | Between 2nd/3rd embryonic week. |
|---|---|
| Features: | Anencephaly and other neural tube defects. |
| Relative risk: | ↑ 3–18×. |

**Cardiac anomalies:**

| Arises: | Between 3rd/6th embryonic week. |
|---|---|
| Features: | Ventricular septal defects, transposition of the great arteries, coarctation of aorta. |

- The majority of malformations have already occurred by the time the mother realizes she is pregnant.
- Congenital anomaly rates have been directly linked with poor glycaemic control.
- The key intervention which affects blood sugar levels during the critical time for malformations is **pre**-pregnancy counselling.

## Pre-pregnancy counselling

NICE (NG3) recommend that we should empower women with diabetes to have a positive experience of pregnancy and childbirth by providing information, advice, and support. Part of the emphasis should be the focus on planned pregnancy; discussions regarding choice of contraception should be part of the annual review from adolescence onwards for women with diabetes. Effective contraception is a must. T1DM per se used to be considered a relative contraindication to prescribing the combined oral contraceptive. This is no longer the case; choice should be based on preference and risk factors. Pre-pregnancy counselling is an opportunity to discuss the risks of pregnancy. It should be stressed that risks can be minimized but not eliminated.

There are limited studies, but those available show that women who attend pre-pregnancy care:
- Book earlier for antenatal care (6/40 vs. 8/40).
- Have lower HbA1c at booking (6.5% vs. 7.6%) (48 vs. 60mmol/mol).
- Are three times less likely to have major malformation, stillbirth, or neonatal death (3% vs. 9% for T1DM).
- Are three times less likely to have a very premature delivery <34 weeks (5% vs. 15% for T1DM).

Issues to be discussed and documented include:
- Contraception until optimum control—HbA1c <6.5% (48mmol/mol).
- High-dose folic acid supplementation—5mg once a day.
- Rubella antibody and thyroid status.
- Retinopathy, nephropathy, and hypertension screening.
- Optimization of blood glucose control—dietary advice, intensify blood testing, and potentially alter insulin regimen.
- Warn of increased risk of hypoglycaemia, particularly in first trimester with lack of awareness. Reinforce advice regarding testing blood sugars especially at times relevant to driving.
- Review medication:
  - Replace ACE inhibitors with methyldopa/labetalol.
  - Stop statins.
  - Stop oral hypoglycaemic agents (metformin and glibenclamide (post first trimester), although outside licensed indication, are now recommended/approved by NICE).
- Lifestyle: smoking, alcohol, exercise BMI.
- Discuss increased risks of complications:
  - Congenital anomaly rate (3–10×).
  - Macrosomia/polyhydramnios.
  - Late pregnancy stillbirth.
  - Birth trauma/caesarean sections.
  - Preterm delivery (3×).
  - Perinatal mortality (4×).
  - Neonatal hypoglycaemia.

## Gestational diabetes mellitus (GDM)

- The entity of gestational diabetes (diabetes first detected during pregnancy) continues to provoke international debate, which has led to variations in diagnostic criteria, resulting in varied treatment practices.
- Two seminal papers have been published: the Australian Carbohydrate Intolerance Study in Pregnant Women Study (ACHOIS), 2005 and the Hyperglycaemia and Outcomes Study (HAPO), 2007.
- Both demonstrated an increase in poor fetal and maternal outcomes with increasing hyperglycaemia above the norm. ACHOIS also showed an improvement in outcome, if treatment to lower hyperglycaemia was initiated.
- In the UK NICE (NG3) has defined GDM as abnormal glucose handling following a 75g oral glucose tolerance test (OGTT).
- All women, at risk of GDM, are to be screened with an OGTT between 24 and 28 weeks.

### Risk factors
- BMI >30kg/m².
- Previous macrosomic baby (>4.5kg).
- Previous GDM.
- First-degree relative with diabetes.
- Ethnic family origin with a high prevalence of diabetes.

For those with previous GDM, screening is brought forward—either through initiation of home blood glucose monitoring (HGBM) as soon as pregnancy is confirmed or via an early OGTT as soon as possible after booking, with repeat at 24–28 weeks if the first was normal.

### Diagnostic criteria

- 75g OGTT—fasting plasma glucose >5.6mmol/L.
- And/or 2-hour plasma glucose ≥ 7.8mmol/L.

### Prescreening advice

- GDM responds to diet and exercise in some women.
- OHGA/insulin will be needed if diet and exercise are insufficient.
- Small increased risk of adverse birth complications if not detected/controlled.
- Additional monitoring and/or interventions may be required during pregnancy and labour.

### Risks of GDM

Once GDM is confirmed the risks can be explained in greater detail. These include:

- Fetal macrosomia.
- Birth trauma (to mother and baby).
- Requirements for induction of labour or caesarean section.
- Transient neonatal morbidity, particularly hypoglycaemia.
- Perinatal death.
- Obesity and/or diabetes in the baby's later life.

### Treatment

- Patients should have access to a dietician. They are advised to follow a healthy diet avoiding simple sugars. Low GI rather than high GI foods. Carbohydrates are essential for a healthy diet, but may have to be spread throughout the day. High-density carbohydrates, e.g. rice, pasta, may have to be eaten in significantly smaller quantities.
- HBGM—target glucose levels are <5.3mmol/L fasting, <7.8mmol/L 1 hour, <6.4mmol/L 2 hour post-prandially.
- Exercise post meals should also be emphasized as part of the treatment.
- If diet and exercise fails, OHGA metformin may be used (outside of current licence indications), but if target blood sugars are not attained within a week insulin should be initiated.
- Insulin should be initiated immediately in those with fasting glucose>7mmol/L.
- Consider glibenclamide who decline insulin or cannot tolerate metformin.

### Maternal implications—postnatal care

- Hypoglycaemic medication can be stopped immediately post delivery. Ensure euglycaemia prior to discharge.
- Women should be advised about symptoms of hyperglycaemia, and benefits of weight control, diet, and exercise.
- They should undertake a test of glucose homeostasis, ideally a fasting plasma glucose at 6–13 weeks. After 13 weeks HbA1c is possible. They will need an annual test of glucose homeostasis thereafter.
- The risk of recurrence of GDM in subsequent pregnancies and lifetime risk of T2DM should be discussed.

## Antenatal care

- Antenatal care for both pre-gestational and gestational pregnancies should ideally be provided by a multidisciplinary team comprising of both an obstetrician and midwife with a specialist interest in diabetes, a consultant diabetologist, diabetes specialist nurse, as well as a specialist dietician.
- NICE provides very precise guidance as to what tests should be offered and at what gestation when screening for maternal well-being, e.g. timing of repeat retinopathy and nephropathy screening, for the pre-gestational mother.
- Glucose homeostasis is assessed at every visit. HbA1c is measured in all women with preexisting diabetes at booking to assess level of

risk. It should also be measured at diagnosis of GDM to exclude preexisting type 2 diabetes. It can be used to assess level of risk in the second and third trimester but not to assess glucose control.

- HBGM records should be reviewed. The majority of centres use a 'downloadable' meter, which can aid understanding of trends, and facilitate remote analysis of blood glucose records. The majority of women are advised to test their fasting, pre-meal and 1-hour post-meal, and bedtime glucose. Targets are equivalent to the criteria for GDM.
- Hypoglycaemia and its treatment should be discussed. Increased insulin sensitivity is common in the first trimester as is hypoglycaemic unawareness. Aim to keep glucose levels above 4mmol/l.
- Fetal surveillance. All mothers should be offered the same screening as the non-diabetic population. The pregestationals should also be offered a specialist fetal cardiac scan at approximately 20 weeks of gestation as well as the routine anomaly scan. Fetal growth and amniotic fluid volume should be assessed every 4 weeks, minimum from 28–36 weeks using ultrasound. Increased abdominal circumference can be an indication of poor glycaemic control and efforts should be made to tighten up control. However growth may accelerate despite good glycaemic control, and there is evidence that this is influenced by periconceptual glycaemic control. Other tests of fetal well-being should not be routinely offered before 38 weeks. An individualized approach should be considered for those with a risk of fetal growth restriction.

## Delivery

- The obstetrician will use all the information gained from antenatal care when discussing each woman's birthing plan. A formal delivery plan should be agreed and documented at the 36-week visit. For those with pre-gestational diabetes and no other complications, delivery should be planned between 37+0 and 38+6, providing there are no other complications. For those with GDM and no other complications advise delivery by 40+6.
- Early delivery is recommended because of the increased incidence of still births. (CEMACH reported a rate approximately 5× normal.)
- Women with a macrosomic fetus need to be counselled about the increased risk of obstructed labour, particularly shoulder dystocia.

### Labour

- Neonatal hypoglycaemia requiring intervention is reduced if maternal glucose homeostasis is maintained during labour. Monitor sugar hourly and aim for between 4 and 7mmol/L. If this cannot be maintained consider VRIII.
- The documented delivery plan should include a post natal glucose management plan. This will include insulin reductions/or discontinuation. Breast feeding is encouraged with advice on hypoglycaemia avoidance. Metformin and glibenclamide are compatible with breast feeding.

## Neonatal care

- The neonate is at risk of hypoglycaemia post delivery as a consequence of relative maternal hyperglycaemia and fetal hyperinsulinaemia.
- Women are encouraged to feed their infant within 30 minutes of giving birth.
- Routine assessment of the neonate's blood glucose is not undertaken until at least 2 hours post delivery, unless hypoglycaemic symptoms are present. If blood glucose assessment is undertaken immediately post delivery the infant is likely to be hypoglycaemic: this is a normal physiological phenomenon, not exclusive to infants of diabetic mothers. It can lead to unnecessary treatment and admission of an asymptomatic infant to a neonatal unit. However, admission to a neonatal intensive care may be necessary for intravenous dextrose and monitoring for those who are symptomatic and/or unwilling to feed.
- The infant should remain in hospital for 24 hours to ensure stable glucose homeostasis.

# 8.10 Metabolic syndrome and insulin resistance

## Background

The term 'metabolic syndrome' describes the clustering of cardiovascular risk factors, including dyslipidaemia, glucose intolerance/T2DM, and hypertension, with central obesity. It was first described in 1988 by Reaven, and is also variably known as Reaven syndrome, Syndrome X, insulin resistance syndrome, and dysmetabolic syndrome. Its prevalence continues to rise, mirroring the epidemics of obesity and T2DM.

Over time, the diagnostic criteria for the syndrome have been progressively refined, culminating in the 2005 report of the International Diabetes Federation (IDF) (Box 8.1). More detailed parameters for research are also defined and include pro-inflammatory markers.

The syndrome is associated with a fivefold increased risk of developing T2DM and a threefold rise in the rate of heart disease. It has been estimated to affect ~20% of the adult population in developed countries, and 80% of people with T2DM. Its prevalence rises with age and it is present in ~40% of individuals aged >60 years.

However, some have questioned the utility of creating another 'syndrome', asking what value it adds over and above that provided by considering each of its elements separately. In clinical practice the diagnosis of metabolic syndrome is no better at predicting cardiovascular risk than other CVS risk calculator. Others counter that it not only serves to remind clinicians to address the 'whole' cardiovascular risk profile for any given patient, but in addition it focuses attention on the underlying core drivers for these disorders, i.e. central/visceral obesity and insulin resistance. Latterly the concept of ICO (index of central obesity) has been shown to be as effective as race and gender-specific WC. It is a ratio of your waist to height; if the ratio is >0.5, it is an indicator of metabolic syndrome.

## Management

### Primary Intervention

*Weight loss*
- Even moderate weight loss, in the range of 5–10% of body weight, can significantly improve insulin resistance.

*Dietary modification*
- Eating complex carbohydrates, such as wholegrain bread (instead of white), brown rice (instead of white), sugars that are unrefined (instead of refined), and increasing fibre consumption by eating legumes (e.g. beans), whole grains, fruits, and vegetables can all help to reduce insulin resistance.
- Moderate calorie restriction to achieve 5–10% weight loss.

*Exercise*
- Increased physical activity can also reduce insulin resistance.
- Aerobic exercise, such as a brisk 30-minute daily walk, can result in weight loss, lower BP, a more favourable cholesterol profile, and a reduced risk of developing diabetes.
- Most healthcare providers recommend 150 minutes of aerobic exercise each week.
- Exercise may reduce the risk of heart disease even in the absence of accompanying weight loss.

> **Box 8.1  The new IDF definition of the metabolic syndrome**
>
> According to the new IDF definition, for a person to be defined as having the metabolic syndrome they must have:
> - Central obesity (defined as waist circumference ≥94cm for white ♂ and ≥80cm for white ♀, with ethnicity specific values for other groups).
> - Plus any two of the following four factors:
>   - Raised triglyceride level: ≥150mg/dL (1.7mmol/L) or specific treatment for this lipid abnormality.
>   - Reduced HDL cholesterol: <40mg/dL (1.03mmol/L) in ♂ and <50mg/dL (1.29mmol/L) in ♀ or specific treatment for this lipid abnormality.
>   - Raised BP: SBP ≥130mmHg or DBP ≥85mmHg, or treatment of previously diagnosed hypertension.
>   - Raised fasting plasma glucose (FPG) ≥100mg/dL (5.6mmol/L), or previously diagnosed T2DM.
> - If >5.6mmol/L or 100mg/dL OGTT is strongly recommended but it is not necessary to define presence of the syndrome.
>
> Reproduced with permission from International Diabetes Federation. The IDF consensus worldwide definition of the Metabolic Syndrome. Brussels: International Diabetes Federation; [2006].

## Secondary Prevention

*Correction of dyslipidaemia*
- Aim of treatment is to reduce TG, raise HDL, and reduce LDL cholesterol.
- The most effective drugs to treat the dyslipidaemia of the metabolic syndrome (hypertriglyceridaemia with low levels of HDL-cholesterol) are the fibrates.
- Statins have been shown to be beneficial in trials, predominantly by reducing LDL and ApoB.
- Co-administration of cholesterol and statins can be associated with statins.

*Treatment of hypertension*
- Lifestyle modifications, including decreasing salt intake, are recommended for the hypertension of the metabolic syndrome, although antihypertensive drugs are usually required to control BP.
- ACE inhibitors and ARBs are often the agents of choice as, in addition to their BP lowering effect, some trials would suggest an additional benefit above their blood pressure-lowering effect.

*Smoking cessation*
- A priority in all patients with obesity, T2DM, or the metabolic syndrome.
- Patients should be counselled about the additional cardiovascular risk and informed of available 'quitting strategies' (e.g. nicotine replacement, NHS 'quit smoking' helpline).
- There is no 'specific' drug treatment for metabolic syndrome itself. Multiple studies investigating the use of insulin sensitisers (e.g. metformin, glitazones) have been undertaken with variable results and are currently not recommended.

# Chapter 9

# Gastroenterology and hepatology

# 9.1 Basic science

## Normal nutrition

Nutrition is the mechanism by which the body aims to restore the balance between the energy expenditure of resting metabolism, thermoregulation, and physical work of the human body.

### Lipids

Stores of triglyceride (TG) are the major fuel source for the human body as a whole. Their calorific value is more than twice that of glycogen. TGs are also important constituents of:

- Hormone synthesis
- Cell membranes
- Micronutrient transport.

The ability to utilize TG as fuel is largely dependent upon the population of functional mitochondria, which reduces with age and during ill health. See Fig. 9.1.

### Protein

Protein consists of compounds of any of the 20 amino acids found in humans. A 75kg male will contain 12kg protein and 2kg of nitrogen—at times of excess protein intake this is catabolized to nitrogenous compounds for excretion (since there is no storage mechanism for protein in contrast to carbohydrate and fat). Nitrogen balance is the difference between intake (dietary amino acids and proteins) and loss (urine, stool, skin, and body fluids). Inadequate protein intake causes net loss of protein initially from liver and, latterly, skeletal muscle mass. During times of low calorie intake there is a rise in total protein requirement and this is proportional to the size of the energy deficit. Similarly, improving energy intake (in whatever form) reduces the need for protein and restores the nitrogen balance. See Fig. 9.2.

### Carbohydrate

There is no **absolute** dietary requirement for carbohydrate (CHO) since glucose can be synthesized from endogenous amino acids and glycerol. CHO is, however, the principal energy resource for:

- Bone marrow
- Erythrocytes
- Leucocytes
- Peripheral nerves

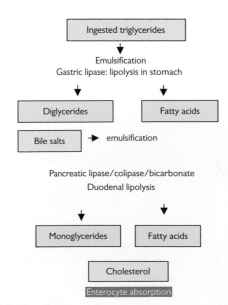

Fig. 9.1 Lipid metabolism.

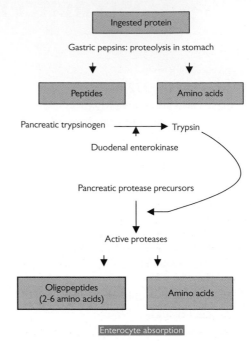

Fig. 9.2 Protein metabolism.

- Renal medulla
- Eye
- Brain.

Dietary CHO intake is also important in terms of its interaction with protein metabolism mediated by insulin, which acts as an inhibitor to muscle protein breakdown and promotes protein synthesis. See Fig. 9.3.

### Minerals

Inorganic nutrients which are required to maintain water homeostasis and normal cell function.

Deficiencies have important clinical sequelae:

- **Sodium**—myopathy (low intravascular volume).
- **Potassium**—myopathy, paraesthesiae, cardiac arrhythmia.
- **Magnesium**—myopathy, tetany, cardiac arrhythmia, hypocalcaemia.
- **Calcium**—osteomalacia, tetany, rickets.
- **Phosphorous**—myopathy, fatigue, leucocyte and platelet dysfunction, cardiac failure.

Trace elements (inorganic nutrients which are required in much smaller quantities): chromium, copper, iodine, iron, zinc, manganese, and selenium.

NB: neither urinary nor serum levels necessarily reflect total body stores and should be interpreted in the clinical context.

### Vitamins

- Organic compounds which are required for normal metabolic processes.
- Serum levels generally reflect total body stores.
- Deficiencies result in specific clinical problems:
  - A (retinol): night blindness.
  - $B_1$ (thiamine): cardiac failure, peripheral neuropathy.
  - $B_2$ (riboflavin): glossitis.
  - $B_3$ (niacin): dermatitis, dementia, diarrhoea (pellagra).

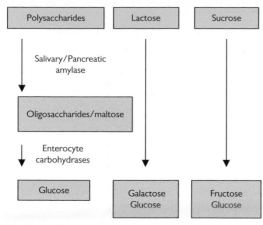

Fig. 9.3 Carbohydrate metabolism.

- B$_5$ (pantothenic acid): fatigue.
- B$_6$ (pyridoxine): glossitis, seizures.
- B$_7$ (biotin): alopecia, dermatitis, seizures.
- B$_9$ (folic acid): megaloblastic anaemia, glossitis, diarrhoea.
- B$_{12}$ (cobalamin): megaloblastic anaemia, ataxia, reduced vibration/position sense.
- C (ascorbic acid): purpura, gingivitis, weakness (scurvy).
- D (ergocalciferol): osteomalacia, osteoporosis, tetany.
- E (α-tocopherol): retinopathy, neuropathy.
- K (phylloquinone): bruising, bleeding (coagulopathy).

# Normal gastrointestinal physiology

Intestinal tract physiology is a complex mechanism by which ingested food is processed to optimize the release of the essential nutrients before absorption and effective transport to the cells of the target organ. The exocrine component of digestion is contributed to by the salivary glands, stomach, pancreas, and biliary system. Each produces specific secretions that are vital to normal digestion and have the capacity to influence absorption and motility in the GI tract.

## Digestion
*Salivary glands*
- Amylase: proteolysis.

*Stomach*
- HCl:
  - Optimum pH for pepsin and lipase.
  - Facilitates inorganic iron absorption.
  - Inhibits gastrin release.
  - Protects against ingested microorganisms.
  - Stimulates pancreatic HCO$_3$ release.
- Pepsin:
  - Protein hydrolysis.
  - Vitamin B$_{12}$ release from protein.
- Lipase: TG hydrolysis
- Intrinsic factor (IF): vitamin B$_{12}$ binding for ileal absorption.
- Mucin: mucosal protection.

*Pancreas*
- Amylase: metabolizes dietary starch/glycogen.
- Lipase: TG hydrolysis.
- Protease:
  - Trypsin, chymotrypsin, and elastase.
  - Carboxypeptidase A/B.
  - Protein metabolism.

Exocrine pancreatic secretion is enhanced by:
- Gastric distension.
- Gastric emptying.
- Duodenal gastric acid, pepsin, and lipase.
And mediated by:
- Hormonal (secretin and cholecystokinin).
- Vagal control.

*Bile salts*
- Important in TG emulsification.

## Absorption
*Fat*
- 40% of human energy requirement is supplied by lipid (mostly TG).
- Gastric acid lyses TGs to fatty acids (FAs) and diglycerides (DGs).
- Phospholipid (ingested and bile-derived) promotes emulsification into micelles.
- Lipase acts to form monoglycerides (MGs) and FAs.
- Most absorbed in proximal jejunum.
- 95% ingested fat is absorbed by adults.

*Protein*
- 10–15% energy requirement.
- Proteolysis begins with pepsin acting at gastric pH to release peptides and amino acids.
- Pancreatic protease action releases trypsin, chymotrypsin, and elastase.
- Release of ingested vitamin B$_{12}$ enables IF binding.
- Assists disaccharide absorption.
- Release of:
  - Amino acids: Na-dependent transporter absorption.
  - Peptides (2–6 amino acids): absorbed directly across epithelium via H$^+$-dependent peptide transporter.
- Peptide utilization by enterocytes.
- Release of amino acids into portal circulation.
- Absorption occurs throughout small intestine (>40% absorbed in ileum).

## Carbohydrate
- 45% total energy requirement is derived from absorbed dietary CHO.
- 50% of dietary CHO is comprised of cereal and plant-derived starch.
- Others:
  - Lactose (milk)
  - Glucose (fruit/veg)
  - Sucrose (fruit/veg)
  - Fructose (fruit/veg).
- Hydrolysed by salivary and pancreatic amylase.
- Disaccharides hydrolysed by enterocyte hydrolase.
- Release of:
  - Glucose
  - Galactose
  - Fructose.
- Readily absorbed at brush border epithelium.
- Not all ingested CHO is absorbed in small bowel.
- Colonic bacterial fermentation results in the release of:
  - Short-chain FA release
  - Hydrogen
  - Methane.

**Vitamins:**

*Fat soluble*

- Vitamin A:
  - Milk/egg yolk/fish oils.
  - Passive diffusion in chylomicrons.
- Vitamin D:
  - Fish oils.
  - Endogenous from skin exposure to UV.
  - Passive diffusion into lymphatics.
- Vitamin E: passive absorption into lymphatics.
- Vitamin K:
  - Liver.
  - Green vegetables.
  - Absorption is dependent on bile salts.

*Water soluble*

- Vitamin $B_{12}$:
  - Liver, kidney, fish, eggs, milk.
  - Absent from vegetables.
  Released from food by gastric HCl and trypsin.
  - Bound to IF in intestinal tract.
  - Absorbed in terminal ileum.
- Vitamin $B_1$ (thiamine):
  - Beans, pulses, nuts.
  - Na-dependent active transport.
  - Absorption into circulation inhibited by ethanol.
- Vitamin C:
  - Fruit.
  - Active Na-dependent absorption across small intestinal enterocytes.
- Folic acid:
  - Spinach, liver, peanuts, beans.
  - Absorption is dependent on hydrolysis at brush border of enterocyte (inhibited by ethanol).
  - Na/pH-dependent absorption.

*Minerals*

- Calcium:
  - Milk/cheese.
  - Active absorption in duodenum.
  - Passive absorption throughout small intestine.
  - Increased by Vitamin D.
- Magnesium:
  - Vegetables.
  - Absorption greatest in ileum >jejunum.
- Iron:
  - Meat/myoglobin
  - Absorbed in proximal small intestine
  - Best absorbed as $Fe^{2+}$
  - Gastric acid increases $Fe^{3+}$ absorption
  - Absorption increased in:
  Fe deficiency
  Pregnancy
  Hypoxia.

*Trace elements*

- Zinc:
  - Meat/shellfish.
  - Enterohepatic circulation.
  - Absorbed in distal ileum.
- Copper:
  - Green vegetables/fish.
  - Absorbed from stomach and small intestine.

**Motility**

**Oesophageal:** pharyngeal contraction propels the bolus through a relaxed upper oesophageal sphincter (UOS) followed by a wave of progressive circular contraction through the body and relaxation of the lower oesophageal sphincter (LOS) with subsequent LOS contraction.

**Gastric:** main peristaltic function is the controlled delivery of fragmented digested food to duodenum. This is also regulated by the LOS and pyloric sphincter. Gastric peristalsis is thought to originate in the greater curve of the mid-body (gastric pacemaker).

After ingestion of a meal there is proximal gastric relaxation with the commencement of the antral 'milling' contractions against a closed pylorus. The pyloric sphincter allows particles of sufficiently fine size to pass into the duodenum.

The principal neural control to gastric motility is afforded via the vagus nerve.

**Small intestinal:** motility is governed by the enteric nervous system (ENS) as a complex interplay between sensory and motor function. ENS may be modulated by autonomic nervous control. Vagal control is thought to be important in terms of secretory function, absorption, and motility. Spinal sensory nerve synapses with the ENS, at present poorly understood, may yet prove to yield more complex regulatory function.

Normal small intestinal motility is disturbed in:

- IBS (clustered contractions).
- Acute illness (ileus).
- Pregnancy (delayed transit).
- Diabetes (slow or rapid transit).
- Drugs (slow or rapid transit).
- Obstruction (high amplitude contractions).
- Pseudo-obstruction (failure of transit).
- Scleroderma (failure of transit).
- Neurological syndromes (failure of transit).
- Myopathic syndromes (failure of transit).

**Colonic:** motility mediated mostly by the ENS which is modulated by:

- Sympathetic
- Parasympathetic
- Extrinsic afferent pathways.

The ENS contains more neural cells than the combined sum of the sympathetic and parasympathetic nervous systems. Each class of nerve cell within the ENS has precise synaptic relationships and functions that remain poorly understood. Nevertheless, aside from motility, the ENS is probably central to the coordination of complex functional and humoral responses of the gut to luminal content.

The ileo-colonic junction appears to regulate colonic filling:

- Prevents reflux/bacterial translocation.
- Proximal colon distension increases emptying.

The preparatory phase of defecation occurs from up to 60 minutes in advance. In the last 15 minutes, pressure waves in distal colon lead to rectal distension and defecatory urge.

## Background

Investigation of the patient with intestinal symptoms or the search for occult GI pathology in the asymptomatic individual generally requires the use of several diagnostic modalities.

## Endoscopy

- Requires informed consent. If a patient is unable to provide consent, an 'incapacity form' must be signed by the responsible consultant (i.e. the consent of a family member is **not** valid).
- Endoscopy performed under sedation is variably cited as carrying a 30-day mortality of 1 in 2000. Recommendations for safe endoscopic practice under sedation include:
  - Relating risk of procedure to patient.
  - Using minimal sedation.
  - Adequate resuscitation before emergency endoscopy.
  - Continuous monitoring both throughout and after the procedure.

### Upper GI tract endoscopy

*Indications*
*Diagnostic*
- Dyspepsia/abdominal pain.
- Haematemesis/melaena.
- Weight loss.
- Iron deficiency anaemia.
- Persistent vomiting.

*Clinical concern of:*
- Peptic ulcer disease.
- Occult GI bleeding.
- Malabsorption (coeliac disease, Whipple disease, giardiasis).
- Upper GI malignancy.
- Upper GI Crohn disease.

*Therapeutic*
- Control of upper GI bleeding (ulcers/varices).
- Dilatation of oesophageal/pyloric strictures.
- Palliation of upper GI cancers.
- Placement of percutaneous gastrostomy (PEG) feeding tubes.

*Complications*
- Cardiorespiratory (arrhythmia, MI, respiratory arrest).
- Death (<0.01%).
- Infection (aspiration pneumonia, endocarditis, hepatitis B/C, HIV, retropharyngeal abscess).
- Bleeding (very rare: <0.1%).
- Perforation (0.03% in diagnostic endoscopy and 2–3% in therapeutic).

*Antibiotic prophylaxis*
- Prosthetic heart valves.
- Previous endocarditis.
- Recent vascular graft (<12 months).
- Neutropaenia.

### Enteroscopy

Push (conventional) 2.5m endoscope will reach into the proximal jejunum:
- Often used in investigation of occult GI bleeding.

Video capsule enteroscopy:
- Visualization of entire length of small intestine.
- No capacity for therapy/biopsy.
- Indicated in otherwise unexplained anaemia.
- Safe procedure (occasional retention of capsule).

### Colonoscopy

*Indications*

*Diagnostic*
- Diarrhoea (± blood).
- Rectal bleeding.
- Assessing extent of Crohn disease/ulcerative colitis (UC).
- Iron deficiency anaemia.
- Surveillance for cancer.

*Will usefully screen for:*
- Neoplasia.
- Vascular lesions (angiodysplasia; see Fig. 9.4).
- Inflammatory bowel disease (IBD).
- Microscopic colitis (lymphocytic colitis, collagenous colitis).

*Therapeutic*
- Polypectomy.
- Thermal therapy to vascular/neoplastic lesions.
- Dilatation/stenting of colonic strictures.

*Complications*
- Death (0.07%).
- Renal failure/electrolyte imbalance during bowel preparation (volume depletion).
- Cardiovascular (MI, arrhythmias).
- Stroke.
- Perforation (0.1–0.2%, more common after polypectomy and in patients with diverticulosis/colitis).
  - Treatment: conservative (antibiotics).
  - May require laparotomy.

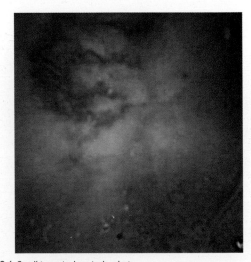

Fig. 9.4 Small intestinal angiodysplasia.
Reproduced with permission of Dr Jeremy Woodward.

- Bleeding (<0.25%).
- Rare complications:
  - Splenic rupture/haematoma.
  - Pneumothorax/pneumomediastinum.
  - Volvulus.

## Radiology

### Plain abdominal X-ray
- Sub-diaphragmatic gas: suggests intestinal perforation.
- Dilated loops of bowel: suggests intestinal obstruction or fulminant colitis.
- Oedematous colonic mucosa = colitis.
- Radio-opacities:
  - Calcification in chronic pancreatitis.
  - Biliary/ureteric /renal calculi.

### Contrast
*Barium swallow/meal*
- Indication: dysphagia.
- If endoscopy is contraindicated.

*Small bowel contrast studies*
- Small intestinal barium follow-through.
- Inferior detail to MR/CT enteroclysis or capsule enteroscopy.
- Indications: suspected Crohn disease, coeliac disease, tumours (lymphoma, adenocarcinoma, hamartoma (Peutz–Jeghers syndrome)), tuberculosis, jejunal diverticulosis.

*Barium enema*
- Lower GI symptoms where colonoscopy is otherwise incomplete.
- CT colonography is likely to replace barium enema as a colonic diagnostic modality.

## Abdominal computed tomography
- If USS not technically possible or diagnostic doubt exists.
- Particularly useful for identifying retroperitoneal disease.
- Other uses:
  - Oesophago-gastric disease
  - Tumour staging
  - Small bowel disease (tumours, IBD)
  - Colonic disease (tumours, IBD)
  - Pancreatic disease (tumours, pancreatitis)
  - Hepatic disease.

### CT colonography
- Ideal for excluding colonic carcinoma in elderly frail patients.
- Sensitivity 85% for carcinoma (~70% Ba enema).

## Ultrasound
- Remains operator-dependent.
- Indications: abdominal pain, jaundice, abnormal LFTs, hepatomegaly, ascites, abdominal mass.
- Body habitus (obesity) makes views suboptimal.

## Magnetic resonance imaging
- Investigation of choice in complex pelvic/perianal Crohn disease.
- Complements CT in the staging of rectal carcinoma prior to surgery.
- Useful in characterizing focal liver lesions and distinguishing adenoma from focal nodular hyperplasia (FNH) or tumour.
- Magnetic resonance cholangiopancreatography (MRCP) is displacing endoscopic retrograde cholangiopancreatography (ERCP) as the primary diagnostic tool in pancreatobiliary disease. See Fig. 9.5.

## Isotope scans
- Indium labelled white cell scan—Crohn activity.
- Technetium red cell scan—obscure GI bleeding.
- $C_{13}$ urea breath test: a useful non-invasive way of testing for the presence or success of eradication of *Helicobacter pylori*.

## Mesenteric angiography
See Fig. 9.6 and Section 9.6.

## Oesophageal pH monitoring
Indicated prior to gastro-oesophageal reflux surgery.

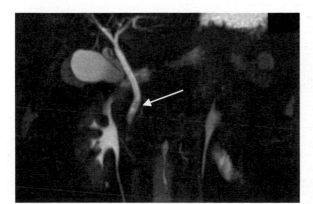

**Fig. 9.5** MRCP demonstrating normal calibre common bile duct with distal filling defect (arrowed) caused by stones.
Reproduced with permission of Dr Jeremy Woodward.

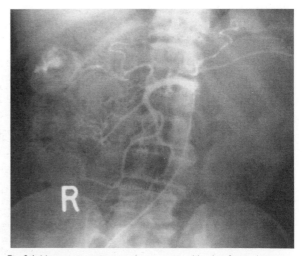

**Fig. 9.6** Mesenteric angiogram showing active bleeding from a lesion in the region of the hepatic flexure.
Reproduced with permission of www.surgical-tutor.org.uk.

# Oesophageal manometry

Indicated where suspicion of achalasia.

# Non-invasive tests

- **Serology:**
  - Tissue transglutaminase antibody (coeliac disease)
  - pANCA (PSC/UC)
  - ASCA (Crohn)
  - ASMA (Autoimmune hepatitis)
  - AMA (PBC).

- **Lactose hydrogen breath test:** lactose intolerance.
- **Glucose hydrogen breath test:** small bowel bacterial overgrowth.
- **Serum 7αOH cholestenone:** bile salt malabsorption.
- **Faecal elastase:** exocrine pancreatic function.
- **Schilling test:** $B_{12}$ malabsorption.
- **Faecal calprotectin:**
  - A stable macrophage-derived protein detectable in stool.
  - High sensitivity for intestinal disease but lacking in specificity.
  - Raised calprotectin seen in inflammatory, infective, and neoplastic intestinal disease.

# 9.3 Malabsorption and malnutrition

## Nutrition in health

Balance between the energy expenditure of the human body and the energy intake provided by nutrients.

## Malnutrition

A state of disequilibrium caused by any condition which results in **inadequate nutrient intake**.

## Malabsorption

A pathophysiological process that leads to specific or generalized **abnormalities in nutrient absorption**. Any malabsorptive condition may eventually result in nutritional deficiencies that amount to a state of malnutrition.

## Clinical assessment of nutritional status

### History
- Weight loss:
  - Mild: <5%
  - Moderate: <10%
  - Severe: >10%.
- Diet: reduced intake.
- Symptoms of malabsorption.
- Reduced physical ability.

### Physical examination
- Body mass index (BMI).
- Hydration.
- Skin-fold thickness.
- Muscle power.
- Signs of specific nutrient deficiencies.
- Ascites/peripheral oedema.

The clinical nutritional rating score achieved defines those at risk of clinical complications.

### Serum albumin
- Protein malnutrition causes reduced albumin synthesis.
- Low serum albumin appears to correlate with poor clinical outcome.

**But** other causes of reduced serum albumin exist:
- Systemic inflammation.
- Protein-losing enteropathy, e.g. IBD.
- Cardiac failure.
- Nephrotic syndrome.
- Wounds/burns.
- Cancer.

## Malabsorption as a cause of malnutrition

Patients with reduced capacity to absorb nutrients by virtue of reduced gut length or intestinal disease usually pose complex clinical management issues.

Global nutritional evaluation is required:
- Assessment of fluid loss and estimation of electrolyte loss.
- Evaluation of weight loss.
- Assessment of specific nutrient deficiencies:
  - Anaemia: Fe, folate, vitamin $B_{12}$

- Prothrombin time: vitamin K
- Electrolytes
- Trace elements
- Vitamins
- Bone mineral density.

## Causes of generalized malabsorption

- Intestinal: amyloidosis, coeliac disease, Crohn disease.
- Infections: Whipple disease, giardiasis, TB, HIV.
- Ischaemia.
- Tumours: intestinal lymphoma and neuroendocrine.
- Previous small bowel resections.
- Cardiovascular: cardiac failure, portal hypertension.
- Endocrine: diabetes, hyperthyroidism, Addison disease.
- Connective tissue disease: MCTD, SLE, scleroderma.

While intestinal disease tends to result in a generalized malabsorptive state, other system disease often results in **specific** malabsorptive problems:
- Gastric: pernicious anaemia.
- Pancreatic: pancreatitis, cystic fibrosis, tumours.
- Liver: cirrhosis/chronic liver disease.
- Biliary: PBC, PSC, tumours.

## Causes of specific nutrient malabsorption

*Fat*
- Liver/biliary disease: reduced luminal bile acid.
- Pancreatic insufficiency:
  - Malabsorption: intestinal lymphangiectasia
  - Coeliac disease
  - Crohn disease
  - Rapid transit: hyperthyroidism
  - Autonomic neuropathy.

*Protein and carbohydrate*
- Pancreatic insufficiency.
- Reduced mucosal absorption:
  - Crohn disease
  - Coeliac disease.

*Vitamin $B_{12}$*
- Autoimmune gastritis.
- Pernicious anaemia.
- Small bowel bacterial overgrowth.
- Terminal ileal Crohn disease/resection.

*Folate*
- Proximal small bowel disease:
  - Coeliac disease
  - Whipple disease.
- Alcohol excess

*Fat-soluble vitamins: A D E K*
- Bile salt deficiency:
  - Liver disease
  - Biliary disease
  - Bacterial overgrowth.

*Calcium*

- Small intestinal disease: coeliac.
- Previous gastric resection:
  - Reduced calcium absorption.
  - Reduced vitamin D.

*Iron*

- Previous gastric resection.
- Small intestinal disease: coeliac.

## Clinical features of malabsorption

- Ascites/oedema: protein loss/malabsorption.
- Tetany/myopathy: low calcium/magnesium/phosphate/ potassium.
- Bone pain: calcium/vitamin D deficiency.
- Bruising: vitamin C (Fig. 9.7)/K deficiency.
- Glossitis: iron/folate/vitamin B/C.
- Dermatitis: zinc/niacin.
- Koilonychia (Fig. 9.8): iron.
- Night blindness: vitamin A.
- Peripheral neuropathy: vitamin $B_{12}$.

### Treatment

*Control diarrhoea*

- PPI: reduce gastric secretions.
- Octreotide: reduce small intestinal secretions.
- Loperamide.
- Codeine.

*Maintain fluid/electrolyte balance*

Especially important in those patients with <100cm of remaining small intestine ('short gut syndrome').

- Oral isotonic rehydration therapy (1–2L/day):
  - Ideally 90–120mmol/L Na.
  - May significantly reduce ileostomy fluid loss.
- Serum magnesium: normal level does not exclude deficiency.
- Plasma calcium:
  - Normal level does not exclude deficiency.
  - Routinely treat with 2g calcium/day.
- Zinc: deficiency is common.
- Iron: consider IV iron.

*Nutritional support*

In the malnourished patient and even in profound short gut syndrome, enteral nutrition may be sufficiently effective in providing the

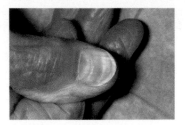
**Fig. 9.8** Koilonychia.
Reproduced from Longmore et al., *Oxford Handbook of Clinical Medicine*, Eighth Edition, 2010, p. 321, with permission from Oxford University Press.

deficient minerals and calories and defer the requirement for parenteral feeding.

*Parenteral support*

Where the earlier listed parameters cannot be achieved by enteral support, intravenous therapy should be considered.

This is especially important when:

- Urine output <1L/day.
- Ongoing mineral deficiency (despite replacement).
- Consider IM $B_{12}$ and IV/IM vitamin K.

Parenteral nutrition (PN) may be the most appropriate route to improving the quality of life of the enterally fed patient.

Long-term requirement for TPN may best be provided to the patient at home with the relevant support.

It is delivered through a central venous catheter during an 8–12-hour period overnight.

PN for 'benign' intestinal disease is associated with 87% survival at 12 months but 6% mortality from PN-associated complications.

These include:

- Line sepsis
- Venous thrombosis
- Chronic liver disease
- Cholelithiasis
- Metabolic bone disease.

## Small intestinal diseases resulting in malabsorption

### Coeliac disease

- Characterized by villous atrophy of the small intestinal mucosa following exposure to ingested gluten (in wheat) or related proteins (in rye and barley) and results in malabsorption of nutrients (Box 9.1).
- Associated with specific HLA class II DQ haplotypes (principally DQ2). The products of these genes present gluten-derived gliadin peptides to intestinal mucosal T cells in coeliac patients.
- In addition, modification of gliadin by the host enzyme tissue transglutaminase (tTG) enhances the T-cell response to gliadin in coeliac

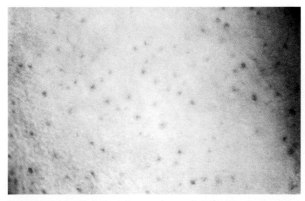
**Fig. 9.7** Perifollicular haemorrhage in vitamin C deficiency.
Source: CDC. This image is in the public domain. http://phil.cdc.gov/phil/details.asp (ID# 6238)

| Box 9.1 Other causes of villous atrophy | |
| --- | --- |
| Milk intolerance | Post-gastroenteritis |
| Peptic duodenitis | Giardiasis |
| Zollinger–Ellison syndrome | Crohn disease |
| Bacterial overgrowth | Eosinophilic enteritis |
| Radiotherapy | Tropical sprue |
| Chemotherapy | Malnutrition |
| Small intestinal lymphoma | Graft vs. host disease |
| Hypogammaglobulinaemia | α chain disease |

patients. This has led to tTG being adopted as a sensitive serological test to complement the diagnostic evaluation of patients.

### Epidemiology

- Marked geographical variation: highest incidence in Europe: 1 case per 100–200/population.
- Especially prevalent in Celtic populations (Northern Ireland: 1 case per 122/population).
- ♀ preponderance 2:1.

The true prevalence of coeliac disease is uncertain as many patients are asymptomatic and, therefore, remain undiagnosed.

### Pathogenesis

Coeliac disease is considered an immune disorder, but there is complex interplay between genetic, immune, and environmental factors. Disease onset is triggered following exposure of the small intestine of the genetically susceptible host to gliadin.

- Up to 20% first-degree relatives affected.
- 70% concordance in monozygotic twins.
- 95% of coeliac patients are HLA DQ2, however:
  - Not all people with DQ2 develop disease.
  - DQ2 is present in 25–30% of European population.

Autoantibodies:

- Anti-gliadin IgA/IgG—non-specific for coeliac and found without clinical disease.
- Antiendomysial IgA (EMA)—highly specific for coeliac.
- tTG is the autoantigen within the endomysium (connective tissue structure around smooth muscle) that acts as the target.

Cell mediated immune response:

- Release of interferon γ and TNFα.
- Activation of CD4 lymphocytes in the lamina propria.
- Increase in intraepithelial lymphocyte population (CD8).

The length of small intestinal involvement is variable and correlates with severity of malabsorption. Where there is total involvement of the length of the small intestine, clinically significant malabsorption results. In less severe disease, it is not uncommon for the distal ileum to be histologically normal even in the presence of severe duodenal villous atrophy. Conversely, distal ileal involvement does not occur without the characteristic duodenal disease.

The histopathological changes of the small intestinal mucosa seen in other enteropathies may mimic that seen in coeliac disease.

### Clinical picture

Many patients at diagnosis have few (if any) symptoms and the condition is often identified during the course of screening relatives of patients or patients with associated autoimmune conditions such as hypothyroidism, diabetes or Down syndrome. In others, coeliac disease is found to account for biochemical or haematological abnormalities such as iron deficiency or hypocalcaemia, even without prominent clinical features. See Tables 9.1 and 9.2.

**Table 9.1 Clinical features of coeliac disease**

| Children | Adults |
| --- | --- |
| Abdominal pain | Diarrhoea |
| Steatorrhoea | Steatorrhoea |
| Watery diarrhoea | Flatulence |
| Vomiting | Abdominal bloating |
| Failure to thrive | Aphthous stomatitis |
| Short stature | Weight loss |
| Muscle wasting | Fatigue |
| Anaemia | Anaemia |
| Rickets | Hypokalaemia |

**Table 9.2 Extra-intestinal manifestations of coeliac disease and their likely cause**

| Manifestation | Cause |
| --- | --- |
| Anaemia/pallor | Low ferritin/folate |
| Koilonychia | Low ferritin |
| Finger clubbing | Unknown cause |
| Osteopenia/pathological fractures | Low Ca/vitamin D |
| Myopathy | Low K$^+$ |
| Tetany | Low Ca |
| Peripheral neuropathy/ataxia | Low B$_{12}$/thiamine |
| Amenorrhoea/infertility | Pituitary dysfunction |
| Peripheral oedema/ascites | Low total protein |
| Petechiae/bruising | Low vitamin K |
| Dermatitis herpetiformis | Unknown cause |
| Fever | T-cell lymphoma |
| Lymphadenopathy | T-cell lymphoma |

### Diagnosis

#### Serology

IgA anti-endomysial antibodies (EMAs):

- >90% sensitivity/~100% specificity overall.
- Sensitivity ∝ severity of disease (total vs. partial villous atrophy: 100 vs. 31%).
- Indirect IF technique.
- Become negative as coeliac disease is treated.
- False negative in IgA deficiency (~2%).

IgA anti-tissue transglutaminase (tTG) antibody:

- Sensitivity and specificity both ~95%.
- ELISA assay.
- Less costly/more convenient than EMA.
- False negative in IgA deficiency (~2%).

Anti-gliadin antibodies IgG/IgA (AGA):

- Only modest sensitivity/specificity.
- Poor predictive value.
- IgG AGA can be diagnostically useful in those patients with IgA deficiency.

#### Small intestinal histology

Small intestinal biopsy is generally recommended before dietary gluten restriction in order to confirm the characteristic features of coeliac disease (villous atrophy, lymphocytic infiltrate (lamina propria and intraepithelial) and crypt hyperplasia).

#### Radiology

Small bowel contrast studies are useful to exclude other clinical conditions (e.g. Crohn disease, scleroderma, jejunal diverticulosis), or to identify complications of coeliac disease.

#### Recognized complications of coeliac disease

- T-cell lymphoma
- Adenocarcinoma
- Ulcerative jejunoileitis
- Stricture.

#### Differential diagnoses

Any cause of malabsorption and steatorrhoea:

- Pancreatic insufficiency
- Cholestatic liver disease
- Terminal ileal disease
- Small bowel bacterial overgrowth

- Whipple disease
- Mycobacterial enteritis
- Giardiasis
- Hypogammaglobulinaemia
- Viral gastroenteritis
- Collagenous sprue.

See Table 9.3 for associated diseases.

### Treatment

#### Gluten-free diet

- 70% will experience symptomatic clinical improvement within 2 weeks.
- Histological resolution may take up to 2 years.

Where there is no response to dietary exclusion of gluten, possible explanations include:

- Inadequate gluten exclusion.
- Another condition causing villous atrophy.
- Refractory sprue: requires immunosuppressive therapy: prednisolone ± azathioprine.

#### Nutrient supplementation

- Iron/folate in anaemia (rarely $B_{12}$).
- Vitamin K (where deficient).
- Ca/Mg (tetany or osteopenia).
- Vitamin D (osteopenia).
- Copper/zinc replacement (where deficient).

## Whipple disease

Rare condition of (predominantly) white middle-aged men due to infection with the actinomycete bacterium *Tropheryma whippelii*. Box 9.2 lists characteristic clinical features of Whipple disease. The resulting chronic multisystem disease almost always affects the small intestine but also:

- Joints
- Cardiovascular system
- Central nervous system.

### Diagnosis

Histological examination with periodic acid–Schiff (PAS) staining of (several) small intestinal mucosal biopsies is usually sufficient to demonstrate the presence of the bacterium within the macrophages of the lamina propria. PCR assays are also available and electron microscopy is sometimes required.

### Treatment

Combination trimethoprim—sulphamethoxazole (Septrin®) is especially effective. A few cases have been reported to relapse despite treatment (some with important CNS sequelae) and it is this that has prompted the recommendation for induction of treatment with a third-generation cephalosporin (e.g. ceftriaxone), followed by 12 months of septrin.

## 'Tropical sprue'

Malabsorption and diarrhoea occurring in tropical countries can occur as a consequence of a recognizable infectious enteropathy that is associated with histopathological changes similar to that seen in coeliac disease (villous atrophy, crypt hyperplasia, and lymphocytic infiltrate).

Such enteropathogens include:

- *Giardia*: the most common enteropathogen worldwide.
- *Isospora*: restricted to the tropics.
- *Cyclospora*: tropics and subtropics.
- *Cryptosporidium*: usually self-limiting but a major cause of morbidity in the immunocompromised.
- *Microsporidium*.
- Helminths (e.g. *Strongyloides*).
- Viruses (e.g. rotavirus, adenovirus, HIV).
- Bacteria (e.g. *Escherichia coli*, *Shigella*, *Salmonella*, *Mycobacterium tuberculosis*).

Tropical sprue, however, is a clinical malabsorptive disease state that occurs in people in defined areas in the tropics (South-East Asia, India, and Caribbean) for which no viral, parasitic, or bacterial cause can be determined. The condition is recognized both in indigenous people and in visitors to the regions.

### Clinical course

Acute illness (1st week):

- Watery diarrhoea
- Fever
- Malaise.

Chronic illness (over ensuing months/years):

- Chronic diarrhoea.
- Steatorrhoea.
- Weight loss.
- Lactose intolerance.
- $B_{12}$/folate deficiency:
  - Anaemia.
  - Glossitis.
  - Stomatitis.
  - Subacute combined degeneration of the cord.
- Hypoproteinaemia: peripheral oedema.
- Vitamin A deficiency: night blindness.

### Characteristic pathological features

- Atrophic gastritis:
  - Reduced gastric acid.
  - Reduced intrinsic factor—low $B_{12}$.
- Enteropathy:
  - Villous atrophy.
  - Small intestinal inflammatory infiltrate in lamina propria/epithelium.
  - Thickened basement membrane.
- Colonopathy: impaired sodium/water absorption.

### Diagnosis

- Small intestinal mucosa shows partial villous atrophy.
- Exclude coeliac disease.

| Table 9.3 Diseases associated with coeliac disease | |
| --- | --- |
| Dermatitis herpetiformis | Diabetes mellitus |
| Thyroid disease | IgA deficiency |
| Crohn disease | Ulcerative colitis |
| IgA nephropathy | Rheumatoid arthritis |
| Sarcoidosis | Down syndrome |
| Fibrosing alveolitis | Sjögren syndrome |
| SLE | Polymyositis |
| Myasthenia gravis | Addison disease |

| Box 9.2 Characteristic clinical features of Whipple disease | |
| --- | --- |
| • Malabsorption | • Fever |
| • Weight loss | • Lymphadenopathy |
| • Diarrhoea | • Arthralgia |
| • Abdominal pain | • Skin hyperpigmentation |
| • Dementia | • Myocarditis |
| • Ataxia | • Pericarditis |
| • Cranial nerve lesions | • Endocarditis |

- Exclude parasitic/bacterial infection:
  - Stool cultures.
  - Jejunal biopsy/jejunal fluid aspiration.
- Small intestinal radiology:
  - Jejunal mucosal fold thickening.
  - Jejunal dilatation.
  - Slow small intestinal gut transit time.

### Treatment

- Water and electrolyte replacement.
- Iron/folate/B$_{12}$ replacement.
- Tetracycline 250mg four times a day (for several months).

## Eosinophilic gastroenteritis

Rare condition that is characterized by an eosinophilic infiltration of any layer of the intestinal wall in any part of the intestinal tract from oesophagus to rectum (most commonly stomach and small bowel). See Box 9.3 for clinical features.

### Clinical picture

- GI symptoms:
  - Abdominal pain
  - Nausea/vomiting
  - Diarrhoea
  - Weight loss.
- Eosinophilic infiltrate in the GI tract.
- Absence of eosinophilic infiltration in other organs outside of the GI tract.
- Absence of parasitic infection.
- Peripheral blood eosinophilia is present in 80% (but is not necessary for diagnosis).

### Diagnosis

- Peripheral blood eosinophilia.
- Exclusion of parasitic infection.
- Endoscopic evaluation and intestinal mucosal biopsies.
- NB: eosinophilic infiltration of the **distal** oesophagus occurs most often in reflux oesophagitis. True eosinophilic oesophagitis should be suspected where there is **mid** or **proximal** oesophageal involvement ± luminal narrowing.

### Radiology

- Thickened intestinal wall.
- Lymphadenopathy.

### Treatment

- Antihelminthic: mebendazole should be considered where there is clinical risk of parasitic infection (e.g. travel/pets).
- Sodium chromoglycate can be useful.

---

### Box 9.3 Clinical features of eosinophilic gastroenteritis

- Anaemia
- Protein-losing enteropathy
- Malabsorption
- Hypoalbuminaemia
- Pancreatitis
- Atopic dermatitis/urticaria
- Pyloric/upper GI obstruction
- Eosinophilic ascites

---

- Corticosteroids are used where chromoglycate/mebendazole has resulted in little clinical improvement.
- Surgery should be avoided where possible since recurrence of disease is common following resection.

### Prognosis

- Typically excellent.
- Intestinal obstruction is the most common complication.

## Small intestinal infections resulting in malabsorption

See Section 9.7.

## Small intestinal Crohn disease

See Section 9.4.

## Short bowel syndrome

### Management of patients with short bowel

Short bowel refers to those patients with <2m of small bowel remaining.

### Common causes

- Crohn disease
- Mesenteric ischaemia
- Irradiation
- Small bowel volvulus
- Adhesions.

### Clinical problems

- Nutrient malabsorption
- Sodium/water/magnesium depletion
- Vitamin deficiency
- Diarrhoea
- Drug absorption problems
- Gallstones
- Renal stones.

### Treatment

- Exclude infection.
- Oral glucose/saline solution.
- Reduce oral hypotonic fluids to <500mL/day.
- NaCl added to liquid feeds ([Na]~100mmol/L).
- Loperamide/codeine.
- PPI (reduce gastric secretion).
- Correct low Mg.

### Intestinal transplantation

- Indicated where:
  - Significant complications of PN exist.
  - Lack of venous access for PN.
  - PN fails to supply adequate nutrition/hydration.
- Recent advances in transplant medicine have improved outcomes:
  - 80% 1-year survival.
  - 50% 5-year survival.
- Most patients become free of PN.

Early referral appears to improve outcome but most patients in the UK are referred too late for consideration of surgery.

# 9.4 Inflammatory bowel disease

## Background

These chronic inflammatory conditions of the GI tract are characterized by a relapsing and remitting illness from diagnosis throughout the patient's lifetime. Ulcerative colitis (UC) is a confluent colitis extending proximally from the rectum to a variable extent (i.e. proctitis or pancolitis). Crohn disease (CD), however, may affect *any part* of the gastrointestinal tract (usually segmentally) from oral to rectal mucosa.

## Epidemiology

- Important cause of GI disease worldwide.
- Incidence exhibits geographical variation (higher in Northern than Southern Europe), and has been reported as 11–33 new cases per 100,000 population per year.
- Prevalence (probably underestimated) may be as high as 400 per 100,000 population.
- Presentation: any age, most are 15–40 years but a significant proportion first present aged >60.
- Seasonal variation exists with clinical presentation twice as common in winter than summer months.

Ileocolonic distribution is the most common enteric site for CD (50%) (Fig. 9.9) whereas UC affects the colon only and typically extends proximally from the rectal mucosa **confluently** without intervening normal mucosa (unlike Crohn colitis). There are a number of histopathological criteria upon which CD may be inferred as the likeliest diagnosis in an inflammatory colitis (e.g. the presence of granuloma), but often the colitis is 'indeterminate' where it is difficult to make the distinction between CD and UC.

## Aetiology

The precise cause of IBD is unknown. Recent progress has been made towards understanding the contributions of host genetic and gut luminal environmental factors that are associated with susceptibility to disease.

- 15% of patients will have a relative with IBD. Concordance for disease in monozygotic twins is greater for CD (67%) than UC (20%).
- Mutations of *NOD2/CARD15* gene on chromosome 16 have been shown to be associated with ileal CD, and are prevalent in around 30–40% of cases. A series of other CD susceptibility genes have now been defined.

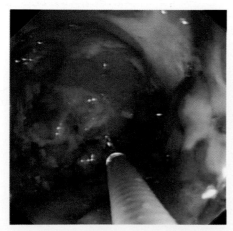

**Fig. 9.9** Crohn disease: An endoscopic view of the terminal ileum showing inflammation and ulceration.

Reproduced from Walsh et al., *Oxford Case Histories in Gastroenterology and Hepatology*, 2010, with permission from Oxford University Press.

- There is good evidence to suggest that the intestinal bacterial flora may be an important key in the trigger for inflammatory change, but no single microbial agent has been confirmed
- Smoking has been consistently shown to be associated not only with susceptibility to CD (doubles the risk), but also with: severity of inflammatory disease, frequency of relapse, requirement for surgery, and a higher risk of recurrence following operation. Conversely, ex- or non-smokers have an increased susceptibility to UC.
- Previous appendicectomy reduces the risk of UC by 70% and independent of smoking history.

## Clinical presentation

Typical symptoms include abdominal pain and increased frequency and liquid volume of bowel motion (diarrhoea). Colitis (CD/UC) is more typically associated with bloody diarrhoea. Small bowel CD gives rise to diarrhoea, steatorrhoea, anorexia, weight loss, and abdominal pain. CD can be associated with complex disease such as stricturing or fistula communication to either distant segments of the enteric tract or to other viscera (e.g. bladder, vagina). Management of such disease can be very challenging with requirement for close surgical and medical collaboration.

### Extraintestinal manifestations

IBD may be associated with a number of other important inflammatory conditions outside of the GI tract:

*Arthropathy*

- Finger clubbing.
- Peripheral arthropathy (seen in 20% of CD):
  - Pauciarticular (<4 joints) = type 1.
  - Polyarticular (>5 joints) = type 2.
- Associated with colonic disease.
- Clinical improvement after ileocaecal resection.
- Rheumatoid factor negative.
- Spondylitis.
- Sacroiliitis.
- Axial arthropathy (less common).

**NB:** osteoporosis in IBD may result from inflammatory activity/malabsorption, or secondary to corticosteroid therapy. Symptoms from osteoporosis/osteonecrosis may mimic the inflammatory arthropathy described earlier. DXA scanning is a key tool in determining those patients who will benefit from therapy (calcium, vitamin D, bisphosphonates).

*Ocular*

- Scleritis/episcleritis (Fig. 9.10):
  - Associated with active GI disease.
  - May result in lasting visual loss.
- Uveitis:
  - Headaches, blurred vision, photophobia.

*Cutaneous*

- Mouth ulcers (especially in CD; Fig. 9.11).
- Erythema nodosum (Fig. 9.12):
  - Tender subcutaneous nodules.
  - Typically pre-tibial.
  - Associated with arthropathy.
- Pyoderma gangrenosum (Fig. 9.13):
  - Initially a pustular lesion.
  - Develops into ulcerating lesion.
  - Typically lower leg after minor trauma.

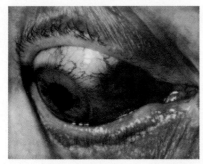

**Fig. 9.10** Episcleritis.

Image reprinted with permission from Medscape Reference (http://emedicine.medscape.com/), 2013, available at: http://emedicine.medscape.com/article/1918545-overview.

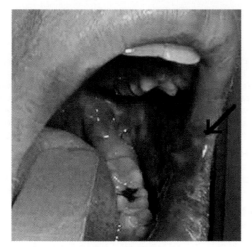

**Fig. 9.11** Crohn disease of the lips with ulceration at the angle of the mouth.

GASTROLAB/Science Photo Library

- Psoriasis is probably more common.
- Granulomatous skin inflammation.

*Hepatobiliary*
- Gallstones: 25% IBD.
- Primary sclerosing cholangitis (PSC): especially associated with UC (also colonic CD).

*Renal—calculi:*
- Oxalate/urate.
- Especially in small intestinal CD.

*Genitourinary*
- Penile and vulval involvement (well-recognized complication of CD).

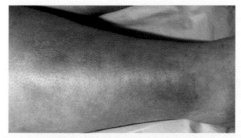

**Fig. 9.12** Erythema nodosum with smooth tender erythematous nodules on both shins.

Reproduced from Burge and Wallis, *Oxford Handbook of Medical Dermatology*, 2010, with permission from Oxford University Press.

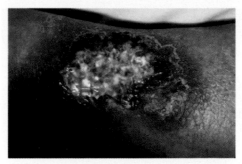

**Fig. 9.13** Typical pyoderma gangrenosum with a purplish undermined border.

Reproduced from Burge S and Wallis D, *Oxford Handbook of Medical Dermatology*, 2010, Figure 15.5, page 277, with permission from Oxford University Press.

## Evaluation of IBD

### History and examination

Consider alternative differential diagnoses of bloody diarrhoea.

*Exclude infective diarrhoea*

This is as vital in newly diagnosed IBD as in the setting of a relapse of established colitis since a significant proportion will have concurrent infection (e.g. clostridial colitis).

### Colonoscopy

Careful colonoscopic evaluation (Figs 9.14 and 9.15) serves to exclude colorectal malignancy which is more prevalent in patients with IBD. Biopsy can be undertaken for histological diagnosis.

### Enteroscopy

Small intestinal CD can be remarkably difficult to diagnose. The lack of sensitivity of small bowel barium studies for inflammatory disease means that direct endoscopic appraisal is sometimes required. Conventional push enteroscopy (2.5m endoscope) allows visual appraisal and the capacity for mucosal biopsy but will not allow full small intestinal surveillance without surgical assistance at simultaneous laparotomy. The novel technique of double balloon enteroscopy (DBE) does allow access to all the small intestine via oral or anal approach but at this time is not widely available in most clinical units.

### Wireless capsule endoscopy (WCE)

This modality for small bowel imaging has emerged in recent years as a valuable tool in establishing significant disease where other tests have been non-diagnostic. There are some data to suggest that WCE remains less sensitive than either double balloon enteroscopy or MR enteroclysis but WCE remains nevertheless a less invasive and better tolerated technique than enteroscopy.

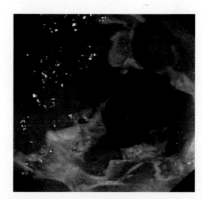

**Fig. 9.14** Colonoscopic appearance of linear and pleomorphic ulceration of Crohn disease.

Reproduced from Warrell et al., *Oxford Textbook of Medicine*, Fifth Edition, 2010, Figure 15.11.2, with permission from Oxford University Press.

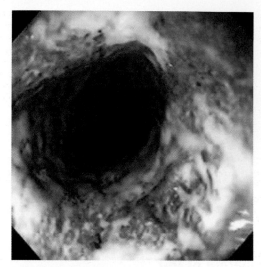

**Fig. 9.15** Ulcerative colitis as visualized with a colonoscope.

Image reprinted with permission from *Medscape Drugs & Diseases* (http://emedicine.medscape.com/), 2015, available at: http://emedicine.medscape.com/article/183084-overview.

## Plain abdominal and contrast radiography

Plain abdominal radiography (Fig. 9.16) represents a simple way of assessing disease extent and also of excluding severe inflammatory disease associated with toxic dilatation (colon diameter >5cm). Inflamed colonic mucosa rarely contains luminal faeces and mucosal thickening, ulceration, and pseudopolyp formation is often visible. If there is clinical suspicion of visceral perforation then the presence of the visible intestinal wall—inner and outer wall (Rigler sign), or an erect chest film (free air under the diaphragm) may be most useful.

Contrast enema studies (Fig. 9.17) may be particularly useful in patients in whom colonoscopy visualization is complicated (e.g. stricture). Small bowel contrast studies lack the sensitivity to exclude inflammatory disease but can be a helpful tool in excluding significant stricturing small intestinal CD.

## CT/MRI abdomen

Abdominal pain, bloating and diarrhoea are included amongst the criteria for irritable bowel syndrome (IBS), but are also typical symptoms in terminal ileal or ileocolonic CD. Inflammatory disease at this site may be distinguished from IBS by computed tomography (CT) cross-sectional imaging usually in conjunction with histopathological confirmation at the time of colonoscopy/terminal ileoscopy. CT can be especially useful in defining complex inflammatory/fistulating

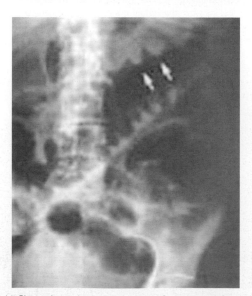

**Fig. 9.16** Plain radiograph of Crohn disease of transverse colon with mucosal oedema and associated dilatation.

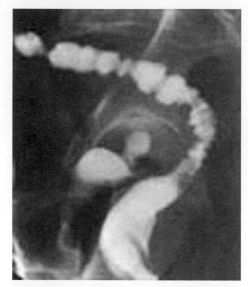

**Fig. 9.17** Contrast enema showing rectovaginal fistula in Crohn disease.

disease. Where the inflammatory process is confined to the pelvis, MRI can provide more valuable detail, particularly where surgical intervention is being considered. MR enteroclysis (real-time images obtained during infusion of contrast via a naso-duodenal tube) has also emerged as a sensitive method for small intestinal imaging.

## Serological markers

C reactive protein (CRP) is typically elevated in active disease and may be used to distinguish IBD from IBS. As CRP and ESR can be high in infective colitis, these markers cannot be reliably used to discriminate.

## Faecal markers

Calprotectin is a protein expressed by neutrophils and macrophages. It is stable in faeces and is a sensitive marker for inflammatory, neoplastic and infectious enterocolitic disease. Although it lacks specificity, high faecal calprotectin has been shown to be associated with active IBD.

# Medical management of IBD

The surgical aspects of management are a vital component of therapy but a detailed description is outside the scope of this text. Nevertheless, a collaborative team of surgeons, physicians, IBD specialist nurses, and dieticians offers the ideal approach to therapy.

## General principles

1. Resuscitation
2. Induction of remission
3. Maintenance of remission.

### Resuscitation

Patients with IBD often present nutritionally deplete. This may be either generalized malnutrition or specific deficiency states e.g. anaemia (iron, vitamin B$_{12}$, folate). Management therefore involves identifying such requirements and providing the relevant supplementation.

### Induction of remission
### Steroids

Conventionally first-line medical therapy for IBD is with corticosteroids. Around 60% of acute IBD will respond to steroid therapy but a significant number will prove either refractory to or dependent upon steroids requiring consideration of other lines of treatment. Topical corticosteroid, given as suppository or enema, may be useful for distal UC and especially so in combination with topical 5ASA.

### Mesalazine (5-aminosalicylic acid (5ASA))

Mesalazine may be used to induce remission in both CD and UC (inhibits T-cell proliferation and TNFα release). Studies in mild–moderately active CD have demonstrated a 25% benefit over placebo. 5ASA has been shown to be similarly effective in treating active UC. Topical 5ASA, can also be effective in inducing remission in active distal UC and is at least as effective as topical corticosteroid.

### Ciclosporin

This drug may be effective in acute severe UC where there has been no improvement with 5–7 days of intravenous corticosteroid therapy. There is evidence to support the use of the lower dose (2mg/kg) and this is associated with a lower incidence of nephrotoxicity.

### Methotrexate (MTX)

May be useful in inducing remission in patients with chronic active CD despite ongoing steroid therapy.

### Anti-TNFα

Increasingly, therapy using a monoclonal antibody against the pro-inflammatory cytokine TNFα is being adopted as an alternative strategy in steroid resistant/dependent disease (CD and UC), either as second- or third-line intervention. Some authorities even advocate their use as first-line therapy prior to steroids. Anti-TNFα strategies for induction of remission may be used most valuably as a bridge to maintenance therapy with thiopurine.

### Acute severe colitis

This condition has been recognized as a medical emergency since the first description of 'idiopathic colitis' by Samuel Wilkes in 1859. Mortality from the condition has fallen from 37% to <1% due in part to advances in medical therapy, improved fluid and electrolyte resuscitation, as well as improved surgical technique.

Conventionally, the first-line approach has been intravenous corticosteroid therapy followed, in non-responders, by intravenous ciclosporin. With the recognition of efficacy of anti-TNFα therapy in UC this may represent a useful alternative strategy as either first or second line.

Despite these advances in medical therapy, a proportion of patients will require colectomy. Prediction of which patients are unlikely to respond to medical therapy may be made on the presence of colonic dilatation, albumin ≤30g/L, and stool frequency >8/day within the first 72 hours.

### Maintenance of remission
### Mesalazine

There is evidence to suggest long-term mesalazine is useful in the maintenance of remission of UC but not CD. Emerging evidence also suggests the use of mesalazine in UC may have a protective effect against colonic neoplasia.

### Thiopurines

For some years now, the thiopurines (azathioprine/6-mercaptopurine) have been used with good effect in the maintenance of remission in IBD following induction of remission with corticosteroids. There is good evidence that frequency of relapse and the requirement for steroid therapy is reduced with this treatment. These drugs are not, however, without significant tolerance issues and pancreatitis, nausea, hepatitis, and neutropaenia are all real concerns that require close clinical supervision and blood monitoring. Functional assay of the enzyme thiopurine methyl transferase (TPMT) prior to commencement of therapy may help to identify those individuals (TPMT deficiency affects 1 in 300) who are at particular risk of toxicity.

As effective as these drugs can be for maintaining remission, there is little evidence to suggest that they are useful in induction of remission from an active inflammatory state.

### MTX/ciclosporin

There is evidence for both methotrexate and cyclosporin in maintenance of remission following induction in both CD and UC respectively.

### Anti-TNFα therapy

Anti-TNFα therapy maintained on a scheduled basis in an attempt to sustain remission is now widely accepted practice for maintaining remission in inflammatory disease otherwise refractory to steroid, mesalazine or thiopurine therapies. The possible consequences of long-term anti-TNFα blockade (including opportunistic infection (TB), demyelinating disease, and neoplasia (hepatosplenic T-cell lymphoma)) remain an area of concern that prompts close clinical surveillance.

Other novel therapies continue to emerge and it is hoped that efficacy can be achieved without compromising patient safety.

## Cancer in IBD

In those patients with extensive or total colitis there is a reported increase in relative risk of colorectal cancer into the longer term.

This becomes apparent after disease duration of 10 years or more (estimated risk: 7% at 20 years, 17% at 30 years). The risk may be highest in those patients in whom disease onset is during childhood.

Surveillance colonoscopy is considered at regular intervals beyond 10 years following diagnosis. The relative risk of colorectal cancer is highest in patients with marked inflammatory mucosal activity and extensive colonic inflammatory involvement and other factors as detailed in the following subsections. Where high-grade dysplasia is found, colectomy is advised.

Patients with extensive colitis (ulcerative colitis or Crohn disease) can be risk stratified as follows:

### Lower risk: 5-yearly colonoscopy

- No endoscopic/histological active inflammation on the previous colonoscopy (histological chronic or quiescent changes acceptable) **or**
- Left-sided colitis (any grade of inflammation) **or**
- CD colitis affecting <50% surface area of the colon (any grade of inflammation).

### Intermediate risk: 3-yearly colonoscopy

- Mild endoscopic/histological active inflammation on the previous surveillance colonoscopy **or**
- Presence of post-inflammatory polyps **or**
- Family history of colorectal cancer in a first-degree relative aged 50 years or over.

### Higher risk: yearly colonoscopy

- Moderate or severe endoscopic/histological active inflammation on the previous surveillance colonoscopy **or**
- Stricture within past 5 years **or**
- Confirmed dysplasia within past 5 years in a patient who declines surgery **or**
- Primary sclerosing cholangitis (Fig. 9.18)/post orthotopic liver transplant for PSC **or**
- Family history of colorectal cancer in a first-degree relative aged <50 years.

Following colectomy and ileoanal pouch anastomosis recommendations for pouch surveillance are as follows:

### Post-colectomy surveillance

- Higher-risk post-colectomy patients: consider yearly flexible sigmoidoscopy of pouch/rectal mucosa in patients with:
  - Previous rectal dysplasia or dysplasia **or**
  - Colorectal cancer at the time of pouch surgery **or**
  - Primary sclerosing cholangitis **or**
  - Type C mucosa in the pouch (mucosa exhibiting permanent persistent atrophy and severe inflammation).
- Biopsies should be taken from pre-pouch ileum, the pouch–anal anastomosis, and the body of the pouch with four biopsies from each site. Pouch surveillance should be started early after pouch formation.
- There is increasing evidence to support a reduced risk of colorectal malignancy in IBD in those treated with long-term maintenance 5ASA therapy.

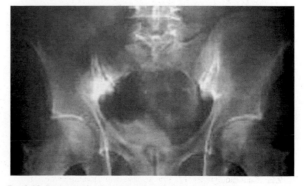

**Fig. 9.18** Radiograph of periarticular sclerosis in sacroiliitis.

# 9.5 Acute upper gastrointestinal haemorrhage

## Background

- GI haemorrhage from a source proximal to the ligament of Treitz (suspensory muscle at duodenal–jejunal junction).
- Common medical emergency (see Section 1.10).
- Incidence: 160/100,000 population/year.

## Mortality

- Remains ~10%.
- Only marginal improvement since advent of endoscopic treatment.
- Rising cause of mortality in the elderly.
- Mortality and morbidity remain highest in those patients with **recurrent** haemorrhage. Most recurrent bleeds (95%) occur within 72 hours of admission to hospital.
- Trained endoscopic medical and nursing support essential.
- Multidisciplinary involvement from surgical, anaesthetic, and critical care medical teams.

## Source of bleed

### Clinical

- Fresh haematemesis or coffee ground vomit or melaena = upper GI.
- Rectal bleeding = lower GI (but up to 5% of upper GI bleeds will present with fresh blood per rectum).
- Biochemical: raised blood urea with normal creatinine = upper GI.

### Upper GI haemorrhage

- Peptic ulcer (50%).
- Gastroduodenal erosions (25%).
- Oesophagitis (10%).
- GO junction (Mallory–Weiss) tears (5%).
- Oesophageal varices (4%).
- Vascular malformations (4%).
- Tumours (2%).

## Clinical assessment

Simultaneous resuscitation and assessment of clinical significance of bleed (prognosis) based on history, examination, and blood results.
Clinical factors associated with significant upper GI haemorrhage:

- Shock (BP <100mmHg/HR >100bpm).
- Passage of fresh red blood.
- Age >60 years.
- Haemoglobin <10g/dL.
- Significant comorbid disease.
- Variceal or large peptic ulcer bleed.
- Onset in hospital.
- Recurrent bleeding.
- Fresh haematemesis associated with shock or Hb drop >2g/dL in 24 hours.

## History

- Age.
- Comorbidity.

- Pre-existing liver disease/EtOH abuse.
- Previous peptic ulcer disease (PUD).
- NSAID/aspirin use.
- Warfarin/antiplatelet agents.

## Examination

- Tachycardia.
- Hypotension/postural hypotension.
- Peripheral vasoconstriction.
- Signs of chronic liver disease (spider naevi, ascites, caput medusa, splenomegaly).
- Rectal examination.

## Bloods

- FBC/U&E/LFT.
- Coagulation: PT/aPTT.
- Cross match 4–6 units.

## Resuscitation

- Position: if reduced conscious level consider head down (in recovery position) as cerebral perfusion improved. **NB:** avoid supine position due to risk of aspiration.
- Oxygen.
- IV access: two or more large-bore sites.
- If haemodynamic shock, consider central venous access.
- CVP monitoring :
  - Guides fluid replacement.
  - Especially important in patients with organ failure, elderly, and those with cardiovascular disease.
  - Sudden CVP drop = possible rebleed.
- Careful fluid balance: urinary catheter.
- CXR.
- ECG.

## Management

**Airway**: consider Guedel airway or intubation (especially where conscious level is reduced)
**IV fluid** replacement:

1. Crystalloid (convenient and inexpensive, no disadvantage over colloid):
   - Avoid saline in liver disease.
2. Packed red cells (PRCs) given in brisk bleeding:
   - If important comorbidity (e.g. IHD) then transfuse to Hb >10g/dL.
   - Where no comorbidity: PRCs may be reasonably withheld where Hb >8g/dL.
   - Give PRC if Hb <10g/dL and postural hypotension.
3. Blood products. Prescribe FFP (or factor concentrates)/vitamin K/platelets as indicated to correct coagulation and platelet count.

Consider **immediate referral** to

- Gastroenterologist
- Surgeon
- Anaesthetist.

# Peptic ulcer disease

## Epidemiology

- Affects~10% of the population of Western countries during the course of a lifetime.
- Recognition of aetiological role of *Helicobacter pylori* has led to the development of effective eradication therapy.
- Rate of complications (including bleeding and perforation) has not, however, changed significantly. This is particularly true of the elderly for whom PUD complications are rising in incidence. There is some evidence to suggest that the use of NSAIDs has contributed to this.
- Cigarette smoking appears to be a risk factor. Interestingly, no such association has been clearly demonstrated with alcohol consumption.

## Clinical features

- Epigastric pain (dyspepsia) is frequently reported and typically starts 2–3 hours postprandially. The pain may then resolve on eating.
- Anorexia and weight loss are not uncommon features.
- Many patients, even with complications of PUD, do not report preceding symptoms.

It is most common for complications to occur in the elderly on NSAIDs.

## Investigation

Endoscopy has become the gold standard for diagnostic evaluation of clinically suspected PUD and provides the opportunity for therapeutic intervention. Endoscopic control of acute GI bleeding can be achieved in 90% of cases.

In gastric ulceration (where >80% are located on lesser curve), endoscopy also allows the discrimination between benign and malignant ulcers by histopathological analysis of biopsies. By contrast, duodenal ulcers are rarely neoplastic and biopsy is not routinely recommended.

There is evidence that if initial endoscopic evaluation of a benign gastric ulcer has been thorough (more than six biopsies and cytology) then no further endoscopic follow-up is necessary.

## Management

### Modalities for detection of Helicobacter pylori

- *Campylobacter*-like organism (CLO) test: detects urease activity within gastric biopsy.
- C$^{13}$ urea breath test: relies on urease activity to result in labelled $CO_2$ on exhaled breath.
- Serology: presence of *H. pylori* antibodies.
- Stool antigen.

Careful assessment for the presence of *H. pylori* should be made in all cases of PUD and eradication therapy prescribed where indicated.

### Alarm symptoms meriting endoscopic evaluation

- Weight loss
- Vomiting
- Dysphagia.

The management of dyspepsia (potentially related to uncomplicated PUD) does not always warrant endoscopic evaluation. Published UK guidelines (NICE/SIGN) for dyspeptic patients <65 years without 'alarm symptoms' recommend non-invasive testing and treatment for *H. pylori* in the first instance.

## Proton-pump inhibition

- Inherent component of the strategy for *H. pylori* eradication.
- Used widely for healing of both gastric (GU) and duodenal (DU) peptic ulcer disease.
- PPI once daily for 4–8 weeks can achieve healing in 80–100% of DU and 70–85% of GU.
- PPIs heal PUD more often and with greater speed than H$_2$ receptor antagonists.

Most patients with PUD will require short-term PPI as part of a regimen for *H. pylori* eradication.

Long-term PPI may be required for those with hypersecretory conditions (Zollinger–Ellison syndrome), those on clinically indicated long-term NSAID, and certain patients with complicated PUD.

**Intravenous PPI**: there is evidence to suggest a bolus of IV PPI (e.g. omeprazole) followed by a continuous infusion over the next 72 hours in patients with acute bleeding from PUD reduces the risk of recurrent bleeding. There may be justification in starting pre-emptive therapy in PUD bleeds where immediate endoscopy is not proposed.

A clinical risk score in acute peptic ulcer bleeding has been devised by Rockall et al. (1996). This provides a useful guide to:

- Risk of re-bleeding.
- Likelihood of requirement of surgery.
- 30-day mortality.

It incorporates endoscopic features that are associated with re-bleeding and poor outcome.

- Total scores <3: re-bleeding and mortality is virtually nil.
- Scores >9: 30 day mortality nears 100%.

## Endoscopy

**Timing:** endoscopy should, where possible, be deferred until adequate fluid resuscitation has taken place. Loss of postural BP drop can be a useful guide to the correction of hypovolaemia.

Endoscopic therapy in the setting of GI haemorrhage complicating PUD is confined to those with active bleeding or stigmata of recent haemorrhage.

Endoscopic stigmata of recent haemorrhage (Fig. 9.19):

- Visible vessel within ulcer.
- Blood clot within ulcer.
- Black spots in ulcer crater.

## Post endoscopy management

**IV PPI infusion**: re-bleeding may be reduced by continuous treatment for 72 hours.

Without the clinical suspicion of re-bleeding, there is no good evidence to suggest that repeat endoscopy is warranted or that it confers reduced risk of re-bleeding. If, however, the index endoscopy did not permit delivery of therapy or adequate haemostasis (e.g. due to suboptimal views) then a second procedure may be considered appropriate.

The patient should remain fasted where there is uncertainty regarding haemostasis (recurrent or continued bleeding).

Where satisfactory control has been established, it is reasonable to reintroduce clear fluid intake within 12–24 hours.

Careful clinical assessment following endoscopy is essential to be alerted to early re-bleeding.

With the clinical suspicion of re-bleeding, a decision is required in respect of repeat endoscopy or surgery. Surgical intervention (over repeat endoscopy) for recurrent bleeding appears to be associated with more complications but there does not appear to be any difference in 30-day mortality.

In peptic ulcer bleeds unrelated to NSAID usage, it remains important to treat and ensure successful eradication of *H. pylori*.

# Mallory–Weiss tear

- Mucosal tears occurring in the region of the gastro-oesophageal junction. Mainly gastric mucosal tears (only 10–20% occur in the oesophageal mucosa).
- Account for up to 10% of all upper GI haemorrhages.
- Up to 30% are associated with a history of retching.
- Bleeding stops spontaneously in up to 90% of patients.
- Re-bleeding occurs in <5%.
- Endoscopic confirmation of non-bleeding tears allows supportive management and prompt discharge from hospital.

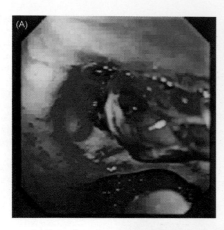
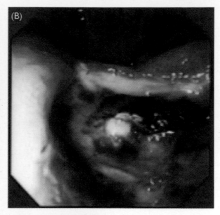
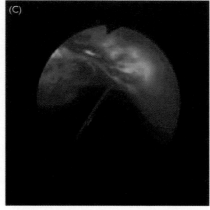

**Fig. 9.19** Endoscopic stigmata associated with significant risk of peptic ulcer re-bleed (% risk). (A) Adherent clot (33%). (B) Non-bleeding visible vessel (50%). (C) Bleeding vessel (90%).

- Where active bleeding or recent haemorrhage stigmata are identified, endoscopic therapy (diathermy/sclerotherapy) is appropriate.
- Where bleeding is refractory to endoscopic therapy, selective angiography with vasopressin infusion or embolization may be indicated and is effective in the majority.
- Surgical intervention for the management of complications is only rarely required.

# Gastro-oesophageal reflux disease

- Constellation of clinical symptoms (heartburn, regurgitation, and dysphagia) which correspond to episodes of reflux of gastric secretions into the distal oesophagus.
- Reflux oesophagitis is an endoscopic diagnosis made in patients with visible mucosal lesions secondary to gastro-oesophageal reflux disease (GORD) (present in 50–80% of GORD patients).
- Some patients (even those with endoscopically severe reflux oesophagitis) will be asymptomatic.
- ♂:♀= 3:1 (oesophagitis).
- ♂:♀= 10:1 (Barrett oesophagus—see Barrett oesophagus and adenocarcinoma).
- Occurs in 50–80% of women during pregnancy.

There is an inverse relationship between the incidence of hospitalizations for GORD (rising) and peptic ulcer disease (falling) leading some authorities to suggest a protective relationship of *H. pylori* against GORD.

**Clinical symptoms**
- Heartburn:
  - Retrosternal burning discomfort radiating into neck.
  - Typical onset after meals, during exercise and lying.
  - Often relieved by drinking water or taking an antacid.
- Regurgitation: involuntary reflux of gastric contents into pharynx.
- Dysphagia:
  - Occurs in >30% patients with GORD.
  - Can occur without endoscopic abnormality.
  - May be caused by peptic stricture or mucosal inflammation.

*Atypical symptoms of GORD*
- Laryngitis: 10% of all patients with laryngitis have clinically significant GORD.
- Asthma: 77% of asthmatics report heartburn. Treatment of GORD in these patients improves respiratory symptoms.
- Cough: 10–40% of patients with chronic cough will have significant GORD.
- Chest pain: 30% of patients undergoing coronary angiography for chest pain will have normal coronary anatomy. Many of these patients have abnormal acid exposure on oesophageal pH studies that correspond with episodes of chest pain.

**Clinical course**
Most patients with endoscopically significant oesophagitis can be healed with medical therapy. Recurrence occurs in up to 80% on discontinuation of therapy.

A minority may develop oesophageal strictures (8–20%), significant bleeding (<2%), or oesophageal perforation (very rare).

### Differential diagnosis

- Oesophageal candidiasis.
- Herpetic (simplex/CMV) oesophagitis.
- Peptic ulcer disease/dyspepsia.
- Biliary colic.
- Coronary artery disease.
- Oesophageal dysmotility/achalasia.
- Iatrogenic oesophagitis (bisphosphonate/NSAID).

### Management

Diagnosis of reflux oesophagitis is achieved by endoscopy, however only 30–40% of patients with GORD will have endoscopically evident mucosal lesions. Endoscopy is, therefore, a poorly sensitive modality for evaluating the patient with reflux symptoms.

Ambulatory oesophageal pH monitoring over 24 hours is the most widely used technique for establishing GO reflux and to correlate events with reported symptoms.

pH monitoring is unnecessary in the majority of patients but can be a useful way of assessing those refractory to medical antacid therapy for whom antireflux surgery is being considered.

### Antacid medical therapy

- PPIs suppress acid more effectively than $H_2$ receptor antagonists with a reduction in gastric acid secretion of 90% (cf. 50–70%).
- Higher doses of PPI are likely to be more effective.
- There is a rationale for twice daily dosing where once daily is ineffective.
- There is a requirement for maintenance of PPI in the majority of GORD patients since 80% experience recurrence of symptoms on discontinuation of therapy.

### Antireflux surgery

Results in a profound clinical benefit in experienced hands.
Complications include:

- Mortality: 0.2%.
- Dysphagia: 12%.

---

## Oesophageal peptic strictures

- Complicate 8–20% of patients with oesophagitis.
- Managed safely and effectively by endoscopic dilatation (50% of strictures will require repeat dilatation).
- Complications of dilatation include:
  - Significant bleeding (requiring transfusion): 0.5%.
  - Perforation: 0.4%.

Long-term maintenance PPI in these patients has been shown to be cost-effective in reducing both number of interventions and complications.

---

## Barrett oesophagus and adenocarcinoma

Specialized intestinal metaplastic change of the oesophagus (Barrett) is an important consequence of GORD. Histopathologically, this epithelial change is recognized as a transformation to a villous architecture with goblet cells. This results in the potential for dysplastic change and the widely held belief that Barrett represents an intermediate step in the development of oesophageal adenocarcinoma. See Fig. 9.20.

The cause of Barrett change is uncertain but there is a clear clinical association with GORD.

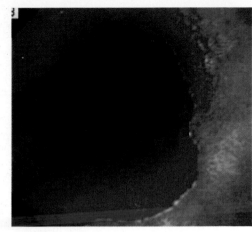

**Fig. 9.20** Barrett oesophagus.
Reproduced from Bloom et al., *Oxford Handbook of Gastroenterology and Hepatology* (2 ed.), 2011, with permission from Oxford University Press.

### Risk factors

GORD symptoms have also been reported as being associated with an increased risk for oesophageal adenocarcinoma (odds ratio (OR) 7.7 (5.3–11.4)) over asymptomatic patients. Where severe reflux symptoms are longstanding (>20 years) there is an even greater risk (OR 43.5 (18.3–103.5)).

Obesity (another reported independent risk factor for adenocarcinoma) appears to compound the risk associated with reflux symptoms with a relative risk (RR) for malignancy of 180.

Nevertheless, the incidence of adenocarcinoma is considered very small, even in the highest risk category.

### Long segment Barrett

- Definition: extending >3cm proximal to the squamo-columnar junction.
- Prevalence is reported as 1% (although higher in GORD and ♂; ♂:♀ = 10:1).
- Incidence of adenocarcinoma is ~0.5% per year. The potential for malignant change in short segment Barrett (<3cm) is considered much smaller.

### Management

- Control of reflux symptoms.
- Risk reduction for adenocarcinoma.

*In vitro* and *in vivo* studies have reported increased cell proliferation on exposure to acid and this has provided the momentum for acid suppressive therapy in patients with Barrett. Nevertheless, there is no clinical evidence to suggest that this reduces the risk of adenocarcinoma or results in regression of metaplasia. The available evidence supports PPI therapy titrated against reflux symptoms irrespective of the presence of Barrett.

### Endoscopic surveillance for Barrett

Quadrantic biopsies every 2cm through the Barrett segment is recommended to exclude significant dysplasia and examined endoscopically under narrow band imaging.

Barrett without dysplasia: where surveillance is considered clinically appropriate endoscopic review is undertaken every 2 years. In low-grade dysplasia:

- Repeat biopsies should be taken after a period of 3 months of acid suppressive therapy since inflammatory change confounds the reporting of dysplasia.
- 6-monthly endoscopies.

In high-grade dysplasia:
- Reported as associated with adenocarcinoma in 25% of patients over a 4-year follow-up.
- Coexistent adenocarcinoma in patients undertaking oesophagectomy for high-grade dysplasia is reported as 47%.
- Management options considered appropriate include: oesophagectomy, endoscopic surveillance, and mucosal resection/radiofrequency ablation (HALO procedure).
- Oesophagectomy carries an operative mortality of 3–10%.
- Surveillance in high-grade dysplasia appears a reasonable strategy since up to 75% will remain histologically stable or even downgrade.
- Subsequent confirmation of carcinoma complicating high-grade dysplasia is associated in the majority with surgically curable disease.

- Endoscopic therapeutic options include thermal or chemical ablation of the relevant epithelium.
- Oesophageal perforation and stricturing are significant complications of such therapy.
- Photodynamic therapy (PDT) is reported as successful in downgrading high-grade dysplastic Barrett in 90% of patients.
- Localized endoscopic mucosal resection of focal lesions is an option in patients otherwise unfit for surgery.

## Reference

Rockall TA, Logan RF, Devlin HB, *et al*. Risk assessment after acute upper gastrointestinal haemorrhage. *Gut* 1996; 38(3): 316–21.

## Background

Lower GI haemorrhage is defined as abnormal intraluminal blood loss from a source distal to the ligament of Treitz.

## Clinical features

Whilst left-sided colonic bleeding often clinically manifests as fresh rectal bleeding, more proximal colonic sources of blood loss result in the passage of altered blood or melaena. Right-sided colonic lesions may remain clinically silent and present with iron deficiency anaemia alone, or symptoms consequent upon this (e.g. worsening angina, exertional breathlessness, or syncopal episodes).

Rarely, upper GI haemorrhage can be so torrential as to result in fresh rectal bleeding thereby mimicking a lower GI bleed.

Although lower GI bleeding is common, most patients will not require hospital admission. Nevertheless, acute lower GI bleeding remains an important cause of hospital admission and is also an important cause of morbidity and mortality.

Mortality (10–20%) is associated with:

- Increasing age.
- Comorbidity.
- Recent surgery.
- Sepsis.
- Multiorgan failure.
- Large volume blood loss (transfusion >5 units packed red cells (PRCs)).

Average age of patients with lower GI bleeding: 60 years.

## Causes of lower GI bleeding

- Aetiology is dependent on the age of the patient.
- 10–20% of patients have no demonstrable cause.
- In those with identifiable aetiology:
  - Diverticular disease (60%)
  - Colonic inflammation (15%)
  - Inflammatory bowel disease
  - Ischaemic colitis
  - Infective colitis
  - Anorectal lesions (10%)
  - Haemorrhoidal
  - Anal fissure
  - Fistula-in-ano
  - Colonic tumours (10%)
  - Colorectal carcinoma
  - Adenoma
  - Vascular lesions (<5%)
  - Angiodysplasia.

## Management of massive lower GI blood loss

### Definition

- Passage of a large volume of red blood through the rectum.
- Haemodynamic instability and shock: SBP <90mmHg.
- Initial decrease in Hb to ≤6g/dL.
- Transfusion of ≥2 units of PRCs.
- Bleeding that continues for 3 days.
- Significant re-bleeding within 1 week.

## Resuscitation

The principles of emergency resuscitation are common to both lower and upper GI tract bleeds. See Section 1.10.

- Airway/oxygen.
- IV access (two large-bore cannulae).
- IV fluid replacement (colloid/crystalloid).
- Monitor fluid balance:
  - Pulse
  - BP
  - Urine output (urinary catheter).
- Cross match (± transfuse).
- Correction of coagulation as needed.

### History/examination

- Previous episodes of GI bleeding.
- Significant medical history:
  - Peptic ulcer disease
  - Liver disease
  - Coagulopathy
  - IBD.
- Medications (e.g. NSAIDs/warfarin).

### Symptoms

1. Abdominal pain:
   - Rectal bleeding.
   - Diarrhoea.
   - Mucus discharge in young patients = likely IBD.
2. Abdominal pain:
   - Rectal bleeding.
   - Diarrhoea in elderly patients = ischaemic colitis or diverticular disease.
3. Stools streaked with blood:
   - Perianal pain.
   - Blood drops on the toilet paper/bowl associated with perianal pathology (e.g. anal fissure or haemorrhoids).

## Diagnosis

### Red cell-labelled scintigraphy

- Sensitive diagnostic tool (86%) for localizing bleeding but relies on **active** bleeding at the time of scanning.
- Can detect haemorrhage at rates as low as 0.1mL/min (reportedly 10× more sensitive than mesenteric angiography in detecting ongoing bleeding).
- The low specificity (50%), however, has led many investigators to recommend that scintigraphic imaging be used primarily as a **screening** examination to select patients for mesenteric angiography.
- Furthermore, due to the high false localization rate of scintigraphy (10–60%), segmental resection on the basis of this test alone is not recommended.
- Its role in the diagnosis and treatment of patients who present with lower GI bleeding, therefore, remains controversial.

Immediate 'blush' (<2 minutes) on scintigraphy is associated with a 75% positive predictive value for mesenteric angiography, whereas delayed blush (>2 minutes) is associated with a 93% negative predictive value for angiography (these patients are best assessed by colonoscopy).

### Mesenteric angiography

This has allowed the distinction of diverticular disease and angiodysplasia as the most common causes of lower GI tract bleeding.

Angiography remains particularly useful in defining the precise locality of the source of active bleeding and thereby allows targeted therapy by either selective embolization or limited surgical resection (NB: embolization carries a significant risk of mesenteric ischaemia).

It is therefore an especially valuable diagnostic tool in massive lower GI haemorrhage.

### Colonoscopy

Lower GI tract endoscopy potentially allows:

- Establishment of a diagnosis.
- Therapeutic intervention (thermal or sclerotherapy)
- A diagnosis can be made in 75–90% of patients.
- Colonoscopy may be impeded by the poor views resulting from active luminal haemorrhage, as well as complicated by the real risk of colonic perforation.
- May be most useful for identifying pathology following the resuscitation of a patient in whom active lower GI bleeding has been controlled.

Where no lower GI source of bleeding is identified, the upper GI tract should also be endoscopically assessed.

## Treatment

### Angiography/selective vasopressin infusion

Emergency angiography may be indicated in selected patients with massive ongoing lower GI bleeding. Bleeding is localized in ~70% of patients and allows the potential for selective arterial embolization or selective mesenteric vasopressin infusion.

Angiography can also facilitate monitoring of the clinical response to titrated doses of vasopressin.

Selective mesenteric vasopressin infusions may be successful in controlling bleeding in >90% of patients, but 50% of these experience re-bleeding following cessation of vasopressin therapy.

Emergency angiography and vasopressin infusion have been shown to improve operative morbidity, mortality, and outcome.

### Surgery

- 10% of patients presenting with lower GI bleeding will require emergency surgery.
- Indicated where the patient continues to bleed despite non-operative therapy.
- **Segmental colectomy:**
  - Indicated if the bleeding point is localized by preoperative diagnostic studies.
  - 10% mortality.
  - 7% post-op re-bleeding.
- **Subtotal colectomy:**
  - Procedure of choice if the bleeding point is determined as colonic but cannot be localized by preoperative or intraoperative diagnostic studies.
  - Associated with higher perioperative morbidity (~30%) and mortality (20%).
  - Postoperative diarrhoea is a significant problem in elderly patients.

## Specific management principles

### Colorectal neoplasia

- Colorectal adenocarcinoma is the third most common cancer in the UK.
- Colorectal carcinoma causes occult bleeding and patients usually present with anaemia and related clinical symptoms.
- 5–20% cause massive lower GI bleeding.
- Surgery dependent on:
  - Stage of disease.
  - Comorbidity/anaesthetic risk.

- Bleeding tumours (benign or malignant) may be endoscopically resectable.
- Post-polypectomy haemorrhage is reported to occur up to 1 month following colonoscopic resection (incidence <3%). This is managed by electrocoagulation of polypectomy/bleeding site.

### Diverticulosis

- Common condition in Western societies.
- ~50% of adults >60 years have radiological evidence of diverticulosis.
- Diverticula are most commonly located in the sigmoid and descending colon.
- Up to 20% of patients with diverticular disease experience bleeding.
- In 5%, bleeding from diverticular disease can be massive.
- Haemorrhage from diverticular disease usually stops spontaneously (80%).
- Although diverticulosis is a left colonic condition, ~50% of diverticular **bleeding** originates from a diverticulum located proximal to the splenic flexure.
- If recurrent or persistent diverticular bleeding occurs then segmental resection may be considered.
- Other important complications of diverticular disease include:
  - Perforation (and paracolic abscess formation).
  - Stricture (± colonic obstruction).

### IBD

- Massive lower GI bleeding due to IBD is rare.
- UC causes bloody diarrhoea in most cases.
- Up to 50% of UC patients have mild–moderate lower GI bleeding.
- 4% of UC patients have massive haemorrhage.
- Lower GI bleeding in Crohn disease is not as common:
  - Massive bleeding (1–2%).
  - More common in Crohn colitis than ileal disease.

*Management of severe lower GI bleeding/IBD*

- Fluid resuscitation.
- Cross match (± transfuse).
- Exclude sepsis (blood cultures/CT).
- Exclude perforation (AXR/CT).
- Early surgical input.
- Consider:
  - Broad-spectrum antibiotics.
  - IV corticosteroid (once sepsis excluded).

### Colonic angiodysplasia

- Arteriovenous malformations in the mucosa/submucosa.
- Usually found in the caecum and ascending colon.
- Typically affect elderly patients (>60 years).
- If mesenteric angiography is performed at the time of active bleeding, extravasation of contrast media is visualized.
- Unlike diverticular bleeding, angiodysplasia tends to cause slow but repeated episodes of bleeding resulting in anaemia and related clinical symptoms.
- Easily recognized at colonoscopy as 1.5–2mm red patches in the mucosa.
- Actively bleeding lesions can be treated with colonoscopic sclerotherapy or electrothermocoagulation.
- Even small lesions may be clinically significant, but rarely cause massive lower GI haemorrhage.
- Infrequently, angiodysplastic bleeds require emergency surgery or interventional radiological management.

**Ischaemic colitis**

- Disease of the elderly population.
- Frequently involves the vascular watershed areas:
  - Splenic flexure
  - Rectosigmoid junction.
- Symptoms: abdominal pain/bloody diarrhoea.
- Ischaemia causes mucosal oedema and bleeding.
- Not usually associated with significant lower GI blood loss.
- In most cases, the precipitating event cannot be identified.

**Anorectal disease**

- Benign anorectal disease (e.g. haemorrhoids, anal fissures or anorectal fistulas) typically results in intermittent rectal bleeding although massive rectal bleeding has also been reported.
- Patients who have rectal varices with portal hypertension may develop painless but catastrophic lower GI bleeding. Management can be difficult but transjugular intrahepatic porto-systemic shunting (TIPSS) may be necessary.

NB: the presence of benign anorectal disease does not exclude the possibility of bleeding from the more proximal lower GI tract.

# Unexplained lower GI tract bleeding

Patients who experience episodic lower GI bleeding without a diagnosis should be considered for:

- Elective mesenteric angiography.
- Repeat upper and lower endoscopy.
- Enteroscopy (push/double balloon).
- Capsule endoscopy.
- Meckel scan.
- CT/MR enteroclysis.

Elective evaluation may identify uncommon lesions or undiagnosed arteriovenous malformations.

# Rare causes of lower GI bleeding

- Chronic radiation enteritis/proctitis
- Ischemic colitis/mesenteric vascular insufficiency
- Small bowel diverticulosis
- Meckel diverticulum
- Colonic/rectal varices
- Portal colopathy
- Solitary rectal ulcer syndrome
- Diversion colitis
- Dieulafoy lesion of colon or small bowel
- Vasculitides
- Small bowel ulceration
- Intussusception
- Endometriosis
- GI bleeding in runners.

# 9.7 Gastrointestinal infections

## Background

Infectious diarrhoeal illness is an important cause of death in developing countries and results in significant morbidity elsewhere in the world. Most mortality is related to dehydration.

Infectious enteritic disease is a particular problem in the immunocompromised host (e.g. *Cryptosporidium* and HIV), but the principles of disease management referred to in this section relate to the immunocompetent host.

As with any infectious illness a careful history of recent and previous **travel** and other infectious **contacts** is paramount.

## Classification of infectious pathogens

1. Toxigenic
2. Invasive
3. Viral.

## Enterotoxins

### Cholera

- Severe diarrhoeal illness.
- Gram-negative rod producing an enterotoxin.
- Vomiting and abdominal distension.
- Profuse diarrhoea leads to water and electrolyte loss.
- Can cause death within 3–4 hours.
- Occurs in epidemics/pandemics (especially Indian subcontinent/Asia) and sporadic outbreaks.
- Contaminated water and food is the source of infection.
- Person-to-person infection is uncommon.
- Low gastric acidity (seen in malnutrition) is a predisposing factor.
- Enterotoxin drives osmotic fluid loss: 'rice water' stool (isotonic with plasma).
- $K^+/HCO_3$ loss.
- Vaccines available.
- Treatment:
  - Oral/IV rehydration + $K^+/HCO_3$.
  - Ciprofloxacin.
  - Tetracycline.

### Escherichia coli
#### Enteropathogenic E. coli

- Adheres to and destructs intestinal mucosa.

#### Enterotoxigenic E. coli

- Toxin similar to *Vibrio cholerae*.
- Incubation of 24–48 hours.
- Severe diarrhoea.
- Treatment:
  - IV fluid replacement.
  - (Antibiotics rarely).

#### Enterohaemorrhagic E. coli (E. coli 0157)

- Most common pathogen in bloody diarrhoea in USA.
- Incubation 1–14 days.
- Bloody diarrhoea.
- Friable erythematous inflamed mucosa.
- AXR: mucosal 'thumb-printing' similar to IBD.
- Illness last <7 days.

- Treatment: antibiotics do not appear to confer clinical benefit and may precipitate haemolytic uraemic syndrome.

## Invasive enteropathogens

- Invade the intestinal epithelium.
- Target the lower intestine:
  - Distal ileum
  - Colon.
- Mucosal ulceration and inflammatory change seen.

### Pathogens (diagnosed on stool culture)
*Salmonella*

- Poultry, eggs, dairy, meat.
- Incubation <48 hours.
- Pain/diarrhoeal illness/fever lasting 4 days.
- Colitis: mucosal ulceration and crypt abscesses.
- Treatment: no evidence for improved outcome with antibiotics.
- Beware toxic megacolon/colonic perforation.

*Shigella*

- 'Dysentery.'
- Oral infection: highly contagious.
- Inflammatory, exudative diarrhoea: blood/pus.
- Histologically/clinically may mimic IBD.
- Arthritis: following enteric illness (especially HLA B27).
- Illness: 7 days (severe: 3 weeks).
- Treatment: ampicillin/ciprofloxacin (in those with persistent diarrhoea).

*Yersinia*

- Gram-negative rod.
- Invades through epithelium over Peyer patches.
- Acute diarrhoeal illness.
- Reactive arthritis.
- Erythema nodosum/multiforme.
- Treatment: no evidence for antibiotics.

*Campylobacter*

- C. jejuni/C. fetus.
- Major cause of diarrhoea.
- Incubation <72 hours.
- Clinical picture:
  - Dysentery (asymptomatic excretion).
  - Diarrhoea (± blood).
  - Fever.
  - Abdominal pain.
- Illness: 7 days.
- Relapse: 25%.
- Treatment (if dysentery/fever):
  - Azithromycin.
  - Ciprofloxacin.
- Most spontaneously resolve.

## Viral

### Rotavirus

- Faecal–oral transmission.
- 35% of childhood diarrhoeal illness.

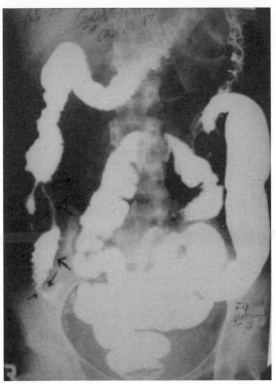

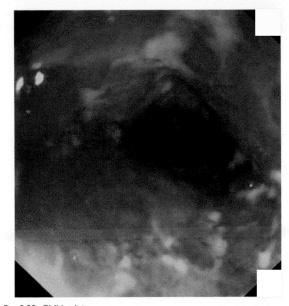

**Fig. 9.22** CMV colitis.
*Coloproctology*, 32, 5, 2010, 268, 'Proktitis – aus gastroenterologischer Sicht', Escher M, with kind permission from Springer Science and Business Media.

**Fig. 9.21** Contrast barium enema image demonstrates marked narrowing of the caecum, ascending colon and terminal ileum. Dilatation of the small intestine proximal to the narrowed segment of ileum is also seen. Reproduced with permission of *Journal of Clinical Imaging Science*.

- Vomiting and diarrhoea for 5–7 days.
- Treatment: rehydration.
- Breast milk appears to have a protective role.
- Vaccine license withdrawn (intussception).

### Cytomegalovirus (CMV)

- Colitis most commonly affects immunocompromised host (e.g. HIV, solid-organ transplant recipient).
- Presentation: fever, anorexia, weight loss, abdominal pain, diarrhoea (may be bloody). See Fig. 9.21.
- Treatment: antiviral (e.g. ganciclovir, foscarnet).
- Reduce immunosuppression burden (if applicable).

## Others: tuberculosis

- Clinical features: pain, fever, weight loss.
- RIF mass in 60% patients.
- Most frequently affects ileocaecum/jejunum (Fig. 9.22).
- Diagnosis: made at laparotomy.
- Treatment: antituberculous medication.

## Bacterial food poisoning

Enteric illness derived from consumption of bacterial derived toxins.

### Clostridium perfringens
- Type A:
  - 24-hour self-limiting diarrhoeal illness.
  - No treatment required.

- Type C:
  - Severe, necrotizing disease of the small intestine (enteritis necroticans/'pigbel').
  - Associated with intestinal perforation and high mortality (40%).

### Staphylococcus aureus
- Clinical features: vomiting, pain, diarrhoea.
- 24-hour illness.
- No treatment required.

### Listeria
- Milk, dairy, seafood, raw meat.
- Systemic illness.
- Diarrhoea and fever.
- Especially affects immunocompromised/pregnant.

### Bacillus cereus
- Two toxins, two syndromes.
- Diarrhoea/vomiting.

## Pseudomembranous colitis

### Clostridium difficile
- Spore-forming organism.
- Found widely in environment.
- Transferable pathogen.
- Hospital epidemics carry high morbidity and mortality.
- Antibiotic treatment predisposes to enteric infection especially:
  - Clindamycin
  - Ampicillin
  - Cephalosporin.
- Spectrum of clinical severity:
  - Asymptomatic carrier state.
  - Mild diarrhoeal illness.
  - PMC.

- 75–90% antibiotic-associated diarrhoea is C. diff toxin-negative.
- Clinical features:
  - Abdominal pain.
  - Diarrhoea: frequency 20–30× daily.
  - Fever.
  - Leucocytosis.
  - Hypoalbuminaemia (protein-losing enteropathy).
- AXR: mucosal oedema/colonic dilatation
- Stool—C. diff toxin:
  - Toxin A enterotoxin
  - Toxin B cytotoxin.

## Treatment

- Supportive:
  - Discontinue antibiotic.
  - IV fluid replacement.
  - Electrolyte correction.
  - Isolation of inpatients.
- Antimicrobial:
  - Vancomycin 125mg four times daily for 7–14 days.
  - Metronidazole 250mg three times daily for 7–14 days.
- Other:
  - Cholestyramine 4g three times daily for 5–10 days.
- Recurrence (16% relapse rate after initial treatment):
  - Vancomycin and metronidazole for 14 days.
  - Cholestyramine.
  - Lactobacillus.
  - Vancomycin 125mg four times daily for 6 weeks.
  - Vancomycin and rifampicin for 14 days.
  - IV immunoglobulin 400mg/kg.
- Where persistent diarrhoea or severe disease consider:
  - Teicoplanin
  - Fusidic acid
  - IV metronidazole:
- Colectomy—occasionally required < 1%. Indications:
  - Organ failure
  - Toxic megacolon
  - Peritonitis.

## Entamoeba histolytica

- Predominant distribution: central and southern America, Africa and the Indian subcontinent
- Clinical features:
  - Asymptomatic (90%).

- Amoebic colitis (bloody diarrhoea).
  - Liver abscess.
  - Acute necrotizing colitis (rare).
- Diagnosis:
  - Colonoscopy/biopsy.
  - Microscopy of hot stool (30–60% sensitive).
  - ELISA for antigen in stool.
- Treatment:
  - Paronomycin (luminal disease).
  - Metronidazole+paronomycin (invasive colitis/liver abscess).

NB. Take care not to miss concomitant amoebic illness in IBD as steroid treatment predisposes to colonic perforation with amoebic colitis.

## Giardia lamblia

- Affects more children than adults.
- Important cause of severe malabsorption and malnutrition.
- Clinical features:
  - Asymptomatic
  - Severe malnutrition
  - Diarrhoea
  - Fatigue
  - Bloating
  - Weight loss
  - Fever
  - Vomiting.
- Diagnosis:
  - Stool ELISA (90–100% sensitive).
  - Stool microscopy (50% sensitive).
  - Duodenal biopsy (80% sensitive but also helpful in excluding other conditions).
- Treatment:
  - Metronidazole 250mg three times a day for 5 days.
  - Tinidazole.
  - Paronomycin.

NB: lactose intolerance following infection is very common and recurrent giardiasis should be confirmed by repeat testing in the individual before retreatment.

## Cryptosporidium

- Infectious enterocolitis in the immunocompromised.
- Diagnosis: stool microscopy.
- Stool ELISA.
- Treatment: no consistently effective treatment.

# 9.8 Gastrointestinal cancer

## Background

Cancers of the GI tract are a common cause of cancer death worldwide (Fig. 9.23).

## Oesophageal cancer

- One of the ten most common cancers worldwide.
- 2% of all cancers, incidence: 3.3/100,000.
- Squamous cell carcinoma is the most common worldwide (Fig. 9.24).
- Rising incidence of distal oesophageal/gastro-oesophageal adenocarcinoma (especially in the USA and Europe).
- Prognosis: overall 5-year survival of 10%. Even for those undergoing 'curative' resection, and despite advances in surgical techniques and perioperative management, the 5-year survival is only 20%.
- Palliative therapy plays a vital role in the management of symptoms.

### Barrett oesophagus

(See Section 9.5.) 5–15% of patients having endoscopy (for any reason) will be shown to have intestinal metaplasia of the distal oesophageal epithelium: Barrett oesophagus. The metaplastic change is almost certainly associated with gastro-oesophageal reflux and a corresponding higher incidence of adenocarcinoma (RR: 7.7).

Annual incidence of adenocarcinoma in Barrett is reported as 0.5–0.8%, representing a 30–60-fold increased risk from the general population. It is for this reason that surveillance endoscopy and biopsies are recommended where the segment is >3cm in length. The emergence of dysplasia in a segment of Barrett has important implications for the patient and the therapeutic options include endoscopic mucosal resection (EMR), photodynamic therapy (PDT), or distal oesophagectomy.

## Clinical presentation

Most patients present with either locally advanced or metastatic disease. Typical signs/symptoms include:

- Dysphagia
- Vomiting/regurgitation
- Weight loss
- Anaemia.

## Investigation

1. Endoscopy/biopsy—to histologically confirm the diagnosis/site.
2. Staging: CT/endoscopic ultrasound (EUS).

Current TNM classification and staging is as shown in Tables 9.4 and 9.5

### Treatment

Dependent on TNM stage:

- Tis/T1 N0 M0: PDT/surgery/EMR.
- (T2 or T3) N0 M0: surgery ± chemo/radiotherapy.
- (T1, T2, or T3) N1 M0: surgery ± chemo/radiotherapy.
- T4 (any N, any M): palliative therapy.

See Fig. 9.25.

#### Surgery

Surgical treatment of oesophageal cancer is considered where:

- Diagnosis of oesophageal cancer in a candidate for surgical resection.
- High-grade dysplasia is present in a patient with Barrett oesophagus (and where EMR is impossible or contraindicated).

Surgical treatment is contraindicated in the following:

- Metastasis to N2 (coeliac, cervical, supraclavicular) nodes or solid organs (e.g. liver, lungs).
- Invasion of adjacent structures (e.g. recurrent laryngeal nerve, tracheobronchial tree, aorta, pericardium).
- Severe associated comorbid conditions (e.g. cardiovascular disease, respiratory disease).
- Impaired cardiac or respiratory function.

#### Neoadjuvant chemoradiation therapy

- Aim: preoperative treatment to facilitate response to surgical resection.

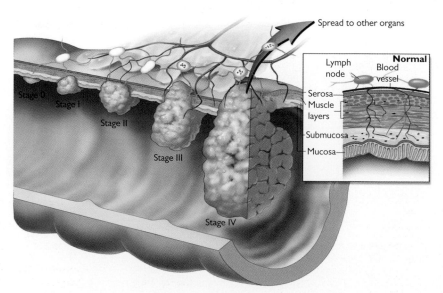

**Fig. 9.23** TNM classification of GI tumours.
Image courtesy of Terese Winslow.

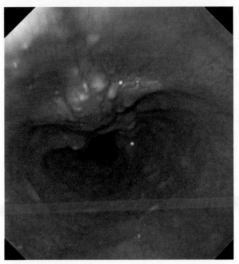

**Fig. 9.24** Endoscopic view of squamous cell carcinoma of mid-oesophagus.

- Eradicate micro metastasis.
- Survival advantage in T3 N1 with preoperative neoadjuvant cisplatin/5FU 5-year survival rates of 23% compared with 17% (Allum et al., 2008).

*Non-surgical therapy*
Reserved for oesophageal carcinoma patients who are not candidates for surgery.

The principal symptom goal is palliation of dysphagia. Treatment modalities include:

- Chemotherapy: a response rate of 48% has been reported in advanced oesophagogastric disease to a combination of epirubicin, oxaliplatin, capecitabine with 46.8% 1-year survival (Cunningham et al., 2008).
- Radiation therapy:
  - Relieves dysphagia in about 50% of patients.
  - May be a useful adjunct in palliation especially for recurrent bleeding.
  - Pre- or postoperatively has not been shown to improve survival.
- Laser therapy (for temporary relief; multiple sessions are usually required).

| Table 9.5 Staging of oesophageal cancer | | | |
|---|---|---|---|
| **Stage 0** | Tis | N0 | M0 |
| **Stage I** | T1 | N0 | M0 |
| **Stage IIA** | T2 T3 | N0 | M0 |
| **Stage IIB** | T1 T2 | N1 | M0 |
| **Stage III** | T3 | N1 | M0 |
| | T4 | Any N | M0 |
| **Stage IV** | Any T | Any N | M1 |
| **Stage IVA** | Any T | Any N | M1a |
| **Stage IVB** | Any T | Any N | M1b |

Tis: carcinoma *in situ*.

- Stent placement.
- PDT, alone or with laser thermal ablation.

## Gastric cancer

Second most common cancer worldwide (Fig. 9.26)

- 'Distal' gastric adenocarcinoma (by contrast to gastro-oesophageal junction adenocarcinoma) is falling in incidence, possibly as a result of widespread *Helicobacter pylori* eradication. There is little doubt that *H. pylori* resulting in chronic gastritis can result in an atrophic gastritis that has potential to dysplastic change and ultimately carcinoma.
- Incidence of GO junction adenocarcinoma (Fig. 9.27) is rising, especially in young adults.
- Majority of patients present between the ages of 65–74 years, with annual mortality rates of up to 6.1/100,000 population in USA/Europe whilst Russia and Far East carry a considerably higher mortality burden (>30/100,000).

### Clinical presentation

- Dependent on site:
  - Dysphagia in proximal tumours.
  - Gastric outflow obstruction in distal tumours (may result in vomiting).
  - Weight loss.
  - Iron deficiency anaemia.
- May be clinically silent.

### Staging

- TNM: (as for oesophageal cancer; Table 9.5).

| Table 9.4 TNM classification of oesophageal cancer | |
|---|---|
| **Oesophagus** | |
| T1 | Lamina propria, submucosa |
| T2 | Muscularis propria |
| T3 | Adventitia |
| T4 | Adjacent structures |
| N1 | Regional |
| M1 | Distant metastasis |
| | Tumour of **lower thoracic** oesophagus |
| M1a | Coeliac nodes |
| M1b | Other distant metastasis |
| | Tumour of **upper thoracic** oesophagus |
| M1a | Cervical nodes |
| M1b | Other distant metastasis |
| | Tumour of **mid-thoracic** oesophagus |
| M1b | Distant metastasis including non-regional lymph nodes |

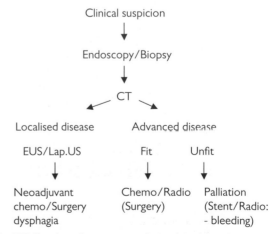

**Fig. 9.25** Flowchart of management of oesophageal carcinoma.

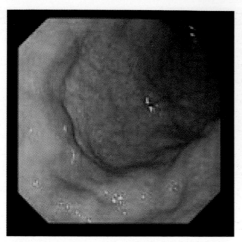

Fig. 9.26 Endoscopic view of infiltrating gastric carcinoma (linitis plastica).

- Modalities: CT/MRI/EUS.
- Treatment algorithm: as for oesophageal cancer (Fig. 9.25).
- Surgery especially useful for debulking symptomatic tumours.

### Prognosis
- T1 N0 5-year survival: 78–95%.
- 75% of patients will have local LN involvement or distant metastases at the time of diagnosis (5-year survival: 7–17%).

### Gastric lymphoma
- 3–6% of all gastric malignancies.
- 95% are NHL.
- 35% are low-grade MALToma (mucosal associated lymphoid tissue).
- RR of lymphoma with *H. pylori* = 6.

### Treatment
- High-grade lymphoma: surgery/chemo/radiotherapy:
  - Localized—5-year survival: 80–95%.

- Nodal involvement both sides of diaphragm—5-year survival: 10–30%.
- MALToma—eradication of H. pylori in HP positive patients ± chemo/radiotherapy: 5-year survival >90%.

## Pancreatic cancer

- Third most frequent GI cancer (after colorectal and oesophagogastric).
- Incidence: 8.8/100,000 per year.
- Extremely poor prognosis.
- 5-year survival rates: 1–5%.
- Clinical presentation:
  - Steatorrhoea/malabsorption.
  - Painless obstructive jaundice.
  - Weight loss.
- Staging: CT (Fig. 9.28).
- Resection (Whipple disease):
  - In selected patients (15%), may afford a long-term survival benefit (in 20%).
  - Median post-op survival: 15–19 months.
- Most patients will be unsuitable for surgery: median survival 4–10 months.
- Endoscopic biliary stenting may be a useful palliative measure in the jaundiced patient.
- Obtain oncology opinion: adjuvant/palliative chemoradiotherapy.

There appear to be survival benefits for adjuvant chemotherapy postoperatively as well as reducing the risk of local recurrence.

There is evidence to suggest there may be a small survival advantage to palliative chemotherapy in unresectable disease.

## Small intestinal neoplasm

This is an uncommon disease, however most (60%) are malignant. Nevertheless, small intestinal malignancies represent only 1–3% of GI tract cancers overall. See Box 9.4.

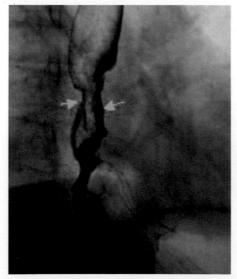

Fig. 9.27 Barium swallow showing distal oesophageal stricture in gastro-oesophageal (GO) junction adenocarcinoma.

Reproduced from Gardiner et al., *Training in Surgery: The essential curriculum for the MRCS (Oxford Specialty Training: Training In)*, 2009, Figure 4.5, page 79, with permission from Oxford University Press.

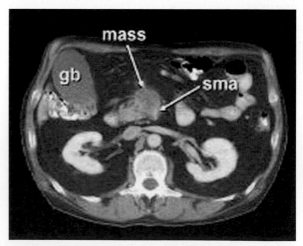

Fig. 9.28 CT image of pancreatic mass (adenocarcinoma) intimately associated with the superior mesenteric artery (SMA).

Image reprinted with permission from Richard A Erickson, MD, FACP, FACG, Scott & White Clinic and Hospital and Texas A&M University Health Science Center, originally published in Dragovich T, Erickson RA, Larson CR, Shabahang M, Pancreatic Cancer, Medscape Reference, updated October 14, 2013, available at: http://emedicine.medscape.com/article/280605-overview.

## Box 9.4 Clinical features of small intestinal neoplasms

- Small bowel obstruction.
- Abdominal pain.
- Volvulus.
- GI bleeding.
- Jaundice (ampullary lesions).
- Carcinoid syndrome (with liver metastases).
- Cachexia.
- Ascites.
- Hepatomegaly.

## Box 9.5 Peutz–Jeghers syndrome

- Autosomal dominant.
- Mucocutaneous pigmentation.
- Multiple hamartomatous polyposis.
- Complicated by GI bleeding and obstruction.
- Often diagnosed age <25 years.
- Increased risk of carcinoma (small and large bowel).
- Colonoscopic/enteroscopic surveillance required.

50% of benign lesions remain asymptomatic whereas 70–90% of malignancies are associated with symptoms.

### Malignant neoplasms

Adenocarcinoma is the most common small bowel malignancy (35–50%):

- Arises from benign adenomatous neoplasms.
- More common in:
  - Crohn disease
  - Coeliac disease
  - HNPCC
  - Peutz–Jeghers syndrome (Box 9.5).

### Carcinoid

Carcinoid tumours represent the second most common small intestinal malignancy (20–40%). The small bowel, in particular the ileum, is the most common site for carcinoid tumours overall. Small intestinal carcinoid tends to present late with lymphadenopathy, liver metastases, and carcinoid syndrome. The discovery of early, potentially resectable disease is usually incidental. See Box 9.6.

### Treatment

All carcinoid tumours should be evaluated for suitability for curative surgical resection. Other options include:

- Palliative resection.
- Somatostatin analogue.
- Chemoembolization of liver metastases.
- Chemo/radiotherapy.

### Lymphoma

The small intestine (and the stomach) remains the most common extra-nodal site for lymphoma. Small intestinal T-cell lymphoma is an important complication of coeliac disease.

## Box 9.6 Clinical features of carcinoid syndrome

- Flushing
- Diarrhoea
- Abdominal pain
- Bronchoconstriction
- Pellagra (niacin deficiency)

## Box 9.7 5-year survival after resection for small intestinal adenocarcinoma

- Limited to mucosa 100%
- Serosa 50%
- Lymph nodes 45%
- Distant metastases 0%

### Diagnosis

Small intestinal tumours are notoriously difficult to diagnose.

- CEA: not elevated until significant hepatic metastatic disease present.
- 5HIAA: not elevated unless there is extensive liver metastases from primary carcinoid (high first-pass metabolism).
- Enteroclysis: MR/CT are reasonably sensitive modalities for diagnosing small intestinal tumours and perform consistently better than conventional barium studies.
- Wireless video capsule endoscopy is emerging as a useful way of directly visualizing the entire small intestinal tract but does not allow tissue sampling.
- Enteroscopy, and in particular double balloon enteroscopy (allowing panenteroscopy), is useful where identified lesions require histopathological appraisal.

### Prognosis

Most are amenable to surgical resection, and prognosis is related to completeness of resection and the presence of lymph node involvement (Box 9.7).

## Benign

- Adenomas account for 30% of all benign small intestinal tumours and have malignant potential.
- Leiomyomas account for 40% and can be complicated by both haemorrhage and malignant transformation.
- Lipomas, where of sufficient size, may cause intestinal obstruction.

## Colorectal cancer

- Second most common cause of cancer death in UK (17,000 deaths per annum) (Figs 9.29 and 9.30).
- Incidence: 30,000 cases per annum.
- Aetiology:
  1. Dietary evidence:
     - High fat/red meat (increased risk).
     - High vegetable/fibre (reduced risk).
  2. Family history:
     - Familial adenomatous polyposis (FAP).
     - HNPCC (6% of all colonic adenocarcinoma).
  3. IBD:
     - Patients with IBD are at increased risk of colorectal cancer (CRC).
     - (Risk is greatest in those with pan-colitis or disease duration >10 years.)

### Clinical presentation

- Rectal bleeding.
- Change in bowel habit.
- Iron deficiency anaemia.
- 80% rectal cancers are palpable.
- Colonoscopy:
  - Sensitive (but not 100%).
  - Not always 100% complete.

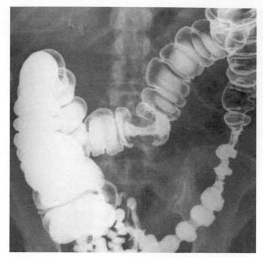

**Fig. 9.29** Double contrast barium enema showing an 'apple-core' stricture resulting from an adenocarcinoma in the transverse colon.

- Screening can produce significant reduction in mortality.
- Adjuvant radio/chemotherapy have important roles.
- MDT decision is required before treatment commences.

## Screening for colorectal cancer

A UK population screening programme is currently being implemented:
- Targeted at both men and women aged between 60 and 69.
- FOB (faecal occult blood) testing via kits sent to the patient's home every 2 years.

In addition:

*Family history of CRC*
- Moderate risk of CRC: colonoscopy at 50 years.

*FAP*
- 1% of all CRC.
- Mutation of APC gene.
- Multiple polyps through colon (Fig. 9.30).
- CRC inevitable (mean 40 years).
- Screening of those with gene mutation: colonoscopy every 2 years.
- When polyps evident—surgery.

*HNPCC*
- 5% of all CRC.
- Mutation of mismatch repair gene.

- Criteria: three relatives with CRC (two consecutive generations, CRC <50 years).
- Once criteria fulfilled:
  - Colonoscopy every 2 years from 20 years

*Sporadic adenoma*
- Associated with 40% risk at 3 years of further adenoma.
- Probable increased risk of CRC.
- Probably the basis for efficacy in population screening.
- Follow-up colonoscopy at 3 yearly intervals IBD.
- Higher risk of CRC than general population.
- Cumulative risk:
  - 2% at 10 years.
  - 8% at 20 years.
  - 18% by 30 years.
- Left-sided colitis/pan-colitis >10 years duration.

*Colonoscopy every 3 years*
- Colitis >20 years **or** indeterminate dysplasia.

*Colonoscopy annually*
- High-grade dysplasia.
- Colectomy should be advised.
- 40% chance of invasive CRC.

## Staging
- After diagnosis it is important to establish the extent of disease (both locally and distant spread).
- Dukes staging (5-year survival post-op):
  - Dukes A: confined to mucosa (>90%).
  - Dukes B: extension into muscularis propria (60–85%).
  - Dukes C: regional lymphadenopathy (40%).
  - Dukes D: distant metastases (5–10%).
- CT: good sensitivity for liver and lung lesions.
- MRI: useful in predicting histological spread in rectal tumours.
- Full colonoscopy in staging distal colon tumours—5% CRC have a synchronous proximal CRC.

## Treatment
*Localized disease*
- Surgery (segmental resection).
- Prophylactic heparin.
- Prophylactic antibiotics.
- Adjuvant chemotherapy for Dukes C and high-risk Dukes B.
- Neo-adjuvant radiotherapy for rectal cancer (pre-op) reduces risk of local recurrence.
- Follow up:

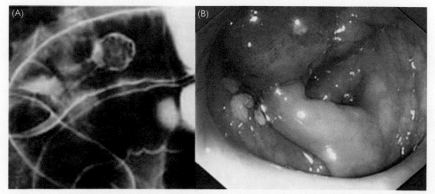

**Fig. 9.30** Pedunculated polyp in transverse colon: double contrast barium enema (A), endoscopic appearance (B).

- Colonoscopy at 3 years post-resection, then 5-yearly intervals.
- CT liver/CEA monitoring may improve survival.

### Advanced disease

Liver metastases—survival improved after resection for operable liver metastases.

Some evidence for:
- Cryoablation
- Radiofrequency ablation.

There are reports of 40% long-term survival in oligometastatic disease.

### Inoperable disease
- Palliative defunctioning may relieve symptoms.
- Palliative radiotherapy for rectal cancer.
- Palliative chemotherapy.

## Future

Modification of cancer process through:
- Biological therapy.
- Gene therapy.

## References

Allum WH, Fogarty PJ, Stenning SP, et al. Long term results of the MRC OEO2 randomized trial of surgery with or without preoperative chemotherapy in resectable esophageal cancer. [Abstract 9] American Society of Clinical Oncology 2008 Gastrointestinal Cancers Symposium, 25–27 January 2008, Orlando, FL.

Cunningham D, Starling N, Rao S, et al. Capecitabine and oxaliplatin for advanced esophagogastric cancer. N Engl J Med 2008; 358: 36–46.

# 9.9 Miscellaneous gastrointestinal problems

## Chronic abdominal pain

Chronic abdominal pain may be caused by one of several problems, of which functional disease remains an important clinical challenge in terms of both diagnosis and management (Box 9.8).

The clinical imperative is to exclude pathological organic causes for the patient's symptoms (Box 9.9).

Once the diagnostic criteria for functional abdominal pain (**ROME II** criteria, see Box 9.10) are fulfilled, it is unusual for other pathology to be identified.

### Psychosocial factors

Functional abdominal pain is not uncommonly associated with other functional systemic symptoms which in turn may be associated with psychological disorders. Many patients have anxiety, depression, or somatization disorders (although they may deny these on questioning).

A history of profound loss/bereavement (parent, spouse, child, stillbirth, abortion) or sexual/physical abuse is a common underlying feature albeit rarely volunteered by the patient.

### Diagnosis

- Thorough history and examination.
- ROME II criteria fulfilled.
- Normal bloods: FBC, U&E, LFT, ESR/CRP.
- Coeliac serology negative.
- FOB/faecal calprotectin (surrogate marker for IBD) negative.

### Treatment

- Reassurance and empathy (through a trusting patient–physician relationship and good rapport).
- Education (in terms of understanding functional abdominal pain).
- Recognition of psychosocial factors and involvement of mental health professionals (where accepted).
- Diary of symptoms and associated triggers (allows the patient to take responsibility and control over their illness). Those with symptoms that are mainly related to psychological distress will gain the most from psychological treatment (cognitive behavioural therapy/gut-directed hypnotherapy).
- Tricyclic and SSRI antidepressants in low dose can be useful. The lag time for clinical effect may be several weeks.
- Nutritional/lifestyle advice (balance energy intake and energy expenditure).

---

**Box 9.8 Functional causes of chronic abdominal pain**

- Irritable bowel syndrome
- Functional dyspepsia
- Functional abdominal pain
- Functional biliary/sphincter of Oddi pain

---

**Box 9.9 Organic causes of chronic abdominal pain**

- Inflammatory bowel disease
- Chronic pancreatitis
- Mesenteric ischaemia
- Endometriosis
- Pelvic inflammatory disease
- Intra-abdominal neoplasm

---

**Box 9.10 Rome II criteria**

*Require >6 months of:*

- Continuous abdominal pain.
- Not related to eating, defaecation or menses.
- Loss of daily functioning.
- Not malingering.
- Insufficient criteria to fulfil other functional disorders.

Adapted with permission of Rome Foundation, Inc.

---

## Irritable bowel syndrome

IBS is characterized by

- Recurrent abdominal pain.
- Diarrhoea and/or constipation.
- Abdominal bloating.

Whilst it is a common complaint, it should not be regarded as trivial, as such patients often require frequent reassurance and extensive investigation.

Additionally, it is common for this group of patients to report other systemic symptoms (Box 9.11).

Since diagnosis is so often arbitrary, the impetus for clinical guidelines has provided the basis for the Rome II diagnostic criteria of functional gastrointestinal disorders (Box 9.12).

### Pathophysiology

Abnormal gut visceral sensitivity/hyper-reactivity. Psycho-visceral tension is relayed through the hypothalamic–pituitary–adrenal system, the activation of which is exaggerated at times of chronic unremitting stress and results in the physical symptoms associated with IBS.

Personal loss is a common source of such stress and is often found to underpin symptoms. Failure of the physician to recognize this loss and the ensuing needs of the patient often results in a breakdown of the doctor–patient relationship and frustration on both sides.

### Diagnosis

Whilst patients will often fulfil the Rome II criteria for IBS, in the absence of structural or metabolic abnormalities, other symptoms supporting the diagnosis include:

---

**Box 9.11 IBS systemic symptoms**

| | |
|---|---|
| - Lassitude | - Arthralgia |
| - Anorexia | - Dyspareunia |
| - Back pain | - Heartburn |
| - Headache | - Chest pain |
| - Insomnia | - Myalgia |
| - Depression | - Anxiety |

---

**Box 9.12 Rome II diagnostic criteria for IBS**

Abdominal pain of ≥12 weeks within 12 months associated with:

- Relief by defecation.
- Onset with change in frequency/consistency of stool.

Additionally:

- Urgency
  - Frequency
  - Incomplete evacuation
  - Abdominal bloating
  - Mucus PR

Adapted with permission of Rome Foundation, Inc.

| Box 9.13 Features which are not consistent with IBS |
| --- |
| • Old age |
| • Fever |
| • Weight loss |
| • Rectal bleeding |
| • Dehydration |

| Box 9.14 Infections causing diarrhoeal illness | |
| --- | --- |
| *Escherichia coli* | *Adenovirus* |
| *Salmonella* | *Rotavirus* |
| *Shigella* | *Cryptosporidium* |
| *Clostridium difficile* | *Entamoeba* |
| *Campylobacter* | *Giardia* |

• Long, relapsing history.
• Significant life events.
• Association with other systemic symptoms.
• Anxiety/depression.
• Conviction of 'organic' cause (e.g. allergy, food toxicity).
Also see Box 9.13.

### Investigation
• FBC, ESR.
• Proctoscopy.
• Diarrhoea-predominant:
  • Vitamin $B_{12}$
  • Folate
  • Ferritin
  • Tissue transglutaminase antibody.
• Constipation-predominant:
  • Colonic transit studies
  • Endo-anal ultrasound
  • Anorectal manometry.

### Treatment
• Anti-spasmodic—mebeverine/peppermint.
• Anti-diarrhoeal—loperamide.
• Anti-constipating—methylcellulose/Fybogel®.
• Anti-depressant—amitriptyline/fluoxetine.
If IBS can be recognized to be caused or associated with psychological stress then allaying fears/reassuring the patient may go further than resolving the physical symptoms than the provision of prescription medication.

## Diarrhoea

• Definition: increased fluidity of stool.
• Typically associated with an increase in faecal volume (>300mL/24 hours).
Whilst such symptoms, when transient, are very common, persistent (chronic) diarrhoea or diarrhoea associated with rectal bleeding, weight loss, or other systemic symptoms, will require further investigation.

### Pathophysiology
Around 10L of fluid/day (a combination of ingested volume and secretions) is presented to the intestinal tract from the stomach and pancreatobiliary systems.
99% of this is efficiently resorbed (in health) by the intestinal tract, mostly across the small intestine (85%).
Loss of efficiency of this physiological function, even to a minimal extent, may result in diarrhoea.

### Acute vs. chronic
**Acute**, short-lived diarrhoeal illness (<4 weeks) is usually due to infection. It may also arise as a result of prescribed medication (Box 9.14).
**Chronic** diarrhoea, by contrast, is often a result of a non-infectious disease process (NB: certain infections may result in chronic symptoms, e.g. *Giardia*).
Chronic diarrhoea may be usefully categorized as:
1. Chronic watery diarrhoea (secretory or osmotic; Box 9.15).
2. Chronic fatty diarrhoea (steatorrhoea; Box 9.16).

| Box 9.15 Causes of chronic watery diarrhoea |
| --- |
| • Enterotoxins (e.g. cholera, *Clostridium difficile*). |
| • Drugs (e.g. antibiotics, NSAID, PPI). |
| • Laxative abuse. |
| • Malignancy: |
|   • Carcinoid |
|   • Phaeochromocytoma |
|   • Gastrinoma |
|   • Intestinal lymphoma |
|   • Adenocarcinoma. |
| • Endocrine: hyperthyroidism. |
| • Addison disease. |
| • Diffuse intestinal mucosal disease: |
|   • Inflammatory bowel disease |
|   • Vasculitis. |
| • Previous intestinal resection: reduced Na/water/bile salt resorption. |
| • Disordered motility: previous vagotomy. |
| • Diabetes. |
| • Hyperthyroidism. |
| • Irritable bowel syndrome. |
| • Scleroderma. |
| • Amyloidosis. |

### Chronic watery diarrhoea
Arises as a result of:
• Disordered electrolyte transport resulting in increased secretions or reduced absorption (**secretory**) or
• Inflammatory intestinal disease (Box 9.17) or (less commonly).
• Ingestion of an osmotically active substance (**osmotic**).
**Osmotic** diarrhoea follows the ingestion of an osmotically active substance (e.g. lactulose, mannitol, sorbitol, magnesium) that is poorly absorbed and results in reduced intestinal water resorption. A well-recognized example of an osmotic diarrhoeal condition is that seen in patients with lactase deficiency.

### Lactase deficiency
Lactase (the disaccharidase enzyme produced on the brush border of the small intestine) tends to diminish through adult life (although lactase levels are maintained into adulthood in those from the Northern European gene pool).
The resulting lactase deficiency may result in lactose malabsorption (intolerance) and osmotic diarrhoea.
Importantly, osmotic diarrhoea is distinguished by its resolution on fasting, whereas secretory or inflammatory diarrhoea typically persists despite fasting.

| Box 9.16 Causes of steatorrhoea |
| --- |
| • Coeliac disease. |
| • Whipple disease. |
| • Short bowel syndrome (post-resection). |
| • Small bowel bacterial overgrowth. |
| • Mesenteric ischaemia. |

Box 9.17 Inflammatory intestinal diseases that result in diarrhoeal illness

- Inflammatory bowel disease:
  - Ulcerative colitis
  - Crohn disease.
- Infections:
  - Clostridial colitis
  - Viral enterocolitis: CMV
  - Tuberculosis
  - *Yersinia*.
- Diverticulitis.
- Ischaemic enterocolitis.
- Radiation enterocolitis.

## Chronic fatty diarrhoea (steatorrhoea)

Steatorrhoea is an increase in stool volume which occurs as a result of fat malabsorption. Clinically, this may be distinguished from other causes of diarrhoea by the reporting of pale stool colour, offensive odour, and difficulty in flushing away such faecal material.

Any condition which results in dietary fat malabsorption or mal-digestion may cause steatorrhoeal symptoms.

### History

- Duration of symptoms.
- Weight loss.
- Bloody diarrhoea.
- Clinical symptoms of dehydration.
- Nocturnal symptoms (organic disease).
- Prescribed drugs.
- Diet: poorly absorbed CHO (e.g. sorbitol).
- Foreign travel.
- IBS ROME II criteria.

### Investigation

- Stool microscopy and culture.
- Coeliac serology.
- Thyroid function.
- 7α hydroxycholestenone-bile acid malabsorption.
- Colonoscopy.
- Upper GI endoscopy and duodenal biopsy.
- Glucose hydrogen breath test.
- Lactose hydrogen breath test.
- Small bowel MRI/CT enteroclysis.
- Capsule endoscopy.
- Faecal elastase + pancreatic imaging.
- Faecal calprotectin.
- Urinary 5HIAA/catecholamines.
- Gut hormones.
- Mesenteric angiography.
- Laxative screen.

## Constipation

- Most common in the very young and elderly.
- Usually resolves without need for medical intervention.

It is important to exclude systemic or structural abnormalities:

*Systemic disorders*
- Hypothyroidism
- Diabetes mellitus
- Hypercalcaemia.

*Neurological disorders*
- Multiple sclerosis
- Parkinson disease
- Spinal cord lesions.

*Structural disorders*
- Obstruction:
  - Anal atresia
  - Intestinal obstruction.
- Smooth muscle disorders:
  - Hereditary myopathy
  - Systemic sclerosis.
- Enteric nerves:
  - Hirschsprung disease
  - Paraneoplastic
  - Trypanosomiasis.
- Anorectal floor:
  - Rectal prolapse
  - Pelvic floor weakness.

*Psychological causes*
- Depression
- Eating disorders
- Denied evacuation.

### Investigation

- Exclude systemic disorders: FBC, ESR, TFT, Ca.
- Exclude structural disorders:
  - Colonoscopy
  - Barium enema.
- Physiological investigation: anorectal manometry (Box 9.18).

*Colonic transit times*
- 20 radio-opaque markers are swallowed and a single radiograph taken 5 days later.
- Retention of more than four markers after 5 days indicates slow gut transit.

### Treatment

- Laxatives:
  - Stimulant (senna/bisacodyl)
  - Osmotic (lactulose)
  - Bulking (Fybogel®).
- Enemas/suppositories.
- Defecation training and biofeedback.
- Colectomy (in selected individuals).

## Dysphagia

**Definition:** difficulty in propagating swallowed food.

- Occasional oesophageal symptoms are a frequent occurrence in the general population but are rarely an indicator of significant underlying disease.
- Persistent or progressive dysphagia does, however, require further clinical evaluation and investigation (Box 9.19).

It is important to recognize that a number of neuromuscular diseases result in dysphagia (Box 9.20) as a result of loss of function of

Box 9.18 Physiological criteria for functional constipation

- Manometric evidence to support failure of relaxation of pelvic floor muscles during defecation.
- Evidence of adequate propulsive force.
- Evidence of incomplete evacuation.

| Box 9.19 Pathologies associated with dysphagia |
| --- |

- Gastro-oesophageal reflux disease (GORD).
- Benign oesophageal strictures: rings (Schatzki).
- Peptic (secondary to GORD).
- Oesophageal carcinoma.
- Oesophageal diverticulum.
- Aortic aneurysm.
- Achalasia.
- Scleroderma.

| Box 9.20 Neurological causes of dysphagia |
| --- |

- Cerebrovascular disease
- Parkinson disease
- Multiple sclerosis
- Myotonic dystrophy
- Myasthenia gravis

| Box 9.21 Causes of odynophagia |
| --- |

- Reflux oesophagitis
- Medication-induced oesophagitis
  - Bisphosphonate
  - NSAID
  - KCl
  - $FeSO_4$
  - Antiretroviral agents
- Oesophageal carcinoma
- Oesophageal infections
- Candidiasis
- Herpes simplex
- CMV
- HIV

the pharynx and upper oesophageal sphincter (part of the normal swallow mechanism).

Odynophagia is defined as **pain** on swallowing which may or may not be associated with dysphagia. Odynophagia results from any one of a number of causes of oesophageal insult (Box 9.21).

### Management
Depends on underlying cause:
- GORD:
  - High-dose acid suppression with proton pump inhibition.
  - Mechanical dilatation (balloon/bougie) at time of endoscopy if peptic stricture present.
- Oesophageal carcinoma:
  - Managed according to the stage of disease and taking into account the individual's comorbid state.
  - Recognize and withdraw culprit **medication**.
- Infection:
  - Careful diagnostic definition and appropriate antimicrobial therapy.
  - Consider the possibility of underlying immunocompromise (e.g. HIV or myeloma).
  - 'High' dysphagia (with/without aspiration) should always prompt evaluation for underlying neuromuscular disease.

# 9.10 Normal liver and biliary function

## Hepatic function

The liver performs many important physiological functions (Table 9.6):

- Post-prandially, >50% of the glucose absorbed is taken up by the liver and either stored as glycogen or converted to lactate (released into the circulation). The liver uses amino acids for plasma and hepatic protein synthesis, and the excess amino acids undergo catabolism to urea.
- In the fasting state, the liver is able to release glucose either from glycogen breakdown or from gluconeogenesis utilizing amino acids released from other tissues, e.g. muscle. Liver amino acid release, endogenous protein synthesis, and synthesis of urea are inhibited during the fasting state.
- The liver is a major regulator of lipid metabolism during both the fed and fasting states. It both **produces** very low-density lipoproteins and **metabolizes** high- and low-density lipoproteins.
- The liver also plays a very important role in the metabolism of drugs, alcohol, bilirubin, and bile salts
- Vitamin K is essential to allow the liver to synthesize the coagulation factors II, VII, IX, and X

### Hepatocytes

- Account for ~80% of the hepatic mass.
- Are involved in:
  - Protein storage and synthesis.
  - Transformation of carbohydrates.
  - Synthesis of bile salts, phospholipids, and cholesterol.
  - Detoxification, modification and excretion of both endogenous and exogenous substances.
- Initiate bile formation and secretion

A number of non-parenchymal hepatic cell types also serve important roles in many aspects of hepatic function:

### Kupffer cells

- Also known as liver monocytes.
- Major phagocytes within the liver.
- Able to remove:
  - Bacteria
  - Viruses
  - Endotoxin
  - Antigen-antibody complexes
  - Damaged or ageing RBCs.
- Also have the ability to synthesize a broad range of inflammatory mediators that may act locally or systemically.

### Hepatic stellate cells (HSCs)

- Located in the perisinusoidal space.
- The major cells involved in the secretion of extracellular matrix during hepatic fibrosis and the development of cirrhosis. Activated HSC undergo a transdifferentiation from a quiescent vitamin-A storing cell to a contractile, proliferative myofibroblast, resulting in increased matrix secretion.
- In addition to their ability to deposit matrix, they also secrete collagenases and metalloproteinase inhibitors and are therefore intrinsically involved in both the synthesis and degradation of liver extracellular matrix.
- Recent evidence suggests that HSCs may also play an important role in orchestrating elements of the hepatic **immune response**. HSCs are able to secrete chemokines (thus amplifying inflammatory cell infiltration) and have also been shown to directly interact with lymphocyte subsets.

### Endothelial cells

- Line the hepatic sinusoids (sinusoidal blood vessels).
- These hepatic capillary vessels differ from capillary beds found elsewhere in the body as they have no basement membrane visible by electron microscopy.
- Hepatic endothelial cells have large fenestrae allowing the free passage of particles and fluid across the perisinusoidal space to hepatocytes.

## Biliary anatomy and function

- The biliary tree originates from the biliary canaliculae which are formed by hepatocytes, and the intrahepatic bile ducts derived from these canaliculae progressively join to form the left and right hepatic ducts. These ducts converge as they emerge from the liver to form the common hepatic duct, which then forms the common bile duct after joining the cystic duct.
- The distal common bile duct usually then joins the pancreatic duct before entering the duodenum. The gall bladder is located under the right lobe of the liver and is joined by the cystic duct to the common hepatic duct. The ampulla of Vater, also known as the hepatopancreatic ampulla, is formed by the union of the pancreatic duct and the common bile duct.
- The liver is able to secrete around 1–2L of bile per day.
- Bile salts are composed of both a hydrophilic and hydrophobic component, meaning they are more likely to aggregate to form micelles.
- Maintenance of common bile duct pressure is achieved by rhythmic contraction and relaxation of the ampullary sphincter. In the fasting state, this pressure exceeds gall bladder pressure resulting in the flow of bile into the gall bladder. This concentrates it ~10-fold by the resorption of electrolytes and water.
- During feeding, cholecystokinin is released from the duodenal mucosa and this causes contraction of the gallbladder and also reduces sphincter pressure resulting in flow of bile into the duodenum.
- Bile helps to emulsify fats, facilitating their absorption in the small intestine. Since bile promotes the absorption of fats, it plays an important role in the absorption of the fat soluble vitamins: A, D, E, and K.
- In addition to its digestive role, bile serves as a route of excretion for the haemoglobin breakdown product, bilirubin.

| Table 9.6 Functions of the liver | |
|---|---|
| **Synthesis of proteins** | **Metabolism of nutrients** |
| Coagulation factors | Carbohydrate |
| Albumin | Lipids |
| Complement factors | Protein |
| Transferrin | **Storage** |
| Caeruloplasmin | Vitamins A, D, and $B_{12}$ |
| Haptoglobin | Copper |
| Protease inhibitors | Iron |
| **Excretion** | |
| Bilirubin | |
| Bile salts | |

# 9.11 Variceal disease

## Background

Portal hypertension is defined as prolonged elevation of the portal venous pressure. Normal values for portal venous pressure are **2–5mmHg**, however patients who develop complications of portal hypertension tend to have portal venous pressures >12mmHg.

## Aetiology

Increased portal vascular resistance is usually the major cause of portal hypertension. Vascular obstruction at various sites in the portal venous system may occur:

1. Extrahepatic post-sinusoidale.g. Budd–Chiari syndrome.
2. Intrahepatic post-sinusoidale.g. veno-occlusive disease.
3. Sinusoidale.g. cirrhosis (90% of portal hypertension in Westernized countries).
4. Intrahepatic pre-sinusoidale.g. schistosomiasis (commonest cause of portal hypertension worldwide, but rare outside endemic areas).
5. Extrahepatic pre-sinusoidal,e.g. portal vein thrombosis.

Increases in portal vascular resistance reduce the portal flow to the liver, and collateral vessels open up in the GI tract (particularly around the oesophagus, stomach, and rectum). This leads to an increased proportion of portal blood being shunted directly to the systemic circulation (i.e. diverted away from the liver).

## Clinical features

- Oesophageal, gastric, and rectal varices may cause severe haemorrhage.
- Splenomegaly with hypersplenism often leads to thrombocytopenia (occasionally leucopenia).
- Collateral vessels on anterior abdominal wall (caput medusae).

## Diagnosis

- Endoscopy of upper GI tract (± lower GI tract) may reveal varices.
- USS may demonstrate splenomegaly and collateral vessels. USS Doppler is also very useful to define patency of portal vein.
- Triple-phase abdominal CT can demonstrate splenomegaly, varices, liver contour, and vascular anatomy, e.g. portal vein thrombosis or hepatic vein thrombosis (Budd–Chiari syndrome).
- Venography and magnetic resonance venography (MRV) may be used to further delineate portal/hepatic venous anatomy.
- Hepatic wedge pressure measurements used (rarely) to confirm portal hypertension and to differentiate pre-sinusoidal from sinusoidal portal hypertension.

## Complications

- Bleeding from varices or portal hypertensive gastropathy (PHG).
- Ascites formation.
- Hepatic encephalopathy.
- Hypersplenism.
- Renal failure.

### Variceal bleeding

Usually secondary to oesophageal or gastric varices (bleeding rarely occurs at other sites, e.g. rectum).

Increased varix size, endoscopic features such as variceal red spots, liver failure, increased portal pressure, and drugs which cause muscosal erosion (e.g. NSAIDs) all predispose to increased risk of bleeding.

## Treatment

See Section 1.10.

- Aggressive resuscitation with blood and blood products to restore circulating volume and reverse clotting abnormalities/replace platelets.
- Early liaison with the anaesthetics team who are experts in managing the airway in torrential upper GI bleeding and can expedite endotracheal intubation in very unstable (either haemodynamically or in terms of major risk of aspiration) patients.
- Early endoscopy (once stabilized haemodynamically and haematological parameters acceptable) to confirm source of haemorrhage and to commence specific therapy.
  - NB: 20% of these patients have a non-variceal bleeding point.
- Administration of intravenous antibiotics (e.g. third-generation cephalosporin).

There is now evidence that survival and re-bleeding rates from variceal haemorrhage are reduced by the administration of antibiotics (whether or not there is evidence of infection).

### Local therapies for variceal bleeding
*Banding*

- Mainstay of initial treatment and can be performed at the time of the first endoscopy.
- Multiple bands may be applied endoscopically to bleeding oesophageal (but not gastric) varices (Fig. 9.31).
- Used in the prevention of recurrent variceal bleeding.
- Fewer side effects than sclerotherapy.

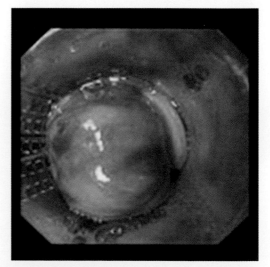

Fig. 9.31 Banding of an oesophageal varix at upper endoscopy. Photograph courtesy of Professor PC Hayes.

*Sclerotherapy*

- Still practised in some units for acute variceal bleeding and to prevent recurrent bleeding.
- Sclerosing agent is injected into the varices and repeated until they are eradicated.
- Side effects include:
  - Oesophageal ulceration, perforation, and strictures.
  - Transient chest/abdominal pain.
  - Transient dysphagia and fever.

## Transjugular intrahepatic portosystemic stent shunt (TIPSS)

- Used in the management of acute and recurrent variceal bleeding.
- Involves radiologically guided stent placement (via the internal jugular vein) between the portal vein and the hepatic vein, thereby reducing portal pressure by providing a portosystemic shunt.
- Prior patency of the portal vein is a prerequisite for the TIPSS procedure to be successful and should be assessed angiographically.
- Coagulation and platelet count should be corrected prior to the procedure and antibiotic cover given.
- Successful TIPSS insertion stops and prevents further variceal bleeding in many cases. Side effects include hepatic encephalopathy and blockage of the shunt (although the latest generation of stents have much lower occlusion rates).

## Balloon tamponade using a Minnesota/Sengstaken tube

- The Minnesota/Sengstaken tube (Fig. 9.32) is used to tamponade acutely bleeding varices and is a very useful interim measure to achieve haemostasis and to buy time whilst trying to stabilize a patient prior to definitive therapy such as therapeutic endoscopy or TIPSS insertion.

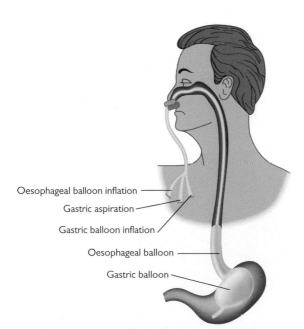

Oesophageal balloon inflation

Gastric aspiration

Gastric balloon inflation

Oesophageal balloon

Gastric balloon

**Fig. 9.32** Sengstaken tube.

- It is passed through the mouth and its presence in the stomach checked by CXR and auscultation of the upper abdomen whilst injecting air into the stomach.
- It has two balloons (oesophageal and gastric) and the aim is to inflate the gastric balloon in the stomach and then with traction on the gastric balloon, exert a tamponade effect on the varices in the fundus of the stomach.
- Gastric balloon inflation must be stopped if the patient experiences pain as inadvertent inflation in the oesophagus can result in oesophageal rupture.
- In most cases the inflated gastric balloon is enough to control bleeding. The oesophageal balloon is only very rarely inflated (if continued bleeding despite traction on the gastric balloon) as it can cause pressure necrosis of the oesophagus and if used should be deflated for ~10 minutes every 3 hours to avoid damage to the oesophageal mucosa.
- Extra lumens on the Minnesota tube also allow aspiration of the stomach and oesophagus.

## Oesophageal transection

With increasing availability of TIPSS, oesophageal transection is now very rarely performed for variceal bleeding. This operation may be indicated when other interventions have failed to control bleeding and TIPSS is unavailable. The operative morbidity and mortality in this setting is usually high.

## Portosystemic shunt surgery

This type of operation is now rarely performed and is usually only utilized when other treatment options have failed. Surgery should only be offered to patients with good underlying hepatic function.

## Pharmacological reduction of portal pressure for acute variceal bleeding

- Variceal banding and TIPSS form the mainstay of current management of acute variceal bleeding. Pharmacological treatment should be regarded as **adjunctive** and **secondary** to the more definitive endoscopic and TIPSS procedures.
- **Terlipressin** (vasopressin analogue) has been shown to be effective in achieving haemostasis and improving survival in the **absence** of endoscopic therapy (used temporarily until more definitive endoscopic therapy or TIPSS can be instituted). However, meta-analysis of terlipressin in **combination** with endoscopic therapy did not show any benefit compared to endoscopic therapy alone.
- Terlipressin is commonly used to reduce portal pressure and is normally administered for a further 24 hours after the bleeding stops.
- Serious side effects of terlipressin include:
  - Exacerbation of ischaemic heart disease.
  - Mesenteric ischaemia.
  - Compromise of limb perfusion in patients with peripheral vascular disease.

If terlipressin administration results in chest pain, abdominal pain, or peripheral vascular insufficiency it should be stopped immediately.

## Primary prophylaxis/prevention of variceal bleeding

- Propranolol (dose 80–160mg/day) or carvedilol (target dose 12.5mg/day) can be used for primary prevention.
- Recent evidence suggests that endoscopic variceal banding is equally efficacious in the primary prophylaxis of variceal bleeding.
- Poor compliance with beta-blockers is not uncommon and so entry of patients into variceal banding programmes for primary prophylaxis is becoming increasingly common.

# 9.12 Hepatic tumours

## Case history

A 54-year-old man with a history of heavy alcohol use (for the past 30 years) and chronic hepatitis C infection (probably contracted during a brief period of intravenous drug use in his late teens) is referred by his GP with mild weight loss and general malaise.

He is seen in the liver clinic and his blood investigations suggest he may be cirrhotic with hypoalbuminaemia, thrombocytopenia, and a mildly prolonged prothrombin time. His alphafetoprotein level (αFP) is normal but liver ultrasound shows a 9 × 5cm mass in the right lobe of the liver.

Hepatocellular cancer (HCC) is a primary cancer of hepatocytes.

## Epidemiology

- Fifth most common cancer in the world.
- >1/2 million new cases/annum and the incidence is rising in the Western world.
- Highest prevalence areas are Eastern Asia and Sub-Saharan Africa.

## Aetiology

- Cirrhosis is premalignant irrespective of aetiology (although cancer may sporadically occur in non-cirrhotic livers).
- HCC is a particular problem in chronic viral hepatitis and haemochromatosis.
- Relative risk of cancer is increased:
  - 20-fold in those with chronic hepatitis B.
  - 24-fold in those with hepatitis C.
  - 135-fold in patients co-infected with both hepatitis B+C.
- In the context of existing chronic viral disease, HIV co-infection may also promote the risk of HCC, as may heavy alcohol consumption.
- Increasing age, ♂ sex, and consumption of aflatoxin are also associated with risk of cancer development.

## Clinical features

- The development of HCC in a cirrhotic patient is frequently asymptomatic.
- There may be evidence of decompensation or liver damage, new right upper quadrant discomfort, or symptoms/signs associated with portal vein invasion or thrombosis (e.g. variceal bleeding, ascites).
- Commonly, patients have non-specific symptoms associated with malignancy such as decreased appetite and weight loss.

## Diagnosis

- Made on the basis of classical imaging appearances (Fig. 9.33) and, where relevant, biopsy.
- The high incidence of HCC in those with existing liver disease/cirrhosis has promoted the concept of HCC surveillance in 'at-risk' groups (see British Society of Gastroenterology surveillance criteria: <http://www.bsg.org>).
- Curative therapy invariably depends on the detection of small HCCs in livers with relatively good underlying function.
- Because cirrhosis is a major risk factor for HCC, the majority of patients have poor underlying liver function and therapeutic approaches are severely limited.

- Usual method of surveillance is ultrasound scanning every 6 months undertaken by a skilled operator.
- Serum αFP level is also measured as a tumour marker, however αFP is not specific for HCC and may be raised in cirrhotic disease with regenerative activity, and is an unreliable surveillance test.
- A rising or very high αFP in an individual should prompt vigorous radiological assessment for an underlying HCC.

### Diagnostic Criteria (American Association for the Study of Liver Diseases—AASLD)

- A lesion >2cm with classical imaging features on CT or MRI is considered diagnostic, without recourse to biopsy.
- Lesions 1–2cm with typical imaging features can also be confidently diagnosed without biopsy.
- If the imaging features are atypical then a biopsy is required.
- If the lesion is <1cm, regular 3-monthly surveillance imaging is advised.
- The imaging used to identify HCC includes triple-phase contrast CT ± MRI.

NB: these guidelines are relevant for work-up in a tertiary/specialist centre where expert cross-sectional hepatobiliary radiology and other relevant specialist expertise is available.

## Treatment

- Curative treatment is by resection or by liver transplantation.
- Stratification of patients for specific treatments is dependent on tumour size/number and underlying liver function.
- For those with well-preserved liver function (Childs A—see Table 9.7) and a single lesion in a resectable position then **resection** is the treatment of choice.
- In patients with solitary tumours ≤5cm in size, or if the patient has ≤3 lesions (none >3cm) with decompensated liver disease (Childs B+C) then **liver transplantation** is the treatment of choice.
- Unfortunately, the majority of patients present with more advanced lesions or disseminated disease.

Treatment at this stage is aimed at retarding tumour growth or is palliative/symptomatic.

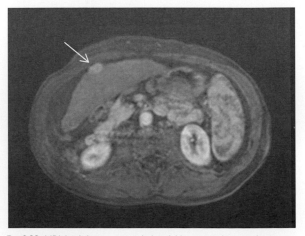

Fig. 9.33 MRI (gadolinium, arterial phase) Hypervascular, exophytic hepatocellular carcinoma arising from anterior surface of right lobe of liver (arrow).
Image courtesy of Dr D Cookson.

| Table 9.7 Child–Pugh classification of chronic liver disease | | | |
|---|---|---|---|
| Measure | 1 point | 2 points | 3 points |
| Bilirubin (μmol/L) | <34 | 34–50 | >50 |
| Albumin (g/L) | >35 | 28–35 | <28 |
| INR | <1.7 | 1.71–2.2 | >2.2 |
| Ascites | None | Suppressed with medication | Refractory |
| Hepatic encephalopathy | None | Grade I–II | Grade III–IV |
| Points | Class | 1-year survival | 2-year survival |
| 5–6 | A | 100% | 85% |
| 7–9 | B | 81% | 57% |
| 10–15 | C | 45% | 35% |

Reproduced from R. N. H. Pugh et al., 'Transection of the oesophagus for bleeding oesophageal varices', *British Journal of Surgery*, 60, 8, pp. 646–649. Copyright 1973 with permission from Wiley and British Journal of Surgery Society Ltd.

- Treatment options include:
  - Transarterial chemoembolization.
  - Percutaneous ablation by radiofrequency ablation (RFA).
  - Ethanol injections.
- Assessment of patients for surgical resection or transplantation involves full staging including chest and abdominal CT and appropriate cardiorespiratory assessment for anaesthetic risk. If not already undertaken, screening should be performed to try to identify underlying causes of chronic liver disease.

## Prognosis

- Currently poor.
- Only a minority of patients have disease suitable for resection/ transplantation.
- Early disease: untreated median survival is 13 months.
- Advanced disease: untreated median survival <1 month.

## Fibrolamellar carcinoma

- Variant of HCC, more often arises in non-cirrhotic liver.
- More frequently observed in young people with an equal sex distribution.

- Rare.
- Frequently presents with discomfort or a feeling of fullness in the right upper quadrant.
- Treatment is by transplantation or surgical resection.

## Cholangiocarcinoma

An aggressive carcinoma of the intra- or extrahepatic bile ducts.

### Epidemiology
- Uncommon, although associated with:
  - Clonorchis sinensis (liver fluke found in Far East).
  - Primary sclerosing cholangitis (West).
- Sporadic disease increasing in incidence in the West.

### Clinical features
- Presentation is usually with signs of biliary blockage with classical features of obstructive jaundice.

### Diagnosis
- Diagnosis is usually made on CT or MRI scan.

### Treatment
- Treatment is by resection (but similar to HCC only a minority of patients are suitable for resection).
- Alternatively patients are treated palliatively by having the lesion stented at ERCP or PTC.

### Prognosis
- The outlook overall is very poor.

## Other hepatic tumours

Uncommon tumours of the liver which may present with a mass or right upper quadrant discomfort include:
- Haemangiosarcoma (rare) associated with use of thorotrast (thorium dioxide) for neurological investigations in the past.
- Haemangioendothelioma.
- Hepatoblastoma(children).

# 9.13 Acute (fulminant) liver failure

## Background

Acute liver failure (ALF) is a rare condition characterized by rapid deterioration of liver function resulting in altered mentation (encephalopathy) and coagulopathy in patients without pre-existing liver disease. ALF is associated with a very high morbidity and mortality. Before the advent of liver transplantation, most case series suggested <15% survival.

## Definition

ALF is defined as occurring within 8 weeks of the onset of symptoms, in the absence of evidence of pre-existing liver disease (to differentiate the syndrome from cases in which hepatic encephalopathy is secondary to decompensation of chronic liver disease).

## Epidemiology

- A rare syndrome.
- The major cause in the UK and USA is accidental or intentional paracetamol poisoning.
- In the developing world, acute hepatitis B viral infection is the predominant cause of ALF because of the high prevalence of HBV.

## Aetiology

The causes of ALF in the UK include:
- Drugs (60%):
  - Major cause is paracetamol.
  - Others (ecstasy, antituberculous drugs, anticonvulsants).
- Viral (30%): hepatitis A, B, D, E, and non-A–E 'viral hepatitis'.
- Miscellaneous (<5%):
  - Wilson disease
  - Shock and cardiac failure
  - Budd–Chiari syndrome
  - Acute fatty liver of pregnancy
  - Leptospirosis.
- Poisons (<5%):
  - Carbon tetrachloride
  - *Amanita phalloides* (death cap mushroom).

## Pathophysiology

- Massive hepatocyte apoptosis, necrosis, and inflammation seen in the explanted liver or from biopsies taken by the transjugular route (ALF patients have severe coagulopathy) (Fig. 9.34).
- Once there has been loss of a critical mass of functioning hepatocytes, ALF ensues frequently complicated by multi-organ failure.

## Diagnosis and initial evaluation

- All patients with clinical or laboratory evidence of moderate–severe hepatic dysfunction should have immediate measurement of **prothrombin** time and careful evaluation for subtle alterations in **mentation**.
- As ALF can progress very rapidly with changes in conscious level occurring hour by hour, patients should be transferred to an intensive care environment as soon as possible.
- Early contact with a centre which offers liver transplantation is mandatory.

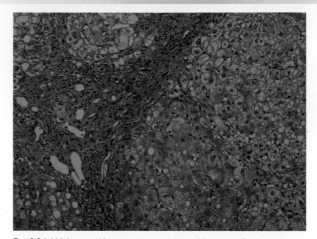

Fig. 9.34 Widespread hepatocyte necrosis and hepatic inflammation secondary to paracetamol poisoning.
Photomicrograph courtesy of Dr T Kendall.

## History

- Careful history for possible drug ingestion, exposure to viral infections, and other toxins.
- If patient is severely encephalopathic history may be entirely from family (or unavailable).

## Clinical features

- Make note of encephalopathy grade (can be subtle in initial stages: poor concentration, yawning and hiccups, slurred speech, inversion of normal sleep pattern, and decreased alertness). This can progress through to altered behaviour such as aggression, convulsions, drowsiness, and coma.
- Look for stigmata of chronic liver disease. Signs of cirrhosis should **not** be present in ALF. The presence of evidence of chronic liver disease has significant implications for management.
- Jaundice is often seen at presentation (absent in Reye syndrome).
- Fetor hepaticus (sweet, faecal smell to breath).
- Right upper quadrant tenderness.
- Hepatomegaly often not present (although may occur in early viral hepatitis, malignant infiltration, acute Budd–Chiari syndrome or congestive heart failure).
- Asterixis is characteristic.
- Raised intracranial pressure secondary to cerebral oedema (abnormally reacting, unequal, or fixed pupils, episodes of hypertension and bradycardia, hyperventilation, general or local myoclonus, focal fits or decerebrate posturing, profuse sweats).
- Papilloedema (rarely occurs, late sign).
- Oedema and ascites (late signs).

## Laboratory investigations

Initial laboratory analysis should include:
- Prothrombin time/INR (measured at least twice daily).
- Full biochemical profile including U&E (plus bicarbonate, calcium, magnesium, and phosphate), creatinine, and amylase.
- Glucose (hypoglycaemia may be present and require correction).
- Liver function tests (plasma ALT is often very high after paracetamol overdose, decreases with progression of liver damage and is of no prognostic value).

- ABG and lactate.
- FBC.
- Group and save.
- HIV status (no longer a contraindication to liver transplantation but may have implications for drug therapy post transplant).

## Aetiological screen

- Toxicology screen of urine and blood (including blood paracetamol level).
- Viral serology: anti-HAV IgM, HBSAg, anti-HBc IgM, anti-HCV, anti-HEV (if clinically indicated).
- Other viruses: CMV, EBV, herpes simplex virus.
- Autoantibodies: ANA, AMA, ASMA, anti-LKM, immunoglobulin levels.
- Caeruloplasmin, serum copper, urinary copper.
- Pregnancy test.
- Ultrasound and Doppler of liver and peri-hepatic vasculature including hepatic veins.
- Transjugular liver biopsy may be indicated in certain conditions such as metastatic liver disease, lymphoma, autoimmune hepatitis, or herpes simplex hepatitis. >70% necrosis on liver biopsy has prognostic significance.

## Management

- Any patient with acute liver injury and hepatic encephalopathy or a rising PT should be cared for in a HDU or ICU.
- Expedient transfer to an ICU in a hospital with a liver transplant service is the optimal environment to manage ALF.
- The outcome is related to aetiology, degree of encephalopathy, and related complications.

Regularly assess the following:
- Cardiorespiratory: pulse, BP, respiratory rate.
- Consider central venous pressure measurement. Ideally the CVP line should be placed by an experienced operator without correction of deranged clotting (if no active bleeding problems) as the prothrombin time (uncorrected) is the laboratory investigation of greatest prognostic value.
- Neurological:
  - GCS score and encephalopathy grade.
  - Pupils (size, reactivity, equality), papilloedema.
  - Plantar responses.
- Fluid status:
  - Accurate fluid balance—keep well hydrated with IV/oral fluids and catheterize.
- Sepsis screening:
  - Monitor temperature.
  - Regular cultures (blood, urine, sputum, cannula sites).
  - CXR.
  - Early empirical broad-spectrum antibiotic therapy.
- Biochemical/haematological parameters:
  - ABGs including lactate and pH.
  - Full blood profile at least 12-hourly.
  - 2-hourly blood glucose measurements in acute phase.

## Complications

ALF can rapidly lead to multi-organ failure so prompt identification of the potentially life-threatening complications of ALF is essential.

Increasing grade of encephalopathy correlates with increased likelihood of complications (Box 9.22).

---

**Box 9.22 Complications of ALF**
- Encephalopathy
- Renal failure
- Cerebral oedema with increased intracranial pressure
- Bleeding
- Hypotension
- Pancreatitis
- Respiratory failure
- Hypothermia
- Sepsis
- Acidosis
- Metabolic disorders (hypoglycaemia, hypokalaemia, hypomagnesaemia, hypocalcaemia, hypophosphataemia)

---

## Treatment

- Liver transplantation remains the only definitive therapy for patients who are unable to achieve regeneration of sufficient hepatocyte mass to sustain life.
- Survival in patients with ALF who are not transplanted is dismal (~10%).
- Currently patients who undergo liver transplantation for ALF have a 1-year survival of ~70–80%.
- NAC (N-acetylcysteine) therapy (prolonged beyond the standard antidote course) may improve outcome in paracetamol-induced ALF.

### Key concepts in the management of ALF

- Any signs of encephalopathy (even Grade I) contact anaesthetic team immediately as the patient may deteriorate very rapidly.
- Rising PT/PT >50 seconds, hypoglycaemia, acidosis, renal dysfunction, or any grade of encephalopathy: discuss early with a liver transplant centre.
- **If in doubt, discuss with a liver transplant unit**.
- In the UK, criteria for listing for liver transplantation have been developed to try and identify patients who are unlikely to survive without a liver transplant. Early transfer of a patient to a liver transplant unit before these criteria are met allows time for the transplant team to make as full an assessment of the patient as possible. This also increases the time available to procure a donor liver if the patient is listed.
- Many patients are intubated for transfer by a 'shock team' to try and ensure as safe a transfer as possible.

## Poor prognostic factors—general

- Age <10 or >40 years.
- Hepatitis D or E viruses.
- Halothane and idiosyncratic drug reactions.
- Jaundice for >1 week before onset of encephalopathy.
- PT >50 seconds.
- Bilirubin >300mmol/L.
- Worsening encephalopathy.

## Poor prognostic factors—paracetamol overdose

- pH <7.3 in an arterial sample.
- PT >100 seconds.
- Elevated creatinine.
- High-grade encephalopathy.

# 9.14 Haemochromatosis

## Case history

A 48-year-old man has found out that his brother who lives in Australia has been diagnosed with haemochromatosis. His GP has checked his bloods and his ferritin level is 4400ng/mL and his transferrin saturation is 93%.

On examination he has a pigmented appearance, palmar erythema, and spider naevi.

Total body iron is increased in haemochromatosis, with the excess iron causing damage to a number of organs including the liver. Hereditary haemochromatosis is used to describe the primary condition. Secondary iron loading may complicate other diseases.

## Hereditary haemochromatosis (HH)

- Iron overload results in deposition of iron throughout the body, with potentially deleterious effects on the liver, pancreas, heart, and endocrine glands.
- In the liver there is deposition of iron within hepatocytes (Fig. 9.35), formation of fibrous septae with nodules, and macronodular cirrhosis may develop.
- Excess hepatic iron may also occur in cirrhosis secondary to alcohol, but is mild.

### Epidemiology

- Haemochromatosis represents one of the most common inheritable genetic defects, particularly in people of Northern European extraction, with ~1 in 10 people carrying the defective gene.
- ~1 in 400 Northern Europeans have HH.

### Pathophysiology

- Increased absorption of iron in the diet.
- Inherited in an autosomal recessive fashion and most often caused by a faulty gene on chromosome 6.
- This gene is named *HFE* and two different mutations in the *HFE* gene are associated with >93% of cases.
- ~78% of affected individuals have two copies of the C282Y mutation (one inherited from each parent), while ~4% have a single copy of the mutation and one normal *HFE* gene.
- ~6% have either 1 or 2 copies of the second mutation (H63D), while a further 5% are known as compound heterozygotes and

have one copy of each mutation. The remaining 7% of cases are likely to involve different *HFE* mutations, or mutations in other genes.
- Interestingly, <50% of C282Y homozygotes develop clinical features of haemochromatosis suggesting other factors are involved.
- Loss of iron secondary to pregnancy and menstruation may be protective in women, as 90% of HH patients are male.

### Clinical features

- Presentation usually occurs in men >40 years old with signs of cirrhosis, diabetes mellitus, or cardiac failure.
- A darkish colour to the skin can occur (hence its name 'bronzed diabetes' when first described by Armand Trousseau in 1865).
- Other features include:
  - Endocrine organ dysfunction (e.g. adrenal, parathyroid, pituitary).
  - Hypogonadism (loss of libido and impotence).
  - Arthritis (degenerative osteoarthritis and chondrocalcinosis).

### Investigation

- Serum ferritin is markedly increased.
- Plasma iron and serum transferrin saturation also increased (transferrin saturation >45% may indicate HH).
- Liver biopsy confirms the diagnosis and demonstrates excess iron deposition predominantly in hepatocytes and may show liver fibrosis or cirrhosis. Hepatic iron content can also be determined directly.
- HFE genotyping for the C282Y and H63D mutations is also performed.

### Management

- Regular **venesection** until normalization of serum iron (measured by serum ferritin) is achieved. Venesection is then undertaken as required to maintain a normal serum ferritin.
- Management of complications (e.g. cirrhosis and diabetes mellitus).
- Screening for HCC is of particular importance.
- First-degree family members should be screened for haemochromatosis by assessing iron indices (serum ferritin and transferrin saturation), liver function tests, and genetic screening.
- Liver biopsy is indicated in asymptomatic relatives if there is evidence of abnormal iron storage (indicated by a serum ferritin >1000mcg/L, transferrin saturation >45% and/or abnormal liver function tests), as these findings can be associated with significant liver disease. MRI may also be useful in this setting to allow a non-invasive assessment of iron overload. Furthermore, asymptomatic disease should be treated by venesection when the serum ferritin rises above normal.

### Prognosis

- In comparison to other types of cirrhosis HH has a relatively good prognosis.
- 75% of patients are alive 5 years after diagnosis (many patients have well-preserved hepatic function at the time of diagnosis, and this improves with treatment).
- Screening for HCC is important as it is the main cause of death (~1/3 of patients with haemochromatosis and cirrhosis develop HCC, irrespective of treatment).
- Patients should undergo 6-monthly liver ultrasound and αFP measurement as HCC surveillance.

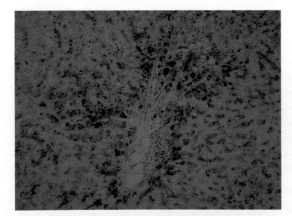

Fig. 9.35 Iron staining (blue) of hepatocytes in haemochromatosis. Photomicrograph courtesy of Dr T Kendall.

## Secondary haemochromatosis (acquired iron overload)

- Causes:
  - Sideroblastic anaemia
  - Chronic haemolytic disorders
  - Multiple blood transfusions
  - Dietary iron overload
  - Porphyria cutanea tarda
  - Alcoholic cirrhosis (occasionally).
- Clinical features may be similar to haemochromatosis but history and examination often suggest the true diagnosis of secondary haemochromatosis.

# 9.15 Wilson disease (hepatolenticular degeneration)

## Case history

A 19-year-old woman is referred by her GP to the neurology team with a 5-month history of increasingly troublesome asymmetric tremor. The patient also feels she has become increasingly clumsy with her hands. Her mother thinks her daughter's personality has also changed and she describes her as 'moodier' in the last 6 months.

Wilson disease results in accumulation of excess copper in the body, which manifests as neurological symptoms and liver disease.

## Epidemiology

- Incidence: ~1 in 30,000 in most parts of the world.
- Estimated heterozygous carrier rate of ~1 in 100.

## Pathophysiology

- Autosomal recessive.
- Normally copper is absorbed from the diet, taken into the liver and stored and incorporated into caeruloplasmin, which is secreted into the blood.
- Excess build-up of copper in the body is normally prevented by excretion in the bile. In Wilson disease the excretion of copper into bile is impaired. Total body copper then builds up with resultant damage to various organs including the liver, basal ganglia, kidneys, eyes, and skeleton.
- In the vast majority of cases there is a failure of synthesis of caeruloplasmin. However, 5% of patients have normal serum caeruloplasmin levels and this is not the primary pathogenic problem.
- The gene responsible for disease (*ATP7B*) resides on chromosome 13 and is expressed primarily in liver, kidney, and placenta. The gene encodes a P-type ATPase that transports copper into bile and incorporates it into caeruloplasmin. Mutant forms of ATP7B protein expressed in people with Wilson disease inhibit the release of copper into bile.
- >200 different mutations have been described and a large majority of cases are compound heterozygotes with two different mutations in the Wilson gene.

## Clinical features

- Symptoms typically appear aged between 5 and 30 years, although the overall age at presentation can be broad.
- Liver disease occurs mainly in childhood and early adolescence (10–14 years) while neurological damage tends to present in later adolescence (19–22 years). Patients can, however, present with a combination of manifestations.
- ~45% of affected individuals present with liver disease, 35% with neurological signs and symptoms, and 10% with psychiatric disturbances.
- Neuropsychiatric symptoms include:
  - Mood disorders or psychosis.
  - Early dementia.
  - Asterixis and so-called 'juvenile parkinsonism' (including ataxia, dyskinesia, and rigidity).
- Other manifestations include renal tubular acidosis, renal calculi, haemolysis, Kayser–Fleischer (KF) rings (see Fig. 9.36), sunflower cataracts, cardiomyopathy, cardiac arrhythmias, osteoporosis, and hidradenitis suppurativa.

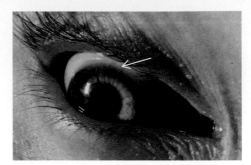

Fig. 9.36 Kayser–Fleischer ring (arrowed) in Wilson disease. Reproduced from Bloom et al., *Oxford Handbook of Gastroenterology and Hepatology*, Second Edition, 2011, plate 16, with permission from Oxford University Press.

- Liver disease can mimic many forms of liver disease and patients may present with hepatitis, a recurrent hepatitic picture or liver failure.
- Investigate for Wilson disease if:
  - Recurrent acute hepatitis of unknown aetiology, particularly if accompanied by haemolysis.
  - Idiopathic chronic liver disease in someone <40 years old.

## Investigation

- Screening tests include measurement of 24-hour urinary copper, serum copper, and serum caeruloplasmin.
  - NB: caeruloplasmin levels can be low in advanced hepatic failure of any cause, and are normal in 5% of Wilson disease patients.
- KF rings represent the most useful clinical pointer to the diagnosis (slit-lamp examination may be required). These consist of copper deposits in Descemet's membrane (where the cornea meets the sclera) and in earlier stages the slit-lamp demonstrates golden brown or greenish-yellow crescents. In later stages, KF rings can be seen with the naked eye and are brownish in colour. KF rings can disappear with treatment but are also rarely found in other forms of chronic liver disease such as primary biliary cirrhosis.
- The definitive diagnostic test is percutaneous liver biopsy with quantitative assay of copper.
- Usually a combination of various laboratory parameters is necessary to firmly establish the diagnosis. Serum copper concentration is high, urinary copper excretion is high, and there is a very high hepatic copper content.

## Management

- Wilson disease is treated with lifelong use of chelating agents (copper-binding agents) such as **penicillamine** or trientine hydrochloride. Zinc can also be used to treat patients with Wilson disease. Penicillamine should be avoided in pregnancy because of known teratogenicity. A sufficient dose of penicillamine must be given to produce cupriuresis and it is possible to reduce the dose once the disease is in remission. Treatment is lifelong and it is important to check that copper reaccumulation does not occur. Copper-chelating treatment should not be stopped abruptly as this may precipitate ALF.

- **Liver transplantation** is required in some cases of acute hepatic failure or cirrhosis secondary to Wilson disease. Hepatic transplantation should be reserved only for patients with severe liver failure and never used for neurological indications.

## Prognosis

- Prognosis is excellent if treatment is commenced prior to irreversible damage.

- Screening of children and siblings of patients with Wilson disease is imperative, and treatment should be instituted if any are found to have the disease (even if asymptomatic).
- Hepatocellular carcinoma is rare in Wilson disease.

# 9.16 Alpha-1 antitrypsin deficiency

## Case history

A 37-year-old man is reviewed by the respiratory team and diagnosed with severe emphysema. It is noted that his cumulative pack-years of smoking has not been remarkable and to have developed severe emphysema with his smoking history is felt to be unusual. In addition he is noted to have deranged LFTs with raised transaminases.

Alpha-1 antitrypsin (A1AT) is produced in the liver and is a serine protease inhibitor. A1AT deficiency is an inherited disorder associated with retention of A1AT in the liver and low serum levels of A1AT.

## Epidemiology

People of Northern European, Iberian, and Saudi Arabian ancestry are at the highest risk for A1AT deficiency, and it is rarely found in African Americans or Asians.

## Pathophysiology

- A1AT deficiency is an inherited disorder caused by a defective gene on chromosome 14.
- A1AT is the predominant serine protease inhibitor (PI) found in the blood, and inhibits tissue proteinases such as neutrophil elastase and various other proteinases.
- Genetic mutations that cause A1AT deficiency interfere with A1AT synthesis, export from hepatocytes, and the ability of A1AT to inhibit proteinases.
- A1AT can be analysed in blood samples by isoelectric focusing analysis (where the protein is passing along a pH gradient).
- Everyone inherits two copies of chromosome 14, and a normal individual is designated PiMM (Pi represents protease inhibitor).
- The two most important abnormal variants of A1AT are designated S and Z (both these variants are secondary to genetic mutations in the A1AT gene).
- Individuals may inherit two of these abnormal genes, e.g. PiZZ, PiSS, or PiSZ, or they may inherit one normal copy and one abnormal copy of the gene, e.g. PiMZ (heterozygous carrier of the disease).
- ~95% of all A1AT deficiency states resulting in clinical manifestations are made up of PiZZ homozygotes.
- In individuals with the PiZZ phenotype, A1AT levels are <15% normal and patients are likely to develop emphysema at a young age.

- The Z variant of A1AT results from a single point mutation and gives rise to a variant version of the protein that is unstable and polymerizes within the endoplasmic reticulum and cannot be secreted into the blood.
- This retention of A1AT in the hepatocyte leads to liver damage and unopposed activity of elastase in the lungs, with resultant development of emphysema.
- In individuals with PiSS, PiMZ, and PiSZ phenotypes, serum levels of A1AT are reduced to 35–60% of normal. The relationship of these genotypes to hepatic disease is uncertain.

## Clinical features

- Bimodal pattern.
- Children can develop neonatal hepatitis and prolonged cholestasis in infancy.
- Most adults are identified by their chest symptoms secondary to development of chronic obstructive pulmonary disease (accelerated by cigarette smoking).
- Adult liver complications include chronic hepatitis, cirrhosis with/without portal hypertension, and hepatocellular carcinoma.

## Diagnosis

- Diagnosis is determined by low plasma A1AT concentration and the PiZZ genotype.
- Liver biopsy can demonstrate A1AT containing globules (these can be seen on PAS stain and identified immunohistochemically) but is not necessary to make the diagnosis.

## Treatment

- All patients should be advised strongly not to smoke because of the increased risk of severe, early-onset emphysema.
- For severe liver disease the only available treatment is liver transplantation. This offers an effective cure by correcting the phenotype of the recipient and normalizing the serum levels of A1AT.

## Screening

- Genetic counselling for affected families is recommended. Screening tests (plasma A1AT levels and genotyping) should also be performed to identify relatives at risk.

## Case history

A 29-year-old woman presents to the emergency department with jaundice and feeling unwell. She has a history of heavy alcohol intake since her teens. Over the last 5–6 years she has been drinking a bottle of vodka per day. She last drank alcohol 2 days prior to admission.

On examination she is deeply jaundiced, tremulous, has tender hepatomegaly and multiple spider naevi (Fig. 9.37). Her admission temperature is 37.9°C and initial blood tests show a leucocytosis with a neutrophil count of 24, bilirubin 422μmol/l, ALT 55, ALP 450, GGT 723, urea 1.4, and INR 1.8.

Chronic alcohol consumption can lead to a range of liver abnormalities from simple fatty liver (steatosis) (Fig. 9.38), to steatohepatitis, cirrhosis, and hepatocellular carcinoma. Alcoholic fatty liver generally has a good prognosis and usually resolves after ~3 months of abstinence. Alcoholic steatohepatitis (ASH) and alcoholic liver cirrhosis are, however, serious conditions with high mortality rates.

## Epidemiology

- Alcoholic liver disease (ALD) is the most common cause of cirrhosis in the West.
- ALD and its complications represent one of the most frequent causes of death in the Western world.

## Pathogenesis

- Complex; we still have a poor understanding of disease pathogenesis.
- Metabolism of alcohol occurs almost exclusively in the liver and multiple factors appear to be involved in the development of ALD. Genetic influences, oxidative stress, the innate immune system, pro-inflammatory cytokines such as TNFα, and endotoxin have all been implicated as factors playing a role in the development of alcohol-induced hepatocyte dysfunction, necrosis, and apoptosis.
- Many theories have been derived from animal models, and whether these can be applied to human ALD is still unclear.

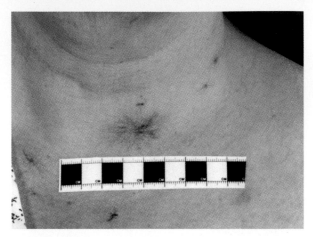

**Fig. 9.38** Spider naevi.
Photograph courtesy of Professor PC Hayes.

- Coexistent liver disorders such as hepatitis C and haemochromatosis will accelerate liver disease in combination with excessive alcohol use.

## Clinical features

### Alcoholic steatohepatitis (ASH)

- This term covers a spectrum of disease from subclinical liver inflammation to liver failure.
- Patients with severe ASH have a high mortality.

Presenting features of patients with ASH include:
- Low-grade fever.
- Jaundice.
- Hepatomegaly (may be tender).
- Anorexia.
- Ascites (~50% of cases) (Fig. 9.39).

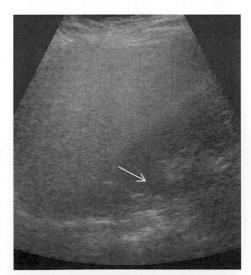

**Fig. 9.37** Ultrasound image showing diffusely echogenic right lobe of liver. Appearances are consistent with diffuse hepatic steatosis. Note the hypoechoic cortex of adjacent normal right kidney (arrowed).
Image courtesy of Dr D Cookson.

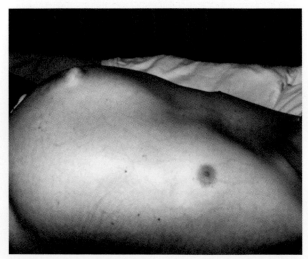

**Fig. 9.39** Ascites, umbilical protrusion, and prominent superficial veins.
Photograph courtesy of Professor PC Hayes.

- Leucocytosis (common).
- Features of cirrhosis.
- Blood analysis may show particularly:
  - Raised GGT (in addition to derangement of other liver function tests).
  - High MCV (in absence of anaemia).

Alanine aminotransferase can be normal or only moderately raised.

Scoring systems such as the Glasgow alcoholic hepatitis score (GAHS) can be used to estimate the severity of ASH (factors measured include age, WCC, urea, prothrombin time, and bilirubin).

## Treatment of acute ASH

### General management of severe ASH

- Management of alcohol withdrawal (benzodiazepines and abstinence).
- Adequate fluid replacement (oral/IV), but avoid over-hydration as this may lower plasma sodium, increase ascites, and precipitate variceal haemorrhage.
- Thiamine.
- Nutritional support.
- Vitamin K (parenteral) is commonly given in patients with a prolonged prothrombin time although may be ineffective and should not be continued if there is no improvement in the INR.
- Low threshold for admission to a critical care bed if unstable.
- Ensure adequate airway protection in patients with encephalopathy.

Poor understanding of disease pathogenesis has hampered development of targeted therapies. Few treatments have consistently been shown to be of benefit and there is no firm consensus among practising hepatologists.

### Corticosteroids

- Corticosteroids have been studied intensively and there remains controversy as to their efficacy in ASH. Overall meta-analyses indicate short-term benefit in patients with severe ASH.
- Mortality with treatment remains high, however, particularly in patients who have concurrent renal impairment, and treatment is contraindicated in a relatively large group of patients with infection and GI bleeding.

### Nutritional supplementation

- Most studies have demonstrated that nutritional supplementation (ideally by enteral feeding) improves liver function and histology.
- There is no clear evidence of nutritional supplementation consistently reducing mortality, but some studies suggest that nutritional therapy could have a role in the improvement of medium- to long-term survival in patients with severe ASH.

### Pentoxifylline

- This medication is a non-selective phosphodiesterase inhibitor. It has a moderate anticytokine effect secondary to decreased transcription of the *TNF* gene.
- One randomized, controlled trial has suggested that pentoxifylline reduces mortality in ASH.
- Further trials will be required, however, to delineate whether pentoxifylline should become standard therapy for patients with ASH.

## Treatment of hepatorenal syndrome in patients with ASH

- The development of hepatorenal syndrome (HRS) in patients with severe ASH is a very ominous sign with survival <10% even with intensive supportive management
- One of the biggest advances in the management of patients with advanced liver disease and HRS in recent years has been the use of **albumin** infusions combined with splanchnic vasoconstrictor agents (e.g. **terlipressin**). This combination of treatments appears to significantly improve survival of cirrhotic patients with HRS.
- Despite no randomized trials specifically looking at albumin infusions and splanchnic vasoconstrictors in patients with ASH, the high mortality observed in ASH patients with HRS suggests that this strategy might have a significant and beneficial effect on patient survival.

## Alcoholic liver cirrhosis

- The bulk of the alcoholic liver disease burden is represented in the form of advanced fibrosis or cirrhosis rather than ASH.
- Patients with histologically advanced ALD can be asymptomatic and may only have mild derangement of, or even normal, liver function tests.

### Treatment

- Independent of the stage of disease, abstinence from alcohol is the cornerstone of treatment.
- Survival in patients with well-compensated or decompensated ALD improves with abstinence.
- Medical management of patients with advanced ALD includes the prevention and treatment of the complications of liver failure, portal hypertension, and hepatocellular carcinoma.
- Liver transplantation is the only definitive therapy for patients with severe ALD.
- Several studies have shown that patients who undergo liver transplantation for cirrhotic ALD have a comparable 5-year survival to patients transplanted for other aetiologies.

# 9.18 Hepatitis

## Viral hepatitis

### Hepatitis A

#### Case history
A 24-year-old man has just returned to the UK from a backpacking trip in South America. He has had fever and nausea for the past 5 days and has now become jaundiced with dark urine.

#### Epidemiology and transmission
Hepatitis A virus (HAV):

- Is a non-enveloped ssRNA virus.
- Is most commonly transmitted by the faecal–oral route (such as contaminated food), and can be highly infectious.
- Overcrowded conditions with poor sanitation facilitates spread.
- Infected individuals excrete virus in the faeces for around 2–3 weeks prior to the onset of illness and for ~2 weeks thereafter.
- Can be sexually transmitted, especially during oro–anal contact.

There is no chronic carrier state, as the immune system develops antibodies against HAV that confer immunity.

#### Clinical features

- Infected individuals often have asymptomatic incubation periods of around 3–4 weeks.
- Active disease commonly starts with systemic upset such as anorexia, fever, nausea, vomiting, and diarrhoea.
- The patient may develop right upper quadrant pain (secondary to liver capsule stretch) and splenomegaly.
- Following the onset of jaundice a prolonged cholestatic phase can occur with pale stools and dark urine.
- Recovery usually occurs within the next 1–3 months.

#### Diagnosis

- Anti-HAV IgM is diagnostic of acute HAV infection and is already present in the blood at the beginning of the clinical illness.
- Anti-HAV IgG is of no diagnostic use as HAV infection occurs commonly and anti-HAV IgG persists for years after infection (presence indicates immunity to HAV).

#### Prognosis

- Acute liver failure is a rare event in HAV infection.
- HAV infection in patients co-infected with hepatitis C or chronic hepatitis B may result in serious or life-threatening disease.

#### Prevention

- Good sanitation and reducing overcrowding.
- Immunization with an inactive virus vaccine can result in substantial protection and should be considered in patients with chronic liver disease (hepatitis B and C) and in people whose sexual activity puts them at risk.
- Travellers to areas where HAV is endemic should also be vaccinated. Individuals given an initial dose of vaccine followed by a booster 6–12 months later can expect up to 10 years of protection.
- Immediate protection can be provided by immune serum globulin if given soon after HAV exposure.

### Hepatitis B

#### Case history
A 42-year-old man is referred to the clinic. He was born in Hong Kong, but came to the UK aged 6 months. He was found to have deranged LFTs at a routine insurance medical. His ALT is 105 and the rest of his liver function tests are normal. Hepatitis serology shows him to be hepatitis B surface antigen positive and e antigen negative, with an HBV PCR value of 1100IU/mL.

Hepatitis B virus (HBV) is a DNA virus and is one of few known non-retroviral viruses which utilizes reverse transcription as part of its replication process (Fig. 9.40). Chronic HBV infection can cause cirrhosis and predisposes people to the development of hepatocellular carcinoma (even in the absence of cirrhosis).

#### Epidemiology

- Chronic hepatitis B is a massive worldwide health problem affecting ~300 million people.
- 3–6% of the world's population are infected with HBV, and ~1/3 have been exposed.
- Chronic carrier rates vary from 10–20% in Africa, Asia, and the Middle East where most infections are acquired in infancy, to 2% in North America and Europe.

#### Transmission

- Mainly by exposure to bodily fluids containing the virus.
- Vertical transmission from mother to child at the time of birth is a major source of infection worldwide.
- May occur following administration of contaminated blood products, intravenous drug abuse, or tattooing and acupuncture with inadequately sterilized needles.
- Unprotected sexual contact, particularly in male homosexuals.

#### Clinical features and prognosis
HBV infection may be either acute (self-limiting) or progress to chronic infection. People with self-limited infection clear the virus within weeks to months (Fig. 9.41).

- Acute hepatitis B infection can be asymptomatic, but in other cases may lead to malaise, anorexia, GI disturbance, myalgia, dark urine, and then jaundice.

These symptoms usually last a few weeks and then resolve.

- Rarely, acute hepatitis B can result in fulminant hepatic failure with a high mortality.
- In general, older individuals have a higher chance of spontaneously clearing the infection. >95% of people who become infected as adults will clear the virus and develop protective immunity to hepatitis B. The remaining 5–10% develop chronic infection which is usually lifelong (although later recovery can occur).
- Vertical transmission (naïve immune system) is most likely to lead to chronic HBV due to non-clearance of virus. Only 5%

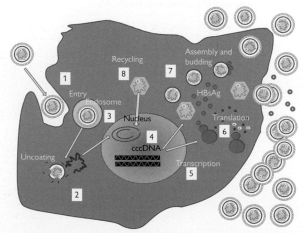

**Fig. 9.40** Schematic diagram of hepatitis B viral replication.

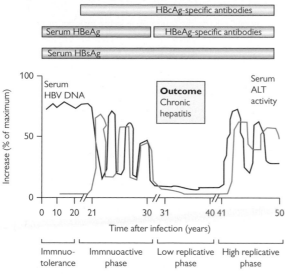

Fig. 9.41 Timeline of hepatitis B infection and serological markers.

of newborns who contract HBV from their mother at the time of birth will clear the virus, the rest becoming chronic carriers of HBV.

### Chronic HBV infection
- Variable clinical course.
- Patients who are chronically infected who do not have active liver disease or viral replication (inactive carriers) tend to run a benign course with a very low chance of progression to cirrhosis.
- In contrast, patients with continuing active viral replication, HBV DNA at high levels, and hepatitis B e antigen (HBeAg) positivity have progressive hepatic damage, and cirrhosis and end-stage liver disease may ensue.
- HBeAg loss does not always result in permanent resolution of disease, and flares of disease can occur, particularly in patients treated with immunosuppressants.
- Chronic carriage of HBV is associated with a 10-fold increased risk of developing HCC. Patients co-infected with hepatitis C and older men with cirrhosis are at the highest risk.
- In areas of the world where HBV is endemic, HCC is the leading cause of cancer-related death. HBV carriers should, therefore, undergo HCC surveillance with 6-monthly ultrasound and αFP measurements.
- Co-infection with hepatitis D virus (HDV) further increases the risk of cirrhosis and liver cancer.

### Investigations
- The assays used for investigation of HBV infection detect either viral antigens or antibodies produced by the immune system. Interpretation of these assays can be complex.
- In acute HBV infection the hepatitis B surface antigen (HBsAg) is the first detectable viral antigen to appear. HBsAg is usually a reliable marker of HBV infection, but early in an infection this antigen may not be present and may also be undetectable later in the infection as it is being cleared by the host. Therefore during this window, when the host remains infected but is successfully clearing the virus, a negative test for HBsAg should prompt testing for IgM antibodies to the hepatitis B core antigen (anti-HBc IgM), which may be the only serologic evidence of disease.
- Antibody to HBsAg (anti-HBs) usually appears after approximately 3-6 months and persists for many years or even permanently. Anti-HBs implies either a previous infection (in which case anti-HBc IgG is usually present), or previous vaccination (anti-HBc IgG is not present).

- In acute HBV infection the HBeAg appears transiently at the outset of the illness and is followed by synthesis of anti-HBe antibody. HBeAg positivity reflects active replication of the virus in the liver.
- Chronic hepatitis B is defined as the persistence of HBsAg in the serum of a patient for at least 6 months.
- In rare cases anti-HBc IgG alone will be the only indicator of chronic infection.
- Chronic HBV carriers can be subdivided into:
  - Patients with evidence of active replication, typically associated with higher viral loads and abnormal transaminases.
  - Patients in the non-replicative state, associated with lower viral loads and decreased markers of hepatic inflammation.
- Clinical outcome of HBV infection correlates with HBeAg status. Conversion to eAg negative, eAb positive typically results in reduced hepatic inflammation, with decreased levels of HBV DNA in the blood and normalizing transaminases: 'the inactive carrier' state.
- Mutant strains (eAg-negative) of HBV exist and can be associated with more aggressive liver disease.
- PCR is used to detect HBV DNA in blood (seldom needed for diagnosis but is useful in the selection of patients for treatment, and in monitoring response to therapy).

### Management
#### Acute hepatitis B
- Mainly supportive with close monitoring for the development of acute liver failure.
- Antivirals may be helpful in severe cases.

#### Chronic hepatitis B
Treatment is given to suppress viral replication and prevent progression of liver disease:
- Not routinely recommended for patients with normal transaminases.
- Recommended for patients with evidence of active hepatic damage (raised ALT).

Liver biopsy pre-treatment is the gold standard to assess the degree of necro-inflammatory activity and fibrosis. Data with regard to treatment is constantly evolving. The ultimate goal is to prevent chronicity and the development of cirrhosis, hepatic failure, and hepatocellular carcinoma.

Outcomes tend to focus on the decrease in HBV DNA levels, rate of normalization of liver enzymes or seroconversion (eAg-positive → eAg-negative and positive eAb).

Available treatments include:
- Interferon α (both pegylated and non-pegylated).
- Lamivudine.
- Adefovir, entecavir, and telbivudine and tenofovir.

These should be instituted and monitored by a specialist.

Whether combination therapy using two or more agents will translate into better treatment response rates is still unclear.

#### Prevention
- A recombinant HBV **vaccine** containing HBsAg is available (Engerix®) and results in active immunization in 95% of healthy people. It should be used in those at particular risk of infection (such as hospital staff, close contacts of infected individuals, patients with chronic renal and liver disease, newborns of infected mothers, male homosexuals, and parenteral drug users).
- Postexposure prophylaxis consists of a single dose of hepatitis B immune globulin (HBIG) injected intramuscularly (given within 24 hours–1 week following exposure to infected blood) and followed immediately by a HBV vaccination course.
- Many countries now routinely vaccinate against HBV.

Babies born to HBV-infected mothers should be given HBIG immediately after birth and commenced on a course of vaccination to prevent transmission. In endemic countries where rates of HBV infection are high, vaccination of newborns has not only reduced the risk of infection, but has also resulted in a marked reduction in the incidence of childhood hepatocellular carcinoma.

## Hepatitis C

### Case history

A 42-year-old man is referred by his GP for investigation of raised ALT and GGT levels. Of note is that he injected drugs intravenously 20 years ago and has a heavy alcohol intake of 70 units/week.

On examination he has spider naevi, gynaecomastia, and splenomegaly.

Hepatitis C (HCV) is an infectious, blood-borne viral disease caused by a small (50nm) RNA-containing flavivirus. HCV infection can result in hepatic inflammation (often asymptomatic), chronic hepatitis, cirrhosis, and HCC.

### Epidemiology

- ~150–200 million people worldwide are infected.
- Most common indication for liver transplantation in the USA.

### Transmission

- Blood-to-blood contact (inoculation with blood or blood products, intravenous drug use).
- HCV was responsible for >90% of post-transfusion hepatitis before serological testing allowed the screening of blood donors. This is the reason for the high incidence of hepatitis C infection in haemophilia patients.
- Vertical transmission and spread by sexual contact may occur but is less common than in HBV infection.

### Acute hepatitis C

- First 6 months after infection, incidence unknown.
- Usually asymptomatic and spontaneous recovery occurs in 30–50% of patients with symptomatic infection, usually within 3 months.
- It is currently advised that treatment should start between 3 and 6 months after diagnosis of acute hepatitis C, if the infection has not resolved spontaneously.

### Chronic hepatitis C

- Infection persisting >6 months, is often asymptomatic.
- Generalized symptoms include fatigue, myalgia, arthralgia, and weight loss.
- Occurs in 70–80% of infected patients and is associated with a significant risk of progression to cirrhosis and HCC.
- Older age at HCV acquisition, ♂ gender, heavy alcohol consumption, and HIV co-infection are associated with more rapid disease progression.
- Intrahepatic cholangiocarcinomas (especially in Asia) are a known complication.
- Extrahepatic manifestations include:
  - Porphyria cutanea tarda
  - Thyroiditis
  - Cryoglobulinaemia
  - Glomerulonephritis (specifically membranoproliferative GN)
  - Sicca syndrome
  - Thrombocytopenia
  - Vasculitis
  - Arthritis
  - Lichen planus
  - Diabetes mellitus
  - B-cell lymphoproliferative disorders.
- Liver function tests may be normal but often show variable elevations of ALT, AST, and GGT.
- Screening for HCC should be performed in patients with chronic HCV and cirrhosis.

### Diagnosis

- Rarely made during the acute phase as the majority of people infected experience no symptoms.
- Detection of antibodies to HCV.
- Anti-HCV antibodies indicate exposure to the virus, but do not determine if ongoing infection is present. HCV PCR is now routinely performed to test for the presence of the HCV itself.
- HCV PCR can measure both viral load and HCV genotype (this is important as it determines the duration of treatment and likelihood of response to antiviral therapy).

### Treatment of chronic hepatitis C

- Very low rate of spontaneous viral clearance (0.5–0.74%/year).
- Current treatment of choice is combination therapy:
  - Pegylated interferon alpha (IFN-α) and ribavirin.
  - 12–48 weeks, depending on genotype.
- Sustained cure rates (sustained viral response, SVR) of up to 80% are achievable in people with genotypes 2 and 3, and around 50% in those with genotype 1.
- However, it should be noted that data with regard to treatment is constantly evolving. Treatment of hepatitis C should be instituted and monitored by a specialist.
- Main side effects:
  - Haemolytic anaemia (ribavirin).
  - Miscarriage when given to women or their male partners (adequate contraception is essential) (ribavirin).
  - Flu-like symptoms (these tend to become less severe after the first month of treatment).
  - Depression (including suicidal ideation). Patients who experience depression should be considered for treatment with antidepressants and for referral to a specialist.
  - Thyroid dysfunction (both hypo- and hyperthyroid) (IFN-α).

### Prevention

- No available vaccine for HCV.
- Advise vaccination for hepatitis B and A in patients with HCV.
- Avoid activities which could result in percutaneous or mucous membrane exposure to infected blood (sharing razors or toothbrushes).
- Injecting drug users should be advised not to share needles.
- Patients should also be advised that drinking alcohol (even in moderation) can accelerate progression of liver disease.

## Hepatitis D

### Case history

A 42-year-old man, who is a known HBV carrier, is admitted with new-onset jaundice and abdominal/leg swelling. Examination reveals gross ascites, peripheral oedema, and splenomegaly.

Hepatitis D virus (HDV) is a small circular RNA virus and is a subviral satellite as it can propagate *only* in the presence of HBV.

### Epidemiology and transmission

- Endemic areas include Africa, South America, and the Mediterranean basin.
- Same sources and transmission routes as HBV.
- Transmission can occur:
  - Simultaneous infection with HBV (co-infection).
  - In an individual previously infected with HBV (superinfection).

### Clinical features, investigation, and treatment

- More severe hepatic complications (hepatitis, liver failure, HCC) compared to infection with HBV alone.
- Diagnosis is made by detection of anti-HDV antibody.
- Superinfection can lead to chronic infection with both viruses.

*Co-infection*
- Treatment is mainly supportive.

*Superinfection*
- Antiviral therapy (IFN-α) for chronic infection.

Patients with decompensated liver disease secondary to HBV and HDV infection may require liver transplantation.

No HDV vaccine is available; however, HBV vaccination is effective against HDV.

## Hepatitis E

### Case history

A 33-year-old, pregnant, Indian woman has recently arrived in the UK from New Delhi to visit family in the UK. She develops malaise, anorexia, and abdominal pain.

On examination she is jaundiced, pyrexial and has hepatomegaly.

Hepatitis E virus (HEV) particles are non-enveloped and contain a single-strand of positive-sense RNA.

### Epidemiology and transmission

- Prevalent in most developing countries (widespread in India, northern and central Africa, Southeast Asia, and Central America).
- Excreted in stools, spread mainly through faecal contamination of water supplies or food.
- Increasingly being reported as a source of sporadic acute hepatitis in developed countries, including the UK.

### Clinical features, investigation, and treatment

- Most common in adults aged 15–40 years.
- Clinical illness resembles acute HAV infection.
- Usually a self-limiting disease, chronic infection does not normally occur (however chronic infection can occur in the post-liver transplant setting). Mortality rates are low (~2%).
- Can occasionally develop into acute liver failure (pregnant women (especially those in 3rd trimester) are particularly susceptible, with a high mortality of ~20%).
- Diagnosis is by detection of anti-HEV antibodies or detection of the virus by RT-PCR.
- Supportive management.
- No vaccination currently available.

## Non-A–E hepatitis (seronegative hepatitis)

- Hepatitis thought to be secondary to a virus but not HAV, HBV, HCV, or HEV.
- Causes:
  - Epstein–Barr virus (EBV)
  - Cytomegalovirus (CMV)
  - Herpes simplex virus (HSV)
  - Acute HIV infection
  - Measles
  - Chicken pox
  - Rubella
  - Yellow fever.

## Autoimmune hepatitis

### Case history

A 45-year-old woman is referred to the medical outpatient department with jaundice, arthralgia, and malaise.

On examination she is jaundiced, has palmar erythema and multiple spider naevi. In her past medical history she has received treatment for thyrotoxicosis. Initial blood tests reveal a bilirubin level of 180µmol/L and ALT of 1620IU/L.

Autoimmune hepatitis (AIH) is a form of chronic hepatitis with an often insidious onset.

### Epidemiology, pathogenesis, and genetics

- ♀ >♂ (similar to other autoimmune diseases).
- The anomalous presentation of human leukocyte antigen (HLA) class II on the surface of hepatocytes (influenced by genetic predisposition, viral, and environmental factors) is thought to lead to a cell-mediated immune response against the liver, resulting in AIH and hepatocyte death
- A number of subtypes have been proposed.

The clinical utility of distinguishing subtypes is limited; however, the terms have been useful as clinical descriptors. The two main subtypes are:

1. **Type 1 (classical):**
   - Most common form worldwide.
   - Characterized by positive antinuclear or anti-smooth muscle antibodies (neither of these antibodies are cytotoxic), and raised IgG.
   - Commonly associated with other autoimmune disorders such as Graves disease

2. **Type 2:**
   - Characterized by the presence of anti-LKM1 (liver-kidney microsomal) antibodies and a lack of antinuclear and anti-smooth muscle antibodies.
   - Occurs mainly in children and teenagers and can give rise to severe disease.

### Clinical presentation and physical signs

- Often insidious (but can be acute)
- Jaundice
- Fatigue
- Arthralgia
- Anorexia
- Vitiligo
- Amenorrhoea
- Fever
- Jaundice
- Signs of chronic liver disease.

*Conditions associated with autoimmune hepatitis*

- Thyrotoxicosis
- Myxoedema
- Hashimoto thyroiditis
- Urticaria
- Migrating polyarthritis
- Ulcerative colitis
- Coombs-positive haemolytic anaemia
- Nephrotic syndrome/glomerulonephritis
- Lymphadenopathy
- Pleurisy and transient pulmonary infiltrates.

### Diagnosis

- Best achieved with a combination of clinical and laboratory findings.
- Serological testing for specific auto-antibodies can suggest AIH but these auto-antibodies are heterogenous and are also found in healthy people.
- Increasing evidence suggests overlap syndromes with primary biliary cirrhosis and primary sclerosing cholangitis. Such patients may present with both a hepatitic and cholestatic biochemical picture, and histological features and auto-antibody profile of the separate diseases listed.
- Liver biopsy confirmation is required.

### Laboratory analysis

- Deranged LFTs.
- Positive auto-antibodies:

- Antinuclear or anti-smooth muscle antibodies (ANA, SMA)
- Anti-liver-kidney microsomal antibody
- (Anti-LKM1).
- Raised IgG.

### Liver biopsy

Histological confirmation is required to make the diagnosis, and classically demonstrates interface hepatitis with lymphoplasmacytic infiltrate with/without fibrosis/cirrhosis.

### Complications

- AIH can progress to cirrhosis and liver failure requiring liver transplantation.
- HCC can occur (but is uncommon).

### Treatment

- Corticosteroid treatment is lifesaving, particularly during florid and symptomatic disease.
- **Prednisolone** 30–40mg/day with a gradual dose reduction (as patient and liver function tests improve).
- Once control of the disease with corticosteroids has been achieved **azathioprine** is normally introduced and overlapped with corticosteroids to allow the dose of prednisolone to be reduced gradually.
- In some cases, patients can be maintained on azathioprine monotherapy. A significant proportion of patients do, however, require both long-term, low-dose corticosteroids and azathioprine for disease remission.
- Patients with osteoporosis should be treated with calcium and vitamin D supplementation, and may require bisphosphonates such as alendronate.
- Indications for liver transplantation include chronic end-stage liver disease refractory to medical therapy, and also in cases where AIH presents as acute (fulminant) liver failure.

### Prognosis

- Variable: some patients run a fairly indolent course, while others experience frequent exacerbations requiring high doses of immunosuppressive therapy, and progress to cirrhosis and liver failure.
- With treatment, however, even patients with cirrhosis have a good outcome (90% survival at 10 years).

## Gallstones

### Case history

A 60-year-old man is admitted to the emergency department with a 6-week history of intermittent epigastric pain. The episodes of pain last 4–6 hours and are associated with nausea and vomiting.

Blood tests demonstrate abnormal LFTs (obstructive pattern). Abdominal ultrasound scan demonstrates a gallstone within a dilated common bile duct.

Gallstones are the most common disorder of the biliary tree.

### Pathology

- Classified into cholesterol, pigment, or mixed stones.
- Cholesterol stones: most common in the Westernized world.
- Pigment stones: more common in developing countries.
- Gallstones result from a chemical imbalance (cause unknown) in bile that causes precipitation of one or more of the components.

### Epidemiology

- 10–15% of adults in the Western world will develop gallstones and 1–4% per year will develop symptoms.

### Risk factors for gallstones

- Increasing age
- Female sex
- Obesity
- Rapid weight loss
- Total parenteral nutrition (TPN)
- Pregnancy
- Family history
- Haemolysis
- Diabetes (metabolic syndrome)
- Loss of bile salts (terminal ileitis, ileal resection)
- Cirrhosis.

### Clinical features

- Majority of gallstones are asymptomatic.
- Bilary colic and cholecystitis are the most common presentations (Box 9.23).

### Diagnosis

- Abdominal pain: commonly felt in the epigastric region or right upper quadrant (RUQ), and may radiate to the back, right shoulder, lower chest, and left upper quadrant.
- Abdominal pain >6-8 hours tends to suggest the development of a complication such as cholecystitis or pancreatitis. Furthermore, tenderness in the RUQ and inflammatory signs (fever, leucocytosis) would suggest acute cholecystitis.

---

**Box 9.23 Problems caused by gallstones**

- Biliary colic (56%)
- Cholecystitis (36%)
- Jaundice
- Ascending cholangitis
- Pancreatitis
- Bouveret syndrome (gastric outlet obstruction)
- Gallstone ileus
- Mirizzi syndrome (gallstone impacted in the cystic duct causing stricturing in the common hepatic duct)
- Gallbladder cancer

---

- LFT derangement may suggest the presence of a stone in the bile duct.
- Plasma amylase should be measured to detect pancreatitis.
- Ultrasonography is a key test to investigate for the presence of gallstones, bile duct dilatation, and thickening of the gallbladder wall (secondary to cholecystitis) (Fig. 9.42).
  - NB: the absence of stones on ultrasound does not exclude their existence. If a high index of clinical suspicion remains an interval ultrasound or MRCP should be undertaken.
- CXR can also be useful to exclude a perforated viscus or lower lobe pneumonia.

### Management

- Analgesia (e.g. morphine, diclofenac).
- Maintenance of fluid balance with IV fluids.
- Broad-spectrum antibiotics for cholecystitis and cholangitis (blood cultures should be taken prior to antibiotic therapy).
- Symptomatic gallstones are best treated **surgically**:
  - Cholecystectomy (laparoscopic or open).
  - It is recommended that all patients admitted to hospital as an emergency with symptomatic gallstones should be offered cholecystectomy on the index admission.
  - Urgent surgery is required when cholecystitis progresses despite medical treatment or when complications such as perforation or empyema develop.
- Therapeutic **ERCP** with stone removal and sphincterotomy is the treatment of choice in choledocholithiasis (gallstones in the common bile duct), particularly in patients >60 years old.
  - Surgical treatment of choledocholithiasis is performed less frequently than therapeutic ERCP due to its higher morbidity and mortality.
- **Ursodeoxycholic acid** (dissolution therapy) does not reduce symptoms from gallstones but may be of benefit in preventing gallstone formation in high risk groups (e.g. in the weight loss period following bariatric surgery).

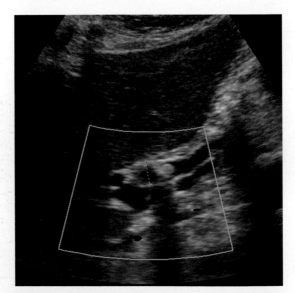

**Fig. 9.42** Duplex ultrasound image of a single acoustically shadowing calculus within the common bile duct.

Image courtesy of Dr D Cookson.

# Primary biliary cirrhosis

## Case history

A previously fit and well 51-year-old woman has bloods checked including LFTs at a routine insurance medical. Her blood tests show bilirubin 14, ALT 83, ALP 620, GGT 452, albumin 38, and INR of 1.0.

On examination she is well and the only finding is xanthelasma.

Primary biliary cirrhosis (PBC) is a slowly-progressive chronic liver disease which causes destruction of the bile ducts within the liver and mainly affects women. The cause is currently unknown, although PBC is suspected to be an autoimmune disease.

## Epidemiology

- Peak incidence in the 5th decade.
- Rare in people <25 years old.
- Most prevalent in Northern Europeans.
- More common in first-degree relatives of patients than in unrelated people.

## Pathology

- Characterized by portal inflammation and immune-mediated destruction of intrahepatic bile ducts.
- Over time, loss of intrahepatic bile ducts results in reduced bile secretion and hepatic injury, development of cirrhosis, and eventual liver failure.

## Clinical features

- ~50% of patients are asymptomatic at diagnosis.
- Most common presenting symptoms are pruritis and fatigue.
- Xanthelasma is seen in ~10%.
- Jaundice is a late feature.
- Other common findings include:
  - Osteopenia.
  - Hyperlipidaemia (Fig. 9.43).
  - Thyroid disease (particularly hypothyroidism).
  - Coexisting autoimmune diseases (including Sjögren syndrome and scleroderma).
  - Steatorrhoea and malabsorption of fat-soluble vitamins and calcium (prolonged cholestasis).
  - Encephalopathy, ascites or variceal haemorrhage (less commonly).
- Patients with longstanding histologically-advanced disease are at increased risk of hepatocellular carcinoma.

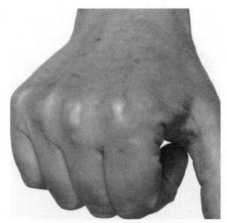

**Fig. 9.43** Tendon xanthomata indicating hyperlipidaemia in a patient with primary biliary cirrhosis.
Reproduced from Longmore et al., *Oxford Handbook of Clinical Medicine*, Seventh Edition, 2010, Figure 3, page 36, with permission from Oxford University Press.

- Other associated diseases include:
  - Coeliac disease
  - Sarcoidosis
  - Interstitial pneumonitis
  - Renal tubular acidosis
  - Autoimmune thrombocytopenia
  - Haemolytic anaemia.

## Diagnosis

Based on three criteria:
1. Presence of anti-mitochondrial antibodies (AMA, type M2).
2. Elevation of LFTs (usually ALP) for >6 months.
3. Compatible liver biopsy findings.

A probable diagnosis of PBC requires two of the three criteria, a definite diagnosis requires all three.

- Some clinicians believe that liver biopsy is unnecessary, however it can allow disease staging.
- NB: 5–10% of patients have no detectable AMA antibodies but have identical disease to AMA-positive patients.

## Treatment of symptoms and complications

- Pruritis can be treated with **cholestyramine. Rifampicin** can be used if cholestyramine is ineffective.
- If neither of these therapies are effective, the opioid antagonists **naloxone** and **naltrexone** can be used. **Plasmapheresis** is reserved for extreme cases.
- Patients with osteoporosis should be treated with calcium and vitamin D supplementation and may require bisphosphonates such as alendronate.

## Treatment of PBC

- Many patients are treated with **ursodeoxycholic acid**. This improves LFTs and may retard histological progression, but overall has not yet been shown convincingly to decrease mortality or liver transplantation rates.
- Liver **transplantation** is the only effective therapy for PBC patients with liver failure, and this procedure has markedly improved survival (92% and 85%, 1- and 5-year survival respectively).

# Sclerosing cholangitis

## Case history

A 54-year-old man presents with jaundice, anorexia, weight loss, and steatorrhoea. Examination reveals stigmata of chronic liver disease. Initial blood tests reveal a bilirubin 104μmol/L, ALP 468IU/L, GGT 589IU/L, low albumin, and mildly prolonged prothrombin time.

Sclerosing cholangitis can be classified as primary or secondary and is characterized by inflammation, fibrotic obliteration, and destruction of the intrahepatic and/or extrahepatic bile ducts. The cause of primary sclerosing cholangitis (PSC) is unknown, and in 70–80% of cases is associated with inflammatory bowel disease (IBD; the majority of which is ulcerative colitis). PSC is also occasionally associated with some autoimmune disorders.

## Epidemiology

- ♂ >♀.
- Normally presents age 30–60 years (although can present in children).

## Clinical features

- Patients may present with pruritis, fluctuating jaundice, RUQ pain, and intermittent fevers.
- A proportion of patients can present with signs of cirrhosis.
- Some patients with IBD are diagnosed when raised serum ALP and GGT are noted on routine blood testing.
- Steatorrhoea (secondary to malabsorption of fat and fat-soluble vitamins A, D, and K).

- Strongly associated with the development of cholangiocarcinoma so progressive jaundice, weight loss, and anorexia should raise suspicion for this complication.
- PSC patients with IBD have an increased risk of colon cancer.

**Diagnosis**

- LFTs usually show cholestasis (elevated serum bilirubin, ALP, and GGT, with slight elevations in serum AST/ALT)
- Prothrombin time may also be prolonged prior to the development of cirrhosis (secondary to decreased vitamin K absorption), which should correct with intravenous vitamin K. Alternatively, with disease progression and the development of cirrhosis, serum albumin decreases and this also prolongs the PT.
- Cholangiography (either MRCP or ERCP) which typically demonstrates narrowed irregular obstruction and beading of the intra- and extrahepatic bile ducts. Disease may be present throughout the whole of the biliary tree or may be limited to the intra- or extrahepatic regions of the biliary system.
- Liver biopsy, if undertaken, may show typical 'onion skin' lesions (concentric layers of fibrotic tissue surrounding a bile duct).
- Main differential diagnoses include IgG4-associated cholangitis/ autoimmune pancreatitis and cholangiocarcinoma

**Management**

- Currently no specific therapy exists.
- Episodes of cholangitis should be treated aggressively with antibiotics, and patients may require cyclical antibiotics as prophylaxis against episodes of biliary sepsis.
- **Ursodeoxycholic acid** (URSO) has been shown to lower elevated liver enzymes in PSC but has not been shown to impact on survival. It should be given in patients with IBD and PSC as this reduces the risk of colon cancer.
- Patients may also require medications to relieve itch.
- When a single dominant biliary stricture is present, **stenting** can sometimes be performed at ERCP (by a skilled operator).
- If concern exists regarding underlying cholangiocarcinoma as a cause of the stricture then **surgical** resection may be performed.
- Patients with osteoporosis should be treated with calcium and vitamin D supplementation and may require bisphosphonates such as alendronate.
- In advanced PSC, liver **transplantation** is the only effective treatment.

# 9.20 Non-alcoholic fatty liver disease

## Case history

A 51-year-old businessman has to undergo a medical as part of his private health insurance. He feels well and is asymptomatic, however routine bloods checked at the time of the medical show that some of his LFTs are deranged: ALT 72IU/L, GGT 176IU/L, his random glucose is 12.6mmol/L, and random cholesterol 9.2mmol/L. Furthermore his BMI is 33 and his BP is elevated at 168/101mmHg. He smokes 20 cigarettes per day and does not drink alcohol.

Non-alcoholic fatty liver disease (NAFLD) is fat accumulation within the liver which is not secondary to excess alcohol intake. NAFLD is related to insulin resistance and the metabolic syndrome (obesity, combined hyperlipidaemia, type 2 diabetes mellitus, and hypertension). In a minority of patients hepatic steatosis is associated with an inflammatory infiltrate and progression to fibrosis, and this condition is known as **NASH** (non-alcoholic steatohepatitis).

## Epidemiology

In the Western world NAFLD is reaching epidemic proportions, affecting 1 in 3 adults in the US population.

## Pathophysiology

- NAFLD is a spectrum of disease activity.
- Patients may simply have fatty liver throughout their lives, or may progress to develop inflammation within the liver associated with steatosis, so called NASH.
- Why some patients progress along this spectrum from steatosis to steatohepatitis and others do not is currently unknown. Postulated mechanisms include a 'second hit' hypothesis whereby oxidative stress or endotoxin-mediated cytokine release occurs within the liver stimulating the development of inflammatory infiltrates.
- ~20% of patients with NASH may go on to develop cirrhosis.

## Clinical features

- Most patients with NAFLD have few or no symptoms directly related to the liver.
- Patients are more likely to have symptoms related to the cause of NAFLD such as diabetes mellitus or obesity.
- Rarely patients complain of RUQ discomfort.
- NAFLD is commonly diagnosed as a result of abnormal LFTs picked up on routine blood testing.
- NASH may lead to cirrhosis, and liver transplantation is the only treatment for NASH-induced end-stage liver failure.
- Many patients may, however, be precluded from transplantation secondary to significant comorbidities related to other manifestations of the metabolic syndrome (e.g. major cardiac disease or end-stage complications of diabetes mellitus).

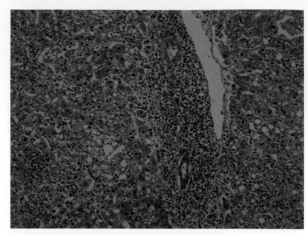

**Fig. 9.44** Non-alcoholic steatohepatitis on liver biopsy. Photomicrograph courtesy of Dr T Kendall.

## Diagnosis and investigations

- Mildly deranged LFTs are common, particularly increases in GGT.
- Raised transaminases can suggest the development of NASH.
- Liver ultrasound may show increased echogenicity consistent with steatosis.
- Liver biopsy (Fig. 9.44) is the most useful test when trying to distinguish NASH from other forms of liver disease, and is used to assess disease severity in terms of degree of inflammation and resultant hepatic fibrosis.
- Full lipid profile and fasting blood glucose is required.
- A screen should also be done to exclude other causes of liver disease (e.g. virology, auto-antibodies, and metabolic screen). Thyroid function should also be checked as hypothyroidism is more common in patients with NASH.

## Treatment

- The mainstay of treatment is intensive management of the **metabolic syndrome** (should be led by an endocrinologist/ diabetologist).
- This includes:
  - Weight loss (if obese).
  - Tight control of diabetes mellitus.
  - Tight BP control.
  - Reduction in alcohol intake.
  - Advice to stop smoking and increase exercise.
- Trials are currently underway examining whether thioglitazones (insulin sensitizer), angiotensin receptor antagonists, or antioxidants may be effective treatments in the management of NAFLD.

# Chapter 10

# Genetics

# 10.1 Karyotype, mitosis, and meiosis

## The human karyotype

- 46 chromosomes (23 pairs) are present in all nucleated cells (Fig. 10.1).
- The autosomes are in pairs, numbered 1–22.
- Females have two X sex chromosomes (46,XX), and men have one X and one Y sex chromosome (46,XY).
- Chromosomes have a short arm (p) and long arm (q).
- Euchromatin contains the active genes.
- All chromosomes show normal variation of DNA sequences.

## Lyonization

- Lyonization is inactivation of one X chromosome in every cell where there are at least two X chromosomes.
- Inactivation only occurs in somatic cells.
- Random process whether paternal or maternal X is inactivated, but is subsequently fixed for all descendants of that cell.
- X inactivation affects most but not all genes on the X chromosome.
- Exceptions are those genes which have homologues on the Y chromosomes, in the pseudo-autosomal region.
- Inactive X remains condensed during most of interphase and can be seen as Barr body or X chromatin.
- If the cell has more than two X chromosomes then the extra Xs are also inactivated.
- The randomness of X inactivation accounts for some females being affected with X-linked recessive disorders.

## Mitosis

- Occurs in somatic cells.
- One cell produces two identical daughter cells (Fig. 10.2).

| Interphase | • Includes gap 1 (G1), S, and gap 2 (G2) phases.<br>• Replication of DNA occurs during S phase. |
|---|---|
| Prophase | • Each chromosome consists of a pair (sister chromatids), held together at the centromere.<br>• Centriole divides and migrates to opposite poles of the cell. |
| Metaphase | • Chromosomes move to the equatorial plate and attach to spindle fibre by centromere. |
| Anaphase | • Chromatids pulled toward opposite cell poles. |
| Telophase | • Cytoplasm divides.<br>• Nuclear membrane reforms. |

## Meiosis

- Occurs in gonads.
- Two successive divisions.
- DNA replicates only once, before the first division (S phase).
- Somatic diploid chromosomal complement halved to a haploid number. (Fig. 10.3).

### First meiotic division (reduction division)
*Prophase*
- Leptotene (pair of sister chromatids formed).
- Zygotene (pairing of homologous chromosomes, as bivalents).
- Pachytene (cross-over occurs).
- Diplotene (bivalents start separating).
- Diakinesis (chromosome thickening, spindle fibres form).

*Metaphase*
- Chromosomes move to equatorial plate.

*Anaphase*
- Bivalents separate, one going to each pole.
- Cytoplasm divides.

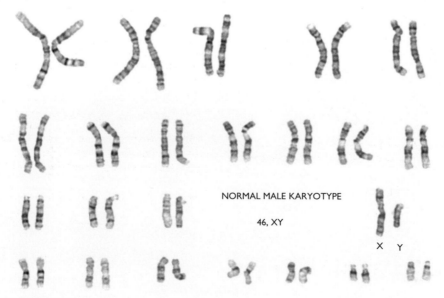

NORMAL MALE KARYOTYPE

46, XY

X   Y

Fig. 10.1 Normal male 46, XY karyotype.

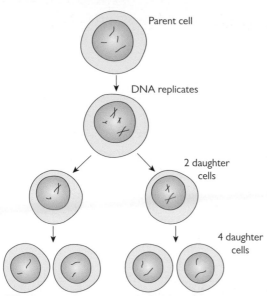

**Fig. 10.2** Mitosis.

Reproduced from Gardiner *et al.*, *Oxford Specialty Training: Training in Paediatrics*, 2009, Figure 12.2, page 248, with permission from Oxford University Press.

- Each cell now has 23 chromosomes, each of which is a chromatid pair.
- Chromatids differ only as a result of crossing-over.

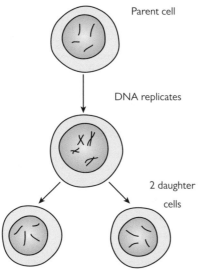

**Fig. 10.3** Meiosis.

Reproduced from Gardiner *et al.*, *Oxford Specialty Training: Training in Paediatrics*, 2009, Figure 12.3, page 248, with permission from Oxford University Press.

### Second meiotic division (resembles mitosis)

- Second meiotic division follows first meiotic division with no interphase.
- Centromeres now divide.
- Sister chromatids pass to opposite poles.

## Non-disjunction

- Failure of sister chromatids to disjoin at anaphase in either mitosis or meiosis.
- Causes aneuploidy with two cells produced, one with extra copy (trisomy) and one with missing copy (monosomy) of a chromosome.
- Related to increasing maternal age.
- For example, Down syndrome (trisomy 21), Edward syndrome (trisomy 18), Patau syndrome (trisomy 13).

## Spermatogenesis

- Occurs from time of sexual maturity onwards.
- In seminiferous tubules.
- Primary spermatocyte undergoes first meiotic division to produce two secondary spermatocytes, each with 23 chromosomes (Fig. 10.3).
- Following the second meiotic division, two spermatids are formed.
- Spermatogenesis produces four sperm per meiotic division.
- Production of a mature sperm takes 61 days.
- Numerous replications increase chances for mutation, particularly in older men.

## Oogenesis

- Mostly complete by birth.
- Primary oocytes form by the end of first trimester and remain in suspended prophase (dictyotene) until sexual maturity.
- Oocyte released into fallopian tube after first meiotic division.
- Completion of first meiotic division may take over 40 years.
- First meiotic division results in formation of the first polar body.
- Second meiotic division is completed at fertilization, resulting in an embryo and second polar body.
- Oogenesis produces only one ovum.
- Long resting phase during the first meiotic division may be a factor in increased risk of separation failure of homologous chromosomes during meiosis (non-disjunction) in older mothers.

## Chromosomal rearrangements

- Balanced rearrangements are common, 1 in 500.
- Unbalanced rearrangements have additional/missing genetic material, causing fetal loss or physical/mental handicap.

## Background

There are several different types of inheritance patterns with different underlying mechanisms. These may involve single nuclear genes (autosomal dominant, autosomal recessive, X-linked recessive, X-linked dominant), single mitochondrial genes (see Section 10.3), chromosomal rearrangements or imprinting (see Section 10.4), and multifactorial inheritance.

## Autosomal dominant

- Vertical transmission, from one generation to the next.
- ♀ and ♂ equally affected.
- ♂ to ♂ transmission possible.
- Heterozygotes are phenotypically affected.
- Each child has a 50% chance of inheriting the gene mutation.
- Variable penetrance (frequency of developing the phenotype) and variable expression (severity of disease) due to modifiers (genetic and environmental).
- Anticipation is a worsening of disease severity in successive generations.
- Examples: dominant polycystic kidney disease, myotonic dystrophy, Marfan syndrome, Huntington disease, neurofibromatosis type 1, familial adenomatous polyposis, familial breast cancer.

## Autosomal recessive

- Usually affected siblings in one generation only, unless consanguineous family or high population carrier frequency.
- ♀ and ♂ equally affected.
- Heterozygotes usually unaffected, i.e. healthy carriers.
- Heterozygotes may have a survival advantage, e.g. sickle cell trait and malaria protection.
- When both parents are carriers, each child has a 1 in 4 chance of developing phenotype, unaffected offspring have 2 in 3 carrier risk.
- All offspring of affected individuals will be obligate carriers.
- Examples: cystic fibrosis, thalassaemia, most inborn errors of metabolism, alpha1-antitrypsin deficiency.

## X-linked recessive

- ♂ more severely affected than ♀.
- ♀ may be affected if skewed X inactivation or has Turner syndrome (45,XO).
- No ♂ to ♂ transmission.
- For carrier ♀, each son and each daughter has 50% chance of inheriting the gene mutation.
- For affected ♂, all sons will be unaffected and all daughters will be carriers.
- Examples: Duchenne muscular dystrophy, haemophilia, red–green colour blindness, fragile X syndrome, Alport syndrome.

## X-linked dominant

- Often lethal in ♂.
- Heterozygote ♀ affected and more severe if skewed X inactivation or has Turner syndrome (45,XO).
- No ♂ to ♂ transmission.
- For carrier ♀, each son and each daughter has 50% chance of inheriting the gene mutation.
- For surviving affected ♂, all sons will be unaffected and all daughters will be affected.
- ♂ born with features of severe X-linked dominant condition that is normally lethal may have Klinefelter syndrome (47,XXY) or somatic mosaicism.
- Examples: X-linked hypophosphatasia, incontinentia pigmenti, Rett syndrome.

## Mitochondrial disease

See section 10.3.

## Chromosomal rearrangements

See Section 10.1.

## Imprinting

See Section 10.4.

## Multifactorial

- Development of disease depends on genetic and environmental factors.
- Risk greatest amongst close relatives and decreases with increasing distance of relationship.
- Risks to relatives greater if proband severely affected.
- If two or more affected relatives, increased risk to relatives.
- Examples: ischaemic heart disease, type 1 diabetes, schizophrenia.

## Types of DNA mutation

Some mutations are clearly pathogenic, e.g. deltaF508 (a deletion of phenylalanine at codon position 508 of the *CFTR* gene) in cystic fibrosis. However, many mutations are now described which may represent normal variation within the general population (polymorphisms). If there is any doubt, mutation results should be discussed with a clinical or molecular geneticist.

### Mis-sense mutations

- A mutation that results in an altered amino acid sequence in the encoded protein. The protein is of normal length.
- Not all mis-sense mutations are pathogenic.

### Protein truncating mutations

- Mutations that result in a shortened protein are nearly always pathogenic.

*Nonsense mutations*

- Single nucleotide substitutions that encode 'stop' codons.

*Frameshift mutations*

- Base pair deletions or insertions that alter the reading frame, producing a premature 'stop' codon.

### Splice site mutation

- A base pair change(s) that alters the position of splicing between exons and introns.

### Large deletions or duplications

- May involve more than one gene

### Trinucleotide expansion

- See Section 10.4.

## References

Firth H, Hurst J. *Oxford Desk Reference in Clinical Genetics*. Oxford: Oxford University Press, 2005.

Tobias ES, Connor M, Ferguson-Smith M. *Essential Medical Genetics*, 6th edition. Oxford: Wiley-Blackwell, 2011.

# 10.3 Mitochondrial disease

## Background

- Mitochondrial diseases can be difficult to diagnose.
- Mitochondrial disorders can be coded for by the nuclear or mitochondrial genome (Fig. 10.4).
- The incidence of mitochondrial respiratory chain diseases is:
  - Under age 6 = 1 in 1000.
  - Under age 16 = 1 in 21,000.
  - Adults = 1 in 8000.

Mitochondrial DNA (mtDNA) is a circular double-stranded molecule encoding 37 genes, 13 of which encode components of the oxidative phosphorylation (OXPHOS) system. Typical cells can contain up to 1000 mitochondria each with one or several copies of the mtDNA genome.

The organs most affected by mitochondrial diseases are those affecting high-energy tissue such as the central nervous system, muscle, pancreas, liver, and kidneys.

## Terminology

- Homoplasmy = only one type of mtDNA in the cell (Fig. 10.5).
- Heteroplasmy = several different types of mtDNA either in the cell, organ, or individual.

- Threshold effect = abnormal mutational load above a threshold level, resulting in greatly impaired function and the severity of clinical symptoms increases sharply.
- Tissue variation is when the level of mutant mtDNA varies in different tissues.
- Selection is where there is preferential accumulation of mutant mtDNA load in certain tissues.

## Mitochondrial inheritance

- The disorder can affect ♂ and ♀ equally.
- mtDNA is almost exclusively maternally inherited.
- Any paternal mitochondria entering at fertilization from sperm is later eliminated.
- ♂ to ♂ transmission is possible but exceedingly rare.
- Mutation rates for mtDNA are 10–20× that of nuclear DNA, probably due to replication repair system errors.
- Variable penetrance (frequency of developing the phenotype) and variable expression (severity of disease) are due to genetic and environmental modifiers.
- Point mutations are usually maternally inherited.
- Deletions and duplications are commonly sporadic occurrences.

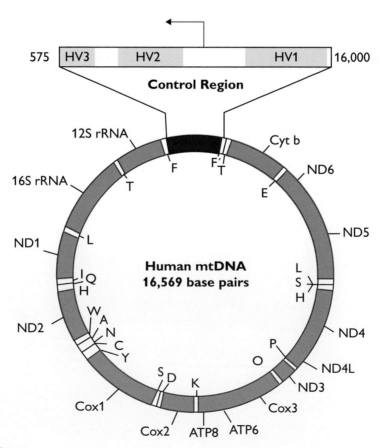

Fig. 10.4 The mitochondrial genome.

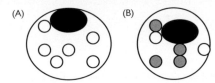

Homoplasmic wild type mtDNA (A) and heteroplasmic mutant mtDNA with wild type mtDNA (B)

**Fig. 10.5** Examples of cellular homoplasmy and heteroplasmy (nucleus = black oval; mitochondria = circles).

- If a mother is heteroplasmic, the proportion of affected mtDNA in her offspring can vary greatly.

## References

Collier J, Longmore M, Amarakone K (eds). *Oxford Handbook of Clinical Specialties*, 9th edition. Oxford: Oxford University Press, 2013.

Firth H, Hurst J. *Oxford Desk Reference in Clinical Genetics*. Oxford: Oxford University Press, 2005.

Harper P. *Practical Genetic Counselling*, 7th edition. Boca Raton, FL: CRC Press, 2010.

Lyons Jones K, Smith DW. *Smith's Recognizable Patterns of Human Malformation*, 7th edition. Philadelphia, PA: Saunders, 2013.

Tobias ES, Connor M, Ferguson-Smith M. *Essential Medical Genetics*, 6th edition. Oxford: Wiley-Blackwell, 2011.

## Trinucleotide repeats

~10% of the human genome is composed of repetitive DNA repeats which are usually inherited in a stable form. Certain trinucleotide repeats become unstable and prone to dramatic expansion affecting the expression of neighbouring genes.

### Trinucleotide repeat expansion diseases

Interestingly, trinucleotide repeat expansion has to date been implicated only in conditions with a neurological component, for example:

- Huntington disease
- Myotonic dystrophy
- Fragile X syndrome
- Friedrich ataxia
- Spinocerebellar ataxia.

*Anticipation*

Inherited diseases can occur at an earlier age in successive generations. This is called 'anticipation'. One biological explanation of anticipation is the unstable expansion of DNA trinucleotide repeat sequences. The instability of these repeats means that different members of the same family can show different repeat lengths which positively correlate with clinical severity.

*Parent of origin effect*

Some trinucleotide repeats can rapidly expand over the course of one generation depending on the parent of origin:

- Juvenile Huntington disease can occur following paternal inheritance of a trinucleotide repeat.
- Congenital myotonic dystrophy can occur following maternal inheritance of a trinucleotide repeat.

*Mutation carriers*

Fragile X syndrome is an X-linked recessive condition that predominantly manifests as learning difficulties in boys and also some girls. Female carriers of a 'premutation' (small expansion only) are at 25% risk of developing premature ovarian failure. Male 'premutation' carriers are at risk of tremor, ataxia, and cognitive impairment in older age. Expansion is more unstable if inherited maternally. See Section 10.13.

### Anticipation without trinucleotide repeat expansion

Many other conditions display an earlier onset of disease in successive generations without any evidence of trinucleotide repeat expansion, e.g. familial rheumatoid arthritis, inflammatory bowel disease, and familial leukaemia. This may in part be due to statistical ascertainment bias, earlier diagnosis through improved care, or other, as yet unknown, biological mechanisms.

### Genetic testing

Molecular genetic testing is widely available for many trinucleotide disorders.

## Imprinting

Genomic imprinting is a genetic mechanism by which genes are selectively expressed from the maternal or paternal homologue of a chromosome. Imprints are erased during the early development of the male and female germ cells and then reset prior to germ cell maturation. The imprint remains throughout life. Imprinting defects are more common following *in vitro* fertilization (IVF), with Beckwith–Wiedemann syndrome being particularly more common.

Imprinted genes can be altered in different ways to produce a non-functioning copy of a gene with a resultant phenotype:

- Mutated.
- Silenced.
- Deleted.
- Uniparental disomy (UPD): each chromosome of a pair has been inherited exclusively from one parent, usually by non-disjunction.

### Imprinting and human disease

In humans, >50 genes are known to be imprinted and often have roles in growth and development. Some examples of imprinted genes and their phenotypes are:

- Prader–Willi syndrome (loss of paternal gene expression at chromosome 15q11–q13).
- Angelman syndrome (loss of maternal gene expression at chromosome 15q11–q13).
- Beckwith–Wiedemann syndrome (loss of maternally or paternally expressed genes at chromosome 11p15.5).
- Albright hereditary osteodystrophy or pseudohypoparathyroidism (loss of maternally or paternally expressed gene at chromosomes 20q13.32).
- Russell–Silver syndrome (abnormalities at imprinted domain on chromosome 11p15.5 or loss of paternal gene expression on chromosome 7).

### Genetic testing for imprinting disorders

- For a microdeletion, fluorescent *in situ* hybridization (FISH) studies may be used.
- Analysis may be undertaken using DNA from the affected patient to look for abnormal methylation patterns suggestive of an imprinting defect.
- To look for uniparental disomy, DNA is required from both the affected patient and usually also the parents.
- Direct molecular genetic analysis to look for a specific gene mutation of an imprinting centre locus.

## References

Collier J, Longmore M, Amarakone K (eds). *Oxford Handbook of Clinical Specialties*, 9th edition. Oxford: Oxford University Press, 2013.

Firth H, Hurst J. *Oxford Desk Reference in Clinical Genetics*. Oxford: Oxford University Press, 2005.

Harper P. *Practical Genetic Counselling*, 7th edition. Boca Raton, FL: CRC Press, 2010.

Lyons Jones K, Smith DW. *Smith's Recognizable Patterns of Human Malformation*, 7th edition. Philadelphia, PA: Saunders, 2013.

Tobias ES, Connor M, Ferguson-Smith M. *Essential Medical Genetics*, 6th edition. Oxford: Wiley-Blackwell, 2011.

# 10.5 Investigative techniques in genetic medicine

## Background

Peripheral blood leucocytes are typically used to study chromosomes and DNA. However, almost any growing tissue can be used e.g. skin fibroblasts, amniocytes, or cells from chorionic villi. DNA may also be extracted from archived histopathological material and Guthrie blood spots, although analysis may be limited.

## Samples for genetic analysis

### Blood samples

- Karyotype: 5–10mL blood in lithium-heparin blood tube.
- DNA: 5–10mL blood in EDTA blood tube.

### Skin biopsy

- Punch biopsy (3–5mm) placed in transport medium for fibroblast culture.
- Can be used for karyotype, biochemical assays, and DNA analysis.

### Amniocytes and chorionic villi

- See under 'Chorionic villus sampling'.

## DNA analysis

The lymphocytes from a 10mL blood sample (EDTA tube) yield ~300mcg of DNA, sufficient for multiple DNA analyses. DNA can be stored frozen for very many years.

### Polymerase chain reaction (PCR)

- Used to amplify a DNA sequence of interest.
- Two oligonucleotide primers are used which are complementary to the DNA sequence of interest.
- Firstly, the double-stranded DNA is denatured by heat into single-stranded DNA fragments.
- The reaction is then cooled to allow annealing (binding) of primers to the target DNA sequence.
- Heat-stable *Taq* DNA polymerase then extends the primers along the template target sequence.
- After one cycle there are two copies of double-stranded DNA, after two cycles there are four copies and so on.
- Typically a PCR reaction involves 25–30 cycles, thus allowing millions of DNA amplifications.

### DNA sequencing

- Di-deoxy sequencing allows identification of the exact nucleotide sequence of DNA.
- The region of interest is amplified by a PCR reaction. This builds a new DNA chain complementary to the region of interest.
- The reaction is carried out in one tube, containing all four nucleotides and all four di-deoxy nucleotides (adenine, cytosine, guanine, thymine), each tagged with a different fluorescent marker.
- The di-deoxy nucleotides are incorporated into the growing chain and where incorporated stop the addition of any further nucleotides.
- The fragments are electrophoresed and the DNA sequence is determined by fluorescence: DNA fragments of different sizes will contain different 'end' bases (the tagged di-deoxy nucleotides). Identifying fragments by size and fluorescence allows the base sequence to be determined.
- DNA sequencing can be used to identify point mutations, small deletions, and insertions.

## Southern blotting

- DNA is cut into fragments using a restriction enzyme that recognizes a specific DNA sequence.
- The fragments are separated according to size by gel electrophoresis and transferred (blotted) to filter paper.
- A labelled probe is then used to bind to its complementary sequence on the blot and can be identified by autoradiography.
- Southern blotting requires relatively large amounts of good-quality DNA and is time-consuming.
- Southern blotting can be used for detection of large DNA expansion mutations (e.g. triplet repeats), which cannot be detected by PCR

## Multiplex ligation-dependent probe amplification (MLPA)

- This is a high-resolution method to detect copy number variation in genomic sequences, e.g. large gene deletions and duplications.
- Often gene analysis now involves DNA sequencing and MLPA to identify different types of mutation.
- MLPA can also be used instead of FISH for the analysis of telomeres.

## Next-generation sequencing

- High-throughput sequencing, producing thousands or millions of DNA sequences simultaneously.
- These methods are intended to lower the cost of DNA sequencing.

## Chromosome analysis

### Karyotyping (chromosome analysis)

- Samples are cultured.
- Cell division is then stopped in metaphase.
- Chromosomes stained with Giemsa, i.e. G-banding.
- Alternating light (euchromatin) and dark (heterochromatin) bands are characteristic for each chromosome pair using light microscopy.
- The resolution of G-banding is ~5Mbases.

### Fluorescent *in situ* hybridization (FISH)

- Technique used to detect the presence of specific DNA sequences on chromosomes.
- Uses fluorescent probes and light microscopy.

### Haematological malignancies and solid tumours

- Haematological neoplasms and paediatric solid tumours can be characterized by acquired genetic rearrangements detectable using karyotype analysis.
- Used to provide information about diagnosis, e.g. Philadelphia chromosome (9;22 translocation) in CML, for prognosis and remission.

## Molecular cytogenetics

Technology using molecular DNA analysis has recently been developed to determine genomic copy number.

### Array-CGH (comparative genomic hybridization)

- Patient and control DNA are given different fluorescent labels and hybridized to arrays containing thousands of genomic clones.

- The fluorescent signals are compared to determine whether there is a change in genomic copy number (deletions or duplications) of patient DNA relative to control DNA.
- The resolution is much greater than routine karyotyping and FISH.
- However, it cannot detect apparently balanced rearrangements.
- A number of variants have been identified with as yet unknown significance. Therefore, this technology is still being used with caution in determining results.
- In the future, this technology is likely to significantly increase the ability to diagnose chromosome abnormalities as a cause of mental retardation and congenital defects (Vissers et al., 2003).

### Quantitative fluorescence polymerase chain reaction (QF-PCR)

- QF-PCR is used to test for gene dosage, i.e. the number of copies of a given gene present in a sample.
- Examples of its use includes testing for aneuploidy of whole chromosomes, e.g. 13, 18, 21, X, Y in a chorionic villus sample (CVS) or amniotic fluid.
- Markers of DNA from the sample are amplified, labelled with fluorescent tags, and measured by electrophoresis.

---

## Genetic testing and prenatal diagnosis

### Free fetal DNA

- Enrichment of fetal cells circulating in maternal blood can now be analysed for gender determination (used in X-linked disorders) and also aneuploidy, as early as 6 weeks' gestation.
- Fetal DNA comprises 2–10% of total DNA in maternal blood

### Chorionic villus sampling (CVS)

- Under ultrasound guidance, needle inserted transadominally through uterine wall for biopsy of chorionic villi.
- From 11 weeks' gestation.
- Miscarriage risk 1% above normal population risk.
- Can be used for fetal karyotype, biochemical assays, and DNA analysis.

### Amniocentesis

- Under ultrasound guidance, needle inserted transabdominally through uterine wall for aspiration of amniotic fluid.
- From 15 weeks' gestation.
- Miscarriage risk 1% above normal population risk.
- Can be used for fetal karyotype, biochemical assays, and DNA analysis.

### Pre-implantation genetic diagnosis (PGD)

PGD is a form of genetic diagnosis performed prior to implantation.

- The patient's oocytes are fertilized *in vitro* and, at the eight-cell stage of embryogenesis, a single cell is removed and analysed for the genetic condition in question.
- The diagnosis itself can be carried out using several techniques, e.g. FISH and PCR

---

## References

Firth H, Hurst J. *Oxford Desk Reference in Clinical Genetics*. Oxford: Oxford University Press, 2005.

Vissers LEM, de Vries BBA, Osoegawa K, *et al*. Array-based comparative genomic hybridisation for the genome-wide detection of submicroscopic chromosomal abnormalities. *Am J Hum Genet* 2003; 73: 1261–70.

# 10.6 Down syndrome

## Background

Down syndrome (named after John Langdon Down, British physician who first described the condition in the 1860s) is a congenital disorder resulting from an extra copy (trisomy) of chromosome 21. The mechanisms by which increased dosage of genes on chromosome 21 leads to Down syndrome are as yet unknown (Roizen & Patterson, 2003). However, neuropathological changes associated with dementia in Down syndrome are typical of Alzheimer disease.

## Epidemiology

- Incidence: 1/650–1/1000.
- All ethnic groups.
- ♂ = ♀.
- Commonest genetic cause of severe learning difficulty.

## Genetics

Trisomy 21 can occur due to the following mechanisms:
- Chromosome 21 non-disjunction (see Section 10.1 and Fig. 10.6) (95%). The risk of chromosome non-disjunction increases with advancing maternal age:
  - At 18 years of age the risk is 1:1500.
  - At 38 years of age the risk is 1:150.
- Robertsonian translocation (= translocation of chromosome 21 onto another chromosome, usually chromosome 14 (Fig. 10.7), less commonly 13, 15, 21, or 22) (2%). 50% are familial.
- Mosaicism; some cells normal, some have trisomy 21, due to post-zygotic non-disjunction (2%). The phenotype may be milder.
- Other chromosome rearrangements (1%).

## Clinical presentation

Clinical features are variable. Trisomy 21 may present pre- or postnatally.

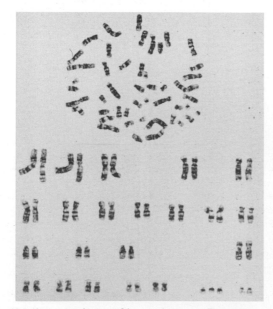

Fig. 10.6 Karyotype of trisomy 21—non-disjunction. Three copies of chromosome 21 are present in this individual (bottom right).

## Pre-natal features

- Miscarriage.
- Abnormal maternal serum screening: increased human chorionic gonadotropin (hCG) (assayed as part of the routine second trimester 'triple test'—together with alpha-fetoprotein and oestriol), increased inhibin-A (in addition to the triple test).
- Ultrasound scanning: increased nuchal translucency, nasal bone hypoplasia, cardiac defect, double stomach bubble (secondary to duodenal atresia).

## Post-natal features

- Hypotonia and feeding problems in infancy.
- Dysmorphism.
- Congenital anomalies, particularly congenital heart defects.

## Physical signs

- Dysmorphism.
- Upslanting palpebral fissures, epicanthic folds (Fig. 10.8).
- Brushfield spots on iris.
- Protruding tongue.
- Small ears.
- Brachycephaly.
- Single palmar creases (Fig. 10.9), clinodactyly, sandal gap.
- Evidence of congenital heart defect.
- Evidence of gastrointestinal obstruction.

## Diagnosis

- Routine karyotyping is essential to determine the aetiology. Only need parental karyotype if the child has a chromosomal rearrangement causing trisomy 21. Pre-natal cytogenetic testing is available.
- Skin biopsy if mosaic Down syndrome suspected.
- Echocardiogram.
- Thyroid function.

## Complications

- Congenital heart defects (40–50%), ventricular septal defect is the most common, followed by combined AV septal defects, atrial septal defect, patent ductus arteriosus and tetralogy of Fallot.
- Short stature.
- Hypothyroidism (20–40%).
- Diabetes mellitus (1%).
- Leukaemia, especially acute lymphocytic (2%).
- Obstructive sleep apnoea.
- Duodenal atresia/stenosis, Hirschsprung disease.
- Behavioural problems (10%).
- Seizures (8%).
- Dementia, mean age 50 years+.
- Atlantoaxial subluxation (15% on X-ray, few symptomatic).
- Eyes (refractive errors).
- Learning difficulties, average IQ 45–48, adults will require daily supervision.

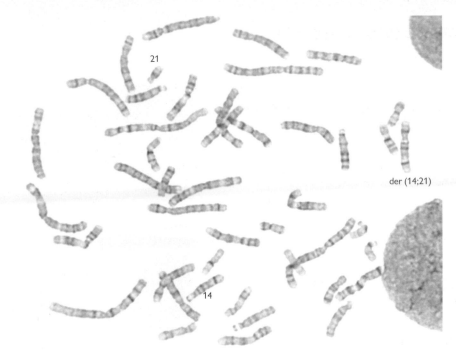

21

der (14;21)

14

**Fig. 10.7** Translocation of chromosome 21 onto 14 causing trisomy 21. During meiosis gametes may form containing the (14:21) chromosome plus a normal chromosome 21. These will give rise to trisomy 21 in the offspring.

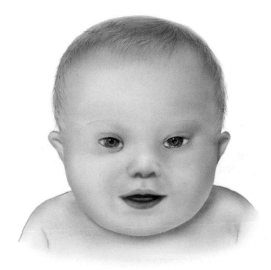

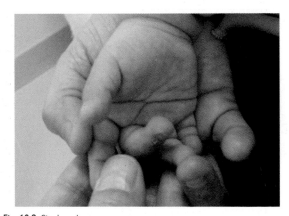

**Fig. 10.9** Single palmar crease.
Reproduced from Gardiner et al., *Oxford Specialty Training: Training in Paediatrics*, 2009, Figure 12.15, page 254, with permission from Oxford University Press.

**Fig. 10.8** A drawing of the facial features of Down syndrome.
Source: Centers for Disease Control and Prevention, National Center on Birth Defects and Developmental Disabilities, http://www.cdc.gov/ncbddd/birthdefects/DownSyndrome.html

### Life expectancy

- Median age at death is 49 years.
- Congenital heart disease is the major factor in increased mortality.

## Treatment

- Will depend on time of presentation and specific complications.
- Surgical correction for congenital heart and gastrointestinal defects.
- Referral to local child development centre.

### Genetic counselling

- Recurrence risks (RR) depend on the cause of trisomy 21: for non-disjunction: women aged <39 years RR= 0.8%; for women aged >39 years RR is the age-related risk.
- After two pregnancies with trisomy 21, there is ~10% recurrence risk; consider parental mosaicism.
- Robertsonian translocation: if *de novo* the recurrence risk is low; if inherited the recurrence risk is up to 50%.

## Reference

Roizen NJ, Patterson D. Down's syndrome. *Lancet* 2003; *361*:1281–9.

# 10.7 Klinefelter syndrome

## Background

Klinefelter syndrome is due to an extra copy of an X chromosome in males (47,XXY). Adult males have hypergonadotropic hypogonadism and are invariably infertile. However, lifespan is normal and many males may never be diagnosed.

## Epidemiology

- Incidence: ~1/600–1/800 ♂ births.
- There is a significant maternal age effect with incidence 1/300 at maternal age 43 years.

## Genetics

- Cases occur sporadically.
- The extra X chromosome is of maternal origin in 56%.
- It usually arises by non-disjunction.
- Mosaicism may occur, e.g. 46,XY/47,XXY; some of these ♂ are fertile
- There is an increased incidence of chromosome abnormalities in conceptuses fathered by 47,XXY ♂ following intracytoplasmic sperm injection (ICSI) with IVF.

## Clinical presentation

- 47,XXY may present antenatally following CVS or amniocentesis.
- Babies appear normal.
- Increased incidence of undescended testes.
- Delayed puberty.
- Gynaecomastia.
- Infertility.

## Physical signs

- ♂ tend to have a taller final height (186cm 47,XXY vs. 176cm 46,XY).
- Gynaecomastia (Fig. 10.10).
- Increased carrying angle at elbow.
- Centripetal obesity.
- Hypogonadism.
- Normal IQ range.

## Diagnosis

- Routine karyotype.

## Complications

- IQ: usually only lower by 10–15 points compared to siblings. Overall intelligence is normal as an adult although ~60% will need

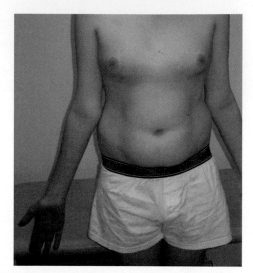

Fig. 10.10 Body habitus in Klinefelter syndrome. Note gynaecomastia, wide carrying angle, and centripetal obesity.

some degree of additional educational help. The majority of patients tend to be passive and good natured.
- Cancer risk: there is no good evidence for a general increased risk of cancer although there is a 3% risk increase in breast cancer. There is a <1% risk of primary germ cell tumour.
- In adult life there is an increased risk of diabetes and cardiovascular disease.
- Hypogonadism: delayed puberty, gynaecomastia, infertility.
- Osteoporosis.

## Treatment

- Hormone replacement with intramuscular or transdermal testosterone improves libido, facial hair, self-esteem, and may reduce the risk of osteoporosis.
- Management of infertility, sperm donation, and adoption. ICSI may be offered to the few patients that have viable sperm.
- Surgery for gynaecomastia.
- Genetic counselling: prenatal diagnosis should be offered to parents with a previously affected child although recurrence risk is <1%.

### Surveillance

- From 10 years of age: follicle-stimulating hormone, luteinizing hormone, testosterone measurements.
- Height, weight and development.

# 10.8 Turner syndrome

## Background

Turner syndrome is due to the deficiency of all or part of one X chromosome.

## Epidemiology

- Incidence: 1/2500 live ♀ births.
- Sporadic.

## Genetics

- Most 45,X is due to loss of the paternal X chromosome.
- Mosaic forms (42%) may have a milder phenotype.
- Short stature in Turner syndrome is due to loss of 'growth' genes on the X chromosome.

## Clinical presentation

Turner syndrome has a very variable phenotype and presents with diverse clinical features in different age groups:

### Pre-natal
- Miscarriage.
- Increased nuchal translucency.
- Hydrops fetalis.

### Newborn
- Oedema of hands and feet.
- Congenital heart defect.

### Childhood
- Short stature.

### Teenage
- Primary amenorrhoea.

### Adulthood
- Infertility.

## Physical signs

- Short stature.
- Webbed neck (Figs 10.11 and 10.12).
- Low hairline.
- Broad ('shield') chest with widely spaced nipples.
- Wide carrying angle of elbow.
- Oedema of hands and feet, especially in infancy.
- Short 4th and 5th metacarpals.
- Evidence of congenital heart disease: heart murmur, delayed femoral pulses, hypertension.

## Diagnosis

- Karyotype.

## Complications

- Recurrent otitis media (60%).
- Congenital heart defect (15–50%): coarctation of the aorta, bicuspid aortic valve, ventricular septal defect.

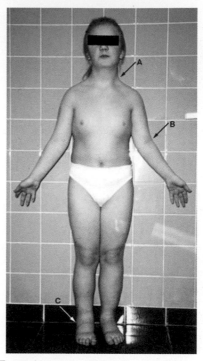

**Fig. 10.11** Turner phenotype in childhood.

Reprinted by permission from Macmillan Publishers Ltd: *Nature Clinical Practice Endocrinology & Metabolism*, Gawlik and Malecka–Tendera, 'Hormonal therapy in a patient with a delayed diagnosis of Turner's syndrome', 4, 173–177, © 2008.

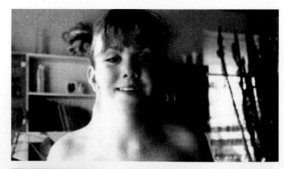

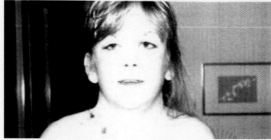

**Fig. 10.12** Girl with Turner syndrome before and immediately after her operation for neck-webbing.

Source: Johannes Nielsen, http://www.aaa.dk/TURNER/ENGELSK/TURN_ORI.HTM#baby

- Renal anomalies (30%): horseshoe kidney, agenesis.
- Autoimmune disease: hypothyroidism, diabetes mellitus.
- Ovarian dysgenesis (most are infertile).
- Infertility.
- Osteoporosis (secondary to decreased oestrogen).
- Gonadoblastoma in the presence of a 46,XY cell line in mosaic Turner syndrome.
- Intelligence is usually within normal range.
- Life expectancy is reduced due to obesity, ischaemic heart disease, and aortic dissection.

## Treatment

- Removal of testicular tissue if any 46,XY cell line present.

- Consider growth hormone therapy.
- Commence oestrogens at time of puberty.
- Ovum donation.

**Genetic counselling**

- The recurrence risk for parents of an affected child is negligible.

**Surveillance**

- Hearing.
- Growth.
- Blood pressure.
- Autoimmune disease.
- Thyroid function.
- Aortic root, especially in pregnancy by echocardiogram.

# 10.9 Neurofibromatosis

## Background

The neurofibromatoses can be distinguished according to type and distribution of hamartomatous lesions (Figs 10.13 and 10.14). Neurofibromatosis type 1 (NF1) is a common and well-known disorder first described by von Recklinghausen in 1849 (see also Section 7.14) (Fig. 10.15). Neurofibromatosis type 2 (NF2) is a much rarer condition and characterized by the formation of VIIIth cranial nerve vestibular schwannomas.

## Neurofibromatosis type 1

### Epidemiology
- Incidence: 1/2500–1/4000.
- ♂ = ♀.
- There is considerable phenotypic variability between members of the same family.

### Genetics
- Autosomal dominant inheritance.
- NF1 is caused by mutations in the *NF1* gene on chromosome 17q11.2, encoding neurofibromin.
- *NF1* gene mutations are found in ~80% patients fulfilling diagnostic criteria (see 'Diagnostic criteria').
- Neurofibromin is a tumour suppressor involved in cell cycle regulation.
- 50% of cases are *de novo* (new mutations).
- Penetrance is 100%.

### Clinical presentation
Patients with NF1 usually present in childhood with café-au-lait (CAL) patches or in adulthood with neurofibromas.

### Physical signs

*NF1 diagnostic criteria*
Patients must have **two or more** of the following:
- CAL patches (six or more >5mm prepubertal, >15mm in an adult) (>99% of individuals have this feature).
- Axillary or inguinal freckling (85%).
- Neurofibromas (two or more cutaneous/subcutaneous) (>99%).
- Plexiform neurofibromas (one or more) (30–50%).
- Lisch nodules—benign iris hamartomas seen with slit lamp (two or more) (95%).
- Optic pathway glioma (15% total, 5% symptomatic).

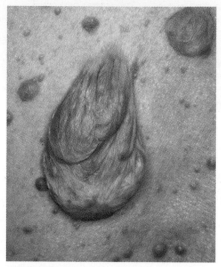

Fig. 10.14 Skin lesions in neurofibromatosis.

- Bony dysplasia (sphenoid wing/long bone or pseudarthrosis) (2%).
- First-degree relative with NF1.

### Diagnosis
NF1 is a clinical diagnosis made when the diagnostic criteria are fulfilled. MRI head/spine only if focal neurological signs or epilepsy.

*Genetic testing*
Molecular DNA analysis is usually reserved for:
- Borderline cases.
- Known family mutation.
- Pre-natal testing.

### Complications
- Mild cognitive impairment (30–60%).
- Scoliosis (11%).
- Malignant peripheral nerve sheath tumours (8–13% lifetime risk).
- Cerebral gliomas (2%).

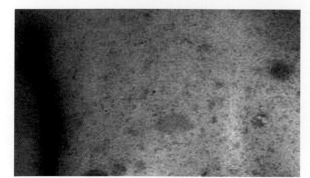

Fig. 10.13 Skin lesions in neurofibromatosis.

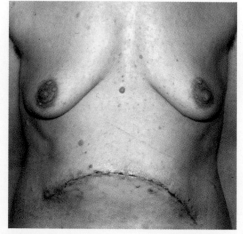

Fig. 10.15 Neurofibromatosis type 1.

- Raised blood pressure may be due to benign essential hypertension, renal artery stenosis, or phaeochromocytoma (2%).

## Treatment
- Consider removal of neurofibromas if symptomatic.

*Surveillance*
- Annual systems review including skin, spine, and neurology.
- Annual development and ophthalmology assessment in childhood.
- Blood pressure.

*Genetic counselling*
- If parent affected, recurrence risk is 50% for each offspring.
- If parent unaffected or *de novo* mutation, recurrence risk is <1%.
- If parent has segmental NF1 there is a low recurrence risk.

# Neurofibromatosis type 2

## Epidemiology
- Incidence: 1/40,000–1/100,000.

## Genetics
- Autosomal dominant inheritance.
- NF2 is caused by mutations in the *NF2* gene on chromosome 22q12.2, encoding merlin, a tumour suppressor.
- 50% of patients with NF2 are *de novo* (new mutations).

## Clinical presentation
- Typically bilateral vestibular schwannomas, deafness, and tinnitus.

## Physical signs
- CAL patches: 4% of patients have more than three, none have more than six.
- In contrast to NF1, plexiform neurofibromas, axillary freckling, and Lisch nodules are rare.

*NF2 diagnostic criteria*
Patients must have **one** of the following:
- Bilateral vestibular schwannoma.
- A parent, sibling, or child with NF2 and either:
  - A unilateral vestibular Schwannoma *or*
  - Two or more of: meningioma, glioma, schwannoma, posterior subcapsular lenticular opacities, cerebral calcification.
- Unilateral vestibular Schwannoma and two or more of: meningioma, glioma, schwannoma, posterior subcapsular opacities, cerebral calcification.
- Multiple meningiomas (two or more) and one or more of: glioma, schwannoma, posterior subcapsular opacities, cerebral calcification.

## Diagnosis
- Clinical diagnostic criteria fulfilled.

*Genetic testing*
- Molecular DNA analysis is available.

## Complications
- CNS tumours and surgical sequelae.

## Treatment
*Surveillance*
- First-degree relatives should have baseline MRI brain and annual assessment.
- Refer for genetic counselling.

# 10.10 Tuberous sclerosis

## Background

Tuberous sclerosis is a multisystem disorder with a highly variable clinical presentation. The high degree of variability has led to the condition now being called tuberous sclerosis complex (TSC).

## Epidemiology

- Incidence: ~1/10,000.
- ♂ = ♀.

## Genetics

- Autosomal dominant inheritance.
- *TSC1* on chromosome 9q (75% cases): encodes hamartin.
- *TSC2* on chromosome 16 (25% cases): encodes tuberin.
- Hamartin and tuberin dimerize to form a tumour suppressor that acts as an inhibitor of the 'mammalian target of rapamycin' (mTOR) pathway, critical in cell cycle growth and proliferation.
- Over 60% of cases are due to a new spontaneous mutation.
- Penetrance is 100% but with variable severity.
- A small minority of patients have a contiguous deletion involving *TSC2* and the adjacent autosomal dominant polycystic kidney disease (*ADPKD*) gene on chromosome 16. This subset of patients often develop early-onset renal cystic disease and hypertension. ~5% of these patients go on to develop end-stage renal failure.

## Clinical presentation

- The most common presentation is in childhood with epilepsy (90%), developmental delay (80%), or infantile spasms (30%).
- Intellectual impairment is common (but variable).
- Increasing numbers are being diagnosed in adulthood.

## Physical signs

- Facial angiofibromas (adenoma sebaceum) or forehead plaques.
- Subungal fibromas (Fig. 10.16).
- Hypopigmented macules (ash-leaf shaped, fluoresce under ultraviolet (Woods) light).
- Shagreen patch (roughened patches of skin, usually over lumbar spine—Fig. 10.17).

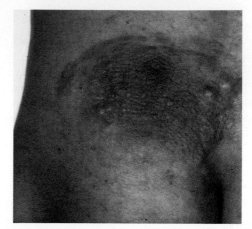

Fig. 10.17 Shagreen patch (to left of lower lumbar spine).

## Diagnosis

Diagnostic criteria have been developed for TSC which require two major features or one major and two minor features.

### Major clinical diagnostic features

- Developmental delay
- Epilepsy
- Subependymal nodules/hamartomas/cortical tubers
- Periventricular calcification
- Facial angiofibromas or forehead plaques
- Subungal fibromas
- Hypopigmented macules
- Shagreen patch
- Renal angiomyolipomas
- Cardiac rhabdomyoamas (as neonates) (30–70%).

### Minor clinical diagnostic features

- Renal cysts (40%)
- Dental pits (Fig. 10.18)
- Bone cysts
- Rectal polyp hamartomas
- Retinal hamartomas
- Hepatic hamartomas (15%).

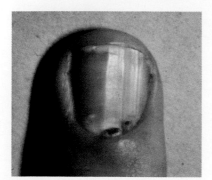

Fig. 10.16 Subungual fibroma.

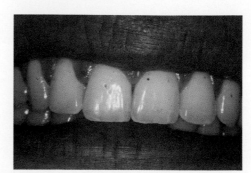

Fig. 10.18 Dental pits in TSC.

### Genetic testing

● Gene mutations are found in ~80% patients fulfilling diagnostic criteria. Molecular DNA analysis is available for:
● Borderline cases where there is a known family mutation.
● Pre-natal testing.
● Predictive testing.

## Complications

● Sporadic mutation patients with *TSC1* mutations have a milder condition compared to *TSC2* patients. Otherwise there is little difference between the genotypes in their complication rates.

The lesions of TSC are often asymptomatic but the main complications are:

● Intractable seizures.
● Severe developmental delay.
● Intracranial hypertension secondary to subependymal giant cell astrocytomas.
● Enlarging renal angiomyolipomas (Figs 10.19 and 10.20) and haematuria.
● Cystic lung disease (lymphangiomyomatosis) in ♀.

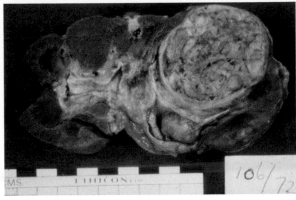

**Fig. 10.20** Renal angiomyolipomata in TSC.

## Treatment

Annual systems review is directed towards preventative management in the following systems:
● Neurological
● Ophthalmological
● Cardiac
● Dermatological
● Developmental
● Renal.

### Genetic counselling

● If parent affected, recurrence risk is 50% for each offspring.
● If parent unaffected or *de novo* mutation, recurrence risk is <1%.

### Differential diagnosis TSC

● Isolated cardiac rhabdomyomas: 30–80% diagnosed prenatally will have TSC.
● Periventricular heterotopia: rare X-linked disorder associated with normal intelligence, seizures, and non-calcified periventricular nodules.
● Isolated renal angiomyolipomas, usually unilateral and more common in ♀.

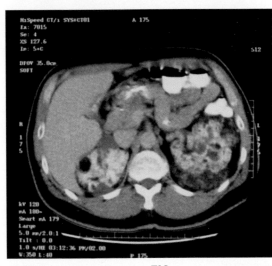

**Fig. 10.19** Renal angiomyolipomata in TSC.

# 10.11 Myotonic dystrophy

## Background

Myotonic dystrophy is the most common heritable neuromuscular disorder, inherited in an autosomal dominant manner. It is also known as dystrophica myotonica, DM1, or Steinert disease.

## Epidemiology

- Incidence: 1/8000.
- ♂ = ♀.

## Genetics

- Myotonic dystrophy is caused by CTG triplet repeat expansion in the non-coding region of the *DMPK* gene (DM1) gene on chromosome 19q13.3, encoding myotonin.
- Triplet repeat expansion is detected in 98% of patients.
- Onset of symptoms is earlier in successive generations due to increasing size of triplet repeat expansion (anticipation).
- As a general rule, prognosis cannot be predicted using molecular analysis alone except in congenital myotonic dystrophy when there is gross (>1000) repeat expansion.
- Normal myotonin is required for intercellular conduction.
- The effect of the CTG repeat is complex but may affect adjacent genes and RNA processing.

## Clinical presentation

- Clinical presentation of myotonic dystrophy is extremely variable, even within families.
- Varies from severe respiratory insufficiency in infancy to cataracts alone in adulthood.
- Most common age of symptom onset is 20–30 years.

## Physical signs

- Frontal balding (Fig. 10.21).
- Myotonia: elicited by inability to rapidly relax clenched fist or by tapping thenar eminence.
- Facial muscles: ptosis, inability to frown, clench teeth, smile.
- Peripheral muscles: reduced power in sternocleidomastoids, distal arm and leg; reflexes may still be present if only mild disease presentation.
- Bradycardia/heart block.
- Lens opacities.
- Testicular atrophy in men.

## Diagnosis

- Molecular DNA analysis is routinely available for myotonic dystrophy. Pre-natal diagnosis is available.
- Urine dipstick for glucose.
- ECG: conduction defects.
- Ophthalmology assessment.
- Sleep studies.
- Consider electromyogram if there is diagnostic uncertainty and normal molecular analysis.

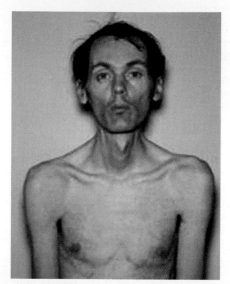

Fig. 10.21 40-year-old patient with en:myotonic dystrophy presenting with bilateral cataracts and complete heart block.
Source: Herbert L. Fred, MD, Hendrik A. van Dijk, http://cnx.org/content/m14898/latest/

## Complications

- Myopathy: poor mobility, difficulty swallowing.
- Lens opacities/cataracts.
- Cardiac conduction defects/ventricular arrhythmias.
- Gastrointestinal dysfunction.
- Increased risk of diabetes mellitus.
- Obstructive sleep apnoea and daytime hypersomnolence.
- In pregnancy: higher miscarriage rate, polyhydramnios, prematurity, failure to progress in labour, postpartum haemorrhage:
  - ⚠ Adverse response to general anaesthetics: (prolonged recovery, aspiration, dysrhythmias).
  - ⚠ May lead to malignant hyperpyrexia.
- Mean age of death 60 years.
- Mortality most commonly due to pneumonia and cardiac dysrhythmias.

### Congenital myotonic dystrophy

There is a risk of congenital myotonic dystrophy in babies born to affected mothers. This is due to gross triplet repeat expansion. Congenital myotonic dystrophy presents with hypotonia, respiratory and feeding difficulties, and has 25% mortality. Surviving children have learning difficulties.

## Treatment

- May require pacemaker.
- May require non-invasive positive pressure ventilation (NIPPV) for obstructive sleep apnoea.
- MedicAlert badge.
- Caution with sedatives, opiates, general anaesthetics.

### Genetic counselling

- Offspring risk of an affected individual is 50%.
- Predictive testing for at-risk relatives is available. Referral to clinical genetics is recommended to discuss implications including psychosocial and insurance issues.

### Surveillance

- Annual ECG, urine dipstick for glucose and optician.
- Ability to drive.

### Differential diagnosis

- Proximal myotonic myopathy (DM2): autosomal dominant, proximal myopathy, muscle pain, mild myotonia.
- Distal myopathies: inclusion body myositis, limb girdle myopathies.
- Congenital non-progressive myotonias: improve with exercise.
- Hyperkalaemic periodic paralysis (also autosomal dominant inheritance).

# 10.12 Friedreich ataxia

## Background

Friedreich ataxia is an autosomal recessive disorder and is the most common inherited ataxia. The dorsal root ganglia, dorsal columns, corticospinal tracts, and heart are predominantly affected.

## Epidemiology

- Incidence: 1/30,000–1/50,000.
- Gender: ♂ = ♀.

## Genetics

- GAA trinucleotide repeat in intron 1 of the *FXN* gene on chromosome 9q: 96% of cases.
- Other inactivating *FXN* gene mutations: 4% of cases.
- Carrier frequency in the general population: 1/65–1/110.
- *FXN* gene mutations cause reduced levels of frataxin.
- This probably causes disease by iron accumulation in mitochondria leading to increased free radicals and cell damage.

## Clinical presentation

- A slowly progressive ataxia.
- Mean age of onset 10–15 years.
- May present in adulthood with milder disease.

## Physical signs

- Dysarthria.
- Spasticity in lower limbs.
- Muscle weakness.
- Absent/reduced lower limb reflexes with extensor plantars.
- Reduction/loss of vibration sense and proprioception (dorsal columns).
- Progressive gait and limb ataxia.
- Pes cavus (Fig. 10.22).
- Scoliosis.
- Optic nerve atrophy.
- Evidence of cardiomyopathy.

## Diagnosis

- Molecular DNA analysis of the *FXN* gene.
- Carrier testing for at-risk relatives and prenatal diagnosis is possible.

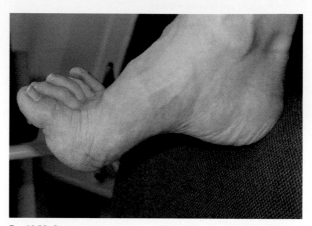

Fig. 10.22 Severe pes cavus in a patient with Friedreich ataxia.

## Complications

- Average age of death is <40 years, most commonly due to cardiomyopathy.
- Diabetes mellitus (30%).

## Treatment

- Prostheses/walking aids/wheelchairs for mobility.
- Speech, occupational, and physical therapy.
- Antispasmodic medication.
- Orthopaedic interventions for scoliosis and foot deformities.
- Consider antiarrhythmic agents and pacemaker insertion.
- Genetic counselling for at-risk family members.

Surveillance includes:
- Bi-annual ECG and echocardiogram.
- Annual monitoring for diabetes mellitus.

Conditions predisposing to pes cavus and/or kyphoscoliosis include:
- Friedreich ataxia
- Hereditary spastic paraplegia
- Charcot–Marie–Tooth disease
- Neurofibromatosis
- Syringomyelia
- Poliomyelitis.

### Differential diagnosis

- Roussy–Levy syndrome: Charcot–Marie–Tooth disease type I with ataxia, tremor, autosomal dominant.
- Spastic paraparesis.
- Spinocerebellar ataxias.
- Ataxia with vitamin E deficiency.

# 10.13 Fragile X syndrome

## Background

Fragile X is the commonest form of inherited learning disorder in males.

## Epidemiology

- Prevalence: 1/5700 ♂ with a full fragile X A (FRAXA) mutation.
- ♂ affected: ♀ are carriers but may be variably affected because of skewed X inactivation.
- There is no maternal age effect but the allele (repeat) expansion is unstable and increases in length in successive generations (anticipation).
- Some individuals carry smaller expansions (see Table 10.1).

## Genetics

### FRAXA

- Fragile X A (FRAXA) is caused by a CGG triplet repeat expansion within the *FMR1* gene on the X chromosome at Xq27.3.
- With full mutations the *FMR1* gene is methylated and no FMR1 protein is translated. Onset of symptoms is earlier in successive generations due to anticipation.
- There is a strong correlation between the amount of fragile X protein (FMRP) made and intellectual function.

## Clinical presentation

*Full mutations in males*

- IQ is significantly reduced in methylated-full mutation ♂ to approximately 41.
- Developmental delay with hypotonia is common.
- Speech and language varies from no speech to mild delay. Rare individuals have normal, fluent, speech.
- Behaviour is characterized by overactivity, impulsiveness, reduced concentration, and poor social interaction, often punctuated by aggression. Autistic spectrum features are common.
- Many children have some degree of minor joint laxity.
- Macrocephaly, large ears.
- Macro-orchidism in adult ♂.

*Full mutations in females*

- ♀ are less affected because the normal X produces FMRP.
- Level of FMRP correlates with IQ.
- Up to 50% of full-mutation ♀ have some learning or behavioural difficulty. Verbal skills tend to be better than physical skills.

| Table 10.1 Allele size in FRAXA | |
|---|---|
| Normal individuals | <45 repeats |
| Intermediate alleles | 45–54 repeats |
| Premutation ♀ and normal transmitting ♂ | 55–200 repeats |
| Affected ♂ and full mutation carrier ♀ | >200 repeats |

## Premutation alleles

- Children with learning problems and premutation alleles should be fully investigated to exclude other causes.
- ♂ and occasionally ♀ may develop a progressive tremor and ataxia syndrome (FXTAS) associated with cerebellar tremor, ataxia, and cerebral atrophy leading to cognitive decline. The prevalence is unknown.
- ♀ with premutations are at risk of premature menopause (~25% stop menstruating by age 40).

## Intermediate alleles

Transmitted intermediate alleles are remarkably stable in the absence of a family history of fragile X. Intermediate alleles may become full mutations in successive generations but by definition, only premutation alleles have the potential to expand to full manifesting mutations across one generation. Nolin et al. (2003) found that ~20% of alleles in the range 49–54 were unstable and could contract or expand.

## Diagnosis

- Molecular DNA analysis of FRAXA repeat size and methylation status.
- Carrier testing for at-risk relatives and prenatal diagnosis is possible.

## Management

- Referral to a developmental paediatrician is essential to plan learning support and community liaison. Some but not all can manage mainstream schools.
- Recurrent otitis media leading to conductive deafness occurs in 60–80% of children.
- Seizures are uncommon (20%) in children.
- Adult life often requires a degree of supported living.

### Genetic counselling

- 50% of ♂ born to carrier ♀ will be at risk of being severely affected.
- Cascade screening of adult members is indicated.
- ♂ with a full mutation or premutation will pass this on to all daughters only. The repeat size is likely to stay stable.
- ♀ with a premutation are at equal risk of it expanding into a full mutation or remaining a premutation.

## Prenatal testing

- Possible by CVS at 12 weeks. Phenotype prediction in a ♀ fetus carrying a full mutation is not possible.

## Reference

Nolin SL. Familial transmission of the fragile X CGG repeat in females with a premutation or intermediate alleles. *Am J Human Genet* 2003; 72: 454–64.

# 10.14 Prader–Willi syndrome

## Background

Prader–Willi syndrome (PWS) is the most recognized form of inherited childhood obesity.

## Epidemiology

- Incidence: 1/10,000–15,000.
- All ethnic groups.
- ♂ = ♀.

## Genetics

- PWS results from a lack of expression of an imprinted **paternal** allele (*SNRPN*) on chromosome 15q11–13.
- This is due to a deletion of the paternal allele (~70%), or maternal origin of both chromosomes 15 (uniparental disomy (UPD), ~25%), or an imprinting centre defect (~5%).
- Imprinting results in inactivation of the maternally-inherited *SNRPN* locus and so normal development is dependent on paternal allele expression.

## Clinical presentation

Clinical features are variable:
- Breech presentation *in utero*.
- Feeding problems in infancy.
- Failure to thrive initially.
- Hyperphagia.
- Truncal obesity.
- Morbid obesity developing between ages 1–6 years.

## Physical signs

- Almond-shaped palpebral fissures.
- Down-turned corners of the mouth.
- Small hands and feet.
- Hypotonia.
- Microcephaly.
- Hypogonadotropic hypogonadism (♂ and ♀).
- Mental disability (IQ evenly distributed around 60).
- Short stature.
- Dental malocclusion (40%).
- Cryptorchidism (80%).
- Labial hypoplasia.
- Micropenis.
- Strabismus (40–95%).

## Diagnosis

- Chromosome (FISH analysis) and DNA diagnosis demonstrating microdeletion of band 15q13–15, UPD, or defective DNA methylation (~5%). Abnormal methylation in the absence of a deletion or UPD is indicative of an imprinting centre defect.
- Methylation analysis of the *SNPRN* locus on chromosome 15q detects 99% of cases of PWS.

## Complications

- Sexual activity is uncommon. Fertility is rare in men and uncommon in women.
- Day time sleepiness is common (50–90%).
- Respiratory problems and sleep apnoea requiring anaesthetic precautions.
- Congestive heart failure due to morbid obesity.
- Diabetes mellitus (15%).
- Older children and adults are often depressed.

## Treatment

- Emphasis is on weight management to avoid morbidity and early mortality.
- Monitoring for cognitive, behavioural, and motor problems.
- Management of strabismus.
- Monitoring for sleep apnoea.
- Most adult patients with PWS require support and few will live independently. Performance in solving mazes or codes is substantially above verbal performance.
- Referral to local child development centre.

### Genetic counselling
- Deletion, UPD, or defective DNA methylation are sporadic events with a low recurrence risk for parents of affected children.
- Imprinting defects have up to a 50% chance of recurrence.
- Prenatal testing is possible at 12 weeks by CVS or later at 16–18 weeks by amniocentesis.
- Affected ♀ have up to 50% risk of having a child with Angelman syndrome, depending on the underlying genetic cause of PWS.

# 10.15 Angelman syndrome

## Background

Angelman syndrome (AS) is a behavioural disorder characterized by seizures, severe developmental delay, absent speech, and ataxia.

## Epidemiology

- Incidence: 1/12,000–40,000.
- All ethnic groups.
- ♂ = ♀.

## Genetics

- AS results from a lack of expression of an imprinted **maternal** allele (*SNRPN*) on chromosome 15q11–13. In PWS, the lack of expression of a paternally inherited allele causes the syndrome (see Section 10.14).
- Normal imprinting results in inactivation of the paternally inherited *SNRPN* locus. Normal development is therefore dependent on maternal allele expression.
- Lack of the required maternal expression results from a deletion of the maternal allele, paternal origin of both chromosomes 15 (UPD), an imprinting centre defect, or a mutation in the E3 ubiquitin protein ligase gene (*UBE3A*).
- Patients with a deletion are the most severely affected whilst UPD and imprinting centre defect patients are the least affected.

## Clinical presentation

- Severe developmental delay.
- Profound speech delay. Many children do not speak more than 3–4 words.
- Seizures.
- Specific behaviour with excitability and inappropriate laughter.
- Movement and balance problems.
- Wide-based ataxic gait.
- Sleep disorder.
- Less commonly, hypopigmentation.

## Physical signs

- Microcephaly
- Jerky gait
- Increased muscle tone
- Down-turned corners of the mouth
- Wide mouth
- Deep-set eyes
- Prominent chin
- Hypotonia
- Happy and sociable affect.

## Diagnosis

- Chromosome (FISH analysis) and DNA diagnosis demonstrating microdeletion of band 15q13–15.
- Most often this is due to a deletion of the maternal allele (~70%); UPD (~2–5%), or an imprinting centre defect (~2–5%). Methylation is abnormal in all three situations.
- Abnormal methylation in the absence of a deletion or UPD is indicative of an imprinting centre defect.
- Methylation analysis of the *SNPRN* locus on chromosome 15q detects ~80% of cases of PWS.
- AS may also result from a mutation in the *UBE3A* gene (20%). Methylation is normal in this case.
- There is only a 44% pick-up rate of *UBE3A* gene mutations in methylation-normal, sporadic cases.
- An EEG may show characteristic 2–3Hz amplitude slow wave bursts said to be typical of AS.

## Complications

- Almost all patients develop seizures (90%) with a deletion, 20% if UPD. Usual onset is by the second year.
- Scoliosis occurs in 40% of adults.
- Loss of mobility and contractures.
- Early motor skills are compromised by ataxia and walking is often delayed until 3–4 years.

## Treatment

- Monitoring for cognitive, behavioural, and motor problems.
- Many children are able to learn some language by sign, e.g. Makaton.
- Most adult patients with AS require close supervision in secure environment.
- Referral to local child development centre.

### Genetic counselling

- An interstitial maternal deletion, UPD, or defective DNA methylation are sporadic events with a low recurrence risk of <1% for parents of affected children.
- Females carrying a *UBE3A* mutation have a 50% risk of AS in each pregnancy. Paternal transmission is silent.
- AS patients without a FISH deletion or UPD can have a recurrence risk as high as 50% due to phenocopy of an abnormal AS gene.
- At-risk family members should be advised if an imprinting centre defect is suspected.
- Prenatal testing is possible at 12 weeks by CVS or later by 16–18 weeks by amniocentesis.

## Background

Ehlers–Danlos syndrome (EDS) is subdivided into several subtypes (types I–VIII) with different inheritance patterns and collagen gene mutations. The most common and/or significant EDS types (I–IV and VI) are described here.

## Epidemiology

- Prevalence: ~1/5000.
- EDS type III (hypermobility) = most common, usually mild.
- EDS type IV = uncommon, but is a serious disorder.

## Genetics

- Classical EDS (types I, II): AD, COL5A1 and COL5A2 gene mutations, encoding type V collagen.
- Hypermobility EDS (type III): AD, gene unknown.
- Vascular EDS (type IV): AD, COL3A1 gene mutations, encoding type III collagen.
- Kyphoscoliosis EDS (type VI): AR, PLOD1 gene mutations causing lysyl hydroxylase deficiency.

## Clinical presentation

Patients may present with:
- Skin: fragility, easy bruising, thin atrophic scars.
- Joints: hypermobility, premature osteoarthritis.
- Intestinal perforation or bladder/uterine/arterial rupture (type IV).

## Physical signs

### Classical EDS (types I, II)
- Skin: soft, thin atrophic scars (Fig. 10.23), bruising.
- Joints: hyperextensible (Fig. 10.24).
- Varicose veins.

### Hypermobility (type III)
- Skin: soft.
- Joints: hyperextensible, recurrent dislocations.

### Vascular (type IV)
- Subcutaneous fat loss.
- Face: pinched nose, thin lips, hollowed cheeks.
- Skin thin and translucent, veins often visible.
- Limited large joint hyperextensibility.

### Kyphoscoliosis (type VI)
- Skin: soft and hyperextensible (Fig. 10.25).
- Joints: hypermobile.
- Muscle hypotonia.
- Scoliosis.

## Diagnosis

- Based on medical history, family history, and clinical features.
- Consider skin biopsy for electron microscopy analysis and fibroblast culture for collagen studies.

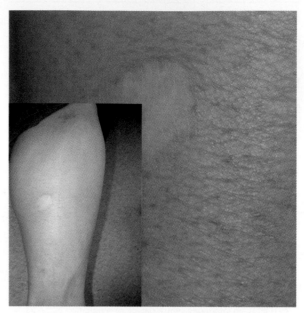

**Fig. 10.23** Typical 'paper' scar in classical EDS. Multiple cutaneous neurofibromata, axillary freckling, and large abdominal scar after removal of a phaeochromocytoma.

- Echocardiogram for mitral valve prolapse and aortic root diameter.
- Genetic testing: mutation analysis is available for vascular EDS (type IV) and kyphoscoliosis EDS (type VI).

## Complications

- Aortic root dilatation (EDS types I, II 33%; type III 20%).
- Premature osteoarthritis.
- Premature labour, postpartum haemorrhage (types I, II).
- Optic globe rupture (type VI).

### EDS type IV
- Uterine, bowel, and arterial rupture.
- Complications occur in at least 25% of individuals after 20 years of age and 80% before 40 years of age.
- Arterial repair not always technically possible.
- Shortened life expectancy, median 48 years.

## Treatment

- There is no specific treatment to alter the progression of EDS.
- Modified management in pregnancy and during labour.

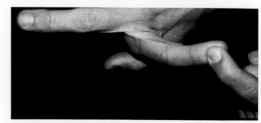

**Fig. 10.24** Hyperextension of joints in EDS.

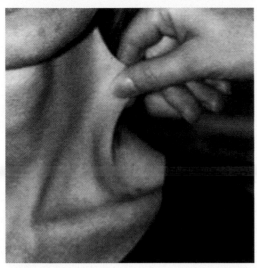

**Fig. 10.25** Skin hyperextension in EDS.

- Offer clinical genetics/counselling advice.
- Physiotherapy.
- Encourage non-weight bearing exercises, e.g. swimming, cycling.
- Genetic counselling.

**Surveillance**
- Varies with different subtypes of EDS.
- Echocardiogram if evidence of aortic root dilatation.
- Blood pressure (EDS IV).

## Differential diagnosis

- Benign joint hypermobility syndrome.
- Cutis laxa: loose skin, abnormality of elastic fibres.
- Marfan syndrome: hypermobile joints, lens dislocation, aortic root dilatation dissection.
- Rare EDS subtypes, e.g. arthrochalasia (type VIIA and B) with congenital hip dislocation; dermatosparaxis (type VIIC) with severe skin fragility; X-linked EDS (type V).

# Chapter 11

# Haematology

## Haematopoiesis

### The stem cell and haematopoietic progenitors

Haematopoietic tissue is characterized by constant and limitless cell turnover. It is estimated that $6 \times 10^9$ new mature blood cells per kilogram of body weight are produced daily in adult marrow and released into the blood circulation, to replace the cells removed or lost. Blood formation relies on haematopoietic stem cells (HSCs) whose frequency is 1–10 per $10^6$ marrow cells. HSCs are characterized by three major properties:

1. Self-renewal capacity.
2. Multilineage differentiation into all blood cells.
3. Capacity to reconstitute haematopoiesis when injected into lethally irradiated recipients.

Differentiation pathways of HSCs into the cellular constituents of blood are outlined in Fig. 11.1.

### The role of the marrow microenvironment

The survival, proliferation, and differentiation of haematopoietic progenitors require an appropriate environment. In normal adults, bone marrow is the organ of haematopoiesis where the extracellular matrix and marrow stroma cells play a major role in the regulation of haematopoiesis.

The cellular compartment of the stroma includes:

1. Mesenchymal stem cells and their progeny (osteoblasts, adipocytes, fibroblasts).
2. Monocyte-derived macrophages and osteoclasts.
3. Vascular endothelial cells.

Stromal cells form discrete cellular spaces, with specialized functions, called '**haematopoietic niches**'. There are three different types of niches:

- The **bony niche**: close to the endosteal regions, is lined with osteoblasts and hosts the primitive HSCs.
- The **stromal niche**: located in more central regions of the marrow, consists of fibroblasts, macrophages, adipocytes, and endothelial cells. It contains haematopoietic progenitors.
- The **adipocyte niche** is the area of yellow marrow and is thought to provide the nutrients for the highly proliferating mature cells.

The fate of haematopoietic progenitor cells regarding cell proliferation, differentiation, and maturation is largely determined by the niche environment. The regulatory mechanisms involve:

- Cell contact interactions, mediated by integrins, selectins, and other adhesion molecules.
- Stimulation by haematopoietic growth factors, cytokines, and chemokines

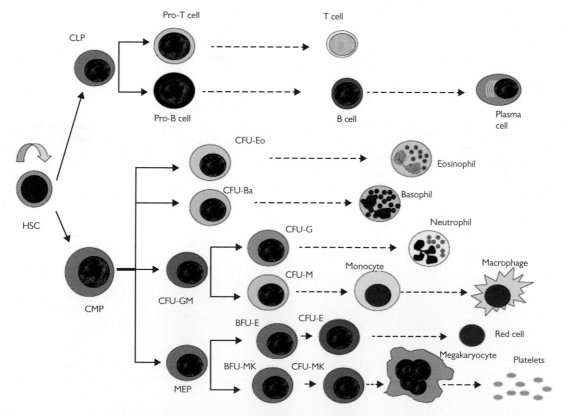

**Fig. 11.1** The first step in HSC differentiation is the production of the common lymphoid precursor (CLP) and the common myeloid precursor (CMP) cells. These precursors retain the capacity for self-renewal, but unlike HSC they are committed to the lymphoid and myeloid lineage, respectively. The first precursors (colony-forming units or CFUs) derived from the differentiation of CLP and CMP also retain self-renewal capacity, but show commitment in the generation of a specific cell lineage. Thus, the CLP gives rise to B-cell precursors and precursors for T cells, NK cells, and lymphoplasmacytoid dendritic cells. The CMP provides granulocyte-monocyte precursor cells (CFU-GM) which can differentiate either into the granulocyte (CFU-G) or monocyte precursor (CFU-M). The CMP also differentiates into the CFU-Bas, the progenitor of basophils, and the CFU-Eo, the progenitor of eosinophils. Finally, the CMP also gives rise to the common precursor of the megakaryocytic and the erythroid lineages (MEP). MEP differentiates into the erythroid (burst forming unit erythroid, BFU-E and CFU-E) and the megakaryocytic precursors (BFU-Meg and CFU-Meg).

## Haematopoietic growth factors

*Erythropoietin (EPO)*

- Glycoprotein hormone produced mainly by peritubular cells of the kidneys. The most important humoral factor in erythropoiesis.
- Hypoxia inducible factor-1 (HIF-1) enhances EPO production in response to hypoxia. CFU-E and the more mature erythroid precursors express EPO receptors (EPO-R), but the intensity of expression declines with maturation.
- EPO prevents apoptosis in erythroid precursors and induces their maturation.
- Other important mediators in erythropoiesis are interleukin 3 (IL-3), IL-6, thrombopoietin, and the stem cell factor (SCF).

## Factors for myelopoiesis

- **Granulocyte-monocyte colony-stimulating factor** (GM-CSF) induces the production and activation of monocytes, granulocytes, and eosinophils
- **Granulocyte colony-stimulating factor** (G-CSF) induces the proliferation and differentiation of granulocyte precursors. G-CSF is used in the clinical setting to increase the number of neutrophils in the peripheral blood and mobilize HSCs into the peripheral blood. It also stimulates chemotaxis, adhesion, and phagocytic activity of neutrophils.
- **Thrombopoietin** (TPO) is a glycoprotein produced in the liver, kidneys, and other tissues. It binds the c-MPL receptors on megakaryocytes and induces proliferation, maturation, and platelet formation. Other important factors in thrombopoiesis are IL-3, IL-6, IL-11, and the leukaemia inhibitory factor (LIF).

## Peripheral blood cells

- **Red blood cells (RBCs)**: are the final stage of erythroid lineage differentiation. The normal RBCs are biconcave discs with a central pallor area, which normally does not exceed one-third of the cell diameter. The mean diameter of RBC is 8μm. RBCs lose their nucleus during the maturation of late erythroblasts, but retain some RNA for the first 1–2 days of their life. These young RBCs are called reticulocytes.
- **Granulocytes** include neutrophils, eosinophils and basophils. Neutrophils have a segmented nucleus and faint pink cytoplasm with fine granules. The cytoplasmic granules contain enzymes such as myeloperoxidase, lysozyme, collagenase, lactoferrin. The main function of neutrophils is phagocytosis and killing of microorganisms. The eosinophils have bilobed nucleus and large eosinophilic granules. Eosinophils are involved in parasitic infections and allergies. The basophils are characterized by large, basophilic cytoplasmic granules, which may obscure the nucleus. They have a role in allergies.
- **Monocytes:** are the largest cells found in a normal blood smear. They circulate in the peripheral blood for a short period of few days and then migrate to tissues and act as phagocytes (known as macrophages after passage through the vascular endothelium). Some monocytes give rise to tissue dendritic cells, which are specialized antigen-presenting cells.

- **Lymphocytes**: they circulate between blood, marrow and lymphoid organs. T cells comprise 70–80%, B cells 5–15%, and NK cells 5–10% of the peripheral blood lymphocytic population.

# Haemoglobin

Haemoglobin (Hb) is the most abundant protein in RBCs.

- Main physiological role is to transfer and release $O_2$ from lungs to peripheral tissues.
- In addition, Hb facilitates $CO_2$ exchange, while free plasma Hb also seems to participate in vascular tone modulation, via interaction with nitric oxide (NO).
- The Hb molecule contains two pairs of polypeptides called globins. Each globin is attached to a haem, a molecule made of protoporphyrin and iron. The iron provides the $O_2$ binding sites.

## Globin genes

Six different types of normal globins participate in Hb synthesis, the α, β, γ, δ, ε, and ζ globins (Table 11.1). The α and γ genes are both duplicated (α1/α2 and Aγ/Gγ).

Hb in a normal adult consists of Hb A (α2β2) 96–97%, Hb A2 (α2δ2) <3.5% and Hb F (α2γ2) 0–1%.

## Affinity for oxygen

The $O_2$ saturation of Hb follows a sigmoid curve pattern in relation to partial pressure of $O_2$ (p$O_2$). Additionally, some other factors may shift the curve towards increased or decreased affinity to $O_2$:

- ↓ pH causes ↓ affinity—right shift (Bohr effect).
- ↑ 2,3-DPG causes ↓ affinity.
- ↑ temperature causes ↓ affinity.
- ↑ $CO_2$ causes ↓ affinity.
- Some haemoglobinopathies have ↑ or ↓ affinity.
- Pyruvate kinase deficiency causes ↓ affinity (indirectly through ↑ 2,3-DPG).

# Haemostasis

Haemostasis is the prevention of blood loss after vascular injury. The mechanisms of haemostasis involve blood vessels, platelets, and the coagulation cascade. The first step after injury is vasoconstriction, immediately followed by platelet plug formation on the damaged endothelium. The activation of the coagulation cascade results in fibrin production, which stabilizes the plug and forms the fibrin clot. Haemostasis is a strictly balanced and regulated process and failures may result in haemorrhage or thrombosis.

## The vessel

The vascular endothelial cell has a significant role in the regulation of vascular tone, platelet activation, and coagulation cascade. Vascular endothelial cells produce several anticoagulants to prevent thrombosis on the intact vessel:

- Prostacyclin and NO are both vasodilators produced by the endothelial cells and block platelet adhesion and activation.

Table 11.1 Haemoglobins during development. Different globin genes are expressed in humans during embryonic, fetal, and adult life, resulting in different Hb molecules. This diversity serves the particular requirements for $O_2$ delivery in different developmental stages. Embryonic Hbs and fetal Hb (Hb F) have a higher $O_2$ affinity to enable placental $O_2$ transfer from the maternal to fetal circulation

| Phase | Site of erythropoiesis | Globin genes expressed | Hb molecules |
|---|---|---|---|
| 0–8 weeks | Yolk sac | ζ and ε Later α and γ appear | Hb Gower-1 (ζ2ε2) Hb Portland (ζ2γ2) and Gower-2 (α2ε2) |
| 8–20 weeks | Fetal liver | α and γ | Fetal Hb F (α2γ2) |
| After 20th week | Fetal spleen | α and β | Adult Hb A (α2β2) starts to appear |
| From 35th week | Fetal spleen | α and δ | Hb A2 (α2δ2) appears, but remains at low levels throughout fetal and adult life |
| After birth | Bone marrow | Mainly α and β | Hb A replaces Hb F almost completely within first 30 weeks of postnatal life |

- Surface CD39 digests ADP, hence blocking platelet activation.
- Thrombomodulin is expressed on the endothelial surface and participates in activation of protein C.
- The endothelial cells are also a source of tissue factor pathway inhibitor (TFPI).

On the other hand, endothelial cells produce prothrombotic molecules such as von Willebrand factor (VWF). Finally, endothelial cells are involved in fibrinolysis, producing proteins such as the tissue-type plasminogen activator.

### The platelets

Platelets are small (mean diameter 1.5–3µm), anuclear cytoplasmic fragments of the mature megakaryocytes. They circulate in the peripheral blood for only 8–12 days, because of their limited synthetic capacity.

Following vascular damage, platelets adhere and aggregate on exposed collagen forming a plug, which helps to control haemorrhage, but most importantly facilitates the generation of thrombin. Platelets have an important haemostatic role in arterial vessels and the microvasculature, where the high shear flow conditions create an optimal environment for their activation. VWF binds both exposed vascular collagen and platelet glycoproteins GPIb and GPIIb/IIIa and mediates platelet vascular adhesion and aggregation. The platelets initially form a monolayer on the damaged endothelium, change their shape, degranulate, and release molecules with important roles in further aggregation and plug formation including VWF, thromboxanes, thrombin, calcium, and ADP. The platelet membrane provides a phospholipid surface on which the coagulation reactions occur.

### The coagulation factors

Coagulation factors include:

- Proenzymes: they are converted into their active enzyme at certain stages of coagulation (prothrombin, factors XII, XI, VII, IX, X, prokallikrein, protein C, and factor XIII).
- Co-factors (tissue factor (TF), high-molecular-weight kininogen (HMWK), factor V, protein S).
- Normal inhibitors (antithrombin, protein C, TFPI).

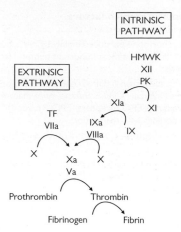

**Fig. 11.2** Cascade model of coagulation pathways.

- Fibrinogen: cleaved by thrombin to produce fibrin.

Prothrombin, factors VII, IX, X, and proteins C and S require vitamin K for their synthesis.

The classical concept of coagulation cascade describes two reaction pathways which appear to occur independently and meet in a common pathway ending in the generation of thrombin (Fig. 11.2).

Although the cascade model offers a good understanding of coagulation and is useful in the laboratory diagnostic approach, it cannot explain several *in vivo* aspects of the haemostatic process. A newer, cell-based model suggests that coagulation occurs on cell membranes, at the site of endothelial injury (Fig. 11.3). The cell-based model of coagulation offers a more rational explanation of clinical aspects, such as the bleeding tendency in haemophilia (lack of factor VIII or IX).

**Inhibitors of coagulation:** required to prevent uncontrolled thrombin generation, after initiation of the cascade.

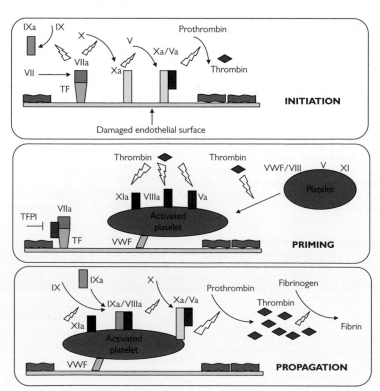

**Fig. 11.3** Cell-based model of coagulation.

- Protein C is a proenzyme, which is converted to activated protein C (APC) by thrombomodulin-bound thrombin. APC and its co-factor protein S inactivate factors Va and VIIIa and control further thrombin generation.
- Antithrombin is a serine protease with inhibitory activity against thrombin and factors Xa, IXa, XIa, and XIIa. Heparin enhances significantly the antithrombin activity.
- TFPI is an inhibitor of TF/VIIa complex.

## Fibrinolysis

The fibrinolytic system degrades fibrin when it is no longer needed, and ensures clot dissolution and a patent vessel lumen.

The proenzyme plasminogen can be converted into plasmin by two activators: tissue-type plasminogen activator (tPA) and urokinase-type plasminogen activator (uPA). Plasmin degrades fibrin into Y, D, and E fragments. The D fragments are linked with one E fragment to form D-dimers. Laboratory assays detect and quantify D-dimers in the plasma and are used in the clinical evaluation of conditions with active thrombosis and fibrinolysis, such as disseminated intravascular coagulation. Two plasminogen activator inhibitors (PAI-1 and PAI-2) counteract plasmin formation and $\alpha$2-antiplasmin binds the enzyme itself and deactivates it.

## The intrinsic pathway

- Starts with the activation of factor XI by HMWK, prekallikrein, and factor XII on negatively charged surfaces.
- In the presence of $Ca^{2+}$, factor XIa generates IXa from its proenzyme.
- Factors IXa and VIIIa form the tenase complex (IXa/VIIIa) with strong catalytic activity on factor X, in the presence of phospholipids and $Ca^{2+}$, producing Xa.
- The factors Xa and Va complex (prothrombinase) finally converts the prothrombin to thrombin.

- The activated partial thromboplastin time (aPTT) uses kaolin as negatively charged surface and added phospholipids to activate the cascade. aPTT is the preferable test to evaluate the intrinsic pathway.

## The extrinsic pathway

- Requires the presence of tissue factor (TF), which forms a complex with factor VIIa (TF/VIIa).
- This complex can activate factor X in the presence of $Ca^{2+}$ and in this stage the two pathways meet. Additionally, factor Xa can convert more factor VII to VIIa.
- The prothrombin time (PT) test uses exogenous TF to activate the cascade and is the preferable test to evaluate the extrinsic pathway.

Three overlapping phases are recognized (Fig. 11.3).

- **Initiation phase**: endothelial injury exposes TF to plasma. Factor VII binds TF and is activated to form the TF/VIIa complex. The TF/VIIa activates factors IX and X. If Xa leaves, the site of injury is rapidly deactivated. Some Xa remains on site and activates factor V on the vascular surface. At this point, the Xa/Va complex (prothrombinase) is able to convert small amounts of prothrombin to thrombin.
- **Priming phase**: thrombin produced in priming phase adheres to platelets, further activating them and the factors VIII, V, and XI on the platelet surface.
- **Propagation phase:** factor IXa produced by TF/VIIa and factor XIa, forms the tenase complex with VIIIa on the platelet surface and induce significant activation of factor X. This creates the prothrombinase complex (Xa/Va) resulting in a burst of thrombin generation and sufficient fibrin production to produce fibrin clot.

# 11.2 Anaemia

## Background

Anaemia can be defined as a condition of low red blood cell (RBC) mass and insufficient oxygen delivery to peripheral tissues. The routine measurement of the RBC mass is impractical. Therefore, the Hb concentration, haematocrit (Hct), and the RBC count are used for the assessment of anaemia. These parameters are provided by automated analysers together with the RBC indices, which are useful for the investigation of anaemia. The mean corpuscular volume (MCV), Hb, and RBC count are measured directly and used for the calculation of Hct, mean cell Hb (MCH), and mean cell haemoglobin concentration (MCHC). The RBC distribution width (RDW) provides an estimation of the RBC size variation. The use of Hb, Hct and RBC count has some limitations and does not always predict precisely the RBC mass. For instance, low plasma volume or acute blood loss may produce normal values for Hb, Hct, and RBC count and mask the presence of anaemia.

## Approach to anaemia

### History and clinical examination

- Symptoms arise either from the underlying condition or from tissue hypoxia and the additional cardiovascular and pulmonary effort needed to compensate for the anaemia.
- The degree of anaemia and the period of time it takes to develop dictate the severity of symptoms.
- Mild to moderate anaemia may not produce any symptoms, especially in young adults.
- Severe anaemia usually presents with fatigue, exertional dyspnoea, and palpitations. Tachycardia, dizziness, and loss of consciousness may occur with acute anaemia.
- Chronic anaemia may present with headache, vertigo, drowsiness, angina, impaired mental function, or even abnormal behaviour.
- Pallor is a feature of anaemia—most prominent on the oral mucosa. Jaundice, ecchymoses, petechiae, hair loss, thin and fragile nails, leg ulcers, cheilitis, and glossitis are other important findings in the skin and the mucosa.
- The family history, dietary habits, fever, bleeding or bruising history, and exposure to occupational hazards are important aspects in the investigation of anaemia.
- Dysphagia, gastrointestinal bleeding, haematuria, hepatomegaly, splenomegaly, and lymph node enlargement may also help to elucidate the cause of anaemia.

### Aetiology of anaemia

Normal RBCs have a lifespan of 100–120 days following release into the peripheral blood. After this period, they are removed from the circulation and replaced by young cells. Marrow erythropoiesis allows for normal RBC loss and can also compensate for small amounts of chronic blood loss, provided adequate nutrients are available to sustain the generation of new cells. Anaemia will develop when:

- There is acute or chronic blood loss of significant amount (haemorrhage).
- The rate of RBC destruction is increased, i.e. there is significant decrease of the normal lifespan of RBCs (haemolytic anaemia).
- Marrow erythropoiesis is insufficient due to nutritional deficiencies, marrow infiltration (leukaemia, lymphoma, metastatic carcinoma, or fibrosis), marrow hypoplasia, marrow dysplasia, and systemic diseases.

### Laboratory approach to anaemia

Anaemia + abnormal white blood cell (WBC) count and platelet count is suggestive of bone marrow pathology. Cytopenia is associated with marrow infiltration, myelodysplasia, or aplastic anaemia.

Apart from these parameters, examination of the reticulocyte count and the RBC indices is fundamental in the assessment of anaemia.

**The reticulocyte count** provides information on the rate of RBC replacement by young cells. Normally, about 1% of the RBCs are replaced by reticulocytes daily. Thus, the normal reticulocyte count ranges from 0.5–2% or $25–100 \times 10^9$/L.

- An **increased reticulocyte count** represents increased marrow erythropoiesis. It can be found after blood loss, in successful replacement therapy with iron or folate/vitamin B$_{12}$, and in haemolytic anaemias.
- An inappropriately **low reticulocyte count** usually represents impaired erythropoiesis.

**The MCV** reflects the average RBC size. Anaemia can be classified according to MCV values as:

- Microcytic (MCV <80fL).
- Normocytic (MCV 80–99fL).
- Macrocytic (MCV ≥100fL).

(Exact ranges may vary between laboratories.)

The combination of MCV, reticulocyte count, and RDW facilitates the diagnosis of anaemia (Fig. 11.4).

Examination of the **peripheral blood smear** (Fig. 11.5) reveals morphological features of the RBCs that cannot be deduced from the RBC indices. This may suggest the exact diagnosis, and also provides information on the WBC and platelet morphology.

**Bone marrow biopsy** may be indicated if abnormalities from the other cell lineages are found.

## Iron metabolism

Iron is an essential element for enzymes involved in several metabolic processes (cytochromes, catalases, peroxidases). It is also necessary for the oxygen carrier molecules, namely haemoglobin and myoglobin. The total amount of body iron in adults is 2–3g and most of it is used by the RBCs and the erythroid precursors. The marrow macrophages offer most of the iron needed for the daily erythropoiesis. This iron derives from the aged, phagocytosed RBCs. Small amounts of iron (1–2mg) lost daily—through menstruation and epithelial apoptosis—are replaced from dietary intake.

Excess of unbound iron leads to free radical production and is toxic for the cells. Therefore, the iron intestinal absorption, transport, cellular intake, and storage are strictly regulated by a series of complex mechanisms (Fig. 11.6).

Ferritin, a multimeric polypeptide, binds iron and controls its release, protecting the cell from the free iron toxicity. Haemosiderin is a compound of degraded ferritin and organelles, unable to mobilize iron effectively. The liver is the organ with the largest iron storage capacity, while significant amounts are found in the myocardium and the skeletal muscles.

## Microcytic anaemia

The microcytic anaemias result from reduced haemoglobin synthesis, most commonly due to iron deficiency. Other conditions with microcytic anaemia include the thalassaemias, lead poisoning, and congenital sideroblastic anaemias.

### Iron deficiency anaemia
*Epidemiology*

- Iron deficiency is the most common nutritional deficiency, affecting a large but variable portion of the population, depending on age, sex, and dietary habits.
- The prevalence in young men is around 1% and increases in up to 4% with aging.
- More common in young, menstruating teenagers and women (5–11%), infants (9%), and in pregnancy.

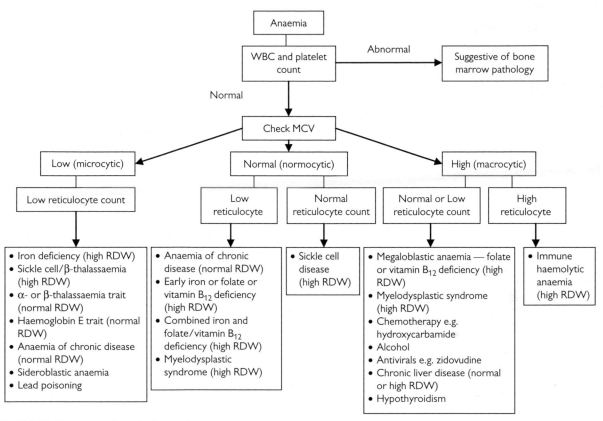

Fig. 11.4 Decision tree for diagnosis of anaemia.

- Prevalence also higher in social groups living in chronic poverty and in the developing world.

*Aetiology*

The iron deficiency arises from increased blood loss, pregnancy, rapid growth, or inadequate iron intake:

**Blood loss** is the most common cause. The finding of iron deficiency should always initiate investigation to unveil the underlying disease. The blood loss may arise from:

- The gastrointestinal tract: haemorrhoids, duodenal or gastric ulcers, gastritis, oesophageal hernia, diverticuli, schistosomiasis, carcinoma (most typically of the caecum).
- Menstruation: the most common cause for young women.
- Massive haemorrhage.

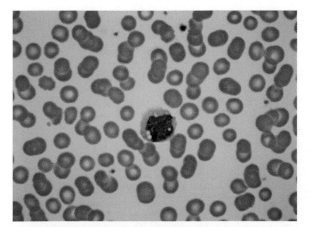

Fig. 11.5 Normal red cells and a monocyte.
Image supplied courtesy of Professor Barbara Bain.

- Haematuria and haemoglobinuria: paroxysmal nocturnal haemoglobinuria, prosthetic heart valves.
- Blood donation.
- Iatrogenic: repeated blood tests in inpatients, especially in ICUs.

**Pregnancy** requires ~1000mg additional iron for normal fetal development and the expansion of the maternal total RBC mass and plasma volume. Iron deficiency develops in 30–50% of mothers in Western countries and ≤80% in the developing world. The iron loss in lactation is 1–2mg daily.

**Growth** requires increased iron requirements, particularly in premature infants and young teenagers

**Inadequate iron intake** is usually related to poor diet (poverty), impaired absorption due to gastrectomy or achlorhydria (atrophic gastritis), or malabsorption due to coeliac disease, which should always be considered in refractory or recurrent iron deficiency or where there is more than one haematinic deficiency.

*Clinical features*

Three stages are recognized during depletion of iron stores and development of anaemia:

1. Iron stores in liver and bone marrow are depleted, but still enough iron to sustain erythropoiesis with normal Hb levels. The ferritin levels are low.

2. Decrease in transferrin saturation plus a few microcytes in the blood smear. Hb is not below normal and the MCV is not low. Some patients at this stage may already complain of tiredness.

3. Anaemia, microcytosis, and hypochromia.

**Symptoms** result from the anaemia and from the epithelial cell damage, due to insufficiency of several enzymes.

- Fatigue (the most common reason to check Hb).
- Weakness.
- Irritability, abnormal behaviour.
- Dysphagia with pharyngeal or oesophageal webs (Plummer–Vinson syndrome).

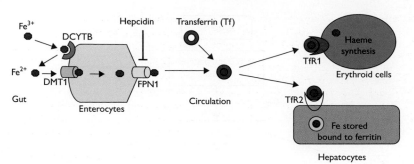

**Fig. 11.6** Overview of iron metabolism.

DCYTB (duodenal cytochrome B) catalyses reduction of $Fe^{3+}$ to $Fe^{2+}$.

DMT1 is divalent metal transporter 1.

FPN1 (ferroportin-1) is negatively regulated by hepcidin, an antimicrobial peptide, recently shown to be an important negative regulator of iron transporters. The haemochromatosis gene product (HFE) is among the proteins that affect hepcidin and indirectly control cell iron intake. HFE mutations are related to inappropriate iron uptake and are a cause of hereditary haemochromatosis.

TfR1 (transferrin receptor 1) is expressed on erythroid cells; TfR2 is expressed on hepatocytes. The expression of TfRs and other proteins involved in iron metabolism is regulated at translational (mRNA) level by iron responsive proteins (IRPs). In iron-deplete conditions, IRPs bind to the iron translation elements (IREs) of the mRNA molecules and induce translation of the protein. The presence of iron prevents IRPs from binding to IREs.

**Pica syndrome**: very rare, abnormal eating behaviour, characteristic of iron deficiency anaemia. Patients tend to eat ice, paper, chalk, or other bizarre items.

**Signs:**
- Pallor when Hb <9g/dL.
- Thin, fragile nails, koilonychia (spoon-like nails).
- Angular cheilitis, stomatitis.
- Sore tongue with papillary atrophy.
- Retinal haemorrhages.
- Impaired growth in infancy.

*Laboratory findings*

Depend on the severity of iron deficiency and anaemia. The **FBC and the blood film** (Fig. 11.7) reveal:
- Low reticulocyte count.
- Microcytosis and hypochromia (low MCV, MCH, MCHC).
- Anisocytosis is an early finding (high RDW).
- Poikilocytosis with pencil cells, tiny microcytes, elliptocytes.
- Thrombocytosis is common.

Bone marrow examination:
- Confirms empty iron stores and sideroblasts (erythroid precursors with iron granules) <10%.

Biochemical iron metabolism studies reveal:
- Low serum iron.

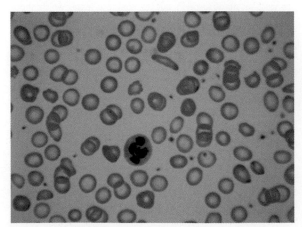

**Fig. 11.7** Blood film in iron deficiency anaemia: microcytosis, hypochromia, anisocytosis, and poikilocytosis.

Image supplied courtesy of Professor Barbara Bain.

- The total iron binding capacity (TIBC) is increased.
- The ratio of iron/TIBC gives the iron saturation, which is <16% in iron deficiency anaemia.
- Very low serum ferritin: best single predictor of body iron (but can be elevated as part of acute phase response).
- The serum soluble transferrin receptor (TfR) is significantly elevated.

*Treatment*
- Investigation and treatment of any underlying disease.
- Oral iron supplementation (1.5–2mg/kg of elementary iron daily), aiming to replenish the iron stores.

Patients with severe symptomatic anaemia, intolerance of oral iron, impaired absorption, or continuous significant blood loss may require intravenous iron therapy.

## Megaloblastic anaemia

The most common of the macrocytic anaemias (MCV >100fL), it is caused by impaired purine and pyrimidine synthesis due to folate and/or vitamin $B_{12}$ deficiency. DNA does not replicate but protein synthesis, including Hb synthesis, is preserved. This asynchrony of maturation between the nucleus and the cytoplasm is the essential feature of megaloblastic erythropoiesis but it also affects myelopoiesis.

### Pathophysiology

**Folate** coenzymes transfer single-carbon units during purine and pyrimidine synthesis. Methylenetetrahydrofolate (methylTHF) is required for the methylation of deoxyuridylate to thymidylate by thymidylate synthetase, a necessary step in the DNA synthesis.

**Vitamin $B_{12}$** is required for at least two reactions:
1. Methylation of homocysteine to methionine by methionine synthetase, also dependant on folate. Thus, vitamin $B_{12}$ deficiency disturbs folate metabolism.
2. Conversion of the methylmalonyl CoA to succinyl CoA by the enzyme methylmalonyl CoA synthetase.

Therefore, folate deficiency and indirectly vitamin $B_{12}$ deficiency impair DNA synthesis.

### Aetiology

**Vitamin $B_{12}$** is found only in foods of animal origin.
- Average daily intake = 5mcg, requirement = 2.4mcg.
- Body stores are 3–5mg (several years supply).
- Deficiency of vitamin $B_{12}$ usually results from impaired absorption—unlikely to occur through poor dietary intake (except in vegans).

Vitamin $B_{12}$ requires the R-binder protein, found in the saliva and gastric fluid, for its passage through the stomach. It is released from the

R-binder by pancreatic enzymes in the alkaline environment of the duodenum/jejunum. It then binds to intrinsic factor (IF), a protein produced by the gastric parietal cells, and travels to the distal ileum in complex with IF, where it is finally absorbed.

The most common causes of vitamin $B_{12}$ deficiency are:

- **Pernicious anaemia**: immune-mediated disorder with gastric atrophy and lack of IF. Coexists with other autoimmune disorders (e.g. Addison disease, Sjögren syndrome, Graves disease), increased risk of gastric carcinoma.
- Total or partial gastrectomy.
- Pancreatic insufficiency.
- Zollinger–Ellison syndrome.
- Abnormal intestinal flora: bacterial overgrowth in blind loop syndrome, rarely fish tapeworm.
- Crohn disease.
- Rare inherited disorders of the vitamin $B_{12}$ protein carriers.

**Folate** is found mostly in vegetables and the body stores are more readily depleted. Folate deficiency can occur from both poor dietary intake and impaired absorption. The most common causes are:

- Poor diet.
- Alcohol abuse.
- Malabsorption in coeliac disease, tropical sprue, Crohn disease.
- Increased requirements in pregnancy and chronic haemolytic anaemias.
- Drugs: anticonvulsants.

### Clinical features

- The inability of the erythroid precursors to mature normally results in **ineffective erythropoiesis**, a condition of erythroid hyperplasia with early cell destruction and mild haemolysis. The slightly increased levels of bilirubin together with pallor give the typical **lemon yellow skin** colour seen in patients with megaloblastic anaemia. Cheilitis, glossitis, and spontaneous bruising are also typical.
- Apart from megaloblastic anaemia, vitamin $B_{12}$ deficiency presents with neurological manifestations, including sensory neuropathy, loss of tendon reflexes, ataxia, gait disturbances, optic neuritis and visual changes, cognitive and emotional changes, lethargy, seizures, and dementia. Patients can occasionally develop neuropathy with normal FBC.
- Folate deficiency rarely causes neurological dysfunction, although folate deficiency in pregnancy may be responsible for severe neural tube defects (anencephaly and spina bifida).
- However, most cases are now detected early with minimal clinical features.

### Laboratory features

The characteristic findings of megaloblastic anaemia in the peripheral blood (Fig. 11.8) are:

- Increased MCV (often >110fL) and macrocytosis. Both may precede the presentation of anaemia.

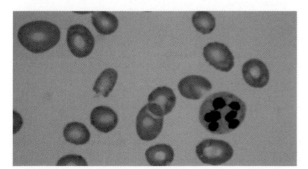

**Fig. 11.8** Hypersegmented neutrophil, macrocytosis, oval macrocytes and basophilic stippling in vitamin $B_{12}$ deficiency.
Image supplied courtesy of Professor Barbara Bain.

- Low reticulocyte count.
- Anisocytosis (high RDW).
- Poikilocytosis with tear-drop cells, oval cells, fragmentation, and nucleated RBCs especially in advanced anaemia.
- Howell–Jolly bodies.
- Cabot rings in the RBCs.
- **Hypersegmented neutrophils**.

The marrow is hypercellular with relative increase of the early erythroid over the myeloid precursors. Megaloblastic changes affect all three lineages:

- Erythroblasts: **asynchrony of nuclear and cytoplasmic maturation** with loose, open chromatin and well-matured and haemoglobinized cytoplasm. Nuclear bridges, binuclear cells, and karyorrhexis are also seen.
- **Giant metamyelocytes**.
- Abnormal nuclear maturation of the megakaryocytes.

Biochemical studies reveal:

- High lactate dehydrogenase (LDH).
- Low serum vitamin $B_{12}$ and/or low folate.
- High homocysteine.

### Other investigations

- **Schilling test** can identify whether low $B_{12}$ is due to malabsorption or lack of IF: radioactive $B_{12}$ is given ± IF; if urinary excretion is greater when co-administered with IF, then IF deficiency is likely.
- Antibodies to gastric parietal cells and IF (the latter more specific) in pernicious anaemia.

### Treatment

- Usually only the deficient vitamin is given.
- Vitamin $B_{12}$ injections: hydroxocobalamin 1mg IM 3× week for 2 weeks, then 1mg every 3 months.
- Folate is given orally 1–5mg daily.

The reticulocyte count increases after 2–3 days, and the anaemia completely resolves by 8 weeks. However, any neurological dysfunction can take >6 months to resolve and some severe changes may be irreversible.

## Haemolytic anaemia

Haemolysis is the premature destruction of the RBCs with a decrease of their normal life-span (100–120 days). Haemolytic anaemia develops when the bone marrow is unable to compensate for the RBC loss.

Haemolytic anaemia is caused by:

- Hereditary disorders:
  - RBC membrane disorders
  - Enzymopathies
  - Haemoglobinopathies
- Acquired disorders:
  - Immune haemolysis
  - Hypersplenism
  - Non-immune RBC destruction
  - Paroxysmal nocturnal haemoglobinuria

Clinical and laboratory features depend largely on the aetiology and the possible underlying disease (extravascular vs. intravascular or immune vs. non-immune). Generally, the haemolytic anaemias are characterized by:

- Increased reticulocyte count, LDH, and bilirubin.
- Haptoglobulin is very low.
- Blood film may reveal RBC morphological abnormalities, including polychromasia (high reticulocyte count), spherocytosis, and fragmentation, depending on the cause.

# Hereditary haemolytic anaemias

## Hereditary spherocytosis (HS)

An inherited RBC membrane disorder characterized by anaemia, jaundice, splenomegaly, and correction of the anaemia after splenectomy.

### Epidemiology

- Prevalence = 1 per 5000.
- The most common type of hereditary haemolytic anaemia.
- Positive family history in 75%; important for diagnosis.
- Usually AD, less commonly AR.

### Pathogenesis

HS results from mutations affecting proteins with a structural role in the erythrocyte membrane: spectrin, ankyrin, band 3, and protein 4.2. Affected RBCs have a destabilized surface lipid bilayer. During their passage through the spleen they lose part of their surface and become spherocytes. After repeated passages and further membrane loss, they are finally phagocytosed by the splenic macrophages.

### Clinical features

- Variable clinical severity from asymptomatic carriers to severe haemolytic anaemia.
- Patients with mild forms of HS have only increased reticulocytes, spherocytes in the blood smear, and normal Hb. The diagnosis may escape until very late in adulthood, when usually **splenomegaly or cholelithiasis** is found.
- Moderate HS is the most common type (60–70%), presenting with **anaemia**, splenomegaly (75%), and gallstones (60%). Jaundice is not a constant finding. Degree of anaemia depends on the severity of haemolysis and the spleen size. Pregnancy may exaggerate haemolysis so that blood transfusions are needed. Patients may also experience aplastic crises after infection with parvovirus B19.
- Severe HS is uncommon and diagnosed early in life. It may present with **neonatal jaundice** requiring exchange transfusion or even with hydrops fetalis.

### Laboratory findings

- Anaemia with high reticulocyte count.
- Spherocytes and/or microspherocytes (Fig. 11.9).
- Anisocytosis (high RDW).
- High MCHC, usually normal MCV.
- Negative DAT (direct antiglobulin test).
- Abnormal osmotic fragility test (80–90%).
- Marrow: erythroid hyperplasia.

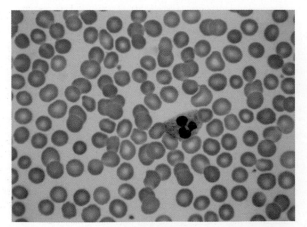

**Fig. 11.9** Hereditary spherocytosis: moderate numbers of spherocytes. Image supplied courtesy of Professor Barbara Bain.

### Diagnosis

The diagnosis usually relies on typical clinical features, positive family history, and laboratory testing. When the presentation of HS is atypical, exclusion of other types of haemolytic anaemia and studies of RBC membrane proteins using gel electrophoresis may be required.

### Treatment

- Folate replacement therapy is recommended, at least for moderate and severe HS.
- Splenectomy depends on symptom severity. It is indicated for all children with severe HS, where it significantly controls the symptoms, the incidence of cholelithiasis, blood transfusion requirements, and growth impairment. Splenectomy is also indicated in many cases of moderate HS, but in few cases of mild HS. In these patients anaemia and symptoms resolve completely. The main drawback of splenectomy is the life-threatening infections from *Streptococcus pneumoniae* or other encapsulated organisms. For this reason, splenectomy should be delayed until the age of 5 years and combined with pre-operative vaccination and lifelong antibiotic prophylaxis.

## Hereditary elliptocytosis (HE)

- A clinically heterogeneous group of RBC membrane disorders, characterized by the presence of elliptocytes (oval-shaped or elongated RBC) in the blood smear.
- HE results from genetic defects of spectrin (60%), protein 4.1, and glycophorin C.
- Estimated prevalence is 1 per 5000, but it is significantly higher in endemic areas of malaria.
- The **common form of HE** is an AD condition, usually diagnosed when elliptocytes are found incidentally in a routine blood test. It rarely causes mild haemolysis, and elliptocytosis (15–90% of the RBCs) is the only finding. It is a benign condition and does not require treatment.
- Homozygous or double heterozygous HE may produce chronic haemolytic anaemia of variable severity.
- Similarly, **hereditary pyropoikilocytosis** is a cause of severe haemolytic anaemia. Osmotic fragility test may be abnormal in these severe forms. Splenectomy improves Hb levels.

## Pyruvate kinase (PK) deficiency

- Common cause of non-spherocytic, hereditary haemolytic anaemia.
- AR: >150 mutations described to date in PK deficiency.
- Estimated prevalence 1:20,000 in Caucasian population.
- PK catalyses the conversion of phosphoenolpyruvate to pyruvate, a glycolytic reaction which provides the RBC with ATP. Blockage of the reaction leads to 2,3-DPG accumulation with right shift of the haemoglobin saturation curve and finally to ATP depletion and haemolysis.
- Clinical manifestations of variable severity develop in the homozygous and the double heterozygous conditions. Severe forms of PK deficiency present with neonatal jaundice, requiring exchange transfusion, and rarely with hydrops fetalis. The phenotype of PK deficiency becomes milder with ageing during childhood and constant in adult life. The patients are susceptible to aplastic crisis after infection with parvovirus B19.
- Common lab findings:
  - Anaemia (Hb 6–12g/dL), with high reticulocyte count, poikilocytosis, acanthocytosis, anisocytosis, and nucleated RBCs.
  - High unconjugated bilirubin and LDH.
- Folate supplementation is needed in significant chronic haemolysis. Splenectomy may improve the Hb levels in severe forms of PKD.

## Glucose-6-phosphate dehydrogenenase (G6PD) deficiency

An X-linked (Xq28) inherited cause of haemolytic anaemia, affecting more than 400 million people worldwide.

### Pathophysiology

The RBCs depend on G6PD for the generation of reduced glutathione (GSH), a molecule that protects the cell from oxidative damage. G6PD deficiency results in accumulation of oxidants under stress conditions, oxidation of haemoglobin and other cellular proteins, and finally haemolysis. The oxidation of haemoglobin reduces its solubility and creates intracellular precipitations, called **Heinz bodies**.

### Genetics

Men have only one G6PD gene, and will thus suffer from this disorder. Heterozygous females have half the enzyme activity, but may be affected due to random X-inactivation of the second gene in the female embryo, or if homozygous.

The wild-type enzyme is G6PD B. More than 400 variants with different degrees of enzymatic deficiency and haemolysis have been described and classified into five classes.

- The G6PD A− variant is found in 10–15% of African Americans and causes moderate haemolysis (class III).
- The Mediterranean G6PD variant affects the white population of the Mediterranean basin and causes moderate to severe haemolysis (class II).
- Class I variants are uncommon and occur across all populations. They cause severe enzymatic deficiency (<10% of normal) and significant haemolysis.

### Clinical manifestations

- **Acute haemolytic episodes** following exposure to certain conditions of oxidative stress characterize G6PD A− and the Mediterranean variant. Patients present with pallor, jaundice, and haemoglobinuria (dark urine). Laboratory testing confirms severe anaemia, increased reticulocytes with microspherocytes, RBC fragmentation, and Heinz bodies in the blood smear. LDH and unconjugated bilirubin are elevated, haptoglobulins low, and the DAT negative. The diagnosis of G6PD deficiency is confirmed using functional enzymatic assays.
- Conditions of oxidative stress that induce haemolysis in G6PD deficiency include **infections**, **drugs** (e.g. primaquine in G6PD A−), **diabetic acidosis**, and **favism** (consumption of fava beans). **Neonatal jaundice** develops in the Mediterranean and the class I variants.
- **Chronic non-spherocytic haemolytic anaemia** in steady-state (absence of oxidative stress) occurs in the severe class I variants.

### Management

- Patients with G6PD A− and the Mediterranean variant should avoid drugs and conditions that trigger haemolytic episodes.
- Neonatal jaundice may require phototherapy or exchange transfusion.
- The rare cases of chronic haemolytic anaemia may need folate supplementation and occasionally blood transfusion. Splenectomy has not been proved beneficial in this group of patients.

## Immune haemolytic anaemia

Immune haemolytic anaemia (IHA) is caused by IgG and/or IgM antibodies against RBC antigens, which trigger complement and/or reticuloendothelial system macrophage-mediated haemolysis.

IHA can be classified into:

- Autoimmune haemolytic anaemia (AIHA): antibodies are directed against self-antigens.
- Alloimmune haemolytic anaemia: previous exposure to allogeneic RBCs is needed. This usually occurs after blood transfusions, pregnancy and transplantation. The alloantibodies do not recognized self-antigens. The main forms of alloimmune haemolytic anaemia are haemolytic transfusion reactions and haemolytic disease of the newborn.
- Drug-induced haemolysis.

Regardless of the type of IHA, the mechanisms of RBC destruction are similar:

- RBCs coated with IgG antibodies (especially IgG1 and IgG3) are recognized by the Fc receptors of the splenic macrophages and phagocytosed.
- A heavy coat of IgG also activates complement, thus C3b also binds the RBCs. This enhances phagocytosis by Kupffer cells in the liver, which express complement receptors.
- If IgM mediated, although macrophages lack IgM Fc receptors, IgM strongly activates the classical pathway of complement and the coated RBCs are destroyed in the liver.
- Additionally, intense complement activation may overcome the protection offered to RBCs by the surface regulatory proteins CD55 and CD59 and may cause direct, intravascular haemolysis.

### Autoimmune haemolytic anaemia

- Annual incidence = 1–3 cases per 100,000.
- AIHA can be idiopathic (50–70%) or secondary to an underlying disease. It may be caused by warm, cold, or mixed autoantibodies.

**Warm autoantibodies**, usually IgG (with or without coexistent IgA and IgM), are active at 37°C and are responsible for 50–70% of AIHA.

- Secondary AIHA from warm autoantibodies arises from:
  - Autoimmune diseases: SLE, RA, scleroderma, and UC.
  - Haematological malignancy: chronic lymphocytic leukaemia (CLL), lymphomas, Waldenström macroglobulinaemia.
  - Solid organ tumours.
- Patients may present with pallor, jaundice, haemoglobinuria, fever, and symptoms of anaemia. Splenomegaly and lymphadenopathy are suggestive of an underlying lymphoproliferative disorder.
- Laboratory investigation shows low Hb, increased reticulocytes, mild macrocytosis, and few spherocytes. DAT is positive for IgG and/or C3b, IgA, IgM. The indirect antiglobulin test (IAT) detects autoantibody in the serum. Warm autoantibodies are usually panagglutinins and react with all RBCs in the diagnostic antibody panel.
- The treatment of the underlying disease will generally control the haemolysis in secondary AIHA from warm autoantibodies, although in some cases it may exaggerate it (e.g. fludarabine in CLL). Corticosteroids may be needed along with other treatments.
- Idiopathic AIHA may require only folate replacement if it is well-compensated. When anaemia develops, corticosteroids (e.g. prednisolone 1mg/kg) are the first-line treatment. In unresponsive patients, intravenous immunoglobulins, immunosuppression (cyclophosphamide or azathioprine), rituximab (antiCD20 mAb), or splenectomy should be considered.

**Cold autoantibodies** are most active at 4–18°C and may cause cold agglutinin disease (CAS) or paroxysmal cold haemoglobinuria (PCH).

### CAS

- Older adults—idiopathic or secondary to lymphomas.
- Children or young adults—*Mycoplasma pneumoniae* and infectious mononucleosis or other viral illness cause a transient, secondary form of CAS.
- Cold autoantibodies are usually IgM, coat the RBCs and bind complement after exposure of hands and feet to low temperatures. When blood returns with the circulation to the body (37°C), they dissociate from the RBCs, but complement remains and mediates phagocytosis in the liver. DAT is only positive for C3b.
- Idiopathic CAS or CAS secondary to lymphoma requires avoidance of low temperature. Treatment with corticosteroids is useful in high-titre IgM only. Splenectomy is ineffective.

Cyclophosphamide, chlorambucil, and interferon-alpha (IFNα) are helpful in severe haemolysis. Rituximab has been reported as beneficial in some cases. Treatment of the underlying lymphoma is also necessary.

- Transient CAS is self-limiting and corticosteroids are rarely indicated and only in severe haemolysis.

*PCH*

- Previously associated with syphilis, but nowadays usually follows viral illness in children.
- The responsible autoantibody is a biphasic IgG (Donath–Landsteiner autoantibody), which binds complement at a low temperature (4°C) and activates the complement cascade at a higher temperature (37°C).
- PCH may present with severe **intravascular haemolysis**: fever, rigors, back pain, abdominal cramps, and haemoglobinuria. Avoidance of low temperatures and supportive transfusion may be necessary. Corticosteroids are not useful in PCH.

### Drug-induced haemolysis

Drugs can induce immune and non-immune mediated haemolysis. Drug-induced immune haemolysis accounts for about 10–20% of AIHA cases.

Three major mechanisms have been recognized:

1. Formation of autoantibodies: methyldopa is the typical example. These are true autoantibodies and react with the RBC in a drug-independent manner.
2. Drug adsorption on the RBC membrane and reaction of the autoantibody with the drug itself (penicillin type).
3. Neoantigen mechanism, originally described with quinidine. The drug is attached on the RBC surface and the autoantibody binds a new antigen formed by components of both the drug and the cell membrane.

Some drugs may cause haemolysis by multiple mechanisms. For instance, cephalosporins may induce both neoantigen formation and drug adsorption mediated haemolysis.

Drug discontinuation is indicated if there is clinical evidence of significant haemolytic anaemia and this is usually sufficient to control haemolysis. An isolated positive DAT is not an indication per se for discontinuation of the drug.

### Non-immune mediated haemolytic anaemia

RBC destruction by non-immune mechanisms occurs in several conditions:

- Infections:
  - Parasites: malaria, leishmaniasis, trypanosomiasis
  - Bacteria: *Clostridium perfrigens* sepsis
- Toxins and venoms:
  - Arsenic, lead
  - Snake venoms
- Burns
- Metallic heart valves and grafts
- Microangiopathic haemolytic anaemia:
  - Thrombotic thrombocytopenic purpura (TTP) and haemolytic uraemic syndrome (HUS)
  - Disseminated intravascular coagulation
  - HELLP syndrome
  - Malignant hypertension
- Hypersplenism

### Paroxysmal nocturnal haemoglobinuria (PNH)

This is an acquired, clonal disorder of the HSC, associated with intravascular haemolysis, thrombosis, and aplastic anaemia.

PNH is a rare disease and has an estimated prevalence of 1–10 cases per million.

*Pathogenesis*

- PNH results from a somatic mutation of the phosphatidylinositol glycan complementation class A gene (*PIGA*) in a HSC. Thus, the PNH clone includes cells from all three cell lineages.

- The *PIGA* gene is located on the X chromosome and a single mutation leads to GPI deficiency phenotype in both sexes, because of X-inactivation in the female.
- *PIGA* is responsible, with other genes, for the biosynthesis of the glycosylphosphatidylinositol (GPI) anchor molecule.
- Several cell surface molecules are GPI-anchored, explaining why a single mutation affects the expression of a number of molecules.
- The decrease of expression can be partial (PNH type I and II) or complete (PNH type III).
- The heterogeneous clinical manifestations in PNH arise from the absence of different GPI-anchored molecules. For instance, CD55 (decay accelerating factor or DAF) and CD59 control the activation of the complement cascade on the cell surface. PNH RBCs are more susceptible to complement-mediated haemolysis, due to decreased CD55 and CD59 expression and have a shorter life-span compared to normal cells. The lack of CD55 and CD59 expression on platelets may also contribute to the pathogenesis of thrombosis. The binding of NO by free haemoglobin may also relate to platelet activation and possibly to oesophageal dysfunction and painful dysphagia.
- It is not clear how the PNH clone dominates normal haematopoiesis. It is speculated that an immune-mediated suppression of normal haematopoiesis exists, from which the PNH clone can escape. This also offers some explanation about the relation of PNH with aplastic anaemia.

*Clinical manifestations*

1. **Haemolysis** is a cardinal feature of PNH.
   - Most patients have subclinical, low-degree haemolysis, which may precede diagnosis.
   - Haemolysis is exaggerated during sleep and the patients typically present with dark urine in the morning (nocturnal haemoglobinuria). A possible explanation of the worsening haemolysis during sleep is the $CO_2$ increase and the pH drop, which may activate the alternative pathway of the complement cascade.
   - Episodic, severe exacerbation of intravascular haemolysis is a serious complication. Its occurrence is unpredictable or triggered by other conditions, usually infections. Patients develop anaemia, abdominal pain with tenderness and rebound, lumbar pain, fever, headache, and drowsiness.
   - Back pain and dysphagia may occur. Gallstones can develop.
   - Haemoglobinuria causes **acute renal impairment** and despite appropriate treatment repeated episodes may damage the kidneys irreversibly and result in chronic kidney disease.
2. **Thrombotic events** are another devastating feature of PNH and are responsible for 50% of its mortality. Abdominal and cerebral veins are commonly affected. Thrombosis of the mesenteric veins may present with severe pain, resembling an 'acute abdomen'. Hepatic vein thrombosis (Budd–Chiari syndrome) occurs in 30%. Cerebral vein thrombosis may present with severe, refractory headache.
3. **Aplastic anaemia** develops in 25–58% of patients. The complications of pancytopenia are responsible for ~10% of deaths in PNH.
4. **Transformation to AML or MDS** occurs in 1–5%, in the context of aplastic anaemia.
5. Finally, PNH spontaneously resolves in 15% of cases.

*Laboratory findings and diagnosis*

- **Anaemia** can be severe (Hb <7g/dL) with mild macrocytosis and reticulocytosis, especially during acute haemolytic episodes.
- Significant iron loss from haemoglobinuria is uncommon, but it may cause iron deficiency with microcytosis and hypochromia. Check for urinary haemosiderin.
- Leucopenia and thrombocytopenia occur in aplastic anaemia.
- Serum LDH is markedly elevated, more than 20-fold during severe episodes of haemolysis.
- Unconjugated bilirubin is also high and haptoglobin low.

- The marrow shows normoblastic hyperplasia. A hypoplastic marrow is suggestive of aplastic anaemia or transformation to MDS.
- The diagnosis of PNH was traditionally based on the **Ham test**, which exposes RBCs to acidified conditions, and the **sucrose lysis test**. Both take advantage of the increased sensitivity of PNH RBCs to complement activation. **Flow cytometry** of peripheral blood facilitates the diagnosis by demonstrating reduced or absent GPI-anchored surface molecules (CD55 and CD59) on both RBCs and granulocytes.

*Treatment*

- Folate replacement is needed in chronic haemolysis.
- Iron should be replaced in iron-deficient patients, although haemolysis worsens in some cases.

- ~50% of patients with anaemia respond to androgens. The use of steroids is controversial.
- Lifelong anticoagulation with warfarin should follow the first episode of thrombosis.
- Allogeneic bone marrow transplantation, mostly from HLA-matched sibling donors has been used, mainly in patients with aplastic anaemia. In one series of patients the survival rate was 56% at 2 years. The indications for bone marrow transplantation are similar to those for aplastic anaemia.

Eculizumab is a humanized antibody against the C5 protein of complement. It eliminates extravascular haemolysis and blood transfusion requirements, and it appears to reduce the risk for thrombotic complications.

## Acquired aplastic anaemia

Acquired aplastic anaemia (AA) is a disease characterized by pancytopenia in the peripheral blood and a hypocellular bone marrow, in the absence of an abnormal infiltrate or increased reticulin.

### Epidemiology

- Rare, with an annual incidence of 2 per 1 million population.
- More common in East Asia.
- Age at presentation follows a bimodal pattern, with a peak between 15 to 25 years and a second peak after 60 years.

### Aetiology

In about 70% of patients with AA, the identification of a cause is not possible (**idiopathic AA**). Secondary AA (10–20%) relates to certain conditions:

- **Irradiation**.
- **Drugs:** cytotoxic chemotherapy, chloramphenicol, NSAIDs, D-penicillamine, anticonvulsants.
- **Chemicals:** benzene and derivatives, insecticides.
- **Post-hepatitis AA**: serology for hepatitis A, B, and C is usually negative.
- **Other viruses**: EBV, CMV.
- **Paroxysmal nocturnal haemoglobinuria**.
- **Autoimmune diseases**: SLE.
- **Pregnancy**.

### Clinical presentation

The symptoms and signs of AA result from the underlying anaemia, leucopenia, and thrombocytopenia:

- Anaemia causes fatigue, shortness of breath, and angina.
- Gum bleeding, epistaxis, petechiae, and bruising are the usual manifestations of the bleeding diathesis. Visual disturbances are caused by extensive retinal haemorrhage. Cerebral haemorrhage may be a fatal complication and is common if the platelet count is $<10 \times 10^9/L$.
- Prolonged periods of neutropaenia predispose to bacterial and fungal infections.

Examination reveals signs from the complications of pancytopenia. Lymphadenopathy or organomegaly are not found. Clinical examination should also exclude findings suggestive of congenital syndromes of bone marrow failure.

### Laboratory findings and diagnosis

- **FBC:** confirms cytopenia with low Hb, WBC count, platelets (PLT), and reticulocytes. Usually the lymphocyte count is preserved.
- Examination of the **blood film** will help to exclude other causes of pancytopenia, namely acute leukaemias, hairy cell leukaemia, myelodysplastic syndromes, and myelofibrosis.
- **Bone marrow** aspirate and trephine must reveal:
  - Hypocellular marrow (<25% of the normal cellularity) with a variable degree of residual haematopoiesis (Fig. 11.10).
  - Erythroid precursors, megakaryocytes, and myeloid cells are reduced or absent. Blasts should not be increased in AA. Lymphocytes and plasma cells may appear prominent.
- **Severe AA** is defined by decreased marrow cellularity (<25% of the normal) and at least two of the following: neutrophil count $<0.5 \times 10^9/L$, PLT $<20 \times 10^9/L$, and reticulocytes $<20 \times 10^9/L$.
- **Very severe AA** is defined as for severe AA but the neutrophil count is $<0.2 \times 10^9/L$.
- Investigation to exclude other causes of pancytopenia must include vitamin $B_{12}$/folate, cytogenetics, screening for

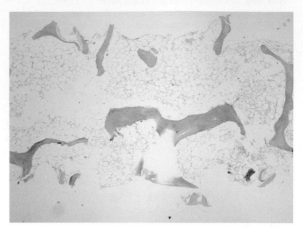

**Fig. 11.10** Bone marrow biopsy in aplastic anaemia shows markedly reduced cellularity.
Image courtesy of Professor Maria Bai.

paroxysmal nocturnal haemoglobinuria, and autoantibody screen.

### Management and prognosis

*Allogeneic stem cell transplantation (SCT)*

- The treatment of choice for young patients (<40 years old) with an available HLA-matched donor and severe disease refractory to conventional immunosuppression.
- Long-term survival and cure rates are 75–90%.
- Complicated by a relatively high risk of graft failure (10%), acute GVHD grade II–IV (20%), and chronic GVHD (25%).
- The transplant conditioning regimens used in AA are highly immunosuppressive, but non-myeloablative. Fanconi anaemia and other congenital types of AA should be carefully excluded before allogeneic SCT, because they require less toxic conditioning.

*Immunosuppressive therapy*

- May be used in patients not eligible for allogeneic SCT. This group usually includes transfusion-dependent patients without severe AA, older patients (>40 years), and those who lack a HLA-matched stem cell donor.
- The immunosuppressive regime is a **ciclosporin** (CSA) and **antithymocyte globulin** (ATG) combination.
- The response rates are 60–80% and 5-year survival is around 70%. ATG is given IV over a 5-day period and because it has considerable immediate toxicity should be administrated in centres with specific expertise. Fever, rigors, anaphylactic reaction, rash, hypotension, and fluid retention are common side effects of ATG infusion. The response to ATG and CSA therapy becomes apparent after the first 3 months.
- Corticosteroids should not be used for the treatment of AA. They have no efficacy and increase the incidence of bacterial and fungal infections.
- Patients who have failed therapy with ATG and CSA may receive a course of high-dose cyclophosphamide without stem cell support, or mycophenolate mofetil (MMF), preferably within clinical trials.

*Supportive treatment*

- All patients with AA will need blood and platelet transfusion to support their counts. A platelet count $>10 \times 10^9/L$, or if there is infection $>20 \times 10^9/L$, should be the aim in order to avoid cerebral haemorrhage or other fatal bleeding. Alloimmunization often leads to platelet refractoriness. Other complications of regular transfusions include infections, allergic reactions, and iron overload that may require chelation therapy.

• Bacterial and fungal infections (aspergillosis) are a serious risk and common cause of death, particularly for patients with severe AA and prolonged periods of neutropaenia. Consider prophylactic treatment with ciprofloxacin and itraconazole. If infection occurs it will require aggressive hospital treatment with broad-spectrum antibiotics and antifungals. *Pneumocystis jirovecii* pneumonia and viral infections are more common following allogeneic SCT.

# Congenital aplastic anaemia

Bone marrow failure and AA may accompany a heterogeneous group of congenital disorders. These conditions are responsible for 10–20% of bone marrow failure cases and may present at birth or later in adult life.

## Fanconi anaemia (FA)

FA is a congenital pancytopenia associated with somatic abnormalities and increased susceptibility to cancer. It is usually an autosomal recessive disorder.

### Epidemiology
• The frequency of heterozygote carriers is ~1 per 300.
• Mean age at diagnosis is 7–9 years.

### Clinical presentation
Physical abnormalities in 2/3 of cases, including:
• Skin hyperpigmentation (café au lait spots) or hypopigmentation (vitiligo).
• Skeletal malformations and low stature.
• Genitourinary, gastrointestinal, ocular, cardiac, and central nervous system abnormalities.

The cytopenia, involving initially one or two lineages, presents within the first decade of life. FA patients have a high incidence of myelodysplastic syndromes or acute leukaemia, increasing with age. Solid tumours, typically squamous carcinoma of the head and neck, are also common. Most young adults with FA die from bone marrow failure or cancer.

### Laboratory findings and diagnosis
• Increased **chromosomal breakage** is a diagnostic feature of FA. This may occur spontaneously, but it is more profound after exposure of the cells to DNA cross-linking agents such as mitomycin-C and diepoxybutane.

• FA has a heterogeneous genetic basis. At least 11 genes are recognized, encoding protein members of the Fanconi group, involved in DNA damage repair mechanisms.

### Treatment
• **Anabolic steroids (oxymetholone)** may correct pancytopenia in 50–70% of patients, but are not definitive treatment.
• **Allogeneic SCT** is the treatment of choice in FA. The use of sibling HLA-matched donors results in 70–80% survival at 2 years.
• Gene therapy trials in FA have been encouraging, showing transient improvement in some patients.

## Dyskeratosis congenita (DC)
• Inherited disorder characterized by skin pigmentation, nail dystrophy, and mucosal leucoplakia. Bone marrow failure usually develops during the first two decades of life and it is a leading cause of death, together with pulmonary dysfunction and malignancies.
• In X-linked DC the gene *DCK1* at Xq28 is affected. *DCK1* encodes the nuclear protein dyskerin, which associates with the RNA component of telomerase (TERC).
• AD form of DC is associated with TERC mutations.
• Oxymetholone and haematopoietic growth factors (G-CSF and erythropoietin) improve counts in DC. Allogeneic SCT may correct bone marrow failure in DC, but pulmonary comorbidity significantly increases the rate of transplant-related mortality.

## Blackman–Diamond anaemia (BDA)
• A congenital condition characterized by anaemia, RBC aplasia, and somatic abnormalities.
• BDA has a heterogeneous genetic background.
• Physical abnormalities involve head and neck, arms and hands, genitourinary system, and heart. Low stature in 1/3.
• Initial treatment involves corticosteroids. Almost 80% of patients initially respond: if remission is sustained, survival at 40 years is 90–100% (60% if don't; treated with regular blood transfusions and iron chelation therapy).
• Allogeneic SCT is a curative option for patients with an HLA-matched sibling donor.

# 11.4 Haemoglobinopathies

## Thalassaemias

- A group of genetic disorders resulting from impaired synthesis of the normal human haemoglobins.
- α- and β-thalassaemia are the most common forms and characterized by reduced synthesis of the respective α- and β-globin chains of normal haemoglobin A.

### α-Thalassaemia

- Commonly found in Southeast Asia and sporadically in countries of the Mediterranean basin.
- There are two α-globin genes on chromosome 16, so unaffected people have four copies in total. In α-thalassaemia, one or more of the α-globin genes is deleted.
- Depending on the number of affected genes, α-thalassaemia is classified into different types:

| α+ trait | 1 affected gene (−α/αα) |
|---|---|
| Homozygous α+ | 1 affected gene on each chromosome (−α/−α) |
| α⁰ | Both genes on the same chromosome are deleted or mutated (−−/αα) |
| Haemoglobin H disease | Only 1 α gene is functional (−−/−α) |

- The γ-globin chains in excess in the RBC form a tetramer (γ4-**haemoglobin Bart**), while the excess of β-globin chains form **haemoglobin H** (β4).

**α+ trait:** usually silent carriers with normal red cell indices or a mild thalassaemic picture with slightly low Hb, MCV, and MCH.

**α⁰ and the homozygous α+ thalassaemia**: variable thalassaemic picture with low MCV and MCH and mild anaemia. Hb Bart at birth ranges from 2% in α+ trait to 5–15% in α⁰ and homozygous α+.

**Haemoglobin H disease**: intracellular haemoglobin H is thought to induce RBC membrane damage and RBC destruction (haemolysis). Most individuals do not require treatment. They are usually anaemic (Hb 7–10g/dL), with low MCV (58–64fL) and MCH (18pg), reticulocytes 5–10%, and splenomegaly. Haemoglobin electrophoresis at alkaline pH reveals Hb H 1–40%. If α-globin production is very low the patients may require occasional transfusions or, in the case of hypersplenism, splenectomy.

**Hydrops fetalis syndrome** is the most severe form of α-thalassaemia; all four α-globin genes are affected. Hb Bart is the main haemoglobin found. This condition is incompatible with life beyond the late intrauterine period. The fetus has severe anaemia (Hb 3–8g/dL), hepatosplenomegaly, cardiac failure with generalized oedema, and extramedullary haematopoiesis. This condition is associated with preeclampsia, polyhydramnios, haemorrhage, and other severe pregnancy complications.

### β-Thalassaemia

- Mutations affect the β-globin gene **expression** (chromosome 11) resulting in reduced production of β-globin chains and intracellular excess of the α-globin chains.
- This causes premature death of erythroid precursors in the marrow and severe anaemia due to **ineffective erythropoiesis** and **haemolysis**.
- Approximately 200 different mutations have been described, mostly point mutations—rarely deletions—which affect β-globin chain production to varying degrees.

*Prevalence and geographic distribution*

- One of the most common single-gene recessive inherited disorders.
- Approximately 3% of the world population carry a β-thalassaemia gene.

- The carrier prevalence is higher in the Mediterranean region, mostly in Italy (6–13%), Greece (5–15%), Cyprus (15%), Turkey, and northwest Africa. Relatively high frequencies are also found in areas of India, Pakistan, and the Caribbean.

*Clinical forms and diagnosis*

Heterozygous β-thalassaemia results in a mild clinical form, **β-thalassaemia minor** (β-thalassaemia trait), which manifests with mild anaemia (Hb almost always >10g/dL), hypochromia, and microcytosis (MCV 63–77fL), target cells, basophilic stippling, and increased reticulocytes (Fig. 11.11). Haemoglobin A2 (α2δ2) is >3.5%. Increased HbF is usual. This condition rarely requires treatment.

**β-thalassaemia intermedia** is usually a homozygous or compound heterozygous condition where patients do not require regular transfusions. It results when at least one gene encodes reduced β-globin chain synthesis or when there is interaction of β-thalassaemia with other thalassaemic disorders, e.g. haemoglobin E. Patients present with anaemia (Hb 6–12g/dL), hypochromia and microcytosis, target cells, and basophilic stippling. Hb F may be 70–80% and Hb A 10–20%. The amount of Hb A2 varies.

**β-thalassaemia major (Cooley anaemia)** is the most severe clinical form, in which β-globin chain production is entirely or virtually absent. The patients have severe anaemia and are transfusion dependent. The blood film shows a marked thalassaemic picture with hypochromia and microcytosis, target cells, basophilic stippling, anisopoikilocytosis, and nucleated red cells (Fig. 11.12). Haemoglobin electrophoresis shows Hb F 98%, Hb A2 2%, and no or little Hb A.

Molecular genotype testing further facilitates diagnosis and prenatal diagnosis of β-thalassaemia.

*Clinical features of β-thalassaemia major*

β-thalassaemia major presents with **severe anaemia** early in life (2–36 months). Without adequate transfusion therapy, the erythroid precursor mass expands strikingly to compensate for anaemia, resulting in **bone deformities** (Fig. 11.13), **splenomegaly**, and **extramedullary haematopoiesis**.

In the pre-transfusion era, children appeared normal at birth, but soon developed pallor, jaundice, and a bulky abdomen due to massive splenomegaly. Marrow expansion caused skull bone deformities and a characteristic facial appearance. Survival was short. Regular blood transfusion controls many manifestations of β-thalassaemia and improved the survival up to the third decade of life. However,

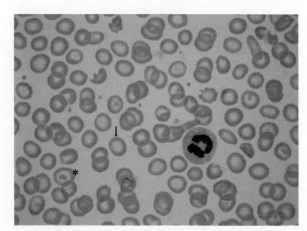

**Fig. 11.11** Blood film in β-thalassaemia minor: microcytosis and hypochromia (arrow), anisocytosis, target cells (star) and poikilocytosis. Image supplied courtesy of Professor Barbara Bain.

446

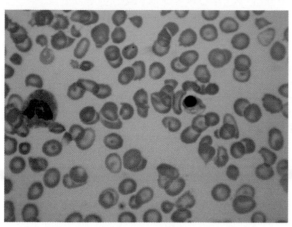

**Fig. 11.12** Blood film in a 4-month-old child with β-thalassaemia major, before transfusion therapy showing anaemia, anisocytosis, poikilocytosis including target cells, and one micronormoblast with defective haemoglobinization.

Image supplied courtesy of Professor Barbara Bain.

transfusions cause severe complications such as **infections** and **alloimmunization**, but most importantly **iron overload** and **secondary haemochromatosis**.

The iron overload in β-thalassaemia results mainly from blood transfusions (~200mg per unit) but also from increased intestinal

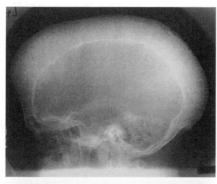

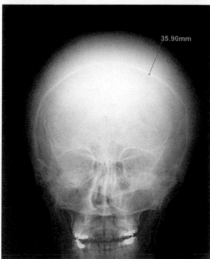

35.90mm

**Fig. 11.13** Skull lesions in a patient with β-thalassaemia major and inadequate transfusion therapy: plain films show gross widening of the diploid space of the skull vault ('hair-brush' pattern) due to extramedullary haemopoiesis.

iron absorption. Iron accumulation in the heart, liver, and endocrine glands is responsible for most of the morbidity and mortality in treated β-thalassaemia. **Cardiac failure, arrhythmias, and liver cirrhosis** are usual complications and leading causes of death.

Endocrinopathies include **growth impairment, hypogonadotropic hypogonadism** and **delayed puberty** mostly in males, **diabetes mellitus, osteoporosis, hypoparathyrodism** and **hypothyroidism.** These are more common in patients receiving inadequate iron chelation therapy. **Cholelithiasis** (4–23%) and **thrombotic complications** (4–10%) are seen with both β-thalassaemia intermedia or major.

*Management*

The management of β-thalassaemia involves regular blood transfusion and iron chelation therapy. Transfusions should aim for Hb 9–10g/dL in order to suppress marrow expansion and support normal growth. Chelation therapy should start after the first 10–15 units of blood are given, to avoid the consequences of iron overload.

Serum ferritin levels, MRI, and liver biopsy are used to estimate the degree of tissue haemochromatosis and the effectiveness of chelation.

**Deferoxamine** (desferrioxamine) was the first iron chelator introduced in the management of thalassaemia. It can be given only by parenteral infusion (subcutaneous or intravenous) using a pump, over 8–12 hours daily for 5–7 days per week. Retinopathy, optic nerve damage, and ototoxicity are systemic side effects of deferoxamine therapy. Compliance with therapy is often suboptimal.

**Deferiprone** is an oral iron chelator, and is probably more effective in reducing cardiac iron overload than deferoxamine, reversing iron-induced cardiomyopathy in some patients. There is also evidence of synergistic effect of the combination with deferoxamine. Agranulocytosis is a rare (1%) but serious complication. Other side effects include nausea, vomiting, anorexia, hepatitis, and arthropathy.

**Deferasirox** is a newer, oral chelation agent with non-inferior efficacy compared to deferoxamine. Gastrointestinal and renal toxicity has been reported.

**Haematopoietic stem cell transplantation** is the only curative approach. It has proven highly effective and safe for young, low-risk patients (low liver damage, effective pre-transplant iron chelation therapy) with an HLA-matched sibling donor.

Potentially affected families should be offered **pre-conceptual counselling**. Antenatal/neonatal testing enables early diagnosis.

# Sickle cell anaemia (Hb SS)

Sickle cell anaemia (SCA):
- Autosomal recessive haemoglobin disorder.
- Single mutation in the sixth codon of the β-globin gene (GAG → GTG). As a result, a valine substitutes for glutamic acid and the abnormal haemoglobin S is produced.
- SCA is common in tropical Africa, Mediterranean countries, Saudi Arabia, and parts of India.

## Pathophysiology

The deoxygenated haemoglobin S polymerizes in the red cells, especially under certain conditions. Low oxygen, high haemoglobin S concentration, low temperature, and low haemoglobin F or A2 concentration favour polymerization. The haemoglobin S polymers form fibres and cause the sickle-like shape of red cells.

Sickle cells have impairment of membrane function and adherence properties, plus decreased deformability. **Vascular occlusion** is a principal feature of SCA. The underlying mechanism is thought to be complex and involves the structural deformity of the sickle cells, abnormal adhesion to vascular endothelium, but also activation of platelets and neutrophils, coagulation factors, and inflammatory mediators. Both intravascular and extravascular **haemolysis** occur and usually result in Hb 6–10g/dL during steady-phase SCA.

## Laboratory findings and diagnosis

Anaemia (Hb 6–10g/dL) with normal MCV and MCH, increased reticulocytes (10–20%) and presence of sickle cells, target cells,

Howell–Jolly bodies, and basophilic stippling is the usual picture. The haemoglobin electrophoresis shows Hb S 80–100%. There is also laboratory evidence of chronic haemolytic anaemia.

## Clinical features and management

- The clinical features of SCA are produced by vascular occlusive events, anaemia, and end-organ damage.
- Infants normally have high amount of Hb F and are protected for the first 6 months. The first complications of SCA are noted within the first 6–12 months of postnatal life.
- The clinical presentation is highly variable. Patients may experience long periods of asymptomatic steady-state disease, which is interrupted by acute events.
- Penicillin prophylaxis should be provided, and patients kept under annual review.

### Acute events

The vascular occlusive events have abrupt onset and can result in several clinical syndromes. Sometimes a triggering condition is recognized. Infections, dehydration, exposure to cold, and physical or emotional stress are the most common.

- **Painful crises.** Severe painful attacks usually involve the ribs, spine, large bones of the upper and lower limbs, and the abdomen. The painful crises are attributed to vaso-occlusion and infarcts of the bone marrow or obstruction of the mesenteric vessels. Hydration and adequate analgesia to control the pain are the main therapies. If there is a recognizable triggering condition (e.g. infection) specific treatment is also required.
- **Strokes** are a devastating complication of SCA and affect 5–20% of children and young adults. Strokes present suddenly with hemiparesis, sensory deficits, seizures, or altered consciousness. There is a high recurrence rate and patients require aggressive treatment to avoid repetitive events and disability. Regular transfusion schedules and/or exchange transfusions to maintain Hb S <30% for several years is needed. Transcranial Doppler ultrasonography and MRI may reveal lesions in asymptomatic patients and predict strokes.
- **Acute chest syndrome** presents with chest pain, fever, tachypnoea, hypoxemia, pulmonary infiltrates, leucocytosis, and haemolytic anaemia. Infection from *Streptococcus pneumoniae* or atypical organisms is documented in many cases. Lung embolism with fat from the infarcted marrow may also cause acute chest syndrome. Management includes correction of hypoxemia, analgesia, antibiotics, hydration, and exchange transfusion.
- **Aplastic crisis** is usually triggered by parvovirus B19. It is a self-limiting condition and requires only supportive treatment (transfusions).
- **Priapism** occurs in 5–45%. Affected men may require regular transfusions or a programme of exchange transfusion for prevention.
- **Dactylitis** is painful, swollen fingers and toes caused by ischaemia of the metacarpal and metatarsal bones, usually in children aged up to 2 years old.
- **Splenic sequestration** is a life-threatening complication, which mostly affects children. Large amounts of blood are suddenly trapped in the spleen leading to severe acute anaemia (Hb 2g/dL).
- **Infections** from *Streptococcus pneumoniae* can be quite severe due to functional hyposplenism and mortality rates up to 35% have been reported. *Salmonella* species are the main causative bacteria of osteomyelitis in SCA. Penicillin prophylaxis and vaccination reduce the incidence of severe infections.

### End-organ damage

- **Bones and joints.** Plain radiographs show abnormal bone architecture and MRI reveals high signal, which corresponds to ischaemia and avascular necrosis. The vertebrae present 'fish bone' deformity. Fingers and toes may be shortened because of dactylitis in childhood. Osteonecrosis, avascular necrosis

of femoral or humeral heads, arthropathy, and fractures are also seen.

- **Cardiac failure** may result from chronic anaemia, iron overload, and infarcts.
- **Pulmonary function** tests are usually impaired. Pulmonary hypertension is found is some patients and correlates with short survival.
- **Renal impairment** arises from a constellation of kidney pathologies; CKD develops in about 4% of patients.
- **Hepatitis** from viral infections and haemosiderosis may result in cirrhosis. **Choledocholithiasis** and related complications occur in 10–60%, especially in older patients.
- **The spleen** is enlarged in children but the size decreases following repetitive vaso-occlusion and adults have an atrophic spleen and hyposplenism.
- **Retinopathy** is caused by vaso-occlusion and the subsequent neovascularization of the retina.
- **Leg ulcers** are a typical complication of SCA. Management and healing is usually very problematic.
- **Pregnancy.** SCA can lead to severe complications of pregnancy. Pregnancy can be responsible for a significant proportion of maternal and fetal mortality, even in developed countries.

### Other therapies

#### Induction of haemoglobin F synthesis

The presence of significant intracellular amounts of Hb F ($\alpha2\gamma2$) can prevent Hb S polymerization and clinical expression of sickle cell phenotype. Thus, several treatment strategies aim to induce Hb F synthesis:

- 5-azacytidine is a chemotherapeutic agent that can block DNA methylation, when given in low doses. It produces up to sixfold increase of the $\gamma$-globin gene expression and had been used in SCA. It was withdrawn because it is potentially carcinogenic.
- Hydroxycarbamide (previously hydroxyurea) appears to be safe in terms of carcinogenesis. It is thought to increase the number of early erythroid precursors with high Hb F content in the marrow, although the mechanism of action is probably more complex. Treatment with hydroxycarbamide decreases the incidence of painful crises, acute chest syndrome, transfusions, and hospitalization and increases survival in adults with SCA.
- Erythropoietin may have a synergistic effect in the increase of Hb F, but the clinical benefit is unclear.

#### Allogeneic stem cell transplantation (SCT)

SCT could be considered in patients with severe complications, such as stroke or repeated acute chest syndrome and painful crises. Event-free survival around 90% and transplant-related mortality of 10% have been reported.

## Haemoglobin C disease

- Haemoglobin C results from the substitution of glutamic acid in the sixth position of $\beta$-globin by lysine.
- The homozygous condition produces mild to moderate haemolytic anaemia.
- The spleen is enlarged, but splenic function is preserved. Hb C does not cause severe veno-occlusive events or end-organ damage. Similarly to other chronic haemolytic anaemias, cholelithiasis is common.
- The peripheral blood smear reveals microcytosis, many **target cells**, irregularly contracted cells and polychromasia (increased reticulocytes).

## Sickle cell/haemoglobin C disease

- Compound heterozygosity of Hb S and Hb C produces a sickling syndrome similar to SCA but less severe (Fig. 11.14).
- This condition is more common in the black population of West Africa and the Caribbean.

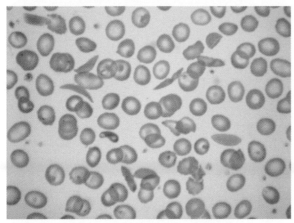

**Fig. 11.14** Sickle cells.
Image supplied courtesy of Professor Barbara Bain.

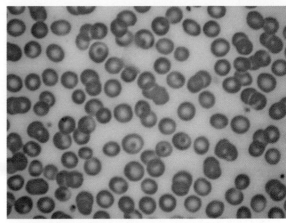

**Fig. 11.15** Haemoglobin C trait: several target cells are present.
Image supplied courtesy of Professor Barbara Bain.

- Episodes of abdominal pain are the most common veno-occlusive events. The spleen is enlarged in children, but its size may decrease during adulthood, and severe, life-threatening infections due to hyposplenism may occur. **Retinopathy, avascular necrosis of the shoulder,** and **pregnancy complications** are seen in increased frequency compared to SCA.
- Mild to moderate anaemia (Hb ~10g/dL), normal or low MCV, normal or high MCHC, and many **target cells** are typical laboratory findings (Fig. 11.15).
- Hb S plus β-thalassaemia can also cause sickle cell disease.

## Causes of target cells

- Liver disease.
- Post-splenectomy.
- Thalassaemias, haemoglobin C disease.

# 11.5 Acute leukaemias

## Background

Acute leukaemias are a heterogeneous group of malignant blood disorders, which result from abnormal cell proliferation and differentiation with maturation arrest at the stage of immature myeloid or lymphoid cells. The leukaemic cells or blasts accumulate in the bone marrow and circulate in peripheral blood. The marrow infiltration with blasts results in haematopoietic insufficiency and cytopenia.

Acute leukaemias are divided into two main categories, based on the origin of blasts: the acute myeloid and the acute lymphoblastic leukaemias. On rare occasions, blasts may have both myeloid and lymphoid features (biphenotypic leukaemia).

## Acute myeloid leukaemia

In acute myeloid leukaemias (AMLs), the blasts are of myeloid or monocytic origin. In some cases (10%), blasts arise from the erythroid or megakaryocytic lineages.

### Epidemiology

- 70% of acute leukaemias.
- AML occurs in any age but is more common in the elderly. Median age at diagnosis is 60 years.
- The annual incidence is 2.4 per 100,000, but increases to 12.6 per 100,000 for individuals >65 years.

### Aetiology

AML may develop **'de novo'**, secondary to exposure to leukaemogenic drugs or by **transformation** from another blood disorder. Risk factors associated with increased incidence of AML include:

- Benzene
- Irradiation
- Cytotoxic chemotherapy

### Clinical presentation

The principal clinical manifestations of AML result from bone marrow failure and the related cytopenia:

- Patients present with symptoms and signs of **anaemia**, such as dyspnoea on exertion, easy tiredness, and pallor.
- **Bacterial and fungal infections** occur at diagnosis or during the course of AML, especially in prolonged neutropaenia.
- **Haemorrhagic complications** related to thrombocytopenia include gum or nose bleeding, easy bruising, menorrhagia, and occasionally severe intracranial or gastrointestinal bleeding.
- Organomegaly or lymphadenopathy is found in 50%.
- Blast accumulation in extramedullary sites (chloromas) may affect virtually any organ, most frequently the skin, orbits, sinuses, testes, and bones.
- A high blast count (>50 × 10⁹/L) may cause **hyperviscosity symptoms** due to leucostasis, presenting with dyspnoea, respiratory failure, headache, visual disturbances, confusion, seizures, and coma.

### Diagnosis and classification

The initial diagnosis of AML is usually unproblematic. It relies on the typical morphological features of blasts found in the peripheral blood film and marrow smear examination. The number of circulating blasts in the peripheral blood (Fig. 11.16) is variable, but usually high (sometimes >100 × 10⁹/L). The presence of at least 20% blasts in the marrow is typically required for the diagnosis of AML, although in most cases the marrow is heavily infiltrated with blasts.

The previous FAB (French–American–British) classification of AML rested on morphological criteria after Wright–Giemsa and cytochemical staining. The most recent classification proposed by WHO (used here) incorporates morphology, flow cytometry, and

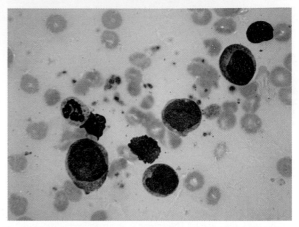

**Fig. 11.16** Myeloblasts in the peripheral blood (in FAB M2 AML)—large, immature, myeloid cells.
Image supplied courtesy of Professor Barbara Bain.

cytogenetic features in a unified clinicopathological definition of the different types of leukaemia.

### AML with balanced translocations and inversions

*AML with t(8;21)(q22;q22) (RUNX1-RUNX1T1)*

- Accounts for 5–12% of AML cases in younger adults.
- The marrow in AML with t(8;21) has morphological features of myeloid maturation. Large blasts with basophilic cytoplasm and numerous large azurophilic granules are seen in some cases.
- These patients have a favourable prognosis and achieve high rates of complete remission (CR) and long overall survival (OS) with chemotherapy based on high-dose cytarabine.

*AML with inv(16) or t(16;16) (CBFB-MYH11)*

- This group includes 5–8% of AML.
- The blasts show myeloid and monocytic differentiation and abnormal eosinophil precursors are found in the marrow. It was previously described as acute myelomonocytic leukaemia with abnormal eosinophils (M4 Eo).
- Chemotherapy based on high-dose cytarabine therapy offers high CR rates (80%) and long OS.

*Acute promyelocytic leukaemia (APL) (M3, FAB)*

- Accounts for 5–10% of all AML cases.
- Characterized by the presence of the **t(15;17)(q22;q12)** translocation. The retinoid acid receptor alpha gene (*RARA*) at 17q12 is translocated close to the *PML* gene at 15q22 (Fig. 11.17).

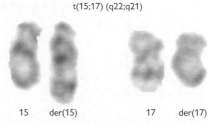

t(15;17) (q22;q21)

15    der(15)        17    der(17)

**Fig. 11.17** The reciprocal translocation t(15;17)(q22;q21) in APL. The derivative chromosome—der(15)—contains the fusion gene *PML-RARA* which is central to the pathogenesis of APL.
Image courtesy of Dr. Alistair Reid.

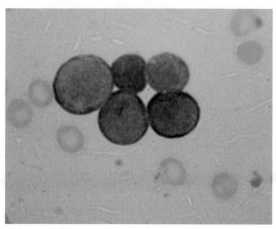

**Fig. 11.18** Myeloblasts with Auer rods: peroxidase staining. Image supplied courtesy of Professor Barbara Bain.

The fusion gene **PML-RARA** is responsible for the inhibition of terminal differentiation and apoptosis of the leukaemic cells. Treatment with **all-*trans*-retinoic acid (ATRA)** unblocks the differentiation arrest and induces CR in most patients with APL.

- The blast equivalents in APL are abnormal **promyelocytes**, with distinctive morphological features:
  - Usually larger than the normal promyelocytes.
  - The nucleus has an irregular shape and is often bilobed.
  - Cytoplasm contains numerous, large, bright pink, or purplish granules.
  - **Auer rods** (Fig. 11.18)—cytoplasmic inclusions formed by fusion of granules—are typically present in large numbers within the promyelocytes ('faggot cells').
- APL affects young adults; median age 31 years.
- WBC count usually ranges from 5–15 × 10⁹/L, with the exception of M3v where the WBC count is usually high >50 × 10⁹/L.
- About 80–90% of patients with APL present with **severe coagulopathy and bleeding diathesis** due to thrombocytopenia, disseminated intravascular coagulation (DIC), fibrinolysis, and proteolysis. The mechanism of coagulopathy in APL is unclear. It is believed that the abnormal promyelocytes release mediators with strong procoagulant activity, such as tissue factor, lysosomal neutrophilic enzymes, and annexin II. The patients require treatment with fresh frozen plasma (FFP), cryoprecipitate, fibrinogen, and platelet transfusion.
- The use of ATRA in combination with chemotherapy (e.g. idarubicin and mitoxantrone) induces molecular CR (Box 11.1) in >90% of APL with undetectable *PML-RARA* using polymerase chain reaction (PCR).

---

**Box 11.1 Haematological malignancy and response to therapy**

Stratification of response to treatment between patients is of great importance both for an individual's prognosis and also in clinical trials, where they may act as surrogate endpoints. CR = complete remission, which may be (sub)defined as:

1. Morphological CR: normalization of FBC, blast <5% in bone marrow.
2. Cytogenetic CR: absence of chromosomal markers, e.g. Philadelphia (Ph) chromosome.
3. Molecular CR: absence of molecular markers. Persisted negative results may indicate cure.

---

- The **differentiation syndrome** (previously referred to as ATRA syndrome) occurs in 5% of patients treated with ATRA and it is a potentially fatal complication. It is characterized by fever and fluid leakage through the small vessels leading to fluid retention, peripheral oedema, weight increase, effusions, pulmonary oedema, and hypotension. It resolves after discontinuation of ATRA and treatment with high-dose dexamethasone.
- Arsenic trioxide is an effective treatment for relapsed APL.
- Autologous or allogeneic SCT should be considered only after second CR.

*AML with t(9;11)(q22;q23); MLLT3-MLL*
Rare (2% in adults), intermediate prognosis AML with monoblastic and promonocytic morphology.

*AML with t(6;9)(p23;q34); DEK-NUP214*
Rare (<2%), presents with cytopenias, poor prognosis AML.

*AML with inv(3)(q21;q26.6) or t(3;3)(q21;26.6); RPN1-EVI1*
Aggressive disease with poor prognosis.

*AML with t(1;22)(p13;q13); RBM15-MKL1*
Common in infants with Down syndrome, with morphology and immunophenotype of megakaryoblastic AML.

### AML with gene mutations
Apart from recurrent translocations and inversions, specific mutations are found in AML and define response to treatment and prognosis. The most important are:
- *FLT3-ITD* mutation defines a poor prognosis subgroup among AML patients with normal cytogenetics.
- *NPM1* mutation is related to better prognosis.
- *CEBPA* mutations are related to longer OS.
- *KIT* mutations: generally higher relapse rates and shorter OS.

### AML with myelodysplasia-related changes and therapy-related myeloid neoplasms
These two groups are generally associated with a poor prognosis.

### AML not otherwise specified
Other leukaemias that do not have these three specific chromosomal rearrangements are often still classified according to the FAB classification:

*AML minimally differentiated (M0 FAB)*
- The blasts may resemble lymphoblasts so immunophenotyping is essential to confirm the diagnosis. It includes 5% of AML.

*AML without maturation (M1 FAB)*
- The blasts may have peroxidase-positive granules or Auer rods. Immunophenotyping confirms myeloid antigens. It comprises 10% of AML.

*AML with maturation (M2 FAB)*
- There is evidence of myeloid maturation in the marrow and neutrophils ≥10%.

*Acute myelomonocytic leukaemia (M4 FAB)*
- Both myeloblasts (≥20%) and monocytic precursors (≥20%) are seen.

*Acute monoblastic (M5a FAB) and acute monocytic leukaemia (M5b FAB)*
- Most leukaemic cells are of monocytic lineage. This type of AML can present with **gingival infiltration** (Fig. 11.19), extramedullary disease in the liver, spleen, and lymph nodes (54%), and CNS involvement (22%). DIC may also be seen.

*Acute erythroid leukaemias (M6 FAB)*
- There is a mixed erythroid and myeloid blast (≥30%) population. It affects older patients (>50 years), presenting with organomegaly. It has poor response to treatment.

*Acute megakaryocytic leukaemia (M7 FAB)*
- >50% blasts are of megakaryocytic lineage.

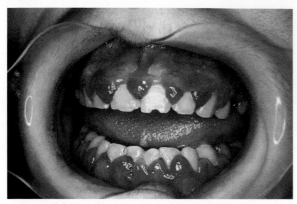

**Fig. 11.19** Gingival hypertrophy caused by malignant infiltration in AML (M5 FAB). Other causes of gum hyperplasia include: drugs (phenytoin, nifedipine, ciclosporin, oral contraceptives), scurvy, pregnancy, familial.

*AML and MDS therapy-related*
- Includes cases associated with previous exposure to chemotherapy and/or irradiation. Prognosis is generally poor.

**Prognostic factors and risk stratification**

Clinical and biological parameters may predict the response to chemotherapy, relapse risk and survival in AML patients. Risk stratification is critical for the definition of treatment strategies in each patient with AML.

*Favourable prognostic factors*
- Age <60 years.
- AML with t(15;17) or t(8;21) or inv(16)/t(16;16).

*Unfavourable prognostic factors*
- Age >60 years.
- High WBC >100 × $10^9$/L.
- Secondary AML.
- Biphenotypic acute leukaemia.
- Failure of induction therapy or relapsed AML.
- Complex cytogenetics (≥3 unrelated abnormalities).
- Cytogenetics: −7, −5, 5q, 3q abnormalities, Ph+.
- Mutations of the *FLT3* gene.

In most clinical trials, the cytogenetic characterization is used to define risk groups that predict relapse risk and survival. Good-risk AML (20%) includes APL and AML with t(8;21) or inv(16)/t(16;16). Poor-risk AML (30%) is defined from the presence of a complex karyotype or 7, 5, 5q, Philadelphia chromosome, 3q, and 11q23 abnormalities. This group may also include patients with other unfavourable prognostic factors. The majority of AML patients do not fit into these two groups and have intermediate-risk AML (50%).

**Treatment**

1. **Induction chemotherapy.** 80–90% of patients with AML other than APL achieve CR with chemotherapy based on anthracyclines and cytarabine. However, about 10% fail to achieve response and a similar number of patients die from complications at this early stage.

2. **Consolidation therapy**. The second goal in the treatment of AML should be the sustained CR and long-term survival. There are two treatment options for patients in first CR: further chemotherapy and allogeneic SCT. Good risk AML should be treated with chemotherapy during first CR. Allogeneic SCT is not recommended unless leukaemia relapses. Patients younger than 45 years, with intermediate-risk AML and a sibling HLA-matched donor available should be offered allogeneic SCT (OS 60% at 5 years). Reduced intensity conditioned (RIC) allogeneic SCT is an option for older patients with same characteristics. High-risk

AML has a poor outcome and aggressive treatment with sibling or unrelated donor allogeneic SCT should be considered (OS survival 20% at 5 years).

3. **Relapsed AML** is treated with re-induction chemotherapy and about 30% of the patients achieve long-term OS with allogeneic SCT.

# Acute lymphoblastic leukaemia

Acute lymphoblastic leukaemia (ALL) is a malignancy of immature B or T lymphocyte precursors (lymphoblasts).

**Epidemiology**
- Annual incidence is 1.5 per 100,000.
- The most common leukaemia in children (80%).
- 2/3 of children are 2–6 years old.
- Median age in adults = 50 years.
- Rare in individuals aged >70 years.
- ♀:♂ ratio = 1.4:1.

**Aetiology**

Aetiology is unknown. Exposure, including intrauterine exposure, to irradiation and chemicals may increase the risk for development of ALL.

**Clinical presentation**

The symptoms and signs of ALL arise from the accumulation of lymphoblasts in the bone marrow, lymphoid organs and tissues, and in other extramedullary sites:
- Bone marrow infiltration results in **anaemia**, **neutropaenia**, and **thrombocytopenia**. Patients may present with pallor, tiredness, infections, petechiae or bleeding. **Bone pain** is a common presenting feature of ALL.
- Generalized **lymphadenopathy** with painless, movable lymph nodes, **hepatomegaly** and **splenomegaly** are also common.
- **CNS** and **testes** are the most frequent sites of extramedullary involvement:
  - Lumbar puncture and cerebrospinal fluid (CSF) examination is standard practice at diagnosis and reveals blasts in 5–15% of cases. The CNS is considered a 'sanctuary' site for lymphoblasts and specific CNS treatment is required to prevent later relapse as overt CNS disease.
  - Testicular involvement is found in 25% of boys with ALL. However, in the era of modern intensive chemotherapy, the testes are not considered a 'sanctuary' site of involvement responsible for relapse.
- Rare clinical manifestations of ALL include arthralgias, pericardial effusion, eosinophilia, skin nodules, and renal impairment.

**Diagnosis and classification**
- The diagnosis of ALL is made from the presence of lymphoblasts in the peripheral blood (Fig. 11.20) and in the bone marrow.
- Increased WBC count due to the presence of lymphoblasts is found in 80%.

The FAB classification describes three morphological types of lymphoblasts:
- **L1 type** lymphoblasts are small cells, with regular size nucleus, homogeneous chromatin, and scanty cytoplasm.
- **L2 type** lymphoblasts are larger cells, with irregular size nucleus, more prominent nucleoli, and variable amount of cytoplasm.
- **L3 type** lymphoblasts are medium-sized cells with morphological features of Burkitt lymphoma cells (basophilic with multiple vacuoles). However, Burkitt lymphoma/L3 ALL is not included within the ALL in the WHO classification.

**Immunophenotype**
- Immunophenotyping using flow cytometry is very important for the diagnosis and characterization of ALL. Expression of specific

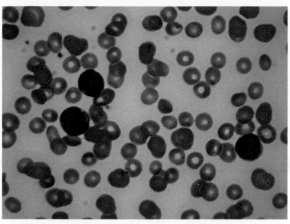

**Fig. 11.20** Lymphoblasts in the peripheral blood (FAB L1 ALL). Image supplied courtesy of Professor Barbara Bain.

lymphoblast surface antigens corresponds with different stages in the lymphoid cell differentiation and enables identification of lymphoblast subsets.

- ~75% of adult ALL cases are of B-cell origin.
- B lymphoblasts express CD19, CD20, CD22, CD24, and CD79a.
- T lymphoblasts express combinations of CD1a, CD2, CD3, CD4, CD5, CD7, and CD8.
- **'Common' ALL** lymphoblasts express CD10 antigen.

### Genetics

- Immunoglobulin gene or T-cell receptor gene rearrangements, using molecular methods (PCR) are detectable in cases of ALL. These sensitive studies can be used to define molecular CR post-treatment and also monitor minimal residual disease (MRD).
- The most clinically important cytogenetic abnormality in ALL is the **Philadelphia chromosome (Ph)—t(9;22) (q34;q11.2)**. This produces a *BCR-ABL1* fusion gene, which usually encodes a 190kD kinase, *different* from the one found in CML. It usually accompanies B-lineage ALL with L1 or L2 morphology and often CD10 expression. Ph+ ALL has a high relapse risk and poor prognosis.
- Other cytogenetic events in ALL include t(8;14), t(4;11), t(12;21), abnormal 9p, −7, and +8.

### Prognostic factors and risk stratification

The identification of adverse prognostic factors in ALL guides the approach to treatment in an individual patient.

*Adverse prognostic factors*

- Age. CR rates decline significantly in older patients. Most clinical trials define age >35 years as an adverse prognostic feature.
- WBC >30 × 10⁹/L in B-lineage ALL, >100 × 10⁹/L in T-ALL.
- B-lineage ALL CD10- or T-lineage ALL CD1a-, surface CD3-.
- Ph+ ALL has the highest relapse risk.
- CNS disease or mediastinal mass.

- CR achieved in >4 weeks.
- MRD positive post-treatment.

In adult ALL, patients are classified into standard or high-risk categories, based on the listed prognostic factors. Patients with Ph+ ALL have the worst prognosis.

### Treatment

1. **Induction chemotherapy.** This is the first phase of the treatment, aiming to induce CR. Treatment protocols for adult ALL use combinations of anthracyclines (daunorubicin), cyclophosphamide, vincristine, cytarabine, L-asparaginase, and prednisolone. About 80–90% of patients will achieve morphological CR. Treatment or prophylaxis for CNS disease with intrathecal injections of methotrexate and cytarabine are also given.

2. **Intensification chemotherapy** includes high-dose methotrexate and cytarabine in order to overcome chemoresistance and also to achieve adequate drug concentrations in the CSF. After this phase, patients have three treatment options: (a) further consolidation and then maintenance chemotherapy, (b) autologous SCT and (c) allogeneic SCT.

   a. **Consolidation and maintenance chemotherapy** usually consists of two or three courses of standard chemotherapy, followed by low-dose mercaptopurine and methotrexate for a long period of time, usually 24 months.

   b. **Autologous SCT** may follow high-dose chemotherapy. It is a safe procedure (transplant-related mortality (TRM) 3%) which offers long-term progression-free survival (PFS) around 50%. This approach is an option for patients ineligible or without an indication for allogeneic SCT. A survival advantage over standard and maintenance chemotherapy is not proven (UKALL12 has shown better survival rate for maintenance chemotherapy compared to autologous transplant), but patients avoid treatment for a prolonged period of time and this may offer better quality of life.

   c. **Allogeneic SCT** has the potential advantage of graft versus leukaemia alloimmune response. The best results with allogeneic SCT in adult ALL are obtained in first CR. Allogeneic SCT significantly decreases the relapse risk but TRM (20–30%) may offset any survival benefit. As a result, it is unclear whether standard-risk patients with an HLA-matched sibling donor achieve longer OS (44% at 5 years) compared to the other treatment options. On the contrary, patients with high-risk ALL have a high relapse risk and short PFS and OS (14% and 20% at 5 years respectively) with chemotherapy alone or autologous SCT. Allogeneic SCT offers long-term disease-free survival (DFS) and OS in about 50%. Allogeneic SCT may also rescue 20–30% of patients with relapsed ALL in second or later CR.

3. **Ph+ ALL.** Despite the poor prognosis of Ph+ ALL disease, combination of tyrosine kinase inhibitors (TKIs; imatinib and dasatinib) with conventional chemotherapy results in clinical CR in almost all patients (94%) and molecular CR in half of them. Furthermore, patients treated with combination of TKI and chemotherapy have much lower relapse rate after allogeneic SCT and better outcome compared to historical controls. TKIs can be used as maintenance treatment in selected patients post-allogeneic SCT or in relapse.

# 11.6 Myelodysplastic syndromes

## Background

- Myelodysplastic syndromes (MDS) are a group of **clonal disorders of the haematopoietic stem cell**, characterized by dysplastic changes in bone marrow cells and ineffective haematopoiesis.
- The abnormal clone involves all three blood cell lineages thus resulting in variable grade of peripheral blood cytopenia, which most commonly involves the RBC series but can also be associated with defective granulopoiesis and/or thrombocytopoiesis.
- The number of myeloblasts in the marrow is increased in some groups. The stem cell abnormalities predispose to the transformation into AML.

## Epidemiology

- MDS is a disease of the elderly, with a median age at presentation of 60–75 years.
- The annual incidence in this population is 3/100,000 but increases to 15–50/100,000 for those >70 years old.

## Aetiology

The aetiology of MDS is largely unknown. Therapy-related MDS develops after exposure to chemotherapy, mostly alkylating agents and/or radiotherapy.

## Clinical presentation

- Most patients present with asymptomatic anaemia detected at a routine blood test or with non-specific symptoms such as fatigue, weakness, dizziness, and shortness of breath on exertion.
- Bacterial infections, mainly of the skin, or easy bleeding and bruising may suggest the presence of neutropaenia and thrombocytopenia respectively.
- MDS may present with isolated neutropaenia but isolated thrombocytopenia is rare.
- Some patients may develop vasculitis, arthritis, or other autoimmune manifestations. In general, lymphadenopathy and organomegaly are not typical findings in MDS.

## Diagnosis

Morphological examination of the peripheral blood film and marrow is critical for the diagnosis of MDS. The anaemia in MDS is often macrocytic and the reticulocyte count is low. The marrow is usually hypercellular or normocellular but can also be hypocellular (in about 20% of the cases).

### Blood film morphology

Dysplastic morphological changes:
- RBC macrocytosis, anisocytosis, poikilocytosis, dimorphic population, and basophilic stippling are common findings.
- Also, agranular neutrophils, pseudo-Pelger cells (Fig. 11.21), hypersegmented neutrophils, agranular or giant platelets may be seen.

### Bone marrow morphology

- Hypercellular, dysplastic cellularity usually affecting all three cell lineages.
- Dys**erythro**poiesis is characterized by erythroblasts with megaloblastic changes, multiple nuclei with an irregular outline,

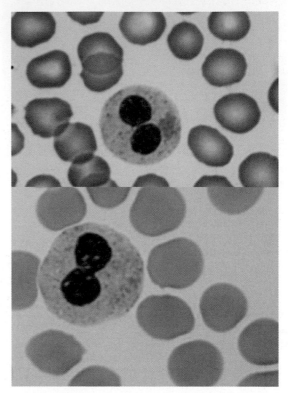

**Fig. 11.21** Pseudo-Pelger cells: bilobed neutrophils in MDS. 'Pelger–Huët anomaly' is the term given to similar cells seen in the peripheral blood—found as an inherited trait and are functionally normal.

Image supplied courtesy of Professor Barbara Bain.

internuclear bridging, ring sideroblasts, cytoplasm vacuolization, and positive PAS staining.
- Dys**granulo**poiesis is characterized by reduced granules in the cytoplasm, hypo- or hypersegmented nucleus.
- The percentage of the myeloblasts is increased in some groups, but still <20%.
- Megakaryocytes may have a hypolobulated nucleus or many nuclei. Small size megakaryocytes (micromegakaryocytes) may also found.

## Differential diagnosis

Other causes of marrow dysplasia should be excluded prior to diagnosis of MDS. These may include vitamin $B_{12}$ or folate deficiency, viral infections, cytotoxic chemotherapy, and toxins (benzene, lead).

Aplastic anaemia and paroxysmal nocturnal haemoglobinuria may present with hypocellular marrow and morphological abnormalities similar to those seen in MDS.

## Classification

The WHO classification is based on findings from blood, marrow, and cytogenetics:
- **Refractory cytopenias with unilineage dysplasia (RCUD):** refractory anaemia (RA), refractory neutropaenia (RN), refractory thrombocytopenia (RT), <5% blasts in the marrow.

- **Refractory anaemia with ringed sideroblasts (RARS):** anaemia, <5% blasts in the marrow, no Auer rods, ±15% ringed sideroblasts.
- **Refractory cytopenia with multilineage dysplasia (RCMD):** cytopenia and marrow dysplasia involving at least two lineages, but marrow blasts <5%.
- **Refractory anaemia with excess of blasts-1 (RAEB-1):** cytopenias, blasts 5–9% in the marrow.
- **Refractory anaemia with excess of blasts-2 (RAEB-2):** as RAEB-1, but blasts 10–19% in the blood or marrow.
- **Myelodysplastic syndrome unclassified (MDS-U)**.
- **MDS associated with isolated del(5q):** the previous FAB classification included also chronic myelomonocytic leukaemia in the MDS.

## Genetics

Cytogenetic abnormalities of the marrow cells are common in the MDS.
- A complex karyotype is present in 10–20% of primary MDS and in up to 90% in therapy-related MDS.
- Monosomy 5 and/or 7 is found in 5–20% primary and in up to 55% of therapy-related MDS respectively, and has a high risk for transformation to AML and poor prognosis.
- An isolated 5q deletion is common in middle-aged women and is characterized by anaemia, thrombocytosis, and megakaryocytes with a hypolobulated nucleus. The risk for transformation is low and the prognosis is good.
- Isolated −Y and del(20q) are also predictive of a favourable prognosis.

## Management

- The management of MDS is problematic.
- DNA methyltransferase inhibitors azacitidine and decitabine improve cytopenias in the majority of patients (>70%) although CR achieved in 15–20%. There is survival advantage even in high-risk patients.
- Supportive treatment with blood and platelet transfusions is usually needed.
- Haematopoietic growth factors (granulocyte colony stimulating factor and erythropoietin) are used to correct cytopenias and are effective in up to 70% of low-risk cases.
- Low-dose chemotherapy (cytosine arabinoside) has been used with unsatisfactory results.
- Patients with RAEB may receive AML-type chemotherapy based on anthracyclines and cytarabine. It is expected that 40–60% of patients will achieve remission, however PFS at 1 year is 10–15%.
- Allogeneic SCT is the only curative option for eligible patients. The PFS after allogeneic SCT using myeloablative conditioning may be 30–40%, however increased transplant-related mortality (TRM) (30–50%) and a high relapse rate (20–40%) compromise the outcome of the patients. Reduced-intensity conditioned SCT has lower TRM and better short-term outcome but the long-term outcome is still largely unknown.

## Prognostic factors and outcome

- The international prognostic scoring system (IPSS) uses the percentage of blasts in the marrow, the karyotype, and the number of cytopenias to predict the outcome of patients with MDS.

- Patients with RA or RARS carry a lower risk for transformation to AML and the median overall survival is ~6 years.
- Up to 1/3 of patients with RAEB will eventually transform to AML, while the remainder develop severe complications due to marrow failure. The outcome of these groups is poor with median OS around 12 months.

## Chronic myelomonocytic leukaemia

Chronic myelomonocytic leukaemia (CMML) is a clonal stem cell disorder characterized by monocytosis in the peripheral blood and evidence of myeloproliferative and dysplastic haematopoiesis in the marrow. The previous FAB classification included CMML in the MDS. The WHO classification describes CMML within the myelodysplastic/myeloproliferative diseases, on the basis of the coexistence of clinical and pathological findings of dysplasia and myeloproliferation.

### Epidemiology
- 20–30% of MDS in the FAB classification.
- Median age at diagnosis 65–75 years.
- Male predominance (2.5:1).

### Diagnosis
- Persistent peripheral blood monocytosis $>1 \times 10^9$/L.
- No Philadelphia chromosome or *BCR-ABL*.
- Blasts <20% in the marrow.
- Dysplasia in one or more myeloid lineages in the marrow.

CMML subcategories include CMML-1 (blasts <5% in the blood, <10% in the marrow), CMML-2 (blasts 5–19% in the blood, 10–19% in the marrow), and CMML with eosinophilia (eosinophils $>1.5 \times 10^9$/L in the blood).

Chromosomal abnormalities are found in 1/3 of the patients at diagnosis. The pattern is similar to MDS.

### Clinical presentation
- Fatigue, fevers, night sweats, weight loss.
- Leucocytosis (48%). Hyperleucocytosis and leucostasis may occur. Leucopenia uncommon (12%).
- Infections (neutropaenia), bleeding (thrombocytopenia).
- Splenomegaly (38%), hepatomegaly, enlarged lymph nodes.
- Skin infiltrates.
- Serous effusions (pleural, pericardial, ascites).

### Management
- Supportive treatment includes blood and platelet transfusions and erythropoietin. This is usually combined with hydroxycarbamide.
- Low- or intermediate-dose chemotherapy (topotecan, cytarabine) may induce short-duration remission.
- Allogeneic SCT is the only curative approach for the young, eligible patients. The estimated DFS and OS reported at 5 years ranges from 18–39% and from 21–43% respectively. The TRM is up to 48%.

### Prognosis
The prognosis is poor:
- CMML-1: median survival 20 months with 18% AML transformation at 2 years.
- CMML-2: median survival 15 months with 50% AML transformation at 2 years.

## Chronic myeloid leukaemia

- Chronic myeloid leukaemia (CML) is a malignant, clonal disease of the haematopoietic stem cell, characterized by the presence of the Philadelphia (Ph) chromosome.
- The Ph chromosome results from a reciprocal translocation between chromosomes 9q34 and 22q11 generating a chimeric fusion gene *BCR-ABL1*. This encodes an abnormal 210kd tyrosine kinase protein, responsible for the neoplastic phenotype.

### Epidemiology
- Annual incidence: 1–2 per 100,000.
- Median age at diagnosis: 55 years, but all age groups may be affected.

### Aetiology
Aetiology is unknown, although exposure to radiation, chemicals, and probably topoisomerase-II interactive drugs account for some cases.

### Clinical presentation
- Three phases: chronic—stable; accelerated—difficult to control; blast—transformation to acute leukaemia.
- Most patients with CML (80%) are diagnosed in the chronic phase and about 40% of them are asymptomatic.
- The incidental finding of leucocytosis alone may lead to diagnosis.
- Symptoms can include fatigue, loss of appetite, night sweats, weight loss, symptomatic anaemia, and gout. Splenomegaly or hepatosplenomegaly are characteristic and can be associated with abdominal discomfort or pain.
- Excessive leucocytosis may result in hyperviscosity syndrome.
- The onset of blastic phase can be accompanied by lymphadenopathy, bone pain, extramedullary localizations (chloromas), and CNS involvement.

### Clinical course
1. Patients with CML in **chronic phase** usually have a good performance status and manageable symptoms and disease complications, especially if a good control of the blood counts is achieved. The chronic phase may last from months to several years with an average of 3–4 years.
2. Untreated, CML invariably progresses to the blastic phase. In most cases, clinical and laboratory findings suggest a gradual progression, called **accelerated phase**. However, in about 20% of the cases, the blastic phase occurs abruptly.
3. **Blast transformation phase** is characterized by transformation to acute leukaemia. In the majority of cases blasts are of myeloid origin but lymphoblasts can be identified in up to 1/3 of patients. Rare forms of biphenotypic blasts are observed. Survival is 3–6 months.

### Laboratory findings of chronic phase CML
- Leucocytosis: cells at all stages of myeloid maturation are present in the blood film with a prevalence of mature neutrophils (Fig. 11.22). Blasts must be <10%.
- Basophilia (but <20%).
- Eosinophilia.
- Normocytic anaemia, although normal or increased (rarely) Hb may be found.
- Platelet count is normal or sometimes increased, and can be >1000 × $10^9$/L.
- Hyperuricaemia.
- Increased serum vitamin $B_{12}$ levels.

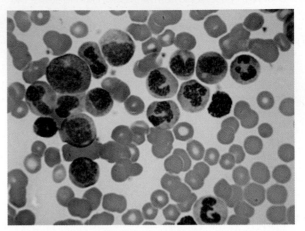

**Fig. 11.22** Blood film in chronic phase CML. Myeloid cells from different stages of differentiation, eosinophils and basophils.
Image supplied courtesy of Professor Barbara Bain.

- Markedly hypercellular bone marrow in biopsy, mostly due to increased myeloid precursors of all stages of maturation. Myeloblasts must be <10%. Myeloid:erythroid ratio is markedly increased (10:1). Megakaryocytes are relatively small, hypolobated, and increased in numbers. A degree of marrow fibrosis may exist.
- The Ph chromosome is found in 90–95% of the cases (Fig. 11.23). In the remaining 5–10% the diagnosis requires molecular analysis to document *BCR-ABL1* fusion by FISH or the transcript by PCR (the fusion gene still exists but is not detectable at the chromosomal level).
- Cases lacking Ph chromosome or bcr-abl are called atypical CML and are not responsive to tyrosine kinase inhibitors.

### Diagnosis
The diagnosis of **chronic phase** CML is confirmed by the detection of Ph chromosome or a *BCR-ABL1* gene, in the context of the clinical and laboratory evidence just described.

The diagnosis of **accelerated phase** (WHO) is made when one or more of the following are found:
- Blasts 10–19% of leucocytes in blood or marrow.
- Basophils ≥20%.
- Persistent thrombocythaemia (>1000 × $10^9$/L) or thrombocytopenia (<100 × $10^9$/L) unresponsive to treatment.
- Increasing splenomegaly or WBC count unresponsive to treatment.
- Cytogenetic evidence of clonal evolution.

The diagnosis of **blast phase** CML (WHO) is made when one or more of the following occur:
- Blasts are ≥20% in blood or marrow.
- Chloromas.
- Large foci or clusters of blasts in the bone marrow biopsy.

### Treatment
- Control of the WBC count and hyperuricaemia may require treatment, especially in the presence of leucostasis. Fertility issues and storage of autologous peripheral blood stem cells should also be arranged at diagnosis.
- **Hydroxycarbamide** (previously hydroxyurea) is useful for the control of the blood count and symptoms, but does not alter the natural course of CML.

456

**46, XY, t(9;22) (q34.1;q11.2)**

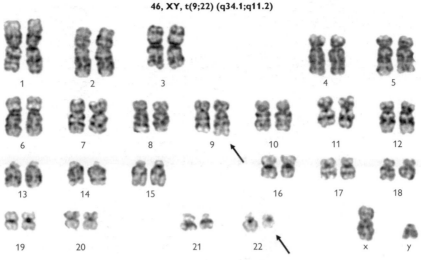

**Fig. 11.23** Philadelphia chromosome (karyotype).
Image courtesy of Dr Alistair Reid.

- Although interferon alpha (IFNa) alone or in combination with other agents was previously the treatment of choice for CML patients ineligible for SCT, it has now been virtually abandoned, its use superseded by TKIs.
- **Imatinib.** The development of specific ABL TKIs such as imatinib has **revolutionized the treatment of CML:**
  - Imatinib is an oral agent that binds in the ATP pocket of the BCR/ABL1 kinase molecule and inhibits the phosphorylation of its substrates.
  - Large randomized trials have shown remarkable efficacy with low toxicity and have established imatinib as the first-line treatment for all patients with CML diagnosed in chronic phase. The IRIS trial compared the previous standard treatment (consisting of IFNa and low-dose cytarabine combination) with imatinib 400mg daily. Imatinib was proved superior in terms of haematological and cytogenetic response, progression to acceleration/blast phase, and toxicity. After a follow-up of 54 months the complete hae-matological response (CHR), complete cytogenetic response (CCyR: 0% Ph+ metaphases), and major cytogenetic response (MCyR: <35% Ph+ metaphases) rates were 98%, 92%, and 86% respectively.
  - Common side effects of imatinib include myelosuppression, gastrointestinal symptoms, superficial facial oedema, muscle cramps, and hepatotoxicity.
  - Patients intolerant of or refractory to imatinib should be treated with alternative TKIs.
  - Resistance to imatinib may develop and some patient will lose their response. Mutations of the *BCR/ABL1* gene are thought to offer resistance, but other mechanisms such as gene amplification may be responsible as well.
- **Dasatinib and nilotinib** are newer tyrosine kinase inhibitors that may overcome resistance to imatinib in some patients. CHR in chronic phase CML patients who have failed treatment with imatinib is 80–90% and 1/3 of them achieve CCyR.
- **Allogeneic SCT** is the only curative option thus far ascertained for CML:
  - The TRM and disease relapse remain the main obstacles and compromise the results of allogeneic SCT, in contrast to low-toxicity therapy with imatinib.
  - Older age, accelerated phase or blastic phase CML, use of matched unrelated donors, a male patient with female donor, and time of transplant >12 months post-diagnosis are predic-tors of poor outcome after allogeneic SCT.

- OS for low-risk patients is ~80% at 2 years but declines to 25% for the high-risk group.
- Donor lymphocyte infusion is a highly effective treat-ment for relapsed CML post-allogeneic SCT, with 60–90% response rates.
- Reduced intensity conditioned allogeneic SCT is a newer approach, with reduced early toxicity (TRM <10% at 100 days) and is applicable to older patients as well. Higher relapse rates are expected, which may be reduced with the pre-emptive use of DLI.
- Currently, patients failing imatinib therapy or losing response or progressing to advanced phase are treated with allogeneic SCT. Some controversy exists as to whether a young patient with an available sibling donor should be selected for a transplant rather than imatinib.
- **Leucapheresis** for leucostasis, priapism.

## Chronic lymphoid leukaemias

### B-cell chronic lymphocytic leukaemia (CLL)

B-cell CLL is a neoplastic disorder characterized by the abnormal proliferation of small B lymphocytes.

*Epidemiology*
- Most common (90%) of the CLLs.
- The annual incidence is 3/100,000.
- Median age at diagnosis is 70 years.
- Twice as common in men than women.

*Clinical presentation*
- ~50% of patients are asymptomatic at diagnosis with incidental finding of lymphocytosis on routine blood tests.
- CLL can present with enlarged lymph nodes, splenomegaly, and hepatomegaly.
- Recurrent infections from the related immunodeficiency.
- ~20% of the patients have constitutional symptoms (fever, sweat, weight loss, fatigue).
- Extranodal disease and pleural effusions are uncommon manifes-tations, usually of advanced disease.

*Common laboratory findings*
- Lymphocytosis (>5 × 10⁹/L) with small lymphocytes and various numbers (but <55%) of larger cell with predominant nucleoli (prolymphocytes).

- Anaemia.
- Thrombocytopenia.
- Low immunoglobulin levels.
- DAT positive (20%), but only half exhibit signs of haemolysis.
- Blood film: lymphocytosis of small/medium cells and smear cells.
- Bone marrow: infiltration with nodular, interstitial, or diffuse pattern.

*Pathogenesis and genetics*
- The aetiology of CLL is unknown. 10% of cases are familial.
- In some cases (40–60%) the immunoglobulin VH gene has no somatic mutations and this relates to worse prognosis.
- Cytogenetic abnormalities indicative of poor prognosis: trisomy 12, del 13q, del 11q, del 6q, del 17p.

*Diagnosis*
The diagnosis is based on:
- Peripheral blood lymphocytosis (>5 × $10^9$/L).
- Morphological features in the blood film (Fig. 11.24) and marrow
- Immunophenotype of CLL lymphocytes: CD5+, CD23+, sIgM/D weakly +, CD79b weakly + and FMC7−. There is light chain restriction (kappa or lambda). The immunophenotyping is essential to differentiate CLL from other lymphomas and leukaemias.

*Clinical staging*
The clinical staging according to Binet or Rai system provide prognostic information and indications for treatment

*Rai staging system*
- **0** Lymphocytosis only.
- **I** Lymphocytosis and lymphadenopathy.
- **II** Lymphocytosis and splenomegaly ± hepatomegaly ± lymphadenopathy.
- **III** Lymphocytosis with anaemia (Hb <11g/dL) ± lymphadenopathy/splenomegaly/hepatomegaly.
- **IV** Lymphocytosis with thrombocytopenia (<100 × $10^9$/L) ± anaemia/lymphadenopathy/hepatosplenomegaly.

*Binet staging system*
- **A** Lymphocytosis and <3 areas of lymph node involvement. No splenomegaly/hepatomegaly/anaemia/thrombocytopenia.
- **B** Lymphocytosis with ≥3 areas of lymph node involvement ± splenomegaly/hepatomegaly. No anaemia/thrombocytopenia.
- **C** Lymphocytosis with anaemia or thrombocytopenia regardless of spleno/hepatomegaly, lymphadenopathy.

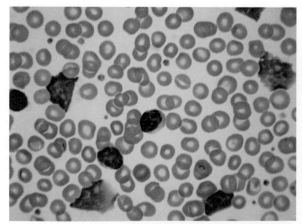

**Fig. 11.24** Blood film in CLL: small lymphocytes and several smear cells (the result of lymphocyte rupture during preparation of blood film). Image supplied courtesy of Professor Barbara Bain.

*Treatment*
Asymptomatic patients with CLL do not require treatment but should remain on active monitoring.
Indications for treatment in CLL include:
- Worsening anaemia or thrombocytopenia due to marrow failure (Binet stage C).
- Massive lymphadenopathy (>10cm) or massive splenomegaly (>6 cm).
- Systemic symptoms.
- Doubling of lymphocytosis in <6 months.
- Autoimmune anaemia or thrombocytopenia.

**Chlorambucil** is the most commonly used alkylating agent in CLL, alone or in combination with prednisolone. Response rates are 40–60%, but CR is <10%. **Cyclophosphamide** is an alternative agent, usually combined with chemotherapy and steroids (COP or CHOP).

**Fludarabine** is a purine analogue that produces higher response rates (70–80%) as a single agent and CR in 30% of patients. When fludarabine and cyclophosphamide are combined with the monoclonal anti-CD20 antibody **rituximab**, 67% of the patients achieve CR and 57% molecular CR, using a PCR method to monitor residual disease.

**Alemtuzumab** (Campath®, anti-CD52 monoclonal antibody) produces response in 81% and CR in 19%. It is effective even in fludarabine-resistant patients and those with p53 mutations/dysfunction.

**Allogeneic SCT** is curative in CLL, but only a small subset of patients will be eligible. The use of reduce intensity conditioning (RIC) relates to low TRM (10–20%) and OS 72% at 2 years.

## B-prolymphocytic leukaemia (B-PLL)
B-PLL is a rare disease (1% of the lymphoid leukaemias) characterized by the presence of malignant prolymphocytes in the blood, marrow, and spleen.

*Common clinical and laboratory findings*
- Marked splenomegaly.
- High blood lymphocyte count (>100 × $10^9$/L).
- Anaemia/thrombocytopenia.

*Diagnosis*
- **Morphology:** medium size lymphocytes with predominant nucleoli.
- **Immunophenotype:** in contrast to CLL, CD23 is negative and CD5 positive only in 30%. The prolymphocytes express the typical B-cell markers.

*Treatment and prognosis*
Chemotherapy similar to CLL is usually used, but the prognosis of B-PLL is poor.

## Hairy cell leukaemia (HCL)
Hairy cell leukaemia (HCL) is a B-cell malignant disorder characterized by the presence of hairy lymphocytes in the blood, bone marrow infiltration, and splenomegaly. HCL is rare, with annual incidence 2.9 and 0.6 per million in men and women respectively.

*Common clinical and laboratory findings*
- Pancytopenia (70–80%).
- Splenomegaly (90%).
- Infections, mostly due to neutropaenia and deficiency of the cellular immunity. Bacteria (50%), but also unusual organisms such us *Mycobacterium kansasii*, *Pneumocystis jirovecii*, *Toxoplasma*, and viruses are usually responsible.
- Autoimmune disorders (vasculitis, polyarthritis).
- Lymphocytes with abundant light grey cytoplasm and fine cytoplasmic projections (hairy cells—Fig. 11.25).
- Lymphocytes positive in staining with tartrate resistant acid phosphatase (TRAP).

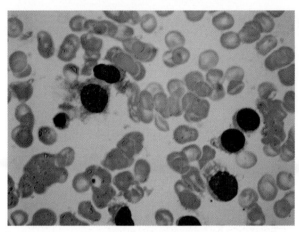

Fig. 11.25 Hairy cell leukaemia: bone marrow aspirate.
Image supplied courtesy of Professor Barbara Bain.

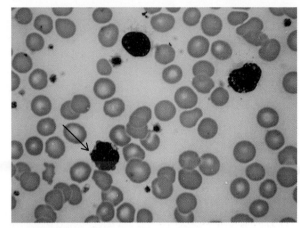

Fig. 11.26 Adult T-cell leukaemia/lymphoma: 'flower cells' (arrowed).
Image supplied courtesy of Professor Barbara Bain.

- Bone marrow infiltration and difficulty in obtaining marrow aspirate ('dry tap').

*Treatment and prognosis*
- **Pentostatin and cladribine** are purine analogues with significant efficacy in HCL. They produce CR in 60–90% of the patients and myelosuppression is the most common toxicity.
- Patients treated with purine analogues have a very good prognosis with estimated 10-year survival rate similar to general population.
- **INFα** induces response, but HCL relapses after discontinuation of the drug. INFα is given subcutaneously and many patients will not tolerate the side effects (flu-like symptoms, thyroiditis, cardiovascular complications and worsening of autoimmune phenomena).
- **Rituximab (anti-CD20 antibody)** is effective in combination with purine analogues in relapsed disease.
- **Splenectomy** was a common option in the past. It may correct cytopenia but does not offer any survival benefit and is currently not indicated for treatment of HCL.

**Adult T-cell leukaemia/lymphoma (ATLL)**
ATLL is a rare malignant disease, which is caused by infection from the human T-cell leukaemia virus 1 (HTLV-1). The disease is common in geographical areas with high prevalence of HTLV-1 infection, such as southern Japan, the Caribbean, and parts of central Africa.

*Common clinical and laboratory findings*
- Some patients have an indolent presentation, but in the majority ATLL has an acute, aggressive course.
- Lymphadenopathy.
- Organomegaly.
- Skin infiltration.
- Osteolytic bone lesions and hypercalcaemia.
- Multilobulated lymphocytes in the blood known as 'flower cells' (Fig. 11.26)

*Prognosis*
Response to chemotherapy is poor and the survival short in the acute forms of ATLL. Infections such as *Pneumocystis jirovecii* (previously known as *Pneumocystis carinii*) pneumonia are a leading cause of death.

# 11.8 Myeloproliferative disorders

## Background

Myeloproliferative disorders (MPD) are is a group of conditions characterized by uncontrolled (clonal) proliferation of myeloid stem cells:

- Polycythaemia (rubra) vera (PV).
- Essential thrombocythaemia (ET).
- Primary myelofibrosis (PM).
- CML (see Chronic myeloid leukaemia).

All are characterized by the over-production of cells with a normal appearance. Constitutional symptoms (fever, night sweats, lethargy, weight loss, anorexia, etc.) are common. There may be transition from one disease to another (especially to myelofibrosis) and all can transform to acute myeloid leukaemia.

Other, rarer MPD include: chronic neutrophilic leukaemia, chronic eosinophilic leukaemia, mastocytosis, and unclassified MPD.

## Polycythaemia vera

PV is a clonal stem cell disorder characterized by increased RBC mass (erythrocytosis) and hypercellular marrow with trilineage hyperplasia. The erythropoiesis in PV is spontaneously increased and independent from the mechanisms that normally control it.

### Epidemiology and aetiology

- The median age at diagnosis is 60 years.
- Annual incidence is 2.8 per 100,000.
- PV equally affects men and women.
- The aetiology is unknown.

### Clinical presentation

- Many patients are asymptomatic at diagnosis.
- Thrombotic and/or haemorrhagic events are the most common presenting features of PV. Coronary and cerebral vascular events, disturbances of the microvasculature such as erythromelalgia (painful burning sensation in the skin), and bleeding from the skin and GI tract are seen.
- Splenomegaly, sometimes with splenic pain, and hepatomegaly are common findings, as well as constitutional symptoms, pruritis, and gout. Facial plethora is also typical.
- PV may transform to myelofibrosis (2–3%) or acute leukaemia (1–2%).

### Laboratory findings

- Increased hematocrit/Hb.
- Oxygen saturations >92%.
- High WBC and PLT count.
- Low serum ferritin.
- Low serum EPO levels.
- High serum vitamin $B_{12}$.

### The JAK2 V617F mutation

Recently, new diagnostic criteria have been proposed for the MPD, which include the presence of Janus kinase 2 (JAK2) gene mutations. The JAK2 V617F mutation has been demonstrated in >95% of patients with PV. This kinase is critical for the intracellular signalling of several cytokines, including EPO, G-CSF, and IL-3. The mutation results in cytokine-independent intracellular signalling and activation of mitogenic molecules.

### Diagnosis

The diagnosis of PV requires the two major criteria and one minor criterion or the first major and two minor criteria.

The **diagnostic criteria** for PV are:

- **Major criteria:**
  - Haemoglobin >18.5g/dL in men or >16.5g/dL in women or other evidence of increased RBC volume.
  - Presence of JAK2V617F mutation or functionally similar mutation such as JAK2 exon 12 mutation.
- **Minor criteria:**
  - Bone marrow biopsy showing hypercellularity for age with trilineage growth with prominent erythroid, granulocytic, and megakaryocytic proliferation.
  - Serum erythropoietin (EPO) below reference range level.
  - Endogenous erythroid colony formation.

### Differential diagnosis

Common causes of secondary erythrocytosis:

*Congenital*

- Hb with high affinity to oxygen.

*Acquired (increased EPO)*

- Hypoxia:
  - Chronic lung disease
  - Cardiopulmonary shunt
  - Smoking.
- Renal hypoxia:
  - Polycystic renal disease
  - Renal artery stenosis.
- Exogenous EPO (athletes).
- Pathological EPO production (tumours):
  - Hepatocellular carcinoma
  - Meningioma
  - Renal carcinoma
  - Phaeochromocytoma
  - Uterine leiomyomas.
- Reduced plasma volume (smoking, diuretics, alcohol, hypertension).

### Treatment

- Aim to prevent and manage complications (haemorrhage, thrombosis) without increasing risk of transformation.
- Age >65 years, history of thrombosis, or risk factors for cardiovascular disease indicate patient groups with higher risk for thrombosis or haemorrhage.
- **Venesection.** Mainstay of treatment is venesection to a haematocrit <0.45 and **aspirin**; cytoreductive treatment is only required if there is thrombocytosis or PV is too difficult to control with venesection alone.
- **Hydroxycarbamide** (hydroxyurea) effectively controls the complications of PV and it is indicated mostly in patients with increased risk for thrombosis, thrombocythaemia, progressive splenomegaly, or constitutional symptoms not controlled by venesection. Avoid in young patients: possibility of leukaemia or myelofibrosis with long-term use.
- **Busulfan** is associated with high risk for transformation to leukaemia but can still be useful in elderly patients.
- **Interferon alpha (INFα)** is the drug of choice for young patients (<40 years) and the safest during pregnancy. It effectively reduces haematocrit (in 30–90%), symptoms and splenomegaly. Cost, parenteral route of administration, and intolerance due to side effects are the major obstacles to its use.
- **Low-dose aspirin** (75mg OD) reduces the risk for severe thrombotic complications and controls symptoms from the microvasculature. All patients should use it, unless contraindicated (history of major bleeding).

# Essential thrombocythaemia

ET is characterized by a sustained increase of the platelet count in the blood—without an underlying cause—and increased numbers of mature, large, megakaryocytes in the marrow. ET is a clonal stem cell disorder. The *JAK2* V617F mutation is found in 50–60%.

## Epidemiology

● The median age at diagnosis is 50–60 years.
● The annual incidence of ET is 1–3 per 100,000.

## Clinical presentation

● Many patients with ET are asymptomatic at diagnosis and may remain so for years.
● ET usually presents with thrombosis (arterial or venous). Haemorrhage is less common, unless the PLT count is very high (>1500 × 10$^9$/L).
● PLT count >1000 × 10$^9$/L, risk factors for cardiovascular disease, age >60 years and previous history of thrombosis significantly increase the incidence of thrombotic events.
● Inherent risk for transformation to myelofibrosis (4–15% in 15 years) or acute leukaemia/MDS (<5%).

## Diagnosis

● Sustained platelet count ≥450 × 10$^9$/L.
● Bone marrow biopsy specimen showing proliferation mainly of the megakaryocytic lineage with increased numbers of enlarged, mature megakaryocytes. No significant increase or left-shift or neutrophil granulopoiesis or erythropoiesis.
● Exclusion of PV, primary myelofibrosis, CML, MDS, or other myeloid neoplasm.
● Demonstration of *JAK2V617F* mutation or other clonal marker or no evidence or reactive thrombocytosis.

## Treatment

● Antiplatelet drugs and cytoreductive agents are used to reduce thrombotic complications and control symptoms in ET. Vigorous control of reversible risk factors is also needed.
● **Low-dose aspirin** (75mg OD) alone is safe (low incidence of bleeding) and effective in reducing thrombosis and symptoms of the microvasculature in low-risk patients.
● **Hydroxycarbamide** in combination with aspirin should be offered to high-risk patients aiming a PLT count <400 × 10$^9$/L.
● **IFNα** may be used in pregnancy for patients with intolerance to hydroxycarbamide.
● **Anagrelide** is an antiplatelet agent that reduces platelet aggregation and counts. It may be used in intolerance/toxicity or refractoriness to hydroxycarbamide. Main side effects include headaches, palpitations, cardiomyopathy, dizziness, CCF, and severe anaemia.

# Primary myelofibrosis

PM is a clonal myeloproliferative disorder characterized by marrow fibrosis and extramedullary haematopoiesis. The *JAK2* V617F mutation is found in 40–60%.

## Epidemiology

● The median age at diagnosis is ~60 years.
● The annual incidence of CIM is 0.4–1.4 per 100,000.

## Clinical presentation

● 1/3 of patients are asymptomatic at diagnosis.
● PM may present with constitutional symptoms, manifestations of extramedullary haematopoiesis (pleural/pericardial effusions, spine compression), splenomegaly (90%), hepatomegaly (50%), and complications of cytopenia (infection, bleeding). Thrombocytosis may cause vascular events.

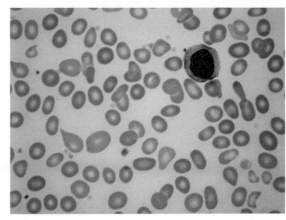

**Fig. 11.27** Myelofibrosis: tear-drop cells (dacrocytes) and a blast in peripheral blood.
Image supplied courtesy of Professor Barbara Bain.

● Leukaemic transformation occurs in 20% and accounts for most of the mortality of the disease.

## Laboratory findings

● Anaemia.
● Leucopenia or leucocytosis.
● Thrombocytopenia or thrombocytosis.
● Leucoerythroblastosis (presence of immature granulocytes and nucleated red cells in the blood).
● Dacrocytes and poikilocytosis in the blood film (Fig. 11.27).
● **Bone marrow** (Fig. 11.28):
  ● Hypercellular or fibrotic marrow.
  ● Megakaryocyte hyperplasia and atypia.
  ● Increased bone marrow reticulin and/or collagen fibrosis.
  ● New bone formation.

## Diagnosis

Exclusion of other causes of marrow fibrosis plus the clinical, laboratory, and histopathological findings of the disease.

## Treatment

● **Allogeneic SCT** is the only curative option in PM, but eligibility is confined to young patients with a suitable donor.
● **Erythropoietin** injections may increase Hb in 50%.

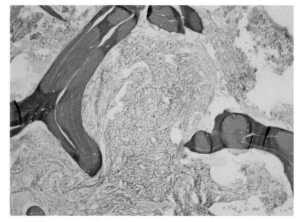

**Fig. 11.28** Bone marrow trephine in myelofibrosis: reticulin staining.
Image courtesy of Professor Maria Bai.

- **Androgens or corticosteroids** have similar response rates.
- **Thalidomide** in low doses (50mg daily) is well tolerated and in combination with steroids may correct cytopenia and control symptoms in 40–70%.
- **Hydroxycarbamide** is useful in the control of leucocytosis or thrombocytosis.

- **Splenectomy** may offer symptomatic relief and improvement of anaemia in 50%, but may exaggerate hepatomegaly, thrombocytosis, and transformation to acute leukaemia. Perioperative mortality is about 30%.
- **Splenic irradiation** may be employed in patients with contraindications for surgery. It is usually complicated by myelosuppression.

# 11.9 Lymphomas

## Hodgkin lymphoma

Hodgkin lymphoma (HL) is a lymphoproliferative malignancy that usually affects young adults, presenting with solitary or extensive lymphadenopathy. HL is a curable disease even in advanced stages, with overall cure rate around 80%.

### Epidemiology

- Men:women ratio = 1.4:1.
- **Bimodal age distribution**: 15–39 years and >50 years.
- **Epstein–Barr virus (EBV)** genome and proteins (EBNA and LMP1) are expressed in about 50%. Other lymphotropic viruses may be involved in the EBV-negative cases.

### Clinical presentation

**Lymphadenopathy** is apparent in almost all patients. It affects the cervical and supraclavicular nodes (60–70%), the mediastinum (60%), para-aortic (34%), axillary (25%), and inguinal nodes (16%). **The spread pattern** of affected lymph nodes in HL is characteristically contiguous. **Splenomegaly** is found in 10% of patients. **Extranodal disease** (<10%) may affect any organ, most commonly the bone marrow, lungs, and liver.

**B-symptoms** at presentation have prognostic significance. These include unexplained low-grade fever or high spikes (PelEbstein pattern), night sweats, and weight loss (>10%).

Pain in the lymph nodes after consumption of alcohol, bone pain in the case of extranodal disease, pruritus and fatigue are common symptoms, but lack prognostic significance.

### Diagnosis—histopathology

The diagnosis of HL is confirmed by biopsy of an involved lymph node (Fig. 11.29). The neoplastic population in HL is of B-cell origin and composed by the mononuclear **Hodgkin cell** and the multinucleated **Reed–Sternberg** cell (HRS cell). Typically, this is a large, binucleated or multinucleated cell with prominent eosinophilic nucleoli and abundant slightly basophilic cytoplasm. The HRS cells are a small minority of the cellular component, surrounded by a heterogeneous cellular background of reactive, non-neoplastic T lymphocytes, eosinophils, neutrophils, histiocytes, and plasma cells in various numbers. The Reed–Sternberg cell is not specific for HL and not sufficient alone to establish the diagnosis. Immunophenotyping is also helpful for the diagnosis and histological classification of HL.

The histological subtypes of HL (WHO) are

- **Nodular lymphocyte predominant HL (5%):** very good prognosis for early clinical stages.
- **Classical Hodgkin lymphoma (CHL) (95%):**

  **Nodular sclerosis CHL (70%):** collagen bands divide the lymph node, favourable prognosis (Fig. 11.30).

  **Mixed cellularity CHL (20%):** B-symptoms and advanced stages at presentation are common.

  **Lymphocyte-rich classical CHL (<5%):** favourable prognosis.

  **Lymphocyte-depleted CHL (<5%):** aggressive course, poor prognosis.

### Clinical staging

The Cotswold classification staging system was proposed in the early 1990s. It is based on the previous Ann Arbor system, but involves further sub-staging of the disease. Laparotomy, splenectomy, and lymphangiography performed for staging purposes in previous decades have been abandoned. CT/PET scans of neck, thorax, abdomen, and pelvis is now the main imaging used for staging and response assessment in the course (interim) or completion of treatment. PET relies on uptake of 2-fluoro-2-deoxy-D-glucose (FDG) by metabolically active lymphoma tissue and offers disease detection with higher sensitivity. PET scan significantly facilitates the detection of residual disease.

*Cotswold classification staging system*

- **Stage I:** involvement of a single lymph node region or lymphoid structure (organ or site).
- **Stage II:** involvement of ≥2 lymph node regions in the same side of the diaphragm.
- **Stage III:** involvement of lymph node regions or structures in both sides of the diaphragm.

  **Stage III1:** limited to the upper abdomen with or without splenic hilar, coeliac, or portal nodes.

  **Stage III2:** with para-aortic, iliac or mesenteric nodes.

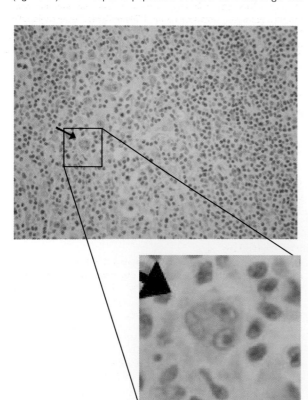

**Fig. 11.29** Bone marrow biopsy in HL: the Reed–Sternberg cell (arrow) in an appropriate pleomorphic background.

Image courtesy of Professor Maria Bai.

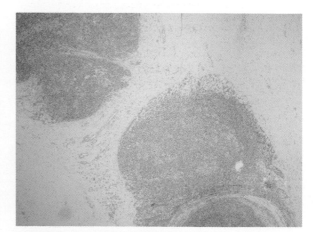

**Fig. 11.30** Nodular sclerosis lymph node biopsy: collagen band (centre of image) divides the lymphoid tissue.

Image courtesy of Professor Maria Bai.

- **Stage IV:** involvement of extranodal sites (but not those designated E).
- **Designations:**
  - A: no B-symptoms.
  - B: fever, drenching sweats, weight loss.
  - X: bulky disease, >1/3 of mediastinum width, >10cm maximum dimension of nodal mass.
  - E: involvement of a single site contiguous or proximal to a known nodal site.
  - CS: clinical stage.
  - PS: pathological stage.

## Prognostic factors

Although most patients with HL will be cured using chemotherapy with or without radiotherapy, the late effects of the treatment may significantly compromise their long-term outcome. Prognostic systems for disease recurrence have been developed and used to optimize treatment in HL.

Criteria of unfavourable prognosis proposed by the German Hodgkin Lymphoma Study Group (GHSG)

- Mediastinal mass ratio (MMR) ≥0.35.
- Age ≥ 50 years.
- High erythrocyte sedimentation rate (ESR).
- Involvement of ≥4 sites.

The European Organisation for Research and Treatment of Cancer (EORTC) suggests similar prognostic criteria.

An International Collaborative Study has identified seven parameters with prognostic significance for patients with advanced stage or bulky disease:

- Age ≥45 years.
- Stage IV.
- Male sex.
- WBC count >15 × 10$^9$/L.
- Lymphocytes <0.6 × 10$^9$/L.
- Albumin <40g/L.
- Haemoglobin <10.5g/dL.

Patients with none of these factors have PFS and OS of 84% and 89% at 5 years respectively. On the contrary, a score ≥5 relates to a PFS and OS of 42% and 56% at 5 years respectively.

## Treatment

**Limited-stage Hodgkin lymphoma.** This group includes stage I–IIA HL without bulky disease. Cure rates over 95% are achievable. The current treatment approaches has changed significantly over the last decades. The use of extensive field radiotherapy has been abandoned, mainly due to the long-term toxicity. Instead, three to six courses of chemotherapy (e.g. ABVD: doxorubicin, bleomycin, vincristine, dacarbazine) with or without involved field radiotherapy is usually given. Recent studies suggest that the chemotherapy alone is less toxic and offers long-term PFS, while radiotherapy can be reserved for relapse. Early-stage HL with bulky disease should be probably treated with combined modalities.

**Advanced stage HL.** ABVD chemotherapy is established as standard treatment in advanced stage HL. Several trials has shown superior efficacy for ABVD over the initially used MOPP regimen (mechlorethamine, vincristine, procarbazine, and prednisone). The GHSG and other groups have developed more intense regimens for patients with advanced HL (e.g. BEACOPP: bleomycin, etoposide, doxorubicin, cyclophosphamide, vincristine, procarbazine, and prednisone). Although a better tumour control is shown, toxic deaths may offset outcome advantage.

**High-dose therapy and autologous SCT** may induce long-term OS in 50–70% of patients with chemosensitive refractory/relapsed HL and has been established as standard practice. TRM is relatively low (5–10%). Allogeneic SCT offers 50% OS at 2 years with 20% TRM during the first year. Reduced intensity conditioning (RIC) has been used, especially in heavily treated patients, with low toxicity. There is evidence of graft versus lymphoma effect and donor lymphocyte infusions were given after relapse with response.

**Other treatment options** for patients relapsed after autologous SCT are limited. These include chemotherapy (gemcitabine, vinorelbine), monoclonal antibodies (anti-CD30), and immunotherapy.

# Non-Hodgkin lymphomas

Non-Hodgkin lymphomas (NHL) include all lymphoid malignancies arising from the lymphoid tissue, except for HL. They comprise 5% of all cancers in Western countries. NHL are a heterogeneous group of entities, which are separated into B-cell, T-cell, and NK-cell neoplasms, depending on the cell of origin. Despite considerable diversity, NHL share some common clinical and pathological features.

## Aetiology

The exact aetiology of many NHL is unknown. However, some conditions relate to significantly higher risk for development of lymphomas.

- **Immunosuppression:** patients receiving immunosuppressive therapy following bone marrow or solid organ transplantation have a risk of developing post-transplant lymphoproliferative disorders (PTLDs).
- **Infections:** HIV infection relates to 60–100 fold risk for NHL, usually diffuse large B-cell lymphoma (DLBCL) or Burkitt lymphoma. HTLV-I causes adult T-cell leukaemia/lymphoma. EBV relates to endemic Burkitt lymphoma. *Helicobacter pylori* infection may cause mucosa-associated lymphoid tissue (MALT) lymphoma, particularly of the stomach.
- **Autoimmune diseases:** patients with rheumatoid arthritis, lupus, Sjögren syndrome and coeliac disease have a higher risk for NHL.

## Clinical presentation and staging

Two-thirds of patients with NHL will present with lymphadenopathy. Extranodal disease is also common, affecting virtually any organ, most often the GI tract, skin, and bone marrow. Enlarged lymph nodes and extranodal masses may cause obstructive phenomena. The CNS may be affected primarily or as part of dissemination of the disease. Pleural or pericardial effusion and ascites may arise. B-symptoms are common in advanced clinical stages. Abnormal laboratory findings in NHL include autoimmune haemolysis, increased levels of serum LDH and beta-2-microglobulin (B2M), and the presence of monoclonal immunoglobulin on serum protein electrophoresis. Although originally developed for HL, the Ann Arbor staging system is used for NHL as well. CT and/or PET scanning and bone marrow biopsy should be part of the diagnostic workup.

## Diagnosis

Affected lymph node or lymphomatous tissue biopsy is needed for the confirmation of diagnosis. Immunohistochemistry and cytogenetic studies are usually necessary.

## Classification of NHL

The histological classification of NHL proposed by WHO describes specific disease entities under two large categories, based on the origin of the neoplastic cell. These categories are: (1) the mature B-cell neoplasms and (2) the mature T-cell and NK-cell neoplasms.

Some of these entities (chronic lymphoid leukaemias and multiple myeloma and related diseases) are discussed elsewhere in this chapter.

## B-cell lymphomas

This group comprises 90% of NHL. It is believed that B-cell lymphomas arise from B lymphocytes at various stages of differentiation, although for many types of NHL the normal B-cell counterpart has not been identified.

*Follicular lymphoma (FL)*

*Epidemiology*

- 35% of all NHL.
- Most common type of indolent NHL (70%).
- Median age at presentation: 60 years.

*Clinical presentation*

Most patients with FL are asymptomatic at diagnosis, although may have widespread lymphadenopathy and splenomegaly. However, 1/3 of them will have only localized nodal disease. The bone marrow is involved in 50%. Peripheral blood and the Waldeyer ring may also be affected. Extranodal disease is rare and involves the GI tract and skin. FL is usually a low-grade malignancy at diagnosis. However, in many cases FL will transform to a more aggressive, high-grade lymphoma. The risk of transformation is estimated at around 20% at 5 years. These patients need aggressive therapy and have poorer prognosis.

*Morphology*

FL is thought to arise from germinal centre cells. The infiltration typically follows a follicular or diffuse/follicular pattern. Two types of neoplastic cells are seen: **centrocytes**, which are always present and usually the predominant cell population and **centroblasts**. Histological grading (grade 1 to 3) is based on the number of centroblasts. The histology of high-grade transformation is similar to that of diffuse large B-cell lymphomas. See Fig. 11.31.

*Immunophenotype and genetics*

FL cells are positive for B-cell markers (sIgM, CD19, CD20, CD22, CD79a) and also for CD10 and the BCL6 nuclear protein. **BCL2 protein expression** is found in 75–100%, depending on the histological grade. It relates to **t(14;18)(q32;q21)** translocation, which is the most common chromosomal abnormality (70–95%). Mutations of the **TP53** gene encoding p53 protein have been associated with the high-grade transformation, at least in some cases.

*Prognostic indices*

The Follicular Lymphoma International Prognostic Index (FLIPI) incorporates five parameters:

- Age >60 years.
- Disease stage III or IV.
- Hb <12g/dL.
- >4 nodal sites of involvement.
- Elevated LDH.

Patients may score low (score 0–1), intermediate (score 2), or high risk (score ≥3) with OS at 5 years of 91%, 78%, and 52% respectively.

*Treatment*

Patients with early stage FL (stage IA and IIA) may achieve long remissions with involved field radiotherapy (IFRT). For stage IA patients, PFS of 66% at 15 years has been reported. The relapse rate after IFRT for stage I/II is 46% at 10 years and it rarely occurs thereafter. Observation only is acceptable for early stage FL and not inferior to radiotherapy, if this is the patient's choice.

For asymptomatic patients with advanced disease (≥stage II) a 'watchful waiting' approach has been proven equally effective in terms of OS, when compared to early treatment with low- or high-intensity chemotherapy. Symptomatic patients should be treated with rituximab combined with chemotherapy (e.g. R-CVP rituximab, cyclophosphamide, vincristine, and prednisone). Rituximab maintenance increases the PFS after induction chemotherapy.

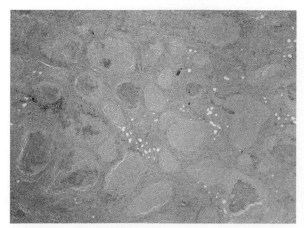

**Fig. 11.31** Follicular lymphoma: lymph node biopsy.
Image courtesy of Professor Maria Bai.

Autologous SCT has a role in relapsed FL with prolongation of DFS, although immune-chemotherapy is the treatment of choice in relapse. Autologous SCT after first remission, produces longer DFS compared to conventional chemotherapy (in non-randomized comparisons) but its effect on OS is unclear. A high incidence of secondary malignancies (3.5–9%), mostly MDS and AML, has also a serious impact on OS rates.

Conventional allogeneic SCT has low relapse rates (20%) but the effect on OS is largely offset from the toxic deaths (TRM 30%). RIC allogeneic SCT is a safer approach with PFS 60% at 5 years.

Radioimmunotherapy (RIT) is an attractive newer approach, especially in older patients, which combines monoclonal anti-CD20 antibodies and the radionuclides yttrium-90 (ibritumomab) or iodine-131 (tositumomab).

### Mantle cell lymphoma (MCL)

*Epidemiology*

- 5% of all NHL.
- It mostly affects males, median age: 63 years.

*Clinical presentation*

Most patients present with stage IV disease (70%). MCL involves the lymph nodes (75–100%), the spleen (35–75%), and the bone marrow (60–90%). Malignant cells in the peripheral blood are seen in 25% of the patients. MCL characteristically involves the GI tract (25%) with multiple lymphomatous polyposis. Half of the patients present with B-symptoms. CNS involvement is rare.

*Morphology*

The normal counterpart of the MCL malignant cell is thought to be a naïve B cell of the follicle mantle zone. The malignant cells are usually monomorphous or pleomorphic, small to medium size lymphocytes with irregular nuclear contour, resembling centrocytes, although blastoid variants are also well recognized.

*Immunophenotype and genetics*

The tumour cells are positive for B-cell markers such as CD19, IgM, FMC7, and CD20. CD5 is positive (typically) but CD23 is negative, in contrast to CLL.

MCL cells express **cyclin-D1**, as a result of the **t(11;14) (q13;q32)** translocation.

*Treatment and prognosis*

- Although MCL has the morphological features of an indolent lymphoma, it is an aggressive disease with poor prognosis.
- The addition of rituximab to CHOP chemotherapy (cyclophosphamide, doxorubicin, vincristine, and prednisolone) has improved outcome compared to CHOP alone.
- More recent studies in young patients (<65 years) show longer PFS and OS with addition of high-dose Ara-C regimens (e.g. R-CHOP/R-DHAP) followed by autologous or allogeneic SCT.
- For elderly patients R-CHOP or similar (R-CVP) is used.
- Rituximab-bendamustine produces similar, if not better results to R-CHOP
- For advanced stage patients, ineligible for autologous or allogeneic SCT, maintenance with rituximab significantly prolongs remissions.
- Relapses are treated with rituximab plus fludarabine, cyclophosphamide/mitoxantrone or rbendamustine.
- Bortezomib, lenalidomide, temsirolimus, and Bruton kinase inhibitors may be used in advanced relapses.

### Diffuse large B-cell lymphoma (DLBCL)

*Epidemiology*

- 30–40% of all adult B-cell lymphomas.
- The most common type of aggressive NHL.
- Median age at diagnosis: 65 years.

*Clinical presentation*

Most patients present with rapidly progressive lymphadenopathy. DLBCL affects extranodal sites in 40% of the patients and in some cases this is the primary manifestation of the disease. Common sites of extranodal involvement include GI tract, skin, CNS, testis, lungs, bones, liver, and kidneys. Primary testicular, mediastinal, and CNS DLBCL are relatively uncommon, distinct clinicopathological entities with increased risk of relapse, and need for more aggressive treatments.

*Morphology*
DLBCL have heterogeneous morphology. Four common morphological variants can be recognized: (1) centroblastic, (2) immunoblastic, (3) T-cell/histiocyte rich, and (4) anaplastic.

*Immunophenotype and genetics*
Lymphocytes are positive for B-cell markers (CD19, CD20, CD22, CD79a). The BCL-2 protein is expressed in 30–50%. Markers of cell proliferation, such as Ki-67 are positive in >90% of the cells. The t(14;18)(q32;q21) translocation that relates to BCL-2 expression is found in 20–30%.

*Prognostic indices*
The International Prognostic Index (IPI) has strong predictive value for the response rates to treatment and OS. IPI is composed of five parameters:

- Age >60 years.
- LDH >normal.
- Performance status 2–4.
- Stage III or IV.
- >1 extranodal site.

Risk score: low (0–1), low intermediate (2), high intermediate (3), and high (4–5).

*Treatment*
The **R-CHOP** regimen (rituximab plus cyclophosphamide, doxorubicin, vincristine, and prednisolone) has been established as standard first-line treatment in patients with DLBCL. CR rates are 44–87% depending on the IPI risk group. More than 50% of patients with DLBCL will be cured with this approach. Patients with localized disease may benefit from a combination of R-CHOP and IFRT. Patients with involvement of the paranasal sinuses, testis, and mediastinum have an increased risk of CNS relapse and should receive prophylactic intrathecal methotrexate injections.

Patients with relapsed DLBCL are treated with **DHAP** (cisplatin, cytarabine, and dexamethasone) or similar chemotherapy, followed by high-dose therapy and **autologous SCT**. About 50% of them will achieve long-term CR and OS with TRM around 5%.

### Burkitt lymphoma (BL)
BL is a highly aggressive form of B-cell NHL. Three clinical variants are described: endemic, sporadic, and immunodeficiency associated.

*Epidemiology and aetiology*
**Endemic BL** was originally described in African children who live in areas of endemic malaria. It mostly affects boys (♀: ♂ ratio 2:1), aged 4–7 years. EBV is detected in 100% of the cases and plays a significant role in pathogenesis.

S**poradic BL** occurs worldwide and affects both children and adults. Neoplastic cells are EBV+ in 15–30% or less in some series. **Immunodeficiency associated BL** is nearly entirely found in HIV+ individuals. Before the introduction of highly active antiretroviral therapy (HAART), HIV+ adults had 1000-fold higher incidence of BL, compared to the general population and it represented 40% of all NHL.

*Clinical presentation*
In general, BL affects mostly extranodal sites. Endemic BL characteristically presents with large tumours affecting the jaw and other facial bones (Fig. 11.32). These children can also present with large abdominal masses involving the GI tract, kidneys, and ovaries. Sporadic BL usually involves the gut, ovaries, kidneys, Waldeyer ring, and breasts. Pleural effusions and ascites are common. Lymphadenopathy is a clinical feature mostly seen in adult patients. Advanced clinical stage, bulky disease, and increased LDH levels relate to higher risk for CNS involvement.

In some variants, the bone marrow is heavily infiltrated and Burkitt cells are seen in the peripheral blood (Fig. 11.33). These cases were

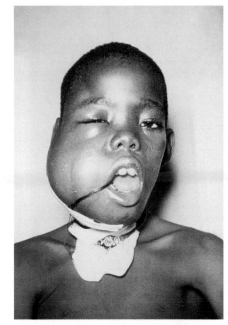

**Fig. 11.32** Endemic Burkitt lymphoma: facial bone and jaw infiltration. Courtesy of CDC/Robert S. Craig. This image is in the public domain. http://phil.cdc.gov/phil/details.asp (ID# 6050)

previously classified as acute lymphoblastic leukaemia, L3 type in the FAB classification. In the HIV+ population, BL may be the first AIDS defining criterion. It involves the bone marrow, lymph nodes, and abdominal extranodal sites.

*Morphology*
The malignant cells are medium-sized, with **deeply basophilic cytoplasm** and **abundant lipid vacuoles**. The nucleus is round, with multiple basophilic nucleoli. The BL cells have high proliferation capacity and mitotic as well as apoptotic figures are commonly seen. The infiltrate consists of uniform malignant cells and numerous scattered macrophages that produce the characteristic 'starry-sky pattern' (Fig. 11.34).

*Immunophenotype and genetics*
BL cells express B-cell-related antigens such as sIgM, CD19, CD20, CD22, and also CD10 and BCL6. CD34, CD5, and CD23 antigens are not expressed. The translocation **t(8;14)(q24;q32)** is found in 80% and t(2;8) or t(8;22) is found in the remaining 20% of cases. With these events, the **MYC gene** is translocated close to the promoters

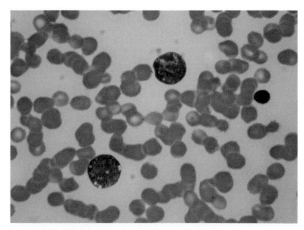

**Fig. 11.33** Burkitt lymphoma cells (peripheral blood). Image supplied courtesy of Professor Barbara Bain.

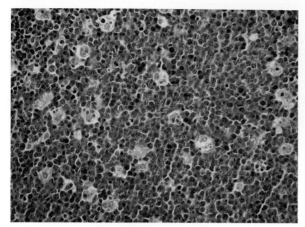

**Fig. 11.34** Burkitt lymphoma: 'starry sky' pattern of lymph node infiltration. Image courtesy of Professor Maria Bai.

of one of the Ig genes and is expressed under their influence. MYC overexpression is thought to contribute to lymphomatogenesis in BL.

### Treatment

Short-term, high-intensity chemotherapy combined with CNS prophylaxis offer CR and long-term OS in 75–90% of the children with BL. With similar approaches, adult patients achieve CR in 65–100% and long-term OS in 50–70%. Commonly used chemotherapy protocols are the CODOX-M/IVAC (cyclophophamide, vincristine, doxorubicin, high-dose methotrexate, and intrathecal therapy/ifosfamide, etoposide, high-dose cytarabine, and intrathecal therapy), the similar COP/COPADM protocol (prednisone, vincristine, cyclophosphamide, cytarabine, methotrexate and doxorubicin), and the hyper-CVAD protocol (hyperfractionated cyclophosphamide, vincristine, doxorubicin, and dexamethasone) combined with intrathecal therapy.

## T-cell lymphomas

Mature T-cell and NK-cell malignancies represent 20% of all NHL. Some entities present mainly with a leukaemic picture and are discussed elsewhere in this chapter.

### Peripheral T-cell lymphomas

This is a heterogeneous group of clinical and pathological entities, which includes 3–4% of all NHL. They occur in adult patients presenting with lymphadenopathy, splenomegaly, hepatomegaly, and marrow involvement. B-symptoms are common. The immunophenotype of the malignant cells is usually CD3+, CD2+, CD5+, CD4+, CD8−.

Peripheral T-cell lymphomas have a suboptimal response to combination chemotherapy. CR may be achieved but the relapse rates are very high. The OS at 5years is 20–30%.

### Anaplastic large cell lymphoma (ALCL)

#### Epidemiology
- 3% of all adult NHL.
- 20–30% of paediatric NHL.

#### Clinical presentation
ALCL are aggressive lymphomas and most patients (75%) present with advanced stage disease. Lymphadenopathy and systemic symptoms comprise the typical clinical pattern, although extranodal involvement of skin, bones, soft tissues, lung, and liver is also seen.

#### Morphology
Several morphological variants are described. The common variant ALCL (70%) is characterized by pleomorphic, large cells that invade the lymphoid sinuses.

#### Immunophenotype and genetics
Expression of the **CD30 antigen** (previously known as Ki-1) is the most notable feature of the ALCL immunophenotype. The majority of cases of ALCL (60–85%) are positive for the **ALK protein** (anaplastic large cell lymphoma kinase). This relates to translocations involving the *ALK* gene locus on chromosome 2. The most common translocation is t(2;5), which results in gene overexpression with both nuclear and cytoplasmic positive staining for ALK protein using immunohistochemistry. The ALK protein expression is specific feature of ALCL.

#### Treatment
Despite the aggressive clinical presentation, ALCL responds to combination chemotherapy. The IPI may predict the outcome in ALCL. In addition, ALK-negative cases have shorter OS.

**Brentuximab vedotin** is an anti-CD30 antibody conjugated to the potent antimicrotubuline agent monomethylauristatin E (MMAE). It achieves >80% response rates, including 57% CR, in relapsed/refractory ALCL with 12 months' median duration.

### Mycosis fungoides (MF) and Sézary syndrome (SS)
MF and SS are T-cell lymphomas that present mainly with cutaneous disease.

#### Epidemiology
- MF represents 3% of all NHL.
- More common in black and in male individuals.
- Rare in individuals aged <30 years.

#### Clinical presentation
MF has a long natural history, usually over 4–10 years. It evolves from a premalignant phase, where non-specific eczematous eruptions or atopic dermatitis is seen. The first diagnostic lesions of MF are patches that involve sun protected sites and may be associated with pruritus. Plaques resembling psoriasis that regress with ultraviolet radiation may also develop. Hyperkeratosis of the palms and soles may also be seen in this phase. If untreated, MF progresses to the tumour phase with skin nodules in previously unaffected areas that may ulcerate and become secondarily infected. Lymphadenopathy and visceral organ infiltration follows. The MF may also evolve into generalized erythroderma, alone or in combination with tumours and plaques.

SS is the leukaemic variant of MF, characterized by malignant T cells in the peripheral blood, (Sézary cells) erythroderma, lymphadenopathy, and visceral organ infiltration in the terminal stages. Sézary cells are recognized in the peripheral blood from their typical **cerebriform nucleus**. The bone marrow is involved only in the late phase of the disease.

#### Immunophenotype and genetics
Lymphoma cells express CD2, CD3, CD5, CD7, CD25, and TCRbeta. The TCR receptor genes are clonally rearranged. This can be of clinical importance, since molecular studies applied in tissue biopsies can differentiate MF from polyclonal T-cell infiltrates or be used to monitor residual disease.

#### Treatment
In the early phase of MF, treatment aims at the control of the skin lesions and prevention of evolution to tumour phase disease. Topical treatment modalities include chemotherapy (nitrogen mustard, BCNU), phototherapy (PUVA), and electron beam therapy. Single agent or combination chemotherapy is used in advanced or relapsed tumour stage disease. Extracorporeal photopheresis alone or in combination with other treatment has been used in tumour stage MF and SS. Small series of patients have been treated with allogeneic SCT in tumour stages. Tumour stage MF has a poor prognosis with a median OS of 2.5 years in cases of lymph node or visceral involvement.

## Multiple myeloma

Multiple myeloma (MM) is a malignant disorder in which plasma cells infiltrate the bone marrow and produce a paraprotein, usually a monoclonal immunoglobulin—IgG/IgA or light chains. The paraprotein is found in the serum and/or urine.

### Epidemiology

- MM accounts for ~10% of haematological malignancies.
- Its annual incidence is 3–4/100,000 and is significantly higher in the black population.
- The median age at diagnosis is around 65 years.
- MM is slightly more common in men.

### Aetiology

Aetiology is unknown. However, individuals with monoclonal gammopathy of undetermined significance (MGUS) have 1% annual risk of developing MM.

### Pathogenesis and genetics

Myeloma plasma cells accumulate in the marrow and develop a complex network of interactions with osteoclasts, endothelial cells, other stromal cells, and the marrow matrix, mediated by cytokines, adhesion molecules, and cell–cell contact. This network supports growth and survival of the myeloma cells and is also the basis for many complications of MM such as osteoclast activation and bone destruction.

Primary genetic abnormalities are thought to occur in development of MM and include:

- Chromosomal rearrangements involving the highly expressed IGH gene in chromosome 14q32 (40%).
- Hyperdiploidy (60%).

In the evolution of MM secondary genetic events occur, such as p53 deletion, RAS or MYC upregulation.

### Clinical presentation and complications

- **Anaemia** (Hb <12g/dL) is present in 70% at diagnosis but develops in virtually all patients during the course of MM.
- **Skeletal disease**. Bone pain due to osteolytic lesions is the most characteristic clinical feature of MM. The vertebrae, ribs, skull, hips, pelvis, and humeri can be affected (Fig. 11.35). Unexplained back or rib pain, persisting for months before diagnosis, is typical. Large lesions may result in pathological fractures, commonly vertebral collapse. Plain XRs reveal osteolytic lesions and osteopenia.
- **Hypercalcaemia** occurs in >30% as a consequence of osteoclast activation. It causes drowsiness, confusion, polyuria, polydipsia, constipation, long QT, and renal impairment. Severe hypercalcaemia is an emergency.
- **Infections.** Both humoral (immune paresis: low normal serum immunoglobulins) and cellular immunity are impaired in MM. Patients may present with recurrent bacterial chest and urinary tract infections. At diagnosis, encapsulated organisms such as *Streptococcus pneumonia* and *Haemophilus influenzae* are the most common pathogens. After chemotherapy, severe infections by Gram-negative bacilli and *Staphylococcus aureus* are a leading cause of death. Herpes zoster reactivation can occur, sometimes with two or more episodes in the same patient.
- **Renal impairment**. Mainly due to the excretion of large amounts of free light chains in the urine, the resultant protein deposition in the renal tubules causing cast nephropathy. Other contributing conditions include dehydration, hypercalcaemia, nephrotoxic drugs or contrast media, infections, amyloid, or plasma cell kidney infiltration. Patients with light

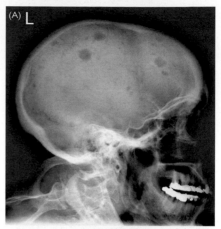

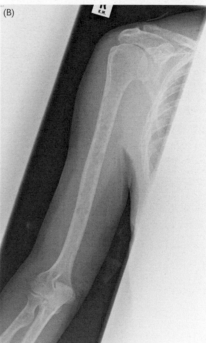

**Fig. 11.35** Multiple myeloma: osteolytic lesions of the skull (A); several osteolytic lesions of the right humerus (B).

chain myeloma are at greater risk of renal impairment. Serum creatinine >130μmol/L is found in 30% at diagnosis, reversible in 50% of patients, especially if it relates to hypercalcaemia or dehydration.

- **Spinal cord compression** is a severe complication of MM (and a medical emergency) caused by a myelomatous mass or collapsed vertebra compressing the spinal cord (Fig. 11.36). It usually presents with severe back pain, muscle weakness, urinary frequency/retention, constipation, or sensory loss. Examination may reveal a sensory level. MRI spine is the preferred diagnostic imaging technique.
- **Other manifestations** of MM include hyperviscosity syndrome, bleeding due to haemostatic abnormalities, and peripheral neuropathy.

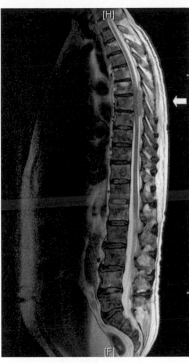

**Fig. 11.36** MRI spine in multiple myeloma: several lesions of the vertebrae bodies and cord compression caused by a soft tissue mass (plasmacytoma) in C6–C8 level.

## Laboratory investigation and findings

- At diagnosis, FBC may reveal anaemia, but the WBC and platelet counts are usually normal. **Plasma cell leukaemia** is defined as $>2 \times 10^9/L$ or >20% plasma cells in the peripheral blood and it can occur *de novo* or secondary to MM. Rarely, in plasma cell leukaemia, leucocytosis can occur. Thrombocytopenia occurs as a result of extensive plasma cell infiltration of the marrow.
- The ESR is increased in MM. The blood film shows increased **rouleaux formation** (Fig. 11.37).
- Biochemical studies may reveal increased serum creatinine, calcium, and B2M. CRP and LDH may also be elevated. ALP is normal, except when there is a fracture, liver amyloidosis, or other liver disease.

- Serum protein electrophoresis and immunofixation detect monoclonal immunoglobulin (paraprotein), usually IgG or IgA. Levels of normal immunoglobulins in the serum are low (hence hypogammaglobulinaemia should prompt a search for MM). In 30% of cases, myeloma cells produce only light chains, which are excreted and detected in the urine (Bence Jones protein). Rarely, no paraprotein is secreted (non-secretory MM).
- In almost all cases free light chains can be detected in the serum, even in cases where paraprotein or Bence Jones protein is undetectable. Serum free light chains can be used instead of urine test to monitor light chain myeloma.
- The plain radiological survey of the skeleton reveals lytic bone lesions, more prominent in the spine, sternum, ribs, skull, humeri, and femora. MRI has increased sensitivity in detecting spine lesions and cord compression.

### Diagnosis

The diagnostic criteria of symptomatic MM (WHO) are:
- Bone marrow plasma cells >10% or plasmacytoma (Fig. 11.38).
- Serum paraprotein IgG >30g/L, IgA >25g/L, or urine Bence Jones protein >1g/24 hours.
- Organ or tissue impairment (CRAB: hyper**c**alcaemia, **r**enal insufficiency, **a**naemia, **b**one lesions).

The diagnosis of **asymptomatic myeloma** requires marrow plasmacytosis >10% and/or paraprotein at MM levels and absence of any myeloma-related tissue or organ involvement (including lytic lesions) or symptoms.

### Treatment of MM

Only patients with symptomatic MM require treatment. Patients with asymptomatic MM should be actively monitored and there is no evidence to support early treatment. Treatment of MM includes: systemic chemotherapy to control disease and improve survival and treatment of complications and supportive care.

*Chemotherapy for MM*

Chemotherapeutic agents with proven efficacy in MM include conventional chemotherapy (melphalan, cyclophosphamide, anthracyclines) corticosteroids immunoregulatory drugs (thalidomide, lenalidomide, pomalinomide), and the proteasome inhibitors bortezomib and carfilzomib.

- **Induction chemotherapy.** Patients eligible for high-dose therapy and autologous SCT should receive induction chemotherapy that spares the haematopoietic stem cells. Commonly used combinations of a newer agent with steroids and/or conventional chemotherapy: CTD (cyclophosphamide, thalidomide, dexamethasone) or VTD (bortezomib, thalidomide, dexamethasone). Induction chemotherapy is given to maximum response. Patients ineligible for SCT may be treated with melphalan or

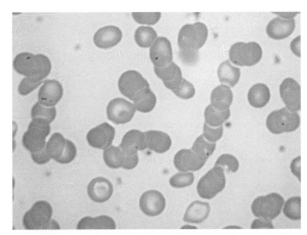

**Fig. 11.37** Blood film in MM: RBC rouleaux.
Image supplied courtesy of Professor Barbara Bain.

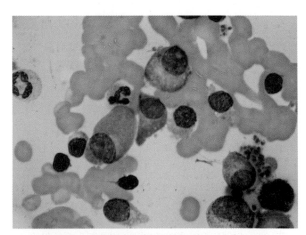

**Fig. 11.38** Bone marrow: myeloma plasma cells.
Image supplied courtesy of Professor Barbara Bain.

cyclophosphamide —plus corticosteroids plus thalidomide or bortezomib.

- **Autologous SCT.** Standard treatment for patients <60 years and should be considered in fit patients 60–70 years or older. High-dose melphalan and autologous SCT is a safe and effective treatment for MM, although all patients relapse. Median PFS after autologous SCT is 20–28 months and the OS is 54–72 months.

- **Allogeneic SCT.** The only potentially curative option but applicable only to young patients, providing they have first achieved at least partial response to chemotherapy/autologous SCT. High transplant-related mortality (30–50%) remains a major barrier. Allogeneic SCT using reduced intensity conditioning (RIC) is safer and may follow an autologous SCT. Donor lymphocyte infusions can be given for residual/relapsed disease.

- **Relapsed/refractory MM.** Patients with relapsed MM may receive re-induction and second high-dose therapy plus autologous SCT. The proteasome inhibitor bortezomib may be used at first relapse. Lenalidomide and pomalinomide are effective even in thalidomide refractory MM, and have a safer toxicity profile.

*Supportive care—treatment of complications*

- **Anaemia.** May require blood transfusion.

- **Bone disease**. Bisphosphonates are part of standard supportive care and should be offered to all myeloma patients. Biphosphonates (zoledronic acid) may reduce bone pain, new lytic lesions and pathological fractures, and are also effective for the management of hypercalcaemia. There is risk of osteonecrosis of the jaw with bisphosphonate use; all patients should have a dental assessment prior to starting bisphosphonates. Vertebroplasty is the percutaneous injection of cement into a fractured vertebral body, under radiological guidance (Fig. 11.39). It effectively reduces the pain and strengthens the bone but does not restore the vertebra to previous size.

- **Hypercalcaemia.** Vigorous hydration ± furosemide (to increase calcium excretion) with fluid balance monitoring, bisphosphonates (zoledronic acid is more effective), MM treatment.

- **Spinal cord compression.** It is a medical emergency. Dexamethasone 8–12mg daily, urgent local radiotherapy administrated within the first 24 hours. Surgery is indicated only if fractured bones compress the cord or in spinal instability.

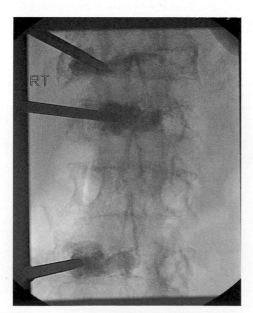

**Fig. 11.39** Vertebroplasty: cement infusion in collapsed vertebrae.

- **Acute renal impairment**. Hydration and correction of hypercalcaemia usually corrects renal function to normal within 48 hours. Unresponsive renal impairment requires advice from a renal physician and possibly dialysis. The role of plasmapheresis in light chain myeloma presenting with renal failure is controversial; trials are in progress.

# Monoclonal gammopathy of undetermined significance

Approximately 2% of individuals aged over 50 years have a low concentration paraprotein in the serum, without symptoms or signs suggestive of MM. The risk rises with age. WHO diagnostic criteria:

- Paraprotein, but less than myeloma levels.
- Marrow plasmacytosis <10%.
- No lytic bone lesions.
- No symptoms related to myeloma.

The annual risk for progression to MM or other related disease is estimated at 1%. Higher level of paraprotein, IgM or IgA paraprotein, and marrow plasma cells >5% have been proposed as predictors of progression. The life expectancy of individuals with MGUS seems to be slightly lower compared to control population. 50% die from another cause. Differential diagnosis from MM is essential. Management includes periodical clinical evaluation with measurement of paraprotein levels and skeletal imaging if indicated.

# Waldenström macroglobulinaemia

Waldenström macroglobulinaemia (WM) is a type of lymphoma with lymphoplasmacytic lymphocytes and presence of IgM paraprotein.

## Epidemiology

- The median age at diagnosis is 65 years.
- The estimated annual incidence is 2.5 per million.
- WM is more common in men than women

## Aetiology
Unknown.

## Clinical presentation and complications

Some patients with WM remain asymptomatic for many years after diagnosis, without any treatment. The clinical manifestations and complications of WM result from the presence of a high concentration of an IgM paraprotein in the serum and the infiltration of the marrow and other organs by malignant lymphocytes, or deposition of IgM paraprotein or amyloid.

- **Anaemia and thrombocytopenia** are common consequences of marrow infiltration.

- **Fatigue, fever, sweats, weight loss** are non-specific, constitutional symptoms caused by the tumour cells.

- **Hepatomegaly, splenomegaly, lymphadenopathy** are found in about 1/3 of the patients.

- **Bleeding diathesis,** mostly with mucosal haemorrhage, is caused by the interference of the serum paraprotein with several coagulation factors and platelet function.

- **Hyperviscosity syndrome**. The blood viscosity increases significantly when increased amounts of the large-size IgM immunoglobulin are present. It occurs in 10–30% of the patients with WM. The hyperviscosity syndrome presents with dizziness, oronasal bleeding, visual disturbances that may relate to retinal bleeding, ataxia, vertigo, confusion, and encephalopathy.

- **Cryoglobulinaemia** presents in 5% of WM with skin ulcers/necrosis, cold urticaria, and Raynaud phenomenon.

- **Organ infiltration** by malignant lymphocytes, including skin (maculopapular lesions, nodules, plaques), lungs (infiltrates, masses, pleural effusions), and kidneys.

- **Amyloidosis**, related to WM usually affects the heart, peripheral nerves, lungs, kidneys, and skin.
- **Peripheral neuropathy** may be caused by IgM paraprotein with autoantibody activity or by amyloid deposition.
- In contrast to myeloma, lytic bone lesions are **not** a feature of WM.

### Laboratory findings
- Bone marrow reveals infiltration by lymphoplasmacytic lymphocytes, sometimes plasma cells. Mast cells are characteristically increased.
- Immunophenotyping demonstrates lymphocyte markers.
- Increased serum B2M, low Hb, thrombocytopenia <100 × 10⁹/L, cryoglobulinaemia, and low serum albumin are findings of adverse prognostic significance.

### Diagnosis
The diagnosis of WM is based on the presence of an IgM paraprotein in the serum and the infiltration of the marrow by lymphoplasmacytoid lymphoma. Although in most cases the amount of IgM paraprotein in the serum is >30g/L, the diagnosis of WM can be made irrespectively of the paraprotein concentration. A typical immunophenotype of blood or marrow lymphoplasmacytoid cells also supports a WM diagnosis and may help to differentiate it from other lymphomas.

### Treatment
- Asymptomatic patients do not require treatment.
- Common indications for treatment are anaemia (Hb <10g/dL) or thrombocytopenia (PLT <100 × 10⁹/L) related to disease, significant organomegaly and/or lymphadenopathy, constitutional symptoms, hyperviscosity syndrome, or coagulopathy.
- **Plasmapheresis** can be effective in the management of hyperviscosity syndrome.

*Chemotherapy for WM*
- The main agents used in the treatment of WM are alkylating agents, purine analogues, corticosteroids, and rituximab. Newer treatments, mostly for relapse/chemoresistance, include thalidomide and bortezomib. Response to chemotherapy can be slow, and the IgM may continue to fall after the course of treatment has ended.
- **Alkylating agents** (chlorambucil, cyclophosphamide, melphalan) alone produce a slow response with minimal toxicity in 60% of the cases with a median estimated survival of 60 months.
- The purine analogues **fludarabine** and **cladribine** are equally effective and produce a response in 60–90% of the previously untreated patients—also effective in relapse.
- **Rituximab** (anti-CD20 mAb) alone may induce response in 30–50% including those who have relapsed after previous treatments. It may be beneficial for peripheral neuropathy. It can transiently aggravate the symptoms of hyperviscosity and should be used with caution.
- **Combination chemotherapy** with the earlier listed agents or also corticosteroids, e.g. CHOP chemotherapy may increase response rates because of the synergistic effect.

- **Autologous SCT** following high-dose chemotherapy is a possible safe approach for younger patients (TRM 5%) and although complete remission is rare and cure never achieved, median event-free survival (EFS) of 70 months and estimated OS 93% at 4 years has been reported.

## Systemic AL amyloidosis

- Amyloid is an amorphous, proteinaceous material, which deposits in several body tissues.
- Systemic AL amyloidosis results from tissue deposition of amyloid derived from monoclonal immunoglobulins or their fragments. The majority of cases are due to clonal plasma cell neoplasms but symptoms are due to light chain deposition not bulk of malignant cells; only 20% have overt myeloma. Monoclonal lambda light chain is the most common type of paraprotein involved in amyloid formation.
- The median age at diagnosis is 65 years.

### Clinical presentation
Depends on the involved organs. Amyloidosis usually presents with nephrotic syndrome, cardiomyopathy, peripheral or autonomic neuropathy, purpura (vessel wall infiltration), carpal tunnel syndrome, macroglossia, and skin infiltration.

### Diagnosis
- Systemic AL amyloidosis should be suspected in the setting of a plasma cell dyscrasia and a clinical syndrome of specific organ involvement with amyloid infiltration.
- The diagnosis requires **biopsy** of an affected organ and **Congo Red staining**, which produces characteristic apple-green birefringence under polarized light. Special stains can confirm if the amyloid is AL light chain or a different type of protein deposition.
- Evaluation of organ involvement and extent of amyloidosis is needed for treatment planning and prognosis. Consider referral to a specialist. SAP scan is a quantitative method using serum amyloid P component labelled with iodine-123. It offers the best imaging for visceral amyloidosis. ECG and echocardiography assess cardiac infiltration and function. Studies for autonomic neuropathy are useful.

### Treatment
Treatment of AL amyloidosis is aimed at the underlying plasma cell disorder. Organ-specific treatment may also be necessary.

Melphalan and high-dose corticosteroids have been widely used with limited response. Eligible patients should be treated with autologous SCT, which may produce higher OS than chemotherapy alone. Patients with single organ involvement are most likely to benefit. Thalidomide plus dexamethasone has been used more recently with good results.

Response to treatment can be monitored by reduction in paraprotein, serum free light chains, and reduction in amyloid deposition on a SAP scan. Response to treatment may be very slow, and in many patients achievement of stable disease is the best that can be expected.

## Hereditary bleeding disorders

Hereditary bleeding disorders are usually caused by deficiency of a single coagulation factor. Although deficiencies of most of the coagulation factors have been recorded, von Willebrand disease, haemophilia A, and haemophilia B account for >96% of the cases.

### Von Willebrand disease

Von Willebrand factor (VWF) is an adhesive glycoprotein which plays a major role during early haemostasis:

- Produced only by megakaryocytes and endothelial cells.
- Secreted into the plasma and the subendothelium, but also stored in large amounts in the secretory granules of platelets and endothelial cells.
- Produced and secreted in the form of large multimer molecules, made of 300kD-subunit dimers. These multimers have highly adhesive properties and some of them can remain attached on the vessel surface. Normally, since the metalloprotease ADATMS13 processes the high-molecular-weight (HMW) multimers into smaller molecules, WVF is present in plasma in a range of multimers measuring 600–20,000kD.
- In the plasma it complexes with and stabilizes factor VIII.
- Upon tissue injury, VWF is released and binds the collagen of the endothelial basement membrane and platelet glycoprotein Ib (GPIb), slowing platelet flow. This is essential for initial adhesion of platelets to the vessel surface.
- VWF also binds strongly to GPIIb/GPIIIa on the platelet surface and participates in platelet plug formation.

Von Willebrand disease (VWD) results from **quantitative** or **qualitative defects** of VWF. It is the commonest inherited bleeding disorder and follows an AR or AD pattern. The different genetic defects, but also the myriad of parameters that affect the levels of VWF in the plasma reflect the heterogeneous clinical severity of VWD.

*Clinical presentation and diagnosis*

Bleeding history is of paramount importance for the diagnosis of VWD. This should assess:

1. **Spontaneous bleeding** and
2. **Response to haemostatic challenges**.

Bleeding manifestations suggestive of VWD include:

- Spontaneous epistaxis lasting >20 minutes.
- Bruising or cutaneous bleeding with trivial trauma.
- Prolonged (>15 minutes) bleeding from trivial wounds or the oral cavity that recurs with 7 days.
- Spontaneous GI bleeding and chronic anaemia.
- Heavy and prolonged bleeding after surgery (tooth extraction, tonsillectomy), menorrhagia, or skin or mucous membrane bleeding requiring medical attention.
- Family history of bleeding is important, as well as the pattern of inheritance.

*Laboratory testing*

- Preliminary screening should include:
  - FBC (thrombocytopenia is found in type 2B VWD).
  - Activated partial thromboplastin time (aPTT, usually prolonged or normal in VWD).
  - Prothrombin time (PT), fibrinogen, and thrombin time (all normal in VWD).
- Specific investigation includes testing for the plasma levels of VWF antigen (VWF:Ag) and factor VIII (FVIII:C) and functional assays. The ristocetin cofactor activity (VWF:RCo), the ristocetin-induced platelet aggregation (RIPA), and the PFA-100® assays measure VWF affinity to platelet ligands. Other functional assays measure VWF's binding affinity to collagen (VWF:CB) and

factor VIII (VWF:FVIII). The analysis of VWF multimers with gel electrophoresis reveals characteristic distribution patterns for some types of VWD.

*Some factors may influence VWF levels*

Genetic defect ↓ or ↑, O blood group ↓, neonates ↑, pregnancy ↑, stress ↑, physical exercise ↑, malignancy ↑, inflammatory diseases ↑, hypothyroidism ↓, hyperthyroidism ↑.

*Classification of VWD*

There are >22 types of VWD, which can be classified as a qualitative (type 2) or quantitative defect (types 1 and 3):

**Type 1**: clinically mild to moderate bleeding disorder, characterized by partial quantitative deficiency of VWF.

- Most common type of VWD; 60–80% of all cases.
- aPTT prolonged or normal.
- VWF:Ag values are low (10–40IU/L).
- FVIII:C are also decreased.
- Patients with VWF:Ag <20IU/L may present with more severe bleeding. Mild phenotype in those with only slightly decreased VWF:Ag levels.

**Type 2A**: qualitative defect associated with absence of HMW multimers on electrophoresis.

**Type 2B**: gain of function defect characterized by increased binding affinity of VWF to GPIb. Patients present with thrombocytopenia (platelets 75–100 × 10⁹/L), which may worsen in pregnancy or with DDAVP® (1-deamino-8-D-arginine vasopressin).

**Type 2M**: qualitative defect with normal HMW multimers.

**Type 2N (Normandy)**: decreased binding affinity for factor VIII. The FVIII:C is low (5–20IU/L) but VWD must not be confused with haemophilia A.

**Type 3**: severe quantitative defect where VWF:Ag is almost absent. Patients present with severe complications with joint and muscle haemorrhage, starting during childhood.

*Treatment*

- **DDAVP**® is a synthetic vasopressin analogue, which releases stored VWF and FVIII and increases their plasma levels. It can be given IV or as a nasal spray. It is effective for type 1 and may reduce the use of blood products. DDAVP® has variable effect on type 2 and no effect on type 3 VWD. Use in type 2B is controversial, since release of abnormal VWF may worsen thrombocytopenia.
- **Tranexamic acid** is an antifibrinolytic drug, which can be used alone or in combination with DDAVP®. It is given intravenously, orally, or as a mouthwash for the management of menorrhagia, epistaxis, mucosal bleeding, or to cover tooth extraction. It should be avoided in urinary tract bleeding, due to the risk of clot obstruction.
- **Blood product** concentrates are used in lack of response to DDAVP®, in severe types of VWD, or to cover major surgery. The products most commonly used are BPL 8Y®, Alphanate®, and Haemate-P®. The use of cryoprecipitate is generally not recommended when appropriate concentrates are available.

### Haemophilia A and B

Haemophilia A and B (Christmas disease) are caused by absent or very low activity of factor VIII and factor IX respectively.

- Both are X-linked recessive congenital disorders.
- The prevalence of haemophilia A is ~100–160 per million male population. Prevalence of haemophilia B is 5× lower.

*Genetics*

The factor VIII gene is located at Xq28 and has 26 exons. The most common genetic defect, found in 45% of patients with severe haemophilia A, is a large inversion and translocation of exons 1–22.

Although >800 other mutations have been described, the genetic defect remains unclear in 5–10% of patients.

The factor IX gene is located at Xq27 and at least 2100 genetic defects have been recorded, mostly point mutations.

As the diseases are X-linked, almost all patients are male, but females can be affected if daughter of carrier mother and affected father, or carrier females may be mildly affected if skewed X-inactivation.

### Pathophysiology

Factor VIII is a glycoprotein produced mainly in the liver with a $t_{1/2}$ of 12 hours in the plasma. It forms a complex with VWF and is protected from proteolytic degradation. Factor IX is a vitamin K-dependant serine protease with a $t_{1/2}$ ~24 hours.

Both factor VIIIa and IXa are needed for the amplification and consolidation of factor Xa activity, which follows its initial activation from the tissue factor/factor VIIa complex. Primary haemostasis and platelet plug formation occur normally, but secondary haemostasis and fibrin formation to stabilize the plug fail in haemophilia due to absence of factor VIIIa or IXa.

### Clinical manifestations

Depend on the amount of factor VIII or IX in the plasma:

- Severe haemophilia: <0.01IU/L (<1% of normal).
- Moderate haemophilia: 0.01–0.05IU/L (1–5% of normal).
- Mild haemophilia: 0.05–0.4IU/L (5–40% of normal).

### Severe haemophilia

- Children with severe haemophilia have a small risk (1–4%) of intracranial bleeding during the 1st week of life. Otherwise, the first manifestations occur when they start to crawl.
- **Major, spontaneous joint haemorrhage** is the hallmark presentation of haemophilia. Knees, elbows, and ankles are commonly involved. The bleeding is followed by oedema and severe pain. Untreated chronic joint haemorrhage is destructive, leading to arthropathy, deformities, and muscle weakness (Fig. 11.40). Joint deformities and muscle wasting in poorly treated haemophilia result in immobility and chronic disability.
- **Spontaneous muscle or soft tissue bleeding with bruising** presents with pain and swelling (Fig. 11.41).
- Mucous surface and GI tract bleeding may be induced by aspirin or NSAIDs.
- **Intracranial bleeding** is the most common fatal complication.
- In general, any bleeding episode in patients with severe haemophilia is considered a serious event and requires prompt treatment.
- Individuals with moderate haemophilia develop joint haemorrhage usually after minor injuries. In mild forms of haemophilia,

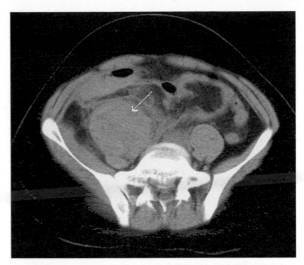

**Fig. 11.41** Severe haemophilia A: large right-sided psoas sheath haematoma (arrow). Bleeding into the psoas muscle or the retroperitoneal space can be of large volume. It may present with abdominal pain and fever resembling an acute abdomen.

475

spontaneous bleeding does not occur and diagnosis may not be made until later in adult life. Tooth extraction, surgery, or trauma followed by excessive bleeding and a prolonged aPTT suggest the diagnosis.

### Diagnosis

- The bleeding presentation and history in haemophilia is typical and highly suggestive of the diagnosis.
- Family history is helpful, although unremarkable in 1/3.
- aPTT is prolonged and levels of factor VIII or IX very low. VWF levels and functional tests normal or slightly high (differentiate haemophilia A from (rare) VWD types 2N and 3).
- Genetic testing of patient (and family) confirms diagnosis.

### Management

- **Replacement therapy** with the missing factor is vital for the management of bleeding episodes in haemophilia. Patients with severe haemophilia A are given intravenous infusions of factor VIII to achieve plasma levels 20–40% of normal in case of minor bleeding. More severe bleeding requires factor VIII levels >50%, while in life-threatening bleeding or to cover major surgery the target is 75–100% of normal. Factor IX is given in a similar fashion in haemophilia B, but at 18–24-hour intervals because of its longer $t_{1/2}$. Early treatment is important for pain relief in joint haemorrhage and for the prevention of arthropathy.
- **Recombinant factors VIII and IX** have now replaced plasma-derived factors used in previous decades. This eliminates the risk of viral infection (hepatitis B and C, and HIV infection), previously the most devastating complications of treatment with factor infusion.
- Patients with mild haemophilia A may be treated with DDAVP® and tranexamic acid, which can effectively cover minor bleeding, minor surgery, and tooth extraction without factor infusion. DDAVP® has no use in haemophilia B.
- **Long-term prophylactic factor infusion** starting in the first 2 years of life was tested in clinical trials, aiming to achieve factor levels >1% and convert severe haemophilia to moderate. This approach decreased joint damage and need for surgery, reduced bleeding episodes, and improved performance status. Cost and need for central vein devices are the main drawbacks. There is no evidence that prophylactic use of factors increase the incidence of inhibitors.
- **Inhibitors** are antibodies against the infused factor. They usually develop in severe haemophilia A (30–50%) but are far less

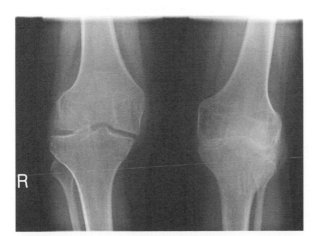

**Fig. 11.40** Arthropathy in a patient with severe haemophilia A and previous repeated haemarthrosis: complete loss of the joint space within the left knee. There are also degenerative changes within the right knee.

common in haemophilia B (3%). Black patients and some geno-types (large deletions) are more susceptible. If the presence of an inhibitor is suspected, a mixing test with normal plasma should be performed—if the aPTT does not correct, the presence of an inhibitor is likely and further investigation is required. Some haemophiliacs have transient, low-titre inhibitors, easily solved with a higher dose of infused factor, whilst the management of high-titre inhibitors can be extremely problematic. Recombinant factor VIIa bypasses the lack of active factor VIII and is used in bleeding episodes and surgery. High-dose immunosuppression is a successful approach in up to 80% of the cases.

- **Gene therapy** may offer a future cure for haemophilia, but concerns regarding effectiveness and safety remain.

## Hereditary disorders of platelet function

Hereditary disorders of the platelet function are rare conditions associated with impaired platelet adhesion, aggregation, or secretion of their granular content.

### Bernard–Soulier syndrome
- AR; absent/reduced GPIb-IX-V complex → impaired interaction with VWF, ↓ platelet adhesion.
- Thrombocytopenia, giant platelets, spontaneous bleeding.
- Platelet aggregation induced by ADP, adrenaline (epinephrine), and collagen is normal. However, RIPA in platelet-rich plasma is absent.
- Bleeding is treated with platelet transfusion. DDAVP® produces transient response in some patients.

### Glanzmann thrombaesthenia
- AR; mutations in genes encoding GPIIb and GPIIIa.
- Reduced or absent platelet aggregation in response to normal stimuli (ADP, collagen).
- Variable phenotype depending on residual amount of functional GPIIb/GPIIIa on the platelets.
- Severe disease presents with mucocutaneous bleeding in infancy, purpura, epistaxis, GI tract bleeding, and haematuria.
- Platelet count and morphology normal. The bleeding time is prolonged, but PT and aPTT are normal. Aggregometry and molecular characterization confirm the diagnosis.
- Platelet transfusion is the treatment of bleeding episodes.

### Storage pool diseases (SPD)
- Heterogeneous group of conditions characterized by impaired secretion of platelet granules and abnormal aggregation after stimulation with ADP and adrenaline (epinephrine).
- The SPD are divided into three groups, based on the affected type of granules: α-granules SPD (α-SPD), dense granules (δ-SPD), or αδ-SPD.
- **Grey platelet syndrome** (α-SPD) is characterized by moderate thrombocytopenia, large platelets that appear grey on May–Grünwald–Giemsa or Wright staining, and marrow fibrosis. Patients present with mucocutaneous bleeding and may require platelet transfusion.
- **Hermansky–Pudlak syndrome** is an AR δ-SPD. It presents with oculocutaneous albinism and easy bruising. Some cases also develop pulmonary fibrosis and granulomatous colitis.
- **Chédiak–Higashi syndrome** is also AR δ-SPD. Presents with bruising, oculocutaneous albinism and ↑ infections.
- **Wiskott–Aldrich syndrome** is a X-linked SPD of immunodeficiency, eczema and thrombocytopenia. The platelets are small and dysfunctional.

## Acquired bleeding disorders

### Disseminated intravascular coagulation
Disseminated intravascular coagulation (DIC) is an acquired pathological and clinical syndrome characterized by systemic activation of coagulation, intravascular formation of fibrin, and consumption of platelets and coagulation factors. The clinical expression of DIC varies from only abnormal laboratory tests to profuse bleeding or widespread microvascular thrombotic events with end-organ dysfunction. DIC is always triggered by an underlying clinical condition.

*Pathogenesis*
See Fig. 11.42.

*Clinical conditions associated with DIC*
- **Infections:** Gram-negative bacteria and Gram-positive encapsulated bacterial sepsis, varicella.
- **Malignancies:** acute promyelocytic leukaemia, prostate and pancreatic cancer.
- **Obstetric complications:** abruptio placenta, amniotic fluid embolism, pre-eclampsia, dead fetus syndrome.
- **Tissue injury and trauma:** head injury, burns, fat embolism, necrotic pancreatitis.
- **Toxins:** snake venoms.
- **Immunological disorders:** blood transfusion reactions, transplant rejection, severe allergic reactions.

*Clinical presentation and diagnosis*
The clinical manifestations of DIC present in the context of an underlying disorder.

**Acute and subacute DIC** is usually seen in bacterial sepsis, in some obstetric complications, in acute promyelocytic leukaemia, and tissue injury:
- Presentation is often through abnormal lab tests alone.
- Mucocutaneous bleeding is the most prominent clinical presentation, due to consumption and exhaustion of platelets and coagulation factors.
- **Waterhouse–Friderichsen syndrome** is a rare condition caused by thromboembolism of vital organs and adrenal necrosis.
- Purpura fulminans is usually seen in children with DIC and is characterized by skin microemboli and necrosis.
- Investigations show a low platelet count which further decreases rapidly, prolonged PT and aPTT and high levels of fibrin-degradation products and D-dimers. Levels of normal anticoagulants (antithrombin, protein C) are low.

**Chronic DIC** accompanies solid tumours and the dead fetus syndrome:

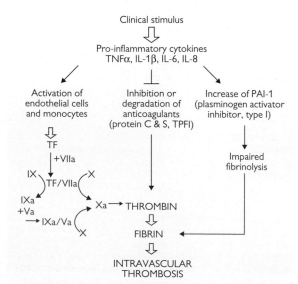

Fig. 11.42 Excessive and unregulated generation of thrombin has a primary role in the pathogenesis of DIC. TFPI: tissue factor plasminogen inhibitor.

- It is typically associated with thromboembolic complications and microangiopathic haemolytic anaemia.
- Thrombocytopenia, red cell fragmentation, hypofibrinogenaemia, and high fibrin-degradation products and D-dimers are the usual laboratory findings.

### Management

Specific treatment and control of the underlying disease is the basis of management. Otherwise, any therapy for DIC fails. Supportive treatment is needed in those with bleeding, overt thrombosis, and organ damage from fibrin deposition.

Replacement therapy with blood products should not be dictated by the laboratory test results, but reserved for significant bleeding:

- Platelet transfusion to aim for a count >20 × $10^9$/L.
- Cryoprecipitate to maintain fibrinogen >1mg/mL.
- FFP (10–15mL/kg) is given if ↑ PT or aPTT.
- Vitamin K replacement may be also necessary.

Patients with obvious thromboembolic complications (e.g. purpura fulminans, DVT in chronic DIC) require anticoagulation therapy with intravenous heparin infusion.

### Idiopathic thrombocytopenic purpura

Idiopathic thrombocytopenic purpura (ITP) is an autoimmune disorder characterized by platelet destruction, thrombocytopenia, and mucocutaneous bleeding.

- The aetiology is unknown.
- ITP develops in the absence of an underlying disease whereas secondary immune thrombocytopenia occurs in the context of autoimmune diseases (SLE), leukaemias and lymphomas, viral infections (hepatitis, HIV), and drug therapy (heparin).
- Acute ITP mostly affects children, resolves within 6 months (in 70%), and generally has an indolent course.
- Chronic ITP is mostly seen in adults.

### Epidemiology

- The annual incidence of ITP is 10 per 100,000, with children involved in 60–70% of the cases ($\female$:$\male$ = 1:1).
- Median age of adult patients is 57 years, $\female$:$\male$ = 2:1.

### Pathogenesis

- The platelet destruction in ITP is immune mediated.
- The presence of antiplatelet IgG autoantibodies against surface glycoproteins, such as GPIIb/GPIIIa, is well documented.
- Genetic factors and infections from viruses or bacteria (*Helicobacter pylori*) are presumed predisposing factors, although the mechanisms of antiplatelet Ab production remain unclear.
- Antibody-coated platelets are recognized by Fcγ receptors on macrophages and other antigen-presenting cells in the spleen or liver and phagocytosed, with platelet epitopes then presented to T$_h$-cells which induce high-affinity antibody production by B cells and platelet destruction. The role of cytotoxic T cells, NK cells, and complement in platelet destruction is unclear.
- Decreased platelet production may also participate in the pathogenesis of ITP.

### Clinical presentation and diagnosis

ITP presents with easy bruising, petechiae, epistaxis, haematuria, and mucosal bleeding. The severity of bleeding depends on the degree of thrombocytopenia:

- PLT count >50 × $10^9$/L rarely produces any symptoms.
- Petechiae or purpura develops when PLTs <20 × $10^9$/L.
- Intracranial haemorrhage and melaena, although uncommon complications at presentation, are associated with PLTs <10 × $10^9$/L and require urgent treatment.

Viral infections may precede ITP in children, but in general ITP develops in previously asymptomatic individuals. ITP remains a diagnosis of exclusion. Clinical and laboratory investigation should exclude conditions of secondary thrombocytopenia. Bone marrow examination is indicated in older patients (>60 years).

### Management

- ITP does not always require treatment.
- Children with ITP should be managed conservatively and require no active treatment: the risk of serious bleeding is extremely low and 80% will recover spontaneously within 8 weeks.
- Adult patients with PLT >50 × $10^9$/L will not require treatment in most cases. Treatment is clearly indicated for those with active bleeding or PLT <20–30 × $10^9$/L. A decision on individual basis should be made if PLT count is 30–50 × $10^9$/L (Table 11.2).

**Corticosteroids** are started together with IVIG. Prednisolone 1mg/Kg is usually given. The dose is then tapered slowly, especially after reaching 10mg daily. Dexamethasone 40mg for 4 days monthly may also produce rapid and lasting response. High-dose methylprednisolone has been used in refractory ITP.

**Intravenous immunoglobulin** (IVIG) (2g/kg) over 2–5 days produces rapid but transient response. IVIG is thought to block the Fcγ receptors of macrophages. It is also a good option for emergency therapy, in combination with high-dose methylprednisolone.

**Anti-D immunoglobulin** is an alternative to IVIG for Rh+ patients. The mechanism of action is not well understood.

**Splenectomy** is an option for patients with relapsing or refractory ITP. However, thrombocytopenia reoccurs in up to 25% and patients have increased risk for severe infections.

**Immunosuppression** with rituximab (anti-CD20), vincristine, and cyclophosphamide produce response rates of 25–50% and are alternatives to splenectomy for refractory ITP.

**Thrombopoietin-receptor agonists (romiplostim and eltrombopag)** are approved in chronic ITP patients failing steroids, IVIG, or splenectomy. Long-term responses are seen in 75% of patients.

### Thrombotic thrombocytopenic purpura

Thrombotic thrombocytopenic purpura (TTP) is a rare disorder, originally described by Moschcowitz in 1924. The clinical manifestations of TTP arise from widespread thrombosis of the microvasculature by platelet-rich thrombi.

### Epidemiology

- Annual incidence of TTP is 3–7 per million.
- $\female$:$\male$ = 2:1.

Allogeneic SCT, drugs (ticlopidine), infections (HIV), and carcinomas have been reported to trigger TTP, however in the vast majority of the cases (85%) the aetiology remains unknown.

### Pathogenesis

Only recently has the pathogenesis of idiopathic TTP been elucidated. The disease results from dysfunctional proteolysis of the HMW multimers of VWF. Under normal circumstances, the metalloproteinase ADAMTS13 is responsible for the proteolytic cleavage of these molecules into smaller size multimers. The presence of autoantibodies against ADAMTS13 and dysfunctional proteolysis is now documented in most cases of idiopathic TTP. The non-cleaved HMW multimers attach to the vascular endothelium and unfold under the high shear conditions of the microvasculature, exposing their active domain for platelet adhesion and aggregation. Severe deficiency of ADAMTS13 appears to be very specific for idiopathic TTP. An AR inherited form of ADAMTS13 insufficiency has been described in rare cases of familial TTP.

### Clinical presentation and diagnosis

Classically, TTP is described as a pentad of clinical features:

1. **Microangiopathic haemolytic anaemia** (MAHA): ↓ Hb, numerous red cell fragments in the blood smear (Fig. 11.43),

| Table 11.2 Recommendations for 'safe' platelet counts in adults | |
|---|---|
| Dentistry | ≥10 × $10^9$/L |
| Dental extractions/regional block | ≥30 × $10^9$/L |
| Minor surgery | ≥50 × $10^9$/L |
| Major surgery | ≥80 × $10^9$/L |

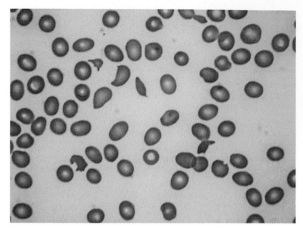

**Fig. 11.43** Blood film in TTP: red cell fragmentation.
Image supplied courtesy of Professor Barbara Bain.

↑ reticulocytes, ↑ nucleated red cells (latter two findings result of marrow reaction to compensate anaemia). The direct Coomb test is negative. ↑ bilirubin and ↑ LDH—the latter attributed both to red cell fragmentation and ischaemic tissue damage.

2. **Thrombocytopenia**: usually <50 × 10⁹/L, rarely complicated by haemorrhagic events. The coagulation screen typically unremarkable but D-dimers are elevated.

3. **Fever**: usually low grade; rigors or high-grade fever should raise the possibility of infection.

4. **Renal impairment**: reported only in 18–58% of the patients and usually mild–moderate.

5. **Neurological dysfunction**: common at presentation (70–100%) and represents thromboembolic disease of the brain microvasculature. Symptoms are diffuse, multifocal, transient but recurrent. Headache, dysarthria, aphasia, hemiparesis, confusion, and coma are common signs at diagnosis. They resolve with treatment, but residual neurological dysfunction is possible.

Presentation is often variable and the complete pentad is only found in 40% of patients.

Other clinical features of TTP include abdominal pain, nausea, and fatigue. Pancreatitis or cardiac events, including sudden death, are complications of the ischaemic tissue damage.

Patients should be tested for ADAMTS13 enzyme level and inhibitor (by specialist centres) to confirm diagnosis and distinguish between congenital/autoimmune TTP.

*Management*
Untreated TTP is nearly always (90%) fatal. Renal failure, cerebral, and myocardial infraction are the leading causes of death. With early diagnosis and treatment long-term survival exceeds 70%.

**Plasma exchange** is the only treatment with proven efficacy. Daily replacement of 1–1.5× of the patient's estimated plasma volume is recommended, at least until the platelet count returns to normal. Plasma therapy alone was shown inferior to plasma exchange. It is now believed that plasma exchange removes the inhibitor of ADAMTS13 and also replaces the deficient enzyme. The use of cryosupernatant plasma instead of FFP was addressed by randomized trials. The cryosupernatant plasma has the theoretical advantage of lacking VWF multimers. However, it remains controversial whether this translates into a clinical benefit.

**Corticosteroids** are used in TTP with little clinical benefit: UK guidelines recommend 3 days of IV methylprednisolone 1mg/kg, and adding aspirin when the platelet count is >50 × 10⁹/L .

**Relapse of TTP** occurs in 30–40% at 10 years. The timing of relapse is unpredictable and multiple relapses are possible. Splenectomy, defibrotide and rituximab are treatment modalities under investigation for this group of patients, in addition to plasma exchange.

## Haemolytic uraemic syndrome
The haemolytic uraemic syndrome (HUS) is characterized by the triad of: **microangiopathic haemolytic anaemia**, **thrombocytopenia**, and **renal impairment**. Unlike TTP, renal impairment is a predominant manifestation.

*Pathogenesis*
There are two main categories of HUS:
● Diarrhoea-associated HUS (D+)—90% of cases.
● Sporadic HUS (D−)—10% of cases.

*D+ HUS*
● 90% of HUS is associated with a preceding diarrhoeal illness which may occur in epidemics.
● Commonest form of AKI in children; no gender bias.
● More common in children <5 years old.
● Seasonal variation, more common in summer.
● Female preponderance in adults.

*Aetiology*
● Preceding diarrhoea is frequently caused by cytotoxin-producing strains of *Escherichia coli*. As few as 50 organisms can cause disease by releasing verocytotoxin or Shiga toxin into the bloodstream.
● The most common strain is O157:H7—although the 2011 German outbreak was caused by the novel strain O104:H4.
● The toxin promotes glomerular endothelial cell activation and ultimately a thrombotic microangiopathy with platelet activation and consumption. Renal histology reveals glomerular thrombosis and necrosis. ADAMTS 13 activity is not affected in HUS.

*Clinical evaluation*
● Prodrome of watery and bloody diarrhoea. Abdominal pain may be severe with haemorrhagic colitis.
● Onset of renal/haematological problems is usually after 6–10 days, by which time the diarrhoea may have resolved.
● AKI is usually oliguric with microscopic haematuria and proteinuria, but may be non-oliguric with macroscopic haematuria.

*Laboratory investigations*
● Thrombocytopenia.
● Anaemia is common; blood films shows fragmented and deformed cells with a reticulocytosis.
● LDH and unconjugated bilirubin are elevated.
● Coomb test is negative.
● Fibrin degradation products are elevated, but PT is normal.
● Neutrophilia may be marked, and is a poor prognostic indicator.
● Urate, urea, and creatinine are raised, and hyponatraemia is often seen at presentation.

*Management*
● No specific treatment is of proven benefit.
● Supportive management comprises careful fluid and electrolyte balance, blood pressure control, nutritional support, and dialysis where required.
● Antibiotics do not offer protection from developing D+ HUS.
● Most patients recover renal function.
● About 5% die during the acute episode, 5% develop ESRF, and 30% have long-term renal impairment with persistent proteinuria.

*D− HUS*
● The onset is typically insidious, although it may present following an upper respiratory tract infection. People of all ages can be affected, and there is no seasonal incidence.
● Severe hypertension is frequent and mortality is higher than with D+ HUS. Renal involvement is usually pronounced with significant proteinuria and uraemia.
● The disease may recur in both native kidneys and allografts, and may recur in a transplanted kidney.

- The cause is unknown. D− HUS can be associated with pregnancy, SLE, HIV, and various drugs including oral contraceptives and calcineurin inhibitors (ciclosporin and tacrolimus).
- D− HUS may be familial and may be inherited as both AR and AD forms.
- Mutations in Factor H, a regulator of the alternative complement pathway, have been identified in about 20% of both sporadic and familial cases of D− HUS, implicating complement-mediated endothelial damage in the pathogenesis of the disease.
- Plasmapheresis is thought to be beneficial in D− HUS, though some patients are treated with FFP alone.

### Acquired haemophilia-A

Acquired haemophilia-A (AHA) is a rare haemorrhagic disorder, which results from the development of factor VIII inhibitors.

- Annual incidence between 0.2 and 1 per million.
- It affects older individuals, with median age 60–70 years.
- AHA may be idiopathic or secondary to pregnancy, autoimmune diseases (SLE, RA, Sjögren), inflammatory bowel disease, allergic drug reactions, dermatological disorders (psoriasis, pemphigus), CLL, lymphomas, multiple myeloma, Waldenström macroglubinaemia, and solid cancers.
- Most patients (80%) present with mucocutaneous bleeding (skin, GI tract, and urinary tract).
- Unlike hereditary haemophilia A, joint haemorrhage is uncommon.
- Life-threatening complications include large retroperitoneal haematomas, intracranial haemorrhage, postpartum and surgery bleeding.
- The mortality rate is 8–22%.

*Diagnosis*

- Prolonged aPTT not corrected by mixing.
- Low factor VIII levels and the presence of inhibitor in a patient without previous or family history of bleeding disorders. Inhibitors in AHA are usually IgG, IgA, or IgM autoantibodies and have different functional properties compared to inhibitors found in hereditary haemophilia-A.

*Treatment*

- Treatment of bleeding episodes in low-titre inhibitor AHA is DDAVP® or human factor VIII. For high-titre inhibitors porcine factor VIII, prothrombin complex concentrate, or recombinant factor VIIa is used.
- Postpartum inhibitors may spontaneously resolve, but other patients will require eradication therapy. Immunosuppressive treatment usually with high-dose steroids and cytotoxic drugs (cyclophosphamide) is given, with response rates up to 70%. Rituximab (anti-CD20) is a less toxic approach and effective at least for low-titre inhibitors.

# Hereditary thrombophilia

= the tendency of some individuals to develop venous thrombosis, related to specific genetic defects. Affected persons develop venous thrombosis or thromboembolism usually when another acquired predisposing factor coexists, e.g. malignancy, surgery, therapy with oral contraceptives, and indwelling venous catheters.

Thrombophilia is a polygenic multifactorial condition. Only about 50% of families will have an identifiable genetic defect. Even in the absence of one of the following abnormalities, a strong family history—e.g. first-degree relative with VTE—is still an indication of increased thrombophilic risk.

### Factor V Leiden

Factor V Leiden results from a single point mutation and substitution of arginine by glutamine at position 506 (R506Q).

- Mutation frequency in the general population = 1–8%.
- Factor V Leiden confers resistance to activated protein C (APC).

- Heterozygotes have a 4× ↑ risk for thrombosis compared to general population, but >50× ↑ for homozygotes.
- Recurrent thromboses in 39% of heterozygotes and require lifelong anticoagulation.
- Thrombotic events are more common when another prothrombotic condition (e.g. OCP therapy) coexists.
- Factor V Leiden also increases the risk of arterial thrombosis and myocardial infarction.

### G20210A prothrombin gene mutation

- Threefold ↑ risk for venous thrombosis.
- Prevalence of the mutation in Europe is 3–4%.
- Risk for thrombosis increases in the homozygous state.
- Factor V Leiden coexists in 40% of G20210A prothrombin gene mutation cases presenting with thrombosis.

### Hereditary protein C deficiency

- AD disorder. Protein C is a vitamin K-dependent serine protease inhibitor of factors Va and VIIIa.
- Protein C deficiency is found in 0.5–4% of patients presenting with their first episode of thrombosis.
- ~75% of those with heterozygous protein C deficiency develop at least one thrombotic event, in most cases without the coexistence of other predisposing factors.
- Aggressive long-term anticoagulation is needed for patients with recurrent thromboses.
- Warfarin-induced skin necrosis is a severe complication associated with protein C deficiency.

### Hereditary protein S deficiency

- AD disorder found in 10% of individuals with hereditary thrombophilia.
- DVT and pulmonary embolism in heterozygous protein S deficiency occurs in 74% and 38% respectively.
- Long-term anticoagulation and control of other prothrombotic conditions is needed.
- Homozygous individuals may present with neonatal purpura fulminans.

### Hereditary antithrombin (AT) deficiency

- AD disorder with absent or dysfunctional AT.
- AT is a natural inhibitor of thrombin, factors Xa, IXa, Xia, and XIIa, plasmin, and kallikrein.
- Low levels of functional AT (<50%) result in ↑ incidence of thrombosis during surgery, pregnancy, and OCP therapy.
- Unfractionated heparin alone is inadequate for the treatment of acute thrombosis and replacement with AT concentrate is needed. Recurrent thrombotic events require long-term anticoagulation therapy with warfarin.

Specialist advice should be obtained about prophylaxis and treatment of VTE in pregnancy in thrombophilic individuals. Warfarin is teratogenic in early pregnancy and must be stopped at a positive pregnancy test.

# Acquired thrombophilia

**Pregnancy** is a prothrombotic condition with sixfold increase of venous thromboembolism, particularly after surgery and immobilization or in coexistence of the factor V Leiden or the G20210A prothrombin gene mutation. Some types of hereditary thrombophilia have also been associated with recurrent fetal loss.

**Oral contraceptives** are a well-known risk factor for venous thrombosis and thromboembolism, especially in cases of hereditary thrombophilia. A dose effect on degree of risk has also been recognized.

**Surgery and trauma.** Orthopaedic surgical operations are among the most thrombogenic procedures. The risk of thrombosis and fatal pulmonary embolism after total knee replacement without prophylaxis is 70% and 2% respectively. Gynaecology and urology surgery and major trauma have also high rates of thrombosis, without prophylaxis.

Other conditions of acquired thrombophilia include malignancies, paroxysmal nocturnal haemoglobinuria, nephrotic syndrome, central venous catheters, immobility, obesity, organ transplantation, the **antiphospholipid syndrome** (APS) and **heparin-induced thrombocytopenia** (HIT).

## Antiphospholipid syndrome

APS is the most common acquired thrombophilic condition. It is principally characterized by recurrent venous/arterial thrombosis or recurrent pregnancy failure, associated with the presence of antiphospholipid antibodies (aPLs).

### Pathogenesis

aPLs against bovine heart extract were first described by Wasserman in 1906, in the serum of patients with syphilis. Later, cardiolipin, a mitochondrial phospholipid, was identified as the target antigen. Lupus anticoagulants (LAs) are antibodies that can prolong phospholipid-dependent tests in vitro. It is now believed that aPLs recognize epitopes on plasma proteins, which bind and form complexes with phospholipids. The β2-glycoprotein-I (β2-GP-I) is a plasma protein target for many aPLs, when it binds negatively charged phospholipids or surfaces. Other proteins with similar properties are prothrombin, annexin V, proteins C and S, thrombomodulin, and the HMW kininogen.

The exact mechanism of disease in APS and the role of the aPLs in it remain largely unclear. It seems that thrombosis is the basis of most clinical manifestations, including fetal loss due to placental vessel thrombosis. Thrombosis is probably triggered by vascular endothelial injury and local activation of platelets and procoagulant factors, increased protein C resistance, and impaired fibrinolysis.

### Clinical manifestations

Incidental aPLs are detected in 1–5% of healthy individuals, without evidence of thrombosis or other manifestation of APS and their prevalence increases with aging. aPLs are detected in 12–34% of the patients with SLE and APS will develop in 50–70% of them at 20 years.

Overall APS can be primary or secondary to autoimmune diseases (SLE, RA, Sjögren syndrome, Behçet syndrome, systemic sclerosis, temporal arteritis), infections (hepatitis C, varicella, syphilis, malaria), lymphomas, and drugs.

- Recurrent **DVT** with or without pulmonary embolism is the most common clinical manifestation of the APS. The thrombosis involves veins of the limbs and the visceral veins but also unusual sites such as the cerebral venous sinuses.
- However, **stroke** is a more common cause of cerebral ischaemia. It accounts for 50% of all arterial thrombosis and occurs mainly in young adults.
- Coronary artery disease presenting with unstable angina and **myocardial infraction**, heart valve abnormalities, peripheral artery embolism, and **gangrene** are less common manifestations of APS.
- **Recurrent pregnancy loss** due to spontaneous abortion or fetal death is a major feature of APS. aPLs are present in up to 42% of the women with recurrent pregnancy loss. In mothers with APS pre-eclampsia is ninefold more common, restricted fetal growth due to placental insufficiency occurs in 30%, and fetal distress in 50%.
- Practically, any organ may be involved in APS. Some other clinical features of APS are thrombocytopenia (40–50%), haemolytic anaemia (14–23%), vitiligo reticularis (11–22%), renal impairment, retinal ischaemia, and hearing loss.
- **Catastrophic APS** is an acute, devastating, and often lethal condition, characterized by simultaneous thrombotic events affecting at least three organs within a period of few days or weeks. The kidneys (78%), lungs (66%), central nervous system (56%), heart (50%), and skin (50%) are usually affected.

Infections, surgery, withdrawal of anticoagulation therapy, and drugs can trigger the catastrophic APS.

### Laboratory findings

- It is essential to check both LA and antiphospholipid antibodies as otherwise diagnosis may be missed.
- ELISA is used for the detection of anti-cardiolipin and anti-β2-GP-I antibodies. It is positive in 80% of APS.
- The aPTT is a common screening test for LA and it is often prolonged with evidence of inhibition in the mix test. However, it is not sensitive and can be normal if fibrinogen and factor VIII are increased due to pregnancy or an acute phase reaction.
- Dilute Russell viper venom time (DRVVT) and the kaolin cephalin time (KCT) are performed in a mixture of patient and normal plasma and found prolonged in the presence of LA.
- Evidence of LA is found in 20% of the APS and although less sensitive it is more specific than anti-cardiolipin and anti-β2-GP-I antibodies.

### Diagnosis

Defined by an international consensus group in 1999:

#### Clinical criteria

- **Thrombosis:**

  ≥1 vascular thrombosis of vein, artery, or small vessel of any organ documented with imaging or histology.

- **Complications of pregnancy:**

  ≥1 death of morphologically normal fetus at or after 10 weeks of gestation.

  ≥1 premature birth of morphologically normal neonate occurring at or before 34 weeks of gestation.

  ≥3 spontaneous abortions before the 10th week of gestation (other causes of abortion should be excluded).

#### Laboratory criteria

- Medium or high titres of IgG and/or IgM anti-cardiolipin antibodies measured by a standardized ELISA for β2-GP-I dependent anti-cardiolipin antibodies or a positive lupus anticoagulant test on two or more occasions at least 6 weeks apart.

### Management

- Individuals with incidental finding of aPLs do not require prophylactic anticoagulation, but it might be temporarily indicated if another prothrombotic condition (e.g. surgery) arose.
- A single episode of DVT can be treated initially with unfractionated or low-molecular-weight heparin (LMWH) and then with warfarin (INR 2–3) for 6 months.
- Recurrent events require long-term if not lifelong therapy. When they occur during adequate warfarin therapy, the target INR should be probably increased to 3–4.
- Aspirin has proved ineffective for the prevention of recurrences.
- Arterial thrombotic events should be treated with long-term warfarin, because of the high recurrence rates and the devastating consequences.
- Low-dose aspirin and heparin is effective therapy for women with recurrent miscarriages.

## Heparin-induced thrombocytopenia

HIT is a life-threatening, immune-mediated disorder, which follows exposure to heparin and results in thrombocytopenia and thrombotic events.

### Pathogenesis

- HIT is caused by IgG antibodies against the platelet factor 4 (PF4), which becomes immunogenic after binding to unfractionated heparin (UFH).
- HIT associated with LMWHs is 10× less common.
- The complexes of heparin, PF4, and IgG bind platelet Fc receptors and cause potent platelet activation. Evidence of increased thrombin generation has been also documented.

### Clinical features

HIT is more common in orthopaedic and cardiovascular surgery, in patients with neurological conditions, and patients undergoing chronic dialysis. It is a rare event during pregnancy and in the paediatric population.

**Thrombocytopenia** is defined by >50% reduction of the baseline platelet count and it is found in almost all patients (95%) with HIT. The nadir platelet count ranges between 15 and $150 \times 10^9$/L. Thrombocytopenia $<15 \times 10^9$/L is unlikely in HIT and other causes such as sepsis, haemodilution, and drugs should be excluded. The timing of thrombocytopenia is typically 5–10 days after the initiation of heparin therapy, although very rapid reduction may be seen if there is exposure to heparin in the previous 100 days. The platelet count in HIT recovers after heparin discontinuation, usually within 4–14 days.

The risk of **thrombosis** in HIT is 30× higher than the general population and it occurs in 35–70% of cases. Thrombosis may happen even after the platelet count recovers $>150 \times 10^9$/L. DVT and pulmonary embolism are the main types of thrombosis, particularly in the postoperative setting. Arterial thrombosis is 4× less common, but involves large limb arteries resulting in acute ischaemia and limb amputation in 5–10% of HIT cases. Myocardial infarction and stroke also occur. Skin lesions and skin necrosis at the sites of heparin injection is an uncommon manifestation.

### Laboratory testing

Antibodies against heparin/PF4 can be measured in the serum of patients with suspected HIT using ELISA. This test is highly sensitive, but has low specificity and many individuals without HIT are found seropositive. However, patients with HIT are rarely seronegative and therefore its negative predictive value is high (95%). Functional assays can detect platelet activation mediated by patient plasma. They are highly sensitive and specific but technically demanding methods.

### Diagnosis

The final diagnosis of HIT should rely on the typical clinical presentation and confirmed with detection of antibodies against PF4/heparin with ELISA or functional assays. The HIT score gives a pre-test probability for diagnosing HIT.

### Management

All forms of heparin should be discontinued in patients with clinical suspicion of HIT, to avoid further platelet activation and thrombin generation. HIT requires alternative anticoagulation therapy for the prevention of the thrombotic complications. UFH-associated HIT cannot be treated with LMWH due to cross reactivity. The upfront use of warfarin has been associated with increased incidence of warfarin-induced skin necrosis and limb gangrene due to venous thrombosis.

Direct-thrombin inhibitors and heparinoids are the anticoagulants used in HIT.

- **Lepuridin** is a direct and irreversible thrombin inhibitor with no cross-reactivity to heparin. It is given with intravenous infusion and is renally excreted. The aPTT is used to monitor its activity, aiming for an aPTT ratio of 1.5–2.5. Lepuridin decreases significantly the incidence of new thrombotic events, but it relates to increased bleeding complications including deaths (1.2%). Its use is problematic in patients with renal impairment. Antibodies against lepuridin develop in 50% after the first use and in 70% after the second.

- **Danaparoid sodium** is a mixture of heparan sulphate, dermatan sulphate, and chondroitin sulphate. It mainly inhibits factor Xa and to a lesser extent thrombin. It is given by intravenous infusion aiming for anti-Xa levels 0.5–0.8U/mL, although monitoring probably is not necessary apart from patients with renal failure. Danaparoid has equivalent efficacy with lepuridin.

Patients with HIT and thrombosis will require oral anticoagulation with warfarin after platelet recovery $>150 \times 10^9$/L. In the beginning, warfarin administration should be covered with lepuridin or danaparoid therapy for at least 5 days and until a therapeutic INR level is achieved for 48 hours.

# Chapter 12

# Infectious diseases

# 12.1 Infectious diseases: an overview

## Background

The specialty of infectious diseases is concerned with the prevention, diagnosis, and treatment of infection. Infectious diseases have particular characteristics that make them a unique and interesting challenge:

### Communicable

Many infections are transmissible from person to person and knowing which these are and how they are transmitted is important in order to prevent the spread of infection. Certain infections are notifiable diseases that should be reported to local public health services. In certain circumstances, screening of contacts to identify undiagnosed infection and to prevent community spread is vital.

### Curable

Many infections are completely curable if the appropriate antimicrobial therapy is given. Understanding how to recognize and treat sepsis, including knowing which antimicrobial to give and how best to give it, is crucial to avoid preventable morbidity and mortality.

### Emergent

The infective agents that affect humans change continuously over time. Some pathogens are no longer seen in the UK due to improvements in standards of living (cholera and typhus) or following introduction of vaccination programmes (smallpox and rubella). However, as old diseases are controlled, new pathogens can appear (HIV, severe acute respiratory syndrome (SARS)) and previously controlled pathogens can become more common (pertussis, tuberculosis (TB)) or spread to new areas (dengue).

### Evolving

All micro-organisms have short reproductive cycles meaning that selection pressure can induce changes in their genetic make-up over relatively short time periods. Misuse of anti-infective drugs can render them ineffective during treatment of an individual patient (e.g. multidrug-resistant TB). Long-term widespread antibiotic misuse can also lead to the evolution of resistant organisms at a population level (e.g. methicillin-resistant *Staphylococcus aureus* (MRSA)), meaning that antimicrobial stewardship is important.

### Globally diverse

Infective agents vary widely in their distribution, both within a country and worldwide. Increasing migration of people means that diseases not present in the UK are being seen more commonly (malaria, typhoid). Knowledge of travel-related infection is important.

### Public

Infection holds an intense fascination in the lay press and outbreaks of disease or discovery of new infective agents can quickly enter the public domain. Avian flu, viral haemorrhagic fevers, and 'superbugs' like MRSA are examples.

## Definitions

- **Infection**: a disease directly caused by a micro-organism.
- **Contagious**: an infectious disease transmissible from person to person (e.g. influenza, HIV, TB).
- **Non-contagious**: an infectious disease not directly transmissible from person to person (e.g. malaria, legionella).
- **Commensal**: an organism present on or within the body which does not usually cause disease.
- **Pathogen**: an organism capable of causing disease.
- **Opportunistic pathogen**: an organism capable of causing disease only in immunocompromised hosts.
- **Pathogenicity**: the capacity to cause disease.

- **Virulence factor**: a microbial gene product that aids it in causing disease.
- **Attack rate**: the proportion of a susceptible population affected following exposure. Some diseases have a high attack rate (e.g. measles), others have a low attack rate (paralysis from polio).
- **Clinical expression**: infections with the same micro-organisms can manifest differently in different hosts. Host genetics, strain variation in the organism, infecting dose, and route of infection all contribute to this variability.
- **Vertical spread**: infection from mother to child *in utero*, during birth, or by breastfeeding (e.g. HIV, hepatitis B virus (HBV), rubella).
- **Horizontal spread**: spread of infection to others, e.g. airborne (influenza), ingestion (typhoid), sexual contact (syphilis), vectors (malaria).
- **Antimicrobial**: a drug with anti-infective properties including those derived from bacteria (antibiotics) and those produced synthetically (sulphonamides and quinolones).
- **Antibiotic**: the strict definition is any drug *derived from a micro-organism* with anti-infective properties (penicillin, cephalosporins, and macrolides), but is often used to describe any antimicrobial agent.

Clinical teams and microbiology labs have a legal duty to notify certain infectious diseases to public health under the Health Protection (Notification) regulations 2010 (see Table 12.1). The notification system enables the early identification and prevention of outbreaks, as well as providing useful epidemiological information.

## Some diseases requiring contact tracing

- **TB**: contact screening, some may require prophylactic antibiotics.
- **Meningococcal disease**: prophylactic antibiotics to close contacts.
- **Sexually transmitted infection**: notification of potentially exposed partners, testing and treatment of infected partners.
- **Hepatitis B**: testing and vaccination of household contacts and sexual partners.

| Table 12.1 Notifiable diseases in the UK | |
|---|---|
| Acute encephalitis | Meningococcal disease |
| Acute poliomyelitis | Meningitis |
| Anthrax | Mumps |
| Botulism | Plague |
| Brucellosis | Rabies |
| Cholera | Rubella |
| Diphtheria | SARS |
| Enteric fever | Scarlet fever |
| Food poisoning | Smallpox |
| Haemolytic uraemic syndrome | Tetanus |
| Infectious bloody diarrhoea | TB |
| Invasive group A streptococcus | Typhus |
| Legionella | Viral haemorrhagic fever |
| Leprosy | Viral hepatitis |
| Malaria | Whooping cough |
| Measles | Yellow fever |

## Clinical scenario

A 29-year-old South African woman diagnosed with pulmonary TB 6 weeks previously has been referred to the medical on-call team because of an ongoing productive cough and weight loss despite standard four-drug TB therapy. Copious acid and alcohol-fast bacilli are seen in a sputum sample obtained earlier today, and culture from her first presentation has recently been reported as showing rifampicin and isoniazid resistance (multidrug-resistant TB). She is refusing admission for further treatment.

## Detention under the Public Health Act

The Public Health Act (1984) permits the removal and detention of a person who poses a risk to the public due to an infectious disease. The need to use this law arises rarely and it should be considered a last resort in any negotiating process. Some believe it may be open to challenge under the European Human Rights Act. A patient with smear-positive pulmonary TB who refuses treatment is one situation where the law might be invoked. Discussion should be made with a consultant in public health (who will issue a warrant for detention) and a consultant in infectious disease (who will normally provide clinical care for the patient once detained). Removal is usually to an isolation room in an infectious diseases unit. Once admitted to hospital, no restraint is permitted—the patient is free to leave, but will be returned by the police. The patient cannot be forced to take medication under this law.

In the earlier clinical scenario, the woman will need to be admitted to a negative pressure isolation room and receive five anti-TB drugs including a parenteral agent. Her inpatient stay will be at least 3 months. HIV testing should be done if not done previously, however this need not be discussed immediately.

In the course of your discussion you should:

- Establish what the patient knows about TB.
- Explain the seriousness of resistant TB to her health.
- Explain that she is infective to her family.
- Give information on what the treatment will involve.
- Explain the need for isolation in hospital.
- Explore all the reasons behind admission being declined. Lack of understanding of the condition, concern about child care or loss of work, fear of prolonged isolation, and fear of toxic or injected drugs are all common reasons why admission might be declined and each should be explored before bringing up the possibility of forced detention.
- Attempt to negotiate solutions that will permit a voluntary stay in hospital.
- If needed, state that forced detention will result if she does not comply. Sometimes, the threat of forced detention is sufficient to ensure compliance.

# 12.2 Diagnostic techniques

## Background

Diagnostic techniques in infectious diseases can be broadly divided into those which directly detect the infective agent (such as microscopy or polymerase chain reaction (PCR)) and those which detect a specific immune response against the infective agent (such as serology). There are strengths and limitations to each technique and these are discussed in the following sections.

## Direct tests

**Microscopy** can be performed in most labs. Although some organisms can be identified using unprepared slides (e.g. *Trichomonas* on a wet film, or malaria on a blood film), the use of staining techniques allows for better identification of different types of micro-organism (e.g. Gram staining for most bacteria, Ziehl–Neelsen staining for mycobacteria, India ink staining for *Cryptococcus*).

- **Advantages:** rapid, inexpensive.
- **Disadvantages:** no information on antimicrobial sensitivity, may not allow specific microbiological diagnosis (e.g. *Staphylococcus aureus* (see Fig. 12.1) cannot be distinguished from *Staphylococcus epidermidis*), may be negative with prior antimicrobial use, does not distinguish between colonization and infection.

The sensitivity of microscopy can be increased by the use of fluorescent stains (e.g. auramine-rhodamine for TB), or augmented by antibodies specific for the pathogen in question (e.g. immunofluorescence for *Legionella* or *Pneumocystis jirovecii*).

**Culture** is also widely available and is carried out using a variety of agar plates or broths, kept at the ideal temperature for growth of the micro-organisms. Some organisms need particular growth media and the lab needs to be informed in advance if they are suspected (e.g. *Neisseria gonorrhoeae*, *Brucella*, or *Corynebacterium diphtheriae*). Some are simply difficult to grow (fastidious) meaning that cultures may need to be kept for prolonged periods of time (*Brucella*, the 'HACEK' group of organisms).

- **Advantages:** allows accurate identification of the pathogen, permits antibiotic sensitivity testing to be performed.
- **Disadvantages:** may be negative with prior antibiotic use, does not distinguish between colonization and infection, often takes >24 hours.

Identification of isolates involves noting growth characteristics, performing biochemical tests based on known metabolic properties of particular bacteria (e.g. *Staphylococcus aureus* possess both catalase and coagulase enzymes), or using specific antisera (e.g. Lancefield grouping in streptococci (Fig.12.2)).

**Sensitivity testing** can be performed on cultured bacteria to ensure an effective antimicrobial is used. Disc testing is a relatively crude assay which can quickly compare the inhibition of bacterial growth by several classes of antibiotics. More information can be obtained by testing the minimum inhibitory concentration (MIC). Serial dilutions of an antibiotic are tested. The lowest concentration of antibiotic inhibiting bacterial growth is the MIC.

**Antigen testing** detects molecules specific for the pathogen in question. This is only available for certain organisms. There are several different types of test available and they can be performed on a range of clinical samples including blood, urine, and cerebrospinal fluid (CSF).

- **Advantages:** rapid, less influenced by recent antimicrobial use than culture, specific for a single pathogen.
- **Disadvantages:** provide no information on sensitivities.

**Toxin detection** can be useful as a surrogate marker for infection by toxin-producing organisms. Toxin detection is commonly used in the diagnosis of *Clostridium difficile*-associated diarrhoea.

**Nucleic acid detection** can very precisely identify organisms by amplifying either RNA or DNA using PCR technology.

- **Advantages:** detects pathogens which cannot be cultured, can provide accurate identification even if organisms are dead.
- **Disadvantages:** expensive, may require specialist equipment or expertise, does not distinguish live and dead organisms.

Nucleic acid-based tests can also provide information on antimicrobial resistance. This is particularly useful in slow-growing organisms (e.g. detection of rifampicin resistance in TB) or organisms that cannot be cultured (e.g. resistance in HBV or HIV). Quantitative tests of viral nucleic acid (viral loads) can be extremely useful in diagnosing infection (e.g. CMV) or in monitoring antiviral treatment (HBV and HIV).

## Indirect tests

**Serology**, or the detection of host antibodies raised against a specific pathogen, has traditionally been used to detect the presence of pathogens that cannot be readily cultured, such as viruses or *Mycoplasma*. The presence of antibodies is not influenced by prior antibiotic use, but there is a lag period of several days or weeks to their development during acute infection. The more rapid nucleic acid-based tests

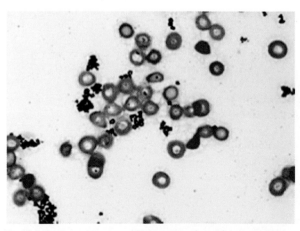

**Fig. 12.1** *Staphylococcus aureus* (Gram-positive (purple) cocci appearing in clumps).
Reproduced with permission from James Donnelly.

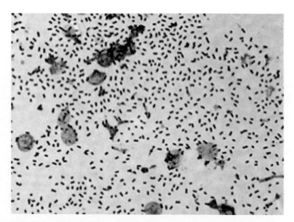

**Fig. 12.2** *Streptococcus pneumoniae* (Gram-positive cocci appearing in chains of two (diplococcic)).
Reproduced with permission from James Donnelly.

have superseded serology in many areas, particularly in diagnosing acute infection. Serology remains particularly useful in chronic infection where it can be used to detect immunity (hepatitis A virus (HAV), HBV, VZV), previous exposure to infection (CMV, hepatitis C virus (HCV), toxoplasmosis), or to identify chronic viral infection (HIV, HBV).

**Cellular responses** are most helpful in detecting mycobacterial infection. The tuberculin skin test can detect T-cell immunity to TB, but is operator dependent and unreliable following BCG or in immunosuppression. Some of these difficulties may be overcome by new γ-interferon release assays where a patient's lymphocytes are exposed *ex vivo* to *Mycobacterium tuberculosis*-specific antigen. If anti-*Mycobacterium tuberculosis* T cells are present, γ-interferon is released which can be quantified and is indicative of prior TB exposure. Neither tuberculin testing nor γ-interferon release assays help distinguish latent from active TB.

## Gram staining

The **Gram stain**, named after Hans Gram who first described the technique in 1884, is the main stain used in medical microbiology. It rapidly differentiates bacteria based on the structure of their cell wall and provides useful information on the likely identity of the bacteria and which antibiotics may be effective.

A sample is prepared on a slide and washed with:
- Crystal violet (purple), which stains bacterial cells purple.
- Iodine, which fixes the crystal violet in the cell wall.
- Acetone, which causes the violet stain to leach out of the cell wall. Stain leaches more readily from Gram-negative bacteria.
- Fuschin or Safranin, which causes cells from which the violet stain has leached out to appear pink (Gram negative (Fig. 12.3)). Cells retaining violet stain appear purple (Gram positive (Fig. 12.4)).

Some bacteria do not stain with a Gram stain (e.g. rickettsia), some can appear Gram variable, and excessive treatment of Gram-positive bacteria can make them appear Gram negative (over-decolourization).

## Examples of common antigen tests

- *Pneumococcus*
- *Legionella*

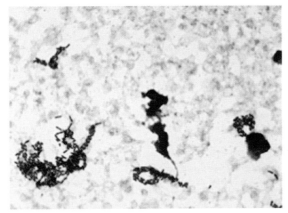

**Fig. 12.3** *Escherichia coli* (Gram-negative (pink) bacilli, with a clump of pink stain deposit in the top right).
Reproduced with permission from James Donnelly.

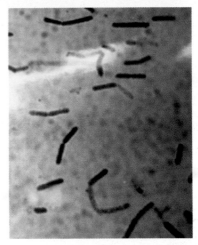

**Fig. 12.4** Gram-positive bacilli (e.g. *Clostridium perfringens*).
Reproduced with permission from James Donnelly.

- Malaria
- *Cryptococcus*
- Hepatitis B surface antigen.

## Getting the most from your microbiology laboratory

- Take appropriate samples, clearly labelled, and sent in the correct containers.
- If you're not sure what to send, speak to your lab.
- Labs may process samples differently depending on clinical details—make sure important details (e.g. including immunocompromise, pregnancy, prosthetic material, penicillin allergy) are clearly documented on the request form.
- Speak to the lab in advance about unusual tests.
- A sample of pus in a universal container is better than a swab of pus.
- For urgent samples notify the lab, ensure the specimen is picked up and provide a clear contact phone or page number.
- You can't get an urgent result on blood cultures—they take time to become positive (usually at least 12 hours).

## Taking blood cultures

- Get a second pair of hands for confused or agitated patients.
- Clean the skin thoroughly with alcohol or chlorhexidine.
- Use a 'no touch' technique.
- Disinfect the bungs—the rubber tops of each bottle.
- Place 8–10mL in each bottle.
- Take 2 sets in severe sepsis.
- Take 3 sets if endocarditis is suspected.
- Send to the lab promptly.
- Take cultures before starting or escalating antibiotics.

# 12.3 Sepsis

## Background

Sepsis is the systemic inflammatory response caused by infection. It is common among emergency medical admissions. The in-hospital mortality rate from sepsis is about 20%, similar to that of myocardial infarction. International guidelines provide consensus on definitions and optimal management of sepsis. Randomized controlled trials (RCTs) have shown benefit in certain patients from treatments such as early goal-directed therapy. However, although not supported by RCT evidence, the mainstay of sepsis management is early recognition, prompt administration of effective antimicrobials, correction of hypoxia and hypovolaemia, and, if necessary, inotropic and ventilatory support.

## Recognition

**Systemic inflammatory response syndrome (SIRS)** is the presence of two or more of:

- Temperature dysregulation (>38°C or <36°C).
- Tachypnoea (respiratory rate >20/minute).
- Tachycardia (pulse >90/minute).
- Abnormal white cell count (WCC) (>12 or <4 × 10⁹/L).

Failure to appreciate the significance of hypothermia or low WCC is a common error in sepsis recognition. Certain patient groups can have 'masked' sepsis whereby the normal physiological responses are blunted. These include those with untreated hypothyroidism, beta-blocker use, extremes of age, and immunocompromised patients. In hospitalized patients, around half of patients with SIRS will develop a form of sepsis: (sepsis in 26%, severe sepsis in 18%, and septic shock in 4%).

**Sepsis** is SIRS plus evidence of infection which can be:

- Clinical (e.g. history of rigors, soft tissue infection).
- Radiological (e.g. consolidation on CXR, see Fig. 12.5).
- Microbiological (e.g. identification of bacteria from a sterile site).

**Severe sepsis** is sepsis associated with organ dysfunction:

- Circulatory (systolic BP <90mmHg, mean arterial pressure <70mmHg, or drop of 40mmHg).
- Metabolic (lactic acidosis).
- Respiratory (hypoxia).
- Neurological (confusion, diminished consciousness).

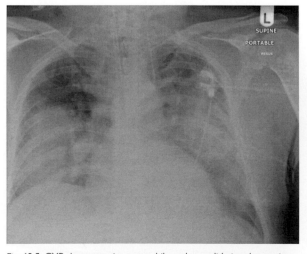

**Fig. 12.5** CXR demonstrating severe bilateral consolidative changes in a mechanically ventilated patient in ITU.

- Haematological (platelets <80 × 10⁹/L, disseminated intravascular coagulation).
- Hepatic (hyperbilirubinaemia, elevated transaminases).
- Renal (urine output <0.5mL/kg/hour, acute renal failure).

Caution has to be exercised in distinguishing organ dysfunction caused by sepsis from that caused by a separate aetiology. Sometimes this can be difficult to determine (e.g. patients on anticoagulation, coexistent renal or hepatic disease).

**Septic shock** is the presence of sepsis plus hypotension despite fluid resuscitation, together with perfusion abnormalities.

## Management

### How severe is the sepsis?

The presence of severe sepsis or septic shock is an emergency requiring prompt action and input from an experienced clinician. Severe sepsis may sometimes be immediately apparent, but often is diagnosed when the results of investigations become available (FBC, coagulation, U&E, LFT, lactate, arterial blood gases). If no severity markers are present, correction of hypoxia and suitable fluids should be given as clinically indicated. For patients with severe sepsis, follow the 'sepsis six' (see The 'sepsis six', this section).

### Where is the infection?

This can usually be determined by history and examination coupled with simple investigations (urinalysis and CXR). Failure to identify a source of sepsis initially is not uncommon and can be due to a primarily bacteraemic illness (such as *Staphylococcus aureus* or *Streptococcus pyogenes*), or a more unusual site of infection (e.g. tonsillitis, endocarditis, infection of prosthetic material, prostatitis, abdominal or pelvic abscess).

### What are the possible causes of this infection?

A travel history should always be sought as this can greatly increase the range of possible pathogens or raise the possibility of antimicrobial resistance patterns not commonly seen in the UK (see Section 12.7). The presence of hospital-acquired infection and immunosuppression are important considerations and are dealt with separately (see Sections 12.6 and 12.8).

### What antimicrobial should I use?

Empirical antimicrobials should cover likely pathogens depending on local epidemiology, while considering allergies and comorbidities of the patient. Errors can be made here by not providing sufficiently broad antimicrobial cover for hospital-acquired infection. If in doubt help should be sought from local specialists in infectious disease or microbiology. Further detail on how to choose an antibiotic regimen is found in Section 12.4.

### Is removal of a focus of infection needed?

Examples would include removing infected cannulae, vascular or urinary catheters, chest drain insertion for empyema, and surgical or radiological abscess drainage.

### Is the patient responding to treatment?

Ensure the patient is in an appropriate clinical environment for the severity of their disease and having frequent observations and input/output charting. Empirical antibiotics should be changed once positive cultures are available, always seeking to use the narrowest spectrum of antibiotics that will be effective. A switch to oral antimicrobials should be made when sepsis criteria have resolved, although certain infections need prolonged intravenous therapy (endocarditis, meningitis, *Staphylococcus aureus* bacteraemia).

### Indicators of poor prognosis in sepsis

- Hypothermia.
- Leucopenia.
- Age >40 years.

- Comorbidity (e.g. immunosuppression, cancer, hepatic or renal failure).
- Staphylococcal bacteraemia (MRSA >MSSA).
- Fungaemia.
- Pseudomonal infection.
- Ineffective first-line antimicrobials.

### Clinical lessons in sepsis *recognition*

- Always look at observations and investigations—you cannot diagnose and categorize sepsis without them.
- Know the sepsis criteria, they help to guide management and predict outcome.
- Hypothermia and low WCCs are poor prognostic signs.
- Patients with early septic shock can look surprisingly 'well', particularly if young. They will appear flushed rather than grey and their peripheries will be warm.

### Clinical lessons in sepsis *management*

- Severe sepsis and septic shock are emergencies. Involve senior medical staff and critical care teams early.
- Assume a patient with rigors is bacteraemic until proven otherwise.
- Assume the septic patient with no obvious source is bacteraemic until proven otherwise. Beware diagnosing 'viral infection' in sepsis, unless you have a good idea of what the virus might be.
- Diarrhoea and vomiting may be symptoms of sepsis, not necessarily of gastroenteritis.

- Correct abnormal physiology—fluid and oxygen are as important as antibiotics.
- Give appropriate antimicrobials promptly. If you're not sure what to give, seek help.

## The 'sepsis six'

1. Give high-flow oxygen.
2. Take blood cultures.
3. Give IV antibiotic.
4. Start IV fluid resuscitation.
5. Check serum lactate.
6. Monitor hourly urine output accurately.

## References

Dellinger RP, Carlet JM, Masur H, *et al.* Surviving sepsis campaign guidelines for the management of severe sepsis. *Crit Care Med* 2004; 32: 858–73.

Levy MM, Fink MP, Marshall JC, *et al.* 2001 SCCM/ESICM/ACCP/ATS/SIS International Sepsis Definitions Conference. *Crit Care Med* 2003; 31: 1250–6.

Rangel-Frausto MS, Pittet D, Costigan M, *et al.* The natural history of the systemic inflammatory response syndrome. A prospective study. *JAMA* 1995; 273: 117–23.

# 12.4 Antibiotics

## Background

Approximately 1/3 of hospital inpatients receive an antibiotic, making them one of the most prescribed classes of medication. The timely delivery of an effective antibiotic can be life-saving. However, widespread and often inappropriate use of antimicrobials has led to increasing antimicrobial resistance and a rise in the complications of antibiotic therapy such as *Clostridium difficile*-associated diarrhoea. The ability to prescribe antibiotics rationally is important for all grades of doctor. This section will deal with common antibacterial agents. Drugs for TB, viral, fungal, protozoal, and helminthic infection are discussed separately.

## Antibiotic pharmacology

All antibiotics work by selective toxicity—they target a biochemical pathway specific for the infective agent, resulting in death of the pathogen but preservation of host cells. The drug should reach a concentration at the site of infection greater than the MIC for the pathogen. Some antibiotics are bactericidal (actively kill bacteria) while others are bacteristatic (prevent replication of bacteria). Generally, in severe infection and in immunocompromised hosts, bactericidal drugs are preferable. Antibiotics exert their effect in one of two main ways:

- **Concentration-dependent killing**: the higher the antibiotic concentration is above the MIC, the greater the killing. These drugs are best given in large doses (to ensure the highest possible peak) infrequently (to minimize build-up of drug and potential toxicity). The classic example is gentamicin.
- **Time-dependent killing**: provided the drug concentration is above the MIC, killing occurs at a constant rate. No difference in killing rate is seen at higher concentrations. These drugs are best given at frequent intervals or by continuous infusion (flucloxacillin or vancomycin), or with infrequent dosing of drug with a long half-life (ceftriaxone).

Many drugs fall between the classes, and these phenomena are usually only clinically relevant in certain severe infections.

## Inhibitors of cell wall synthesis

### Beta-lactam antibiotics

All beta-lactam drugs possess a beta-lactam ring, exert their effect via penicillin binding proteins (PBPs), and impair the production of peptidoglycan, a key component of the bacterial cell wall. Their main class side effect is hypersensitivity. Cross-reactivity exists—between 1% and 10% of patients with true penicillin allergy will also be allergic to cephalosporins.

**Penicillins** can be subdivided into several categories:

- Penicillin is derived from the mould *Penicillium*. It has a rather limited spectrum now, but remains useful in treating group A *Streptococcus* infection, *Neisseria meningitidis*, certain anaerobic infections, and syphilis.
- Penicillinase-stable penicillins (e.g. flucloxacillin) are resistant to breakdown by penicillinases produced by *Staphylococcus aureus*. They are the drug of choice for sensitive *Staphylococcus aureus* infections.
- Aminopenicillins (e.g. amoxicillin) have additional Gram-negative activity and are effective against some coliforms, salmonellae, and *Haemophilus*. They are not active against *Pseudomonas*.
- Anti-pseudomonal penicillins (e.g. piperacillin) have activity against *Pseudomonas*.

**Beta-lactamase inhibitors** (e.g. clavulanic acid) can be combined with beta-lactam antimicrobials to improve their activity against beta-lactamase producing organisms like *Staphylococcus aureus*, coliforms, *Haemophilus*, and anaerobic bacteria. Co-amoxiclav (amoxicillin and clavulanic acid) is the most commonly used and is useful in the treatment of urinary and respiratory infection (including aspiration pneumonia). Piperacillin-tazobactam (Tazocin™) is commonly used in the treatment of severe hospital-acquired infection or neutropaenic sepsis.

**Cephalosporins** are grouped into 'generations'. None are active against enterococci or MRSA.

- First-generation drugs (e.g. cephalexin) have good activity against Gram-positive cocci and some activity against Gram-negative rods. Orally available, they are occasionally used to treat skin or urinary infection in the community.
- Second-generation drugs (e.g. cefuroxime) are similar to the first generation, but have more activity against Gram-negative rods and anaerobes.
- Third-generation drugs (e.g. cefotaxime, ceftriaxone) have reasonable cover for staphylococcal (excluding MRSA) and streptococcal infections, but have excellent Gram-negative activity. They have good central nervous system penetration and are the drugs of choice in suspected meningitis. Some third-generation cephalosporins have anti-pseudomonal activity (e.g. ceftazidime).

**Carbapenems** (e.g. meropenem) are extremely broad-spectrum antibiotics with excellent Gram-positive, Gram-negative (including extended-spectrum beta-lactamase (ESBL) producers), and anaerobic cover. They have no activity against MRSA, enterococci, or agents causing atypical pneumonia.

**Glycopeptides** (e.g. vancomycin and teicoplanin) are large molecules with excellent Gram-positive activity (including MRSA), but no Gram-negative activity. They inhibit cell wall synthesis, but do not act via PBPs. The oral form is not absorbed from the gut, and is thus ineffective for treating systemic infection, but can be used to treat *C. difficile*. There is an association with nephrotoxicity, particularly if administered with an aminoglycoside. Teicoplanin is possibly less nephrotoxic than vancomycin. Monitoring of levels should be performed. In severe infection, continuous infusion is the easiest way to ensure stable, adequate drug levels. We aim for 10–15mg/L for soft tissue infection and 15±5mg/L for bacteraemia. Local guidance should be followed. Over-rapid infusion can result in flushing called 'red man syndrome'. This is not an allergy and can be prevented by slowing the rate of infusion.

## Inhibitors of protein synthesis

Bacterial ribosomes are structurally different from mammalian ribosomes. The following antibiotics bind selectively to bacterial ribosomes (either to 30S or 50S subunits), preventing bacterial protein synthesis.

**Aminoglycosides** (e.g. gentamicin) are potent drugs which can only be given parenterally to produce systemic effects. They have good anti-staphylococcal and Gram-negative activity (including *Pseudomonas*), but no activity against anaerobes or streptococci. Nonetheless, they have synergistic action when combined with penicillins and can be used with penicillins in the treatment of streptococcal or enterococcal endocarditis. They have the potentially severe side effects of nephrotoxicity and ototoxicity and should be used with caution in the elderly, children, and those with renal impairment. Accurate dosing and monitoring of trough levels is crucial.

**Macrolides** (e.g. erythromycin, clarithromycin) have a broad spectrum of activity with fair action against Gram-positive organisms, some Gram-negative organisms, and also *Mycoplasma* and *Chlamydia*. Their main role is in the treatment of atypical pneumonia and non-severe infection in penicillin-allergic patients. The most common side effects are nausea and diarrhoea. QT prolongation can occur and care should be taken when other QT-prolonging agents are used. Macrolides are also enzyme inhibitors and drug interactions are common.

**Tetracyclines** (e.g. doxycycline) also have a broad spectrum of activity including Gram-positive bacteria (including some strains of MRSA) and activity against some unusual pathogens such as psittacosis, Q fever, and *Rickettsia*. Doxycycline is also used in the treatment and prevention of malaria. The main side effects are heartburn and photosensitive rash.

**Clindamycin** is an agent with excellent Gram-positive and anaerobic cover with good bioavailability. In toxin-producing staphylococcal and streptococcal infection it can inhibit toxin production and should be included in any antibiotic regimen where toxic shock or necrotizing fasciitis is suspected. It is associated with *C. difficile* diarrhoea, but probably is no more responsible for this than other broad-spectrum antimicrobials.

**Chloramphenicol** is an inexpensive drug, frequently used in developing countries. Its role in the UK is limited to meningococcal disease where other drug options are not possible. It rarely causes irreversible myelosuppression. Eye drops are safe and commonly used to treat bacterial conjunctivitis.

## Inhibitors of nucleic acid synthesis

**Quinolones** (e.g. ciprofloxacin) inhibit DNA synthesis by acting on bacterial DNA gyrase. They have excellent bioavailability and are the only oral anti-pseudomonal agents. They have good anti-Gram-negative activity, some activity against staphylococci and agents causing atypical pneumonia, but most have no anaerobic cover. They are typically used in complicated urinary tract infection. Newer agents, the extended-spectrum quinolones (e.g. levofloxacin and moxifloxacin), have improved anaerobic and pneumococcal activity. Rare but important side effects include lowering of the seizure threshold and tendon rupture. Newer agents can cause QT prolongation that can result in ventricular dysrhythmias.

**Dihydrofolate reductase inhibitors** (e.g. trimethoprim and sulphonamides) act to prevent folate metabolism, an essential part of nucleic acid synthesis. Trimethoprim and sulphonamides are synergistic in combination and the co-formulation (co-trimoxazole) has a fairly broad spectrum of activity, including *Pneumocystis jirovecii* pneumonia, a fungal infection of the immunocompromised host.

**Rifampicin** is useful for its anti-tuberculous activity, but also can be used in conjunction with other agents to treat staphylococcal infections including some strains of MRSA. Hepatotoxicity is the main unwanted effect.

## Other antimicrobials

**Metronidazole** is an inexpensive drug with excellent anaerobic activity; it is ineffective against aerobes. Patients should be counselled to avoid alcohol whilst on metronidazole because of the risk of a disulfiram-like reaction. Prolonged use is associated with peripheral neuropathy and should be avoided. It is the drug of choice for non-severe *C. difficile* infection.

**Fusidic acid** is an anti-staphylococcal agent, often with activity against MRSA. When used as a single agent, resistance rapidly develops, and it should be combined with a second anti-staphylococcal drug. Hepatitis is the main side effect.

**Nitrofurantoin** is now usually limited to treating cystitis. Nausea is common and it can also cause an acute pulmonary reaction with fever, cough, and breathlessness after a mean time from exposure of 9 days. Chronic therapy is associated with the development of pulmonary fibrosis or neuropathy and should be avoided.

## Newer antibiotics

**Linezolid** is a relatively new agent with good activity against Gram-positive organisms, including MRSA. It has excellent bioavailability and is useful for soft tissue infections and pneumonia caused by MRSA. It is only licensed for use for 14 days or fewer due to risks of myelosuppression, lactic acidosis, peripheral and optic neuropathy.

**Daptomycin** is a new agent with excellent Gram-positive activity including MRSA and vancomycin-resistant enterococci (VRE). It is rapidly bactericidal and can be used for skin and soft tissue infections, bacteraemia, or right heart endocarditis.

**Tigecycline** is a new tetracycline derivative with very broad spectrum of activity including MRSA, resistant Gram-negative organisms, and agents causing atypical pneumonia. However, it does not cover *Pseudomonas*.

## Antibiotics in pregnancy

Many antibiotics are safe, or not known to be harmful, in pregnancy. In any serious infection the risk of suboptimally treated sepsis must be weighed against the possibility of adverse antibiotic effects to the mother and fetus. Discussion with an experienced clinician or microbiologist is recommended.

**The following antibiotics are generally considered safe in pregnancy**: penicillin, amoxicillin, cephalexin, ceftriaxone, clindamycin, erythromycin.

**The following antibiotics should be avoided in pregnancy if possible**: doxycycline, ciprofloxacin, aminoglycosides.

## Antimicrobial resistance

Antimicrobial resistance is an increasing problem worldwide. Patterns of resistance vary widely within Europe. Scandinavian countries, Holland, and Germany see little resistance, but France, Spain, Italy, and Greece have a much higher incidence, particularly of MRSA, ESBL-producing Gram-negative organisms, and penicillin-resistant pneumococcal infection. In the UK, MRSA is common but decreasing in prevalence, while ESBLs are less common but increasing. Rates of pneumococcal resistance remain low.

**Inherent resistance:** certain bacteria are inherently resistant to particular antimicrobials because of a lack of drug target (e.g. enterococci and third-generation cephalosporins, *Mycoplasma* and penicillin) These resistance patterns are *fixed* and not influenced by antimicrobial prescribing.

**Acquired resistance:** resistance can be selected in certain bacteria, either through spontaneous mutation in the genomic DNA, or by acquisition of transmissible genetic elements such as plasmids or transposons. Transmissible elements can cause acquisition of multiple resistance genes and can transfer resistance between different bacterial species.

## Antibiotic allergy

Severe antibiotic allergy is rare, but can be fatal. All patients should be asked about drug allergy and this information should be clearly documented. Patients who report allergy must be questioned over the nature of their reaction. The development of rash within hours of drug administration, bronchospasm, facial or oral swelling, and hypotension are all features of IgE mediated type I allergy (anaphylaxis). A delayed rash (after 7–10 days) is more in keeping with T-cell mediated type IV allergy (delayed hypersensitivity). The risk of re-challenge is greatest with type I hypersensitivity.

The presence and nature of drug allergy should be clearly documented in case notes and the prescription chart. New allergies should be communicated to the patient's GP promptly. Nausea or dizziness is often misinterpreted as allergy. It is usually safe to challenge patients with a very remote or vague history of allergy if they are inpatients.

## Clinical lessons

- Know your local antimicrobial policy.
- Ask about allergies before you prescribe.
- Always clarify whether adverse reactions are allergy or intolerance.
- Document the indication for antibiotic treatment in the case notes.
- Seek help in antimicrobial choice and dosing in severely ill or complex patients.

- Always ensure antibiotics are administered promptly to sick patients. This will involve good communication with nursing staff and, if the required antibiotic is not common ward stock, pharmacy staff.

## Choosing an antibiotic

Many doctors find antibiotics confusing—there are a large number of antibiotics, each with activity against different organisms and each with different side effects. A series of steps should be considered before prescribing any antimicrobial treatment.

### Infection

- Is there an infection? Antimicrobials should not be used to treat asymptomatic bacteriuria (unless pregnant or immunosuppressed), skin and ulcer colonization, or exacerbations of chronic respiratory disease without evidence of infection.
- How severe is it? Sepsis syndrome should always be treated promptly. After appropriate cultures, broad cover is preferred in the very sick which can be de-escalated when the results of cultures are known.
- Where is it? Some drugs penetrate better to certain tissues.
- What is likely to be causing it? Additional antibacterial cover may be required in hospital-acquired infection, immunosuppressed patients, or in returning travellers.

- What are local resistance patterns? Some units or hospitals have higher rates of resistance which may need to be considered.

### Patient

- Do they have an antibiotic allergy?
- Comorbidities? Significant renal or hepatic disease will influence drug choice and dosing.
- Concomitant medication? Beware of patients on warfarin or anti-epileptics. Both can be seriously disturbed by concomitant antibiotic prescribing.

### Drug

- What is the best route? Severe infections should normally be treated with IV drugs. Well-absorbed drugs (ciprofloxacin, linezolid) rarely need to be given intravenously. An early appropriate switch to oral therapy can result in earlier hospital discharge.
- What is the optimum dose? Severe infections should be treated with high doses of antimicrobials (e.g. ceftriaxone 2g twice daily for suspected meningococcal disease).
- Will it cause interactions? Clarithromycin and rifampicin can interact with many medications (e.g. warfarin, anti-epileptics, and immunosuppressants). Check the patient's drug chart before prescribing.

# 12.5 Needlestick injury

## Background

Accidental occupational exposure to fluid potentially infected with blood-borne viruses (BBVs) is common. Typically this exposure is sustained from needle injury, although bites and splashes of blood or other body fluid to the eyes, mouth, or areas of broken skin can also transmit infection.

**Prevention** is the key and can save the significant anxiety and hassle that accompanies needlestick injury:

- Gloves should always be worn during exposure-prone procedures.
- Masks and eye protection should be worn if splashes of body fluid are anticipated.
- Safety needles should be used if available.
- Sharps bins should be immediately available and needles disposed of promptly without re-sheathing.
- Where possible, procedures should be performed in an unhurried manner.
- Seek assistance when patients are confused or intoxicated.
- All doctors should receive vaccination against HBV and be aware of their vaccination status.

### Hepatitis C

Risk of transmission from a single needlestick injury is <3%. No prophylaxis is available for HCV infection. Follow-up with serial PCR and serology is recommended. Spontaneous clearance of acute HCV infection occurs in ~20% of cases. Treatment with interferon is effective, and may be considered in those cases which do not resolve spontaneously.

### Hepatitis B

Risk of transmission to a non-immune source is ~33%. In an immunized individual who has a documented adequate anti-HBs (surface antigen) antibody response, no further action other than a HBV vaccine booster is required. Specific immunoglobulin (HBIG) is only recommended where individuals are non-immune and the source patient has confirmed HBV infection. HBIG should be given along with accelerated HBV vaccine.

### HIV

The risk of transmission from a single needlestick injury from a patient with HIV is ~0.3%. This will be higher for deep injuries and sources with high viral loads, and lower if gloves are worn and if the source has a low viral load. The risk from mucosal splash is ~0.1%. Post-exposure prophylaxis (PEP) with 4 weeks of combination antiretroviral drugs reduces this risk, particularly if taken within a few hours of exposure. Unfortunately PEP can be poorly tolerated, due mainly to GI upset. Many individuals find it difficult to complete treatment. Serious side effects from PEP are, however, very rare and should not discourage individuals from taking therapy where appropriate. Senior advice should be sought on whether PEP should be given, usually from an infectious diseases specialist.

## Management of needlestick injury

### Immediate response

- First-aid with *immediate* irrigation, but not with scrubbing or sucking of the site.

- Splashes to eyes or oral mucosa should be copiously washed with warm water or saline, without swallowing the irrigant.

### The injured person

- The needlestick-injured person should report the incident to their line manager.
- They should present themselves for assessment urgently. This may be via occupational health, A&E department, or infectious diseases unit, depending on local arrangements.
- If no significant injury has occurred, the person can be reassured.
- Where a significant injury has occurred, blood should be obtained for storage and medical details including HBV vaccine status, medical history, and drug history obtained in case PEP is needed. The need for further treatment and follow-up depends on the risk assessment and BBV test results of the source patient.
- An investigation and risk assessment should be undertaken by the manager of the clinical area where the incident occurred.

### The source patient

- A senior member of the team responsible for the source patient should inquire about BBV infection or risk factors for BBV infection and arrange for blood to be taken for BBV testing if the patient is agreeable. Blood should not be taken if the patient chooses not to give consent.
- If the patient is unable to give consent (e.g. is unconscious), blood can be tested but only after approval of a senior doctor. The patient should always be informed of the results of the tests and given appropriate follow-up.
- If the source patient is known to have HIV, details of current antiretroviral therapy are crucial. The normal PEP regimen may be ineffective if the patient is known to have resistant virus.
- Results of BBV testing from the source patient should be passed on to the person responsible for the injured person.

## Clinical lessons

- All blood is potentially infectious, hence the need for universal precautions.
- Know your local needlestick policy in advance.
- Know your HBV vaccine status.
- Always wear gloves when performing procedures.
- Take care with your sharps.
- Do not risk assess your own needlestick injury.
- Patients who have donated blood within the past 3 months, who have engaged in no risk can be considered BBV negative, as this would have been routinely tested before blood donation.
- HIV is rare in injecting drug users in the UK (<4%), but HCV is common (50–80%).

# 12.6 Nosocomial infection

## Background

There are ~100,000 hospital-acquired infections per year in the UK (Box 12.1), equating to 9% of hospital inpatients at any given time. A nosocomial infection will result in, on average, a hospital admission extended by 11 days, an extra £3000 in healthcare costs, and a sevenfold increase in mortality.

## Prevention

Between 15% and 30% of nosocomial infection is thought to be preventable by observing good infection control practices:

- Isolate patients who carry potentially transmissible infections (see Box 12.2).
- Practise good hand hygiene by washing with soap or alcohol gels between every patient contact. *C. difficile* spores are not removed by alcohol, so washing with soap and water is needed.
- Use strict aseptic precautions when performing invasive procedures such as central line or chest drain insertion.
- Remove unnecessary cannulae and catheters.
- Avoid unnecessary antimicrobial use.

## Specific infections

- **Pressure sores** should be preventable with good nursing care, but when present can become infected, particularly in incontinent patients. Infections are often polymicrobial, including anaerobes. Infection is often more extensive than is clinically apparent, particularly in patients with sensory loss (Fig. 12.6).
- **Peripheral venous cannulae** are common sites of infection that can result in cellulitis, abscess, or bacteraemia. Remove cannulae that are no longer being used, that have become painful or have erythematous sites. Flucloxacillin is often sufficient treatment, but vancomycin should be used where MRSA is likely.
- **Urinary tract infection** is usually caused by indwelling catheters. Gram-negative organisms including *Pseudomonas* are the usual culprits, but MRSA or *Candida* can also be present. Antibiotics should not be given in the absence of symptoms. Even in symptomatic infection, removal or change of the catheter alone may suffice.
- **Vascular access devices**, such as central lines or Hickman lines, typically become infected with *Staphylococcus aureus* or coagulase-negative staphylococci (CoNS). Enterococci, Gram-negative organisms, or *Candida* spp. can also be implicated. Taking blood cultures through the line and also from peripheral veins is important to distinguish line infection from bacteraemia. Vancomycin is usually the antibiotic of choice, but should always be replaced by a beta-lactam if a sensitive organism is grown. Seven days of treatment can be given for uncomplicated infection (i.e. no embolic infection or endocarditis, and no positive cultures following line removal). Complicated infection requires longer courses of antimicrobials, depending on the nature of the complication. Removal of the infected line is sometimes not required in

| Box 12.1 Frequency of hospital-acquired infection by site |
| --- |
| - Lower respiratory tract: 23% |
| - Urinary tract: 23% |
| - Wound: 11% |
| - Skin: 10% |
| - Bacteraemia: 6% |
| - Other: 25%. |

| Box 12.2 Common situations that require isolation to prevent nosocomial infection |
| --- |
| - Infectious gastroenteritis. |
| - Smear-positive TB. |
| - Meningococcal disease (for first 24 hours). |
| - Invasive group A streptococcal infection. |
| - Chickenpox and shingles. |
| - Mumps. |
| - Measles. |
| - Influenza. |
| - *Clostridium difficile*-associated diarrhoea. |
| - Colonization with MRSA. |
| - Neutropaenia (usually $<0.5 \times 10^6$/mL). |

CoNS infection, but is necessary in *S. aureus* and fungal infection. Line removal alone is often sufficient to treat CoNS line infection.

- **Hospital-acquired pneumonia** (HAP) can difficult to diagnose. There are no universally agreed diagnostic criteria. Gram-negative organisms and *S. aureus* are more common causes than for community acquired-pneumonia, therefore the British Thoracic Society guidelines for managing community-acquired pneumonia do not apply. Good randomized control trial evidence for the best empirical treatment for HAP is lacking. Optimum treatment will depend on the local microbial ecology, but may include a quinolone or anti-pseudomonal penicillin, plus vancomycin or linezolid if MRSA is a concern.

## Specific organisms

Management of hospital-acquired infection is made more difficult by the increased frequency of resistant organisms in hospital. The prevalence of these organisms varies widely between hospitals and initial antimicrobial therapy should be influenced by local resistance patterns.

### Methicillin-resistant *Staphylococcus aureus* (MRSA)

- MRSA produces a penicillin binding protein (PBP2a) with a reduced affinity to beta-lactam antibiotics. When exposed to beta-lactam antibiotics, PBP2a can continue to function and maintain the integrity of the bacterial cell wall. The gene encoding PBP2a, *mecA*, is present in all strains of MRSA, providing a molecular diagnostic tool.

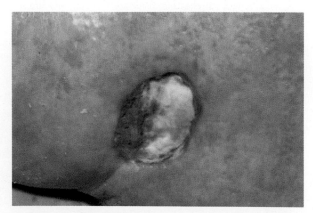

Fig. 12.6 Infected pressure sore.
Reproduced with permission from Dr Andrew Seaton.

- There is now mandatory reporting of MRSA bacteraemia in the UK. Episodes have fallen substantially since 2007 when mandatory surveillance began. In 2011 there were around 1100 episodes in England.
- MRSA decolonization can be achieved by topical chlorhexidine washes, nasal mupirocin, or a combination of oral antibiotics such as rifampicin and doxycycline. However, re-colonization often occurs.
- Vancomycin remains the drug of choice for MRSA infections. Teicoplanin is an alternative.
- Daptomycin, linezolid, and tigecycline and are newer agents with good anti-MRSA activity. They are all effective in treating skin infection. Linezolid is also effective in treating MRSA pneumonia. Daptomycin is licensed to treat bacteraemia and right-sided endocarditis.
- MRSA is variably sensitive to oral agents such as rifampicin, fucidic acid, clindamycin, and trimethoprim.
- Vancomycin intermediate (MIC 4–8mcg/mL) and vancomycin resistant (MIC >16mcg/mL) S. aureus occur, but are very rare. Treatment can be difficult.

### Clostridium difficile-associated diarrhoea (CDAD)

- 2011 saw 19,600 cases of CDAD from England, Wales, and Northern Ireland. This has fallen substantially falling from 57,000 in 2007 when mandatory surveillance began.
- CDAD can be induced by any antibiotic, but cephalosporins, co-amoxiclav, quinolones, and clindamycin are the most associated. Tetracyclines and aminoglycosides are the least associated.
- Elderly patients with severe comorbidity are at increased risk of infection. The use of proton pump inhibitors (PPIs) may predispose to infection.
- Treatment should be based on a severity assessment, with metronidazole used for non-severe disease and oral vancomycin for severe CDAD.
- 15–20% will have recurrence of disease. In those who have already had a relapse, there is a 65% chance of a further relapse after standard therapy.
- The need for isolation is based on the presence of diarrhoea, not the presence of toxin in stool.

## Vancomycin-resistant enterococci (VRE)

- High-level vancomycin resistance is seen due to vancomycin resistance genes (vanA, vanB, vanD). Expression of these genes causes the peptidoglycan chain in the enterococcal cell wall to change from ending in D-alanine to ending in D-lactate. Vancomycin is unable to bind to the altered peptidoglycan. Some VRE are also resistant to teicoplanin.
- Prior exposure to vancomycin or cephalosporins can predispose to carriage in stool. Stool carriage is not a cause of diarrhoea and does not require treatment.

- Bloodstream, urinary, and vascular access-related infections are the most common manifestations.
- Treatment can be difficult. Linezolid or daptomycin may be effective.

## Extended-spectrum beta-lactamases (ESBLs)

- ESBLs are a variety of enzymes that confer resistance to beta-lactam antibiotics, including most penicillins and third-generation cephalosporins such as ceftriaxone. Other resistance mechanisms may also be present so isolates may also be resistant to aminoglycosides and quinolones.
- A range of Gram-negative bacteria can acquire ESBL including Klebsiella and Escherichia coli.
- Risk factors for acquiring ESBL include: length of hospital stay, ITU admission, prior antibiotic administration, and emergency abdominal surgery.
- Carbapenems (e.g. meropenem) are the most effective treatment. Piperacillin-tazobactam or temocillin may be effective. Cephalosporins are not effective, even if in vitro tests suggest activity. High mortality rates are seen if ineffective treatment is given.

## Candidaemia

- Candida is the fourth most common cause of hospital-acquired bloodstream infection.
- Infection usually occurs from a patient's endogenous Candida, found in the GI tract.
- Candida albicans is the most common, but non-albicans candidal species, which can be resistant to fluconazole, are increasing in incidence.
- Candidaemia should always be treated (see Section 12.17).

## Clinical lessons

- Remember to practise good hand hygiene.
- Remove cannulae and urinary catheters promptly when they are no longer needed.
- Don't treat positive culture results from skin, ulcers, or urine in the absence of clinical evidence of infection.
- Hospital-acquired infection often needs different antimicrobial treatment to community-acquired infection—be sure you are giving the correct antibiotics.
- In febrile inpatients:
  - Always look at cannula and central line insertion sites.
  - Always take down bandaging and look at wound sites and pressure areas—they may be hiding the source of the infection.

# 12.7 Travel-related infection

## Background

One in 12 travellers to developing countries will develop an illness requiring medical attention. Most will become unwell within a month of travel. The most common reported causes of imported infection in the UK are listed in Table 12.2. As these are based on formal reports they will underestimate the total burden of disease and will under-report diseases where definitive diagnosis is more difficult (e.g. dengue).

## Assessing the febrile traveller

Life-threatening infection can develop rapidly, particularly with falciparum malaria. The assessment of the febrile traveller hinges on obtaining a detailed travel history, thorough examination, and obtaining country-specific information on infectious agents which may have been encountered, in order to rapidly identify, contain, and treat those infections that can result in serious morbidity.

### Taking a travel history

- **Destination**: note each country visited, including countries travelled through. Disease prevalence can vary within a country so *regional* details are often required. Note whether the trip was to urban or rural areas, and the type of accommodation used.
- **Duration**: document dates of departure and arrival plus the length of time spent in each location.
- **Purpose**: note whether the trip was for business, holiday, voluntary work, or visiting family and who the patient was travelling with.
- **Preparation**: vaccines, malaria prophylaxis, and adherence.
- **Activities and exposures**: animal contacts, insect bites, unusual foods, adventure sports, water sports, and sexual contacts may expand the differential diagnosis.
- **Onset and nature of illness:** when did the disease begin relative to the travel and to the current presentation? List symptoms and their progression.
- **Treatment received:** whether abroad or on return.

### Obtaining country-specific information

Information on endemic diseases or current outbreaks in a particular country can be found at:

- <http://www.travax.nhs.uk>

### Examination

Most travel-related infections have no specific findings on examination. A thorough examination is needed, particularly looking for:

- Eschar (typhus) on legs, inguinal region or axillae.
- Rose spots on torso (typhoid).

### Table 12.2 Most common UK imported infections*

| | |
|---|---|
| *Salmonella* spp. (non-*typhi*) | 1141 |
| Malaria (*falciparum*) | 602 |
| *Campylobacter* | 562 |
| *Salmonella typhi* and *paratyphi* | 220 |
| *Shigella* spp. | 194 |
| Malaria (non-*falciparum*) | 177 |
| *Giardia* | 124 |
| *Legionella* | 70 |
| *Cryptosporidium* | 46 |
| *Entamoeba histolytica* | 26 |

*Cumulative reports to Health Protection Agency (HPA) and Health Protection Scotland for 2005.

- Erythema chronicum migrans (Lyme disease).
- Lymphadenopathy.
- Hepatosplenomegaly.
- Jaundice (malaria, HAV, HBV).
- Conjunctival suffusion (leptospirosis).
- Genital lesions (syphilis, lymphogranuloma venereum).

Signs indicating a severe problem requiring urgent treatment include:

- Tachypnoea (respiratory rate >30/minute).
- Hypotension.
- Meningism, confusion, focal neurology, seizures.
- Unprovoked haemorrhage, petechiae, ecchymoses.

### Initial investigations

After risk assessment for viral haemorrhagic fever (see Box 12.3), the following investigations should be performed in most patients:

- FBC, U&E, LFT, CRP, glucose.
- Malarial films (thick and thin) and antigen testing.
- Blood cultures.
- Urinalysis and urine culture.
- Culture of sputum, and faeces, if applicable.
- CXR.
- Consider serological or nucleic acid testing for viruses (dengue, HIV, HAV, HBV), bacteria (leptospirosis, typhus), and parasites (amoebiasis, schistosomiasis).

## Malaria

Malaria kills 2 million people annually, mostly children. It is present in most tropical and subtropical countries, and is transmitted by the female *Anopheles* mosquito, which bites at dusk. The incubation period is usually ~2 weeks, with most cases occurring within 3 months of exposure.

**Falciparum malaria**, caused by *Plasmodium falciparum*, parasitizes all stages of red blood cells causing both haemolysis leading to anaemia and increased adhesiveness of red cells resulting in their

---

**Box 12.3 ▶ Risk assessment for viral haemorrhagic fever**

Imported viral haemorrhagic fever (VHF) is extremely rare. Four viruses have the potential for nosocomial spread, particularly to front-line medical, nursing, and laboratory staff: **Lassa, Ebola, Marburg**, and **Congo-Crimean haemorrhagic fever** (CCHF). Each carries a high mortality rate. Risk assessment for VHF seeks to identify patients with a potentially fatal illness and limit the possibility for nosocomial spread. As the incubation period of VHF is 3–21 days, all patients whose illness began within 3 weeks of travel to an endemic country should be risk assessed. This should be done rapidly before blood tests are taken. Full details on how to do this are available from the Public Health England website.

A patient in whom VHF is possible should be isolated in a single room and screened for malaria and any other relevant imported infections. If the malaria screen is negative and the fever persists, a VHF screen should be sent. Any patient who has bruising or bleeding should be discussed with the nearest high security infectious diseases unit (HSIDU).

Patients with a high possibility of VHF should be isolated and have an urgent VHF and malaria screen sent. Public health and infection control teams should be notified. Any patient with uncontrolled diarrhoea or vomiting, or bleeding or bruising should be discussed urgently with the nearest HSIDU.

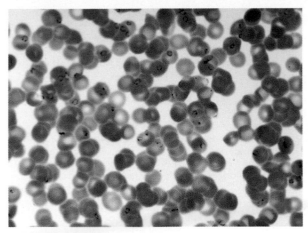

**Fig. 12.7** Blood film of *Plasmodium falciparum*.
Reproduced with permission from James Donnelly.

sequestration in the microvasculature. The resulting tissue hypoperfusion can cause end-organ damage in numerous sites, particularly the brain and kidneys. Death can occur in a previously asymptomatic person in <48 hours. There are 10–20 deaths annually in the UK. Falciparum malaria should always be initially managed in a hospital context by a clinician experienced in its management.

- **Presentation** is non-specific. Fever with no localizing signs is the usual presentation, but cough, headache, or GI upset can be present leading to misdiagnosis of flu or gastroenteritis. Jaundice, confusion, and seizures may also be present in severe disease.
- **Diagnosis** is made by identifying *Plasmodium* trophozoites on a blood film (Fig. 12.7).
- **Assessing severity:** determines prognosis and treatment and should be performed rapidly. If there are features of severe disease, arterial blood gases, lactate, and coagulation screen should be taken. Severe disease may need to be managed in a critical care environment.
- **Treatment**: non-severe forms can be treated with oral **quinine** 600mg three times daily for 7 days. Nausea and tinnitus are common side effects. Severe malaria is treated with IV **artesunate** or **quinine**: a loading dose of 20mg/kg followed by 10mg/kg three times daily. The loading dose is omitted in patients who have already received quinine or mefloquine. There is the potential for cardiac dysrhythmias and hypoglycaemia, so cardiac monitoring and regular blood glucose measurements are needed with IV quinine. Treatment is also for 7 days and step down to oral therapy can be made when clinically stable. Treatment should be combined with a second agent such as doxycycline 100mg twice daily or clindamycin 450mg three times daily to ensure eradication of parasites that may be resistant to quinine.

**Non-falciparum malaria** (or benign malaria) is caused by *Plasmodium vivax*, *Plasmodium ovale*, or *Plasmodium malariae*. These forms infect only immature red cells, typically accounting for <1% of red cells. This results in a much lower parasitaemia than falciparum malaria and therefore a less severe disease. Management is usually an outpatient. Diagnosis is by blood film and treatment is with **chloroquine** 600mg stat, then 300mg at 6 hours, 24 hours, and 48 hours. In *Plasmodium vivax* and *Plasmodium ovale* infection, eradication of liver hypnozoites is needed to prevent recurrence. **Primaquine** (15mg for ovale and 30mg for *vivax*) is given for 14 days. G6PD should be checked prior to administration because of the risk of haemolytic anaemia.

**Prevention** is important. The risk of malaria following 1 month's stay in sub-Saharan Africa is 2.5% if no chemoprophylaxis is taken. Covering skin at night, sleeping under nets, using diethyl toluamide (DEET)-based insect repellent and taking chemoprophylaxis can reduce, but not eliminate, the risk of infection.

## Diagnosing malaria

**Antigen testing** on peripheral blood can rapidly assess whether malaria parasites are present. Some tests differentiate falciparum and non-falciparum infection. They do not give information on severity of infection.

**Thick films** are best to establish a diagnosis of malaria, by maximizing the number of red cells examined.

**Thin films** are best to speciate malaria and give a parasitaemia count which is crucial for guiding treatment.

The first film is positive in 95% of cases. However, taking 3 films over 48–72 hours is recommended to exclude malaria. Results should be available within 1–2 hours.

### Markers of complicated malaria

One or more of:
- Parasitaemia >2%.
- Spontaneous bleeding.
- Disseminated intravascular coagulation.
- Haemoglobin <8g/dL.
- Renal impairment.
- Haemoglobinuria.
- Acidosis pH <7.3.
- Impaired consciousness (always check blood glucose).
- Seizures.
- Hypoglycaemia.
- Acute respiratory distress syndrome.
- Shock.

### Clinical lessons

- Assume a febrile person who has recently been to an endemic area has malaria until proven otherwise.
- Malaria can occur in someone who has correctly taken anti-malarial medication.
- Mixed malaria is rare. Always treat for falciparum malaria if there is uncertainty.

British guidelines on the management of malaria are available from the British Infection Society: <http://www.britishinfection.org>.

# Travellers' diarrhoea

Approximately one-half of travellers to developing countries will develop diarrhoea. Bacteria are the most common causes and ingestion of contaminated food and water is the usual source. The use of stomach acid-suppressing drugs such as PPIs or H2 blockers increases the risk of infection. The vast majority are short, self-limiting episodes and occur within the first 2 weeks of travel. Fluid and electrolyte replacement is the most important intervention. **Ciprofloxacin** is indicated in severe disease, (e.g. high fever, bloody diarrhoea, or protracted symptoms) or in high-risk patients (immunosuppressed, elderly, severe comorbidity). The presence of bloody diarrhoea should raise the possibility of amoebiasis which will not be treated by quinolones. Antimotility agents should be avoided. Post-infective lactose intolerance or irritable bowel syndrome occurs in a minority of patients and it may take weeks for the bowel habit to completely normalize.

### Causes of travellers' diarrhoea

- Enterotoxigenic *Escherichia coli* (ETEC)
- Enteroaggregative *Escherichia coli* (EAEC)
- *Salmonella* (non-typhi)
- *Campylobacter*
- *Shigella*
- Enteric fever
- Cholera
- Giardiaisis
- *Cryptosporidium*
- Rotavirus.

# Enteric fever

Enteric fever is the collective term for the illnesses caused by *Salmonella typhi* and *paratyphi* (intracellular Gram-negative bacilli). Only humans are affected. Following ingestion, *Salmonella* bacilli are taken up into mucosal-associated lymphoid tissue in the intestine where proliferation occurs. The bacteria spread to lymph nodes, liver, and spleen via the bloodstream. Organisms resist killing by tissue macrophages and survive intracellularly within the bone marrow, liver, and spleen. Chronic asymptomatic carriage occurs in <5% cases.

- **Clinical features**: enteric fever is a febrile illness occurring 7–21 days after infection. The presentation is usually non-specific with fever the predominant finding. In the first week of illness, fever rises in a step-wise manner. Rigors, cough, headache, anorexia, abdominal pain, and malaise can also develop, but diarrhoea is usually absent. Rose spots on trunk may occasionally appear during the second week. If untreated, hepatosplenomegaly, intestinal perforation, and GI bleeding ensue. Severe presentations with shock or altered consciousness can occur. Bacteraemia can seed other organs causing pneumonia, osteomyelitis, pericarditis, or cerebral disease. Mortality without treatment is ~15%.
- **Diagnosis** is by blood culture in most cases. Culture of stool or rose spot aspirate will sometimes be positive. Serology is difficult to interpret in the context of prior vaccination. Routine lab tests have no suggestive features—mild anaemia and elevated transaminases are common. The WCC can be high or low.
- **Treatment**: **ciprofloxacin** is the drug of choice in sensitive *Salmonella*, but increasing rates of quinolone resistance means that **ceftriaxone** may be preferred for empirical therapy. Amoxicillin, gentamicin, and azithromycin may also be effective for sensitive organisms. In severe disease (coma or shock), steroids may be of benefit. Even with appropriate treatment defervescence usually takes 4–5 days.
- **Prevention**: avoid contaminated food and water. Vaccination provides only partial protection against typhoid and no protection against paratyphoid.

# Amoebiasis

Amoebiasis is present worldwide, though more common in developing countries. Infection is usually by ingestion of *Entamoeba histolytica* cysts in food or water. Cysts develop into trophozoites in the small intestine. Trophozoites can cause local invasion of the colonic mucosa leading to mucus production and bloody diarrhoea. Penetration of colonic mucosa can lead to dissemination.

- **Intestinal infection**: bloody diarrhoea, often with fever, is the commonest presentation. Severe colitis or perforation occurs rarely. Identification of trophozoites by microscopy in stool can be difficult and antigen testing of stool is more sensitive.
- **Liver abscess** is the most common extra-intestinal manifestation. It typically occurs within 8–20 weeks of travel. Right upper quadrant pain, fever, anorexia, and hepatomegaly are usual. Jaundice is uncommon. Stool microscopy is rarely diagnostic, but serology will be positive in >90%. Ultrasound is helpful, but cannot distinguish amoebic from other forms of liver abscess. Aspiration is only recommended if rupture appears imminent, there is diagnostic uncertainty, or there has been no response to antibiotic treatment. The aspirate has a characteristic anchovy paste appearance.
- **Other extra-intestinal sites**: pulmonary, pericardial and cerebral infections occur rarely.

**Treatment** is with **metronidazole** to kill invasive forms. 400–800mg three times daily for 10 days has ~90% efficacy when combined with **diloxanide furoate** to eliminate trophozoites in the intestinal lumen.

# Dengue

Dengue is a flavivirus with four serotypes. It causes 100 million infections worldwide annually and is spread by *Aedes* mosquitoes. It is endemic through much of the tropics and subtropics. Around 2.5 billion people are at risk of infection.

- **Clinical features:** after an incubation period of 4–14 days a flu-like illness develops with fever, headache (often retro-orbital, and marked myalgia and arthralgia. A maculopapular rash is present in ~50%. The illness last up to a week. Leucopenia, thrombocytopenia, and elevated transaminases are common.
- **Complications**: dengue haemorrhagic fever (DHF) occurs rarely. Previous infection with dengue predisposes to the development of DHF, which therefore is less common in travellers than those in endemic areas. Fever, thrombocytopenia, haemorrhage, and increased vascular permeability are the diagnostic criteria. Shock can occur (dengue shock syndrome), carrying a mortality rate of ~10%, even with supportive treatment.
- **Diagnosis** is primarily clinical but can be confirmed by PCR and serology.
- **Treatment** is supportive. There is no antiviral agent.
- **Prevention** is by avoidance of mosquito bites. Unlike *Anopheles* mosquitoes, *Aedes* bites during the day. There is no effective vaccine available.

# Schistosomiasis

Schistosomiasis (or bilharzia) is a helminthic infection affecting 200 million people globally. It can present with acute infection or chronic complications involving the bladder and urinary tract (*Schistosoma haematobium*) or liver (*Schistosoma mansoni* or *Schistosoma japonicum*). Infection is water-borne. Free-living cercariae in water directly penetrate human skin, migrate to and mature in the vasculature, before seeding capillary beds of the portal, mesenteric, or vesical vessels. Once there, adult worms produce eggs which are excreted in urine or stool. The final part of the life cycle is completed within water snails.

- **Acute infection** has two manifestations:
  1. **Swimmer's itch**, an itchy papular rash on the feet or ankles, follows skin penetration by cercariae.
  2. **Katayama fever**, occurs within 2 months of exposure and reflects migration of schistosomes through the body. Fever, headache, arthralgia, myalgia, cough, and diarrhoea can occur. Lymphadenopathy and hepatosplenomegaly may be found. Eosinophilia is common.
- **Chronic infection** can cause complications in a number of organs, usually after years of infection:
  - Liver: pre-hepatic portal hypertension.
  - Intestine: abdominal pain, diarrhoea, bleeding, ulcers, strictures.
  - Urinary tract: haematuria, ureteric strictures, renal impairment, increased risk of squamous cell carcinoma of bladder.

Diagnosis is by the identification of eggs in urine, stool, or biopsy specimens. Serological testing is useful for screening travellers, but is less useful in endemic regions. Treatment is with **praziquantel**.

# Chikungunya

Chikungunya is an alphavirus transmitted by *Aedes* mosquitoes that has caused large outbreaks of illness in southern India and Mauritius in recent years. It causes a flu-like illness with fever and malaise. Rash is common, but severe joint pains are the most characteristic feature. There is no specific treatment, and person-to-person spread does not occur. Serological testing is available.

# Tick typhus

Tick typhus is the commonest imported rickettsial infection in the UK, usually acquired after a safari in southern or eastern Africa. High fever, headache, myalgia, maculopapular rash, and eschar are the typical features. Treatment with **doxycycline** is extremely effective.

## Legionella

*Legionella* is a potentially serious cause of pneumonia in travellers, particularly if staying in air-conditioned hotels in Europe or the USA. Treatment should be with a **quinolone** or **macrolide.**

## Leptospirosis

Leptospirosis is an infrequent cause of febrile illness in returning travellers (see Section 12.14).

## Penicillin-resistant pneumococcus

Penicillin-resistant pneumococcus is common in certain areas of the world, particularly the USA, Japan, and southern Europe. Empirical treatment of meningitis in travellers returned from these areas should include **vancomycin** in addition to standard doses of **cefotaxime** (2g four times daily) or ceftriaxone (2g twice daily).

## *Giardia*

See Section 12.18.

## Cutaneous larva migrans

Cutaneous larva migrans is a helminthic infection caused by several *Ancylostoma* species. Penetration of exposed skin by larvae present in soil or sand can cause cutaneous infection in humans. Infection occurs in tropical and subtropical countries where cats and dogs are the main reservoir.

- After an incubation period of a few days to weeks, an itchy, painful, red track develops, usually on the feet, ankles, or buttocks, which can be serpiginous, indicating larval migration (Fig. 12.8). There is no fever or systemic upset. Rarely pulmonary involvement can occur with dry cough and migratory infiltrates on CXR.
- Diagnosis is clinical, based on the typical rash.
- Resolution without treatment will occur after several weeks but **albendazole** will shorten the duration of disease.

## Clinical lessons

- Diarrhoea or cough can be a presenting feature of malaria.
- Diarrhoea is an uncommon feature of typhoid.

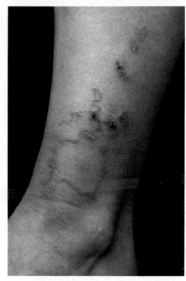

**Fig. 12.8** Cutaneous larva migrans.
Reproduced with permission from Dr Andrew Seaton.

- If bloody diarrhoea is present, think of amoebiasis.
- The febrile patient from sub-Saharan Africa is most likely to have malaria.
- The febrile patient from south Asia is almost equally likely to have enteric fever, malaria, or dengue.

## Reference

Freedman DO, Weld LH, Kozarsky PE, *et al.* Spectrum of disease and relation to place of exposure among ill returned travellers. *N Engl J Med* 2006; 354(2): 119–130.

# 12.8 Immunocompromised hosts

## Background

Immunocompromise is a state in which the function of the immune system is impaired. There are many causes and the severity of the immunodeficiency will depend on the nature and duration of the cause (see Table 12.3).

**Ageing** results in impairment of many facets of the immune system. Fever response can be blunted and T-cell responses diminish. Infections can present non-specifically in the elderly (with confusion or falls) and fever may be absent.

**Pregnancy** results in relative immunosuppression. Infections such as chicken pox, malaria, or listeria can be more serious.

**Antibiotic therapy** can eliminate protective microbial flora causing candidal or *Clostridium difficile* infection.

**Medical devices** such as venous cannulae, urinary catheters, and endotracheal tubes bypass the body's innate immune system, providing an entry route for infection. They should always be removed promptly when no longer needed.

**Infection** can also cause breaches of skin and mucosal barriers. Tinea infection can predispose to cellulitis, zoster rashes can become super-infected with bacteria, and viral upper respiratory infections can lead to pneumonia.

**HIV infection** produces a unique immunodeficiency state with progressive loss of CD4 cells. Opportunistic infection with shingles (Fig. 12.9) or oral candidiasis can occur, but severe infection typically occurs when the CD4 count is $<200 \times 10^6/L$.

**Splenectomy** results in an impaired response, particularly to encapsulated bacteria (pneumococcus, *Haemophilus influenza*, and meningococcus), that can result in rapidly overwhelming sepsis. Vaccination, prophylactic antimicrobials, and patient education are all important components of management.

**Chronic diseases** such as cancers (particularly haematological malignancy), diabetes mellitus, rheumatoid arthritis, systemic lupus erythematosus, chronic kidney disease, cystic fibrosis, and malnutrition all cause multifactorial immunocompromise.

**Chemotherapy** acts against all rapidly dividing cells, which include blood cells. Transient neutropaenia can result after many

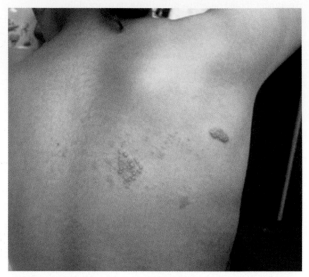

**Fig. 12.9** Shingles.

Reproduced from Gardiner et al., *Oxford Specialty Training: Training in Paediatrics*, 2009, Figure 9.16b, page 202, with permission from Oxford University Press.

different regimens and patients should be educated to present promptly if fever develops. Prophylactic antimicrobials many be needed. Neutropaenic sepsis is a medical emergency.

**Immunosuppressant medication** (such as steroids, azathioprine, mycophenolate mofetil, ciclosporin, or tacrolimus) for treating autoimmune diseases or to prevent transplant rejection can cause profound immunosuppression. The new anti-TNF (tumour necrosis factor) drugs carry a particular risk of TB reactivation.

**Bone marrow transplantation** causes one of the most extreme forms of immunosuppression by eliminating all of the host's cellular immune system. B-cell and neutrophil function can recover in a few weeks, but T-cell function may take 6–12 months to fully recover, if at all.

## Management of neutropaenic sepsis

The presence of fever in a patient with neutropaenia is an emergency. The same principles of managing any septic patient apply; however, deterioration can occur more rapidly.

- Take appropriate specimens, including blood cultures.
- Promptly give IV antibiotics according to local protocol (often gentamicin and piperacillin/tazobactam).
- Where pneumonia is present add a macrolide (although note that CXR may be normal until neutrophil count recovers).
- If no response is seen within 48 hours consider changing antimicrobials (often to meropenem and a glycopeptide).
- Consider viral infection (e.g. influenza, HSV, or respiratory syncytial virus (RSV)) or fungal infection (*Candida* or *Aspergillus*).

| Table 12.3 | Some pathogens affecting the immunocompromised | |
|---|---|---|
| **Viral** | VZV | Elderly, chemotherapy, HIV |
| | CMV | HIV, post-transplant |
| | JC virus | HIV |
| **Bacterial** | Pneumococcus | Splenectomy, HIV, alcoholism |
| | Meningococcus | Splenectomy, complement deficiency |
| | Listeria | Pregnancy, old age, malignancy |
| | TB | Malnutrition, HIV, anti-TNF therapy |
| **Fungal** | Candida | Chemotherapy |
| | Aspergillus | Chemotherapy, post transplant |
| | Cryptococcus | HIV |
| | Pneumocystis | HIV, post transplant |
| **Protozoal** | Toxoplasmosis | HIV |

# 12.9 Pyrexia of unknown origin

## Background

True pyrexia of unknown origin (PUO) is rare now due to improvements in imaging techniques which can detect deep-seated infection or neoplasia that previously went unrecognized in their early stages. Strictly defined, PUO is a fever >38.3°C for >3 weeks, with no diagnosis after 1 week of inpatient investigation.

## Aetiology

The largest case series in recent years showed that no cause is found in ~33% and that three groups account for most of the identified causes:

1. Infective (20%)
2. Inflammatory (24%)
3. Neoplastic (10%).

**Infective**: the most common infective causes are TB, abscesses, endocarditis, and osteomyelitis. Many other infections can cause a PUO including HIV, *Brucella*, Q fever, syphilis, Whipple disease, chronic meningococcaemia, and gonococcaemia.

**Inflammatory**: Still disease (juvenile-onset rheumatoid arthritis), polymyalgia rheumatica, and temporal arteritis are the commonest causes. Sarcoid, systemic lupus erythematosus, and systemic arteritis are included in the rarer inflammatory causes of a PUO.

**Neoplastic**: lymphoma, leukaemia, renal cell carcinoma, hepatocellular carcinoma, and liver metastases can all present as PUO. Atrial myxoma is a much rarer, but well-recognized, cause of PUO.

There are numerous other causes of PUO. The most common of these is probably drug fever. Alcoholic hepatitis, hyperthyroidism, phaeochromocytoma, adrenal insufficiency, periodic fevers (e.g. familial Mediterranean fever), hypothalamic damage, and factitious fever are some of the others.

## Management

Thorough history-taking, examination, and review of case records and prior investigations is the key. Most diagnoses are made by a methodical approach revealing a common entity, rather than a serendipitous finding of an unusual disease. All the common diseases previously listed should be considered. Presence of a significant travel history, animal contact, occupational exposures, or the presence of immunosuppression can broaden the possible differential diagnosis.

A broad panel of simple investigations should initially be requested, with more specialist and invasive procedures reserved for specific epidemiological risk factors (for infection) and identification of organ-specific abnormalities from the initial work-up.

## Prognosis

When no cause is found for PUO, most patients' symptoms will resolve without treatment. A cause will become apparent over time in a minority. Death resulting from an initially undiagnosed PUO is uncommon.

## Some drugs which can cause fever

- Antibacterials, e.g. penicillins, rifampicin, vancomycin, sulphonamides.
- NSAIDs.
- Barbiturates, phenytoin.
- Methyldopa and hydralazine.
- Procainamide.
- Antimalarials.

## Investigating a PUO

### Baseline tests

- FBC, ESR, U&E, LFT, CRP, calcium, phosphate, LDH, thyroid function tests.
- Immunoglobulins, rheumatoid factor, ANA.
- Blood cultures.
- HIV testing.
- Tuberculin testing or interferon release assay.
- Urinalysis and culture.
- CT chest/abdomen/pelvis.

## Targeted investigation

- Biopsy of lymph node or target organ.
- Bone marrow aspirate and trephine.
- Specific microbiological testing depending on epidemiological factors (e.g. brucella, Q fever, etc.).
- Echocardiogram.
- Bone scan.
- MRI scan.
- White cell scan.

## Therapeutic trials

Where a patient is unwell it is often wise to empirically treat for the common community-acquired infections until further information becomes available. Occasionally empirical anti-tuberculous treatment or doxycycline can be given, although this is best avoided where possible. If no cause is identified, empirical steroids may result in symptomatic improvement.

## References

de Kleijn EM, Vandenbroucke JP, van der Meer JW. Fever of unknown origin (FUO). I A. prospective multi-centre study of 167 patients with FUO, using fixed epidemiologic entry criteria. The Netherlands FUO Study Group. *Medicine* 1997; 76: 392–400.

Knockaert DC, Dujardin KS, Bobbaers HJ. Long-term follow-up of patients with undiagnosed fever of unknown origin. *Arch Intern Med* 1996; 156: 618–20.

# 12.10 Infection in injecting drug users

## Background

Inpatient management of injecting drug users is commonly complicated by their delayed presentation to medical services, difficult IV access, and behavioural problems often related to drug intoxication or substance dependence. Appropriate identification and treatment of opiate withdrawal is necessary. Behavioural contracts can be helpful, as can early liaison with community homelessness and addiction teams.

## Blood-borne viruses

The seroprevalence of HIV is low in injecting drug users in the UK (0.4% in Glasgow to 4% in some areas of London).

Hepatitis C seroprevalence is, however, high (although the rate of chronic infection defined by PCR positivity is lower). Those patients who are PCR negative are considered non-infective and at no increased risk of liver disease. Accordingly all patients with positive HCV ELISA should be offered referral to specialist services to assess their HCV, although treatment options may be limited by ongoing injecting habits.

Chronic hepatitis B infection is less common than HCV. All injecting drug users should be offered HBV vaccination and regular screening for BBVs.

## Skin and soft tissue infection

Unhygienic injecting practice and direct injection into muscle or subcutaneous tissues ('skin popping') predispose injecting drug users to skin and soft tissue infections, typically related to a recent injection site. Local abscess formation requiring aspiration or drainage can occur. Following femoral vein injection, subsequent DVT is common. The clot can become seeded by bacteria and act as a source of bacteraemia. This situation requires prolonged LMWH and IV antimicrobials. It is inadvisable to treat DVT in people with substance abuse with outpatient warfarin; 6 weeks of LMWH is an accepted alternative. When IV access proves difficult, oral drugs with good bioavailability such as ciprofloxacin and clindamycin can be combined with good effect.

## Bacteraemia and endocarditis

*Staphylococcus aureus* is the most common cause of bacteraemia in injecting drug users, but polymicrobial infections (particularly with anaerobes) are also common. Complicated bacteraemia with septic DVT, septic arthritis, septic pulmonary emboli (Fig. 12.10), or endocarditis can occur. Septic injecting drug users should be considered bacteraemic until proven otherwise and treated promptly with IV antimicrobials with good anti-staphylococcal cover (such as flucloxacillin, gentamicin, and clindamycin) after obtaining several blood cultures.

Right-sided endocarditis is more common in injecting drug users. Repeated injection of substances such as talc (used to cut heroin), damage the tricuspid valve, which predisposes to seeding by bacteria. *Staphylococcus aureus* is the most common cause. A murmur can be absent given the low flow across the tricuspid valve, and peripheral

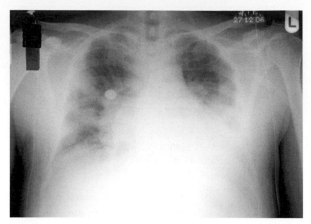

**Fig. 12.10** CXR of septic emboli (wedge-shaped areas of consolidation in right mid-zone).

signs of endocarditis will be absent (such as haematuria or splinter haemorrhages), unless there is also left-sided valve involvement.

The presence of fever and persistent *Staphylococcus aureus* bacteraemia in an injecting drug user with evidence of embolic pulmonary infection fulfils the Duke criteria for definite endocarditis even in the absence of vegetations on echocardiography.

## Infections due to spore-forming bacteria

Rare, but potentially fatal, infections by toxin-producing anaerobic bacilli in the *Clostridium* genus can occur in injecting drug users, notably *Clostridium novyi*, *C. tetani*, and *C. botulinum*. Diagnosis is made on purely clinical grounds.

**Tetanus** is caused by wound contamination of *C. tetani* present in soil. Tetanus toxin (tetanospasmin) causes neuromuscular blockade by preventing inhibitory neurotransmitter release at the neuromuscular junction which leads to increased lower motor neuron activity causing muscle spasm and rigidity. The incubation period is 5–15 days and initial symptoms are sweating, muscle spasm, trismus, dysphagia, and neck stiffness. Agitation, neuromuscular respiratory failure, and cardiovascular instability with dysrhythmias and widely fluctuating blood pressure then develop. Even with supportive care in ICU the mortality is high.

**Botulism** in adults is rare and caused by either ingestion of food contaminated with toxin or *C. botulinum* infection of wounds leading to production of toxin. Botulinum toxin irreversibly blocks presynaptic release of acetylcholine at the neuromuscular junction. The incubation period is 12 hours for food-borne disease and several days for wound botulism. A typical presentation is with descending flaccid paralysis beginning with diplopia, ptosis, and inability to extend the neck, proceeding through dysphonia and dysphagia, to limb weakness and paralysis of respiratory muscles resulting in ventilatory failure and death. Fever and impaired consciousness do not occur. Urgent treatment with botulinum antitoxin, wound debridement, and antibiotic therapy is needed. Recovery is very slow and ventilatory support may be required for weeks.

# 12.11 Bioterrorism

## Background

Bioterrorism is the deliberate release of pathogenic micro-organisms or bacterially derived toxins and can be overt (where warning or declaration of release is given) or covert. Large numbers of casualties can potentially be involved within hours to days of an attack, sufficient to overwhelm standard emergency care facilities. The pathogens involved are not commonly encountered and some familiarity with them is important to promptly recognize and contain a bioterrorist event. Guidelines for the management of suspected or confirmed bioterrorism are available from the PHE. Each institution should have its own protocol contained within its major incident plan.

Organisms are categorized according to severity of illness, ease of transmissibility, and availability of treatment.

## Category A agents

- Easily disseminated or transmitted among people.
- High mortality rate.
- Likely to cause disruption and panic.

## Anthrax

*Bacillus anthracis*, a gram positive bacillus, causes very rare sporadic cases in the UK due to contact, inhalation, or ingestion of spores, usually from animal hides. There are three main forms of disease:
- **Cutaneous:** usually occurs on exposed areas with an enlarging papule that develops a central vesicle. A painless necrotic ulcer with marked surrounding oedema then forms. Systemic upset can occur. Mortality is <1% with appropriate treatment.
- **Inhalational:** the initial illness is non-specific with fever, myalgia, and malaise. After 72 hours progressive breathlessness develops, followed by hypotension, stridor, and shock. Mediastinal widening on CXR or CT chest is classically seen. Even with treatment, the mortality rate is ~50%.
- **Gastrointestinal:** causes intestinal oedema and ulceration. Symptoms include fever, pain and vomiting, followed by bloody diarrhoea, haematemesis and bloody ascites.

Penicillin and doxycycline are effective for natural anthrax, but ciprofloxacin is the drug of choice for anthrax associated with bioterrorism. Combinations of two or three antibiotics plus steroids are advised for inhalational anthrax.

## Smallpox

Smallpox, caused by *Variola major*, was eradicated in 1979. Accordingly, routine vaccination is no longer given and most people are susceptible. After an incubation period of 1–3 weeks, there is abrupt fever, headache, and backache for several days. This is followed by mucosal papules and, a day later, by a macular rash that progresses to papules, vesicles, and pustules over the next week. It can be differentiated from chickenpox by the presence of a single crop of large vesicles predominantly affecting the peripheries. It is extremely infectious and historically carries a mortality rate of >20% in unvaccinated individuals. There is no proven treatment.

## Plague

Plague is caused by *Yersinia pestis*, an aerobic Gram-negative bacillus. There are three clinical forms, all appearing after an incubation period of 2–8 days:
- **Bubonic:** painful lymphadenopathy is preceded by fever, shivers, malaise, and headache. Buboes, extremely painful, non-fluctuant erythematous enlarged lymph nodes, in the inguinal, axillary, or cervical regions are characteristic.
- **Pneumonic:** may occur as a primary illness or secondary to any of the other forms. It is fatal unless early appropriate antimicrobials are given.
- **Septicaemic:** presents with signs and symptoms of severe sepsis—vomiting, diarrhoea, fever, and hypotension without localizing features. Buboes are not present and the diagnosis can be difficult because of the lack of specific features.

Treatment options include streptomycin, gentamicin, doxycycline, co-trimoxazole, and chloramphenicol.

## Tularaemia

Tularaemia is caused by *Francisella tularensis*, a facultative Gram-negative coccobacillus. It is a zoonosis, and transmission is via vectors (ticks and mosquitoes) or from contact with infected animals (typically rabbits, hares, or rodents). Six clinical forms are recognized, all having incubation periods of 2–10 days, including glandular, typhoidal, pneumonic, oropharyngeal, and oculoglandular.

Ulceroglandular infection, however, accounts for ~85% of cases. Without appropriate antibiotic therapy it carries a mortality rate of up to 30%.
- **Ulceroglandular:** presents with fever and erythematous ulcer with central eschar. There is painful regional lymphadenopathy.
- **Pneumonic:** carries the highest mortality rate and is more common in the elderly. It can be indistinguishable from other forms of community-acquired pneumonia.

Streptomycin, gentamicin, and tetracycline are all effective therapies.

## Viral haemorrhagic fever

VHF is very rare in the UK. Only four are readily transmitted and each carries a high mortality rate, although often in the context of limited availability of medical care. Incubation periods are between 3 and 21 days.
- Lassa, an arenavirus transmitted by the multi-mammate rat, causing around 250,000 cases per year in West Africa. Presentation is initially non-specific. Overall the mortality rate is 1%, although 15–20% of those hospitalized die. Ribavirin can be used for treatment.
- Ebola and Marburg are rare filoviruses that cause infrequent outbreaks in Central Africa. No animal reservoirs have been identified and the case fatality rate is 70–90%.
- Congo Crimean haemorrhagic fever is tick-borne and has a shorter incubation period (3–7 days) and a lower mortality rate (10–30%) than other VHF.

### Background

**Viruses** are small (20–400nm) organisms that are unable to self-replicate. They can be classified by morphology under electron microscopy, and by their nucleic acid composition and replication method (Table 12.4).

### Structure

The RNA or DNA of the viral genome is coated in a protein capsid which, in some viruses, is enveloped. Virally encoded molecules may be embedded in the envelope to assist infection of host cells or immune evasion. A virion is the entire viral particle (genome, capsid, and envelope).

### Replication

All viruses depend on a host cell for their replication. Free virions attach to and enter cells, often via cell-specific receptors. Following cell entry, uncoating occurs where the viral nucleic acid separates from the capsid. Some viruses can incorporate into the host genome, inducing latency or oncogenesis. Viral mRNA is transcribed from the viral genome—the precise means by which this is accomplished varies. Viral mRNA is translated on host ribosomes to produce proteins which may be structural components of new virions, enzymes to facilitate replication, or transcriptional regulators to divert host cell mechanisms toward viral proliferation. Newly generated capsid and nucleic acid combine to form virions and are released from the cell by inducing cell lysis or by budding from the host cell. The viral envelope is acquired from the cell membrane during the budding process.

### Antiviral agents

The greater dependence of viral replication on host cell pathways means the production of safe antiviral drugs has proven more difficult than for antibacterial drugs. Consequently, compared with antibacterial agents, there are relatively few antiviral drugs available. The largest group is the antiretroviral drugs (see Section 12.13).

**Aciclovir** is the most commonly used antiviral agent. It is active against herpes viruses, particularly *Herpes simplex 1* and *2* (HSV) and *Varicella zoster* (VZV). HSV is more susceptible to aciclovir than VZV. Aciclovir is phosphorylated intracellularly by viral thymidine kinase. This enzyme is not present in host cells, so the drug is only active in virally infected cells. Cellular enzymes convert the monophosphate form to a triphosphate form that acts as a dGTP analogue and selectively inhibits viral DNA polymerase. Resistance is rare. **Valganciclovir** and **famciclovir** are pro-drugs of acyclovir that have improved bioavailability. The main side effects are GI disturbance (including nausea, vomiting, abdominal pain, and diarrhoea) and renal impairment.

**Ganciclovir** is the principal treatment for CMV infection, although it is also effective against other herpes viruses. It is very poorly bioavailable, although **valganciclovir** is a pro-drug with better oral absorption. Renal impairment and bone marrow suppression are the main adverse effects.

**Foscarnet** and **cidofovir** are also available for the treatment of CMV and other herpes viruses. They have a number of side effects

| Table 12.4 Classification of viruses | | | |
|---|---|---|---|
| **DNA viruses** | | **RNA viruses** | |
| Single-stranded | Double-stranded | Single-stranded | Double-stranded |
| **Naked** | **Naked** | **Naked** | **Naked** |
| *Parvoviridae*<br>  Erythrovirus B19 | *Papovaviridae*<br>  HPV<br>*Adenoviridae*<br>  Adenovirus | *Caliciviridae*<br>  Norovirus<br>*Picornaviridae*<br>  HAV<br>  Polio<br>  Rhinovirus<br>  Coxsackievirus | *Reoviridae*<br>  Rotavirus |
|  | **Enveloped** | **Enveloped** |  |
|  | *Hepadnviridae*<br>  HBV<br>*Herpesviridae*<br>  HSV<br>  VZV<br>  CMV<br>  EBV<br>  HHV-6<br>*Poxviridae*<br>  Orf<br>  Smallpox | *Flaviviridae*<br>  Yellow Fever<br>  Dengue<br>  HCV<br>*Togaviridae*<br>  Rubella<br>*Retroviridae*<br>  HIV-1, HIV-2<br>  HTLV-1<br>*Coronaviridae*<br>  Coronavirus<br>*Filoviridae*<br>  Ebola<br>*Rhabdoviridae*<br>  Rabies<br>*Bunyaviridae*<br>  Crimean-Congo<br>*Orthmyxoviridae*<br>  Influenza<br>*Paramyxoviridae*<br>  Parainfluenxa<br>  RSV<br>  Measles<br>  Mumps<br>*Arenaviridae*<br>  Lassa |  |

and are generally reserved for when other treatments are not effective or contraindicated.

**Ribavirin** had broad antiviral activity *in vitro*. It is used to treat HCV and RSV. Its chief side effect is anaemia. It is available orally, intravenously, or in nebulized form.

**Oseltamivir** (or Tamiflu®) is an oral drug for the treatment of influenza A and B. Its mode of action is to inhibit viral neuraminidase, preventing shedding of virus from infected cells. All hospitalized or at-risk patients with flu should be treated, although treatment is more likely to be effective if given early. **Zanamavir** is an alternative agent that is administered by inhaler. It is the drug of choice for treating flu in immunocompromised patients. An unlicensed IV form is available.

## Epstein–Barr virus

Epstein–Barr virus (EBV) is an extremely common herpes virus infection; 90–95% of adults have serological evidence of prior exposure.

### Clinical features
- Infection is often asymptomatic in children.
- Infectious mononucleosis (glandular fever) occurs in adolescents and adults and presents with fever, malaise, fatigue, nausea, vomiting, and pharyngitis. An erythematous pharynx, bilateral tonsillar enlargement, and white exudates are found on examination (Fig. 12.11). Cervical lymphadenopathy and splenomegaly are common. Palatal petechiae may sometimes be found. The illness usually lasts 1–2 weeks.

### Diagnosis
- Blood investigations show an elevated lymphocyte count, positive heterophile antibody test in 90%, and often show derangement of liver function tests. Atypical lymphocytes may be seen on a blood film.
- EBV serology or PCR will confirm the diagnosis.

### Treatment
- Symptomatic treatment with paracetamol and aspirin gargles. IV fluid may be needed if there is difficulty swallowing.
- Aciclovir is not effective

### Complications
- Rash is common if amoxicillin is given (Fig. 12.12). This is an idiosyncratic reaction and *not* an allergy.
- Splenic rupture is rare (<0.1%) and can happen spontaneously, usually between days 14–21 of illness. Patients with splenomegaly should avoid contact sports for at least 4 weeks.
- Airway obstruction can occur in severe tonsillar enlargement. Steroids and urgent ENT referral are indicated if signs of upper airway obstruction are present.
- Post-viral chronic fatigue may occur in ~10%

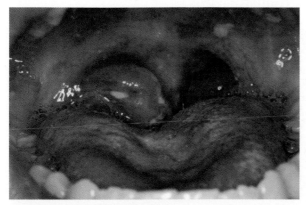

Fig. **12.11** Tonsillar enlargement in EBV.
Reproduced with permission from Dr Andrew Seaton.

## Herpes simplex virus

HSV 1 and 2 cause oral and genital ulcers and encephalitis.

## Varicella zoster virus

VZV causes varicella (chickenpox) and zoster (shingles).

## Heterophile antibody testing

Heterophile antibodies are antibodies that cross-react between species. Human antibodies to EBV can result in agglutination of sheep (Paul Bunnell test) or horse (Monospot test) erythrocytes. The presence of heterophile antibodies in a person with clinical glandular fever is diagnostic of EBV infection.

### Causes of heterophile antibody-*negative* glandular fever
- Early EBV infection (25% negative in 1st week).
- Atypical EBV (5–10% of all EBV infections).
- CMV.
- Acute HIV.
- HHV-6 (human herpes virus 6).
- Toxoplasmosis.

## Mumps

Mumps is a paramyxovirus causing a systemic illness characterized by malaise, fever, and parotitis. Outbreaks still occur in the UK.

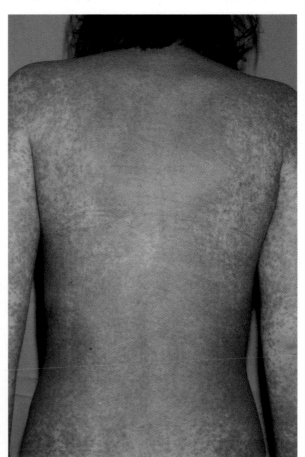

Fig. **12.12** Rash observed when amoxicillin given in acute EBV infection.
Reproduced with permission from Dr Andrew Seaton.

## Clinical features

- The incubation period is 14–18 days.
- Patients are infective for a few days before until a few days after the onset of parotitis.
- Bilateral parotitis is usual, but can be unilateral, and can also affect submandibular salivary glands. Overall the illness tends to last 5–7 days.
- Can present with orchitis or meningitis in the absence of parotitis.
- Occasionally, symptoms are sufficiently severe to require hospital admission, which should be to a single room due to the risk of nosocomial spread. The prognosis, even when complications arise, is excellent.

## Complications

- Orchitis occurs in 20% of ♂, usually a few days after parotitis and accompanied by high fever (often >39°C). Unilateral is more common than bilateral involvement. The risk of sterility is low.
- Oophoritis in ♀ (rare).
- Meningitis (usually follows parotitis by a few days) with fever, headache, neck stiffness, and photophobia. CSF typically shows a lymphocytic picture. Where meningism is present, lumbar puncture should always be performed to exclude bacterial meningitis, even where the clinical diagnosis of mumps is clear.
- Pancreatitis is rare. Raised serum amylase is common in mumps due to the salivary gland involvement and does not signify pancreatitis in the absence of abdominal symptoms.
- Encephalitis is very rare.

## Diagnosis

- Clinical, with confirmation by serology or PCR of oral fluid.

## Treatment

- Symptomatic treatment with paracetamol and NSAID for pain.
- There is no antiviral treatment.
- There is no evidence of efficacy in prophylactic vaccination of contacts.

# Erythrovirus B19

Erythrovirus B19 infection (formerly parvovirus B19) is common in children, causing erythema infectiosum (slapped cheek disease). In adults it is rare, but can cause:

- Fever, rash, and arthritis (particularly in women), which can be mistaken for inflammatory arthritis.
- Anaemia or aplastic crisis in the immunosuppressed.
- Hydrops foetalis if infection occurs during pregnancy.

There is no specific antiviral treatment.

# Measles

Measles is a paramyxovirus. Previously rare in the UK, there has been a recent rise in cases. Worldwide, it causes ~1 million deaths annually.

## Clinical features

- Measles is highly infectious, spread via respiratory droplets, and has an incubation period of 10–14 days.
- There is an initial prodromal illness with fever, conjunctivitis, coryza, and cough lasting 2–3 days.
- Koplik's spots, considered pathognomic for measles, may be present at this time appearing as small white papules on the buccal mucosa.
- A confluent, maculopapular blanching rash follows, beginning on the face and spreading downwards. Fever settles and the rash fades over the next 3 days.
- The period of infectivity is from 5 days before to 4 days after the onset of the characteristic rash.

## Diagnosis

- Clinical, supplemented by serology or PCR of oral fluid.

## Complications

- Primary pneumonia due to measles virus can develop in the immunocompromised.
- Secondary bacterial pneumonia.
- Post-infectious encephalomyelitis.
- Subacute sclerosing panencephalitis.

## Management

- Symptomatic treatment.
- Vitamin A may help in developing countries.
- No specific antiviral therapy is available, but prophylactic vaccination or immunoglobulin can be offered to at-risk contacts.

# Rabies

Rabies is a widespread zoonotic lyssavirus causing fatal encephalitis. Transmission is by the bite of an infected animal, usually a dog, although other mammals can be infected. Rabies is not endemic in the UK so cases are either imported or very rarely acquired from bats. Rabies virus spreads from the bite retrogradely along peripheral nerves to the spinal cord and brainstem. Dissemination then occurs to skin, salivary glands, and internal organs. The median incubation period is 85 days, but can vary depending on the site of bite.

## Clinical features

- Prodrome of flu-like symptoms lasting <1 week.
- Acute neurology which can be *encephalitic* (fever, hyperactivity, salivation, seizures, pharyngeal spasm) or *paralytic* (quadriparesis and sphincter dysfunction).
- Cardiac instability may occur.
- Coma with generalized flaccid paralysis.
- Death usually occurs within 2 weeks of coma—only one case of survival has been described.

## Treatment

- There is no proven treatment.

## Prevention

- Bite avoidance.
- Pre-exposure prophylaxis with rabies vaccine to those at risk.
- Post-exposure prophylaxis in the non-immune with rabies immune globulin followed by 5 doses of vaccine. Post-exposure prophylaxis should be given as soon as possible after the bite (see Table 12.5).

# Cytomegalovirus

CMV is a common herpes virus infection that can cause serious illness in the immunocompromised, particularly in AIDS or post-transplant settings. In HIV infection, CMV disease usually occurs with CD4 counts <50 × 10⁶/L. In post-transplant patients it tends to occur 1–4 months after transplantation, at the time of greatest immunosuppression. Care should be taken not to expose CMV non-immune

| Table 12.5 Rabies post-exposure prophylaxis schedule | | |
|---|---|---|
| | Immunoglobulin | Vaccine |
| Non-immune | 20 units/kg, half around the wound, half IM* | Days 0, 3, 7, 14, 28 |
| Vaccinated | No | Days 0 and 3 |

*Vaccine and immunoglobulin should not be given in the same limb.

immunosuppressed individuals to CMV. Screening of blood products is one way of ensuring this.

### Clinical features (immuno*competent*)

- Asymptomatic infection is very common.
- Heterophile antibody-negative glandular fever is the most common clinical presentation.
- Mild transaminitis can occur during primary infection.
- Colitis occurs rarely in primary infection.
- Congenital infection if primary infection occurs during pregnancy.

### Clinical features (immuno*suppressed*)

Disease is usually due to **reactivation** of previous infection

- Retinitis usually presents with unilateral loss of vision, flashing lights, or floaters in HIV-infected patients. Progression without treatment is usual and can result in irreversible visual loss. Diagnosis is by fundoscopy (Fig. 12.13). Any patient with extraocular disease should be screened for ocular involvement.
- GI disease: any part of the GI tract can be affected, but colitis is the most common presentation.
- Neurological involvement is rare, but can present as encephalitis.
- Pneumonitis.
- Hepatitis.
- Renal graft dysfunction is common during CMV infection although this is often multifactorial.

### Diagnosis

- Serology is of limited use as most people will have evidence of previous exposure.

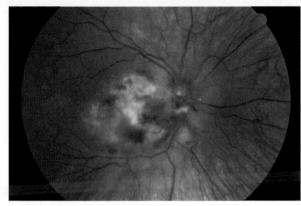

**Fig. 12.13** Fundus, photograph-CMV retinitis.
National Eye Institute, National Institutes of Health (NEI/NIH).

- Nucleic acid detection and quantification by PCR from blood, urine, or CSF.
- Histology can show characteristic owl's eyes inclusion bodies from biopsy specimens.

### Treatment

- Ganciclovir IV (5mg/kg twice daily) is the main treatment. Mild or controlled disease can be treated with oral valganciclovir (900mg twice daily). Intraocular implants can be used to treat eye involvement.
- Foscarnet and cidofovir are alternative options, but are more toxic.
- Restoring immune function is crucial (e.g. antiretroviral therapy in HIV).

# 12.13 HIV and AIDS

## Background

In 1981, small clusters of cases of *Pneumocystis jirovecii* pneumonia (PCP) and Kaposi sarcoma (KS) among otherwise healthy young gay men in California and New York led to the description of acquired immunodeficiency syndrome (AIDS). Two years later the causative agent, human immunodeficiency virus (HIV), was discovered facilitating diagnostic testing. The first antiretroviral agent, zidovudine (AZT), was introduced in 1987. It took a further 8 years for truly effective combination antiretroviral therapy (ART) to revolutionize HIV management, changing it from an inevitably fatal disease to a controllable chronic infection. The estimated life expectancy for a person newly diagnosed with HIV is now nearly 40 years in the absence of HCV co-infection. However, worldwide, only around half of those needing ART currently have access to it.

## Epidemiology

### Global

There are an estimated 34 million people living with HIV, about a tenth of them children. The annual rate of new infections stood at 2.5 million in 2011, with 1.7 million deaths. Although some African countries have achieved control over spread of infection, increasing numbers of new cases are being seen in Eastern Europe, Russia, and India.

### United Kingdom

The end of 2011 saw around 96,000 people living with HIV in the UK. 2011 saw 6280 new cases of HIV. Unlike early in the epidemic, injecting drug users contribute <1% of new cases, with heterosexual transmission now the most common route of spread. The majority of new cases originate from outside the UK, mostly acquired in sub-Saharan Africa. However, HIV-related deaths and new AIDS diagnoses have decreased substantially since 1998. The leading cause of death in HIV-infected patients in the UK is now liver failure, often as a result of HCV.

## Virology

HIV-1 is responsible for the majority of cases in the global pandemic, with HIV-2 still largely being limited to areas of West Africa. HIV-1 is an enveloped, single-stranded RNA virus (Fig. 12.14). Its genome encodes three large genes—*env, gag,* and *pol*—with several smaller genes responsible for transcriptional regulation.

The HIV membrane glycoprotein, gp120, is capable of binding to cells expressing the molecule CD4. These include helper T cells, thymocytes, monocytes, bone marrow progenitor cells, and some neural cells. Efficient binding of gp120 to CD4 is dependent on the presence of co-receptors. Two chemokine receptors, CXCR4 and CCR5, are the chief co-receptors. A polymorphism in CCR5, CCR5 delta 32, commonly found in Caucasian populations, results in absent cell-surface expression of CCR5 which protects against HIV infection.

After the virus binds to CD4, there is fusion of the viral envelope with the cell membrane, after which the HIV nucleic acid enters the cell. The reverse transcriptase enzyme converts viral RNA to DNA and the integrase enzyme allows the viral DNA to insert into the host genome. After transcription and translation, the viral proteins are cleaved into component parts by the protease enzyme. Virions assemble and bud, with a portion of the host cell membrane acting as the viral envelope.

## Pathogenesis

Within 6 weeks of initial infection, HIV induces loss of around 50% of total body CD4 T cells, most of which are resident within lymph nodes in the intestinal mucosa. Following this, there is some immune control mediated by HIV-specific T cells, manifested by a falling viral load. Despite this, however, the HIV-specific T cells are progressively lost, resulting in loss of viral control. CD4 cells are slowly depleted from the peripheral blood (Fig. 12.15). The mechanism for this is multifactorial:

- HIV inhibits T-cell generation in bone marrow and thymus.
- T cells are trapped within lymph nodes.
- Widespread immune activation induces killing of T cells.

Sufficient loss of CD4 T-cell numbers results in the susceptibility to opportunistic infections and neoplasia that characterizes AIDS. Progression to AIDS takes ~10 years on average, but can be within 2–3 years or, in a small minority of patients, >20 years, if at all. CD4 cell loss is reversible, at least in part, by treatment with an effective antiretroviral regimen.

## Diagnosis

Serological testing is technically simple, rapid, and highly accurate. Combined antibody and p24 antigen testing improves sensitivity during acute HIV infection. Standard verbal consent is required, as with any serious communicable disease. The British HIV Association (BHIVA) state that all doctors should have the knowledge and communication skills necessary for pre- and post-test counselling. Non-urgent testing can be referred to specialist counselling services, but increasingly HIV testing is seen as a routine medical test.

Following diagnosis, quantitative PCR testing is performed to give a viral load—the number of copies of viral RNA per mL of blood. The amplified nucleic acid can be used to provide information on the HIV subtype and to identify the presence of mutations which confer resistance to antiretroviral drugs

Flow cytometric analysis of peripheral blood can quantify the number of CD4 T cells, which remains the best prognostic indicator of immune function in HIV. Therapy is usually offered once the CD4 count falls to

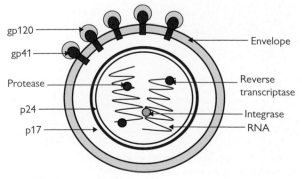

**Fig. 12.14** Structure of HIV.

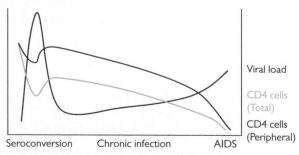

**Fig. 12.15** Natural history of HIV.

<350 × 10$^6$/L, but can be considered prior to this. CD4 counts are quite fluctuant and drop with intercurrent infection or surgery.

### Clinical scenarios

A 28-year-old Zimbabwean woman is admitted to a medical acute admissions unit following a generalized seizure preceded by 4 days of fever and headache. CT scanning shows several ring enhancing mass lesions. You are concerned about toxoplasmosis and think she should have an HIV test.

### HIV testing

HIV is a serious communicable disease and should be tested for only once informed consent has been obtained. BHIVA advises that this counselling can (and should) be performed by doctors where patients present with an illness compatible with HIV infection. Consent forms are not required. Antiretroviral treatment has revolutionized HIV treatment and prognosis is vastly improved. Accordingly, there is now a shift of emphasis to view HIV testing as similar to testing for any other serious but treatable illness in order to prevent delays in diagnosis which are currently still common.

*Pre-test counselling for HIV testing*

- Ensure privacy.
- Explain reasons for testing.
- Stress confidentiality.
- Risk factor assessment.
- Practicalities of testing—how long will it take?
- Establish patient's knowledge and beliefs of HIV.
- Prognosis.
- Follow-up plan—how will the result be delivered, who would the patient want to tell if the result was positive, is there a need for follow-up testing?
- Questions and clarifications.

*Risk factor assessment*

- Patient: IV drug use (IVDU) and sharing of needles/works, blood products, MSM (men who have sex with men), sex worker, travel abroad (especially transfusion, invasive procedures, and sexual contacts in a high prevalence area; NB: time abroad may have been 10–20 years ago).
- Patient's sexual partners: ethnicity, IVDU, MSM, sex workers.
- Ask *specific* questions as tactfully as you can. Acknowledge the difficulty of the subject to the patient and explain why taking a sexual history is necessary. Stress that information given is confidential.
- Establish *timing* of exposures. If the most recent is within the window period of 3 months, recommend follow-up testing.
- Ask about previous BBV testing and if previous results are known to them.

*Pitfalls in HIV testing*

- Fear of bringing up the subject.
- Uncertainty on how to arrange an HIV test. Ask your local lab before you speak to the patient.
- Assuming a patient is HIV negative if they have normal lymphocyte counts or disclose no risk factors.
- Not outlining how the result will be delivered.
- Some patients, particularly some Africans, might assume that any blood test will include HIV testing. If a patient reports a negative HIV test, ask for details on where it was taken and how the result was obtained.

## Clinical manifestations of HIV

**Acute HIV** typically occurs within 3 months of initial infection. It is often asymptomatic, but can present as a glandular fever-like illness with fever, sore throat, macular rash, lymphadenopathy, and sometimes GI upset, arthralgia, and mucosal ulceration. Severe forms can

| Table 12.6 Features of symptomatic HIV | |
|---|---|
| Systemic | Fever, night sweats, fatigue, lymphadenopathy |
| Gastrointestinal | Chronic diarrhoea, anorexia, weight loss, oral ulceration, angular cheilitis |
| Haematological | Any cytopenia, splenomegaly |
| Dermatological | Seborrhoea, oral hairy leucoplakia |
| Infective | Recurrent thrush, HPV, HSV, zoster, tinea, pneumonia |
| Renal | Renal impairment, proteinuria |
| Neurological | Peripheral neuropathy, cognitive impairment |
| GUM | Genital ulceration |

cause lymphocytic meningitis. Antibody tests can be negative early in infection, but p24 antigen and viral RNA testing will be positive.

**Chronic HIV:** following acute infection, an asymptomatic period ensues, often for several years. Eventually patients will become symptomatic (Table 12.6). Initially non-specific symptoms develop, such as fatigue, sweats, diarrhoea, and weight loss. Minor infections such as thrush (Fig. 12.16), shingles, or respiratory infection can occur. Most body systems can be affected and undiagnosed HIV can, therefore, be referred to any medical specialty. The presence of any suggestive features should prompt discussion of HIV testing. Over a quarter of all new diagnoses present with a CD4 count <200 × 10$^6$/L. The majority of these individuals will have presented to medical services in the year prior to diagnosis with symptoms relating to HIV. This group of late-presenters has a significantly higher mortality.

**AIDS** is a clinical diagnosis based on positive HIV serology and presence of one or more AIDS-defining illnesses (Table 12.7). Without ART, death is likely within 18 months. With successful ART, there can be immune recovery and a good prognosis.

## Management of HIV

### General aspects

A new diagnosis of HIV is a difficult time. Not only do patients have to deal with having a potentially fatal illness, but HIV remains very stigmatizing. Issues surrounding disclosure of their status to partners and family, such as isolation, fear of rejection, and loss of sex life are common.

- Give general information about HIV and its management, highlighting the good prognosis with treatment.
- Stress confidentiality, clarify who can be informed of HIV status (e.g. GP), and provide access to counselling for emotional support.
- Give information to reduce the risk of transmission by practising safe sex, not sharing needles or razors, and covering cuts.

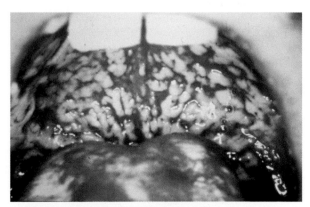

**Fig. 12.16** Acute pseudo-membranous oral candidiasis. Reproduced with permission from Dr John Doran.

| Table 12.7 AIDS-defining illnesses | |
|---|---|
| Positive HIV serology plus one of the following: | |
| Bacterial | TB, MAC, recurrent invasive pneumococcal disease |
| Viral | CMV retinitis or colitis, PML |
| Fungal | Oesophageal candidiasis, cryptococcal meningitis, PCP |
| Protozoal | Cerebral toxoplasmosis, chronic cryptosporidium |
| Neoplastic | KS, non-Hodgkin lymphoma, primary intracerebral lymphoma, invasive cervical cancer |
| Other | Wasting syndrome, dementia |

- Partner notification is essential for identifying undiagnosed cases but can be difficult.
- A full sexual health screen looking for coexistent sexually transmitted infections should be performed in most cases.
- Baseline screening for proteinuria, HBV, HCV, syphilis and, in patients from endemic areas, TB, schistosomiasis, and leishmaniasis.
- ♀ patients should be given contraceptive advice to prevent unplanned pregnancies.

## Disease prevention
- Vaccination for HAV and HBV if non-immune.
- Yearly influenza and 5-yearly pneumococcal vaccines.
- Regular screening for syphilis.
- Examination for anal intraepithelial neoplasia in at-risk men.
- Annual cervical smears for women: increased risk of cervical intraepithelial neoplasia.
- Advise on smoking cessation and alcohol moderation.

## Prevention of opportunistic infection
The risk of opportunistic infection depends on the CD4 count:
- CD4 count <200 × 10⁶/L: daily **co-trimoxazole** (e.g. 480mg once daily) for PCP prophylaxis. This is also effective toxoplasmosis prophylaxis.
- CD4 count <50 × 10⁶/L: *Mycobacterium avium* complex (MAC) prophylaxis with **azithromycin** (e.g. 1.2g weekly).

**ART** should consist of at least three drugs known to be active against the patient's virus, and should aim to achieve an undetectable viral load in blood. Currently, >20 antiretroviral drugs spanning four classes (based on mechanism of action), are available for routine clinical use:
- Nucleoside reverse transcriptase inhibitors (NRTIs): e.g. zidovudine, lamivudine, abacavir, tenofovir, emtricitabine.
- Non-nucleoside reverse transcriptase inhibitors (NNRTIs): e.g. efavirenz, nevirapine.
- Protease inhibitors (PIs): e.g. lopinavir, ritonavir, atazanavir, saquinivir, nelfinavir.
- Fusion inhibitors: e.g. enfuvirtide.

Two newer classes of drugs entering clinical practice are:
- Chemokine co-receptor antagonists (consist of two sub-classes: CCR5 and CXCR4 antagonists).
- Integrase inhibitors.

A typical regimen will include two NRTIs (also called the regimen's backbone) coupled with a PI or NNRTI. Which drugs are chosen will depend on factors such as patient comorbidity, anticipated side effects, other medication, and ease of dosing. Commonly prescribed regimens for treatment-naïve patients include: efavirenz, raltegravir, atazanavir/ritonavir or darunavir/ritonavir with a backbone of lamivudine/abacavir (Kivexa®) or emtricitabine/tenofovir (Truvada®).

Good adherence to ART is the key to good long-term outcomes. Patients must be ready to start taking medication lifelong without missing doses. ART should not be discontinued without consultation with the prescribing doctor. Planned treatment interruptions (drug holidays) are associated with increased mortality and are not advised.

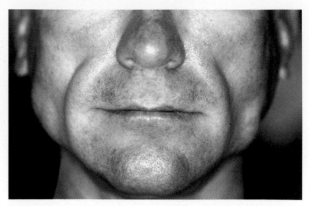

**Fig. 12.17** Facial HIV-associated lipodystrophy in a patient receiving highly active antiretroviral therapy.

Image reprinted with permission from Medscape Reference (http://emedicine.medscape.com/), 2014, available at: http://emedicine.medscape.com/article/1082199-overview

After therapy has begun, a fall in viral load will occur rapidly and an undetectable viral load should occur within 3–6 months. Rising viral loads are usually due to non-compliance, but can also be due to viral resistance or drug interactions decreasing the efficacy of the ART.

Side effects are common with all regimens. Symptoms most commonly reported include: headache, nausea, diarrhoea, malaise and fatigue. These generally settle after a few weeks.

Specific short-term side effects include anaemia (zidovudine), hepatitis or rash (nevirapine), renal impairment (tenofovir), or systemic hypersensitivity (abacavir; associated with HLA B*5701 genotype which must be tested for before commencing treatment).

Immune reconstitution inflammatory syndrome (IRIS) occurs commonly within the first months of therapy and is thought to be caused by the recovering immune system reacting against residual antigen. It can manifest in many ways, but fever, lymphadenopathy, or pulmonary infiltrates are common. Pancreatitis and lactic acidosis are rarer complications or ART which can arise at any time. Longer-term side effects include lipodystrophy (Fig. 12.17), dyslipidaemia, and impaired glucose tolerance. Patients taking protease inhibitors are at increased risk of cardiovascular (CV) disease and CV risk modification is becoming an increasingly important aspect of HIV care.

## Antiretroviral prescribing for non-specialists
Antiretroviral drugs are unfamiliar to most doctors, but small changes or omissions can lead to the development of resistance and loss of future therapeutic options. Interactions exist between ART and many commonly prescribed drugs (e.g. PPIs, statins). If you admit a patient who takes ART:
- Ensure the names, doses, and frequencies of drugs are correct.
- Ensure no doses are missed.
- Check for interactions before giving new drugs.
- Notify the prescribing doctor of the admission and if any changes or cessation of therapy are being considered.
- If in doubt, check with your pharmacist or the patient's HIV treatment team.

## Clinical lessons
- Consider acute HIV in any patient with a monospot negative glandular fever-like illness or lymphocytic meningitis where no other cause is established.
- Do not use a lack of disclosed risk factors or a normal lymphocyte count as a surrogate for HIV testing.
- Any patient with unexplained symptoms of HIV (as detailed in Tables 12.6 and 12.7) should be offered HIV testing.
- Any patient in a high-risk group should be offered testing regardless of symptoms.

## Opportunistic infection

There are many opportunistic infections which have been described due to HIV. All are becoming rarer now due to the availability of ART, but the following are some which are still seen as new presentations of HIV.

**PCP** caused by the fungus *Pneumocystis jirovecii* (previously termed *Pneumocystis carinii*), is the most common AIDS-defining illness in the UK. It typically presents as a subacute illness with progressive exertional breathlessness over weeks to months. It is often accompanied by a non-productive cough and fever. Asthma and interstitial lung disease are the most common misdiagnoses, but features of advanced immunosuppression (such as seborrhoea, oral hairy leucoplakia, weight loss, and oral candida) are usually present with PCP. Chest examination and CXR can be normal early in the disease. Desaturation on exercise is the earliest objective sign. Hypoxia and tachypnoea at rest then develop and increased interstitial lung markings become visible on CXR (Fig. 12.18). The presence of a pleural effusion is unusual in PCP and suggests an alternative pathology. Severe PCP is defined by $PaO_2$ <8kPa breathing room air (see Table 12.8).

Diagnosis is by immunofluorescence or PCR of induced sputum.

Treatment of mild disease can be managed as an outpatient with high-dose oral **co-trimoxazole**, but moderate or severe disease should be managed as an inpatient with **steroids** (e.g. 40mg prednisolone twice daily) and IV co-trimoxazole (30mg/kg four times daily). Co-trimoxazole can be associated with side effects ranging from mild allergic reactions to significant, life-threatening events such as Stevens–Johnson syndrome, myelosuppression, and severe liver damage. Despite appropriate treatment, deterioration can be seen and close observation in a high dependency environment is often needed, in case ventilatory support is required. Treatment with co-trimoxazole and steroids is given for 21 days.

**Toxoplasmosis** is the most common neurological opportunistic infection and is caused by the protozoan *Toxoplasma gondii*. Headache, fever, and focal neurological signs or seizures are the usual presenting features, with multiple ring enhancing lesions seen on brain CT or MRI (Fig. 12.19). These resolve quickly with treatment (**sulphadiazine** and **pyrimethamine** with folate supplementation). Brain biopsy would usually only be considered if the lesions fail to respond to 2 weeks of treatment. Steroids should be given if there is oedema or mass effect. Diagnosis is supported by positive serological tests and PCR of CSF or biopsy specimens.

**Cryptococcal meningitis** is the commonest form of meningitis in AIDS. Caused by the fungus *Cryptococcus neoformans*, it presents with fever and headache. Neck stiffness can be absent. CSF protein and cell count can be elevated with a low glucose, but normal CSF appearances are not unusual. A definitive diagnosis can be made by identifying fungi on an India ink stain of CSF, from antigen testing on blood or CSF, or from CSF culture. Treatment is with **amphotericin** and **flucytosine** (**5-FC**) initially, but can be stepped down to an oral azole (e.g. **fluconazole**).

**Progressive multifocal leucoencephalopathy (PML)** is a demyelinating disease of the brain caused by JC virus. It is uniformly fatal without ART. Presentation is usually subacute with either focal neurological signs or more subtle changes in cognitive function. MRI appearances consist of diffuse, often confluent, increased signal in white matter which is non-enhancing and not associated with oedema (Fig. 12.20). The presence of JC virus in CSF is found in many, but not all, cases. The only proven treatment is **ART**.

**MAC** is rare with CD4 counts >100 × $10^6$/L. Presentation is non-specific with fever, sweats, weight loss, anaemia, hepatosplenomegaly, and diarrhoea. Mediastinal and mesenteric lymphadenopathy can be seen. Diagnosis is by culture from blood, lymph node, bone marrow aspirate, or biopsy specimen. Treatment is usually with three drugs selected from **rifabutin**, **ciprofloxacin**, **azithromycin**, and **ethambutol**.

**Oesophageal candidiasis** causes odynophagia, often with evidence of oral candidiasis (Fig. 12.16). Endoscopy is the definitive investigation but is usually performed only if no improvement is seen with empirical oral **fluconazole**.

**CMV** can cause oesophagitis, colitis, retinitis, and adrenalitis, although pneumonitis is rarer in HIV than other setting of immunosuppression. Retinitis is the most feared complication which can result in visual impairment and blindness (see Fig. 12.13).

| Table 12.8 Severity criteria for PCP | | | |
|---|---|---|---|
| | PaO$_2$(kPa, air) | Treatment | Steroids |
| Mild | >11 | Oral | No |
| Moderate | 8–11 | IV | Yes |
| Severe | < 8 | IV | Yes |

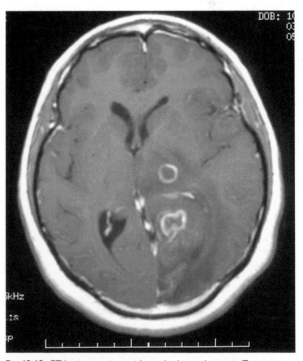

**Fig. 12.19** CT brain in patient with cerebral toxoplasmosis. Two ring-enhancing space-occupying lesions are present with significant oedema, pressure effect, and midline shift.

Reproduced with permission from Dr Andrew Seaton.

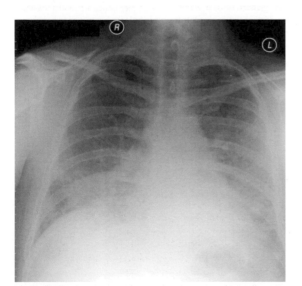

**Fig. 12.18** CXR demonstrating bilateral interstitial opacification in severe PCP infection.

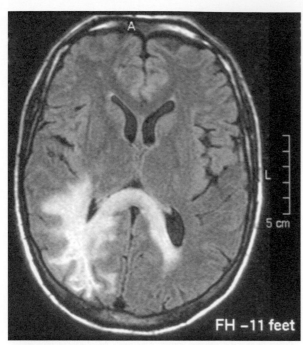

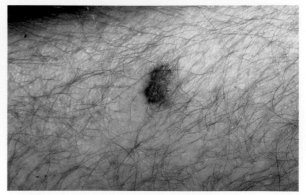

**Fig. 12.21** Kaposi sarcoma lesion.
Reproduced with permission from Dr Andrew Seaton.

**Fig. 12.20** MRI of PML showing high signal intensity in the occipital white matter and corpus callosum.

## Opportunistic neoplasia

**Kaposi sarcoma** is caused by KS herpes virus (or HHV-8) and is more common in homosexual men. It can affect skin, mucosa, or internal organs (often lung or GI tract). Skin lesions can present as plaques or nodules and are purplish in colour (Fig. 12.21). Treatment is with **PI**-based ART.

**Lymphoma** is more common in advanced HIV, particularly non-Hodgkin B-cell lymphoma. Extranodal presentations are common, and lymphoma should be considered in any patient with weight loss, fever, night sweats, and anaemia, where no infective cause has been identified. Two unusual types of lymphoma are seen in advanced HIV: primary effusion lymphoma and multicentric Castleman disease. Prognosis of HIV-associated lymphoma has improved greatly but is generally poorer than that of non-HIV-associated lymphoma.

## Co-infections

**Hepatitis C** co-infection with HIV is common, and progresses more rapidly. Early treatment with 48 weeks of **interferon** and **ribavirin** (regardless of HCV genotype) should be given if possible. Decompensated liver disease is now the leading cause of death in HIV-infected UK patients.

**Hepatitis B** co-infection is less common than HCV in the UK. Antiretroviral agents with anti-HBV activity (such as **lamivudine**, **emtricitabine**, and **tenofovir**) can be used as part of combination ART.

**Tuberculosis:** where possible, ART should be deferred until after completion of anti-tuberculous therapy to avoid drug interactions, superimposed drug toxicities, and the risk of immune reconstitution syndrome. However at very low CD4 counts, delaying HIV therapy is not always possible.

## HIV in pregnancy

Many areas in the UK now offer HIV testing to all pregnant women to prevent vertical transmission of infection. ART is the most effective way to prevent mother-to-child transmission (MTCT). Avoiding breastfeeding is another factor and, if the mother has a significant viral load, a caesarean section may be considered to avoid MTCT at the time of delivery. If the woman has an undetectable viral load at delivery the chance of transmission to the child is <1%, even with a normal vaginal delivery. Although transfer of maternal antibody for up to 18 months makes antibody testing unreliable, detection of viral DNA in neonatal lymphocytes by PCR enables accurate diagnosis even in young infants and babies.

# 12.14 Bacterial infections

## Background

**Bacteria** are unicellular, prokaryotic organisms, mostly a few microns in size. They are classified primarily by morphology and Gram staining (Table 12.9). Genetic techniques for classification, such as phylogenetic analysis of 16S ribosomal RNA, are becoming more widely used.

## Structure

Bacterial genetic information is stored as DNA in a single, coiled chromosome (1–30Mbp in most bacteria) with no surrounding nuclear membrane. Smaller, transferable genetic elements called plasmids can exist in the cytoplasm. Bacteria have no organelles such as mitochondria, and all metabolic and energy generating processes take place in the cytoplasm. The cell wall, which differs in Gram-positive and -negative bacteria, encloses the cytoplasm. Some bacteria possess flagellae, allowing movement along chemical gradients (chemotaxis).

- Gram-*positive* bacteria have a two- or three-layered cell wall comprising of a cytoplasmic membrane, a layer of peptidoglycan, and, in some bacteria, an outer capsule. The cell wall is rich in teichoic acid, a major antigenic molecule in many Gram-positive bacteria.
- Gram-*negative* bacteria have more complex cell walls with an inner and outer cell membrane enclosing a periplasmic space containing a thin layer of peptidoglycan. Lipopolysaccharide (LPS or endotoxin) is the most characteristic molecule in the Gram-negative cell wall. Very small amounts are capable of triggering the sepsis cascade.

## Growth

Most bacteria are capable of rapid independent cell division. This can occur as rapidly as every 20 minutes under optimal conditions. Three forms of growth are seen *in vitro*:

1. Colony formation: bacteria grow as clumps on solid media.
2. Suspension: bacteria grow as a suspension in liquid media.
3. Biofilm: a thin layer of bacteria forms on a surface. Biofilms can form *in vivo* on prosthetic material and can be extremely difficult to eradicate.

Certain bacteria (mostly in the *Clostridium* and *Bacillus* genera) are able to generate spores—highly resistant forms that can survive in a dormant state for months or even years. They are more difficult to eradicate with standard cleaning techniques.

Some bacteria lack typical cell walls and stain poorly by standard methods.

- **Mycoplasma**: the smallest free-living organisms capable of independent growth.
- **Chlamydia**: small, obligate intracellular organisms that have no peptidoglycan in their cell wall. They are unable to produce ATP. They have an infective extracellular form (elementary body) and an intracellular form capable of cell division (reticulate body).
- **Rickettsia:** small, obligate intracellular organisms that are metabolically deficient and can only replicate intracellularly, typically in endothelial cells.

## *Staphylococcus*

Staphylococci are commonly encountered in primary care and hospital practice. They are Gram-positive cocci which form clusters in culture and are further differentiated from streptococci by the production of catalase (an enzyme converting hydrogen peroxide to water and oxygen). *Staphylococcus aureus* produces a coagulase enzyme that distinguishes it from the relatively non-pathogenic coagulase-negative staphylococci (CoNS).

### Staphylococcus aureus

*Staphylococcus aureus* is highly pathogenic with the potential to produce an array of toxins including exotoxin, leucocidin, exfoliative toxin, enterotoxins, and toxic shock syndrome (TSS) toxin. It can cause both minor infection and devastating sepsis in previously well individuals. Asymptomatic nasal carriage occurs in around 50% of people. *S. aureus* resistant to flucloxacillin (MRSA) is becoming an increasing problem worldwide.

### Clinical manifestations

These range from trivial, self-limiting infections to life-threatening and complex presentations:

**Table 12.9 Classification of bacteria with selective examples**

| Gram-Positive | |
| --- | --- |
| **Cocci** | **Bacilli** |
| Staphylococci<br>  S. aureus<br>  S. epidermidis<br>  S. capitis | Corynebacterium<br>  C. diphtheriae |
| | Listeria<br>  L. monocytogenes |
| Streptococci<br>  S. pyogenes<br>  S. agalactiae<br>  S. pneumoniae<br>  S. milleri | Clostridium<br>  C. tetani<br>  C. botulinum<br>  C. perfringens<br>  C. difficile |
| Enterococci<br>  E. faecalis<br>  E. faecium | Bacillus<br>  B. anthracis<br>  B. cereus |
| | Actinomyces |
| | Nocardia |
| **Gram-Negative** | |
| **Cocci** | **Bacilli** |
| Neisseria<br>  N. meningitidis<br>  N. gonorrhoeae | Enterobacteria<br>  Escherichia coli<br>  Klebsiella pneumoniae<br>  Salmonella typhi<br>  Shigella flexneri<br>  Proteus mirabilis<br>  Yersinia pestis<br>  Enterobacter sp |
| Moraxella<br>  M. cattarhalis | |
| | Pseudomonas<br>  P. aeruginosa |
| | Acinetobacter<br>  A. baumanii |
| | Bacteroides<br>  B. fragilis |
| | Campylobacter<br>  C. jejuni |
| | Bordatella<br>  B. pertussis |
| | Pasteurella<br>  P. multicida |
| | Vibrio<br>  V. cholera |
| | Yersinia<br>  Y. pestis |
| | Helicobacter<br>  H. pylori |
| | Haemophilus<br>  H. influenzae<br>  H. ducreyi |
| | Brucella sp |

- **Food poisoning**:
  - Caused by enterotoxin-producing strains.
  - Vomiting and diarrhoea (30 minutes to a few hours after ingestion).
- **Skin and soft-tissue infection**.
- **Abscesses**.
- **Cannulae and central venous catheter infection**.
- **Bone and joint infection**.
- **Bacteraemia**: sepsis with no localizing signs is a common presentation. The mortality is around 20% and roughly 20% will have metastatic complications. There were around 10,000 episodes of *S. aureus* bacteraemia (SAB) annually in England in 2011.
- **Pneumonia**: *S. aureus* tends to cause cavitating pneumonia. Classically, it develops following influenza. It can also cause hospital-acquired pneumonia.
- **Endocarditis**
- **Toxic shock syndrome** (TSS) is a severe multisystem illness caused by a TSS-toxin producing *Staph. aureus* (see Box 12.4). The two main risk groups are menstrual (particularly with use of highly-absorbent tampons) and post-surgical. The diagnosis is clinical. Treatment is predominantly supportive, but the source of infection should be removed and **flucloxacillin** with **clindamycin** (to prevent toxin production) given. Intravenous immunoglobulin (IVIG) may also be effective.

*Treatment*
Flucloxacillin is the most effective treatment for MSSA infection. Macrolides or clindamycin can be used in penicillin allergic patients, although resistance sometime occurs in both MSSA and MRSA. Several agents are now available for severe MRSA infection: vancomycin, linezolid, daptomycin, and tigecycline. Management of bacteraemia requires an appropriate duration of effective therapy (usually at least 14 days), identification of a source of infection (such as endocarditis and bone/joint infection), and removal of potentially infected material.

*Management of Staphylococcus aureus bacteraemia*
- Give effective IV antibiotics for an appropriate duration (usually at least 14 days).
- Remove the source of infection.
- Investigate for deep-seated infection (e.g. endocarditis, discitis, osteomyelitis, infected prostheses or vascular grafts).
- Persistent fever or positive blood cultures 72 hours after starting appropriate treatment suggests metastatic infection or endocarditis.
- Patients with prosthetic material (vascular grafts, prosthetic heart valves or joints) will usually need >14 days of antimicrobial therapy.
- Injecting drug users with bacteraemia and DVT may need >14 days of antibiotics.

---

### Box 12.4 Staphylococcal toxic shock syndrome*

- Fever >38.9°C.
- Systolic BP <90mmHg, postural hypotension.
- Rash: diffuse macular erythema with desquamation at 1–2 weeks, particularly on the palms and soles.
- Three or more of:
  - Vomiting or diarrhoea.
  - Severe myalgia or elevated creatine kinase.
  - Serum creatinine >2× normal.
  - Bilirubin or transaminases >2× normal.
  - Platelets <100 × 10$^9$/L.
  - Altered conscious level.

*CDC diagnostic criteria for epidemiological purposes. Cases where most, but not all features are present should be treated as potential staphylococcal TSS.

---

*Clinical lessons*
- Never assume *Staphylococcus aureus* in blood cultures is a contaminant.
- Bone and joint infection complicating SAB can often present with trivial symptoms that improve with antibiotic therapy. Any new musculoskeletal pain at presentation or during therapy should prompt imaging of the affected area.
- Flucloxacillin is the most effective drug for MSSA infection. Give large doses for severe infections (i.e. 2g four times daily).

### Coagulase-negative staphylococci
Coagulase-negative staphylococci are skin commensals and common contaminants of improperly taken blood cultures. They have a low pathogenicity and tend to cause infections only in immunocompromised hosts where they can cause bacteraemia, infection of prosthetic material and, rarely, endocarditis. Many are resistant to flucloxacillin.

## Streptococci

Streptococci are Gram-positive cocci which form chains and can be distinguished from staphylococci by lack of catalase production. Streptococci are classified by their ability to cause haemolysis of blood agar and by Lancefield groups—a serological classification based on differences in cell wall composition. See Table 12.10.

### *Streptococcus pyogenes*
*Streptococcus pyogenes* (or Group A strep) can cause a range of infections from self-limiting to life-threatening. It is highly sensitive to penicillin which remains the antibiotic of choice. Diagnosis can be assisted by a positive or rising anti-streptolysin (ASO) titre.

### Clinical manifestations
- **Pharyngitis** (strep throat) is common and typically causes unilateral, painful, purulent tonsillitis without cough. It can cause a severe febrile illness with high WCC. Treatment should be for 10 days to prevent post-streptococcal disease.
- **Cellulitis** is also common and typically causes a more demarcated erythema than staphylococcal infection. Erysipelas is a well-demarcated facial cellulitis with a raised edge (Fig. 12.22).
- **Scarlet fever** is characterized by an extensive, fine, blanching macular rash (Fig. 12.23), sometime with an erythematous tongue (strawberry tongue, Fig. 12.24).
- **Bacteraemia** is rare but carries a high mortality rate
- **Streptococcal TSS** is a life-threatening infection caused by streptococcal TSS-toxin producing *Streptococcus pyogenes* (see Box 12.5). It can occur at any age and in previously healthy individuals, presenting as shock, often with fever, preceding flu-like symptoms and pain. It may be associated with necrotizing fasciitis. Diagnosis is clinical. The treatment strategy is threefold: good supportive care, exploration, and debridement of necrotic tissue and antimicrobials. Surgical treatment of necrotizing fasciitis is essential. **Penicillin** and **clindamycin** is the most effective antimicrobial combination. **IVIG** (1mg/kg on day 1 and 0.5mg/kg on days 2 + 3) may also be effective.

### Table 12.10 Classification of common streptococci

| Name | Group | Haemolysis | Commensal |
|---|---|---|---|
| S. pyogenes | A | Beta | Skin, throat |
| S. agalactiae | B | Beta | Vagina |
| S. bovis | D | None | Colon |
| Viridans strep. | None | None/alpha | Mouth |
| S. pneumoniae | None | Alpha | Throat |

Alpha haemolysis is partial haemolysis (often producing a greenish halo around the colony), beta haemolysis is complete clearing of agar around the colony.

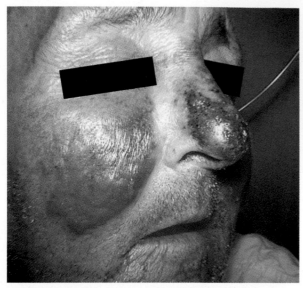

**Fig. 12.22** Erysipelas.

CDC/ Dr. Thomas F. Sellers/ Emory University. This image is in the public domain. (http://phil.cdc.gov/phil/details.asp?pid=2874)

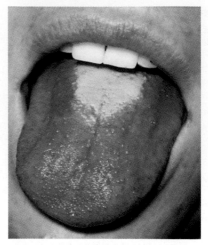

**Fig. 12.24** Scarlet fever.

Foto von Martin Kronawitter, Kellberg. This image is licensed under the Creative Commons Attribution-Share Alike 2.5 Generic (//creativecommons.org/licenses/by-sa/2.5/deed.en) license. (http://en.wikipedia.org/wiki/File:Scharlach.JPG).

**Post-streptococcal disease** is rare and results from infection with specific strains of *Streptococcus pyogenes*:

- **Rheumatic fever** usually occurs 2–4 weeks after pharyngeal infection. The Jones diagnostic criteria describe five major features:
  - Migratory large joint arthritis
  - Carditis
  - Chorea
  - Subcutaneous nodules
  - Erythema marginatum.
- Usually self-limiting, it can cause chronic valvulopathy, particularly mitral stenosis.
- **Glomerulonephritis** is caused by several strains, such as type 12 and 49. It is more common in children. Presentation can vary from microscopic haematuria to nephritic syndrome. Prognosis is usually good.

### Streptococcus pneumoniae

*Streptococcus pneumoniae* (or pneumococcus) is an alpha haemolytic streptococcus that classically grows in pairs (diplococci). There are >80 different types. It commonly causes pneumonia, and can also cause bacteraemia, meningitis, and endocarditis.

### Streptococcus agalactiae

*Streptococcus agalactiae* (or Group B strep) is a leading cause of puerperal sepsis or neonatal infection. In non-pregnant adults it is an uncommon cause of bacteraemia and endocarditis.

### Other streptococci

**Group C and G streptococci** are similar to group A streptococci and are occasional causes of cellulitis or bacteraemia.

**Viridans streptococci** are a variety of alpha haemolytic oral flora that can cause endocarditis, often after dental work.

## Enterococcus

Enterococci are bowel commensals that can cause urinary infection, biliary sepsis, bacteraemia, endocarditis, and line infection. *E. faecalis* and the more resistant *E. faecium* are the most common pathogens. They are inherently resistant to cephalosporins and can easily acquire resistance to a range of antibiotics, including vancomycin (VRE, see Section 12.6).

## Meningococcal disease

Meningococcal disease is due to *Neisseria meningitidis* which causes meningitis and septicaemia. It can be rapidly fatal and requires urgent assessment and treatment if suspected (See Section 14.18).

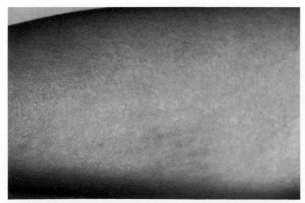

**Fig. 12.23** This patient revealed a scarlet fever rash on the volar surface of the forearm due to group A *Streptococcus* bacteria (magnified on lower image).

CDC. This image is in the public domain. http://phil.cdc.gov/phil/details.asp (image no: 5163).

| Box 12.5 Streptococcal toxic shock syndrome |
| --- |
| • Isolation of group A streptococci* **plus** |
| • Systolic BP <90mmHg. |
| • With two or more of: |
|   • ARDS. |
|   • Coagulopathy. |
|   • Serum creatinine >2× normal. |
|   • Bilirubin or transaminases >2× normal. |
|   • Macular rash. |
|   • Soft tissue necrosis. |
| *Blood cultures will be positive in ~60%. |

# Gonococcal infection

*Neisseria gonorrhoeae* is a Gram-negative diplococcus, usually spread sexually. Its incidence is increasing in the UK.

## Clinical manifestations

- ♂: 90% are symptomatic, usually with urethritis or epididymitis.
- ♀: infection is often asymptomatic. Vaginal discharge and urethritis are the most common symptoms. Pelvic inflammatory disease can occur.
- **Proctitis** and **pharyngitis** can be present in either sex following anal or oral intercourse.
- **Disseminated infection** is rare, and can present with fever, tenosynovitis, a purulent oligoarthritis, and painless papular rash. Not all features need be present.

## Diagnosis

Diagnosis is by urethral or cervical swab for microscopy and culture. Nucleic acid testing by PCR is also possible. Rectal and throat swabs should be taken if indicated. Gonococcus is a fastidious organism and direct plating or use of transport medium should be used to increase the chance of successful culture.

## Treatment

Treatment with **cefixime**, **ceftriaxone**, or **spectinomycin** is recommended. Significant resistance is seen: penicillin (11%), ciprofloxacin (15%), doxycycline (44%). Abstinence from sexual activity for 2 weeks followed by a test of cure, treatment of current partners, and contact tracing is vital for prevention of further spread. Affected patients should have a full sexual health screen.

UK guidelines on management of gonococcal infection can be found at the British Association for Sexual Health and HIC website: <http://www.bashh.org>.

# Pseudomonas aeruginosa

*Pseudomonas aeruginosa* is a common cause of hospital-acquired infection, usually in the immunosuppressed. It possesses a huge diversity of virulence factors and is resistant to many commonly used antibacterial drugs.

## Clinical manifestations

- Hospital-acquired pneumonia.
- Respiratory infection in chronic lung diseases, particularly cystic fibrosis and bronchiectasis.
- Urinary infection (often catheter-related).
- Skin and soft tissue infection (uncommon).
- Bacteraemia (particularly in neutropaenic patients).
- Necrotizing otitis externa.

## Treatment

- In severe infection, treatment with two agents is usually advised.
- **Ciprofloxacin** is the only oral agent available.
- Piperacillin (often given with tazobactam as **Tazocin®**), ceftazidime, meropenem, and aminoglycosides (e.g. gentamicin) are the other active agents.

# Brucellosis

Brucellosis is a zoonotic infection caused by a Gram-negative coccobacillus. The disease is not present in the UK, but endemic in the Middle East, southern Mediterranean, Indian subcontinent, and Latin America. Four species cause infection, *Brucella melitensis* being the most common. Transmission is by ingestion of contaminated unpasteurized milk or cheese, contact with infected animals (vets, farmers, abattoir workers), or exposure in laboratory staff.

## Clinical features

- A subacute febrile illness with sweats, fatigue, anorexia, joint pains, and weight loss. Objective findings other than fever are uncommon.
- Complications include sacroiliitis, epididymo-orchitis, endocarditis, hepatic or splenic abscess, and meningitis.

## Diagnosis

- Culture of blood, bone marrow, or liver biopsy. Cultured *Brucella* is highly infectious and potentially dangerous to lab staff. The microbiology lab should be notified if *Brucella* is suspected clinically.
- Serology.

## Treatment

- **Doxycycline** and **rifampicin** for 6 weeks, or doxycycline for 6 weeks with an aminoglycoside during the first 2–3 weeks

# Bartonella

*Bartonella*, a fastidious Gram-negative bacillus, can cause:

- Cat-scratch disease *(Bartonella henselae)*: presenting as an initial papule at the scratch site with regional lymphadenopathy developing over the next 2 weeks, and persisting for a few months. Dissemination to other organs sometimes occurs. The disease is typically self-limiting.
- Trench fever *(Bartonella quintata)*: a louse-borne infection causing a relapsing febrile illness.
- Endocarditis, often culture-negative, due to *Bartonella henselae* or *Bartonella quintata*. Diagnosis is by serology and treatment with **doxycycline** and **gentamicin** is one suggested regimen.

# Diphtheria

Diphtheria, caused by *Corynebacterium diphtheriae*, a Gram-positive rod with characteristic 'Chinese letter' morphology, is now extremely rare in the UK thanks to the childhood vaccination programme. It is still seen in Eastern Europe, Africa, and Asia.

## Clinical features

- Respiratory disease is most common with a sore throat, cervical lymphadenopathy, and low-grade fever. Grey or white exudates form over the tonsils, merging to form a pseudomembrane. Upper airway obstruction can result.
- Production of diphtheria toxin can cause myocarditis, acute kidney injury, or peripheral neuropathy.

## Diagnosis

- Special media are required for culture. The microbiology lab must be notified if diphtheria is suspected.
- Toxin can be detected but requires specialist testing.

## Treatment

- Prompt administration of diphtheria **antitoxin**.
- Penicillin or erythromycin kills diphtheria but will not prevent disease due to toxin already released.
- Respiratory isolation in hospital and contact tracing are crucial

# Listeria

*Listeria monocytogenes* is a cause of bacteraemia or meningitis, usually in the immunocompromised host. Common risk factors for listeriosis are old age, pregnancy, and underlying neoplasia. Consumption of soft cheeses and pates are the main route of transmission.

# Fusobacterium

*Fusobacterium necrophorum* is an anaerobic constituent of oral flora. It can cause severe parapharyngeal infection and bacteraemia. These two features coupled with jugular vein thrombosis and metastatic spread of infection (commonly to the lungs) is a tetrad known as Lemierre syndrome. The infection is frequently polymicrobial, and treatment should include good anaerobic cover with metronidazole or clindamycin.

## Leptospirosis

Leptospirosis is a zoonotic infection caused by *Leptospira interrogans*. Although found worldwide, the highest prevalence is in tropical countries. Leptospirosis is found in swine, cattle, or dogs, but rodents are the principal carriers. Transmission is by ingestion of leptospirae shed in animal urine, which can survive in water and soil for weeks. Direct invasion through mucosal membranes or skin breaches may also occur. Those most at risk in the UK include sewage workers and participants in water sports.

### Clinical features

- After an incubation period of 7–14 days, a non-specific illness with fever, headache, and myalgia is the most typical presentation. Conjunctival suffusion may be present, a finding unusual in other infectious diseases.
- Laboratory tests reveal non-specific findings, although raised WCC, low platelet count, deranged clotting and liver function tests, and elevated creatine kinase are often seen. A sterile pyuria is common.
- Biphasic illness occurs in <50% of cases, with a recurrence of symptoms thought to be caused by the host immune response. The second phase is characterized by features of aseptic meningitis: severe headache and CSF pleocytosis. Many infections are subclinical or unrecognized, but more severe forms occur and their manifestation depends on the serovar of *Leptospira interrogans* involved. The most severe is Weil disease (caused by serovar icterohaemorrhagiae) which causes both jaundice and acute renal failure. Multiorgan failure can occur and the mortality rate is ~50% in patients who require admission to intensive care.

### Diagnosis

- Leptospira can occasionally be identified from blood or urine by dark field microscopy.
- Most diagnoses are made retrospectively with serology.
- *Leptospira interrogans* can be cultured from blood, urine, or CSF, although special growth medium is required and the lab must be notified if leptospirosis is suspected. Growth *in vitro* is slow, taking 1–2 weeks.

### Treatment

- Oral **doxycycline** is suitable treatment for mild disease.
- Parenteral treatment with **penicillin**, ceftriaxone, or doxycycline is reasonable for severe disease, although there is limited evidence that they reduce mortality.
- Weekly doxycycline 200mg is effective at preventing infection in those at high risk.

## Lyme disease

Lyme disease is a tick-borne infection caused by *Borrelia burgdorferi*, first identified in Lyme, Connecticut, USA, in the 1970s. It is very prevalent in many areas of the USA and continental Europe, but can also be found in the UK particularly around the New Forest and the Scottish Highlands. In the UK, deer and mice are the primary reservoir with the hard tick *Ixodes ricinus* acting as the main vector. Ticks attached for <48 hours are not likely to transmit infection. Prevention is achieved by covering skin appropriately, using a DEET-based insect repellent and rigorous checking for and early removal of attached ticks. In areas of very high prevalence, such as New England, a single dose of doxycycline is recommended for ticks definitely attached for >48 hours. Use of doxycycline prophylaxis is not recommended in the UK. Transmission usually occurs in the summer and early autumn among farmers, forestry workers, and hikers.

### Clinical features

#### Early localized

Erythema chronicum migrans (ECM) is the hallmark lesion but atypical variants can also be seen (Fig. 12.25). ECM begins as a red macule at the site of tick attachment and expands outward. Central sparing to form a ring-like lesion can occur, but not universally. ECM is usually

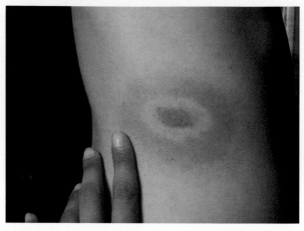

**Fig. 12.25** Erythematous rash in the pattern of a "bull's-eye" from Lyme disease.

From Wikimedia Commons/Hannah Garrison/Original uploader was Jongarrison at en.wikipedia. This image is licensed under the Creative Commons Attribution-Share Alike 2.5 Generic (//creativecommons.org/licenses/by-sa/2.5/deed.en) license. (http://commons.wikimedia.org/wiki/File:Bullseye_Lyme_Disease_Rash.jpg)

found at sites where ticks commonly attach, such as the axillae, groins, or behind the knees. ECM can be accompanied by fever, malaise, myalgia, and headache. Diagnosis of early localized disease is clinical. Serology may remain negative with early treatment. Treatment is with doxycycline 100mg twice daily for 10–21 days, or amoxicillin 500mg three times daily, or cefuroxime 500mg twice daily for 14–21 days.

#### Early disseminated

Lyme disease can occur within 1–2 months after initial infection, although even later presentations can be seen. The risk of dissemination is increased if early local disease is not treated. There are three forms:

- **Musculoskeletal** (60–70%): migratory arthralgia or arthritis, typically a recurring monoarthritis or asymmetrical oligoarthritis. Knees are the most commonly affected joint.
- **Neurological** (10–15%): manifested most commonly by facial nerve palsy, but also by aseptic meningitis, cranial nerve defects, radiculopathy, or polyneuropathy. Neurological involvement is more common in Europe than in the USA.
- **Cardiovascular** (1–4%): conduction deficits, myocarditis, or pericarditis. Rates of 5–10% are seen in the USA. Symptomatic patients and those with high-degree AV block should be managed in hospital. Spontaneous resolution is the norm.

Diagnosis is by positive serology plus a compatible clinical presentation. Synovial fluid should be analysed to establish a diagnosis of Lyme arthritis. Lumbar puncture is required in any patients with neurological involvement to confirm a diagnosis of neuroborreliosis by identifying anti-borrelial antibodies within CSF.

#### Treatment

- Arthritis: 28 days of oral **doxycycline** or **amoxicillin**.
- Mild carditis/unilateral facial palsy (no abnormalities on CSF examination): 14–21 days of doxycycline or amoxicillin.
- All other neurological abnormalities, severe carditis, or ongoing arthritis despite oral treatment: 3-4 weeks of **ceftriaxone**.

#### Late

Lyme disease can present with arthritis and neurological abnormalities months to years after initial exposure and earlier features may not have been present. Seroprevalence in the general population is 3–5% so the presence of positive Lyme serology does not in itself indicate chronic disease. A diagnosis of chronic Lyme disease should incorporate positive serology with confirmatory diagnostic techniques such as western blotting or PCR and a compatible clinical syndrome of objective neurological disease or synovitis. Treatment of chronic neurological disease is with ceftriaxone 2g once daily for 28 days. Doxycycline can be used where disease is musculoskeletal only.

### Post-Lyme syndromes
Chronic symptoms of arthralgia, fibromyalgia, fatigue, or non-specific neurological symptoms are common after Lyme disease or in the presence of positive Lyme serology with no objective arthritis or neurological signs. This is often a difficult scenario for both patients and their doctors, but there is little evidence that antibiotic therapy improves these symptoms. Prolonged antimicrobial treatment can result in significant unnecessary toxicity.

The Infectious Diseases Society of America (IDSA) have published guidelines on the management of Lyme disease: <http://www.cdc. gov/ncidod/dvbid/lyme/IDSA2000.pdf>.

## Syphilis

Syphilis is a chronic multisystem disease caused by *Treponema pallidum*. The incidence in the UK has increased 12-fold since 2000, mostly among MSM, with around 3000 cases annually. Transmission is primarily sexual but can also be transmitted vertically or, very rarely, via blood products. The incubation period is 10–28 days with early syphilis being highly infectious. *Early* disease occurs within 2 years of infection and is defined as primary, secondary, and early latent syphilis. *Late* disease (more than 2 years' duration) is defined as tertiary, quaternary, and late latent syphilis.

- **Latent**: presence of positive serology with no clinical evidence of disease.
- **Primary**: typically a single painless ulcer with a rounded edge and clean base usually located on the glans penis in men, vulva or cervix in women, but can also be on oral or rectal mucosa. It is associated with regional painless lymphadenopathy which heals without scarring within 2 months. It may go unnoticed by the patient.
- **Secondary:** characterized by systemic upset with fever, malaise, and rash occurring weeks to months after initial infection in a quarter of untreated patients. The rash is maculopapular, non-itchy, and affects the whole body including palms and soles (Fig. 12.26). Other features include patchy alopecia, 'snail-track' ulcers on mucosa, or condylomata lata in the perianal area. Painless generalized lymphadenopathy occurs in 50%, with anterior uveitis, hepatitis, or glomerulonephritis occurring more rarely.
- **Tertiary** syphilis occurs ≥2 years after infection and affects skin, mucous membranes, or bone by forming gumma causing skin ulcers, destructive mucosal lesions, or periostitis respectively.
- **Quaternary** syphilis will occur in 10% of untreated patients and affects the cardiovascular or neurological systems. Cardiovascular disease is chiefly an aortitis affecting the ascending portion and arch of the aorta causing aneurysm or aortic incompetence. Neurological disease is classified into meningovascular (aseptic meningitis, cranial nerve palsies, hemiplegia), parenchymatous (cognitive impairment, tremor, seizures, Argyll Robertson pupils) and tabes dorsalis (lightning pains, sensory loss, hypotonia, areflexia, neuropathic ulcers, Charcot joints, and bladder dysfunction).

### Diagnosis
Diagnosis can be made by dark field microscopy in primary infection, but most cases are identified by serology. *Treponema pallidum* cannot be cultured. Serological tests fall into two groups: non-specific (VDRL or RPR) and treponemal-specific (TPPA, FTA). Specific tests become positive first and will be positive lifelong. VDRL titres will fall during successful treatment. Non-specific tests may be negative in late syphilis. False positive non-specific tests can occur transiently in many infections and also in autoimmune disease such as systemic lupus erythematosus.

### Treatment
**Early disease**: IM procaine **penicillin** 750mg for 10 days, two doses of IM benzathine penicillin 2.4g, or oral doxycycline 100mg twice daily for 14 days (see Table 12.11).

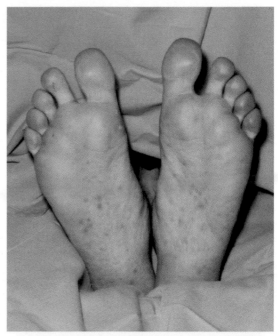
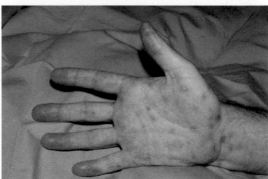
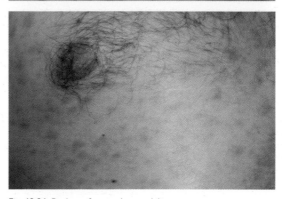

**Fig. 12.26** Rashes of secondary syphilis.
Reproduced with permission from Dr Andrew Seaton.

**Late disease**: IM procaine penicillin 750mg once daily for 17 days, three doses of IM benzathine penicillin 2.4g, or doxycycline 100mg twice daily for 28 days (see Table 12.11).

**Neurosyphilis** requires different treatment with a first-line regimen of procaine **penicillin** 2g IM once daily *plus* oral **probenicid** 500mg four times daily for 17 days, or benzylpenicillin 1.8–2.4g IV 4-hourly for 21 days.

A febrile reaction (Jarisch Herxheimer reaction) can occasionally be seen during treatment, particularly with early disease or neurosyphilis. All patients should have serological follow-up to ensure a

| Table 12.11 Syphilis treatment (other alternative regimens can be given) | | | | |
|---|---|---|---|---|
| Stage | First line | Dose | Duration | Alternatives |
| Early | IM procaine penicillin or IM benzathine penicillin | 750mg once daily<br><br>2.4g once daily | 10 days Day 1 and 8 | Doxycycline 100mg twice daily for 14 days |
| Late | IM procaine penicillin or IM benzathine penicillin | 750mg once daily<br><br>2.4g once daily | 17 days Days 1, 8, and 14 | Doxycycline 100mg twice daily for 28 days |
| Neuro | IM procaine penicillin and oral probenicid | 2g once daily 500mg four times daily | 17 days | Doxycycline 200mg twice daily for 28 days |

falling VDRL titre. Guidelines of syphilis management have been published by the British Association for Sexual Health and HIV (BASHH).

### Syphilis and HIV

All new diagnoses of syphilis should have a full sexual health screen, including HIV testing, and have contact tracing performed. Syphilis can present atypically in the context of HIV infection.

## Other treponemal infections

Yaws (*Treponema pertenue*), bejel (*Treponema pallidum*), and pinta (*Treponema carateum*) are all forms of non-venereal treponemal infection seen only in tropical countries. They typically occur in childhood, are often self-limiting, and usually result in life-long positive *Treponema pallidum* haemagglutination test serology.

- Yaws causes a primary, highly infectious papillomatous lesion on the skin. It occurs in South America, west and central Africa, Indonesia, and the Pacific. Transmission is by direct skin-to-skin contact. Lesions can recur for several years and condylomata and periostitis can develop. Treatment is with penicillin, doxycycline, or erythromycin.
- Bejel, or endemic syphilis, is caused by a serovar of *Treponema pallidum* and leads to skin infections in North Africa and the Middle East. Initially patches appear in the mouth, followed by papules in moist areas such as axillae and perineum. Hyperkeratosis of the palms and soles, and periostitis affecting the shins or nose can occur. Treatment is with penicillin.
- Pinta is confined to Central and South America, causing a papule on limbs, sometimes with smaller satellite lesions developing. Treatment is with penicillin.

# 12.15 Mycobacterial infections

## Background

Mycobacteria are rod-shaped, aerobic bacteria with lipid-rich cell walls giving them a waxy appearance. They do not stain readily with standard stains such as the Gram stain. Once exposed to a suitable stain (e.g. Ziehl–Neelsen or auramine), they do not lose their stain following exposure to acid or alcohol and are therefore known as acid and alcohol-fast bacilli (or AAFB). They grow slowly, taking up to 8 weeks to develop a positive culture.

## Tuberculosis

### Epidemiology

A third of the world's population have been exposed to TB, with 9 million new cases and around 2 million deaths annually. The incidence of TB is rising in the UK and stands at around 7000 cases per year. Cases are not equally distributed with more seen in the elderly, immigrants from Africa and the Indian subcontinent, asylum seekers, HIV infection, and alcohol excess. Treatment with anti-TNF drugs (e.g. etanercept) is a newly described risk factor.

### Pathogenesis

Primary infection with TB is usually asymptomatic. Inhaled bacilli cause pneumonic consolidation, usually of the middle or lower zones, which can drain to hilar lymph nodes. Resolution, sometimes with calcification, normally occurs at this stage. Alternatively, consolidation can progress and cavitate. Infection can spread into the pleural space, or into a blood vessel causing systemic, or miliary, disease (Fig. 12.27). Post-primary TB occurs in later life, often associated with a time of immunosuppression. Ultimately, only ~10% of those infected with the tubercle bacillus will develop symptomatic disease.

### Prevention

TB prevention is achieved through improved housing, infection control (isolating patients during the first 2 weeks of therapy),

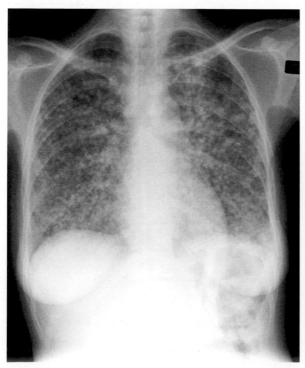

**Fig. 12.27** Chest X-ray of miliary TB.

and, to a degree, vaccination. The BCG vaccine, no longer a routine childhood vaccine in the UK, prevents the development of extrapulmonary infection, but may not prevent pulmonary infection. Chemoprophylaxis for those with a strongly positive tuberculin test in the absence of clinical disease is recommended. Treatment of index cases and contact tracing is important to decrease the extent of disease in the community.

### Clinical features

- **Pulmonary disease** (see Section 18.6).
- **Extrapulmonary TB** can affect any organ, but most commonly involves bone and joints, urinary tract, brain, GI tract, or adrenal glands. Pulmonary disease can coexist. Diagnosis can be difficult and a high index of suspicion must be maintained. Fluid or tissue for microscopy and culture are the mainstay of diagnosis.
- **Tuberculous meningitis** (TBM) usually presents subacutely with malaise, headache, vomiting, and intermittent fever. Seizures and focal neurological signs are common. Diagnosis is by analysis of CSF which can show high protein levels, low CSF glucose, and a lymphocytosis, but may be non-diagnostic. AAFB are occasionally seen. Culture can be positive, but a negative CSF culture does not exclude the diagnosis. It is often a difficult and unpredictable condition to manage. Complications including hydrocephalus, seizures, stroke, and persistent fever can occur. **Steroids** should be given along with anti-tuberculous treatment.

### Investigation

Obtaining sufficient samples (preferably at least three sputum or early morning urine samples on consecutive days) for microscopy and culture is crucial before starting anti-tuberculous therapy. When sputum is not expectorated, or is smear negative and clinical suspicion remains strong, induced sputum or specimens obtained by bronchoscopy can secure a diagnosis. If extrapulmonary TB is suspected, collection of sputum, stool, and early morning urine samples should be performed. Sampling blood, gastric aspirate, synovial fluid, CSF, and bone marrow may be useful. Where symptoms or imaging dictate, biopsy and culture of lymph node, bone, liver, or intestine may be required. Tuberculin skin testing and interferon release assays are not generally helpful for diagnosing active. Testing for coexistent HIV in all cases of TB is advised.

### Treatment

Standard treatment for pulmonary TB involves giving four first-line drugs in most individuals until sensitivities are known, which depends on a positive culture and can take several weeks. In pulmonary TB, providing rifampicin can be used, an intensive phase of at least three drugs is given for 2 months, followed by a 4-month maintenance phase of two drugs. Failure of this regimen is very rare if adherence is good. To improve adherence, combination preparations of rifampicin, isoniazid, and pyrazinamide can be used. Treatment can be given on a daily basis or as thrice weekly directly observed therapy (DOT), if adherence to therapy is poor. DOT is usually supervised by TB liaison nurses. Second-line agents including streptomycin, ciprofloxacin, cycloserine, and prothionamide are reserved for resistant TB, coexistent severe hepatic dysfunction, or drug toxicity. Treatment for certain forms of extrapulmonary TB, or when a rifampicin-based regimen cannot be used, needs to be prolonged, with treatment courses of >1 year sometimes needed.

    **Resistant TB** is an increasingly common global phenomenon, but remains rare in the UK. Isolated isoniazid resistance is found in ~5% of UK TB. Multidrug-resistant TB (MDR-TB) is defined as TB resistant to both rifampicin and isoniazid, with or without other resistances. Treatment of MDR-TB is complex and must be managed by physicians with appropriate clinical experience in appropriate isolation facilities (negative pressure rooms). Extremely drug-resistant tuberculosis (XDR-TB) has recently been identified in South Africa. Resistant to all first-line treatments, quinolones, and at least one of the parenteral agents, it has proven to be almost universally fatal.

### Public health

TB is a notifiable disease and local public health departments should be informed promptly of a new diagnosis. Contact tracing of household or other close contacts is an important part of disease control. In exceptional circumstances, patients who pose a risk to the public and are non-compliant with treatment can be detained under the Public Health Act.

### Clinical lessons

- Always send tissue samples for culture in saline. Formalin will kill mycobacteria and ensure the culture will be negative.
- Sending blood, pleural/ascitic fluid, lymph node or abscess aspirate in a mycobacterium culture bottle will improve the chances of a positive culture.

### Infection control in tuberculosis

- Patients with suspected pulmonary TB who require admission should be admitted to a single room.
- Smear-positive patients are considered infective and if inpatient care is required should be managed in a single room or, ideally, negative pressure room.
- Smear negative patients (requires three samples), most patients who have completed 2 weeks of therapy, and those with extrapulmonary TB are considered non-infectious.
- Patients with suspected or confirmed MDR-TB must be isolated in a negative pressure environment until three negative sputum cultures have been obtained. This may take several months.

## First-line TB treatments

### Rifampicin

- Dose: 450mg (if <50kg) or 600mg (if >50kg) daily.
- Side effects: red discolouration of urine and tears, hepatotoxicity, many drug interactions, fever, headache, GI upset.

### Isoniazid

- Dose: 300mg daily.
- Side effects: hepatotoxicity, rash, peripheral neuropathy (10mg pyridoxine given if at risk of neuropathy).

### Pyrazinamide

- Dose: 1.5g (if <50kg) or 2g (if >50kg) daily.
- Side effects: hepatotoxicity, arthralgia.

### Ethambutol

- Dose: 15mg/kg daily.
- Side effects: optic neuritis, rash.
- Standard regimen: four drugs for 2 months then 4 months with rifampicin and isoniazid.

### Prescribing anti-tuberculous therapy

When treatment is prescribed, the following is needed:
- Accurate weight.
- Baseline renal function and LFT.

- Baseline visual acuity check (if ethambutol used).
- Check for interactions with rifampicin (e.g. oral contraceptive pill).
- Explain potential side effects.
- Explain importance of strict adherence.
- Ensure patient understands how to take medication.
- Notify TB liaison nurse.
- Notify public health.

Once treatment has begun:
- Assess adherence (red urine is a useful indicator).
- Monitor for toxicity (LFT).
- Assess for clinical response (defervescence, clearance of sputum, weight gain).

## Leprosy

Leprosy, caused by *Mycobacterium leprae*, is relatively common in most developing countries and transmitted by respiratory secretions requiring prolonged, close contact. Most infections do not lead to disease. Untreated leprosy can cause significant disfigurement and fear of infection results in stigmatization and social isolation of those infected. The immune response dictates the clinical manifestations of leprosy, which range from tuberculoid (paucibacillary) to lepromatous (multibacillary) with several intermediate stages.

**Tuberculoid**: overactive cellular immune response with few lesions and few viable mycobacteria. Only local nerves are involved. Lesions are well-demarcated, anaesthetic, hypopigmented patches, often around the elbows or knees. Thickening of local nerves may be present and resulting peripheral neuropathy leads to progressive destruction to the hands, feet, or face, depending on the affected nerves.

**Lepromatous**: anergic response, large number of widespread lesions containing many viable organisms. Lesions are symmetrical, hypopigmented macules or papules which enlarge without treatment. Destruction of eyebrows and nasal cartilage occurs, with thickening of facial skin and nasal mucosa. Nerve involvement occurs late in the disease.

Diagnosis is by microscopy of skin smears. *Mycobacterium leprae* cannot be cultured. The lepromin skin test, involving intradermal injection of *Mycobacterium leprae* antigen, favours a diagnosis of tuberculoid leprosy if positive.

Treatment guidelines have been issued by the World Health Organization. Paucibacillary leprosy is treated for 6 months with **rifampicin** and **dapsone**. Multibacillary leprosy is treated for 2 years with rifampicin, dapsone, and clofazimine. BCG vaccination offers some protection against leprosy.

## Other non-tuberculous mycobacteria

Mycobacteria other than TB (MOTT) are commonly found in the environment and rarely cause disease in humans (Table 12.12). Some are capable of infecting immunocompetent hosts such as *Mycobacterium marinum*, an aquatic species that can cause chronic skin infection in exposed persons, e.g. fish enthusiasts (fish-tank granuloma). Others can affect those with chronic pulmonary disease (e.g. *Mycobacterium kansasii* or *Mycobacterium malmoense*) or advanced HIV (*Mycobacterium avium* complex (MAC)).

| Table 12.12 | Distinguishing between MTB and MOTT | | | |
|---|---|---|---|---|
| | Clinical | Culture | γ-INF release | Drug sensitivity |
| **TB** | Should always be considered pathogenic if cultured | Slow >2 weeks | Positive | |
| **MOTT** | May be an environmental contaminant Disease occurs usually in the immunocompromised | Can be rapid <2 weeks | Negative | Isoniazid resistant |

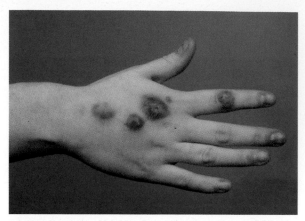

**Fig. 12.28** Fish-tank granuloma (*Mycobacterium marinum* on hand). Reproduced with permission from Dr Andrew Seaton.

Unlike *Mycobacterium tuberculosis*, non-tuberculous mycobacterium can sometimes be considered contaminants of sputum or urine cultures. Treatment should be reserved for those patients where the organism is strongly considered to be causing infection. Combination treatment is usual, although all atypical mycobacteria are inherently resistant to isoniazid. AAFB staining cannot distinguish between *Mycobacterium tuberculosis* and other mycobacteria. Unfortunately, this can lead to weeks of uncertainty after a positive sputum smear before a definite identification is made. Once a culture is growing, nucleic acid analysis can distinguish TB from other mycobacteria more quickly than traditional tests. Certain features can help distinguish TB from atypical mycobacteria.

MAC is an environmental mycobacterium, but can also cause an AIDS-defining illness (see Section 12.13).

**Fish-tank granuloma** is caused by *Mycobacterium marinum* and is typically acquired in those keeping fish. Infection arises on the fingers and hands as cold abscesses at the site of cuts or abrasions and spreads proximally over several weeks (Fig. 12.28). It does not cause systemic illness. Treatment with clarithromycin, co-trimoxazole, or ciprofloxacin monotherapy is possible, or with rifampicin and ethambutol in combination.

# 12.16 Rickettsial infections

## Q fever

Q fever is a zoonosis caused by the highly infectious *Coxiella burnetii*, an obligate intracellular bacterium related to *Rickettsia*. During infection, it undergoes antigenic variation from the virulent phase I form to the less virulent phase II form. Paradoxically, antibodies to the phase II form are identified *early* in infection, with persistently elevated phase I titres indicative of *chronic* disease.

Q fever is rare in the UK, but relatively common in southern European countries. Cattle and sheep are the main hosts, and accordingly farmers, vets, and abattoir workers are the most at risk. Person-to-person spread occurs very infrequently and only during acute infection.

**Acute Q fever** is asymptomatic in ~50% of cases. When symptomatic, it is typically a severe flu-like illness with fever, sweats, fatigue, and myalgia. Less than 5% of cases will require hospitalization. More serious acute forms include pneumonia, granulomatous hepatitis, and meningoencephalitis. Diagnosis is made by identification of elevated or rising phase II IgM antibody titres. Treatment is with 2–3 weeks of **doxycycline** 100mg twice daily although resolution of symptoms without treatment often occurs. Clarithromycin, quinolones, or co-trimoxazole are alternatives. Short courses of antimicrobial treatment will not prevent development of chronic Q fever. Symptoms of fatigue and myalgia quite commonly persist for months following acute Q fever. They do not necessarily indicate the development of chronic Q fever.

**Chronic Q fever** typically presents with many months of non-specific symptoms pertaining to multiple organ systems. The diagnosis is made by identifying a persistently elevated or rising phase I IgG antibody titre. Endocarditis is the most common form of chronic Q fever and is fatal without treatment. It typically affects left-sided valves and often presents with systemic symptoms and without fever. Chronic infection of vascular grafts and bone also occurs. Q fever is an important cause of culture-negative endocarditis and the Duke criteria for the diagnosis of endocarditis have been modified to include serological testing for Q fever. Prolonged treatment with doxycycline and hydroxychloroquine is needed, often with removal of the infected tissue. Despite such measures there is still an appreciable mortality rate.

Certain risk factors predispose to the development of chronic Q fever:

- Valvular heart disease
- Cancer
- Immunosuppression
- Vascular grafts
- Pregnancy.

Endocarditis will result following acute Q fever in ~40% of those with underlying valvopathy without treatment. Prevention of chronic Q fever in these risk groups can be achieved by treatment with hydroxychloroquine and doxycycline for 1 year. A vaccine is available for Q fever, but it has limited efficacy and is not widely used in the UK.

## Rocky Mountain spotted fever

Rocky Mountain spotted fever, a tick-borne illness caused by *Rickettsia rickettsii*, is the most common rickettsial illness in the USA and fatal in 5% of cases. Despite its name, it is most commonly acquired in south eastern and south central states in spring and early summer. It causes a non-specific illness with fever, headache, and myalgia followed by a rash developing after 3–5 days. The rash appears as peripheral macules but becomes petechial and spreads centrally as the illness progresses. The rash can be absent in 10% of cases. Eschars do not develop. Without treatment, diminished conscious level, focal neurological deficits, peripheral gangrene, and organ failure can develop.

Diagnosis is clinical and treatment with **doxycycline** 100mg twice daily should be given pending confirmation with serology.

## Typhus

Typhus is a worldwide group of arthropod-borne rickettsial infections characterized by high fever, rash, myalgia, and headache. An eschar may often be seen (Fig. 12.29). African tick typhus is the most common imported rickettsial infection in the UK. Diagnosis is primarily clinical but can be confirmed by serology. Treatment of all forms is with **doxycycline** 100mg twice daily, and should be started promptly if there is sufficient clinical suspicion, without waiting for serological confirmation. Treatment usually results in defervescence within 48 hours.

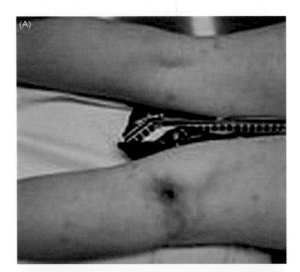

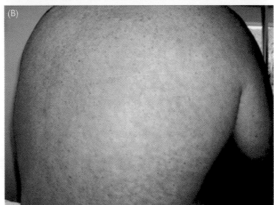

Fig. 12.29 (A) Inoculation eschar on popliteal area and discrete maculopapular elements in patient with lymphangitis infected with Rickettsia sibirica mongolitimonae, Spain, 2011. Cummings KJ, Cox-Ganser J, Riggs MA, Edwards N, Kreiss K. Respirator donning in post-hurricane New Orleans. Emerg Infect Dis [serial on the Internet]. 2007 May [cited 2007 May 1]. Available from http://www.cdc.gov/EID/content/13/5/700.htm

(B) The characteristic rash associated with scrub typhus.

Reproduced with permission of Commonwealth of Australia 2014. http://www.defence.gov.au/health/infocentre/journals/adfhj_apr06/adfhealth_7_1_10-13.html

# 12.17 Systemic fungal infections

## Background

Systemic fungal infections are becoming more common in the UK because of advances in medical therapy. They usually arise in immunocompromised hosts, can be difficult to diagnose, and carry a high mortality rate, particularly if treatment is delayed (Box 12.6).

## Invasive candidiasis

*Candida* is a commensal yeast, the most common species of which is *Candida albicans*, usually sensitive to fluconazole. Other species of *Candida* have variable rates of azole resistance (e.g. *Candida glabrata*, *Candida tropicalis*, or *Candida parapsilosis*). The incidence of these non-*albicans* candidal infections is rising.

### Clinical features
- Sepsis with no localizing signs.
- *Candida* in blood cultures (candidaemia).
- Vascular catheter infection.
- Endocarditis.
- Eye involvement: choroidoretinitis or endophthalmitis can occur in as many as 25% of patients with positive blood culture. Fundoscopy should be performed in all patients with positive cultures.
- Cerebral abscess.
- Renal tract involvement.
- Skin involvement: small pustules or larger nodules can be present.

### Diagnosis
- Gram stain of aspirate or biopsy (particularly useful if skin lesions are present).
- Growth in blood cultures: invasive candidiasis can be present even if cultures are negative. *Candida* species grow relatively slowly and cultures may take several days to become positive. *Candida albicans* can form typical 'germ tubes' in culture, a feature which distinguishes it from non-*albicans Candida* species. Persistently positive cultures suggest the presence of deep-seated infection.
- Antigen (e.g. beta-D-glucan) and PCR tests are being developed but are not yet routine practice.

### Management
- Remove central venous catheters.
- Antifungal agents should always be given, and often need to be given empirically. The choice of agent depends on severity of illness, prior antifungal use, and causative organism:

### Box 12.6 Risk factors for invasive candidal infection
- Prior broad-spectrum antimicrobial use.
- Central venous catheters.
- Total parenteral nutrition.
- Immunosuppressant drugs (including steroids).
- Haematological malignancy.
- Advanced HIV infection.
- Bone marrow or solid organ transplant.
- Haemodialysis.
- GI surgery.
- Intestinal perforation or anastomotic leak.
- Gastric acid suppression.
- Candida colonization at multiple sites.

- *Candida albicans*: **fluconazole** is as effective as other drugs for immunocompetent and clinically stable immunosuppressed patients. In unstable immunosuppressed patients, **amphotericin**, voriconazole, or caspofungin may be needed.
- *Candida glabrata*: fluconazole resistance is common. **Amphotericin**, caspofungin or voriconazole are effective.

There is little good evidence to decide duration of therapy or to support the use of combination antifungal treatments. Two weeks of treatment once blood cultures become negative is recommended by the IDSA for candidaemia. Deep-seated candidal infection requires prolonged treatment.

## Invasive aspergillosis

*Aspergillus* species are ubiquitous environmental moulds that can cause severe infection in immunosuppressed hosts. *Aspergillus fumigatus, Aspergillus flavus,* and *Aspergillus niger* are the most common species to cause systemic infection. Invasive aspergillosis carries a very high mortality. Risk factors are prolonged neutropaenia, bone marrow or solid organ transplantation, and advanced HIV infection.

### Clinical features
- **Pulmonary** disease is the most common manifestation. Cough, haemoptysis, chest pain, and breathlessness may occur, but it can also present as fever unresponsive to antibacterial agents with no respiratory symptoms. CXR is often normal, but CT will be abnormal in >95% cases.
- **Sinus** disease can occur, resulting in local destruction and direct intracranial spread of infection.

Other presentations include **disseminated** disease, which can involve eye, brain, bone, heart valves, and skin.

### Diagnosis
- Stain of aspirate or biopsy can show narrow hyphae with acute-angle branching, although other fungi may also have this appearance. Colonization of sputum or skin can occur in the absence of infection.
- Growth from blood or biopsy cultures.
- Antigen (e.g. galactomannan) and PCR tests are more developed than in candidal infection. Galactomannan detection from serum can occur many days before positive culture or radiological changes appear. A negative test has a good negative predictive value.

### Treatment
- Antifungal agents: **amphotericin**, usually now given as a liposomal preparation, has been the mainstay of treatment for many years, but the newer agents voriconazole is also effective. Fluconazole is ineffective. Treatment is often for weeks or months.
- Surgery is sometimes required to remove sites of infection.
- Reversing immunosuppression by decreasing doses of immunosuppressant regimens or by giving granulocyte colony stimulating factor (G-CSF) should be attempted wherever possible.

## Other fungal infections

***Cryptococcus neoformans*** causes infection in immunocompromised hosts, particularly in advanced HIV (see Section 12.13). Infection in immunocompetent hosts is very rare.

**Mucormycosis** causes a progressive, locally destructive disease in immunocompromised patients, particularly diabetics. The typical presentation is of nasal and sinus infection forming characteristic black, necrotic lesions. The infection can spread directly to the orbits or brain. Prognosis is poor, with amphotericin occasionally effective.

Voriconazole and caspofungin are ineffective. Small series show that posaconazole, a new azole, can be useful.

**Histoplasmosis** is caused by *Histoplasma capsulatum* in inhaled dust. It is found in the USA (Ohio and Mississippi river valleys). Infection is commonly asymptomatic, but acute and chronic pulmonary disease may result. Disseminated disease can sometimes arise. Diagnosis is by culture, antigen testing, or serology, and treatment is **itraconazole**, with **amphotericin** reserved for severe or disseminated cases.

**Coccidioidomycosis** (also known as Valley fever) is caused by *Coccidioides immitis*, present in dust and soil in the southwestern USA and Mexico. Infection is symptomatic in most cases, with minor self-limiting respiratory disease the usual clinical presentation. Chronic pulmonary infection and dissemination can occur, particularly in immunosuppressed hosts. Diagnosis is by microscopy and culture; serology can be useful. Treatment for mild disease is **fluconazole** or itraconazole. Severe disease is treated with **amphotericin**.

# Antifungal drugs

There are three main classes of drugs for use in systemic fungal infection: azoles, amphotericin, and echinocandins

**Triazoles** are the most commonly used antifungal drugs, available in both oral and IV preparations. They inhibit the synthesis of ergosterol (a necessary component of the fungal cell wall) in a cytochrome p450-dependent manner. As they all affect the cytochrome p450 system, significant drug interactions can occur:

- Fluconazole is the oldest drug in the group. It has good bioavailability and a long half-life allowing once-daily dosing. It is effective against sensitive *Candida*, but not *Aspergillus*.

- Itraconazole has more variable bioavailability but is active against some fluconazole-resistant *Candida*.

- Voriconazole is a newer agent, with good activity against aspergillosis and fluconazole-resistant candidal infection.

**Amphotericin B** is a broad-spectrum antifungal agent with activity against most infections due to *Candida* and *Aspergillus*. It inhibits fungal cell wall synthesis by binding to ergosterol. Oral formulations are not systemically absorbed. Two different IV preparations exist:

- Standard amphotericin B (e.g. Fungizone®).

- Lipid formulations of amphotericin B (e.g. AmBisome®, Abelcet®).

A test dose of 1mg is often given prior to administration because of the small risk of anaphylaxis. Doses are titrated upward over the first few days to achieve the optimal dose. Impaired renal function, hypokalaemia, and hypomagnesaemia are common side effects. A decreased GFR will be observed in most patients, but this is rarely clinically significant in the absence of other causes of renal impairment. It is important to ensure normovolaemia when giving amphotericin. Liposomal preparations are associated with fewer adverse events, allowing them to be given in higher doses.

**Caspofungin** is a new antifungal agent, in the echinocandin class, with activity against *Aspergillus* and all species of *Candida*. It has less renal toxicity than amphotericin, and less potential for interaction than the azoles. It is only available intravenously.

# Clinical lessons

- Never regard fungi in blood cultures as a contaminant.
- Watch for drug interactions with triazoles, especially voriconazole.
- Different formulations of amphotericin are not interchangeable. Make sure you know which you are prescribing and that the dose is appropriate.
- Avoid other nephrotoxic drugs and ensure adequate hydration in patients on amphotericin.

527

# 12.18 Protozoal infections

## Background

Protozoa are unicellular eukaryotes that can be found worldwide. They vary considerably in their pathogenicity. Some cause severe disease only in *immunocompromised* hosts (*Toxoplasma* and cryptosporidia), others cause relatively *benign* infections (*Giardia* and *Trichomonas*), but several cause *life-threatening* infections in immunocompetent hosts (malaria, *Leishmania*, and *Trypanosoma*). Globally, the burden of serious infection falls mainly on developing countries. Chronic lack of research and development in anti-protozoal drugs has resulted in a rather limited range of available drugs, many with significant toxicities.

## Classification

There are four groups of medically-relevant protozoa:
- **Amoebae**: *Entamoeba histolytica*, *Acanthamoeba* spp., *Naegleria fowleri*.
- **Ciliates**: *Balantidium coli*.
- **Flagellates**: *Leishmania* spp., *Trypanosoma* spp., *Trichomonas vaginalis*, *Giardia lamblia*.
- **Sporozoa** *Plasmodium* spp., *Toxoplasma gondii*, *Cryptosporidium parvum*, *Isospora belli*, *Babesia* spp.

## Leishmaniasis

*Leishmania* is a genus of intracellular protozoa causing three forms of leishmaniasis—visceral (or kala-azar), mucocutaneous, and cutaneous—all transmitted by sandflies. Most species are zoonotic, with reservoirs primarily in dogs and rodents.
- **Visceral leishmaniasis** is caused by *Leishmania donovani* and is endemic in many areas in Africa, the Indian subcontinent, as well as southern Mediterranean countries. The incubation period varies from 2 weeks to 2 years and the resulting illness begins with fever, sweats, and malaise. Weight loss and hepatosplenomegaly follows, with lymphadenopathy sometimes present. Pancytopenia, low albumin, and raised globulins and inflammatory markers are typical. Diagnosis is by identification of parasites in blood, bone marrow, or splenic aspirates by microscopy or culture. Serology is also available. Treatment with 10 days of liposomal **amphotericin B** has overtaken the traditional 30 days of sodium stibogluconate as the regimen of choice, although amphotericin use is limited by its expense.
- **Cutaneous leishmaniasis** is caused by various species including *Leishmania tropica*, *Leishmania infantum*, and *Leishmania major*. A slowly enlarging, painless cutaneous ulcer at the site of the sandfly bite is the typical presentation (Fig. 12.30). There is no associated lymphadenopathy. Diffuse disease can be seen in *Leishmania aethiopiae* or *Leishmania mexicana* infection, with multiple plaques rather than ulcers. Diagnosis is by Giemsa staining or culture of ulcer smears or skin biopsies. Serology will often be positive. Treatment is with IV **sodium stibogluconate** or **amphotericin B**.
- **Mucocutaneous** leishmaniasis is caused by *Leishmania brasiliensis* and is similar to cutaneous disease, except the ulceration forms at mucocutaneous junctions.

## American trypanosomiasis (Chagas disease)

This is caused by *Trypanosoma cruzi* and transmitted by reduviid bugs in South America. It is associated with poor housing conditions. The majority of infections are asymptomatic.

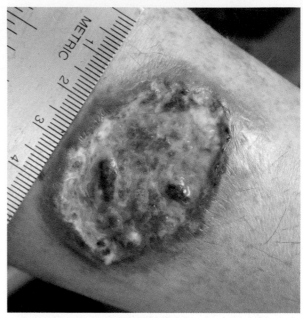

**Fig. 12.30** Leishmaniasis ulcer on left forearm.
This image is in the public domain: Layne Harris, http://en.wikipedia.org/wiki/File:Leishmaniasis_ulcer.jpg

- **Acute** infection occurs more commonly in adults and can cause:
  - Fever and skin lump at the site of insect bite.
  - Unilateral periorbital oedema.
  - Regional adenopathy and hepatosplenomegaly.
  - Myocarditis.
  - Meningo-encephalitis.
- **Chronic** infection typically causes:
  - Dilated cardiomyopathy and conduction defects.
  - Oesophageal or colonic dilatation.

Diagnosis is by blood film in acute infection. Serological testing is available. Anti-trypanosomal drugs (**nifurtimox** or **benznidazole**) can be given in acute infection but result in clinical cure in only ~50% of cases. Treatment of chronic disease is limited to medical therapy for heart failure and dysrhythmia, or surgery for intestinal dilatation.

## African trypanosomiasis (sleeping sickness)

Sleeping sickness is caused by *Trypanosoma brucei* and affects ~500,000 people. There are two forms:
- *Trypanosoma brucei gambesiense* in West Africa.
- *Trypanosoma brucei rhodesiense* in East Africa (with some overlap in central Africa).

Both are transmitted by the tsetse fly and have similar microscopic appearances.

**Clinical features**: both cause an early-stage disease (chancre/painless ulceration, lymphadenopathy, and non-specific systemic upset) and a late-stage disease (with neurological involvement). *Trypanosoma rhodesiense*, however, tends to cause a more severe acute infection and more rapid onset of neurological involvement. Neurological features include headache, apathy, personality changes, seizures, tremor, ataxia, daytime somnolence progressing to coma, and eventually, death.

Gambian disease progresses over months to years, while Rhodesian disease occurs more rapidly over weeks to months.

**Diagnosis** is by finding trypanosomes on a blood film, lymph node aspirate or CSF. Serological tests can be used, but positive tests do not guarantee active infection.

**Treatment** is difficult and involves the use of toxic drugs. **Pentamidine** and **suramin** can be used in early infection. **Melarsoprol** is the main treatment for neurological involvement. It is extremely toxic, carrying a 10% risk of encephalopathy and 5% risk of death. A newer drug, **eflornithine**, may be as effective with a lower mortality rate.

**Prevention** is by vector control and bite avoidance. There is no vaccine or prophylactic treatment available.

## Toxoplasmosis

*Toxoplasma gondii* is a worldwide zoonosis with the domestic cat as the primary host. Infection is very common in the UK, with a sero-prevalence of ~1% per year of age. The sexual cycle occurs in the cat where oocysts are excreted in the faeces and can be ingested by animals or humans. Infection most commonly occurs by ingestion of oocysts, but can also arise from ingestion of meat from animals previously infected with oocysts.

Infection in an immunocompetent individual is typically asymptomatic but can result in a febrile illness with lymphadenopathy and occasionally hepatosplenomegaly. Complete resolution is the rule but complications can, rarely, arise: choroidoretinitis, myocarditis, or pneumonitis. It can cause severe disease in the context of AIDS. Infection occurs during 0.4% of pregnancies and results in fetal infection in 30% of maternal infections. Choroidoretinitis and microcephaly are the most serious fetal complications.

Diagnosis is by serology and no treatment for lymphadenitis is required. Treatment of maternal infection is with **spiramycin** throughout pregnancy, or **pyrimethamine** and **sulphadiazine** with folinic acid supplementation after the first trimester. Treatment and prophylaxis of toxoplasmosis in HIV infection is covered in Section 12.13.

## Giardiasis

Giardiasis is endemic worldwide and caused by ingestion of food or water contaminated with *Giardia lamblia*.

- **Acute** disease is characterized by watery diarrhoea, malaise, nausea, weight loss, abdominal bloating, and flatulence. Fever is rare, and the illness usually lasts >1 week.
- **Chronic** disease can occur without treatment, leading to loose stools, steatorrhoea, weight loss and fatigue.

Diagnosis is made by stool microscopy or antigen testing. Trophozoites are intermittently excreted and several stool specimens should be submitted. Duodenal aspirate or biopsy is the gold standard test, but is reserved for complicated cases. **Metronidazole** 400mg three times daily for 5 days is usually effective.

## *Cryptosporidium*

Cryptosporidia are intracellular protozoans that can cause acute diarrhoea in immunocompetent individuals. They are usually acquired by drinking, or swimming in, untreated water. The illness is self-limiting, and lasts 7–14 days in most cases. No specific treatment is usually needed, but **nitazoxanide** can be used successfully in the immunocompetent. The infection can cause chronic diarrhoea in immuno-compromised patients, particularly those with AIDS.

## *Isospora* and microsporidia

These intestinal sporozoa are rare causes of chronic diarrhoea in immunosuppressed patients, typically AIDS. Diagnosis is by stool microscopy for the identification of oocysts. Treatment can be difficult.

## Babesiosis

Babesiosis is a rare tick-borne infection due to *Babesia divergens* in Europe (including the UK) and *Babesia microti* in the USA. Babesiosis usually results in a non-specific febrile illness, but can cause severe disease in elderly or splenectomized patients. The European form, *Babesia divergens*, causes more severe disease. Diagnosis is by identification of parasites within red cells on a blood film, where appearances can be similar to *Plasmodium falciparum*. Treatment is with **quinine** and **clindamycin**, or atovaquone and azithromycin.

## *Trichomonas vaginalis*

*Trichomonas vaginalis* is the causative agent of trichomoniasis, a sexually transmitted infection causing vaginal or urethral discharge. Diagnosis is by identification of the pear-shaped, highly motile organism on a wet film. Treatment is with **metronidazole.**

## Malaria

Four plasmodium species cause malaria in humans: *Plasmodium falciparum*, *Plasmodium vivax*, *Plasmodium ovale*, and *Plasmodium malariae*. The management of malaria is covered in Section 12.7.

## Amoebiasis

*Entamoeba histolytica* causes amoebic dysentery and amoebic liver abscess. Its management is covered in Section 12.7.

# 12.19 Helminthic infections

## Background

Helminths (worms) are the largest parasites to infect humans and account for a large global burden of disease, principally in tropical countries. Whilst some helminths are found in the UK (*Enterobius vermicularis*, toxocariasis, and hydatid disease), many helminthic infections are imported, with cutaneous larva migrans and schistosomiasis seen reasonably frequently in returning travellers. Helminthic infection stimulates a Th2 immune response, the characteristic finding of which is eosinophilia.

## Classification

- **Cestodes** (flatworms): *Taenia solium, Taenia saginata, Echinococcus granulosus, Diphyllobothrium latum, Hymenolepis nana.*
- **Nematodes** (roundworms): *Ascaris lumbricoides, Ancylostoma* spp., *Necator americanus, Strongyloides stercoralis, Enterobius vermicularis, Trichinella* spp., *Toxocara* spp., *Onchocerca volvulus, Wucheria bancrofti, Loa Loa, Dracunculus medinensis.*
- **Trematodes** (flukes): *Schistosoma* spp., *Clonorchis sinensis, Opisthorchis* spp., *Fasciola hepatica, Fasciolopsis buski, Paragonimiasis westermani.*

## Cestodes

### Taenia solium (cysticercosis)

Ingestion of undercooked pork contaminated with *Taenia solium* eggs can lead to infection in humans. Following ingestion, eggs hatch within the gut, larvae penetrate the bowel mucosa and migrate to subcutaneous tissue and muscle where they can be identified as subcutaneous lumps. The most serious complications occur when larvae migrate to the eye, causing visual disturbance or the brain, causing seizures or raised intracranial pressure. Neurocysticercosis is a common cause of epilepsy in developing countries.

There are international guidelines for the diagnosis and management of suspected neurocysticercosis based on: compatible clinical presentation, epidemiological risk factors, serology of blood or CSF, and typical appearance on brain imaging with CT or MRI. Plain X-ray or CT will sometimes detect calcified cysts in muscle. Treatment with **albendazole** 400mg once daily and **dexamethasone** 2mg three times daily for 10 days is effective at preventing further seizures but elimination of cysts does not always occur, even with treatment.

### Echinococcus granulosus (hydatid disease)

*Echinococcus granulosus* is a dog tapeworm which can infect humans, cattle, sheep, and pigs. It is endemic in Middle Eastern counties and South America. It occurs rarely in the UK. Ingested eggs release an onchosphere which penetrates the gut mucosa and migrates most commonly to the liver, but also lung, spleen, bone, brain, and eye.

Hydatid disease can present in many different ways: hepatomegaly, right upper quadrant pain, an incidental finding on CXR or liver ultrasound, bone or joint pain. Diagnosis is by imaging coupled with serology. Treatment is with **albendazole** or mebendazole, but can be difficult. Surgery is occasionally necessary, but care has to be taken to avoid rupturing cysts into body cavities which can result in severe anaphylaxis.

### Diphyllobothrium latum

Ingestion of raw or undercooked fish can result in infection within the small intestine. The incidence is highest in Scandinavia and Japan. Malabsorption, particularly of vitamin $B_{12}$, can result. Diagnosis is by identification of eggs in stool. Treatment is with **niclosamide** or **praziquantel**.

## Nematodes

### Enterobius vermicularis (pinworm)

Pinworm infection is the most common helminthic infection in the UK, typically affecting primary school children. Humans are the only host and transmission is by ingestion of eggs present in faeces. Most infection is asymptomatic, but pruritus ani or abdominal pain can occur. Infection can also spread to the female genital tract. Diagnosis is by observation of worms (white, thin, and ~10mm long) or eggs in the perianal area. Two doses of **mebendazole** or albendazole 2 weeks apart is effective treatment.

### Ascaris lumbricoides (ascariasis)

Around 1/4 of the world's population are infected with *Ascaris lumbricoides*, an intestinal nematode that can reach up to 40cm in length and which causes 20,000 deaths annually. The highest prevalence is in the tropics, particularly Asia. Transmission is via contaminated food or water. Infection can result in pneumonitis (Loeffler syndrome), GI upset, malnutrition, and intestinal or biliary tract obstruction. Diagnosis can be made by stool microscopy, identification of worms on imaging, or serology. Peripheral eosinophilia is common. **Mebendazole** and albendazole are the main treatments.

### Hookworm

*Ancylostoma duodenale* and *Necator americanus* cause hookworm infection, one of the most common causes of iron deficiency anaemia in the developing world. Larvae present in soil penetrate the feet of the host, migrate to the lung, and then, via the bronchial tree, to the pharynx. Once swallowed, they attach to intestinal mucosa causing damage to villi and resultant blood loss. Stool microscopy can reveal the presence of eggs, but this will only be found several months after initial infection. Absence of eggs on microscopy does not exclude infection. Eosinophilia will usually be present and may be the only indicator of infection. **Mebendazole** or albendazole are the preferred treatments.

## Strongyloidiasis

*Strongyloides stercoralis* is found mostly in the tropics and subtropics. Human infection, via ingestion of larvae in food or water, causes an asymptomatic eosinophilia or mild symptoms in immunocompetent patients, but in the immunocompromised can result in severe disseminated disease. Unlike other helminths, *Strongyloides stercoralis* can replicate in humans, meaning that clinical disease may occur years after exposure. Malnutrition, immunosuppressant drugs, stem cell transplant, or AIDS are all risk factors for severe disease. People who have lived or worked in endemic areas (such as servicemen stationed in the Far East during World War II) should be screened prior to immunosuppressant treatment. Diagnosis is by the identification of larvae in stool and by serology. Larvae can also be found in sputum in disseminated disease. Treatment of severe disease is with **ivermectin,** sometimes in combination with albendazole.

## Trichinellosis

An infection found worldwide. Several species of *Trichinella* cause human infection following the ingestion of cysts in undercooked meat. Pork is the main reservoir of human disease, but wild boar, horse, and bear can also be sources of cysts. After an incubation period of 1–4 weeks, two clinical stages of disease occur:

1. Intestinal infection occurs within a week of ingestion and is associated with abdominal pain, vomiting, and diarrhoea.
2. After the first week, larvae migrate through the blood to skeletal muscle causing fever, severe muscle pain, and swelling. Splinter haemorrhages can be seen. Periocular involvement is common

with chemosis, visual disturbance, and eye pain. A raised creatine kinase and eosinophil count is typical, but specific diagnosis is by serology or muscle biopsy. Rarely, cardiac myositis, meningoencephalitis, or pulmonary disease can develop. **Albendazole** or mebendazole is given for 10 days (sometimes with steroids) in severe disease.

## Toxocariasis (visceral larva migrans)

Toxocariasis is caused by *Toxocara canis* or *Toxocara catis* found in dogs and cats respectively. Transmission is by ingestion of eggs excreted in faeces. Asymptomatic infection can occur, but clinical disease leads to fever, itch, and hepatomegaly. Pulmonary and ocular involvement may also occur. Eosinophilia is common but specific serology is available. Asymptomatic disease does not require treatment. **Albendazole** or mebendazole is effective for severe disease.

## Onchocerciasis (river blindness)

Onchocerciasis, caused by *Onchocerca volvulus*, is a disease causing blindness and occurs in areas of Africa and South America. Humans are the only host. Transmission is by black flies, but is not efficient and travellers must spend many months in an endemic area to acquire infection. After deposition into the skin following an insect bite, larvae mature into adult worms over the next year. After this, adult females (up to 80cm in length) produce several thousand microfilariae per day. Microfilariae migrate through skin and eyes, but cause inflammation when they die. In the skin this can cause an intensely itchy dermatitis and nodules (Calabar swellings), but the chief morbidity is in ocular involvement. Onchocerciasis is one of the leading causes of blindness in the developing world. The severity of disease is proportional to the total microfilarial burden.

Diagnosis of active disease is by identification of microfilaria in skin snips or on slit lamp examination of the eyes. Treatment is with **ivermectin**. Pre-treatment with **steroids** should be given if there is ocular involvement. No drug can safely kill adult filarial worms, and repeated courses of ivermectin are often required.

## Lymphatic filariasis

*Wuchereria bancrofti, Brugia malayi,* and *Brugia timori* all cause lymphatic filariasis in many tropical countries. Transmitted by mosquitoes, microfilariae enter human lymphatics and, over 12 months, mature into adult worms (up to 10cm long). Adult worms can produce up to 10,000 microfilariae/day. Infection is often asymptomatic, but chronic infection can lead to blockage of the lymphatic system, producing lymphoedema of the legs and genitalia. Acute syndromes can cause lymphangitis, fever or tropical pulmonary eosinophilia.

Diagnosis is by examination of a blood smear taken at midnight for the presence of microfilaria. This timing is due to the circadian rhythm of filaria, whereby they are more likely to be found in the peripheral blood at midnight ± 2 hours.

Serological and antigen testing is also available. **Diethylcarbamazine (DEC)** is the preferred treatment.

## Trematodes

### Schistosomiasis
See Section 12.7.

### Paragonimiasis
*Paragonimus westermanii* is the principal cause of paragonimiasis, a pulmonary fluke infection, acquired by ingesting raw fish. It is most common in South East Asia. The incubation period is up to 3 weeks, when abdominal pain occurs as immature flukes pass through the intestine. Following this, they can spread to lung, brain, or skin. Pleuritic pain may occur as larvae penetrate the diaphragm and pleura. Eosinophilic pleural effusion is common at this time. Migration into the parenchyma causes cough, haemoptysis, fever, and chest pain, with peripheral eosinophilia and infiltrates on CXR. Diagnosis is by identification of eggs in sputum or stool, aspirate of pulmonary lesions, and can be supplemented by serology. Treatment is with **praziquantel**.

## Anti-helminthic therapy

Few drugs are available to treat helminthic infections and none of their mechanisms of action have been well-characterized. The three chief classes are:

- **Benzimidazoles** (including albendazole and mebendazole) are active against many cestodes and trematodes. Albendazole is the drug of choice for hydatid disease, neurocysticercosis, or cutaneous larva migrans. All drugs in this class should be avoided in pregnancy.

- **Ivermectin** is active against a range of nematodes, as well as the ectoparasite, scabies. It is the drug of choice for river blindness and strongyloidiasis.

- **Praziquantel** is effective against many trematode infections. It is the drug of choice for schistosomiasis.

# Chapter 13

# Intensive care medicine

# 13.1 Overview

## Definition of intensive care

A widely accepted view of intensive care is that it is a service for patients, with potentially recoverable conditions, who can benefit from more detailed observation and invasive treatment than can be provided in general wards, or high dependency areas (Fig. 13.1).

Intensive care services are vital core entities required by the sickest patients in the hospital and supported by highly skilled multidisciplinary teams.

Intensive care must be viewed as a system that extends beyond the dedicated area (**critical care unit**), also providing resources to support at-risk patients on the ward (**outreach**) and services to facilitate the rehabilitation of patients recovering in hospital and in the primary care setting (**follow-up**) (Box 13.1).

## The critical care unit

### Design, staffing, and quality

- The unit needs to be easily accessible to the areas from which the patients are admitted and close to services that provide support.
- It must be staffed by dedicated and competent senior medical and nursing staff, with many patients requiring 1:1 nursing.
- Evidence-based care, monitoring, and evaluation are crucial parts of intensive care.
- Intensive care supports the use of '**care bundles**', defined as packages of evidence-based clinical interventions accompanied by systematic audit, to ensure the equitable provision of high-quality patient care.
- Examples of care bundles in use include sepsis, tracheostomy, and end of life.

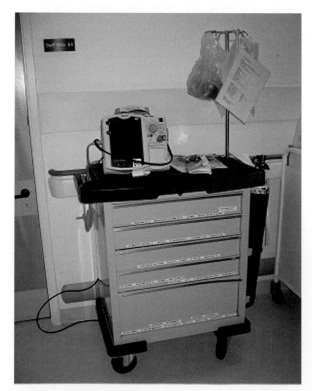

**Fig. 13.1** Resuscitation Trolley

534

---

> **Box 13.1 Key components of an intensive care service**
>
> 1. A fully functioning critical care unit.
> 2. 24/7 outreach services.
> 3. Provision for comprehensive rehabilitation.
> 4. Adequate transfer and transport arrangements.
> 5. 24/7 support services.
> 6. Use of evidence based 'care bundles'.
>
> Reproduced with permission of The Intensive Care Society.

- Infection control is of paramount importance and ICU patients often contract multiresistant organisms, necessitating isolation.
- Dedicated daily microbiology ward rounds take place to guide care.
- Intensive care is an expensive service that costs in the region of £1500 per patient per day in the United Kingdom.

### Levels of care and ICU admission

- **Levels of care** classify the amount of organ support that patients receive in hospital, level 0, 1, 2, and 3 (Box 13.2).
- High dependency care (HDU) provides a level of care intermediate between ward and intensive care and can act as a 'step up' or 'step down' from ICU.
- HDU care can be provided adjacent to the critical care unit or on the unit itself.
- Patients are admitted for ICU care predominantly as a result of **trauma**, **disease**, **adverse events**, or **major surgery**.
- ICU care is usually reserved for those patients requiring **advanced respiratory support** or **level 2 care** and **above**.

### ICU scoring systems

- A number of systems have evolved and the most well known is the **APACHE** score which identifies **disease severity** (Box 13.3).
- Other systems measure workload and resource, compare performance and evaluate research, or provide objectives on patient management (Box 13.4).
- The scoring and identification of the 'at-risk' patient is now a fundamental part of ICU and an integral part of outreach.

> **Box 13.2 Levels of care**
>
> - **Level 0:** patients whose needs can be met through **normal ward care** in an acute hospital.
> - **Level 1:** patients at risk of their condition deteriorating or those recently relocated from higher levels of care whose needs can be met on an **acute ward with support** from the critical care team.
> - **Level 2:** patients requiring more detailed observation or intervention including support for **single failing organ system** or postoperative care and those stepping down from a higher level of care.
> - **Level 3:** patients requiring monitoring and **support for two or more organ systems** one of which may be basic or advanced respiratory support.
>
> *Source:* The Intensive Care Society

Box 13.3 Commonly used calling criteria

1. Respiratory rate >25 or <8 breaths/minute.
2. Oxygen saturation < 90% on ≥35% oxygen.
3. Heart rate >125 or <50bpm.
4. Systolic blood pressure <90 or >200mmHg (or sustained fall >40mmHg from normal value).
5. Sustained alteration in conscious level.
6. Patient looks unwell or you feel worried about their clinical condition.

# Critical care outreach

## Background

- The development of outreach services started with the observation that patients often show abnormal physiology on the general ward in the hours **preceding** cardiorespiratory arrest or emergency admission to the ICU.
- Outreach services were therefore developed to facilitate the delivery of intensive care practice to patients outside ICU.
- Multidisciplinary outreach teams have evolved including METS (medical emergency teams), PART (patient-at-risk team), and PERT (patient emergency response team).
- Teams employ **'track and trigger'** systems such as MEWS (modified early warning system) or PAR score (patient-at-risk score) which allow at-risk patients on the general wards to be 'tracked' and a call to the specialist team 'triggered'.
- Outreach services also provide continuing input from the intensive care service following discharge, which is important for both patients and relatives.
- Studies suggest that early detection of critical illness with timely interaction can reduce morbidity, mortality, and length of stay in medical and surgical patients.
- Outreach teams also help disseminate high-quality practice and education.
- However, not all studies have shown beneficial outcomes following implementation of outreach services

Box 13.4 Commonly used ICU scoring systems

APACHE Acute Physiology and Chronic Health Evaluation
   TISS Therapeutic Intervention Scoring System
   SOFA Sequential Organ Failure Score
   SAPS Simplified Acute Physiology Score
   GCS Glasgow Coma Scale
   PARS Patient-at-Risk Score

*APACHE II: physiological variables measured*

1. Temperature—core
2. Mean arterial pressure
3. Heart rate
4. Respiratory rate
5. Oxygenation
6. Arterial pH
7. Serum sodium
8. Serum potassium
9. Serum creatinine
10. Haematocrit
11. White blood cell count
12. Glasgow Coma Scale score.

Reproduced from Knaus et al., 'APACHE II: A severity of disease classification system', *Critical Care Medicine*, 13, 10, pp. 818–829, copyright 1985, with permission from Wolters Kluwer and the Society of Critical Care Medicine

- A further criticism is that doctors previously responsible for treatment of acute conditions on the general ward may absolve responsibility to outreach teams, de-skill, and ultimately decrease the overall quality of care in the hospital.

## Follow-up

- Clinics now exist in a number of ICUs and can play a significant role in caring for patients recovering from critical illness.
- In addition to the physical and cognitive consequences of an ICU admission, clinics have helped identify and support the huge psychological burden that patients and carers may suffer.

# 13.2 Basic principles of critical illness

## Background

As emphasized in Section 13.1, the key to management of critical illness is **early recognition with timely intervention**.

## Assessment

Some of the principles involved in assessing the unwell patient have already been discussed in Chapter 1 of this book. The following paragraphs emphasize important issues pertinent to the critically ill patient.

### History

- There is no substitute for obtaining an accurate history, examination, and also any advanced directive from a patient, even in an emergency situation.

### Clinical examination

- Whether or not a request for patient assessment is triggered by an abnormal PAR score, it is imperative to measure vital signs including pulse, BP, and temperature and **ensure** respiratory rate is measured.
- Examination of the patient may reveal dysfunction of single or multiple organs.

### Initial monitoring, support, and investigations

In many cases, basic intervention on the general ward may alleviate the problem. However, if a patient is critically unwell, as a baseline, the following should be performed concurrently:

- Ensure correct patient position.
- Place a pulse oximeter, cardiac monitor, and BP cuff.
- Give high-flow, high-concentration $O_2$. Remember **hypoxia kills quickly**.
- Establish intravenous access and send a full set of routine investigations.
- Perform ABG analysis.
- Insert a urinary catheter and measure output.
- Order necessary radiological investigations.
- Involve senior support as appropriate.

## Applied physiology in critical illness

### Cardiac function

Cardiac systolic function is the result of four interrelated variables:
- **Heart rate**.
- **Preload** (filling status of patient).
- **Afterload** (systematic vascular resistance (SVR)).
- **Contractility** (heart pump function).

Their interplay results in **cardiac output (CO)**, which is defined as the volume of blood ejected from the heart per minute. The **stroke volume** is the amount of blood ejected per systolic contraction. Understanding these entities is a pre-requisite to interpreting the different causes of **shock**, where **hypotension** occurs and vital organs are **inadequately perfused** (read **physiological equations** in Box 13.5).

### Clinical manifestation of shock

It is important to realize that an increase in pressure (BP) does not always lead to augmented flow (CO), as this is also dependent on resistance (SVR). This is manifest clinically and may be detected by feeling the peripheries of the shocked patient. If the patient is warm, sweaty, and vasodilated, SVR is low, causing BP to fall. To compensate, the CO may be high, as occurs in sepsis. Conversely, in cardiogenic shock, peripheral vasoconstriction occurs in an attempt to elevate the falling BP, increasing SVR. The patient will be cold

peripherally. The failing heart is inefficient when working against an elevated SVR, so the CO falls further. Treatment with vasodilating drugs may reduce BP, but can improve CO by reducing resistance to flow (Table 13.1; see Section 13.4).

### Oxygen transport and shock

The body is dependent on a continuous supply of $O_2$ from the air to the mitochondria in order to sustain aerobic metabolism. This occurs as a series of steps involving **flow** from the heart and lungs, efficient **transport** across the extravascular matrix, and **extraction** by the tissues. Ultimately, the circulatory transport of $O_2$ from the lungs, **Oxygen delivery (DO$_2$)**, must meet the metabolic demands of the tissues, **oxygen consumption (VO$_2$)**, or circulatory shock occurs. The **extraction ratio VO$_2$/DO$_2$** describes the amount of oxygen consumed as a fraction of delivery and in the normal person is about 25%. In the critically ill patient this may rise to >65% and will be reflected by a fall in mixed venous $O_2$ (SvO$_2$).

$DO_2$ is dependent on the CO, Hb content, the $O_2$, saturation and the Hb–$O_2$ binding capacity. $VO_2$ is also dependent on CO and the difference in $O_2$ content in the arterial and venous systems.

It therefore follows that tissue hypoxia can be caused by poor $O_2$ supply, sluggish CO, a reduction in Hb, increased metabolic demand, or local toxicity, as occurs in endotoxaemia (Box 13.6).

Although vitally important in the treatment of critical illness, improving ventilatory function will only directly augment the first of these factors (Boxes 13.5 and 13.7).

---

**Box 13.5  Important physiological equations**

1. **Cardiac output** = heart rate × stroke volume.
2. **Mean arterial blood pressure** = cardiac output × systemic vascular resistance.
3. **Oxygen delivery (DO$_2$)** = cardiac output × blood $O_2$ content.
4. **Blood $O_2$ content** = haemoglobin × $O_2$ saturation (%) × K (1.34)
   (K: coefficient for haemoglobin-oxygen binding capacity).
5. **Oxygen consumption (VO$_2$)** = cardiac output × (aO$_2$ − vO$_2$)
   (aO$_2$: arterial oxygen content; vO$_2$: venous oxygen content).
6. **Alveolar ventilation (V$_A$)** = respiratory rate × (tidal volume − physiological dead space).
7. **(A–a) gradient** = PAO$_2$ − PaO$_2$ = efficiency of $O_2$ uptake from alveolar gas to arterial blood.

---

**Table 13.1  Types of shock and usual effects on cardiac function**

|  | HR | Preload | Afterload | Contractility |
|---|---|---|---|---|
| Cardiogenic | ↑ | ↑ | ↑ | ↓ |
| Hypovolaemic | ↑ | ↓ | ↑ | ↑ |
| Septic | ↑ | ↓ | ↓ | ↑ |
| Anaphylactic | ↑ | ↓ | ↓ | ↑ |

---

**Box 13.6  Types of hypoxia**

- **Hypoxic hypoxia:** delivery of oxygen to the tissues is reduced.
- **Stagnant hypoxia:** flow is impaired.
- **Anaemic hypoxia:** reduced level of haemoglobin.

Box 13.7 Indicators of inadequate cardiac output

- **Global:**
  - Elevated lactate
  - Reduced mixed venous $O_2$.
- **Regional:**
  - Hyperventilation (drive)
  - Poor capillary refill
  - Poor urine output
  - Confusion
  - Ileus.

## Ventilatory function

The arterial oxygen tension ($PaO_2$) is determined by four factors (also see Box 13.5 and case history):

- **Inspired [$O_2$]/barometric pressure.**
- **Alveolar ventilation.**
- **Alveolar/pulmonary capillary diffusion.**
- **Ventilation/perfusion matching.**

$PaO_2$ can be improved in a number of ways that will be discussed in more detail later in the chapter, namely:

- Use of supplemental $O_2$ with humidification.
- Physiotherapy/positioning.
- Non-invasive ventilation (NIV):
  - CPAP (continuous positive airway pressure)
  - BIPAP (bilevel positive airway pressure).
- Mechanical ventilation.
- Pharmacological: nitric oxide.
- Extracorporeal membrane oxygenation.

# 13.3 Organ support in multi-organ failure

## Daily supportive care

### Overview

- Despite numerous clinical trials of novel ventilatory and pharmacological interventions, very few have ever been shown to provide a mortality benefit to patients in ICU.
- It is increasingly recognized that 'the process of care in ICU' is fundamentally important.
- Daily implementation of evidence-based care bundles such as '**FASTHUG**' and the use of individualized daily physiological targets may be beneficial (Box 13.8).

### Feeding

- No route has proved definitively superior but enteral is favoured over parenteral and may prevent stress ulceration.
- Trials are ongoing to identify the optimal route of feeding in critical care.
- In general provide 25kcal/kg body weight/day.
- Glutamine has been suggested to be beneficial when using total parenteral nutrition (TPN) for prolonged period (>10 days) but a recent trial has reported that this may cause harm.
- Numerous tests exist to confirm nasogastric tube position, but CXR remains the gold standard.

### Analgesia, sedation, and paralysis

- Analgesics and sedatives should be used sparingly but safely and are important in preventing asynchrony with mechanical ventilation.
- They may be used as continuous infusions or bolus injections.
- Commonly used analgesics include the opiates, morphine and fentanyl; sedatives include midazolam and haloperidol.
- Sedation scoring systems exist to ensure accurate dosing occurs and may reduce the overall amount required (Box 13.9).
- Studies suggest that breaks in sedation—'sedation holidays'—may be beneficial.
- There is increasing evidence that long-term use of opiates and sedatives result in poor psychological outcome in critical care patients.
- Long-term use of paralysing agents should be avoided if possible as they can increase risk of critical illness polyneuropathy.

### Thromboprophylaxis

- Studies suggest that rates of deep vein thrombosis are between 13% and 31% in ICU patients not receiving thromboprophylaxis.
- Subcutaneous heparin is therefore advocated unless contraindicated.

### Head-up

- Several studies have shown that elevation of the head of the bed to 30–45° reduces gastro-oesophageal reflux in mechanically ventilated patients.

---

**Box 13.8 FASTHUG care bundle**

**F** Feeding
**A** Analgesia
**S** Sedation
**T** Thromboprophylaxis
**H** Head-up
**U** Ulcer prophylaxis
**G** Glycaemic control
Source: Vincent JL, 'Give your patient a fast hug (at least) once a day', *Critical Care Medicine*, 33(6), PP. 1225–9, 2005.

---

**Box 13.9 The UCLH Sedation Score**

3 Agitated and restless
2 Awake and uncomfortable
1 Aware but calm
0 Roused by voice, remains calm
−1 Roused by movement
−2 Roused by painful stimuli
−3 Unrousable
A Natural sleep
Data from University College London Hospitals

---

- It may also reduce the incidence of ventilator-associated pneumonia (VAP).
- It is important that the patient's **thorax and head** should be elevated.

### Stress ulcer prophylaxis

- This is particularly important for patients receiving steroids, with coagulopathy or history of gastrointestinal haemorrhage.
- Routine use following major surgery or trauma is not usually required.
- H2 antagonists, antacids, and proton pump inhibitors have all been used but the optimal agent is not known.

### Glycaemic control (GC)

- Maintenance of blood glucose levels <10mM/L in ICU patients is thought to be optimal practice.
- Previous studies of tighter glycaemic control (4.4–6.1), which had suggested a mortality benefit were not found to be beneficial.

---

## Other important daily considerations

### Target haemoglobin

- RBC transfusions are administered to augment $O_2$ delivery and avoid deleterious effects of $O_2$ debt.
- However, critically ill patients appear to be at increased risk of immunosuppressive and microcirculatory problems associated with blood transfusion.
- It has been shown that a **restrictive** strategy, with transfusion only given if Hb ≤7g/dL, is associated with improved mortality rate in critically ill patients.
- This strategy may be withheld in patients with significant cardiac disease.
- Treatment of disseminated intravascular coagulation (DIC), which may complicate ICU admission is supportive.

### Catheter-related bloodstream infection (CRBSI)

- ~90% of CRBSI occur with central venous catheters (CVCs).
- It has been approximated that 250,000 CVCs are used each year in the UK, with 30,000 infections per annum, costing £10 million.
- CVC infection is the largest cause of hospital-acquired bacteraemia.
- Mortality rate for CRBSI secondary to CVC is 25% in some patient groups.
- CVC infection occurs via three routes; **intraluminal**, **extraluminal**, or **haematogenous**.
- CVC infection presents locally or systemically.
- If present, the two key questions are:
  - Does the line need removal?
  - Does the patient need antibiotics?

1. Severe sepsis.
2. Persistent fever or bacteraemia despite antimicrobials.
3. Septic thrombosis of a central vein.
4. Septic emboli from the CVC.
5. Infection with organisms of high virulence such as *Staphylococcus aureus, Pseudomonas* species, and yeasts.

- If CVC infection is suspected, assess need for line removal and take peripheral blood cultures.
- If patient is unwell, do not wait for cultures results before starting antibiotics.
- Rates of CVC infection may be improved with meticulous aseptic technique of the operator, advances in design of the device, and high-quality care of the patient and device, pre and post insertion.
- Although it is associated with the least risk of infection, subclavian CVC insertion may be avoided due to risk of pneumothorax (Boxes 13.10 and 13.11).

## Respiratory

### Definition of respiratory failure
- **Type 1:** $PaO_2$ <8kPa with normal/low $PaCO_2$.
- **Type 2:** $PaO_2$ <8kPa and a $PaCO_2$ >6kPa. (Figs 13.2 and 13.3)

Box 13.11 Suggested CVC care bundle

1. Maximal hand hygiene.
2. Maximal barrier precautions upon insertion including prepared trolley, adherent drapes, cap, and gown.
3. Skin antisepsis using 2% chlorhexidine, allowing 30 seconds to dry.
4. Use of internal jugular, subclavian, then femoral vein as preferred route, unless not clinically indicated.
5. Use of sutureless StatLock® at sites liable to movement and BioPatch® at entry site to maintain antisepsis.
6. Daily review of line necessity with prompt removal of unnecessary lines.

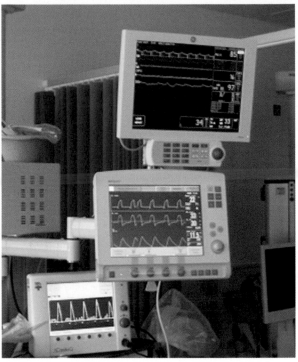

**Fig. 13.2** Critical Care Monitoring.

### NIV vs. invasive ventilation
- NIV is defined as ventilatory support provided via a tight fitting mask or similar interface **as opposed to** invasive support, which is provided via a laryngeal mask, endotracheal tube, or tracheostomy tube (Fig. 13.4).
- Tight fitting masks deliver CPAP, BIPAP, or NIV via the mechanical ventilator (Box 13.12).

### Indications for mechanical ventilation
- The work of breathing usually accounts for 5% of oxygen consumption ($VO_2$). In the critically ill patient this may rise to 30%.

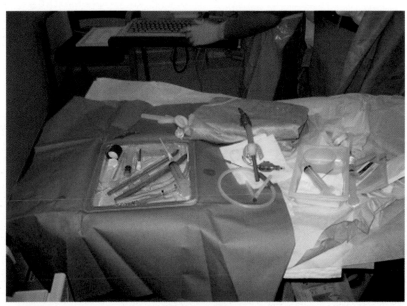

**Fig. 13.3** Percutaneous tracheostomy kit.

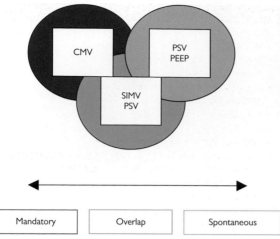

| Mandatory | Overlap | Spontaneous |

Fig. 13.4 Basic non-invasive and invasive ventilation algorithm.

- Invasive mechanical ventilation eliminates the metabolic cost of breathing.
- Mechanical ventilation for the following:
  - Inadequate oxygenation (not corrected by supplemental $O_2$ by mask).
  - Inadequate ventilation (increased $PaCO_2$).
  - Retention of pulmonary secretions (bronchial toilet).
  - Airway protection (obtunded patient, depressed gag reflex).

## Basics of positive pressure mechanical ventilation
- Positive pressure ventilation involves delivering a mechanically generated 'breath' to get $O_2$ in and $CO_2$ out.
- Gas is pumped in during inspiration (Ti) and the patient passively expires during expiration (Te).
- The sum of Ti and Te is the respiratory cycle or 'breath'.
- When patients are intubated, they usually receive continuous mandatory breaths (**CMV**), which are **volume**, **pressure**, or **time** cycled.
- In the different modes, the mechanical ventilator switches from inspiration to expiration when a preset volume, pressure, or time is achieved/delivered.
- Mandatory breaths are delivered during inspiration, to generate a tidal volume (**Vt**), at a set rate (**f**), the quotient of which is the minute volume (**MV**).
- Depending on the type of ventilation used, an **inspiratory flow** rate is set.
- The ratio of the time spent in inspiration: expiration (**I:E ratio**) is usually 1:2.
- Mechanically ventilated patients usually receive positive end-expiratory pressure (**PEEP**), to overcome the loss of physiological PEEP provided by the larynx and vocal cords.
- PEEP is delivered **throughout** the respiratory cycle and is **synonymous to CPAP**, but in the intubated patient.

### Box 13.12 CPAP vs. BIPAP
- CPAP—particularly beneficial:
  - Type 1 respiratory failure.
  - Alveolar oedema.
- BIPAP—particularly beneficial:
  - Type 2 respiratory failure.
  - If started before pH <7.25.
  - If secondary to acute exacerbation of COPD.

### Box 13.13 Bare essentials for intubation: ALSOBLEED
1. **A**irway: oral Guedel airway to lift tongue off posterior pharynx to facilitate mask ventilation during pre-intubation phase.
2. **L**iquids: stop feed and aspirate nasogastric tube.
3. **S**uction: extremely important to avoid pulmonary aspiration.
4. **O**xygen: preoxygenate patient and ensure a source of $O_2$ with a delivery mechanism (ambu-bag and mask) is available.
5. **B**ougie: to facilitate tube insertion in more difficult airway.
6. **L**aryngoscope: have a long and short blade available.
7. **E**ndotracheal tube: for average adult, cuffed oral endotracheal tube 7.0 for women and 8.0 for men.
8. **E**nd-tidal $CO_2$: to confirm correct position of tube.
9. **D**rugs: an induction agent, muscle relaxant, and sedative are usually required.

- Sedation is often required to prevent ventilator-patient asynchrony.
- Once stabilized on CMV, the level of ventilatory support may be reduced (**weaning**) by providing a mixture of synchronized intermittent mandatory breaths (**SIMV**) and spontaneously triggered pressure supported breaths (**PSV**).
- Pressure support is delivered during **inspiration**.
- As patients improve, they may be able to receive pressure-supported breaths alone or breathe spontaneously with or without PEEP. This should be encouraged as respiratory muscle function is maintained (Boxes 13.13–13.17).

### Successful weaning and extubation
- To succeed, the initiating cause of respiratory failure, sepsis, fluid and electrolyte imbalance, and nutritional status should all be treated or optimized.
- Failure to wean is associated with:
  - Ongoing high $VO_2$.
  - Muscle fatigue.
  - Inadequate drive.
  - Inadequate cardiac reserve.
- Weaning screens exist to help select patients for extubation.
- In the unsupported patient, if f/Vt is >200, extubation is likely to be successful.

### Box 13.14 Basic ventilator terminology
Vt Tidal volume
f Respiratory rate (breaths/cycles per minute)
Ti Inspiratory time
Te Expiratory time
Cycle = Ti + Te
I:E ratio Inspiratory:expiratory ratio
$FiO_2$ Inspired $O_2$ concentration
Pi Inspiratory pressure
PAP Peak airway pressure
$P_{PLAT}$ Plateau pressure
PIFR Peak inspiratory flow rate
CMV Continuous mandatory ventilation
SIMV Synchronized intermittent mandatory ventilation
PCV Pressure controlled ventilation
VCV Volume controlled ventilation
PSV Pressure support ventilation
PEEP Positive-end expiratory pressure
CPAP Continuous positive airway pressure
NIV Non-invasive ventilation

---

**Box 13.15 Basic ventilator settings (mode dependent)**

1. Set $FiO_2$.
2. Set Vt at 8–10mL/kg.
3. Set f at 10–15/minute.
4. Set I:E ratio at 1:2.
5. Set PIFR at 40–80L/minute.
6. Set PEEP at 5cmH$_2$O.
7. Set PAP at ≤30cmH$_2$O.

---

- There is some evidence to support extubation to NIV, particularly in patients with COPD.

## Tracheostomy

- Is considered in all patients with prolonged intubation, but ideal time to perform is not currently known.
- Can be performed surgically in theatre but studies suggest morbidity is reduced if carried out on ICU via percutaneous route.
- Facilitates weaning and reduces VAP.

## Useful investigations

- **Radiology:**
  - Routine daily CXRs have now been shown to be of little benefit and should only be taken if clinically indicated.
  - Ultrasound is increasingly used to diagnose pleural effusion.
  - CT may be useful in the diagnosis of respiratory conditions such as ARDS, but involves patient transfer, which may outweigh any benefit.
- **Bronchoscopy:**
  - Is particularly useful in collection of diagnostic samples and relief of endobronchial obstruction.

---

# Renal

## Acute kidney injury in critical care

- Acute kidney injury (AKI; previously called acute renal failure) occurs in 1–25% of critically ill patients.
- Usually due to acute tubular necrosis as a result of circulatory failure and sepsis.
- Coexistent organ failure is common.
- Mortality rate is high (50–80%).
- Renal function recovers in most patients surviving critical illness and only a small number end up needing long-term renal replacement therapy.

## Continuous renal replacement therapy (CRRT)

- Critically ill patients who develop AKI may require CRRT, 'going on the filter' (Box 13.18).
- **C**ontinuous pumped **v**eno-**v**enous **h**aemofiltration (CVVH) or **d**iafiltration (CVVHDF), are usually used.

---

**Box 13.16 Improving oxygenation and $CO_2$ Clearance**

- Depending on ventilatory mode, **other** than increasing $FiO_2$, oxygenation can be improved by increasing alveolar pressure and alveolar ventilation. To achieve this:
  - Increase PEEP.
  - Increase Ti.
  - Increase Vt or Pi.
- Improved $CO_2$ elimination is largely dependent on increasing alveolar ventilation. To achieve this:
  - Increase Vt.
  - Increase f.
  - Decrease deadspace.

---

**Box 13.17 Types of mechanical ventilation and application**

- **Volume cycled:**
  - Vt and f are set.
  - Ventilator cycles when set Vt reached.
  - **Time=Vol/Flow**.
  - Ti can be increased by increasing Vt, reducing PIFR or increasing length of cycle (by decreasing f).
- **Time cycled:**
  - Vt and f are set.
  - Ventilator cycles when set time elapses.
  - Ti can be increased by directly increasing Ti or decreasing f.
  - Increasing Ti will decrease PIFR and reduce PAP.
- **Pressure cycled:**
  - Pi is set to generate Vt.
  - Ventilator cycles when set pressure achieved.
  - Ti can be increased directly to increase Vt and PIFR.

---

- CVVH is **convective** whereas CVVHDF is both **convective** and **diffusive**.
- Both techniques:
  - Based on use of highly permeable membrane (**filter**; Box 13.19).
  - Require a pump to generate **flow rate** and an **extracorporeal circuit**, which may require **anticoagulation**.
  - Large volumes of fluid are removed and replaced (**buffer**).
  - Performed via double-lumen catheter in large central vein.
  - May cause a reduction in core temperature of ~1°C.
  - Can reduce platelet count and impair platelet function.
  - May interfere with cardiac monitor when running.
- Haemodialysis can also be performed in critically ill patients but is more likely to cause haemodynamic instability due to the pump speeds required.

## Choice of replacement fluid (buffer)

- During CVVH/DF, many solutes are removed including **bicarbonate**, which must be replaced.
- **Lactate** is the standard buffer used in replacement fluid, which is metabolized to bicarbonate by the liver.
- In the severely unwell patient, lactate may fail to be metabolized, $H^+$ ions are produced, and a lactic acidosis may arise (Box 13.20).
- '**Lactate-free**' buffer with bicarbonate replacement may be required in these patients.

## Anticoagulation

- May not be required if coagulopathy present.
- If required, unfractionated heparin is usually used (monitor APTT).

---

**Box 13.18 Indications for CRRT in critical illness**

1. Severe metabolic acidosis.
2. Fluid overload.
3. Hyperkalaemia.
4. Oligo/anuria despite circulatory resuscitation.
5. Symptomatic uraemia.
6. Drug overdose with dialysable agent.
7. Concurrent treatment of severe sepsis, ARDS, pancreatitis, hepatic failure, hyperthermia.

## Box 13.19 Problematic filter clotting

- If heparin contraindicated, heparin-induced thrombocytopaenia (HIT) or thrombocytopaenia of other cause present, consider **epoprostenol** (reversible platelet inhibitor).
- Natural anticoagulants antithrombin III and heparin co-factor II may be consumed in critical illness so consider infusion of **FFP**.
- Consider **higher flow rates** on filter.
- Using **sodium citrate** pre-filter, with **calcium infusion** post filter allows citrate to chelate calcium and inhibit calcium-dependent clotting factors.

## Prevention of AKI in critical care

1. Avoid nephrotoxic drugs/alter doses.
2. Avoid iatrogenic haemodynamic instability.
3. Treat elevated IAP (Box 13.21).

## Contrast media nephropathy

- CT with the use of contrast often plays a vital role in the investigation of the critically ill patient.
- Contrast media may cause significant deterioration in renal function in a patient already compromised.
- No agent has been conclusively shown to prevent this happening but a continuous infusion of 1.26% sodium bicarbonate may be useful.
- The best policy is to keep the patient adequately fluid loaded.

# Abdominal/liver

## Intra-abdominal hypertension (IAH) and abdominal compartment syndrome (ACS)

- Are increasingly recognized in critically ill and standardized definitions now exist.
- Causes of raised intra-abdominal pressure (IAP) — see Box 13.21.
- **IAH** is defined as IAP ≥**12**mmHg.
- **ACS** is defined as IAP ≥**20**mmHg, with organ dysfunction/failure.
- Elevated IAP causes diaphragmatic splinting and can dramatically reduce functional residual capacity (FRC) and ventilation.
- It can also precipitate renal failure through multiple mechanisms.
- Abdominal perfusion pressure = MAP − IAP, and as a guide this should be ≥50.
- If IAP is ≥**25** with evidence of **end-organ dysfunction**, surgical decompression can be considered (see Box 13.22 for grades of IAP).
- Bladder pressure is easily measured and is an accurate index of IAP.

## Box 13.20 Lactic acidosis

- Type **A**—inadequate supply of $O_2$ to the tissues:
  - All causes of shock.
  - Severe hypoxia.
  - Severe anaemia.
- Type **B**—where tissues hypoxia is **not** the obvious cause of lactaemia:
  - DKA.
  - Renal, liver failure.
  - Ethanol, methanol, ethylene glycol poisoning.

## Box 13.21 Causes of raised IAP in critical illness

1. Fluid (ascites).
2. Haemorrhage.
3. Tissue oedema (sepsis, ischaemia).
4. Gas (perforated viscus).
5. Abdominal packs.
6. Tumour.

## Box 13.22 Grades of IAP (mm Hg)

I: 12–15
II: 16–20
III: 21–25
IV: >25.

## Acute liver failure/acute on chronic liver failure (ALF/ACLF)

- Although discussed elsewhere in this book (see Section 9.11), the major consequences of ALF/ACLF are very important in critical care including:
  - **Metabolic**: ↓ glucose/↑ lactate.
  - **Immune**: bacteraemia.
  - **Synthetic**: coagulopathy.
  - **Detoxification**: ↑ $NH_3$.
- Mainstay of ICU support includes:
  - Removal of precipitant.
  - Optimization of conditions for liver regeneration, i.e. sepsis.
  - Treating complications.
  - Identify transplantable patients (Box 13.23).
- ACLF is much more common than ALF.
- Severity of ACLF can be assessed by Child–Pugh Score (CPC), model for end-stage liver disease (MELD) or SOFA.
- ALF can be subdivided into hyperacute (<7 days), acute (8–28 days), subacute (5–12 weeks), based on time from **jaundice** to **encephalopathy**.
- Both may be complicated by encephalopathy but ALF has a higher incidence of **cerebral oedema**/intracranial hypertension.
- Invasive cerebral monitoring, early intubation/mechanical ventilation/use of hypertonic saline may be required (also see 'Neurological' topic later in this section).

## Box 13.23 Selection for transplantation in ALF

- **Paracetamol:**
  - Arterial pH <7.3.
- **Or** concurrent findings of
  - Encephalopathy ≥grade III.
  - Creatinine >300mmol/L.
  - INR >6.5.
- **Non-paracetamol:**
  - INR >6.7.
- **Or any 3** of
  - Unfavourable aetiology, i.e. drugs.
  - Age <10 or >40 years.
  - Acute/subacute presentation.
  - Bilirubin >300mmol/L.
  - INR >3.5.

### Extracorporeal liver support

- There has been interest in using this technique for detoxification in ALF/ACLF and the hepatorenal syndrome.
- Whereas renal dialysis primarily removes **water-soluble** toxins, liver dialysis aims to remove **albumin-bound** toxins, which accumulate in liver failure.
- **MARS®** (Molecular Adsorbents Recirculation System) is the best-known technique available, which removes toxins including ammonia, bile acids, bilirubin, copper, iron, and phenols.
- However no RCTs currently exist confirming definitive benefit in the described conditions.

---

## Cardiovascular

### Invasive monitoring

- Many patients in the ICU will require placement of a venous **central line** and **arterial line** to guide therapy.
- Central lines can be inserted into internal jugular, subclavian, or femoral veins and should be inserted using ultrasound guidance.
- They are used to assess right-sided filling pressure and are also useful for measuring central venous oxygenation as discussed previously.
- This makes them particularly useful for guiding volume responsiveness and fluid resuscitation (see later in topic), but also vital for drug administration and parenteral feeding.
- Arterial lines are particularly useful in the cardiovascularly unstable patient and usually mandatory if vasopressors or inotropes are being used.
- They also allow regular measurement of blood arterial oxygen and carbon dioxide tensions and the metabolic status of the patient, without repeated arterial stabs being performed.
- Arterial cannulae are usually sited in the radial artery but pedal, femoral, and brachial sites are also used.
- Compliant tubing connects the cannula to a transducer which converts the detected pulse to a waveform and BP recording.

### Measurement of cardiac output

- There are a number of ways the CO can be measured in critically ill patients involving a techniques such as the Fick principle, dilution, Doppler ultrasound, bioimpedance, and arterial pulse contour analysis.
- The most invasive is by using a **pulmonary artery catheter** (PAC), which uses thermodilution.
- However, a number of studies have now shown that the risk of using a PAC outweighs the benefit and routine use is not suggested.
- The **lithium dilution cardiac output** (LIDCO) technique relies on using a venous bolus injection of lithium chloride (peripherally or centrally) and blood to be withdrawn arterially over a lithium sensor.

**Box 13.24  The fluid challenge and CVP**

1. Measure the baseline CVP.
2. Rapidly administer 200mL of fluid (usually colloid) centrally or peripherally.
3. After 5–10 minutes, re-assess CVP.
4. If the CVP is rises by ≤3cmH$_2$O and falls again in a short time, assume point **a** of graph in Fig. 13.7, the patient is underfilled, continue to fill.
5. If CVP rises by ≤3cmH$_2$O and the effect is **sustained**, assume point **b** of graph, the patient is filled.
6. If CVP rises ≥3cmH$_2$O, assume point **c** of graph, the patient is volume overloaded.
7. The same principles can be used when assessing a ≥10% change in stroke volume while using an oesophageal Doppler.

---

- Software provides pulse contour analysis and 'beat to beat' CO monitoring.
- **Pulse-induced contour cardiac output** (PiCCO) has similarities to PAC and LIDCO and uses a cold centrally administered venous bolus injection and a arterially placed thermistor to measure transpulmonary thermodilution, with software to calculate the CO.
- The **oesophageal Doppler probe** uses ultrasound to detect the velocity of blood in the descending aorta. When combined with the aortic cross-sectional area, the stroke volume is calculated and CO estimated.
- Although this method usually requires some sedation, it is frequently used for CO monitoring as it is less invasive than some of the methods described earlier.
- Other novel non-invasive CO monitoring (NICO) techniques are emerging and suprasternal Doppler, transoesophageal, and transthoracic echocardiography have also been described for CO monitoring.

### Volume responsiveness

- Accurate assessment of the volume responsiveness (or adequacy of cardiac preload) is vitally important in the ICU patient in the haemodynamically unstable patient (see Fig. 13.5).
- The patient should be assessed clinically (as discussed earlier) but invasive monitoring can also be used as a guide.
- The most simple manoeuvre is to perform a straight leg raise, which gives the patient a rapid volume challenge.
- This can be titrated against CVP or stroke volume response using the oesophageal Doppler.
- The fluid challenge (see Box 13.24 and Fig. 13.6) is also a vital tool in volume assessment, the aim again to assess the effect of a rapid fluid bolus on CVP or stroke volume.
- If a patient is oligoanuric, frusemide should not be routinely administered before volume responsiveness is optimized.

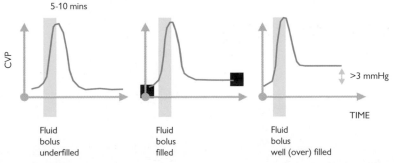

**Fig. 13.5** The Oesophageal Doppler Waveform.

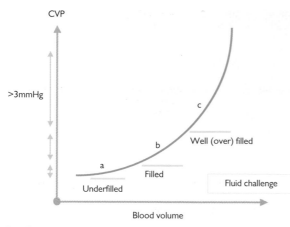

**Fig. 13.6** Fluid challenge.

## Which fluid for volume resuscitation?

- This remains one of the most controversial areas in ICU care.
- Crystalloid, gelatins, albumin, and starches have all been used to expand the plasma volume in hypovolaemia and shock.
- In general, larger volumes of crystalloid then colloid are required for resuscitation, due to rapid redistribution through the extravascular space.
- This has classically led to colloid being favoured over crystalloid, as extravascular accumulation of fluid in critically ill patients is thought to have an increased morbidity.
- Albumin is used in many ICUs, and has been shown to be safe, but is questionably of no additional benefit than any other agent.
- Starches have also favoured but studies have suggested that their use is associated with an increased risk of renal dysfunction and coagulopathy and they have been withdrawn in UK critical care units.
- The choice of maintenance fluid for the ICU patient is also controversial and varies on the volume status and underlying illness.
- It is worthwhile remembering that one of the commonest iatrogenic causes of acidaemia is the over-zealous use of 0.9% sodium chloride.

## Inotropes and vasopressors

- If volume optimization is not successful or relatively contraindicated, i.e. critical pump failure, these agents may be required to treat cardiovascular instability in ICU patients.

- The causes of shock have been discussed earlier (see Section 13.2) but broadly speaking, if pump failure is present, an inotrope will be required and if there is circulatory collapse (as in sepsis/anaphylaxis), a vasopressor is used.
- However, both scenarios may occur in tandem or a result of one another and both agents may be required together.
- The choice of agent is also controversial, but there are few clinical trials to suggest the use of one agent over another.
- A pragmatic choice is to use adrenaline for pump failure with the addition of glyceryl trinitrate (GTN) if there is significantly elevated afterload (SVR). Another option for this scenario is to use dobutamine which has favourable effects on pump function and peripheral vasodilatory qualities.
- Noradrenaline is the usual drug of choice for situations associated with dramatic afterload (SVR) reduction, i.e. sepsis.
- All agents are highly potent and can induce tachyarrhythmias and myocardial instability.

### The oesophageal Doppler waveform
See Fig. 13.5.

# Neurological

### Traumatic brain injury (TBI)

- Trauma is the commonest cause of death before 40 years of age in the Western world
- Head injury is the major cause of death and disability with long-term consequences and profound healthcare and economic implications.
- The head is a fixed bony box with a constant volume with approximate intracranial components of 1600mL volume, of which 80% is parenchyma, 10% CSF, 10% blood.
- The normal intracranial pressure (ICP) is pressure <15cmH$_2$O.
- If the pressure perfusing the arteries of almost any organ is varied, flow through the organ changes very little (**autoregulation**).
- Autoregulation only occurs between certain pressure limits—if the pressure drops too low or is too high, autoregulation fails, and organ perfusion is compromised.
- This concept is of particular importance in TBI where autoregulation is disturbed.
- If the ICP rises, cerebral blood flow is interrupted, reducing the cerebral perfusion pressure (CPP).
- The CPP can be derived from the following equation:
  CPP = MAP − (ICP + CVP)

The CPP should ideally be ≥60 and the ICP ≤20 (Box 13.25).

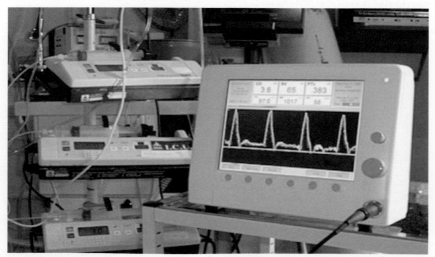

**Fig. 13.7** "The Oesophageal Doppler Waveform"

## Box 13.25 Therapeutic options for ICP >20 or CPP <60

- Sedate and paralyse.
- Consider CSF drainage.
- Hypothermia 35°C.
- Mannitol.
- Hypertonic saline.
- Moderate hyperventilation.
- CT scan.
- Barbiturates or rescue craniotomy.

- Following TBI, as an intracranial mass lesion or oedematous brain expands, some compensation occurs as CSF and blood move into the spinal canal and extracranial vasculature.
- After this, further compensation is impossible and ICP rises dramatically, requiring urgent intervention.

### Management of intracranial hypertension

- Following TBI, a key factor in determining outcome (Table 13.2) is the management of secondary brain injury and inadequate oxygenation of brain tissue.
- Key parameters that can be influenced include brain swelling, decrease in cerebral blood flow, increase in ICP, decrease in $O_2$ delivery, and energy failure (Fig. 13.8).
- In general, all patients should be adequately sedated and may also need paralysing agents if coughing is associated with rises in ICP.
- Brain swelling can be treated in a number of ways.
- Hyperventilation to keep $PaCO_2$ 4.0–4.5kPa may reduce oedema as rising $CO_2$ levels cause vasodilatation.
- Positioning the patient 20° head-up, avoiding tight endotracheal tube ties, and removing hard-collars (once cervical spine # is excluded) are also useful.
- Intravenous mannitol expands circulating volume, decreases blood viscosity, and therefore increases cerebral blood flow and cerebral oxygen delivery.
- Hypertonic 1.8% NaCl is also thought to be beneficial but **both** of these agents may have the **opposite effect** if the blood–brain barrier is breached as a result of TBI.
- Decrease in cerebral blood flow is avoided by ensuring that patients with severe brain injury are kept normovolaemic.
- Free water (5% dextrose solutions) should be avoided as they decrease plasma osmolality and increase the water content of brain tissue.
- In addition, elevated blood sugar levels are associated with a worsening of neurological injury.
- If the CPP target cannot be achieved, vasopressors (usually noradrenaline) or inotropes (adrenaline) may be required.
- Dramatic increases in ICP that are not corrected by standard ventilatory or pharmacological means, can be treated with boluses of mannitol, barbiturates (usually thiopentone), or may require the insertion of a CSF drain or a decompressive craniotomy.
- Oxygen delivery should be optimized by aiming for a target $pO_2$ ≥12kPa.
- Energy failure can be managed by cooling and ensuring normoglycaemia.

### Table 13.2 Outcome of severe head injury

| | |
|---|---|
| Death | 20–40% |
| Persistent vegetative state | 1–10% |
| Severe disability | 5–20% |
| Moderate disability | 20–30% |
| Good recovery | 20–40% (work) |

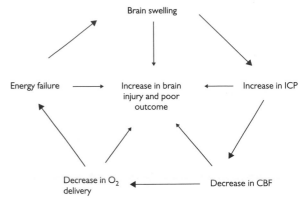

Fig. 13.8 Pathophysiology of traumatic brain injury

- It has been shown in studies that corticosteroids should not be routinely used in the treatment of head injury.

### Monitoring

- ICP monitoring is a central part of critical care management for the severe TBI.
- ICP measurement is necessary to accurately determine CPP but has not been conclusively shown to alter outcome in TBI.
- Generally, it is accepted that maintaining an adequate CPP is most important.
- ICP monitoring should be considered in all patients with severe head injury (GCS score <9) and those patients with moderate head injury (GCS score 9–12) and increased risk (Box 13.26).
- There are a number of ways to measure the ICP but arguably the most accurate is with an intraventricular catheter connected to a pressure transducer.
- They have the added advantage that CSF can be drained in an emergency but do have an infection risk.
- Intraparenchymal 'bolts' can also be used.
- Monitoring of the ICP and CPP is important, but gives little idea of the overall state of the injured brain and does not measure oxygen delivery and usage.

## Box 13.26 The Glasgow Coma Scale score (15 points)

**Best eye response (4):**
No eye opening.
Eye opening to pain.
Eye opening to verbal command.
Eyes open spontaneously.
**Best verbal response (5):**
No verbal response
Incomprehensible sounds.
Inappropriate words.
Confused
Orientated
**Best motor response (6):**
No motor response.
Extension to pain.
Flexion to pain.
Withdrawal from pain.
Localizing pain.
Obeys commands.
Reprinted from the *Lancet*, 2(7872), Teasdale G, Jennett B, Assessment of coma and impaired consciousness. A practical scale, 81–4, 1974, with permission from Elsevier.

- The cerebral metabolic rate for oxygen ($CMRO_2$) can be defined as: $CMRO_2 = CBF \times OEF \times SaO_2$ (CBF = cerebral blood flow; OEF = oxygen extraction fraction).
- Jugular venous bulb oximetry ($SjO_2$), is measured by placing a catheter in the internal jugular vein and directing upwards.
- $SjO_2$ reflects CBF and will fall when there is an imbalance between oxygen consumption and delivery (normal range 50–75%).
- Brain tissue oxygenation ($PtO_2$), intracerebral microdialysis probes to measure pyruvate and lactate, transcranial Doppler USS, continuous cerebral function monitoring via EEG, MRI, PET, and SPECT scanning, have all been described as adding additional value in monitoring the injured brain, but their use is not commonplace.
- The Lund Concept can also be used for the treatment of severe TBI, and is based on basic principles regarding brain volume and cerebral perfusion.

- The concept assumes breakdown of the blood–brain barrier and is ICP-directed and perfusion-directed therapy, not CPP-directed therapy.
- Thus the therapy has two main goals:
  - To reduce or prevent an increase in ICP (ICP-targeted goal).
  - To improve perfusion and oxygenation around contusions (perfusion-targeted goal).
- There are four principles:
  - Reduce the stress response and energy metabolism using sedation, not overfeeding, and avoiding cooling.
  - Reduce capillary hydrostatic pressure by controlling MAP.
  - Maintaining colloid osmotic pressure by targeting serum albumin of ≥40g/dL and plasma Hb of ≥12g/dL.
  - Reducing intracerebral blood volume by using barbiturates (thiopentone).
- Emerging studies suggest that clinical outcome using the concept results in a more favourable outcome than previous CPP-directed approaches.

## Acute lung injury/acute respiratory distress syndrome (ALI/ARDS)

### Epidemiology

- First described by Ashbaugh in 1967, but the incidence of ALI and ARDS has increased and ~200,000 cases per year occur in the USA.
- However, the mortality rate of the condition has improved to 30–40%, thought due to the improved level of support patients now receive in ICU, rather than a specific therapeutic intervention per se.
- In addition, death is not usually related to respiratory failure, but normally due to the underlying condition that manifested as ALI/ARDS in the first instance or late sepsis.

### Aetiology

- Aetiology of ALI/ARDS is diverse and the disorders associated with the condition are divided into those which cause **direct** lung injury, i.e. bronchopneumonia, or **indirect** lung injury, i.e. severe sepsis (Fig. 13.9).
- Environmental factors such as age, sex, smoking history, and pre-existing lung disease may also have an influence.
- More recently, candidate genes have been proposed to alter the progression of ALI/ARDS and the concept of ventilogenomics has arisen, as it is thought that certain genotypes determine

the response of the lung to the injurious effects of mechanical ventilation.

### Pathogenesis and basic science

- Classically, three phases to ALI/ARDS were described; exudative/inflammatory, proliferative, and fibrotic.
- The **exudative** phase is characterized histologically by diffuse alveolar damage (DAD), where the microvascular endothelial and alveolar epithelium of the alveolar–capillary barrier is breached. This leads to the leak of haemorrhagic non-cardiogenic pulmonary oedema fluid into alveoli, promoting fibrinous hyaline membrane formation. Shearing of the epithelium injures type II pneumocytes so that surfactant production is reduced, reducing lung compliance. Intense neutrophilic infiltration also accompanies these changes along with the release of a plethora of pro-inflammatory and pro-fibrotic cytokines, chemokines, and growth factors, from resident and recruited cells.
- Subsequently, **proliferation** of intimal cells, type II cells, and fibroblasts/myofibroblasts proliferate in an attempt to repair the damage.
- During the **fibrotic** phase, myointimal thickening, promoting pulmonary hypertension and mature lung collagen is deposited, the severity of which correlates with an increase in mortality.
- However, this classic theory of pathogenesis has been challenged as there is increasing evidence that there is much overlap between

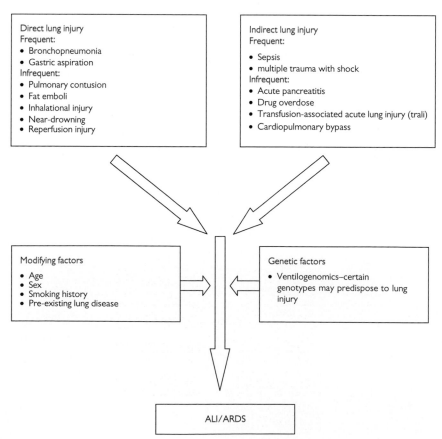

**Fig. 13.9** Management of ALI/ARDS.

## Box 13.27 VAP and VILI

- VAP has a mortality rate of up to 50%.
- Nursing patients in the semi-recumbent position has been shown to decrease VAP.
- Continuous aspiration of subglottic secretions (CASS) may prevent VAP but remains controversial.

the phases of ALI/ARDS and in particular, that fibrosis may be initiated within the first 24 hours after diagnosis

- This may explain why many of the pharmacological therapies described in the following sections, have proved ineffective.
- It is also crucial to be aware that ALI/ARDS can be exacerbated by mechanical ventilation and nosocomial infection leading to ventilator-induced lung injury (VILI) and ventilator-associated pneumonia (VAP) respectively (Box 13.27).

### Diagnosis and clinical evaluation

- ALI/ARDS is diagnosed using the American/European definition of ALI/ARDS.
- Although favoured by many, other observers argue that the diagnosis is too simple and in particular does not take into account the underlying cause or that individual interpretation of the CXR can lead to bias. A further issue is that the PACs, which are fundamental to the diagnosis, are now infrequently used in ICU.
- For this reason, most clinicians use the absence of clinical or **diagnostic evidence of left ventricular dysfunction** to fulfil this part of the definition (Table 13.3).

### Table 13.3

| | Acute lung injury | Acute respiratory distress syndrome |
|---|---|---|
| CXR | Bilateral infiltrates/ airspace shadowing | Bilateral infiltrates/ airspace shadowing |
| Clinical scenario | Acute onset | Acute onset |
| Pulmonary artery wedge pressure | <18mmHg (or no clinical or diagnostic evidence of left ventricular dysfunction) | <18mmHg (or no clinical or diagnostic evidence of left ventricular dysfunction) |
| Oxygenation | $PaO_2/FiO_2$ ratio <300mmHg (<39.9kPa) | $PaO_2/FiO_2$ ratio <200mmHg (<26.6kPa) |

## Specific management of patients with ALI/ARDS

### Ventilatory strategies

- The general supportive measures described earlier in the chapter are extremely pertinent in ALI/ARDS as patients often spend many days on the ICU, but specific ventilatory strategies are also vitally important (Fig. 13.10).
- Classically, patients with ALI/ARDS were ventilated with high tidal volumes of 10–15mL/kg. Increasing concern about VILI led to a landmark ARDSNet study being performed which showed that **reducing tidal volumes to 4–6mL/kg** and setting **inspiratory plateau pressures** (PPLAT) at a **maximum of**

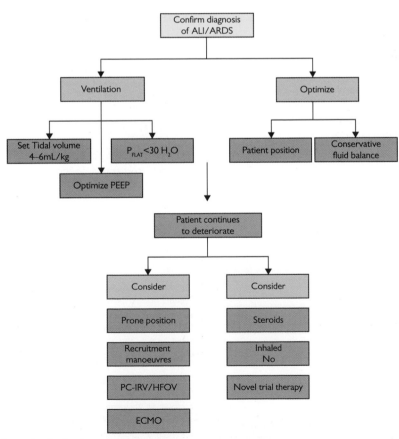

Fig. 13.10 Contributing factors for the development of ALI/ARDS.

**30cm of water** improved survival, although the debate about these parameters is ongoing in the literature.

- In Ashbaugh's initial description of ALI/ARDS, it was noticed that PEEP had beneficial effects, likely due to a favourable effect on recruiting collapsed alveoli, thereby improving oxygenation and increasing lung compliance and also redistributing extravascular lung water and improving ventilation/perfusion matching. To date, trials have not conclusively the optimal level for its use in this condition. A recent ARDSNet study showed no difference in high vs. low levels of PEEP; another study suggests high PEEP accompanied by low tidal volume is optimal. The benefit of PEEP is undoubted, but an overwhelming consensus on the level required remains undecided.

- Short-term variations of PEEP and/or inspiratory pressure via the ventilator, can also be used in the form of **recruitment manoeuvres**, to improve ventilation in ALI/ARDS. Studies have shown them to improve oxygenation and they may be more beneficial in early extrapulmonary.

- A further method for improving alveolar recruitment is **prone positioning** of the patient. Despite generating a number of problems such as potential endotracheal tube displacement, it has been shown to improve oxygenation and recent studies suggest a survival benefit.

- A number of other mechanisms of ventilating the patient with ALI/ARDS exist. The most commonly favoured is pressure controlled inverse ratio ventilation (PC-IRV), where a longer period of the respiratory cycle is spent at PPLAT, promoting a more homogenous ventilation pattern and reducing peak airway pressures. Airway pressure release ventilation (APRV) can also be used.

- High-frequency oscillation ventilation (HFOV) has also been used in this condition but two recent studies have failed to demonstrate a survival benefit.

- Extracorporeal membrane oxygenation (ECMO) has been shown to offer a survival advantage and is now offered in specialist centres around the UK.

### Pharmacological strategies

- Despite numerous trials of pharmacological agents in ALI/ARDS, disappointingly, no agent has shown a mortality benefit. **Steroids** possess both anti-inflammatory and antifibrotic properties and have been used in a variety of study designs. A study did suggest that they might be beneficial in late-phase ARDS but a larger ARDSNet trial did not confirm this, although it suggested they were most beneficial in patients with an early fibrotic phenotype.

- **Surfactant** levels are severely depleted in ALI/ARDS and various trials have used different preparations, administration regimens, and delivery techniques, to assess its effect on this condition. However, improvement in oxygenation has not translated into a survival benefit in these studies.

- **Nitric oxide** (NO) augments hypoxic pulmonary vasoconstriction by selectively vasodilating vessels associated with ventilated alveoli, when delivered exogenously. This effect improves ventilation/perfusion matching and oxygenation in the lung. A number of multicentre studies have shown that NO improves oxygenation but not survival and its use is only as rescue therapy for the severely affected patient. Other agents including $\beta_2$ agonists that may favour alveolar fluid clearance and anticoagulants such as activated protein C (APC) showed promise in preliminary trials but larger trials were not successful.

## Sepsis

### Epidemiology

- Severe sepsis and septic shock, which occur in response to infection are common and associated with substantial use of hospital resources.

- Studies have shown that hospital mortality is 30% for severe sepsis and 50–60% for septic shock. Incidence and mortality is increased in the elderly.

### Clinical manifestation, pathogenesis, and basic science

- As SIRS evolves into severe sepsis and septic shock, circulatory disturbances occur including intravascular volume depletion, peripheral vasodilatation, myocardial depression, and increased metabolic rate, altering the balance between $DO_2$ and $VO_2$, resulting in global tissue hypoxia and shock, as discussed previously. Untreated, tissue dysfunction, multi-organ failure (MOF), and death will occur.

- These events are accompanied and driven by an exaggerated and often overexuberant inflammatory response at the cellular level.

- Stimulation of inflammation leads to activation of macrophages, neutrophils, platelets, endothelium, and the epithelium.

- Pro-inflammatory cytokines and growth factors, free radicals, NO, and proteases are released concurrently and a procoagulant milieu favouring fibrin production is generated.

- The net effect of these events is to cause microvascular obstruction, blood flow redistribution, interstitial oedema, mitochondrial dysfunction, and tissue fibrosis, leading to the clinical manifestations described previously.

- Intense research has failed to identify a final common pathway and one may not exist.

- In addition, there is increasing evidence that genetic predisposition may contribute to the evolution of sepsis.

### Specific management of patients with sepsis

*Early goal-directed therapy (EGDT)*

- During the transition from SIRS to severe sepsis and septic shock (Box 13.28), global tissue hypoxia occurs before MOF.

- Tissue hypoxia is not detected by basic haemodynamic monitoring, but can be predicted using surrogate markers including central venous oxygen saturation ($S_{cv}O_2$), arterial lactate concentration, base deficit, and pH.

- A landmark study showed that mortality in sepsis could be improved by achieving haemodynamic variables and optimizing $S_{cv}O_2$, during the first 6 hours as an inpatient, using fluid (including blood), vasopressors, and inotropes (EGDT).

- This study has helped provide parameters for initial resuscitation, which are an important component of sepsis care bundles that are now widely used (Box 13.29).

- Two large trials are currently ongoing looking at this area in greater detail.

*Pharmacological strategies*

- Prompt recognition of the condition and early treatment with appropriate **antibiotics**, after taking microbiological investigations, is vitally important. However, a number of other agents have been used in an attempt to modify the systemic response in sepsis.

- **Activated protein C (APC)** is an anticoagulant, anti-inflammatory, and profibrinolytic agent. It also may have antifibrotic properties.

- APC was shown to significantly reduce morbidity and mortality in severe sepsis in a landmark trial. However, its usage remained controversial and when a further trial was repeated, the benefit could not be shown so it was withdrawn from use.

- Other anticoagulants have been tried including **antithrombin III**, **tissue factor pathway inhibitor (TFPI)**, and **heparin** but a clear benefit has not been shown with any of these agents.

- Studies have shown that the prevalence of adrenal insufficiency in septic shock is ~50%, so **steroids** in the form of **low-dose hydrocortisone** are often used in the treatment of this condition.

- However, this area also remains contentious and the exact role for steroids in this condition remains controversial.

- If volume resuscitation is inadequate, **vasopressors** may be required to treat the haemodynamic consequences of sepsis, as

**Box 13.28 Definitions for sepsis and organ failure**

*Systemic inflammatory response syndrome (SIRS)*
Two or more of:
- Temperature >38°C or <36°C.
- Heart rate >90bpm.
- Respiratory rate >20 breaths/minute or $PaCO_2$ <4.3kPa
- White blood cell count >12,000/mm³ or <4000/mm³
  **Sepsis**: SIRS caused by infection.
  **Severe sepsis**: sepsis associated with organ dysfunction.
  **Septic shock**: sepsis with hypotension despite adequate fluid resuscitation and with perfusion abnormalities.
Source: Adapted with permission from Wolters Kluwer Health: *Critical Care Medicine*, 'American College of Chest Physicians/Society of Critical Care Medicine Consensus Conference: Definitions for sepsis and organ failure and guidelines for the use of innovative therapies in sepsis', 20, 6, pp. 864–874, 1992.

they potent effects on peripheral vasodilatation. **Noradrenaline** is usually the first-line agent but others including **vasopressin**, **methylene blue**, and **terlipressin** can be used, although none of these agents have been subject to assessment in large randomized controlled trials.

- If sepsis causes significant myocardial depression and low cardiac output is detected, **inotropic support** may be required. **Adrenaline** or **dobutamine** are commonly used agents.

- Many novel agents, which generally have looked at modifying the inflammatory response, have been examined in this condition but none have shown a definite mortality benefit.

- Therapies such as **toll-like receptor blockers**, **anti-tumour necrosis factor antibodies**, and **statins** are under investigation and the results of these studies are awaited with interest.

- Other techniques such as **plasmapheresis** and **early high volume haemofiltration** have been reported as beneficial but these are not routinely used.

# Mass casualty incidents (MCIs)

## Preparedness/disaster management

- Recent natural, accidental, and terrorist global events have brought preparedness and disaster management to the forefront of critical care planning and provision.

- It is generally accepted that better preparation is required for future events and a number of key issues have been identified (Box 13.30).

- Expert observers have suggested a 'when not if' scenario exists for further MCIs including terrorist attacks and an outbreak of pandemic flu in the UK.

## Major incident management and support (MIMMS)

- Multidisciplinary plans for MCIs exist at national and regional level.

- Plans adopt the 'all hazard' approach for MCI irrespective of the nature of the incident.

- A structured approach is used involving **preparation**, **response** (at both medical management and medical support levels), and **recovery** phases.

**Box 13.29 6-hour sepsis bundle targets in EGDT**

- CVP 8–12mmHg.
- MAP ≥65mmHg.
- Urine output ≥0.5mL/kg/hour.
- Central venous (superior vena cava) $O_2$ satn ≥70%
- If central venous $O_2$ satn ≤70%, consider, blood transfusion to keep haemotocrit ≥30% or inotropic/vasopressor support.

**Box 13.30 Key issues for disaster planning**

1. Staff education and training.
2. Portable critical care.
3. Increased demand for device and supplies.
4. Existing ICU patients and ICU admissions unrelated to disaster.
5. Cooperation between ICUs.
6. Budgetary constraints during planning.

- In hospital, preparation includes **construction of MCI plans**, which must comply with national guidelines and be regularly reviewed, **provision for equipment**, and **training**.

- Core components of response at medical management level include **command**, **safety**, **communication**, and **assessment**.

- The command and control structure utilizes a control team (consisting of a senior manager, medical officer, and nursing officer), ambulance liaison, police liaison, and media liaison.

- Vital to the process is the **control room**, which is the first point of contact and is responsible for communication.

- Command structure is divided into Gold (strategic), Silver (tactical), and Bronze (operational).

- Core components of response at medical support level include **triage**, **treatment**, and **transport**.

- On arrival of casualties, trained teams perform expert triage, document and provide a controlled flow of patients.

- Systems have been devised to classify casualties (Table 13.4).

- Treatment employs extrication and basic life support skills, advanced life support techniques, and specific treatments.

- Command and control of the emergency department, theatres and CSSD, ICU bed numbers, imaging, laboratory services, and pharmacy is vital.

- A **consolidation period** will arise where central control continues, information will be disseminated, and staff, relatives, and the media will need to be attended to.

- During the **recovery phase**, the hospital will stand down from the MCI, debriefs occur, and assessment of additional staff and consumable needs, as a result of the MCI, will be calculated.

- Out-of-hospital plans also exist and an example of a triage and assessment system used by the London Ambulance Service to deal with the casualties in the July 7th bombings, using the mnemonic METHANE, is shown in Box 13.31.

**Flu**

- There are three main types of flu:
  - **Seasonal** (normal).
  - **Avian** (H5N1 outbreak).
  - **Pandemic**.

- A pandemic results when three conditions are met:
  - A new influenza virus subtype emerges.
  - It infects humans causing serious illness.
  - It spreads easily and sustainably in humans.

**Table 13.4 Triage of multiple casualties**

| Priority | Colour | Label |
|---|---|---|
| Immediate | Red | PIT1 |
| Urgent | Yellow | P2T2 |
| Delayed | Green | P3T3 |
| Expectant | Black/green | T4 |
| Dead | White/black | T0 |

Box 13.31 Assessment at the scene: METHANE

**M**y call sign/major incident alert
**E**xact location.
**T**ype of incident.
**H**azards at the scene.
**A**ccess.
**N**umber of casualties and severity.
**E**mergency services present or required.

© Crown copyright. Reproduced with permission of Public Health England. This information is licenced under the terms of the Open Government Licence v2.0 (https://www.nationalarchives.gov.uk/doc/open-government-licence/version/2)

- H5N1 is an influenza A virus, the group that show the most antigenic drift and shift, promoting resistance.
- The mortality of H5N1 in birds is 90%.
- H5N1 first passed from birds to humans in 1997.
- The first possible case of human–human transmission was reported in Thailand in 2004.
- It is plausible that H5N1 could mix with seasonal flu virus and acquire the ability to pass between humans.
- In 2009 a new strain of H1N1 influenza was declared to be a **global pandemic** (Stage 6) by the WHO after evidence of spreading in the southern hemisphere.
- Challenging ethical issues can emerge in the event of a pandemic as critical care resources are not finite.
- Secondary bacterial complications occur in pandemics and have a high morbidity and mortality.

# 13.5 Withdrawal of therapy, brainstem death, and organ donation

## Withdrawal of therapy

- A significant proportion of hospital deaths occur in ICU and these deaths need to be managed appropriately.
- The vast majority of deaths in the ICU occur following decisions to withhold or withdraw treatment.
- The majority of ethical authorities agree that there is no moral difference between withholding and withdrawing treatment but many doctors prefer withholding rather than withdrawing treatment.
- It is reasonable to consider a trial of intensive care treatment on the understanding that it will be withdrawn if ineffective.
- Some doctors, nurses, and patients have conscientious objections to treatment withdrawal and their views need to be respected.
- During the processes of withholding or withdrawal, patients and families should be given maximum privacy.
- Key to the process is relief of the patient's pain and distress which usually involves drug therapy by infusion.
- This can be adjusted to relieve the patient's suffering but **never** to intentionally hasten death.
- Organ supportive treatment should be withdrawn as may respiratory support in certain circumstances.
- Medical treatment can be withdrawn on clinical grounds because the treatment will not benefit the patient, but **never for financial reasons or to facilitate ICU bed availability**.
- It is helpful if the wishes of the patient are known but if not, family and friends should be consulted.
- It is recognized that geographical and individual variability exists regarding the reasons for withdrawing and withholding treatment in ICU.
- Further information regarding the decision-making process in ICUs is still required and implementation of common protocols for addressing end of life decisions may be useful.

## Brainstem death

### Overview of brain damage
- Is a generic term that includes patients with the following conditions:
  - Brainstem death.
  - Persistent vegetative state (PVS): cortical damage but **intact** brainstem.
  - Locked-in syndrome: reticular activating system function preserved despite extensive brainstem damage.
- Legally binding guidelines exist for the diagnosis of brainstem death **only**.
- They do not exist for PVS and other forms of coma and withdrawal of care can be legally challenged despite it being in a patient's 'best interests'.

### Death vs. brainstem death
- The definition of death should be regarded as 'irreversible loss of the capacity for consciousness, combined with irreversible capacity to breath'.
- The irreversible cessation of brainstem function (brainstem death) **equates with the death of the individual** (Box 13.32).

---

**Box 13.32** Function of the brainstem

1. All somatic/cranial motor output.
2. All sensory input (except cranial nerves I and II).
3. Respiratory drive.
4. Vasomotor centre.
5. Relays to ascending reticular activating system for generation of consciousness.

---

### Diagnosis of brainstem death
- Requires diagnosis of condition with irreversible brain damage (Box 13.33).
- Requires elimination of secondary causes of coma including:
  - Drugs—muscle relaxants, depressants, etc.
  - No pre-existing hypothermia.
  - No pre-existing metabolic or endocrine disturbances.
- Two doctors perform the tests (Boxes 13.34 and 13.35), which usually will be the consultant in charge of care and a doctor with 5 years of experience on medical register in the UK.
- It is customary to repeat the tests to ensure no observer error and for reassurance.
- No guidance exists for the time interval between the sets of tests but this is usually within hours.
- Each doctor should record preconditions, confirm no exclusion criteria, and detail brainstem tests including pre- and post-apnoea test arterial blood gases.
- The legal time of death is when the first set of tests indicate brainstem death and death is pronounced after the second set of tests are completed.

---

## Organ donation

### Criteria
- A number of criteria exist to guide potential organ donation including:
  - Donation after brainstem death or cardiac death.

---

**Box 13.33** Common causes of brainstem death

1. Spontaneous cerebral haemorrhage or infarction.
2. Cerebral trauma.
3. Cerebral hypoxia.
4. Cerebral infection.

---

**Box 13.34** Brainstem tests

1. The pupils are fixed and dilated and do not react to light.
2. There is no corneal reflex.
3. No vestibulo-occular reflexes.
4. No motor response to pain in a cranial nerve distribution.
5. No gag reflex or reflex response to tracheal stimulation.
6. Positive apnoea test.

## Box 13.35 Performing an apnoea test

1. Disconnect from ventilator.
2. Insufflate oxygen via endotracheal tube.
3. Allow $PaCO_2$ to rise to >6.65kPa or 2kPa above baseline.
4. Confirm no spontaneous respiration.
5. Reconnect ventilator.
6. Avoid hypoxia and hypotension.

## Box 13.36 Organs and tissues that can be donated

*Organs*
1. Kidneys
2. Liver
3. Lung(s)
4. Heart
5. Pancreas
6. Small bowel.

*Tissues*
1. Heart valves
2. Cornea
3. Skin
4. Bone and cartilage
5. Trachea.

- There must be no objection from family.
- Age limit is generally <85 years old.
- Absolute contraindications include HIV, CJD, and known active metastatic cancer.

### Types of donation/donor management

- Different types of donation can be contemplated including:
  - Heart beating donation
  - Non-heart beating donation (NHBD)
  - Tissue donation (Box 13.36).
- In NHBD, an age limit and organ-specific criteria do exist.
- It may be offered to families when a decision has been made to withdraw treatment.
- Once any potential donor is identified, organ function must be optimized so that the family's wishes to donate are fulfilled and the chance of successful transplant is maximized.
- Haemodynamic stability with a well-maintained MAP, with treatment of any potentially correctable abnormal results is desired.

### Other issues

- Any member of the clinical staff or allied health professionals can approach a family to discuss transplantation if criteria are fulfilled including the consultant, the bedside nurse, chaplain, or transplant coordinator.
- No religious groups oppose organ donation.
- Studies have shown that as many as 50% of families give approval if approached.

# Chapter 14

# Neurology and neurosurgery

## Introduction

Neurology, probably more than any other specialty, requires knowledge of anatomy and physiology to help you interpret examination findings. Lesions in the nervous system produce symptoms and signs depending on their location.

After taking the history and performing a neurological examination, the main task is to localize the lesion and reach a reasonable diagnosis. The advances of MRI have not replaced the need of a good diagnostician—the opposite may indeed be true given the increasing number of incidental findings. The neurological evaluation aims to identify the pathophysiology of the symptom and to localize the abnormality. Formulate your hypothesis and arrange sensible tests. Not everyone requires a scan! Furthermore, if tests have been already been performed, aim to review them **after** you have formulated your hypothesis. **Take** the history, **examine**, and then **look** at the scan!

## Neurological history taking

Neurological examination is very valuable, but history taking—possibly in neurology more than other fields of medicine—is the most important part of the neurological evaluation. Spend more time in history taking rather than examining!

Allow the patient to tell you the story in their own words. Usually it is easy to identify the patients for whom you will require collateral history from friends or relatives.

There are many elements to taking a complete neurological history but the most important is timing. Timing indicates pathophysiology:

- Acute onset, without warning, suggests vascular aetiology.
- 'March' of symptoms (progression over seconds) suggests seizure
- Progression over 5–10 minutes is common in migraine aura.
- Gradual evolution of symptoms over weeks and months are the norm for space-occupying lesions.

Knowledge of timing should include symptom onset, periodicity (constant vs. episodic), frequency, and length of symptoms. What induces or exacerbates the symptoms? Are there any relieving factors?

Knowledge of past medical history, family history, medications, and social history are of course vital but there are some specific questions, summarized as follows:

- Weakness.
- Sensory symptoms.
- Loss of consciousness.
- Headache, vision, bladder/bowels, speech, and swallowing.
- Ask about alcohol, think about HIV.

**Quantify** any reported deficits or disability: i.e. 'can walk 10m with a stick' and document the effect in their daily life.

## A few specific situations

### How to approach hemiplegia

Establish if the lesion is . . . :

**Cortical**: test for aphasia, cortical sensory loss (graphesthesia–stereognosis), inattention, apraxia, check for eye deviation (away from the hemiparesis), arm >leg involved suggests middle cerebral artery, or leg >arm suggests anterior cerebral artery territory. History of seizure?

**Subcortical** (basal ganglia–thalamus): face, arm and leg equally involved? Dense sensory loss as in thalamic lesions?

**In the brainstem**: crossed hemiplegia (i.e. left hemiplegia with right brainstem signs), cerebellar signs, nystagmus, facial numbness, dysarthria, and swallowing difficulties.

**In the cord**: all symptoms and signs below the neck, weakness, and loss of vibration on the side of lesion with pin-prick loss on the opposite side.

### How to approach memory complaints

- Lapses of 'working' memory (forgetting a telephone number or why they went to the kitchen) are common and reported more frequently from anxious individuals.
- Episodic memory disturbances, with difficulties acquiring new information (necessary to follow films on TV, the memory of events, times, or places) are frequently seen in cases of Alzheimer disease.
- Semantic memory is the memory of meaning; what we describe as 'lost for words' (unable to name a lobster from a photograph), is commonly seen in semantic dementias, such as progressive aphasias. Again, don't confuse dementia with the occasional language lapses, especially in the elderly, but be concerned with the birdwatcher who cannot name a sparrow.
- Give a name and address, assess immediate recall, and ask again in 5 minutes. Test recent memory (what did the patient do yesterday—confirm with friends/relatives).
- Consider **Mini Mental State Examination** (MMSE; 30 points):
  - 5 for orientation to time (year, month, day, date, season).
  - 5 for orientation to place (country, county, town, hospital, ward).
  - 5 for attention (spell WORLD backwards).
  - 3 for registration (three objects: i.e. keys, pen, ball).
  - 3 for recall of those objects 5 minutes later.
  - 2 for naming a pencil and watch.
  - 1 for repeating 'no ifs, ands or buts'.
  - 3 for following a three-stage command.
  - 1 for following printed command: 'close your eyes'.
  - 1 for writing a sentence.
  - 1 for copying diagram of intersecting pentagons.

### How to approach aphasia

= Poor use or comprehension of language (as opposed to dysarthria: poor articulation but normal grammar and syntax). Most of us use the left hemisphere for our language needs (including most of the left-handed). Aphasia suggests MCA territory dysfunction. Listen to spontaneous speech, ask them to read and write, check repetition, and examine for hemiparesis and hemianopia.

*Broca aphasia (inferior frontal lobe)*

- Slow speech, few words per minute, but can convey meaning successfully (I . . . go . . . home).
- Non-fluent, telegraphic speech, good comprehension, poor phrase repetition.
- Found together with right hemiparesis (arm >leg), right hemisensory loss, patient frustrated!

*Wernicke aphasia (posterior superior temporal lobe)*

- Fluent speech with little content, substitutions of correct word for one related in sound or meaning (paraphasia: dobble for bottle, dox for fox).
- Unable to comprehend, poor repetition.
- Can have right hemianopia but usually motor and sensory function of limbs is normal.

# 14.2 Neurological examination

## Background

Neurological examination confirms the findings of the history and aims to localize pathology and guide further investigation.

It is vital that the examination should be simple, consistent, and reproducible. For simplicity this can be divided into alertness, higher functions, cranial nerves, and limbs.

## Alertness and higher mental functions

### Alertness

The **Glasgow Coma Scale** (GCS) is the most commonly used measure of alertness particularly in head injury but is also valuable as a standardized, objective measure that will identify trends in conscious level (Table 14.1). Its limitations must be borne in mind, e.g. the effects of drugs and alcohol, concurrent systemic disorders like shock, sepsis, and hypoglycaemia, and inadequate use in patients with restricted communication like aphasic stroke, children under 3 years, head and neck trauma.

The GCS is scored between a worst score of 3/15 to best of 15/15, breaking the score down depending on the best response in each category and should be noted as such, e.g. GCS 11/15 E3V3M5.

### Higher mental functions

The most commonly used bedside test is a 10/10 abbreviated mental test score. This is non-specific but quick, easy and useful for identifying trends. A 30/30 MMSE is more sensitive and specific and can identify deficits in different cognitive domains, e.g. recall, orientation, language, etc.

## Cranial nerve and limb examination

It is important to remember that cranial nerve and limb function are controlled both centrally (brain and spinal cord) and peripherally (spinal nerve roots, plexus, peripheral nerves, neuromuscular junction and muscle).

### Cranial nerves (CNs)

Each cranial nerve may be examined in isolation as they each have an individual role. However, the main objective of cranial nerve examination is to localize and to differentiate between a central (UMN and/or central sensory pathway) and a peripheral lesion (LMN and/or peripheral sensory pathway or neuromuscular junction or muscle).

They are often best thought of in groups for convenience of testing and also for localization. The eyes are usually tested together because the functions of the cranial nerves controlling the eyes (II, III, IV and VI) are closely linked. The other cranial nerves are grouped together for examination purposes because of their proximity in the brainstem: pons (middle 4: V, VI, VII, VIII) and medulla (lower 4: IX, X, XI, XII).

### Table 14.1 Glasgow Coma Scale

| Best eye response (4) | Best verbal response (5) | Best motor response (6) |
|---|---|---|
| 1. No eye opening<br>2. Eye opening to pain<br>3. Eye opening to verbal command<br>4. Eyes open spontaneously | 1. No verbal response<br>2. Incomprehensible sounds<br>3. Inappropriate words<br>4. Confused<br>5. Orientated | 1. No motor response<br>2. Extension to pain<br>3. Flexion to pain<br>4. Withdrawal from pain<br>5. Localizing pain<br>6. Obeys commands |

Reprinted from the *Lancet*, 2(7872), Teasdale G, Jennett B, Assessment of coma and impaired consciousness. A practical scale, 81–4, 1974, with permission from Elsevier.

## A practical 'how to':

### Smell

Ask: 'Can you smell coffee?' or 'Have you noticed any change in your sense of smell?'. Smell kits are manufactured but not easily to hand. Remember that noxious smells, e.g. ammonia, are best avoided as they may be irritant and stimulate pain (a function of CN V).

### Eye examination

- Look at the eyes for ptosis, pupillary abnormalities, and other ophthalmic changes, e.g. swelling, pulsation, conjunctival injection, chemosis.

- Visual acuity should be checked in each eye using a Snellen chart at 6m, e.g. 6/60 denotes the ability to see at 6m what a normal person can see at 60m and 6/5 denotes the ability to see at 6m what a normal person can only see at 5m.

- Inattention and visual fields in four quadrants can be grossly assessed with both eyes open and looking into the examiner's eyes. Hold your hands up and out to the side: Ask 'Point to the hand that's waggling or say both if you can see both'. Each eye should then be examined in more detail in each of the four quadrants saying: 'Now tell me as soon as you can see my finger waggling'. A red hatpin can be used as it is more accurate but these are not always readily at hand and by waggling a finger the examiner controls when the test starts.

- Eye movements can be tested by saying 'Follow my finger with your eyes. Let me know if you see double' and moving the finger in a 'H' formation or a 'X' followed by '+' formation

- The examiner should look for any nystagmus which is best elicited by moving the finger in a '+' formation.

- The accommodation reflex of the pupils should be done by holding your finger 10cm from the patient's nose and saying: 'Look in the distance. Now look at my finger'. The pupils will constrict when accommodating to a near object. The light reflexes are sought by shining a pentorch in each eye. Both the direct and consensual reflexes should be elicited. The swinging torch test is carried out to elicit a relative afferent pupillary defect (RAPD). The torch is shone in one eye for 2 seconds and the light is then moved to the other eye. Initial dilatation in the other eye with the light indicates a RAPD (see Section 14.20).

- Eye examination is completed with fundoscopy looking for any disc changes, e.g. swelling (papilloedema), pallor (atrophy). Retinal abnormalities such as exudates, haemorrhages, and abnormal pigmentation should also be noted.

### Pontine nerves (apart from VI—assessed previously)

- The sensory part of CN V can be tested by asking 'Can you feel me touching your face' in each of the three divisions. The two sides should be compared. The motor function of CN V can be tested by asking 'Clench your teeth' and 'Open your mouth against my hand. Stop me closing it'. Your fingers should be placed against the temporo-mandibular joint and below the chin respectively providing some resistance to properly assess this. The corneal reflex should be tested by touching the cornea lightly using a piece of cotton wool with the patient looking away. This should be felt (CN V) and cause a reflex blink (CN VII). This is not a hard sign as some people, e.g. contact lens wearers, may have reduced corneal sensation.

- CN VII can be tested by asking for a few movements including 'Raise your eyebrows, like you're really surprised', 'Screw your eyes shut', 'Smile', and 'Puff out your cheeks'. These movements should also be checked for strength with your fingers providing some resistance. The absence of eyebrow lifting on one side indicates a LMN lesion—but is unhelpful for bilateral lesions.

- CN VIII is formally tested using a 512Hz tuning fork (Rinne and Weber tests) but in the absence of a tuning fork asking 'Tell me the number I'm whispering' in each side whilst rustling fingers in the other ear will suffice. Otoscopy is a vital part of this examination.

### Nerves originating from the medulla (Bulbar)

- Palatal elevation is checked by asking the patient to say 'Aaaah' and looking for a symmetrical elevation of the palate. Uvula deviation can be sought since a unilaterally weak palate results in the uvula being pulled away from the side of the lesion. This is not always helpful however as many uvulae do not always point in the middle to start with. The gag reflex (pharyngeal reflex) is done by touching the soft palate lightly (e.g. with a tongue depressor) and tests CN IX (afferent limb) and CN X (efferent limb).
- To examine CN XII look at the relaxed tongue in the mouth for any asymmetry, wasting, and fasciculations. Fasciculations (indicating a LMN lesion) should only be sought with the tongue in the mouth. Then ask: 'Stick your tongue out. Waggle it from side to side'. A uni-laterally weak tongue will be pushed towards the side of the lesion by the stronger other side. A bilaterally weak tongue will move slowly if at all. Tongue strength can be objectively tested by asking the patient 'Push your tongue into the inside of your cheek' and providing some resistance with your finger touching the outside of the cheek.
- Lastly examine CN XI by asking 'Shrug your shoulders' and 'Push your chin against my hand', testing each side with your own hand providing resistance.

## Limbs

The objective of the limb examination is to identify disorders of the UMN and/or central sensory pathway, the peripheral nervous system (LMN and/or sensory pathway or neuromuscular junction or muscle), the cerebellum and the extrapyramidal system.

## A practical 'how to'

### Inspection

Limb examination starts with inspection including any asymmetry, skin changes, muscle wasting or hypertrophy, fasciculations, tremor at rest. Inspection of the lower limb should also include examination of the gait as this may immediately indicate any ataxia, hemiparesis, festinant gait, freezing, etc.

### Tone

Tone can be examined by moving each joint passively. Cogwheeling can be made more apparent by asking the patient to wave the other limb up and down. In the lower limbs tone is easily tested by rolling the lower limbs (hip and ankle) and by lifting up the relaxed knee.

### Power

The limb movements are usually tested proximally to distally. In the upper limbs: shoulder abduction/adduction, elbow extension/flexion, wrist extension/flexion, finger extension/flexion, finger abduction, and abductor pollicis. In the lower limbs: hip flexion/extension, knee flexion/extension, ankle dorsi/plantarflexion. Other limb movements can also be tested depending on the situation. The golden rules of examination of power are:

1. To compare each side against the other.
2. If possible to compare like with like, e.g. their thumb against your thumb.
3. Always stabilize the proximal joint when testing a more distal joint to prevent a stronger proximal joint from contributing to distal strength.

### Reflexes

Again, the golden rule of comparing each side against the other applies. The deep tendon reflexes that are typically tested are biceps, triceps, supinator, knee, ankle, and plantar. The absence or decrease in reflexes (hyporeflexia) indicates a LMN problem or a sensory problem (afferent pathway) whilst brisk-reflexes (hyper-reflexia) indicates an UMN problem. The presence of more than four beats of ankle clonus indicates hyper-reflexia of the ankle.

### Coordination

Interpretation of deficits in coordination must take into account any weakness. Gait incoordination is termed ataxia and can be caused by cerebellar, sensory, or vestibular problems. This is exemplified by difficulties with tandem gait (heel-to-toe walking). Other cerebellar abnormalities include finger–nose ataxia, dysdiadochokinesis, and impaired heel–shin movements.

### Sensation

Ideally all four sensory modalities should be tested, namely pain, temperature, joint position sense, and vibration sense. The last three are best tested distally to proximally and when a level is reached where that modality is detected then testing can be stopped. Pain (usually using a pin) can be tested either in a dermatomal distribution or in the distribution of an individual named nerve or distally to proximally looking for a sensory level.

## Purpose

- Confirm clinical suspicion.
- Exclude significant or common differentials.
- Disease monitoring (e.g. tumour follow-up).

However, there is no substitute for a carefully taken history and a thorough clinical examination.

## Imaging

### Computed tomography (CT)

*Principle*

Multiple X-rays taken around a single axis of rotation are combined to generate a cross-sectional image of the patient. Intravenous injection of radio-opaque dye (contrast) highlights blood–brain barrier breakdown (BBBB) and blood vessel imaging, both arteries (CT angiography) and veins (CT venography).

*Indications of CT head*

First-line imaging investigation in someone with:

- Acute neurological symptoms (e.g. cerebral or aneurysmal bleed or infarct).
- Evolving neurological signs (e.g. focal neurology or decreased GCS score).
- Suspected head trauma (e.g. skull fracture, subdural bleed).
- See Table 14.2 for comparison with MRI.

### Magnetic resonance imaging (MRI)

*Principle*

Hydrogen atoms (protons) in a magnetic field absorb and release energy in response to electromagnetic pulses. Differences in behaviour of protons in fat and water generate soft tissue contrast.

*Indications*

Definitive imaging modality for characterizing:

- Small, focal abnormalities (e.g. in posterior fossa or spinal cord), due to high spatial resolution.
- Brain parenchymal pathology (e.g. encephalitis, inflammation), due to high sensitivity.

*Contraindications*

- Ferromagnetic (metallic) objects in the body, can lead to considerable artefact or injury (e.g. in the eye or brain).
- Presence of cardiac pacemakers or other implants.

*Commonly used MR sequences*

*T1 weighted ± gadolinium (Gd) contrast*

- Signal intensity: $H_2O$ = low (black); fat = moderate; Gd enhancement = high (white).

- T1 is good for defining normal/abnormal anatomy.
- Gd detects abnormal BBBB (e.g. neoplasm).

*T2 weighted*

- Signal intensity: $H_2O$ = high (white); fat = low (black).
- Good for defining pathology, which tends to show different intensity to normal tissue.

*Fluid attenuated inversion recovery (FLAIR)*

- Similar to T2, but with CSF signal also suppressed.
- Good for inflammation, ischaemia, and especially lesions near CSF spaces (e.g. periventricular lesions in MS or small vessel ischaemia).

*Magnetic resonance angiography (MRV/MRA)*

- Utilizes flow within vessels to image vasculature.
- MRA uses: arterial dissection, aneurysm, vasculitis.
- MRV uses: venous thrombosis, venous stenosis.

*Diffusion-weighted imaging (DWI)*

- Measures changes in motion of water molecules to detect subtle disruption of brain architecture
- Very high sensitivity in detecting early (<7 days) stroke.

### Cerebral angiography

Plain X-ray images using radio-opaque dye injected from a catheter passed (via femoral) into the carotid artery. This is the gold standard for visualization of intracerebral vessels (e.g. in vasculitis) and allows concomitant intervention (e.g. arterial stenting, aneurysm coiling). There is, however, ~1% risk of stroke, increasing with age.

## Electroencephalogram (EEG)

Records spontaneous cortical electrical activity.

EEG is neither required nor particularly helpful for epilepsy diagnosis—a seizure video is much more helpful diagnostically.

*Types*

- Routine or sleep-deprived (outpatient): standard 20-minute recording, usually with provocation (photic stimulation, hyperventilation).
- Ambulatory (outpatient): if having daily seizures with loss of consciousness.
- Video telemetry (inpatient): gold standard test using combined video and EEG.

*Indications*

- To classify epilepsy syndromes.
- To localize seizure onset pre-epilepsy surgery.
- To monitor seizure activity in status (CFAM).
- To confirm encephalopathy/non-convulsive status.
- To support a diagnosis of viral encephalitis/CJD.
- To aid prognosis in coma.
- To characterize sleep disorders like narcolepsy.

**Be warned that:**

- Routine or even sleep-deprived EEG has low sensitivity and specificity for epilepsy.
- Most EEG 'abnormalities' are not epileptiform, and so are a common cause of epilepsy misdiagnosis.

| Table 14.2 Advantages and disadvantages of CT head vs. MRI | |
| CT head | MRI |
| --- | --- |
| **Advantages** | **Advantages** |
| • High sensitivity for acute haemorrhage | • Excellent resolution, multiple sequences and 3-plain views |
| • Cheap and easily available | • Non-ionizing |
| • Short examination time | |
| **Disadvantages** | **Disadvantages** |
| • Low sensitivity for posterior fossa and soft tissue imaging | • Claustrophobia-inducing |
| • Ionizing radiation | • Often less accessible than CT |
| | • Time intensive |
| | • Many contraindications (size, metal, critically ill) |

# 14.4 Coma

## Coma

Normal consciousness depends on adequate functioning of the cerebral cortex and the ascending reticular activating system (ARAS), situated centrally in the brainstem. Decreased conscious level can be graded using a coma scale (see Section 14.2), but the term coma usually refers to a state of complete unresponsiveness from which the patient cannot be roused, i.e. GCS score 3. Because of the proximity of the ARAS to brainstem cardiovascular and respiratory centres, some but not all comatose patients may have coexisting needs for ventilatory and cardiovascular support.

Structural brain lesions can cause coma:

1. If they arise in the brainstem and damage the ARAS locally, or
2. If they arise remotely and cause displacement of the brain with consequent brainstem compression.

Structural lesions affecting the cortex rarely cause coma because the area of cerebral cortex involved in maintaining consciousness is so large. However, insults such as infection, toxins, and metabolic derangement can diffusely injure the brain causing coma.

## Clinical evaluation

A comatose patient represents an emergency. The priority should be to ensure airway, breathing, and circulation are adequate before proceeding to further evaluation. When GCS score is <8 patients often require airway support.

### History
Collateral history is vital in narrowing differential diagnosis (see Table 14.3). Use all available resources: accompanying relatives, previous hospital notes, GP records, MedicAlert bracelet/necklaces and prescriptions.

- Time course: gradual/sudden onset, any fluctuations.
- Preceding illness: fever, neurological symptoms, trauma.
- Comorbidity: diabetes, stroke, renal or hepatic failure.
- Drugs: current medications, alcohol, substance misuse.

### Examination
- Check BP, pulse, respiratory rate, and $O_2$ saturation.
- Blood glucose and temperature vital as they may reveal a reversible cause.
- Survey briefly for signs of trauma, meningism, jaundice, anaemia, rash.
- Neurological examination should aim to grade coma and then look for signs of a structural lesion:
  - Check GCS score and for decorticate/decerebrate posture (Fig. 14.1).
  - Fundoscopy: papilloedema, signs of diabetes, SAH, vasculitis.
  - Pupillary reflex: abnormality can imply a brainstem lesion, herniation of mesial temporal lobe over tentorium, or also substance misuse (e.g. opiates if bilateral).
  - Eye movements: deviation from primary position can imply a focal brain lesion (bilateral, towards lesion) or arise due to CN III or VI palsy (unilateral). Bilateral roving movements imply an intact brainstem; otherwise brainstem can be tested by checking vestibulo-ocular reflex (VOR—Fig. 14.2) or caloric tests.
  - Corneal reflex—brainstem reflex involving CN V and VII
  - Limbs—tone and reflexes may reveal focal pathology. Power, sensation, and coordination cannot be formally tested but any voluntary or involuntary movements should be noted

| Table 14.3 Common causes of coma | | |
|---|---|---|
| **Structural lesion** | | **Diffuse brain injury** |
| **Brainstem** | **Supratentorial** | |
| Infarct | Trauma | Toxins, e.g. carbon monoxide |
| Haemorrhage | SAH | Infection, e.g. encephalitis, post-ictal |
| Central pontine myelinolysis | Sagittal sinus thrombosis | Drugs, e.g. opiates |
| Tumour | Thalamic haemorrhage | Metabolic: uraemia, hypercapnia |

(A) Extension posturing (decerebrate rigidity)

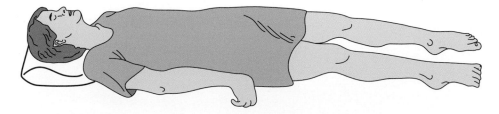

(B) Abnormal flexion (decorticate rigidity)

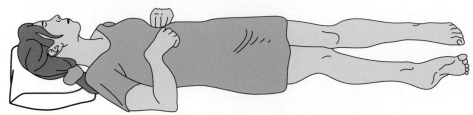

**Fig. 14.1** Abnormal postures indicative of brain injury.

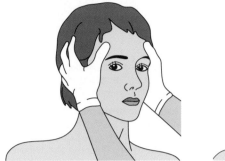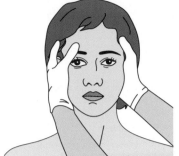

Fig. 14.2 Vestibulo-ocular reflex: on turning the head, eyes should turn in the opposite direction as if fixed on a point in front of the patient.

### Investigations

- FBC, U&E, LFT, Ca, glucose, and ABG.
- Septic screen if infection suspected.
- Neuroimaging: CT good first-line test, MRI if later uncertainty.
- LP if safe and if infection suspected (imaging required **first** if comatose).

- EEG: can provide clue towards structural/diffuse cause and exclude non-convulsive status epilepticus.

## Management

Stabilizing airway, breathing, and circulatory failure may require help from ICU or anaesthetic colleagues.

Further management will depend on investigation results.

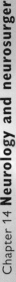

# 14.5 Acquired brain injury

## Background

Acquired brain injury is common, encompassing a range of disorders that results in acute (rapid onset) brain damage:

- Traumatic brain injury (TBI).
- Cerebrovascular disease (stroke, SAH).
- Postanoxic brain injury (cardiac arrest, shock, drowning).
- Infective (meningitis, encephalitis).
- Metabolic (hypoglycaemia).
- Inflammation (vasculitis).

## Pathophysiology

Mechanisms of TBI:

- Diffuse axonal injury—shearing forces by rapid acceleration/deceleration.
- Haematoma (extradural, subdural, SAH, parenchymal).
- Contusion—bruise to the brain.

Mechanisms of cerebral anoxia:

- Insufficient blood flow, e.g. stroke, cardiac arrest.
- Decreased $O_2$-carrying capacity of the blood, e.g. haemorrhage, anaemia, carbon monoxide poisoning.
- Insufficient environmental $O_2$, e.g. at high altitude.

The hippocampus, watershed regions (end-artery areas; poorly-perfused) in the cerebral cortex, cerebellum, basal ganglia, and spinal cord are all particularly sensitive to hypoxia.

## Epidemiology

Overall incidence difficult to estimate since wide range of causes. Stroke and TBI commonest.

- Mild TBI (no evidence of contusion or haematoma) incidence: 180/100,000/year.
- Stroke <65 years incidence: 20/100,000/year.
- Severe brain injury affects 25/100,000/year. 10–20% have prolonged coma or severe disability. 65–85% have good physical (not necessarily cognitive/psychosocial) recovery.

Improved emergency care has meant better survival of brain injury patients, albeit with increased numbers of extremely disabled survivors.

## Clinical evaluation

### Classification of impaired conscious levels

**Locked-in syndrome**: fully conscious but quadriplegic with movement restricted to vertical eye movement and blinking.

**Minimally conscious state**: intermittent/inconsistent evidence of self/environmental awareness, differentiated from reflexive behaviour. Purposeful behaviour can be elicited, including appropriate emotional responses, vocalization, or gestures.

**Persistent vegetative state**: intact brainstem with a destroyed forebrain. Sleep–wake cycles and brainstem reflexes intact but no interaction with the environment. Occasional non-purposeful movements/posture in response to noxious stimuli. May demonstrate startle responses or brief orientation to visual or auditory stimuli, reflexive crying, or smiling.

**Coma**: no sleep–wake cycle, auditory, or visual responses. Motor function limited to reflex and postural responses.

**Brainstem death**: apnoeic coma of known and irreversible cause, normal physiological markers, absence of sedative or muscle relaxant drugs, with no brainstem reflexes.

### Testing for brainstem death

Assessment of pupillary, oculovestibular, corneal, and gag reflexes, with no motor response in the cranial nerve area to somatic stimulation, **and** a positive apnoea test (disconnecting a patient from a ventilator, continuing oxygenation, and allowing $CO_2$ levels to rise while watching for respiratory effort for 10 minutes). Must be carried out by experienced doctors on two separate occasions.

### Investigations

- **Brain imaging**: useful for establishing underlying cause.
- **EEG**: may help to identify subclinical or non-convulsive seizures.
- Intracranial pressure monitoring, study of regional blood flow, and evoked potential testing are also used.

## Management

- Needs-based multidisciplinary care; not pathology-based.
- Supportive treatment: maintaining airway, oxygenation and circulation, fluid balance, nutrition, bladder and bowel care, treatment of metabolic derangement and seizures.
- Prevent secondary complications: pneumonia, pressure sores.
- Recognition and management of psychosocial impairment, e.g. SSRIs for depression, cognitive behavioural therapy for post-concussion syndrome.
- Rehabilitation: early rehabilitation associated with better long-term outcomes. Both hospital-based and home-based rehabilitation helpful.
- TBI: RCT of early corticosteroid and death/disability after head injury—steroid group did worse. Decompressive craniectomy in severe TBI done with malignant brain swelling and is associated with good outcomes in surviving patients.

## Outcome

Poor correlation between degree of acute structural damage on brain imaging and long-term physical recovery. Severe injuries may rapidly and completely recover whilst cognitive and psychosocial impairment can be marked even with minor brain injury.

GCS score, length of coma, and post-traumatic amnesia used as markers of severity of injury but only weakly related to long-term outcome for the individual.

The most important prognostic factors for coma are aetiology, depth and duration of coma, and clinical signs.

### Morbidity

- Gait disorders: UMN or sensory damage, ataxia—may overlap.
- Movement disorders in 10%: mild to severely disabling, e.g. tremor, myoclonus, akinetic-rigid syndrome, dystonia.
- Neuro-ophthalmological: traumatic optic neuropathy 0.5–5%.
- Vascular complications, e.g. haematoma, fistula formation.

### Seizures

Head injury accounts for 7% of all new seizures. Post-traumatic epilepsy can be early (within 1 week) or late (after 1 week). Risk of recurrence after single late seizure is 80%.

Concussive/impact convulsions = tonic posturing with myoclonic jerks within seconds of head injury. These are non-epileptic with no associated structural brain injury, and have good outcome.

*Psychosocial impairment*

Variable abnormality in cognition, attention, and behaviour, often (not always) with EEG, MRI, and neuropathological correlates.

- Memory: impaired laying down of new memories (temporal lobe) and executive function (frontal lobe).
- Post-concussion syndrome (headache, irritability, memory loss, confusion) usually recovers by 1–3 months but 7% with residual symptoms at 1 year.
- Mood: depression common; occurs in 25–50% after TBI.
- Behaviour: due to frontal damage, e.g. impulsivity, apathy.
- Hallucinations.

# 14.6 Encephalopathies

## Background

Diffuse (as opposed to focal) brain disease.

## Aetiology

- Anything disrupting brain function.
- Causes include sepsis, vasculitis, malignancy, and inborn errors of metabolism.
- This section will focus on **metabolic** and **toxic encephalopathy**.

## Metabolic encephalopathy

- Encephalopathy resulting from systemic metabolic dysfunction.
- Neurological deficits are symmetric.
- Pupillary light reflex usually preserved.

Causes include:

| | |
|---|---|
| Liver disease | Hepatic encephalopathy secondary to porto-systemic shunt |
| Renal disease | Uraemic encephalopathy |
| Electrolyte imbalance | Disturbances of Na, K, Ca |
| Endocrine disease | DM<br>Hashimoto encephalopathy<br>Hypoglycaemia<br>Cushing disease |
| Nutritional deficiencies | Wernicke encephalopathy |
| Chest disease | Hypoxia<br>Hypercapnia |

## Toxic encephalopathy

| | |
|---|---|
| Alcohol related | Acute alcohol intoxication<br>Alcohol withdrawal (delirium tremens) |
| Excess or overdose of psychoactive medication | Benzodiazepines<br>Neuroleptics<br>Anticonvulsants<br>Opiates |
| Adverse events from other medication | Immunosuppressants<br>Chemotherapeutic agents<br>Thiazide diuretics |

- Encephalopathy arising from exogenous toxic insult.

Causes include:

## Clinical features

**Early:** poor concentration (e.g. in performing serial 7s), constructional apraxia (cannot draw a star), agitation, confusion, hallucinations, tremor, myoclonus.

**Late:** stupor, coma, seizures.

**Other features:** abnormal respiratory pattern (apnoea, Cheyne–Stokes).

## Clinical evaluation

Identification of underlying cause is critical in providing effective treatment.

The primary aim of clinical evaluation should be directed toward identifying the underlying (hopefully reversible) cause.

**Table 14.4** Systemic stigmata

| Aetiology | Sign |
|---|---|
| Hepatic disease | Jaundice, spider naevi, ascites |
| Renal disease | Anaemia, fistula |
| Sepsis | Fever |
| IV drug use | Needle tracks |
| Hypothyroidism | Dry hair, hypothermia |

### History—ask about:

- Past medical history including pre-existing chest, liver, or kidney disease as well as DM.
- Social history to include alcohol and drug abuse.
- Medication history.

### Examination

- Systemic stigmata can often help identify aetiology (Table 14.4).
- Neurological assessment is directed towards:
  1. Evaluating severity: MMSE and/or GCS.
  2. Identifying any localizing signs.
  3. Identifying aetiological clues, e.g. constricted pupils with opiate overdose, eye movement abnormalities, and disorientation in Wernicke encephalopathy.

### Investigations

*Bloods*

- Biochemistry: U&E, LFT, Mg, Ca, glucose, TFT, CRP.
- Haematology: FBC, ESR, coagulation.
- Arterial blood gas looking for pH as well as $PaO_2$, $PaCO_2$.
- Septic screen: blood and urine cultures.
- Consider full toxicology screen: For advice contact Medical Toxicology Information Services, Tel.: 020 7188 0600, <http://www.medtox.co.uk/>.
- Ammonia (pack bottle in ice, and take straight to lab).

### Imaging

- CXR.
- Brain imaging (CT or MRI): to rule out focal lesion. In general, imaging findings are normal, apart from the late development of cerebral oedema.

### EEG

- To rule out non-convulsive seizures.
- To determine severity of cerebral dysfunction.

### Lumbar puncture

- Should be undertaken only after brain imaging.
- Measure opening pressure and send CSF for biochemistry, microscopy, cytology, lactate, culture.

## Treatment

- Treatment directed toward the underlying cause (Table 14.5).

**Table 14.5** Underlying cause and treatment

| Underlying cause | Treatment |
|---|---|
| Liver failure | Laxatives, neomycin, reduce dietary protein |
| Renal disease | Renal replacement therapy |
| Opiate overdose | Naloxone |
| Wernicke | Thiamine |

# 14.7 Alcohol and the nervous system

## Acute intoxication

Ethanol rapidly crosses the blood–brain barrier resulting in the characteristic features of alcohol intoxication: euphoria, disinhibition, poor coordination, and lethargy. Serum ethanol levels of 50–150mg/dL are sufficient to produce such symptoms in an individual who is not alcoholic (UK driving limit is 80mg/dL) (Fig. 14.3).

⚠ Always consider head injury, hypoglycaemia, or infection as a cause of low GCS score in patients who are intoxicated.

## Alcohol withdrawal

Chronic alcohol ingestion causes CNS inhibition mediated by GABA receptors and the CNS up-regulates excitatory NMDA receptor expression to compensate. The abrupt withdrawal of alcohol can therefore generate an overwhelming excitatory CNS effect called the alcohol withdrawal syndrome (AWS).

The severity of AWS depends on the usual level of ingestion as well as the abruptness of cessation of alcohol.

Onset of AWS usually occurs within 24 hours of alcohol cessation, and peaks by 48 hours.

### Clinical features
- Autonomic: sweating, tachycardia, tremor, pyrexia.
- Psychiatric disturbance: agitation, anxiety, hallucinations.
- Seizures: tonic–clonic, occasionally status epilepticus.

### Management
- Ensure adequate hydration.
- Supplement thiamine to prevent Wernicke—initially with IV therapy, followed by oral maintenance replacement.
- Long-acting benzodiazepines are used for agitation and to prevent seizures. Chlordiazepoxide 25mg four times a day might be prescribed initially with the dose tapered over 1 week.
- Antipsychotics e.g. haloperidol, should be avoided as they lower seizure threshold.

## Wernicke syndrome and Korsakoff syndrome

Malnutrition can occur in patients with alcohol dependence. Thiamine (vitamin B₁) deficiency underlies Wernicke syndrome.

### Clinical features
- Classical triad of ataxia, nystagmus, and ophthalmoplegia.
- Confusion, headache, also vomiting.
- Hypothermia/hypotension can prove fatal.
- High index of suspicion required because of overlap with features of other neurological complications of alcohol.

### Management
- ▶▶ Thiamine replacement (IV Pabrinex® (vitamins B + C): 2 ampoules IV three times daily for 3 days)—give early as IV dextrose or oral carbohydrate can otherwise precipitate deterioration.
- Parenteral thiamine replacement should be followed by maintenance oral replacement.

Offer prophylactic oral thiamine to all alcoholics. Following Wernicke, many patients are left with chronic memory deficits termed Korsakoff syndrome. Typical features are:
- Poor recall of recent events with disorientation and confabulation (production of false memories to fill gaps).
- Anterograde amnesia—inability to learn new knowledge.
- Normal remote memory, intellect, and conscious level.
- Abstinence from alcohol can lead to partial recovery of memory. Overall the prognosis is poor however, because of low rates of long-term abstinence.

## Osmotic demyelination syndromes

Rapid correction of chronic hyponatraemia in alcoholics can cause central pontine (or extra-pontine) myelinolysis. Features range from mild dysarthria to locked-in syndrome.

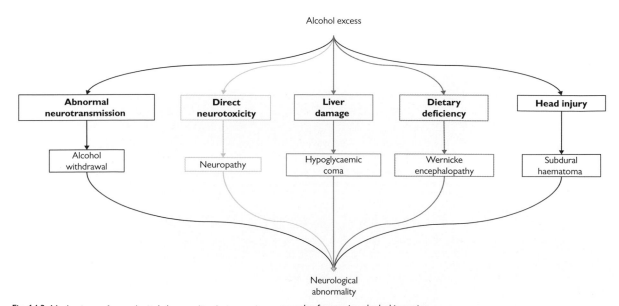

Fig. 14.3 Mechanisms of neurological abnormality that can arise as a result of excessive alcohol ingestion.

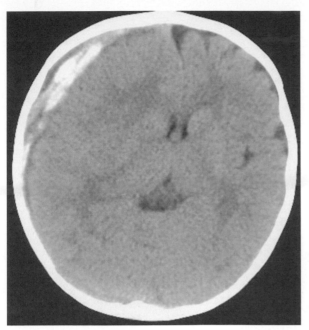

**Fig. 14.4.** Acute right fronto-parietal subdural haemorrhage.

## Cerebellar degeneration

Progressive atrophy of the cerebellar vermis leads to gait ataxia. Abstinence and thiamine can arrest the progression of symptoms.

## Peripheral neuropathy

One of the most common neurological sequelae of chronic alcohol consumption is a sensorimotor neuropathy. It is unclear whether the condition arises from the direct neurotoxic effects of alcohol or results from vitamin deficiency. Paraesthesia/neuropathic pain in the feet can be prominent.

## Myopathy

The cumulative toxic effects of alcohol on skeletal and cardiac muscle are thought to be responsible for the chronic myopathy seen in many alcoholics. Less commonly, an acute myopathy with rhabdomyolysis can be precipitated by an alcohol binge.

## Epilepsy

- Alcohol conveys increased risk of seizures because of AWS, risk of head trauma (think subdural: Fig. 13.4), and alcohol's toxic effect on the brain.
- First seizure in an alcoholic requires structural brain imaging.
- Infection or electrolyte disturbance should be sought in all.
- Anti-epileptics only usually prescribed outside of AWS.

# 14.8 Brainstem disorders

## The basics: the brainstem

- Connects cerebrum to spinal cord and cerebellum.
- Consists of (rostral to caudal): midbrain, pons, medulla.

## Important structures in the brainstem

### Cranial nerve nuclei and related structures

- Midbrain: III, IV.
- Pons: V, VI, VII, VIII.
- Medulla: IX, X, XII.
- Conjugate gaze centres in midbrain (rostral interstitial medial longitudinal fasciculus (riMLF)) and pons (parapontine reticular formation (PPRF))

### Long tracts

- Descending: corticospinal and corticobulbar.
- Ascending: spinothalamics and dorsal columns.

### Cerebellar tracts

- Spinocerebellar, corticocerebellar.

### Reticular formation (RF) and related structures

- In midbrain: involved in maintenance of consciousness.
- In medulla: involved in cardiorespiratory function.

## Brainstem disorders: clinical manifestations

Features arising from:

### Cranial nerve abnormalities

- Diplopia (III, IV, VI).
- Facial numbness and weakness (V, VII).
- Dizziness and vertigo (VIII).
- Dysphagia, dysphonia, dysarthria (IX, X, XII).

### Long tract disruption

- Hemiparesis/quadraparesis.
- Anaesthesia/paraesthesia.
- Crossed signs (e.g. right facial + left limb weakness).

### Cerebellar tract disruption

- Incoordination and ataxia.
- Nystagmus, vomiting.

### RF disruption

- Somnolence.
- Disrupted breathing (e.g. Cheyne–Stokes).

### Disruption of other structures within brainstem

- Internuclear opthalmoplegia (INO): see Fig. 14.5.
- Gaze palsies (riMLF, PPRF).
- Horner syndrome (sympathetic outflow).

The combination of signs localizes the brainstem lesion; e.g. VIth nerve palsy and LMN VIIth implicate a pontine lesion.

## Some brainstem syndromes

### Wallenberg syndrome

See Fig. 14.6.

### Weber syndrome

- Lesion in basal/posterior midbrain (e.g. occlusion posterior cerebral artery).
- Damaged CN III fibres: complete ipsilateral CN III palsy.
- Damaged cerebral peduncle (motor tracts): contralateral hemiplegia (including face).

### One-and-a-half syndrome

- Lesion involving VIth nerve and neighbouring MLF.
- Ipsilateral lateral gaze palsy and contralateral INO.

### Locked-in syndrome

- Lesion in ventral pons, involving descending long tracts.
- Patient is cognitively intact, but completely paralysed, apart from vertical eye movements (midbrain intact).

## Disease processes affecting the brainstem

### Ischaemia

- Commonest cause of brainstem pathology.
- Vertebrobasilar system consists mainly of end-arteries.
- Arterial occlusion through embolus, thrombus, dissection, with clinically evident ischaemia.
- MRI/MRA is investigation of choice.

▶ Prompt expert advice should be sought from a neurologist or stroke specialist.

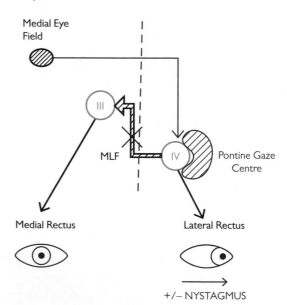

Fig. 14.5 Internuclear ophthalmoplegia.

- Common.
- Lesion in midbrain/pons.
- Internuclear lesion in medial longitudinal fasciculus (MLF) between CN VI nucleus/pontine gaze centre and CN III nucleus.
- Commonly due to demyelinating disease (multiple sclerosis)—to which the MLF is particularly susceptible. Consider cerebrovascular disease in older patients.
- Convergence is normal.
- Eye with failure of adduction (right in the figure) will usually adduct normally if other (left) eye is covered and made to follow a finger, i.e. voluntary gaze directed to **left** (by right frontal eye field).

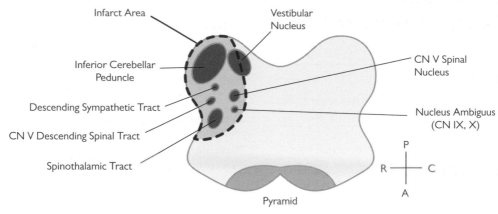

**Fig. 14.6** Wallenberg (lateral medullary) syndrome.
- Dorsolateral lesion within the medulla.
- Commonest brainstem vascular syndrome; from occlusion of basilar artery (classically—albeit less commonly—occlusion of posterior inferior cerebellar artery).

For a right-sided lesion the involved territories are shown in Table 14.6.

| Table 14.6 Clinical features of lateral medullary syndrome, with their respective anatomical correlate | | |
|---|---|---|
| **Affected medullary structure** | **Clinical result** | |
| Vestibular nucleus | Acute presentation with vertigo and vomiting, plus nystagmus. | |
| Descending sympathetic tract | Ipsilateral | Horner syndrome |
| Spinothalamic tract | Contralateral | Loss of pain and temperature sensation **below the neck** |
| Trigeminal nerve (CN V) nucleus and tract | Ipsilateral | Loss of trigeminal nerve (**face**) pain and temperature sensation |
| Nucleus ambiguus (IX, X) | Ipsilateral | Palatal paralysis (dysphagia, hiccups) and loss of gag reflex |
| Inferior cerebellar peduncle | Ipsilateral | Cerebellar signs/ataxia |

## Inflammation
- Multiple sclerosis lesions favour the brainstem, with consequent brainstem symptoms of dizziness, vertigo, ataxia, diplopia, trigeminal neuralgia.
- Sarcoid.

## Mechanical compression
The brainstem is susceptible to compression through the following mechanisms:
- Tumour: from within the brainstem (pontine glioma in children; adults with neurofibromatosis) or from the posterior fossa (medulloblastoma, ependymoma).
- Cerebellar tonsillar herniation: either through raised ICP or Arnold–Chiari malformation.
- Syringobulbia or myelomeningocoele.
- Haemorrhage: secondary to haemangiomata such as with von Hippel–Lindau disease, or with AVMs.

▶ Mechanical compression of the brainstem requires prompt neurosurgical review.

## Infection
- Organisms which can cause a brainstem encephalitis include *Listeria monocytogenes*, HSV, and VZV.
- Adopt a healthy suspicion, especially in immunocompromised or otherwise predisposed individuals.

## Metabolic
- Wernicke encephalopathy: see Section 14.7.
- Central pontine myelinolysis: precipitated by over-zealous correction of hyponatraemia. MRI: central pontine demyelinating lesion. Clinical presentation of tetraplegia, may produce 'locked-in' syndrome.

# 14.9 Common cranial nerve disorders

## Background

Cranial nerve (CN) disorders can be caused by a range of pathologies, depending on location.

## Aetiology

- **Central CN lesions** (within the brain): vascular, tumour, demyelination, infection, motor neurone disease (MND).
- **Peripheral CN lesions** (outside the brain): MND, Guillain–Barré syndrome (GBS), mononeuritis multiplex, neuromuscular junction disorder, myopathy.

## Trigeminal neuralgia

### Epidemiology

♀:♂ = 2:1; age: 30–40 years.

### Pathophysiology

Once thought idiopathic, more recently recognized to arise from compression of the trigeminal nerve (CN V) by an aberrant blood vessel in most cases; 5–10% arise due to a tumour, AVM, or demyelinating plaque.

### Clinical evaluation

*History*

- Excruciating brief pain in the distribution of CN V (usually maxillary or mandibular branches).
- Patients may experience frequent symptoms for periods of days to months, with interspersed intervals of remission.
- Trigger points that produce symptoms are often found in the trigeminal distribution. Patients may resist eating, brushing teeth, or talking for fear of triggering neuralgia.
- Rarely persistent aching or numbness occur in the same area.

*Differential diagnosis*

- Dental pathology.
- Atypical facial pain (more often bilateral and continuous).
- Migraine (episodes more protracted, aura often present).
- Temporal arteritis (especially elderly with systemic upset).
- Trigeminal autonomic cephalalgia.

*On examination*

- Neurological examination is expected to be **normal**.
- ▶ Abnormal CN V sensation or other cranial nerve abnormality should prompt a search for a structural lesion.

*Investigation*

- Dental X-rays may be considered to exclude infection.
- MRI of the trigeminal nerve may highlight an aberrant vessel and will exclude more serious causes.

### Management

*Pharmacological (mainstay of treatment)*

- Carbamazepine most favoured with other anticonvulsants (gabapentin, lamotrigine and topiramate) as second line.

*Surgical*

- Microvascular decompression or ablation of the trigeminal nerve should be considered for refractory cases.

## Bell palsy

Acute CN VII palsy causing unilateral facial weakness.

### Epidemiology

Incidence ~20 per 100,000 per year, ♂ = ♀, middle age.

### Pathophysiology

Herpes simplex virus associated inflammation is thought to be the most likely cause of Bell palsy. Pregnancy and diabetes are both risk factors for Bell palsy.

### Clinical evaluation

*History*

- Unilateral facial weakness which is acute in onset but may take several weeks to reach peak severity.
- May be associated with ear pain.
- Inability to close the affected eye, drooling of saliva, slurring of speech may arise due to facial muscle weakness.
- Also absent taste sensation, intolerance of loud noises and decreased lacrimation (involvement of chorda tympani, nerve to stapedius and greater petrosal CN VII branches).

### On examination

▶ Differentiation between UMN/LMN facial weakness is important as Bell palsy is LMN (Fig. 14.7). Frontalis receives bilateral cortical innervation so is spared in UMN lesions:

- **Bell phenomenon:** eyeball rolls up on attempted eye closure.
- CN VII lesions in the brainstem may cause deficits in adjacent cranial nerves, e.g. lateral rectus palsy or hearing loss.
- Check for herpes zoster of external ear and parotid scars.
- All causes of mononeuritis multiplex (see Section 14.26).
- Specific alternatives include Lyme disease, HIV, otitis media, Ramsay Hunt syndrome, sarcoidosis, lymphoma, tumour (e.g. parotid gland, cholesteatoma).

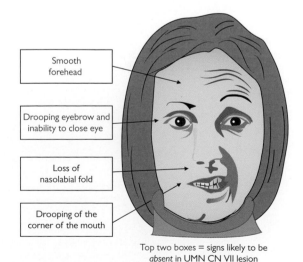

Smooth forehead

Drooping eyebrow and inability to close eye

Loss of nasolabial fold

Drooping of the corner of the mouth

Top two boxes = signs likely to be *absent* in UMN CN VII lesion

Fig. 14.7 Differential diagnosis of Bell palsy.

- UMN causes of CN VII weakness—stroke (affecting cortex/internal capsule/brainstem), tumour or abscess (rare).

### Investigations

- CT/MRI brain ± CSF examination if presentation atypical.

### Management

- If eye closure if reduced, corneal protection must be undertaken, e.g. lubrication, taping the eye shut at night.
- There is good evidence supporting use of corticosteroids (started within 72 hours of symptom onset) to improve recovery, plus possible benefit from the addition of aciclovir in those with severe/complete palsy.
- Psychological support and follow-up is important.
- Prognosis.
- Most recover completely, but ~20% are left with some residual disability (probably 5–10% if treated).

# 14.10 Migraine

## Epidemiology

- ♀ >♂, ~3:1.
- Migraine without aura > migraine with aura, ~3:1.
- Onset usually before the age of 30, often childhood/adolescence; rare after age 50 (consider brain imaging).
- Often family history.
- Rarely underlying structural lesion, e.g. tumour, AVM.
- Occasionally occurs as part of a syndrome e.g. CADASIL (cerebral autosomal dominant arteriopathy with subcortical infarcts and leucoencephalopathy), antiphospholipid syndrome/SLE, mitochondrial disease.

## Symptoms and signs

### Characteristics of headache

- May have prodrome for hours or days before headache, e.g. change in mood, behaviour, cognition, hunger or anorexia, frequent yawning.
- Throbbing or pulsating pain, moderate—severe intensity, unilateral or bilateral.
- Typically lasts 4–72 hours, sometimes longer.
- Associated nausea ± vomiting, photophobia and/or phonophobia.
- Worse with movement/activity (usually have to stop working, exercise etc.).
- Typically prefer to stay still in a dark, quiet room.

### Migraine with aura

- Aura can occur at any time in relation to pain and may persist temporarily after pain resolves.
- The aura evolves over several minutes; in contrast, TIAs are of sudden onset and spectra 'march' over seconds.
- Migraine aura can occur without headache (ancephalgic migraine).
- Most commonly visual, with either +ve symptoms, e.g. flashing lights (photopsia), zig-zags (fortification spectra) or—ve symptoms, e.g. scotoma, hemianopia.
- Visual symptoms are usually homonymous and binocular but can be monocular (retinal migraine).
- The second most common type of aura is sensory (e.g. unilateral paraesthesia or numbness).
- There may be two or more successive auras.

### Other types of aura

- Hemiplegic migraine (unilateral weakness).
- Dysphasia.
- Posterior circulation symptoms—vertebrobasilar migraine (bilateral visual symptoms, ataxia, dysarthria, vertigo, syncope).

- Ophthalmoplegic migraine, typically IIIrd nerve palsy ± pupillary involvement/ptosis.
- Mild confusion, rarely altered level of consciousness.

## Management

### Prevention

Avoid triggers, e.g. too much or too little sleep, alcohol, specific foods, skipping meals.

### Acute attack

Antiemetics and analgesia (consider suppositories if vomiting):
- Paracetamol.
- NSAIDs or 900mg aspirin.
- Triptans (if simple analgesia ineffective):
  - almotriptan, sumatriptan (injectable preparation available).
  - Ineffective if taken before onset of headache (i.e. during prodrome or aura) but do work best when taken early.
  - Contraindications include uncontrolled hypertension and cardiovascular risk factors (e.g. previous stroke).
  - If ineffective try an alternative triptan.

### Prophylaxis

Often consider if more than three disabling migraines per month. Options include:
- β-blockers: atenolol, propranolol.
- Amitriptyline, nortriptyline.
- Sodium valproate.
- Topiramate.
- Methysergide (not for >6 consecutive months as risk of retroperitoneal and pulmonary fibrosis).
- Pizotifen (weight gain).

### Chronic daily headache in migraine

- Medication overuse (e.g. opiates, triptans, or ergots) can lead to transformation of migraine into chronic daily headache. Discontinuation of the medication is central to the treatment of the headache.
- Similarly a series of frequent or severe migraines may result in a chronic daily headache.

### Migraine and the combined oral contraceptive pill (OCP)

- Migraine may worsen or improve with the OCP.
- There is an increased risk of stroke in migraineurs, although the absolute risk remains low. There is also an increased risk of stroke on the OCP. Therefore assess vascular risk factors when considering the OCP with migraine (smoking, BP, diabetes, family history, etc.).
- Provided a female is a non-smoker and is not hypertensive, the risk of stroke in a migraineur on the OCP is small, even in migraine with aura.

# 14.11 Other primary headaches

## Tension-type headache

- Pressing, band-like or tight pain, typically bilateral.
- Last hours to days. Typically worsen as day progresses.
- Featureless (i.e. no nausea, photo—or phonophobia, no aggravation with movement).
- Less severe than migraine, often able to continue activity.
- Episodic tension type headache is common, with most patients not seeking medical attention.
- Neck pain may accompany tension headache, but is seen no more often than with migraine.
- May coexist with migraine; depression, anxiety with sleep disturbances are common in tension-type headaches.
- Treatment—avoid stressors, try relaxation techniques, Amitriptyline 10mg nocte, increasing by 10mg per fortnight as tolerated/required, up to 70mg.

## Cluster headache

- ♂ >♀.
- Presentation—usually 3rd/4th decade.
- Diagnosis is clinical.

### Characteristics of headache

- Excruciating unilateral pain (mainly orbital), peaking within minutes. Usually 45–90 minutes' duration with abrupt onset and cessation.
- Transient ipsilateral autonomic features during attack. May include
  - Conjunctival injection
  - Lacrimation
  - Nasal congestion
  - Rhinorrhoea
  - Ptosis and miosis
  - Eyelid oedema.
- Neurological examination outside of attack should be normal (Horner may rarely persist).

There are clusters of attacks with intervening remissions:

- The cluster attack frequency typically varies between on alternate days to six daily (average 1–2/day).
- Sometimes attacks occur at the same time each day (i.e. circadian periodicity). Nocturnal attacks are particularly common.
- Such a cluster bout may last weeks or months before remitting. These bouts may occur once or twice per year (there may be circannual periodicity).
- Chronic cluster is less common and has no remission.

### Management

- SC sumatriptan 6mg ± 100% oxygen, at high flow rate for acute attacks.

- All patients require prophylaxis.
- Steroids, e.g. 60mg once a day for 5 days, tapering down dose over 2–3 weeks.
- Verapamil is a good preventative medication, often started in conjunction with steroids:
  - Baseline ECG to check PR interval.
  - Start with 40mg three times daily.
  - Increase dose as tolerated/required every 2 weeks (performing ECG before each increment).
- Other prophylactic agents include lithium, methysergide, and topiramate.

### Distinguishing cluster headache from migraine

Cluster headache is much rarer than migraine. The following features of the history are particularly useful in identifying cluster headache:

- Shorter duration of headache.
- Rapid onset/cessation.
- Frequency and circadian periodicity.
- Restless and irritable during attack, i.e. pace about/can't stay still, while patients with migraine stay still.

NB: both types of headache can be triggered by alcohol—within an hour in the case of cluster headaches, after several hours with migraine

## Paroxysmal hemicrania

Like cluster headache, paroxysmal hemicrania causes an excruciating, unilateral headache with associated ipsilateral cranial autonomic features.

However, in contrast to cluster headache, paroxysmal hemicrania is typically characterized by:

- Shorter attacks (usually 10–30 minutes each).
- Higher attack frequency (>5 attacks per day).
- A ♀ preponderance.

In hemicrania continua, moderate continuous unilateral headache is present, with superimposed episodes of more intense pain lasting hours to weeks. Autonomic features usually present but less prominent than paroxysmal hemicrania.

There can be considerable overlap between cluster headache and paroxysmal hemicrania in terms of attack duration and frequency. Paroxysmal hemicrania is less common but important to identify because it responds dramatically to indomethacin. Therefore, if there is diagnostic doubt, a trial of indomethacin should be given.

### Investigations

MRI brain to rule out structural pathology.

### Management

Indomethacin 25mg PO three times daily, titrating up to 75mg three times daily if required. Responds within days of reaching an adequate dose.

## Subarachnoid haemorrhage

### Aetiology
- Ruptured berry aneurysm (85%).
- Other vascular abnormality (e.g. AVM).
- No cause found in 10% (small chance of re-bleed).
- ▶ 25% die within 24 hours, further 25% die in hospital.

### Clinical presentation
Severe explosive headache (often occipital) without warning (may be **only** symptom):
- Typically arises instantaneously or within seconds, but **may** evolve over minutes.
- Usually lasts days or weeks.

Other symptoms/signs **may** include:
- Meningism (may take hours to develop), vomiting, photophobia.
- Reduced loss of consciousness (LOC), restlessness.
- Retinal haemorrhage (subhyaloid).
- Focal neurology, may reflect:
  - Haemorrhage involving the parenchyma (Fig. 14.8).
  - Rupture adjacent to a cranial nerve (usually III).
  - Complication by stroke.

### Complications
- Rebleed—risk reduces with time.
- Vasospasm and ischaemic stroke (highest risk day 5–14).
- Hydrocephalus (therefore re-scan if decreasing GCS score): may require shunt.
- Cerebral salt wasting and hyponatraemia (monitor Na daily).

### Investigations
- CT head—high initial sensitivity (decreases with time; >90% within 24 hours (highest sensitivity in comatose patients); 50% after 1 week.

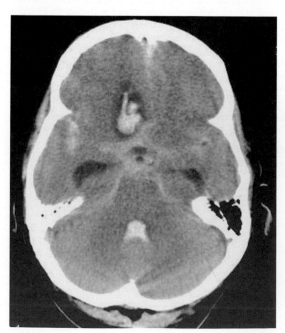

**Fig. 14.8** SAH due to anterior communicating artery aneurysm bleed (notice subarachnoid, parenchymal and intraventricular blood on CT).

- Lumbar puncture mandatory if no blood on CT (and no contraindications):
  - Defer for 12 hours after seizure.
  - Send for spectrophotometry for xanthochromia; must be centrifuged immediately. Almost 100% sensitive for up to 2 weeks.
- Cerebral angiography (IV, MR, or CT).

### Management
- General measures: pain relief, avoid straining (bed rest, laxatives, antiemetics), monitor electrolytes, fluids, BP, GCS.
- Reduce risk of vasospasm: 60mg nimodipine (PO/NG) every 4 hours for 21 days.
- Prevent re-bleed: secure aneurysm (usually endovascular coiling).

### Differential diagnosis of sudden-onset headache
All patients with thunderclap headache should be evaluated for SAH. Other causes include:
- Intracerebral haemorrhage (e.g. posterior fossa bleed) or pituitary bleed (e.g. with pituitary apoplexy).
- Venous sinus thrombosis.
- Primary thunderclap headache (diagnosis of exclusion).
- Phaeochromocytoma.

## Features suggestive of raised intracranial pressure

### Consider urgent scan:
- Worsened by recumbency.
- Aggravated by bending, coughing, straining.
- Nausea, vomiting.
- Visual obscurations.
- Focal abnormalities or papilloedema on examination with space-occupying lesions.
- Remember idiopathic intracranial hypertension.

## Giant cell (temporal) arteritis
- Patchy granulomatous vasculitis affecting medium and large sized arteries (which may occlude).

### Clinical features
- Vast majority: >60 years. ESR typically >60, but can be normal. CRP invariably raised.
- Headache with scalp tenderness. Temporal artery may be hard, tortuous, with absent pulsations and erythema.
- Close association with polymyalgia rheumatica (proximal muscle pain and stiffness).
- Systemic symptoms (e.g. fever, weight loss).
- Jaw claudication (pain on chewing).
- Anterior ischaemic optic neuropathy (usually from ophthalmic artery involvement) causes uniocular visual loss, either partial or complete. Occasionally amaurosis fugax precedes irreversible visual loss.
- Rarer complications include stroke (e.g. from occlusion of carotid or vertebral artery), ischaemic neuropathy of cranial nerves (e.g. IIIrd nerve palsy), and involvement of coronary or mesenteric arteries.
- Temporal artery biopsy should be performed to confirm the diagnosis.

### Treatment
- Prednisolone, initially 60mg od to prevent visual failure.
- Temporal artery biopsy within a few days of starting steroids (can be normal as inflammation patchy).

## Background

Neuro-ophthalmological disorders can originate from eye structures (lens, cornea, retina) or visual and oculomotor pathways in the brain, cranial nerves, and ocular muscles.

## Visual defects

- Visual information travels from the retina via the optic nerve of each eye (Fig. 14.9).

- Temporal retinal information is carried by the nasal (medial) fibres of the optic nerve whilst nasal field information is carried by the lateral fibres. Only information from the temporal visual fields crosses in the optic chiasm.
- The optic tracts carry visual information from half of each eye.
- Prechiasmal lesions cause defects in the ipsilateral eye whilst retrochiasmal lesions affect the contralateral half of both eyes.
- The optic tracts end at the primary visual cortex of the occipital lobes (travelling via the lateral geniculate nuclei and optic radiations).

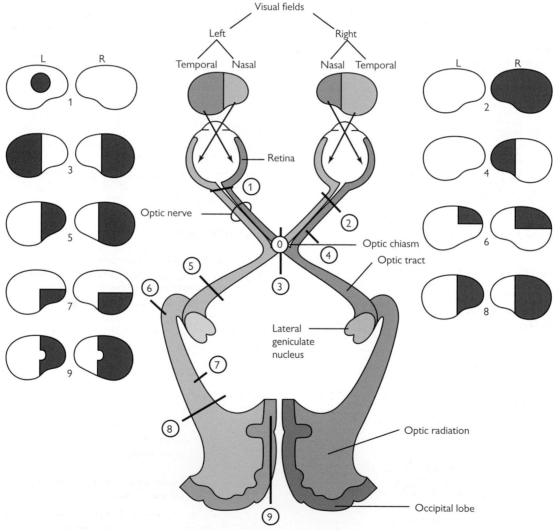

Fig. 14.9 Visual pathways.
1. Central scotoma—optic neuropathy.
2. Monocular blindness—eye defect or optic neuropathy.
3. Bitemporal hemianopia—chiasmal lesion.
4. Right nasal hemianopia—perichiasmal lesion.
5. Right homonymous hemianopia—lesion of optic tract.
6. Right homonymous superior quadrantanopia—left temporal lobe lesion/Meyer loop (inferior part of optic radiation).
7. Right homonymous inferior quadrantinopia—left parietal lobe lesion (superior part of optic radiation).
8. Right homonymous hemianopia—complete lesion of optic radiation.
9. Macula-sparing right homonymous hemianopia.

Reproduced with permission from: S. Paz Maya, P. Lemercier, I. lópez blasco, D. Soriano Mena, J. P. Ruiz Gutierrez, S. Sánchez Rodríguez, G. Silla; Valencia/ES (2013): Sellar and Parasellar Lesions: over and above adenomas (C-2052). Poster presented at ECR 2013. DOI: 10.1594/ecr2013/C-2052

- Neurological lesions causing visual defects can be considered as follows:
  - Monocular
  - Binocular.

## Monocular visual field defects

Lesion anterior to optic chiasm; either eye or optic nerve.

### Optic nerve lesion/optic neuropathy

- Typically causes central scotoma; a complete optic nerve lesion will cause complete unilateral visual loss.
- Inflammatory optic neuropathy is called optic neuritis; if pathology behind the optic disc it is termed retrobulbar neuritis as disc may look normal.
- O/E: test visual fields, acuity, colour vision; possible optic atrophy (pale, well-demarcated disc). Acutely optic neuritis may give appearance of disc inflammation (papillitis).
- Afferent papillary defect, i.e. shining light into affected eye produces no direct or consensual pupillary response. Shining light into unaffected eye will produce direct and consensual responses. In incomplete/milder lesions: relative afferent pupillary defect (RAPD) (described later in this section).

*Causes of optic neuropathy*

- Ischaemic optic neuropathy (associated with atherosclerosis or giant cell arteritis).
- Demyelination (causing optic or retrobulbar neuritis).
- Toxic—tobacco/alcohol/drugs (e.g. ethambutol).
- Leber hereditary optic neuropathy.
- Vitamin $B_{12}$ deficiency.
- Syphilis.
- Optic nerve compression (e.g. Paget disease, orbital or retro-orbital tumour)—look for proptosis.

## Binocular visual field defects

Lesion at or posterior to optic chiasm.

### Bitemporal hemianopia

- Pituitary tumours (functioning or non-functioning) compress the optic chiasm from below and tend to cause a **superior** quadrantanopia initially, although any field defect may result.
- Craniopharygioma compresses the chiasm from above, classically causing an **inferior** quadrantanopia.
- Other causes include space-occupying lesions (SOLs; e.g. aneurysm, meningioma).
- NB: lesions anterior to lateral geniculate nucleus ('pregeniculate') produce loss of red colour vision first.

### Homonymous hemianopia

- Lesion of optic tract, optic radiations, or occipital lobe. The optic radiations can be affected in the temporal or parietal lobes (e.g. SOL, infarct), causing either a superior or inferior homonymous quadrantinopia respectively.
- Occipital lesions secondary to ischaemic events—macular sparing may occur (the occipital pole receives dual blood supply from the posterior and middle cerebral arteries).
- Bilateral occipital nerve lesions cause cortical blindness (Anton syndrome), e.g. bilateral strokes from basilar artery thrombosis; often associated with anosognosia meaning unawareness or denial of symptoms.

### Papilloedema

Optic disc swelling, usually due to raised ICP caused by:
- Brain tumour/abscess/haematoma/CSF obstruction.
- Idiopathic intracranial hypertension (IIH/benign intracranial hypertension).
- Malignant hypertension.

Less common causes of papilloedema:
- Raised CSF protein, e.g. spinal cord tumour, inflammatory polyneuropathy (GBS, chronic inflammatory demyelinating polyneuropathy: CIDP).
- Cyanotic congenital heart disease.

▶ The absence of papilloedema **does not** necessarily exclude raised ICP. Papilloedema due to raised ICP may take several weeks to develop.

*History*
- Headache, nausea, and vomiting.
- Symptoms indicating focal neurological deficit, e.g. diplopia, weakness, sensory symptoms.
- Seizures.

*Examination*
- Check: conscious level and cognition, visual acuity, visual fields, VIth CN palsy (false localizing sign), focal neurological deficit.
- May cause little visual impairment in early stages.
- Initially there is enlargement of the blind spots, later constriction of the visual fields and reduced acuity.
- Visual obscurations: vision becoming grey on standing from a stooped position.

*Investigations*
- CT/MRI brain to exclude SOL.
- If safe to do so may require lumbar puncture for CSF opening pressure (NB IIH), protein, microscopy.
- Unilateral disc swelling may indicate acute papillitis/inflammation of optic disc due to optic neuropathy which may have the same fundoscopic appearances.

## Pupillary disorders

### Holmes–Adie pupil (tonic pupil)

- Caused by 'ciliary ganglionitis'; therefore affects both sympathetic and parasympathetic supply to eye.
- Typically large pupil, very slow to react to light and accommodation . . .
- . . . then slow to dilate when light source removed.
- Vermilliform (worm-like) movements of the iris (seen on slit-lamp examination).
- May be associated with areflexia.

### Argyll Robertson pupil

- Seen in neurosyphilis.
- Usually bilateral, small, irregular, pupils.
- Absent or poor reaction to light.
- Better reaction to accommodation ('accommodates but doesn't react').
- Probably lesion of the internuncial neurons in the midbrain that synapse onto the Edinger–Westphal nucleus.

### Relative afferent pupillary defect (RAPD)

Incomplete (or less severe) optic nerve lesions typically produce a RAPD (typically demyelination).
1. Shine light into the unaffected eye—both pupils constrict.
2. Now swing the light into the affected eye—both pupils dilate slightly. This is due to removal of light from the unaffected eye and the affected eye being slow to detect the light now shining on it.
3. Pupils will not become as constricted as when the light was shone in the unaffected eye.

### Horner syndrome

Caused by an interruption of the sympathetic innervation to the eye.

*Features*
- Partial ptosis.
- Miosis.
- Ipsilateral anhydrosis (and vasodilatation of head and neck).
- 'Apparent' enophthalmos (secondary to ptosis).

*Anatomy of sympathetic supply to eye*
See Fig. 14.10.

*Approach to Horner*
- Examine for lymphadenopathy and scars in neck, wasting of the hand muscles (unilateral—Pancoast's, bilateral—syringomyelia), ipsilateral apical chest signs.
- Preganglionic (lesion proximal to superior cervical ganglion)—Horner pupil dilates with 1% hydroxyamphetamine.
- Postganglionic—Horner pupil fails to dilate.
- Anhydrosis of the whole face indicates lesion proximal to internal carotid.

## Ptosis

### Approach to ptosis
- Is it unilateral or bilateral?
- Are the pupils asymmetrical?—if so is the ipsilateral pupil small (Horner) or large (CN III palsy)?
- Is the ptosis fatiguable? (Myasthenia gravis (MG).)
- Are the eye movements abnormal? (MG, CN III palsy, chronic progressive external ophthalmoplegia (CPEO), oculo-pharyngeal muscular dystrophy (OPMD)).
- Is there facial muscle weakness? (MG, myopathy.)

### Unilateral causes
- CN III palsy (pupil large or normal).
- Horner syndrome (pupil small).
- MG (pupil normal).
- Idiopathic/congenital.

### Bilateral causes
- MG (ptosis unusual in Lambert–Eaton syndrome).
- Muscle disease/myopathy (myotonic dystrophy, OPMD, mitochondrial myopathy with CPEO).
- Bilateral Horner with syringomyelia.
- Syphilis.
- Consider also 'senile' dehiscence of the levator muscle.

## Eye movement disorders

- All eye movements originate in the frontal motor cortex (like all other motor pathways) and cross over in the brainstem to end in the cranial nerve nuclei.
- Three CNs control eye movements: III, IV, and VI
- Each exits the brainstem (either midbrain (III and IV) or pons (VI)) and travels through the subarachnoid space to the cavernous sinus and superior orbital fissure (SOF) to reach the orbit.

### Disorders of conjugate gaze
Lesions are supranuclear if they occur in specific areas along the pathway from the frontal motor cortex up to the CN nuclei. These cause disorders of conjugate gaze, i.e. the ability of both eyes to move in concert.
1. Cortical input: contralateral frontal lobe regulates rapid eye movements (saccades): i.e. right frontal lobe controls saccades to the left. Ipsilateral parieto-occipital lobe regulates slow eye movements (pursuits).
2. Brainstem input: the paramedian pontine reticular formation (PPRF) lies adjacent to the CN VI nucleus and controls ipsilateral horizontal gaze, i.e. the right PPRF controls lateral gaze towards the right. The PPRF coordinates horizontal gaze via the MLF which connects nuclei of CN III on one side to CN VI on the other.
   - A frontal lobe lesion causes a contralateral gaze paresis. The opposite frontal lobe—now unopposed—may push the eyes towards the side of the lesion.

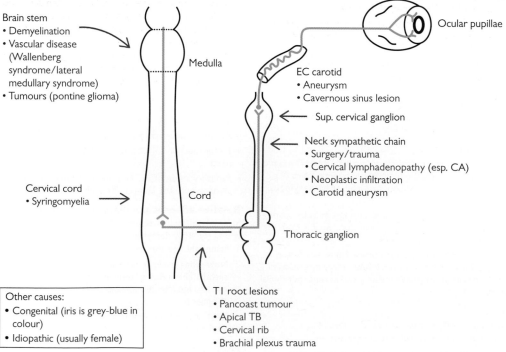

**Fig. 14.10** Anatomy of sympathetic supply to eye and causes of Horner syndrome.

- Brainstem lesions (e.g. tumour, demyelination, stroke) affecting the PPRF cause a horizontal gaze palsy with failure of horizontal movements of both eyes to the side of the lesion acutely causing a deviation of both eyes to the contralateral side.
- Both frontal and brainstem lesions may be associated with a hemiparesis; with a frontal lesion the eyes are deviated away from the hemiparesis; with brainstem lesions the eyes look towards the hemiparesis (because descending motor pathways not yet decussated).

*Internuclear ophthalmoplegia*
See Section 14.8.

## Ophthalmoplegia

= Dysfunction of extraocular muscle(s) causing diplopia.
These nerves can be affected anywhere along their pathway by the following processes:

- Central lesions: in the brainstem at the level of the CN nucleus or the fascicle (e.g. tumour, stroke, demyelination).
- Peripheral lesions.
- Structural causes (skull base tumour, malignant meningitis, aneurysms, tumour).
- Vascular—vasculitis (including giant cell arteritis), diabetic mononeuropathy, hypertension/arteriosclerosis.
- Trauma (often CN IV).
- Raised ICP (typically bilateral CN VI, to a lesser extent IV), i.e. false localizing sign.
- Cavernous sinus or SOF pathology (see later in section).

*Oculomotor (IIIrd) nerve palsy*
A complete III nerve palsy is characterized by:

- Complete ptosis.
- Fixed, dilated pupil (doesn't react to light or accommodation).
- Eye looks 'down and out' (unopposed action of CN III and CN VI respectively).

Partial palsies are more common.

*Causes*

- Compressive lesions (e.g. aneurysm of posterior communicating branch of circle of Willis—'surgical IIIrd') **usually result in pupil involvement** because the parasympathetic fibres travel along the outside of the IIIrd nerve; often painful.
- Hypertension and diabetes (may be painful—pain does not help differentiate from aneurysm) are the commonest causes of **pupil-sparing** ('medical') IIIrd.
- ► Unless the ptosis is complete, and the pupil is **completely spared**, then an aneurysm has to be excluded.

- A 'nuclear' lesion (i.e. at the level of the IIIrd nerve nucleus, within the midbrain) may result in a contralateral superior rectus palsy (fibres to contralateral superior rectus) and bilateral ptosis (levator palpebrae receives bilateral nuclear innervation).

*Trochlear (IVth) nerve palsy*
Weakness of superior oblique → can't look down and in:

- Diplopia (images rotated) is most marked looking down and in (e.g. reading, walking downstairs).
- May demonstrate head tilt away from side of lesion.

*Abducens (VIth) nerve palsy*
Weakness of lateral rectus:

- Horizontal diplopia, worse looking into the distance.
- Head may be turned towards side of lesion.
- Diplopia worse on attempted abduction of affected eye.
- A 'nuclear' lesion is commonly associated with a horizontal gaze palsy on looking towards the side of the lesion (involvement of the PPRF; see earlier) and facial weakness (the fascicles of the CN VII wrap around the VIth nucleus in the pons).

*Combined palsies*
Any of the nerves can be affected, often in combination, with pathology affecting the cavernous sinus, SOF, or orbit:

- Cavernous sinus (e.g. pituitary tumour, thrombosis, carotico-cavernous fistula, aneurysm)—may also affect CN V1, V2, and the sympathetic supply to the eye.
- SOF, e.g. Tolosa–Hunt syndrome—granulomatous inflammatory condition—may cause eye pain, ophthalmoplegia, and numbness in CN V1.

If complex ophthalmoplegia also consider MG (can mimic **any** palsy), thyroid eye disease, muscle disease (OPMD or CPEO), and Wernicke encephalopathy.

*Supranuclear palsies*
Ophthalmoplegia arising from lesions above the level of the cranial nerve nuclei. A few examples:

- Progressive supranuclear palsy (Steele–Richardson–Olzewski syndrome): parkinsonian features + impairment of upgaze (at presentation: later loss of all extraocular movements, and pseudobulbar palsy).
- Parinaud (dorsal midbrain) syndrome; often due to upper midbrain compression by tumours. Combination of up- and downgaze palsies, pupillary retraction, loss of accommodation reflex and eyelid retraction.
- Oculogyric crises: overactivity of basal ganglia may result in fixed upward deviation of the eyes. Commonly precipitated by phenothiazines, metoclopramide.

# 14.14 Vertigo and hearing loss

## Vertigo

Vertigo describes a specific type of dizziness which arises either due to unusual motion (e.g. fairground rides) or due to pathology in the labyrinth, vestibular nerve, or central vestibular structures in the brainstem.

### Clinical evaluation

Try to distinguish vertigo from other forms of dizziness. Attempt to determine a peripheral or central origin.

*History*

- The sufferer has an erroneous perception of movement, either of themselves or their environment, e.g. spinning.
- Vertigo can be difficult to distinguish from other forms of dizziness but clues include:
  - Presence of nausea and vomiting.
  - Symptoms made worse by movement.
- Identifying the tempo of symptoms can be helpful in determining cause. Vertigo is never permanent (because the CNS adapts but patients may have persistent **episodes**).
- Severe episodic vertigo is usually peripheral.
- Other features that may be relevant in determining a differential diagnosis include viral illness, head injury, hearing loss, vascular risk factors, and headache.

*Examination*

- Nystagmus is often seen in vertiginous patients and may help distinguish central from peripheral causes (Fig. 14.11).
- Ataxia common but patient may be reluctant to stand.

*Investigations*

- ▶ MRI is often required to exclude a vascular event especially in patients who are elderly, have vascular risk factors, headache or abnormal cranial nerve examination.
- Audiometry can verify and characterize hearing loss.

### Common causes of vertigo

*Benign paroxysmal positional vertigo (BPPV)*

- The condition's name accurately describes the patient's transient experience of vertigo following rapid changes in head position. Each attack lasts less than a minute.
- BPPV is more common in elderly patients due to the formation of small crystals in the semicircular canals.
- Diagnosis can be made by inducing vertigo: rapidly tilt the sitting patient onto their side (Hallpike manoeuvre).
- Certain repositioning manoeuvres (e.g. Epley) can be performed by specialists to attempt to move the crystals and thus relieve symptoms.

*Vestibular neuritis*

- Benign, self-limiting illness but can be associated with significant disability due to acute severe vertigo, nausea, and vomiting. Hearing is preserved.
- Diagnosis is clinical, consider MRI to exclude differentials.
- The disabling symptoms usually resolve spontaneously in a few days while mild imbalance can persist for 2–3 months.
- Corticosteroids may reduce long-term sequelae.

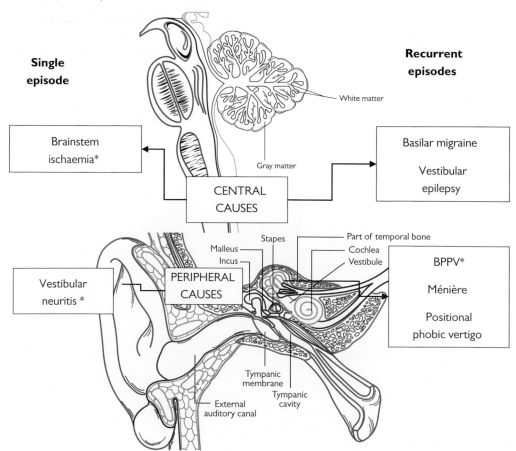

**Fig. 14.11** Some causes of vertigo. * = most common causes.

*Ménière disease*

- An idiopathic condition with onset in middle age.
- Build-up of pressure in the inner ear endolymph causes recurrent severe episodes of vertigo lasting several hours, with unilateral tinnitus, ear fullness, and hearing loss.
- Permanent low-frequency hearing loss can occur.
- No diagnostic test exists.
- Most cases can be managed medically, but those refractory should be referred to ENT for consideration of surgery (ablation of vestibular organ).

*Posterior circulation cerebrovascular disease*

- Acute-onset vertigo can dominate the presentation of an infarct or haemorrhage affecting the brainstem/cerebellum.
- Look for associated gaze palsy, Horner, asymmetrical limb neurology (motor, sensory or ataxia).
- ▶ Urgent MRI/CT vital as cerebellar haemorrhage can cause rapid deterioration requiring surgical intervention.

**Management**

Symptomatic treatments of persistent vertigo include:

- Pharmacological (only short-term use recommended):
  - Antihistamine, e.g. cinnarizine, betahistine.
  - Anticholinergics, e.g. hyoscine.
- Vestibular rehabilitation—exercises that aim to promote CNS adaptation to symptoms, particularly for peripheral causes of vertigo.

## Nystagmus

An involuntary rhythmical oscillation of the eye, nystagmus can occur in vertical, horizontal, or torsional planes. Nystagmus possesses a fast and slow phase—**direction is defined by the direction of the fast phase**. Causes include:

- Congenital.
- Drug-induced, e.g. phenytoin, alcohol.
- Pathology affecting central or peripheral vestibular system.

'Gaze-evoked' is the most common type of nystagmus. It describes the situation where the eyes, on fixing a target, have a tendency to drift back to the central position (slow phase) whereupon the patient makes a corrective saccade (fast phase) to bring the eye back onto the target. This means that the direction of nystagmus will alter depending on the direction of gaze. Drug-induced nystagmus is usually gaze-evoked.

Nystagmus arising from central and peripheral vestibular pathology can sometimes be distinguished clinically:

- Central nystagmus is often gaze-evoked, can be vertical, horizontal, torsional, or any combination, is usually not suppressed by visual fixation and does not fatigue. Upbeat nystagmus tends to indicate lesions of the craniocervical junction while downbeat nystagmus is associated with pontine pathology.
- Peripheral nystagmus tends to be unidirectional (fast phase away from the lesion), always has a horizontal component, and may be suppressed by visual fixation. Sudden changes in head position may worsen nystagmus. During the Hallpike manoeuvre peripheral nystagmus has a latency of a few seconds and fatigues rapidly.

Many patients are unaware of their nystagmus. Occasionally they may be troubled by oscillopsia (jerking of the vision).

## Hearing loss

A common form of physical disability experienced by a considerable proportion of the population especially later in life. Causes of hearing loss tend to be classified according to whether the problem lies in sounds failing to reach the inner ear—conductive—or due to the hearing apparatus failing to successfully transmit messages centrally: sensorineural (Fig. 14.12).

### Clinical evaluation

*History*

- Tempo and duration of symptoms, e.g. gradual/sudden onset.
- Associated features, e.g. earache, itching, discharge, tinnitus, vertigo.
- History of noise exposure including occupation, barotrauma (flying/scuba diving), physical trauma, (head injury).
- Family history of hearing loss.
- Drug history of ototoxins, e.g. aminoglycosides, furosemide.

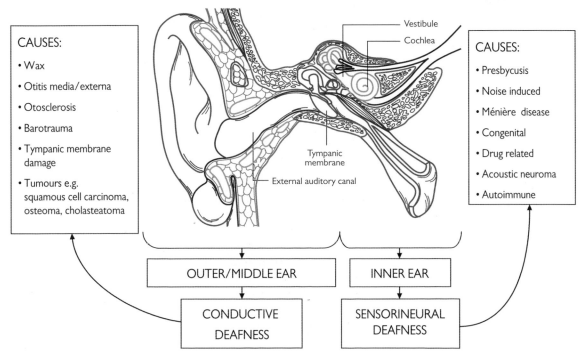

CAUSES:
- Wax
- Otitis media/externa
- Otosclerosis
- Barotrauma
- Tympanic membrane damage
- Tumours e.g. squamous cell carcinoma, osteoma, cholasteatoma

Vestibule
Cochlea
Tympanic membrane
External auditory canal

CAUSES:
- Presbycusis
- Noise induced
- Ménière disease
- Congenital
- Drug related
- Acoustic neuroma
- Autoimmune

OUTER/MIDDLE EAR — INNER EAR

CONDUCTIVE DEAFNESS — SENSORINEURAL DEAFNESS

**Fig. 14.12** Differential diagnosis of hearing loss.

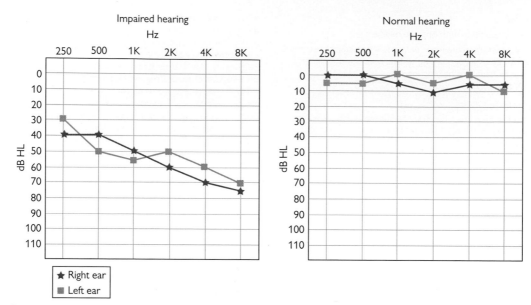

**Fig. 14.13** Pure tone audiometry.
This figure was published in *Neurology and Neurosurgery Illustrated*, KW Lindsay and I Bone, p. 61, Copyright Elsevier, 1997.

*Examination*

- Degree of deafness cannot be quantified by bedside testing but testing ability to hear whispered speech at arm's length is a useful screening test and may help to clarify the presence of asymmetry
- Rinne/Weber tests use a 256 or 512Hz tuning fork to **help** distinguish conductive/sensorineural deafness (not completely reliable):

  **Rinne:** tuning fork base is held on the mastoid until the patient can no longer hear it, then prongs held adjacent to external auditory meatus. The patient should still be able to hear the sound (air conduction normally louder than bone-conduction)—if less implies conductive deafness (or false + ve because sound heard in other ear).

  **Weber:** tuning fork base is placed on the forehead or skull vertex and patients asked in which ear the sound is best heard—normally heard equally by both ears. Unilateral sensorineual deafness: best in normal ear. Unilateral conductive deafness: best in affected ear (has increased sensitivity).

- Otoscopy: look for wax, debris, polyps, or tumours in the auditory canal, and tympanic membrane abnormality.
- Test vestibular function (e.g. balance and nystagmus).

*Investigation*

- Audiometry—pure tone audiometry quantifies the volume required for patient to detect each sound frequency (Fig. 14.13), air/bone conduction is compared, speech sounds are tested separately.
- Examination under microscope by ENT surgeon is recommended in unexplained conductive deafness.
- Electric response audiometry tests the transmission of signals from the cochlea to the brainstem/auditory cortex.
- MRI or CT examining posterior fossa and inner ear are required if sensorineural hearing loss is unilateral.

- Blood glucose, autoimmune/vasculitis screen, TFT (association between deafness and diabetes, thyroid abnormality, and connective tissue disease), and syphilis serology can be performed in unexplained cases.

**Common causes of hearing loss**

- **Otitis media:** commonly caused by viral infection in childhood. Fluid accumulation in middle ear may cause earache and prevent movement of the tympanic membrane. Persistent middle ear effusion occasionally requires drainage.
- **Otosclerosis:** hereditary condition causing bony overgrowth of the ossicles (particularly stapes) which prevents sounds being transmitted to the cochlea.
- **Barotrauma:** sudden pressure changes without equalization can cause rupture of the tympanic membrane.
- **Presbycusis:** most common cause of hearing loss, usually seen in elderly but can occur as early as 40 years. Cochlear degeneration leads to 4kHz loss in particular.
- **Noise induced:** recurrent exposure to loud noise can cause high-frequency (8kHz) sensorineural deafness.
- **Ménière disease** (see earlier): cochlear form of the disease causes episodic low-frequency hearing loss and may result in permanent deficit.

# Tinnitus

The sensation of noise in the ears. Can occur with any ear disorder but commonly in hearing loss that is noise—or drug-induced or related to infection. Highly vascular middle ear tumours or AVM can cause an audible hum, even occasionally heard by the examiner. Unilateral tinnitus and hearing loss—consider acoustic neuroma. **Treatment:** correction of hearing loss, referral for tinnitus masking and treatment of depression.

# 14.15 Seizures and epilepsy

## Three key questions

- **Is it an epileptic seizure?**
- **If so, what type?**
- **Is there an identifiable cause?**

## Seizure differential

- Sudden onset, transient, usually brief (<2 minutes) cerebral event, often with impairment of consciousness.
- Whereas to the general public, seizure only implies convulsion.
- Differential diagnosis: vascular, psychiatric, neurological. See Box 14.1.

### Vascular

*Syncope (transient cerebral hypoperfusion)*

- Vasovagal:
  - Triggers (heat, pain, fear, coughing, micturition).
  - Upright posture.
  - Prodrome (nausea, lightheaded, closing in vision).
  - Loss of consciousness (LOC).
  - Very brief event (<30 seconds).
  - Rapid recovery (if supine).
- Cardiac:
  - Arrhythmia, aortic stenosis, HOCM.
  - Any posture, may be triggered by exertion.
  - No warning before, no confusion after.
  - Abrupt onset and offset.

*Transient ischaemic attack (TIA)*

- Focal neurological symptoms/signs.
- LOC is very rare.
- Vascular risk factors (especially age).

### Psychiatric

- Hyperventilation ± panic attacks:
  - Tingling, chest pain, SOB ± intense dread.
  - Usually some consciousness preserved.
- Non-epileptic attacks (NEAs)—see Section 14.32. Traps for the unwary with PNES:
  - Often deeply unconscious.
  - Often prolonged (>5 minutes), hence often 'status'.
  - May bite 'lip or tip' (of tongue).
  - Often incontinent.
  - Injuries occur including severe, e.g. burns.
  - Can (appear to) occur from sleep.

> ### Box 14.1 Diagnosing epilepsy
> - Epilepsy diagnosis is 99% clinical.
> - EEG/MRI are not diagnostic tools.
> - Always get an eyewitness account (if necessary by phone).
> - The diagnosis is never certain until you have seen an attack in person or on video.
> - Acidosis (just after) or rising CK (2–3 days after) imply tonic–clonic.
> - Don't be afraid to say 'insufficient evidence' for a diagnosis.
> - The diagnosis has significant lifelong implications.
> - The diagnosis should always be confirmed by a Neurologist.

- Psychosis:
  - Hallucinations, bizarre behaviour.

### Neurological

- Migraine:
  - Slower onset, longer duration, mainly aura.
  - If ends in blackout, usually syncopal.
- Sleep disorders:
  - Narcolepsy, parasomnias.
- Metabolic seizures:
  - High glucose, urea, or fever.
  - Low glucose, calcium, or sodium.
  - Alcohol-related.
  - Eclampsia.

## Classifying epilepsy

### Seizures and syndromes

- There are seven classic **seizure types**:
  - Simple partial
  - Complex partial
  - Absences
  - Myoclonus
  - Atonic
  - Tonic
  - Tonic–clonic.
- There are two basic **epilepsy syndrome types**:
  - Generalized epilepsy
  - Focal epilepsy.
- Patients may have two or more seizure types.
- Knowing seizure types determines the syndrome.
- Knowing the syndrome determines investigations, treatment choices, prognosis, and familial risk.

### Seizure types

*Simple partial seizures (auras)*

- Only occur in focal epilepsy syndromes.
- Fully conscious.
- Last for seconds.
- May point to the epileptic focus.

Examples: **frontal** (limb jerking/posturing, head turning); **parietal** (somatosensory); **temporal** (special sense hallucinations except visual, fear, déjà vu, autonomic); **occipital** (lights, colours).

*Complex partial seizures*

- Only occur in focal epilepsy syndromes.
- Partially responsive, often amnestic.
- Longest duration seizure type (1–20 minutes).
- Consist of three stages:
  1. **A**ura
  2. **A**ltered consciousness
  3. **A**utomatisms.
- Automatisms are repetitive actions: lip-smacking, chewing, plucking, fiddling, wandering, humming, speech, spitting.
- If just 'goes blank', it resembles a 'typical absence' (see following subsection).

*Typical absences*

- Only occur in generalized epilepsy syndromes.

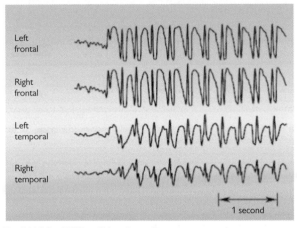

Fig. 14.14 Ictal EEG → 3Hz spike and wave.

- Used to be called 'petit mal' and rarely start in adulthood.
- Last 1–20 seconds (unless 'absence status').
- Full loss of consciousness without significant loss of tone.
- Abrupt onset and offset.
- EEG during an absence shows 3Hz (three per second generalized spike and wave (Fig. 14.14).

*Myoclonus*
- Only occur in generalized epilepsy syndromes.
- Full loss of consciousness, but too brief to realize.
- Shock-like **bilateral** jerks of arms or legs causing spills or falls.
NB: **unilateral** twitching of muscles is often termed myoclonic, but should be called a simple partial motor (clonic) seizure.

*Tonic*
- Occur in focal and generalized syndromes.
- Usually last <2 minutes.
- Rigid limb extension or flexion (symmetric or asymmetric), eye roll, jaw clench (tongue biting), bladder contraction (incontinence), airway contraction (cry, scream, apnoea).

*Tonic–clonic*
- Occur in focal and generalized syndromes.
- Initial muscle rigidity (~30 seconds).
- Then four-limb jerking (30–60 seconds):
  - Initial rapid, small jerks.
  - Evolving to slower, larger jerks.

*After tonic or tonic–clonic may have*
- Postictal stertor (snoring, blowing breath sounds).
- Postictal apnoea.
- Postictal agitated confusion and later psychosis.

*Atonic*
- Occur in focal and generalized syndromes.
- Very brief (<10 seconds) loss of tone and consciousness.
- Typical cause of the 'drop attack'.
- Often associated with learning disability/brain damage.

### Syndrome types
- Generalized epilepsy
- Focal epilepsy.
See Table 14.7.

Table 14.7 Features of generalized vs. focal epilepsy

|  | Generalized epilepsy | Focal epilepsy |
| --- | --- | --- |
| Age of onset (years) | <25 | Any |
| Abnormal MRI | +/− | + |
| Epileptiform interictal EEG | ++ | +/− |
| Photosensitivity | + | +/− |
| Genetic risk | + | +/− |
| Self-remitting | + | + |
| Drug refractory | + | ++ |
| Simple/complex partial | − | +++ |
| Absence | ++ | − |
| Myoclonus | ++ | − |
| Atonic | +/− | +/− |
| Tonic | + | + |
| Tonic–clonic | +++ | ++ |

– Never; +/− rare; + occurs; ++ common; +++ majority.

## Causes

### Acute symptomatic seizures
- Tumour, stroke, limbic encephalitis (viral, autoimmune), venous sinus thrombosis (e.g. pregnancy, thrombophilia), metabolic (diabetes, thyrotoxicosis, uraemia), drug intoxication or withdrawal (especially alcohol), pre-eclampsia.

### Chronic epilepsy
- Syndromes can be divided into:
  - Idiopathic—no structural cause.
  - Cryptogenic—presumed structural cause.
  - Symptomatic—identified structural cause.
- The commonest generalized epilepsy syndromes are idiopathic.
- The commonest focal epilepsy syndromes are symptomatic.

*Idiopathic generalized epilepsy (IGE)*
- Age of onset usually 2–14 years.
- Can be benign (i.e. self-remitting).
- But 50% are juvenile myoclonic epilepsy (JME):
  - Myoclonus, usually soon after waking.
  - Tonic–clonic seizures appear by late teens.
  - Spike/polyspike and wave on EEG (see Fig. 14.14).
  - Highly responsive to sodium valproate (VPA).
  - Lifelong drug treatment required.

*Symptomatic focal epilepsy*
Age of onset depends on cause:
- Commonest cause in younger patients is hippocampal sclerosis—associated with early life insults (e.g. meningitis, febrile fits).
- Commonest cause in middle age is a tumour (Fig. 14.15).
- Commonest cause in older age is cerebrovascular disease.

## Approach to history taking
- Seizure differential is usually between epilepsy, syncope, and psychogenic non-epileptic seizures (PNES).
- Ascertain how many different seizure types there are.

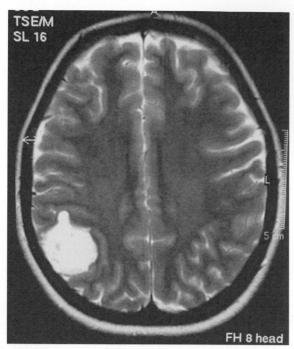

**Fig. 14.15** MRI of right parieto-occipital astrocytoma in a 52-year-old patient presenting with new-onset seizures.

- Then get detailed patient and witness account of each seizure:
  - The prodrome is most helpful for confirming vasovagal syncope (hot, sweaty, nausea, lightheaded, vision closing in, hearing muffled).
  - The ictus is most helpful for confirming PNES (prolonged, waxes and wanes, weeping, backarching, thrashing).
  - Postictal is most helpful for confirming epilepsy (stertorous breathing, agitated confusion, lateral tongue biting, delayed psychosis).
- Tempo hallmarks:
  - Syncope: slow onset, brief ictus, quick recovery.
  - Epilepsy: quick onset, brief ictus, slow recovery.
  - PNES: slow onset, long ictus, slow recovery.
- Ask about other possibly unrecognized seizures:
  - Wake up with blood in mouth/headache/incontinent?
  - Specific auras?
  - Myoclonus ('morning clumsiness', 'flying saucers')?
  - Blank spells with/without automatisms?
- Enquire about possible causes and associations:
  - Birth injury, delayed milestones.
  - Childhood illness, head injury, febrile convulsions.
  - Family history of 'epilepsy' (but need details).
  - Family history of sudden (cardiac) death and IHD.
  - Alcohol consumption.
  - Childhood emotional trauma.
- Document previous investigations (when and where):
  - Imaging (CT or MRI).
  - EEG (routine, sleep, 24-hour).
- Document drugs tried (dose, response, and side effects).
- Detailed social history, especially stress.
- Past medical history especially functional diagnoses or previous presumed 'syncope' (often how PNES presents in teens).
- Find out what they hope to achieve:
  - Complete seizure cessation?
  - Regaining driving licence or employment?
  - Fewer tonic–clonics, reducing mortality risk (SUDEP)?

## Examination

- Standard examination is rarely of major help in diagnosis.
- But it can identify causes of focal epilepsy if focal neurology identified, requiring imaging:
  - Check fundi, EOM, visual fields, drift, plantars, and gait.
  - Broadly assess alertness and cognition.
  - Check BP (lying + standing).
  - Check skin (NF1, tuberous sclerosis, Sturge–Weber).
- If any diagnostic doubt, hyperventilate the patient for 2–3 minutes—this triggers about 70% of PNES.

## Investigations

- Get old notes and reports of old investigations.
- Do an ECG on everyone with lost consciousness.
- Defer special tests until all the information regarding seizure description is available (unless directed by abnormal exam).
- If epileptic seizures likely and cause unknown:
  - Consider MRI (or contrast CT) if cause unknown.
  - Consider EEG if syndromic classification unclear.
- If typical simple syncope (trigger, prodrome, no postictal), ECG is the only test required.
- If syncope likely but atypical (supine, no prodrome, exertional), consider tilt table test ± 24-hour ECG/cardiac referral.
- ECG changes to trigger cardiology referral: QTc >450ms, PR <120ms, inverted T in V1–4, R or left bundle branch block.
- If diagnostic doubt persists, consider 24-hour EEG or up to 5-day admission for video telemetry (video + EEG), both designed to capture an event (also have a single ECG lead).
- **Never assume a previous diagnosis must have been correct.**
- **Always re-evaluate from scratch if poor treatment response.**

## Treatment

### General advice

Document everything in the notes and in writing for the patient. Encourage as normal a lifestyle as possible but:
- All countries have some driving restrictions:
  - In the UK, the patient must inform the DVLA.
  - If first seizure, need 6 months seizure-free (**includes auras**).
  - If epileptic, need 12 months seizure-free to drive again.
- Other safety issues:
  - Should not bathe unsupervised.
  - Common sense regarding working at heights, with machinery or extreme sports.
- Pregnancy and reproduction (see later subsection):
  - Teratogenicity of antiepileptic drugs (AEDs).
  - Interactions of AEDs (especially with various pills).
- SUDEP (sudden unexplained death in epilepsy):
  - Annual incidence 0.1–1% depending on epilepsy severity.
  - Most guidelines advise telling all patients of their risk.
  - Highest risk patients are those with tonic–clonic seizures, especially if nocturnal or poor drug adherence.

### Antiepileptic drugs

- 50% patients get side effects including allergy—minimized by starting at a low dose and increasing every 2 weeks (Table 14.8).
- Tailored to syndrome and individual wherever possible.

First-, second-, and third- line drugs (typical range for maintenance dose):

**Table 14.8** Common AEDs and their side effects

| Commonest AEDs | UK trade name | Important side effects |
|---|---|---|
| Carbamazepine/ oxcarbazepine | Tegretol® (CBZ)/ Trileptal® (OXC) | Rash, ataxia, hyponatraemia |
| Clobazam (CLB) | Frisium® | Sedation |
| Clonazepam (CLN) | Rivotril® | Sedation |
| Levetiracetam (LEV) | Keppra® | Mood swings |
| Lamotrigine (LTG) | Lamictal® | Rash |
| Phenytoin (PHY) | Epanutin® | Cosmetic, ataxia |
| Pregabalin (PRE) | Lyrica® | Weight gain |
| Valproate (VPA) | Epilim® | Weight gain |
| Topiramate (TOP) | Topamax® | Depression |
| Zonisamide (ZON) | Zonigran® | Depression |

**Generalized epilepsies:**
1. VPA (1000–2000mg).
2. LTG (150–300mg), LEV (1000–2000mg).
3. TOP (200–400mg), ZON (200–400mg).

**Focal epilepsies:**
1. LTG, CBZ (400–1200mg), OXC (600–1800mg).
2. LEV, TOP, ZON.
3. VPA, PRE (300-600mg), PHY (300–400mg).
CLB/CLN are used adjunctively in both epilepsy types.

*Drug notes*
- VPA is the most effective AED for idiopathic generalized epilepsy.
- VPA should be avoided where possible in fertile women.
- VPA increases LTG levels by about 50%.
- CBZ, PHY, PRE, and LTG can all exacerbate absences or myoclonus.
- AED levels are mainly performed to check adherence:
  - And where there is clinical suspicion of toxicity.
  - And for PHY where dose-level relations are not linear.
  - And in pregnancy where metabolism may be increased for certain AEDs (LTG, OXC, and possibly LEV).

**Surgery**
- Considered after failure of at least two AEDs at adequate doses.
- Requires a clear target, usually a lesion seen on imaging.
- Outcome partly depends on pathology.
- Best case scenario offers seizure freedom ~75% at 2 years.

**Vagal nerve stimulation**
- Helpful in drug refractory epilepsy without a clear target.
- Generally expect to reduce seizures than seizure freedom.
- Often used in the learning disabled population.

**Ketogenic diet**
- High fat, low carbohydrate diet used in refractory epilepsy.
- Principally used in children, sometimes with great success.

# Prognosis

- Depends on age of onset, syndrome, and cause.
- Some childhood-onset syndromes remit spontaneously.
- Others are expected never to remit (e.g. JME).
- Adult-onset are not expected to remit.
- Most epilepsy (>60%) responds to the first AED tried.
- Most do not die from their epilepsy and do not develop permanent or progressive physical deficits.
- Memory impairment and depression occur in >50% and can be more disabling than the seizures.

# Special circumstances

**First seizure**
- AEDs are not usually started.
- This is because evidence suggests there is no long-term (5-year) benefit for quality of life or achieving seizure freedom.
- Exceptions include patients with focal neurology and epileptogenic foci on EEG or imaging.
- After a second seizure, the risk of a third seizure increases from 30% to 56% (at 5 years).
- Ultimately, the patient should be given sufficient information to make an informed choice.

**Status epilepticus**
(See Section 1.14.)
- Continuous or near-continuous seizure activity.
- May be convulsive or non-convulsive.
- Non-convulsive status may present as confusion or coma.
- Convulsive status is defined as tonic–clonic seizures lasting >30 minutes or occurring serially without regaining consciousness.
- Emergency treatment is advised after 5 minutes (pre-status).
- It is rare in patients on multiple AEDs, so in these patients, always consider non-adherence, alcohol, or NEA.
- There are several markers of epileptic status cf. NEA status:
  - Metabolic acidosis on ABGs.
  - Epileptogenic lesion on brain imaging.
  - Severe mental or physical disability
  'Bad seizures occur in bad brains'
- If epileptic status likely give:
  - First-line: PR diazepam 10mg or buccal midazolam 10mg (community) or IV lorazepam 4mg (hospital) up to twice.
  - Second-line: load with IV PHY 15mg/kg.
  - Third-line: anaesthetize with IV barbiturates, midazolam or propofol (hence need transfer to ITU).
- NB: IV PHY needs cardiac monitoring due to risk of arrhythmia:
  - Identify and treat the trigger for status where possible.
  - Continue PHY at least 300mg daily.
  - Start oral AED if first presentation.

**Post-traumatic epilepsy**
- 2% will go on to develop epilepsy (85% in the 1st year).
- Strongest risk factors for post-traumatic epilepsy:
  - Severity of amnesia
  - Intracerebral bleeding
  - Skull fracture
  - Loss of consciousness (LOC).
- Seizures between 1 hour and 1 week after head injury carry the highest risk of recurrence.
- The increased risk remains even after 20 years.
- Immediate 'concussive fit' carries no increased risk.

**Pregnancy and reproduction**
- Pregnancy should be planned and folic acid 5mg started 3 months before contraceptive measures stop.
There are numerous issues:

*Fertility in epilepsy*
- Decreased fertility in women with epilepsy—if on VPA, check for polycystic ovaries.
- PHY may affect sperm production and motility.

*Reduced efficacy of most hormonal contraceptives with enzyme-inducing AEDs*
- 3 'P's—phenytoin, phenobarbitone, primidone.
- 3 'T's—Tegretol® (CBZ), Trileptal® (OXC), topiramate.

This area is a minefield—seek expert advice and be aware that:
- Oestrogen contraception can fail, even if taken for prolonged periods or if the dose is increased.
- The 'morning-after pill' can fail, even if a higher dose is taken.
- Progesterone-only pills can also fail.
- Only IM Depo-Provera® is (probably) not affected.
- The only entirely safe options are to also use condoms, to switch to the copper coil or abstinence.

*Reduced efficacy of lamotrigine if taking combined oestrogen contraceptive pill—decreases LTG levels by 25–70%*
- Increase LTG dose or switch to a progesterone-only pill.

*Pregnancy in epilepsy—concerns*
1. Risk of worsening mother's seizures:
   - Rare—commonest cause is non-compliance.
   - Some AED levels fall during pregnancy—LTG, OXC:
   - Most need to increase dose after 1st trimester, but not known if this affects teratogenicity.
   - Measuring LTG or OXC levels to pre-empt seizure deterioration is a logical but unproven tactic.
2. Risk to the baby from mother's seizures:
   - Increased stillbirths (×2), cerebral palsy, learning difficulties.
3. Risk to the baby from AEDs (teratogenicity):
   - Psychomotor development, malformations.
   - Greatest risks:
   - On VPA or PHY.
   - On more than one AED, especially if one is VPA.
   - Dose-related.
   - In 1st trimester (the first 12–13 weeks).

*Labour risks*
- 2% increased seizure risk (especially if protracted and mother tired).
- Consider elective caesarean section if having frequent generalized tonic–clonic seizures (GTCS).
- Treat GTCS with IV benzodiazepines.

*Breastfeeding*
- To be encouraged—but monitor for sleepy baby or poor feeding in mothers taking LTG or benzodiazepines.

*Postpartum*
- Risk of haemorrhagic disease of newborn 2–7 days postpartum if on enzyme-inducing AEDs (i.e. any of the 3 'P's and 3 'T's).
- Give mother vitamin K 20mg PO daily in last month of pregnancy.
- Give baby vitamin K 1mg IM on delivery.

## Psychiatric comorbidities
- Depression is very common in epilepsy.
- It may be:
  - Psychosocial as a reaction to epilepsy and its social impact.
  - Biological and due to the process causing seizures.
- The type of depression seen may be different to 'normal' depression (so-called interictal dysphoric disorder).
- SSRIs and SNRIs are safe to give in epilepsy.
- Tricyclics and neuroleptics probably lower seizure threshold.
- Fluoxetine may affect CBZ and PHY levels.
- Start at low dose and cautiously uptitrate as required.
- Postictal psychosis is uncommon and rarely identified—it typically begins the day after serial or severe seizures.
- All AEDs are thought to be associated with an increased suicide risk and patients should be warned of this.

## Stopping AEDs
- Some points to remember:
  - Most adult epilepsy is lifelong, especially if a visible cause.
  - Prior generalized seizures means a risk of SUDEP.
  - A previous high seizure frequency suggests the epilepsy will come back.
  - Once seizure control is lost, it can't always be regained.
  - There are no known long-term issues with modern AEDs.
- Additional issues to discuss with patients:
  - Social impact of a breakthrough seizure, e.g. driving.
  - Psychological impact of a breakthrough seizure.
- Side effects are not a good reason to consider stopping AEDs—a switch to a better tolerated AED is the preferred option.
- Ensure they are truly seizure free before stopping!
- Always reduce drugs slowly, especially the older drugs like phenobarbitone, primidone, benzodiazepines, and phenytoin.
- Advise not to drive during reduction and for 6 months after.

# Acute symptomatic seizures

### Alcohol
- Acute intoxication lowers seizure threshold.
- 50% of withdrawal seizures occur <24 hours after the last drink.
- Inform patient of risks of binge drinking and sudden cessation.
- Alcoholics have atrophied brains and frequent head injuries—always consider intracranial bleed if slow to wake post-fit.
- Consider controlling alcohol intake first before starting AEDs unless epilepsy predated alcohol or structural cause.
- Involve an alcohol liaison team regarding careful detoxification.
- Assess likely engagement and adherence before starting AEDs.
- Monitor LFT if on relevant AEDs.
- LEV or PRE are the safest if there is a risk of liver damage; LTG, OXC, TOP, and ZON could also be used at submaximal doses.

### Tumours or strokes
- AEDs should be offered after a first seizure in these contexts.
- An early seizure (<3 months) after stroke carries a 50% risk of long-term epilepsy; a delayed seizure carries an 85% risk.

### Neurosurgery
- AED prophylaxis is often given after major neurosurgery, but if no seizures occur, it can be discontinued after 2 weeks.

### Encephalitis
- Carries a risk of developing epilepsy, especially if permanent physical or cognitive deficits or MRI scarring.

### Venous sinus thrombosis
- Always consider in pregnant woman with seizures or personal or family history of thrombosis.

### Metabolic derangement
- A common cause of partial status.
- Correct underlying metabolic deficits as soon as able.

# Useful websites
- <http://www.epilepsy.org.uk> (for Epilepsy Action charity).
- <http://www.epilepsysociety.org.uk> (for the Epilepsy Society charity).
- <http://www.stars.org.uk> (syncope support group).
- <http://www.neadtrust.co.uk> (non-epileptic attack support group).
- <http://www.nonepilepticattacks.info> (information about non-epileptic attacks and non-epileptic attack disorder).

## Background

The characteristics of the cerebrospinal fluid (CSF) can be altered by a wide variety of neurological conditions, dealt with in other sections of this chapter. This section focuses on disorders which specifically affect the CSF pressure.

- Most CSF is produced by the choroid plexus.
- Total volume of CSF is variable and depends on factors including age, sex, and obesity.
- Average values range from 140–250mL.
- It is estimated that about 500mL of CSF is formed per day.

## Intracranial hypertension

### Hydrocephalus

The accumulation of increased volumes of CSF, usually accompanied by a rise in intraventricular pressure.

- Hydrocephalus can affect patients at any ages, with both congenital (e.g. Dandy–Walker malformation) and acquired causes (e.g. adhesions following infections, neoplastic lesions blocking the flow of CSF).
- Classified as obstructive or communicating.
- Obstructive hydrocephalus occurs when there is blockage to the flow of CSF (Fig. 14.16).
- Communicating hydrocephalus indicates no obstruction within the ventricular system or its outlet.

#### Signs and symptoms

Symptoms are variable and depend on underlying cause, speed, and age of onset. In a young child whose cranial sutures have not fused, the skull may enlarge significantly, while rapid-onset obstructive hydrocephalus patients tend to have obvious signs and symptoms of raised ICP.

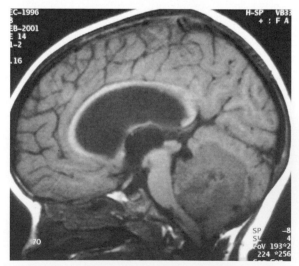

**Fig. 14.16** Obstructive hydrocephalus due to cerebellar tumour.

#### Investigation and treatment

- The investigation of choice is CT or MRI scanning. Depending on the relative size of the ventricles, the lesion may be localized and underlying causes may be visualized.
- Any underlying obstruction is usually treated. Excessive CSF may be diverted away from the CNS by inserting a shunt usually to the peritoneum. Shunts are not without complications, including infection, blockage, or overdrainage. In some patients, a third ventriculostomy may be performed, which enables CSF to bypass the obstruction.

### Idiopathic intracranial hypertension (IIH)

- Originally termed 'benign intracranial hypertension' but because of the potential for serious visual consequences has been renamed.
- Tends to affect overweight women of childbearing age.
- As well as the idiopathic version, similar presentations may occur secondary to a variety of conditions and medications including tetracyclines or nalidixic acid.

#### Presentation

IIH tends to present with headache, nausea, and visual impairment (enlarged blind spot, blurring of vision and visual obscurations). A VIth cranial nerve palsy may be observed and papilloedema is commonly seen.

#### Investigations

- MRI or CT may demonstrate narrowing of the ventricles and can help exclude alternative causes of intracranial hypertension such as cerebral venous thrombosis.
- LP demonstrates raised opening pressure with normal constituents.

#### Treatment

- Weight should be reduced if obese.
- Acetazolamide is a commonly used treatment to reduce the formation of CSF by the choroid plexus.
- If sight is acutely threatened, optic nerve fenestration or lumboperitoneal shunting may be indicated—although with medical treatment most cases remit within a few weeks.

### Normal pressure hydrocephalus

Tends to affect elderly adults who classically present with the triad of:-

1. Urinary difficulties (initially hesitancy and urgency, progressing to incontinence).
2. Gait dyspraxia.
3. Dementia, usually subcortical in nature:
   - Normal pressure hydrocephalus is thought to account for <0.5% of cases of dementia.
   - CT or MR imaging will usually reveal enlarged ventricles.
   - LP shows normal opening pressure (hence its name), although high pressure waves occur at regular intervals if continuous monitoring undertaken.
   - Performing a timed walk and MMSE before and after removal of about 50mL of CSF may indicate the likelihood of a patient's symptoms responding to shunting, which is the treatment of choice.

# Intracranial hypotension

- Most cases are due to spontaneous CSF leaks, which usually occur at the level of the spine and tend to be precipitated by minor trauma.
- Wide variety of presentations, from daily persistent headache with a classical orthostatic pattern, to oculomotor impairment, and thunderclap headache. Severe brain descent may result in diencephalic herniation and coma. Other important complications include subdural haemorrhage and venous sinus thrombosis.
- Investigations include LP demonstrating low opening pressure, MRI of the brain and spine which classically shows meningeal enhancement, and extra arachnoid or extra dural fluid. CT myelography may be useful.
- Treatment ranges from conservative (bed rest and hydration) to medical (IV or oral caffeine) and invasive (epidural blood patch, fibrin glue, or even surgical closure of a leak).
- Spontaneous remission may also occur, and the majority of patients make a full recovery with treatment.

# 14.17 Stroke

## What is a stroke?

- Sudden onset cerebral or spinal focal vascular insult.
- Lasting >24 hours (if not = TIA).

Stroke, like anaemia, is not a diagnosis, but a description.
On 'diagnosing' stroke, the next questions are:

- What is the stroke syndrome?
- What is the stroke mechanism?
- What is the best management?

### Common abbreviations

| ICA | Internal carotid artery |
|---|---|
| ACA, MCA, & PCA | Anterior, middle & posterior cerebral arteries |
| VA & BA | Vertebral & basilar arteries |
| BG | Basal ganglia |
| Bs | Brainstem |
| Cb | Cerebellum |
| GM & WM | Grey & white matter |
| PICA & AICA | Posterior & anterior inferior cerebellar arteries |
| ACom & PCom | Anterior & posterior communicating arteries |
| CoW | Circle of Willis |
| TACS, PACS, & POCS | Total anterior, partial anterior & posterior circulation syndromes |
| LACS | Lacunar syndrome |
| CEA | Carotid endarterectomy |
| TTE/TOE | Transthoracic/transoesophageal echo |

## Vascular anatomy

### Cerebral

Remember arterial disease can affect both 'large' and 'small' vessels:

- Large vessels—ICA, VA, BA, and their immediate branches.
- Small vessels—numerous small perforating arteries supplying Bs, BG, Cb and WM. Occlusion causes small (lacunar) infarcts.

*Anterior circulation*

ICA branches—ACA and MCA:

- ACA mainstem—supplies frontal GM and WM (Fig. 14.17).
- MCA mainstem—supplies parietotemporal GM and WM (Fig. 14.18).
- ACA small deep perforators—supply BG and internal capsule.
- MCA small deep perforators—supply BG, internal capsule and WM.

*Posterior circulation*

VA and BA branches:

- PICA—supplies lateral medulla (see later) + Cb.
- AICA:
  - Supplies medulla, pons and Cb.
  - Gives off artery to CN VIII (→ deafness).
- BA small perforators—supply pons and Cb.
- PCA—supplies midbrain, thalamus, occipital lobe and posterior temporoparietal lobes (although in 30% this is supplied by the ICA via the ACom).

The two circulations are joined anterior–posterior and left–right to form the CoW, allowing some maintenance of blood flow despite occlusion of individual arteries.

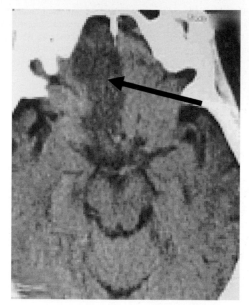

Fig. 14.17 CT head demonstrating infarct in ACA territory (arrow).

## Spinal

- Main supply by anterior spinal artery (ASA).
- Arises from single descending branch of Vas.

*Clinical picture (of spinal stroke)*

- Sudden onset back pain (80%).
- Initial flaccid, areflexic paraparesis.
- Dissociated sensory loss as posterior cord spared:
  - Light touch, pinprick, and temperature affected.
  - Proprioception and vibration spared.

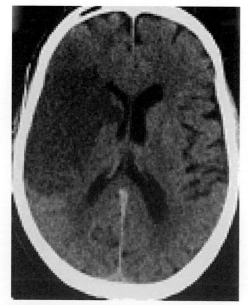

Fig. 14.18 CT head: large right parietal infarct in MCA territory.

- MRI appearances unreliable.
- Consider underlying causes: arrhythmia, shock, aortic dissection.
- Differential diagnosis: GBS, transverse myelitis, cord compression, spinal abscess.
- Deficits may begin to resolve within the first few days.
- Treatment is supportive + physiotherapy.

# Cerebrovascular arterial stroke

## Taking the history
- Time of onset known?
- Instantaneous symptoms?
- Progression?
- Fever, obtunded, stepwise, or prominent headache?
  - Red flags to consider other causes such as infection or carotid/vertebrobasilar dissection
- Possible causes?
  - Trauma—dissection.
  - Heart disease—cardioembolic.
- Vascular risk factors?
- Previous transient events?

## Clinical stroke syndromes

### 'TACS, PACS, POCS, and LACS'
= Bamford (Oxford) Stroke Classification (1991):
- TACS, PACS, POCS = large vessels.
- LACS = small vessels.
- Classification is based on the maximal clinical deficit.
- Useful for epidemiology, treatment, prognostication.

### TACS (total anterior circulation syndrome)
- All three of:
  - Hemiparesis or hemisensory loss.
  - Hemianopia.
  - Higher cortical dysfunction (dysphasia, neglect).
- 20% of strokes.
- Worst outcome (death or permanent disability).

### PACS (partial anterior circulation syndrome)
- 2/3 of:
  - Hemiparesis/hemisensory loss.
  - Hemianopia.
  - Higher cortical dysfunction.
- 35% of strokes.
- Highest early recurrence risk, some functional recovery.

### POCS (posterior circulation syndrome)
- One of
  - Hemianopia/cortical blindness.
  - Gaze paresis.
  - Crossed signs (ipsilateral cranial nerve palsy, contralateral weakness/numbness).
  - Bilateral weakness/numbness.
  - Cerebellar signs.
- 25% of strokes.
- High recurrence risk in first year, good functional outcome.

### LACS (lacunar stroke)
- Four syndromes:
  - Pure motor.
  - Pure sensory.
  - Sensorimotor.
  - Ataxic hemiparesis (an ataxic limb/limbs and ipsilateral pyramidal signs).
- Require absence of dysphasia, neglect, or POCS signs.
- Pure motor or sensory require two of face/arm/leg affected.
- 20% of strokes.
- Most rapid recovery, good functional outcome.

# Stroke mechanisms

## Atherothrombosis and thromboembolism
- Commonest and affects older age group.
- Atheroma develops in large and/or small arteries.
- Slowly developing atheromatous narrowing may be asymptomatic due to collateral formation.
- Embolic occlusion from carotid or vertebrobasilar systems is almost always abruptly symptomatic.

## Cardioembolism
- Consider particularly in young strokes.
- Emboli can occlude large or small arteries.
- Infarction of caudate + putamen ('comma sign') suggests occlusion of MCA perforators, often by an embolus.

*Causes include:*
- Atrial fibrillation—persistent or paroxysmal.
- Mural thrombus (e.g. post-myocardial infarction).
- Endocarditis.
- Patent foramen ovale:
  - Paradoxical venous embolus to brain.
  - Check for evidence of DVT/PE.
  - History of straining (causing reversal of left-to-right shunt).
- Atrial myxoma.

## Dissection
- Commonest identified cause of a young stroke.
- Relevant to large arteries (carotid, vertebral, basilar) only:
  - Enquire about history of neck trauma (hyperextension, twisting, manipulation) and connective tissue disease (Marfan, hypermobility syndrome).
- Tear in arterial vessel wall producing a double lumen.
- Two putative mechanisms:
  1. Occlusion of true lumen by haematoma in false lumen.
  2. Embolism from thrombus at site of tear.
- **ICA dissection:**
  - Periorbital pain.
  - Ipsilateral Horner (compresses sympathetic chain).
  - Ipsilateral hypoglossal palsy (pressure from distended lumen at skull base).
- **Vertebrobasilar:**
  - Neck pain.
  - Ipsilateral Horner (lateral medullary infarct).
  - Bilateral UMN signs in limbs.
- **Aortic:**
  - Cardiac chest pain radiating to back.
  - Unequal brachial BPs.

## Haemodynamic infarction
- Caused by cerebral hypoperfusion.
- From large or small arteries.
- If no pre-existing vascular disease:
  - Bihemispheric infarcts.
  - Watershed distribution (no anastamoses) (Fig. 14.19).

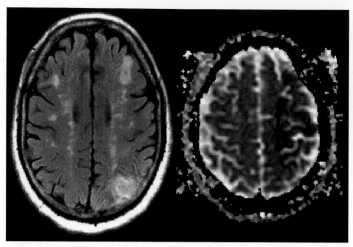

**Fig. 14.19** Magnetic resonance imaging (MRI) scan was obtained in a 62-year-old man with hypertension and diabetes and a history of transient episodes of right-sided weakness and aphasia. The fluid-attenuated inversion recovery (FLAIR) image (left) demonstrates patchy areas of high signal arranged in a linear fashion in the deep white matter, bilaterally. This configuration is typical for deep border-zone, or watershed, infarction, in this case the anterior and posterior middle cerebral artery (MCA) watershed areas. The left-sided infarcts have corresponding low signal on the apparent diffusion coefficient (ADC) map (right), signifying acuity. An old left posterior parietal infarct is noted as well.

Image reprinted with permission from Medscape Reference (http://emedicine.medscape.com/), 2014, available at: http://emedicine.medscape.com/article/338385-overview.

- If pre-existing stenosis:
  - Infarct in territory of stenosis.
  - Minimal hypotension required.
- Causes include: perioperative, LVF, blood loss, sepsis.

### Intracerebral bleed (ICB)
- Clinically indistinguishable from ischaemic stroke.
- Typically older patients.
- Bleeding usually from small rather than large arteries.
- Usually due to uncontrolled hypertension (Fig. 14.20).
- Amyloid angiopathy also a common cause in the elderly.

- Need to exclude underlying tumour or AV malformation (Fig. 14.21)—this often requires re-imaging after 6 weeks.
- Neurosurgical intervention if results in hydrocephalus or brain-stem compression due to posterior fossa bleeding.

## Stroke management

### 1. Immediate
- Is it stroke? (see Differential diagnosis).
- Rule out a bleed ± confirm infarction with CT brain.

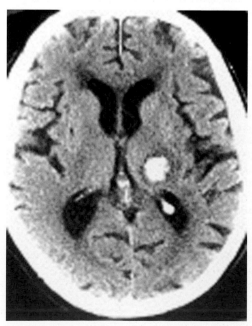

**Fig. 14.20** CT head (with contrast): left thalamic bleed in patient with uncontrolled hypertension.

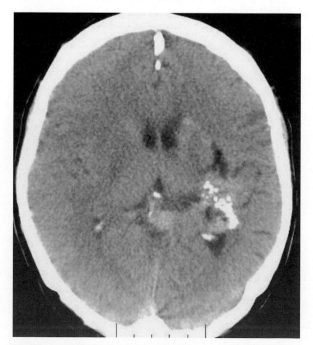

**Fig. 14.21** CT head (with contrast): left-sided arteriovenous malformation.

---

**Box 14.2 Thrombolysis pathway**

- Evidence of benefit if given within 3 hours of onset, haemorrhage definitely excluded and meet NINDS criteria.
- Requires a dedicated stroke service with access to high dependency beds, excellent Emergency department and Radiology links and staff experienced in management of thrombolysis and its complications.
- Contraindications must be excluded (e.g. recent surgery, recent stroke or head injury, prior anticoagulant usage).

---

- If under 3 hours from onset and resources available, contact local stroke team to consider thrombolysis (Box 14.2).
- If resolved <24 hours, follow TIA pathway (Box 14.3).
- Start antiplatelets (delay for 24 hours if thrombolysing).
- Check cholesterol, glucose, ESR.
- Check ECG and if available carotid Dopplers.

**2. Next 24 hours**

- Avoid lowering BP unless evidence of accelerated hypertension (e.g. >220/120mmHg, end-organ damage).
- DVT prophylaxis if immobile—TEDS (full length).
- Monitor and treat complications:
  - Check swallow with sip of water. NBM and NGT early.
  - Hourly neurological nursing observations if possible basilar thrombosis or malignant MCA infarct (see later).
- Consider mechanisms as listed earlier.

**3. Further specialist investigations**

- Consider MRI/MRA/MRV:
  - If dissection or venous sinus thrombosis possible.
  - If diagnosis uncertain and CT unremarkable.
  - If vasculitis suspected from inflammatory markers.
- Consider echocardiogram:
  - TTE only if need to detect mural thrombus and measure left atrial size and LV ejection fraction.
  - TOE only to exclude endocarditis, patent foramen ovale and atrial aneurysms.
- Consider 24-hour ECG/Holter monitor: where paroxysmal arrhythmia suspected.

**4. Young strokes (<65 years)**

- Exclude dissection, cardioembolism.
- Thrombophilia screen if other risk factors present:
  - Protein C&S.
  - Lupus anticoagulant.
  - Antiphospholipid antibodies.
- Review past medical and family history:

---

**Box 14.3 TIA pathway**

- Aspirin 300mg PO stat.
- If anterior circulation symptoms (dysphasia, neglect, hemiparesis), get urgent carotid Dopplers.
- If critical ICA stenosis confirmed (see later), refer for urgent carotid endarterectomy (CEA).
- If ICA stenosis not critical, it may still be clinically relevant, but there is no net benefit from surgery: follow pathway for secondary prevention.
- If posterior circulation symptoms, Dopplers not required unless at a centre offering vertebral angioplasty, or if required to confirm diagnosis or exclude dissection.

---

- Diabetes, deafness, short stature, myopathy or seizures—consider mitochondrial causes e.g. MELAS (**M**itochondrial myopathy, **E**ncephalopathy, **L**actic **A**cidosis, and **S**troke).
- Migraine, dementia, lacunar strokes—consider gene testing for CADASIL (**C**erebral **A**utosomal **D**ominant **A**rteriopathy with **S**ubcortical **I**nfarcts and **L**eucoencephalopathy)—the commonest hereditary stroke disorder.
- Consider vasculitis (rash, systemic features), and Fabry disease (rash neuropathy).

**Secondary prevention**

*Drugs and lifestyle*

- First line is generic clopidogrel 75mg once daily.
- For those intolerant of this, aspirin 75mg + dipyridamole MR 200mg twice a day should be offered.
- Simvastatin 40mg and increased if required to keep cholesterol <4.0 unless haemorrhagic stroke.
- ACE inhibitor to bring SBP <130mmHg—calcium channel antagonist or diuretic if Afro-Caribbean.
- Stop smoking.

*Surgery*

- TIA/stroke recurrence risk is ~10% per year in unoperated severe (70–99%) ICA stenosis.
- CEA reduces 5-year risk of recurrent ipsilateral TIA/stroke by 5% for moderate (50–70%) and 15–20% for severe ICA stenosis.
- Most centres do not offer CEA for 50–60% stenosis.
- MRA may help accuracy if Dopplers show stenosis falls between 60% and 80%.
- Highest risk of recurrent vascular event is in first few weeks, so CEA should be offered as soon as safe and practical.
- Perioperative risks vary according to surgical expertise from about 5–10%.

---

# Differential diagnosis

1. Migrainous aura with/without headache:
   - Hemiplegic.
   - Hemisensory—symptoms **spread** across face or limbs over minutes compared to instantaneous onset in stroke/TIA.
2. Epilepsy:
   - Unwitnessed seizure leading to a Todd paresis.
   - Hemisensory symptoms spread over seconds.
   - Full recovery within 2 days unless structural cause.
3. Multiple sclerosis:
   - Usually progresses over days–weeks, but sometimes rapid.
   - Young age and previous attacks make stroke unlikely.
4. Tumour:
   - Bleed into tumour can be sudden onset and focal.
   - Need repeat imaging at 6 weeks by contrast CT or MRI.
5. Peripheral nerve lesions/plexopathy:
   - Wrist drop, foot drop—remember, stroke **can** affect a single limb.
   - Look for discrete sensorimotor patterns.
6. Cerebral venous sinus thrombosis ('venous stroke'):
   - The great mimic of arterial stroke and SAH.
   - Venous infarction + haemorrhage can cause sudden onset of neurological deficit.
   - Usually have a preceding and prominent (may be 'thunderclap') headache.
   - Atypical appearance for usual arterial territories on imaging.
7. CNS infections:
   - Meningitis/encephalitis can cause acute focal neurology, but fever and prodrome normally present.

8. Functional (psychogenic) hemiparesis:
- Unclear onset with variability of deficit from history.
- Non-pyramidal fluctuating weakness and positive Hoover sign, often with asymptomatic sensory loss, on examination.

NB: TIAs rarely cause:
- Collapse
- Altered awareness/loss of consciousness
- Confusion.

▶ Do not call it a TIA just because it's transient and neurological.

## Notable signs and syndromes

### Amaurosis fugax
- Monocular.
- 'Curtain coming down over one eye'.
- Brief (usually <5 minutes).
- Usually due to embolism via ophthalmic branch of ICA.

### Bilateral ACA territory infarction
- Sudden-onset paraparesis.
- Mimics acute spinal cord or brainstem infarction.
- Look for aneurysm or anatomical variant of ACom.

### Basilar thrombosis
- Sequential bilateral posterior circulation infarcts.
- May cause diffuse pontine infarcts resulting in tetraplegia, clonus, and cranial neuropathies.
- Vertical eye movements and blink typically spared—therefore, can result in 'locked-in syndrome'.
- Usually due to propagation of clot from a dissected vertebral artery, so often affects the young.
- 80–90% mortality, typically because it is diagnosed too late for antiplatelets or anticoagulation to be beneficial.
- In specialist centres, neuroradiological intervention (thrombectomy, intra-arterial thrombolysis) can be lifesaving.

### Crossed brainstem syndromes
- Brainstem infarction interrupts corticospinal pathways that decussate in the medulla and supply the contralateral limbs.
- If it also interrupts cranial nerves and their nuclei, an ipsilateral (LMN) cranial nerve lesion and contralateral (UMN) hemiplegia result.
- **Midbrain:**
  1. Weber—ipsilateral (i/l) IIIrd, contralateral (c/l) hemiparesis.
  2. Nothnagel/Claude—i/l IIIrd, c/l ataxia.
  3. Benedikt—i/l IIIrd, c/l tremor.
- **Pons:**
  1. Millard–Gubler—i/l VIth + VIIth, c/l hemiparesis.
  2. Marie–Foix—i/l ataxia, c/l hemiparesis.
- **Medulla:**
  1. Dejerine (medial medullary syndrome):
     - i/l XIIth, c/l hemiparesis and proprioceptive loss.

2. Wallenberg (lateral medullary syndrome):
- i/l Vth, Horner and ataxia.
- c/l hemiparesis and hypoesthesia.

### Malignant MCA infarction
- Extensive cerebral oedema may develop 2–5 days after large MCA infarct.
- In non-atrophied (i.e. young) brains, there is little room to accommodate expansion—leads almost inevitably to death from raised ICP and coning.
- Hemicraniectomy may save life, but not function.

### Small vessel ischaemic disease
- Atheroma in small, deep penetrating vessels.
- Caused especially by ageing, hypertension, and diabetes.
- Leads to chronic 'lacunar state' which may:
  - Be asymptomatic.
  - Cause subtle cognitive problems and apathy.
  - Produce a small stepped gait with freezing ('vascular parkinsonism').

## FAQs

### 1. When can you use heparin or warfarin?
- Good evidence for warfarin use in AF for secondary prevention of stroke.
- Many clinicians use treatment dose LMWH or IV heparin empirically in evolving vertebrobasilar thrombosis.
- Prophylactic dose LMWH should be considered for DVT prevention if at high risk, or if TEDS contraindicated.

### 2. When do you start warfarin for AF?
- Usually 2 weeks after the stroke to minimize the risk of haemorrhagic transformation of the acute infarct.
- It is almost always safe to start it earlier if TIA or a clinically-resolved small infarct if BP controlled.

### 3. What about haemorrhagic infarction?
- It is not always easy to distinguish from primary ICB.
- If definite bleed into an infarct, should have aspirin (or warfarin if AF), once clinically stable and acute blood resorbed.

### 4. Do lacunar infarctions need carotid Dopplers?
- Yes, as carotid endarterectomy for significant >70% stenosis still reduces the risk of further stroke.

### 5. Do all PFOs need closing?
- Probably no—main indications are young age, large PFO, associated atrial aneurysm, no other risk factors.

## Reference

Bamford J, Sandercock P, Dennis M, *et al*. Classification and natural history of clinically identifiable subtypes of cerebral infarction. *Lancet* 1991; *337*(8756): 1521–6.

## Background

CNS infection can develop in the meninges (meningitis) or the brain/spinal cord parenchyma (encephalitis/myelitis). Myelitis is discussed in the section describing spinal cord disorders (Section 14.23). Additionally, focal infection such as an abscesses or mycotic aneurysm can arise.

## Meningitis

Inflammation of the lining of the CNS.

Most commonly infectious in aetiology (bacterial, tuberculous, viral, fungal), but can also be secondary to systemic inflammation (sarcoid, Behçet disease, lupus) or malignant infiltration.

▶ Acute bacterial meningitis is a life-threatening event, with severe consequences if not identified and treated promptly.

### Epidemiology

- Annual incidence 5 per 100,000 in the UK.
- Children and young adults; incidence also increasing after 3rd decade.

### Clinical evaluation

- A rapid clinical course, altered consciousness and obtundation are highly suggestive. Do not delay—treat immediately if suspected.

*Aims*

- Establish diagnosis.

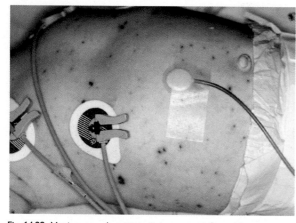

**Fig. 14.22** Meningococcal septicaemia in a young infant with purpura. Reproduced from Lewis-Jones, S., *OSH Paediatric Dermatology*, 2010, Figure 31.3, with permission from Oxford University Press.

- Determine severity and extent.
- Identify predisposing factors.

*History*

- Meningitic triad: headache, fever, neck stiffness.
- Accompanying features: photophobia, nausea, and vomiting.
- Indicators of severe disease: lethargy, confusion, seizures.
- Disease tempo may provide clues to underlying process: acute bacterial (acute onset) vs. chronic fungal or mycobacterial (subacute).
- Predisposing factors: immunodeficiency (including pregnancy), sinusitis, head injury, spinal/cranial surgery, travel history.

*Examination*

- Neck stiffness.
- Kernig sign (performed when supine): neck pain when leg is passively extended.
- Brudzinski sign (performed when supine): neck flexion causes hip and knee flexion
- Fever.
- Signs of increased ICP: papilloedema, focal neurology, decreasing conscious level, coma.
- Signs of systemic infection and sepsis.
- Source of infection: otitis media; URTI.
- Purpural rash suggesting meningococcal septicaemia (Fig. 14.22).

### Investigations

*Lumbar puncture*

- **The most important investigation**, and should be performed at earliest available opportunity **provided safe to do so**.
- Contraindications: papilloedema, SOL, decreased conscious level, focal neurology, clotting derangement, skin infection at LP site.
- If contraindicated, do blood cultures and start empirical antibiotics.

*CSF results*

Immediate CSF results are helpful in pointing towards a particular infectious aetiology (Table 14.9).

### Further tests

- Definitive evidence of the particular infectious agent.
- Exclude differentials (e.g. SAH).

### Management

- Early and continued liaison with microbiologist essential!
- Health Protection Agency requires notification of meningitis: <http://www.hpa.org.uk/infections/topics_az/noids/menu.htm>.

| Table 14.9 Interpretation of cerebrospinal fluid results in suspected meningitis | | | |
|---|---|---|---|
| | **Bacterial meningitis** | **TB meningitis** | **Viral meningitis** |
| Appearance | Turbid | Fibrinous | Clear |
| Predominant cell type | Polymorphs | Mononuclear | Mononuclear |
| Cell count/mm³ | 90–1000 | 10–1000 | 10–1000 |
| Glucose | <1/2 plasma | <1/3 plasma | Often normal, may be reduced |
| Protein (g/L) | <1.5 | 1–5 | <1 |
| Additional tests | Gram stain C/S Latex agglutination | Ziehl-Nielsen C/S PCR | Viral PCR |

*Bacterial meningitis*
- Empirical antibiotic treatment: third-generation cephalosporin (ceftriaxone or cefotaxime) + vancomycin ± rifampicin.
- If *Pneumococcus* or *Haemophilus influenzae* suspected, consider dexamethasone 0.6mg/kg/day in four divided doses.
- More definitive treatment once organism identified (Table 14.10).

*TB meningitis*
- Guided by microbiology, but initiate antituberculous agents, augmented with dexamethasone.

*Viral meningitis*
- Usually supportive treatment, with consideration of aciclovir.

## Complications and prognosis

*Mortality*
- Highest in children and elderly, in pneumococcal cases.
- Overall mortality in treated cases is 10%.
- Poor prognostic indicators: seizures, coma, focal neurology, delay in treatment, underlying medical condition.

*Complications and sequelae*
- Early: cerebral oedema, hydrocephalus, sepsis, seizures.
- Longstanding: focal neurological deficit, learning impairment, seizures.

## Non-infectious causes of meningitis
- Malignancy, sarcoidosis, Behçet, lupus, granulomatosis with poly-angiitis (Wegener).

## Mollaret meningitis
- Recurrent episodes of aseptic meningitis; linked aetiologically with HSV2.

# Encephalitis

Inflammation of the brain parenchyma, most commonly mediated through viral infection. Encephalitis can also refer to parenchymal inflammation secondary to autoimmune or paraneoplastic processes. Focal infections such as staphylococcal or malarial infection can also cause a cerebritis. This section will focus on viral encephalitis.

## Epidemiology/aetiology
- Incidence 7 per 10,0000 per year.
- Highest incidence in infancy, increasing to attain steady-state at 40.
- >100 DNA/RNA viruses associated with encephalitis.
- HSV encephalitis (HSE) most common in UK.
- Japanese encephalitis most common worldwide.
- Others: arboviruses (summer) enteroviruses (winter).

## Pathology
Viraemic invasion of brain parenchyma by neurotropic viruses. Certain viruses have predilections for certain parts of the brain, e.g. HSE and temporal lobes, Japanese encephalitis and basal ganglia.

| Organism | Susceptible groups | Antibiotics |
|---|---|---|
| Haemophilus influen-zae type B | Neonates Adults | Third-generation cephalosporin |
| Neisseria meningitides | Adults | Penicillin G or ampicil-lin or third-generation cephalosporin |
| Pneumococcus | All age groups | Vancomycin + third-generation cephalosporin |
| Listeria | Impaired cell-mediated immunity Pregnancy | Ampicillin or third-generation cephalosporin |
| Group B streptococcus | Children | Ampicillin or penicillin G |

Table 14.10 Common organisms responsible for bacterial meningitis shown with typical at-risk groups and appropriate antimicrobial therapies

## Clinical evaluation
Symptoms can be non-specific, and not dissimilar to meningitis, with greater emphasis on altered cognitive state and consciousness, and focal neurological deficit with less emphasis on neck stiffness.

*History*
- Prodromal URTI.
- Past history of measles (subacute sclerosing panencephalitis (SSPE)).
- Tempo of symptoms (HSE relatively rapid evolution, 24–48 hours).
- Headache.
- Fever.
- Seizures (commonly focal).
- Travel history.

*Examination*
- General confusion, disorientation.
- Focal neurology, including dysphasia and amnesia (HSE).
- More specific features:
  - Rigidity, choreoathetosis (Japanese encephalitis).
  - Rash (human herpesvirus 6 (HHV6), VZV).

## Investigations

*Bloods*
- High WCC.
- Occasionally low serum sodium.
- If differential diagnosis includes other causes of encephalopathy consider: ammonia, autoimmune screen, anti-thyroid peroxidase antibodies, tumour markers).

*CSF*
- Mild pleocytosis of 200/mm³, predominantly lymphocytes.
- High protein.
- Normal or mildly depressed glucose.
- Occasional xanthochromia/RBCs reflective of haemorrhagic necrosis.
- PCR highly sensitive and specific for HSE.

*EEG*
EEG findings will be abnormal, with changes seen diffusely or focally (temporal lobe in HSE).

*MRI*
MRI may show T2-weighted signal change which may be disseminated (SSPE, progressive multifocal leucoencephalopathy (PML)) or confined to certain parts of the brain such as basal ganglia (Japanese encephalitis) or temporal lobes (HSE) (Fig. 14.23).

## Management
- Again, early and continued liaison with microbiologist essential.
- Supportive.
- Antiviral agent: aciclovir as a first-line agent, switching to ganciclovir in cases of suspected HHV6 and ribavirin in postmeasles encephalitis.
- Health Protection Agency will require notification: <http://www.hpa.org.uk/infections/topics_az/noids/menu.htm>.

## Complications and prognosis
Acute encephalitis carries a significant mortality: 30% mortality in treated HSV cases (vs. 70% in untreated cases).

## Subacute sclerosing panencephalitis
- Progressive neurological disorder of childhood.
- Behavioural and cognitive decline, with myoclonus.
- Associated with persistent infection by measles virus.

# Cerebral abscesses

## Pathology
- Direct spread from neighbouring structures (mastoid, sinuses) via bone or draining vessels.

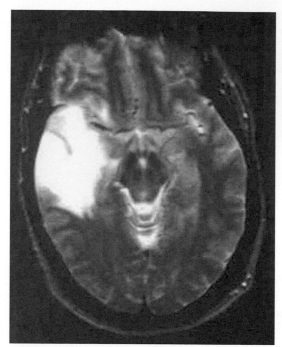

**Fig. 14.23** T2-weighted MRI Brain showing high signal change in encephalitis (predominantly right temporal lobe).
With kind permission from Charles F. Lanzieri.

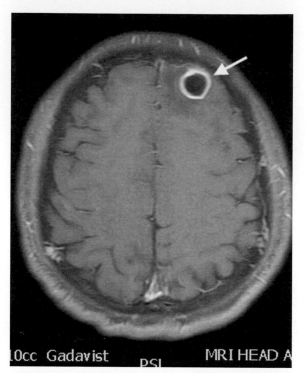

**Fig. 14.24** Brain MRI, T1 with IV contrast. The examination demonstrates the characteristic ring enhancement associated with a brain abscess.
Image reprinted with permission from Medscape Reference (http://emedicine.medscape.com/), 2014, available at: http://emedicine.medscape.com/article/336829-overview.

- Haematogenous spread from remote sources (endocarditis, bronchiectasis).
- In 20% of cerebral abscesses, no source of infection is found.

## Pathogenesis

- Initial poorly defined, localized inflammation surrounding infective focus: cerebritis.
- After a few days, formation of fibrous capsule around infection: abscess.

## Organisms

- 30–60% of abscesses are polymicrobial.
- Commonly isolated organisms include streptococci (especially *Streptococcus milleri*), *Enterobacteriaceae*, anaerobes, *Staphylococcus aureus*, and fungi
- In immunocompromised: *Candida, Aspergillus, Toxoplasma*.

## Clinical presentation

- Dependent on the location and size of the abscess.

*Clinical manifestations (in order of frequency)*

- Headache.
- Drowsiness and confusion.
- Seizures.
- Focal neurology.
- Fever.

If abscess is large enough, there may be

- Signs of increased ICP.
- Meningism.

Look for infective source: otitis media, dental infection, endocarditis, bronchiectasis.

## Investigations

- MRI is the investigation of choice.

- Abscesses are surrounded by a rim of contrast enhancement and oedema (Fig. 14.24).
- MR spectroscopy may help distinguish between abscess and tumour.
- NB: distinguishing between abscess, tumour, and infarct is sometimes difficult on imaging grounds alone. In this situation, a neurosurgical opinion should be sought for a diagnostic aspiration/excision.

*Other investigations*

- CRP and ESR are often elevated.
- Blood cultures.
- Multiple blood cultures and echocardiogram are indicated if endocarditis is suspected.
- In general, LP is contraindicated because of risk of herniation (15–30%).

## Management and prognosis

- Seek microbiology advice.
- Empirical antibiotics can be initiated at the cerebritis stage of the disease: penicillin G, chloramphenicol, metronidazole, with addition of flucloxacillin if *Staph. aureus* suspected.
- If increased ICP is present, symptomatic dexamethasone with referral to neurosurgeons for aspiration/excision.
- Prognosis generally good, 5–10% mortality.
- Epilepsy complicates 30% of cases.

## CNS tumours

- Present with headache (24%), seizure (21%), focal symptoms (21%).
- Neurological signs present in 80%.
- Lone headache without signs only found in 2% of tumours.
- 10% misdiagnosed on CT (2/3 were non-contrast).
- 50% primary, 50% secondary.

## Primary CNS tumours

| Children: | 70% infratentorial | Ependymoma, medulloblastoma, pilocytic astrocytoma |
|-----------|--------------------|----------------------------------------------------|
| Adults: | 70% supratentorial | Oligodendroglioma, astrocytoma, meningioma |

Features of astrocytomas (Fig. 14.25):
- Account for 80% of adult primary CNS tumours.
- Present in middle age.
- Graded I–IV (on basis of histology).
Grade IV = glioblastoma multiforme associations:
- Ventricular and spinal—ependymoma.
- Posterior fossa—medulloblastoma.
- Chemosensitive—oligodendroglioma.
- Radiosensitive—medulloblastoma.

### Treatment
- Low grade—watch and wait:
  - Consider resection as may be curative.
  - Chemo- or radiotherapy for selective cases.

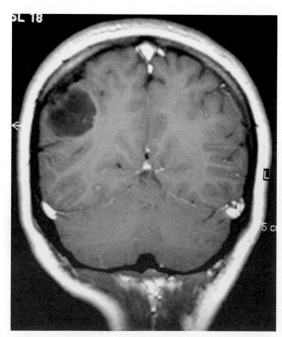

**Fig. 14.25** MRI: right parietal astrocytoma.

- High grade—biopsy or debulking/resection:
  - Then early radiotherapy (ideally targeted).
  - Chemotherapy for recurrence (palliative).

### Prognosis
- Glioblastoma multiforme (GBM) is the most common and most malignant primary brain tumour.
- Survival is 3 months untreated and 9–11 months treated

## Metastatic CNS tumours

### Brain metastases
*Present with:*
- Headache in 50%, especially if in the posterior fossa.
- Seizures/cognitive impairment more frequent than focal symptoms.

*Primary*
- Lung (50%), breast (20%), melanoma (10%).

*Treatment*
- Dexamethasone 16mg/day (reduce surrounding oedema).
- Whole brain radiotherapy if low grade; chemo for SCLC, NHL and germ cell.

### Spinal metastases
*Present with:*
- Pain (80%), LL>UL weakness (75%), sensory signs (50%), sphincter disturbance (50%—usually a late sign).

*Primaries*
- Prostate, breast, lung; also renal, myeloma, NHL.

*Treatment*
- Dexamethasone 16–32mg/day; radiotherapy (especially for pain); surgery if life expectancy >3months, solitary, or very recent paraplegia.

### Carcinomatous meningitis (meningeal metastases)
*Solid tumours*
- Lung (50%), breast (20%), melanoma.

*Non-solid tumours*
- Leukemia, lymphoma.

*Clinical subtypes*
1. Cerebral: raised ICP (headache, seizures, lethargy)
2. Cranial nerves: diplopia, deafness, vertigo, numb face
3. Spinal: radicular pain, weakness, sphincter disturbance

*Differential diagnoses*
- Cerebral metastases, infective (TB, fungal), CNS sarcoid.

*Investigations*
- CSF abnormal in 90% (review CT to ensure safe to LP):
  - Raised pressure, lymphocytes, and protein in >50%.
  - Low glucose (unlike with cerebral metastases).
  - Cytology diagnostic in 50% (at first LP); 90% (by third).
- MRI with contrast:
  - 67% abnormal (50% for contrast CT).

*Prognosis*
- With no treatment, survival <2 months; with treatment, depends on primary.

| Table 14.11 Ten classic paraneoplastic neurological syndromes | |
|---|---|
| **Paraneoplastic syndrome** | **Clinical features** |
| Lambert–Eaton myasthenic syndrome (LEMS) | Myasthenia-like, but with hyporeflexia and dysautonomia |
| Paraneoplastic cerebellar degeneration | Ataxia, vertigo, dysphagia, nystagmus |
| Paraneoplastic limbic encephalitis | Amnesia, seizures, psychiatry, confusion |
| Paraneoplastic brainstem encephalitis | Cranial neuropathies, ataxia, parkinsonism, hypoventilation |
| Stiff person syndrome | Axial + limb stiffness, spasms, startle, anxiety, falls, abnormal EMG |
| Paraneoplastic myelopathy | Cord syndrome |
| Paraneoplastic sensory neuronopathy | Severe sensory ataxia ± pain |
| Paraneoplastic opsoclonus-myoclonus | 'Dancing eyes and feet' ± ataxia |
| Cancer associated retinopathy | Poor night and colour vision, photophobia |
| Paraneoplastic myositis | Poly-/dermatomyositis |

# Paraneoplastic neurological syndromes

- Typically precede cancer diagnosis.
- Different known syndromes of neurological impairment caused by an immune process distant from site of the cancer (Table 14.11).
- Acute (days) to subacute (weeks) onset.
- Severe disability usually within 3 months.

## Diagnosis

- Clinically compatible with a classic syndrome(s).

- Presence of known paraneoplastic antibodies (request 'paraneoplastic Abs' and specify clinical syndrome(s) on request form).

## Management

- Principal aim is to identify and treat underlying cancer.
- PET scan is the single most sensitive test and directs further investigation.
- Immunotherapy (steroids/IVIG/plasma exchange) occasionally used.
- Very early cancer therapy offers the best outcome.

# 14.20 Multiple sclerosis

## Background

- Chronic inflammatory disease of the CNS characterized by multifocal demyelinating sclerotic plaques.
- Multiple sclerosis (MS) is the most common chronically disabling neurological condition affecting young adults in the UK.

## Epidemiology

- Age: usually presents in 3rd or 4th decade (uncommon before adolescence and beyond 60).
- ♀:♂ = 2:1.
- UK prevalence 100–150/100,000.
- Worldwide there is a latitudinal gradient, with rates increasing as one moves away from equator.

## Pathology

White matter plaques; sharply demarcated oval-shaped demyelinating lesions associated with blood–brain barrier breakdown, inflammatory cell infiltration, variable degrees of remyelination, gliosis, and axonal loss.

## Clinical course

80% of MS patients present with relapsing remitting (RR) symptoms. A 'relapse' typically evolves over several days, reaching a plateau for 1–2 weeks, before gradually improving over weeks. Recovery may be complete or partial.

The majority of RR patients (~80% after 20 years) enter a 'secondary progressive' (SP) phase, characterized by a gradual accumulation of disability ± superimposed relapses.

20% present with primary progressive MS (PPMS), characterized by a progressive course from onset without relapses. In contrast to relapsing disease, PPMS usually presents with a chronic progressive myelopathy ± ataxia, affects ♂ and ♀ equally and has an older age of onset.

Fixed disability can therefore be acquired by: (1) incomplete recovery from relapse and (2) disease progression. Overall 50% of MS patients require a walking aid within 15 years of disease onset.

## Symptoms and signs

### Clinical features of relapse

These reflect the anatomical location of the MS plaque. While plaques may occur **anywhere** in the CNS, symptoms/signs frequently result from involvement of:

*Optic nerves*
- Causes optic/retrobular neuritis (usually uniocular).
- Reduced visual acuity and colour vision ± central scotoma.
- Painful eye movements.
- Optic disc normal or swollen → later pale.

*Spinal cord*
- Pyramidal weakness with ↑ tone, ↑ reflexes, ↑ plantars.
- Sensory disturbance, both 'positive' (e.g. dysaesthesia) and 'negative' (e.g. numbness, sensory ataxia).
- Urinary symptoms.

*Brainstem/cerebellum*
- Ataxia and tremor, dysarthria.

- Eye movement disorders:
  - Diplopia.
  - Internuclear ophthalmoplegia.
  - Gaze palsy (often associated with facial weakness).
  - Oscillopsia.
- Facial sensory disturbance.
- Vertigo.
- Limb weakness and/or sensory disturbance.

### Important features from the history

- Attempt to differentiate a new relapse from residual symptoms following a previous relapse (which may wax and wane, e.g. with infection, hot weather, etc.), other paroxysmal symptoms lasting <24 hours etc.
- Is there a past history suggestive of relapses (i.e. patients often don't present until their second or third relapse)?
- Enquire about other common MS symptoms:
  - Lhermitte phenomenon—sensory disturbance ('like an electric shock') travelling down the spine on neck flexion.
  - Uhthoff phenomenon—symptoms (especially those of optic neuritis) worsened by heat (e.g. hot bath, hot weather, even smoking).
  - Stiffness/muscle spasms.
  - Depression, more rarely other psychiatric features.
  - Bowel symptoms, erectile dysfunction.
  - Mild cognitive impairment.
  - Fatigue.

## Investigation

### Preliminary investigation

- FBC, CRP, ESR, urine dipstick and culture.

MS can cause a wide range of symptoms/signs and the differential diagnosis will vary accordingly. **Depending on the presenting features consider:**

- Full septic screen, $B_{12}$, TFT.
- Anticardiolipin and antiphospholipid Abs, autoimmune screen including ANA, RF, ENA, serum C3/C4 levels, immunoglobulins.
- $Ca^{2+}$, LFT, CXR, serum ACE (sarcoid).
- HIV, Lyme, HTLV-1 (tropical spastic paraparesis), and syphilis serology.
- Very-long chain fatty acids (VLCFAs: X-linked adrenoleucodystrophy).

### MRI brain ± spinal cord

- Useful in excluding conditions which mimic MS.
- Brain imaging (T2 and FLAIR) reveals hyperintense lesions (typically involving periventricular white matter, corpus callosum, and posterior fossa structures) in >95% cases (Fig. 14.26).
- Further tests (MRI spinal cord, CSF examination, evoked potentials) are particularly important when brain MRI is borderline/negative.
- MRI lesions may be difficult to distinguish from vascular/age-related changes, although lesions in the spinal cord and corpus callosum are particularly suggestive of MS.
- Gadolinium enhancement is observed with active lesions and lasts ~4 weeks.

### CSF examination

- IgG oligoclonal bands (OCBs)—not matched in the serum—in >90% cases (but not specific).

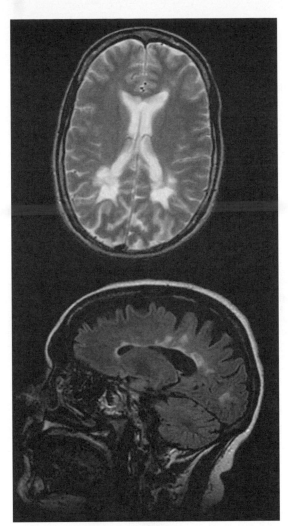

**Fig. 14.26** T2-weighted MRI in a patient with MS. Both images demonstrate the classical periventricular distribution of plaques.

### Evoked potentials

- Visual evoked potentials (VEPs) often provide neurophysiological evidence of demyelination in the optic nerves, even in the absence of a clinical episode of optic neuritis.
- Somatosensory and brainstem auditory evoked potentials are generally less useful diagnostically.

## Diagnosis

Diagnosis is on clinical grounds, supported by paraclinical investigations (MRI, evoked potential studies, CSF examination):
- Diagnosis hinges on establishing **two or more episodes of demyelination affecting separate sites within the CNS**

**at separate times**, e.g. if the patient presents with a relapse and there is a history suggestive of previous relapse(s), particularly if the MRI brain is typical.
- Diagnosis is less straightforward in patients who have only experienced a single clinical episode (i.e. a clinically isolated syndrome, CIS). In this situation imaging may provide evidence of dissemination of lesions in space and time. Therefore, it may be possible to make a diagnosis, particularly in the presence of positive OCBs and VEPs.
- **NB**: an abnormal MRI following a CIS carries a >80% risk of developing MS over 10 years while a normal MRI carries a <15% risk.
- In patients with progressive symptoms it is important to exclude other causes (e.g. compressive lesion of the spinal cord). Spinal cord MRI, CSF examination, and VEPs are extremely useful as the MRI brain is more likely to be normal/equivocal in this setting.

## Management

Coordination between neurologist, MS nurse, GP, physiotherapist, occupational therapist, continence services.

### Acute relapses

- Physiotherapy as required.
- Corticosteroids hasten recovery following a relapse, but don't alter the ultimate recovery from an attack. A typical regimen is IV methyl prednisolone, 1g daily for 3 days, PO methyl prednisolone (e.g. 500mg daily for 5 days, with gastric protection) is a useful alternative.
- Complications of steroids include flushing, worsening of infection, mood change (depression/euphoria/rarely psychosis), osteoporosis, gastric ulceration, worsening glycaemic control in diabetes, avascular necrosis (rare).
- Largely because of the risk of osteoporosis, steroids are reserved for clinically disabling relapses (i.e. causing significant impairment of day-to-day function) and <3 courses per year.

### Symptomatic treatment

- Sensory disturbance (amitriptyline, gabapentin).
- Spasticity: physiotherapy, baclofen, tizanidine, dantrolene, diazepam, intrathecal baclofen, botulinum toxin for focal spasticity.
- Urinary symptoms:
  - Urgency/frequency may occur in the setting of urinary retention, therefore bladder scan to measure residual volume, consider intermittent self-catheterization if >100mL, especially if frequent UTIs.
  - Anticholinergics (e.g. oxybutynin, tolterodine), desmopressin.
- Fatigue (identify/treat coexistent depression, consider amantadine, modafinil).
- Depression (SSRI).
- Erectile dysfunction (sildenafil).

### 'Disease-modifying' immunomodulatory therapies

- Interferon-beta and glatiramer acetate reduce relapse frequency by ~30%, but appear to have little impact on disease progression.
- More powerful therapeutic options include natalizumab, alemtuzumab and mitoxantrone: potentially more efficacious but have less favourable side effect and safety profiles.

## Background

- Parkinson disease (PD) was first described in 1817 by James Parkinson (English physician, 1755–1854) in 'An Essay on the Shaking Palsy'.
- Common, age-related neurodegenerative disorder characterized by bradykinesia, rigidity and tremor.
- Treatment may ameliorate symptoms for many years but needs to be individualized carefully to each patient.

## Epidemiology

- Prevalence: 1% of the population worldwide; increases with age to 3.5% aged 85–89 years.
- ♂:♀ = 1.5:1.
- Median age of onset 65 years: patients presenting <40 years classified as young-onset PD.
- 80% of all parkinsonism.

## Pathology

- Due to loss of dopamine-secreting neurons in the substantia nigra of the basal ganglia. Symptoms arise only after about 60% of these neurons lost.
- Cytoplasmic inclusion (Lewy) bodies seen primarily in substantia nigra but also elsewhere in the nervous system.

## Aetiology

Idiopathic PD is likely to have both genetic and environmental contributions. Only 5% of recognized PD cases are thought to be directly genetic. First-degree relatives of PD sufferers have an elevated risk (about 17%) of developing PD. Environmental risk factors include: the drinking of well water; exposure to industrial plants, pesticides, and quarries; and rural habitation.

## Clinical features

The key features are prominently asymmetrical especially early in the disease course:

- **Resting 3–5Hz pill-rolling tremor:** commonly presents in one upper limb but can involve the mouth, chin, and lower limbs. 20% of patients never develop tremor.
- **Rigidity:** hypertonicity described as 'lead-pipe', i.e. the same increased tone throughout the range of movement with superimposed 'cogwheeling' caused by the coarse rest tremor. It can be exacerbated by synkinesis (simultaneous movement of the other limb). Shoulder pain is common.
- **Bradykinesia:** general slowness of movement. Fine movements will characteristically reduce in speed and amplitude. Also associated with hypomimia (reduced facial expression), hypophonia (quiet voice), micrographia (small handwriting), and a decreased blink rate.

Other signs and symptoms that may be evident include:

- Gait difficulty and postural instability with freezing, poor balance, and loss of righting reflexes. The classical gait is described as 'festinant', characterized by a flexed posture, small steps, and a decreased arm swing.

### Non-motor complications

- **Sialorrhoea:** hypersalivation and drooling affect ≤75%.
- **Autonomic dysfunction:** including sweating, constipation, urinary frequency, seborrhoeic dermatitis, sexual dysfunction, and orthostatic hypotension.
- **Dementia:** may affect up to 1/3 of patients later on in the disease, with common symptoms being poor short-term memory and impaired visuospatial function. Hallucinations may also occur.
- **Depression:** affects up to 40% of PD patients during the course of the disease, possibly due to underlying neurochemical abnormalities.
- **Fatigue and sleep problems** are common and may include restless legs syndrome, periodic leg movements in sleep, REM sleep behaviour disorder, and excessive daytime somnolence.

## Investigation

**Diagnosis is clinical**; the presence of 2/3 key features is estimated to be about 80% specific and 30% sensitive when compared to post-mortem findings. Sustained responsiveness of symptoms to levodopa is helpful but not diagnostic.

- Imaging (using CT or MRI) shows no specific findings in PD but may be useful to exclude differential diagnoses.
- PET and SPECT imaging may show decreased uptake of dopamine but are not widely available.

### Differential diagnosis

- Essential tremor.
- Drug induced.
- Cerebrovascular parkinsonism/small vessel vascular disease.
- Wilson disease (in young patients).
- 'Parkinson Plus' syndromes (see later subsection).
- Huntington disease (Westphal variant).

## Treatment

Effective treatment requires multidisciplinary team input (PD nurse, physiotherapists, occupational therapists, speech and language therapists, as well as medical input).

### Medical treatment

The aim of treatment is to optimize symptoms while minimizing adverse effects. New drugs should be started at a low dose and titrated up slowly. Within 2 years of diagnosis, the majority of patients will require dopaminergic therapy for symptom control. Drug therapy includes:

1. **Levo-dopa with peripheral dopa decarboxylase inhibitor** (e.g. co-careldopa/Sinemet®, co-beneldopa/Madopar®): L-dopa has the greatest antiparkinsonian benefits with the fewest short-term side effects. Start 62.5mg three times daily with meals. Consider domperidone 10–30mgs three times daily if nausea is a problem. Motor complications (fluctuations and dyskinesias) develop in 10% of patients per year of treatment.

2. **Dopamine agonists** (e.g. ropinirole, pramipexole): used initially in younger patients due to risk of longer-term motor complications with L-dopa. Older patients are more likely to get adverse effects with dopamine agonists, e.g. hallucinations, nausea, so levodopa is the initial treatment. Apomorphine is a

short-acting dopamine agonist which can be used as a rescue agent—given subcutaneously—to treat 'off' periods in advanced PD. Ergot derivatives (cabergoline, pergolide) are now largely avoided because of risk of retroperitoneal/pulmonary fibrosis and cardiac valve defects.

3. **Amantadine:** stimulates dopamine release; may be helpful with dyskinesias

4. **Anticholinergics** (trihexyphenidryl/benzhexol, orphenadrine): primarily used for tremor with little effects against other signs and symptoms of PD. They must be used with caution, especially in the elderly who are more prone to the side effects which include dry mouth, confusion, visual problems, etc.

5. **COMT inhibitors** (e.g. tolcapone, entacapone): inhibit the metabolism of dopamine and when used in combination with levodopa increases 'on' time. Liver function tests must be carefully monitored. GI side effects are common.

6. **MAO-B inhibitors** (e.g. selegiline, rasagiline): blocks another pathway in dopamine breakdown

## Treatment problems and their solutions

### Wearing off

- Return of parkinsonian signs/symptoms either predictable (end-of-dose) or unpredictable (when central drug levels within treatment range).
- For end-of-dose try shorter inter-dose intervals of L-dopa, using different preparation (e.g. dispersible levodopa), increasing the dose, or adding in alternative medical treatments (COMT inhibitor/selegiline/amantadine).
- Management of unpredictable wearing off depends on the presence or absence of dyskinesias (involuntary movements). If no dyskinesias, treat similarly to end-of-dose wearing off. If dyskinesias present, more difficult to get a balance and patient preference is important. Increasing dopaminergic input may increase dyskinesias but decreasing the input may increase 'off' time. Patients often prefer to have dyskinesias than off periods.

### Dementia with Lewy bodies (DLB)

- Common form of dementia (10–20%) secondary to widespread accumulation of Lewy bodies in the midbrain and cortex.
- Characterized by visual hallucinations, periods of fluctuating alertness, and parkinsonism.
- Considerable overlap with idiopathic PD; identical histopathological findings and significant number of PD patients with dementia (PDD). Currently, the two diseases are differentiated by time of onset of dementia i.e. parkinsonism preceding dementia by >1 year = PDD otherwise DLB.
- Intermediate release L-dopa preferred over controlled release as it allows more controlled dosing periods. Using smaller doses more frequently also useful.
- Protein-related off periods may occur when the absorption of levodopa is inhibited by large amounts of amino acids after a protein-rich meal, so dietary composition and timing of meals and medications may be important.

### Early morning/'off' period dystonias

- Dystonias (co-contraction of agonist and antagonist muscles in the affected limb) classically affecting the most affected foot.

### 'Parkinson Plus' syndromes

Parkinsonian signs and symptoms are also seen in distinct syndromes:

1. **Multi-system atrophy (MSA)**, which also includes pyramidal, cerebellar and autonomic impairment and results in severe disability within a few years. Incontinence in women and impotence in men are early symptoms. Response to L-dopa is short-lived.

2. **Progressive supranuclear palsy (PSP)**/Steele–Richardson–Olszewski syndrome: initial impairment of downgaze, then upgaze and horizontal movements followed by parkinsonism, prominent axial rigidity, pseudobulbar palsy and memory impairment. Gait disorder and falls are early manifestation. Neck is commonly hyperextended. Characteristic facial appearance with wide-eyed stare. Median survival = 10 years.

3. **Corticobasal degeneration (CBD):** unilateral parkinsonism unresponsive to levodopa with limb apraxia, dystonia, myoclonus, tremor and aphasia. Dementia present in a minority.

   - Occur in the morning before the first dose of antiparkinsonian medication has been taken; may reappear during off periods through the day.
   - Try dispersible L-dopa or dopamine agonist or baclofen.

### Peak dose dyskinesias

- Dyskinesias at peak of therapeutic response in a predictable fashion.
- Probably due to fluctuating dopamine concentration as PD progresses and more dopaminergic neurons are lost.
- Dopamine agonist may provide smoother and sustained dopamine release. Or try amantadine, adjustment of the L-dopa dose and/or interdose interval.

### Hallucinations

- Review PD medication particularly anticholinergics but also dopamine agonists and levodopa; most recent addition usually most relevant.
- If hallucinations remain problematic, an atypical neuroleptic (e.g. quetiapine or clozapine) may be necessary (classic neuroleptics have more parkinsonian effects).

## Non-medical treatment

Surgical deep brain lesioning and stimulation have been used, including thalamotomy/thalamic stimulation for tremor and pallidotomy or pallidal stimulation for tremor, rigidity, bradykinesia, or dyskinesias. Subthalamic stimulation is the most common surgical procedure for PD and has been found to be useful for bradykinesia, tremor, rigidity, and motor fluctuations, with improvements maintained for up to 5 years following surgery.

Neural, stem cell, and neural growth factor transplantation are being developed.

## Outcome

Medical treatment can provide good symptom control for 4–6 years, following which disability tends to progress despite medical input.

If response to treatment not appropriate reconsider the diagnosis:

- Early bladder incontinence or other autonomic symptoms: MSA.
- Marked anterocollis (forward flexion head and neck): MSA.
- Early falls: PSP.
- Early dysarthria and dysphagia: PSP.
- Apraxia, especially unilateral and myoclonus: CBD.
- Early dementia: DLB.

There is an average of 9 years between presentation and death and it is estimated that there is a relative risk of death with PD compared to a matched control population of 1.6–3.0.

## Chorea

Jerky, fidgety, irregular, involuntary movements that move unpredictably between body parts.

### Causes
- Huntington disease.
- Stroke (e.g. caudate or putamen)—acute-onset unilateral chorea (hemibalismus—caused by a lesion of the subthalamic nucleus (e.g. stroke, tumour)—causes unilateral, vigorous proximal movements, often involving the trunk.
- Structural (e.g. tumour).
- Polycythaemia rubra vera.
- SLE, antiphospholipid syndrome.
- Pregnancy, OCP.
- Drugs (dopamine antagonists: tardive dyskinesia).
- Sydenham chorea (post-streptococcal infection).
- Neuroacanthocytosis.
- Wilson disease.

### Management
- Atypical antipsychotic drug (e.g. quetiapine, sulpiride).
- Tetrabenazine.

## Huntington disease

### Clinical presentation
- Onset usually in middle age, but ranges from adolescence to 8th decade.
- Chorea—often florid in early disease, but may later reduce as parkinsonism becomes more prominent.
- Neuropsychiatric/behavioural disturbance + later cognitive impairment.
- Other movement disorders also present:
  - Parkinsonism—may be prominent in juvenile onset disease (Westphal variant).
  - Dystonia, myoclonus, tics.

### Genetics
- AD inheritance with 100% penetrance.
- Family history may be absent due to late presentation (and consider non-paternity).
- Caused by an expanded trinucleotide CAG repeat in huntingtin gene on chromosome 4.
- Exhibits **anticipation** (i.e. further expansion of the repeat causing earlier onset) when paternally inherited.

### Investigations
- Genetic test is diagnostic.
- Imaging often shows marked caudate atrophy.

### Management
- Treatment of movement disorder and psychiatric symptoms, nutritional support.
- Family screening.
- Death at mean of 14 years after onset.

## Dystonia
- Sustained muscle contraction, often resulting in abnormal posturing and tremor.
- Cervical dystonia is the most common form of focal dystonia causing torticollis (head turning), retrocollis (head drawn backwards), antecollis (forwards), or laterocollis (sideways).
- Blepharospasm (forced blinking), oromandibular dystonia (cranial dystonias).
- May be relieved by a 'sensory trick'—'geste antagonistique'—e.g. touching the jaw to relieve torticollis.
- Writers' cramp is an example of a task-specific dystonia—after few seconds of writing develops abnormal posture, e.g. extension of the index finger.
- Treatment— botulinium toxin.

## Tremor

### Essential tremor
= Postural tremor (e.g. holding a drink).
- Bilateral symmetrical tremor of outstretched hands.
- May involve head ('yes–yes'), voice, tongue, jaw.
- Family history in ~50%.
- Often helped by alcohol.
- Very slowly progressive.
- Exclude hyperthyroidism and, in young patients, Wilson disease.

*Treatment*
- Propranolol—at maximum tolerated dose.
- Primidone; starting at 62.5mg once a day if a β-blocker contraindicated.

### Dystonic tremor
In comparison to essential tremor:
- Coarse, often asymmetrical.
- More proximal, changes with different postures.
- When it affects the head it usually causes a 'no–no' tremor (but there may be 'yes–yes' or multidirectional).
- Association with other dystonias (e.g. torticollis).
- May be task-specific (e.g. writing tremor).

*Treatment*
- Trihexyphenidyl starting at 2mg once a day and increasing as tolerated (side effects include drowsiness).
- Other options include clonazepam, β-blocker, gabapentin, botulinum toxin injections.

### Other causes of tremor
- Intention tremor:
  - Seen with cerebellar disease.
  - Amplitude increases on reaching a target.
- Rubral tremor—midbrain tremor seen in MS; may be extremely disabling and involve the head and trunk.
- Hyperthyroidism.
- Drugs (e.g. salbutamol, valproate, ciclosporin, metoclopramide, phenothiazines).
- Physiological tremor.

## Background

In this section, spinal cord disorders are discussed in general with specific attention to cervical myelopathy and transverse myelitis. There are various causes of spinal cord disorder, some of which are discussed elsewhere, e.g. stroke, tumour. They may be confined to the spinal cord and root e.g. myeloradiculopathy, secondary to cervical spondylosis, or may be part of a more widespread disorder, e.g. MS.

Knowledge of the anatomy of spinal cord tracts is key to understanding signs and symptoms of the different cord syndromes—see Fig. 14.27.

## Overview of spinal cord disorders

### Causes

- **Compressive:**
  - Bone and joint disease: cervical spondylosis, rheumatoid arthritis, ankylosing spondylitis, Paget disease.
  - Neoplastic (see Chapter 14—Oncology):
  - Metastatic—usually lung, breast, prostate.
  - Primary CNS tumour (intrinsic or extrinsic).
  - Neoplastic leptomeningitis, e.g. carcinoma, lymphoma, melanoma.

- **Infective:** abscess, Pott disease of spine (spinal TB), HIV, osteomyelitis, tropical spastic paraparesis/HTLV-associated myelopathy.
- **Inflammatory:** multiple sclerosis, sarcoidosis.
- **Vascular:** infarction, dural AVM.
- **Trauma.**
- **Haematoma:** bleeding dyscrasia/injury.
- **Congenital and inherited:** spinal dysraphism (structural abnormality e.g. meningocoele, spina bifida), Arnold–Chiari malformation.
- **Other:**
  - Syringomyelia.
  - Radiation myelopathy.

### Common signs/symptoms suggesting cord disease

Variable depending on site, extent and underlying pathology. May evolve rapidly (minutes to hours), or more slowly (days to weeks).

- Radicular (nerve root) pain at the level of the lesion due to compression of exiting nerve root.
- Spastic para/tetraparesis with increased tone, brisk reflexes, and upgoing plantars (although not always).
- Sensory changes in limbs ± a sensory level.

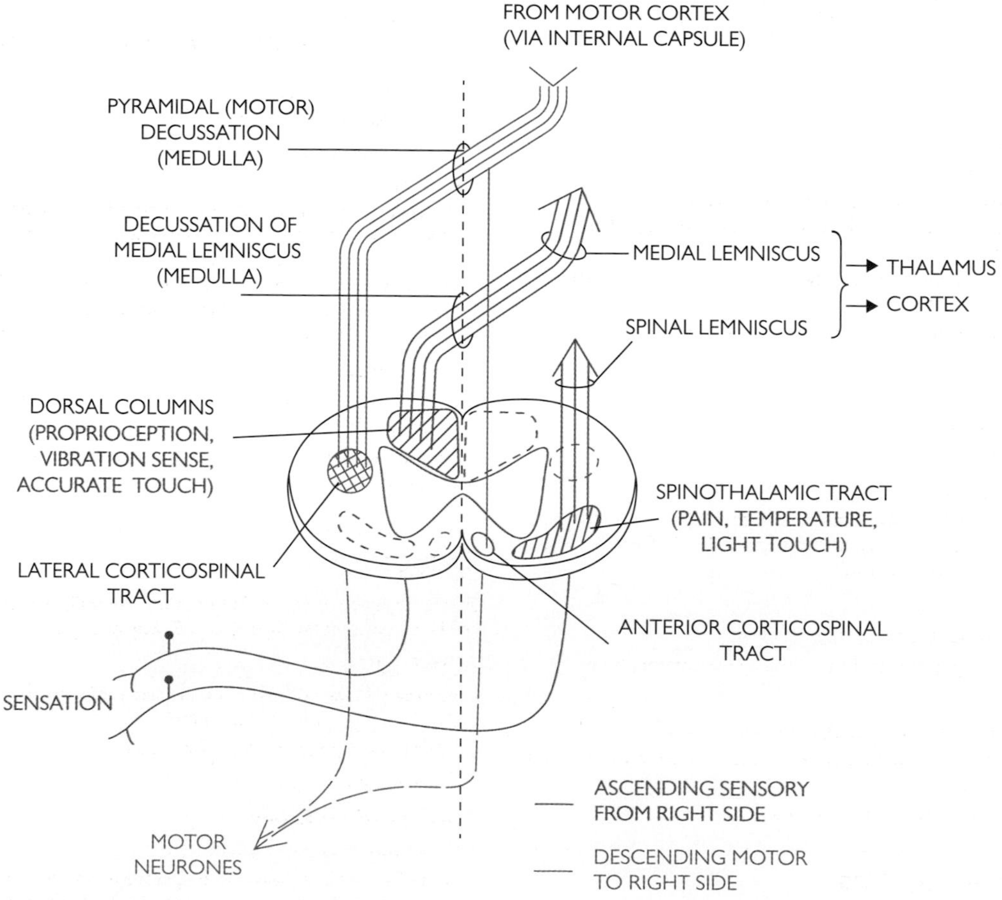

**Fig. 14.27** Spinal cord anatomy.

- Bladder and bowel involvement—urinary frequency and hesitancy early on.
- Reduced anal tone and sensation on examination.

### Specific incomplete spinal cord syndromes

**Anterior cord syndrome**, e.g. spinal stroke: weakness and spinothalamic dissociated sensory loss below the level of the lesion.

**Brown–Sequard syndrome** (cord hemisection): ipsilateral hemiplegia and posterior column sensory loss with contralateral spinothalamic loss (due to differences of decussation of sensory tracts).

**Posterior cord syndrome**, e.g. tabes dorsalis (neurosyphilis): posterior column sensory loss.

### Investigation

Urgent investigation must be arranged. MRI is the imaging modality of choice. Other investigations may include:
- Spinal plain radiographs—bony destruction or deformity.
- Cultures—blood, CSF, possibly operative material.
- FBC and clotting screen.
- Search for any underlying primary malignancy.

▶ Acute spinal cord compression is an emergency. If treatment of a reversible cause is delayed for more than 24 hours, recovery is unlikely.

### Treatment

The initial treatment of metastases causing spinal cord compression is high-dose intravenous corticosteroids. Radiotherapy may also be used. For other causes of spinal cord compression, early referral and discussion of the case with a spinal or neurosurgeon is vital for decisions concerning operative management.

## Cervical myelopathy

### Common causes

- Spondylosis (commonest):
  - Most common cause in patients >50 years.
  - Degenerative change—usually a combination of osteophytic outgrowths and disc degeneration and protrusion in osteoarthritis.
  - Cord impingement commonly at C5/6 and C6/7 (multiple levels may be affected).
  - Posterior columns often remain relatively spared.
- Tumour.
- Syringomyelia.
- Multiple sclerosis.

### Examination

- As noted earlier.

NB: 'inverted reflex'—for example on eliciting a supinator reflex, finger flexion is seen due to areflexia at the level of the lesion and hyper-reflexia below that level.

### Investigation

- Plain C-spine radiographs: rarely useful
- MRI cervical spine: identifies structural/inflammatory lesions

### Treatment

Optimal treatment is unclear. Options are:
- Conservative (cervical collar, analgesia, avoidance of trauma, and physiotherapy).
- Surgical, particularly if defects moderate or severe.

## Transverse myelitis

- Inflammation of the spinal cord; subacute onset.
- 33% of transverse myelitis is associated with viral infection.

- Important to consider MS, but also SLE and neurosarcoid.
- Other causes include TB and syphilis.
- Differential diagnosis: abscess, tumour, ischaemia.

### Epidemiology/aetiology

- Incidence = 0.5 per 100,000 population/year.
- Frequently in association with a respiratory tract infection.
- Most common agents = enterovirus, VZV, HSV-2.
- Others: adenovirus, hepatitis, rubella.
- HIV and HTLV-1 both cause a more indolent myelitis.

### Pathology

Damage to axons can occur directly from viral infection or as a result of the immune response to the virus.

### History

History and examination should be aimed toward excluding differentials and localizing the lesion.
- Evolution over hours to days of paraparesis, bladder symptoms, sensory level.
- Prodromal URTI.
- Previous episodes suggestive of MS.
- Presence of fever.
- Bilateral symptoms.
- Travel history.

### Examination

- Sensory level.
- Associated rash (HSV/VZV).

### Investigations

**CSF**: microscopy and biochemical findings similar to that in aseptic meningitis.
Other CSF tests include:
- Oligoclonal bands (to exclude MS).
- PCR for HSV, VZV, EBV, CMV, HIV.
- Antibodies to HTLV-1.

**MRI** (spine—Fig. 14.28): changes should be most obvious 5 days after symptom-onset. High signal change best seen on T2-weighted scans. Brain MRI may be indicated to exclude MS.

**Other investigations**: these should be aimed at excluding other causes of myelitis, and should include CXR, serum ACE, syphilis serology, and dsDNA

### Management

- If idiopathic/post-infectious/MS-related, consider intravenous methyl-prednisolone.
- If an active viral aetiology is suspected, antiviral therapy could be instituted.

## Syringomyelia

Syrinx = fluid-filled cavity that develops centrally within the cervical cord or brainstem (syringobulbia). Slowly enlarges.

### Aetiology

- Associated with congenital abnormalities of craniocervical junction (Arnold–Chiari malformation).
- Cord trauma (may develop years after).
- Cord tumour.

### Symptoms/pathology

- Onset slowly usually at young age.
- Loss of upper limb pain and temperature sensation (dorsal columns not involved: dissociated sensory loss) in a cape distribution (back and neck)—compression of crossing spinothalamic tract neurons at syrinx level(s).

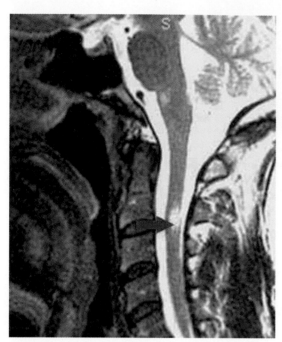

**Fig. 14.28** Intramedullary high signal lesion (arrow pointing) on T2-weighted cervical spine imaging consistent with cord inflammation (myelitis).

- Flaccid weakness and wasting of upper limbs—compression of anterior horn cells (LMN) in cervical cord.
- Eventually spastic paralysis of lower limbs (UMN)—compression of lateral corticospinal tracts.

### Investigations

- Brain and cord imaging (MRI), contrast enhancement can detect tumour.

### Treatment

- Treat any cause, drain syrinx with a shunt.

i) Corticospinal tracts (motor pathways) from the cortex cross in the medulla (except a few fibres forming the anterior corticospinal tract)

ii) Dorsal column sensory neurons enter the dorsal root ganglion then travel upwards on the same side as they entered the cord

iii) Spinothalamic tracts cross within a few segments of entering the cord

# 14.24 Spinal nerve root disorders (radiculopathies)

## Background

Neck/back pain is a common symptom with numerous causes (including nerve root impingement) but is not termed radiculopathy unless in the presence of appropriate symptoms and signs. Damage to the nerve roots occurs through any of a variety of processes.

Radiculopathy should be distinguished from myelopathy (spinal cord disorders) although the same lesion may cause both (myeloradiculopathy).

## Epidemiology

- Affects >2% of the population over their lifetime.
- Major cause of time off work, adverse quality of life, and cost to the health service.

## Causes

### Spondylotic

- Intervertebral disc herniation and degeneration the most common cause: usually degenerative/age-related.
- Most often at L4/5 and L5/S1 interspaces (affecting nerve roots L5 and S1) as mechanical forces are highest here.
- Cervical radiculopathy is much less common, typically C7 (60%) and C6 (25%), whilst thoracic radiculopathy is relatively rare.

### Non-spondylotic

- Infection: may need aspiration for culture and sometimes surgical drainage.
- Tumours: see Chapter 15—Oncology.
- Fractures: compression fracture or dislocation fracture; if benign can be managed conservatively.
- Trauma: even minor trauma (e.g. leaning backwards over the sink at the hairdresser).
- Infection, e.g. Lyme disease:
  - NB: Guillain–Barré syndrome is strictly speaking an acute inflammatory radiculo-neuropathy.
- Vascular (e.g. diabetes or vasculitides); impairing blood supply to the nerve roots.

### Predisposing factors

- Joint disease, e.g. osteoarthritis, rheumatoid arthritis, or ankylosing spondylitis.
- Some individuals are predisposed to have narrow disc spaces or foramina so any impingement on these is more likely to give rise to symptoms.

## Clinical evaluation

### History

- Most common symptom is neck/back pain, which tends to be dermatomal and neuropathic in character.
- In lumbosacral region may result in 'sciatica'; the comparable pain syndrome in the arms due to cervical radiculopathy is known as brachialgia.
- Pain often felt locally in the neck/back (paraspinals) as well as in the limb; may be preceded by a relatively minor injury or movement, such as sneezing.
- Important to consider the less common but potentially serious causes of radiculopathy such as malignancy or chronic infection. Ask about systemic symptoms such as weight loss and fevers, recent infection, immunosuppression and drug abuse.

### Examination

A lesion may often be localized by the pattern of reflexes and myotomes/dermatomes affected (see Tables 14.12 and 14.13):
- Sensory loss or paraesthesia in dermatomal distribution.
- Loss of deep tendon reflex supplied by that nerve root.
- Weakness in the group of muscles innervated by that nerve root.

### Investigation

- MRI: imaging modality of choice; usually not necessary acutely and patients may often be managed without imaging. In 50% people <50 years, asymptomatic disc bulge may be seen which must be interpreted with caution.
- Plain radiographs: may help to identify fracture or subluxation.
- Neurophysiology: electromyography and nerve conduction studies may help in distinguishing a nerve root lesion from a more peripheral problem (e.g. distinguishing C6 root lesion from carpal tunnel syndrome).
- If malignancy or underlying causes other than degenerative diseases suspected, tailor investigations appropriately.

## Treatment

- Natural history of most herniated **lumbar** discs is benign, even with root compression; less clear for cervical radiculopathy.
- Conservative management (initial rest and simple analgesics followed by physical rehabilitation) is often all that is required.
- Traction may be used but the evidence is not robust and often difficult to tolerate.
- If symptoms do not improve more invasive interventions including epidural analgesia, nerve root block or surgical treatment may be considered.

Table 14.12 Symptoms and signs associated with lumbar radiculopathy

| Nerve root | Pain distribution | Dermatomal sensory distribution | Weakness | Reflex loss |
|---|---|---|---|---|
| L1 | Inguinal region | Inguinal region | Hip flexion | Cremasteric |
| L2 | Inguinal region and anterior thigh | Anterior thigh | Hip flexion, hip adduction | Cremasteric, thigh adductor |
| L3 | Anterior thigh and knee | Distal anteromedial thigh including knee | Knee extension, hip flexion, hip adduction | Patellar, thigh adductor |
| L4 | Anterior thigh, medial leg | Medial leg | Ankle dorsiflexion, knee flexion, hip abduction | Patellar |
| L5 | Posterolateral thigh, lateral leg, medial foot | Lateral leg, dorsal foot and great toe | Ankle dorsiflexion, knee flexion, hip abduction | |
| S1 | Posterolateral thigh, lateral foot | Posterolateral leg and lateral foot | Ankle plantarflexion, knee flexion, hip extension | Achilles |

Reprinted from Neurologic Clinics, 25, Devereaux MW, Anatomy and Examination of the Spine, 21, Copyright (2007), with permission from Elsevier

**Table 14.13** Symptoms and signs associated with cervical and thoracic radiculopathy

| Nerve Root | Pain distribution | Dermatomal sensory distribution | Weakness | Reflex loss |
|---|---|---|---|---|
| C4 | Upper neck | **Cape distribution shoulder and arm** | | |
| C5 | Lateral upper arm | Lateral upper arm, over deltoid | Shoulder abduction—deltoid, supraspinatus, infraspin atus, rhomboids | Biceps |
| C6 | Neck to lateral forearm to thumb | Lateral two fingers | Elbow flexion—biceps and brachiora dialis, brachialis | Supinator |
| C7 | Neck to hand to middle finger | **Middle finger** | **Elbow/wrist/finger extension— triceps, wrist flexors, wrist extensors, finger extensors** | Triceps |
| C8 | Neck to shoulder to medial forearm to little finger | **Little finger; medial border hand** | **Finger flexors, finger extensors, flexor carpiulnaris** | Finger flexors |
| T1 | Shoulder/axilla to olecranon | **Dermatomal sensory distribution** | Finger abduction—intrinsic hand muscles | |

Reprinted from *Neurologic Clinics*, 25, Devereaux MW, *Anatomy and Examination of the Spine*, 21, Copyright (2007), with permission from Elsevier

- Maintaining mobility and promoting back strength is important in recovery whether management is conservative or interventional. Physiotherapist input is crucial.

## Lumbar spinal stenosis

- Progressive lower limb and back pain worse with walking/standing (pseudo-claudication).
- Worse walking down incline/stairs.
- Relieved by sitting, leaning forward, or reclining.
- On examination: reduced ankle reflexes (50%) and knee reflexes (25%); mild–moderate weakness L5/S1 distribution; absent vibration sense in feet; patient may stand or walk flexed at waist.
- Investigations: MRI lumbar spine; EMG abnormal in 90%.

- Treatment: moderate benefit from surgery.
- Differential diagnosis: vascular claudication, osteoarthritis of hips and knees, lumbar disc protrusion.

## Conus medullaris and cauda equina syndromes

- Syndrome of pain, perianal/perineal sensory loss, bladder/bowel dysfunction, and leg weakness.
- Causes: same lesions as result in radiculopathy.
- On examination: lower limb weakness, anal sphincter weakness; may have mixed upper and lower motor neurone signs if conus medullaris lesion.
- Investigation and treatment: depend on cause; see earlier.

# 14.25 Motor neurone disease

## Background

Motor neurone disease (MND) is a progressive neurodegenerative condition characterized by a combination of upper and lower motor neurone involvement.

## Epidemiology

- Prevalence ~5/100,000.
- Slight ♂ predominance, with ♂: ♀ ratio of 1.6:1.
- Onset is usually in 50s and 60s.
- Similar incidence worldwide.

## Aetiology

- No exact cause has been identified.
- 90% of cases are sporadic.
- Familial cases have been identified with autosomal dominant inheritance (particularly a mutation in superoxide dismutase gene (*SOD1*); these comprise 20% of familial MND cases).
- Some case clustering has been reported; further investigation may reveal clues as to causation.
- Smoking is a risk factor.

## Pathology

The disease is due to degeneration of both upper and lower motor neurones.

## Signs and symptoms

- Upper motor neurone:
  - Spasticity.
  - Weakness.
  - Brisk reflexes.
  - Upgoing plantars.
- Bulbar upper motor neurone: dysarthria, dysphagia, excess salivation, pseudobulbar affect.
- Lower motor neuron:
  - Weakness—including respiratory muscle.
  - Muscle atrophy.
  - Wasting.
  - Fasciculations.
  - Reduced or absent reflexes.
  - Cramps.

Symptoms may include weakness (initially, usually distal), slurred speech, dysphagia, or altered affect. Hypoventilation may cause early morning headache. 75% of patients present with limb weakness initially, 20% with bulbar signs and symptoms, and the remaining with respiratory impairment.

Sensory abnormalities, sphincteric, smooth, and cardiac muscle, or oculomotor involvement are not classically seen in MND (although up to 1/4 of patients report minor sensory abnormalities, e.g. temperature sensation).

Emotional involvement—particularly emotional lability—is recognized, especially in association with pseudobulbar palsy.

Dementia, commonly of a frontal lobe type, is seen in association with MND.

Signs and symptoms may initially present in one region but typically spread.

## Investigation

- Diagnosis of MND is essentially clinical and may require monitoring of a patient over several months to monitor disease progression. Diagnostic criteria have been drawn up (El Escorial criteria).
- Blood tests do not really have a role, although CK may be elevated 2–3× the upper limit of normal in about 1/2 of patients.
- Imaging may be useful to exclude other conditions, e.g. cervical myelopathy or a brainstem lesions causing bulbar pathology. Imaging modality of choice = MRI brain and spine.
- EMG/NCS—EMG shows fibrillation + fasciculation.

## Classification

- Amyotrophic lateral sclerosis (UMN and LMN involvement).
- Progressive muscular atrophy (LMN).
- Primary lateral sclerosis (UMN).
- Progressive bulbar palsy (LMN innervating mouth, face, and throat).
- Pseudobulbar palsy (UMN innervating mouth, face, and throat).

## Treatment

- Medical treatment is limited and the main aim of management of MND should focus around quality of life.
- Riluzole is a glutamate antagonist which may be used in MND. It is thought to reduce glutamate excitotoxicity, and slows down disease progression (albeit by a few months only). Otherwise, medical treatment is primarily symptomatic (e.g. antispasticity agents, antibiotics in event of infection, etc.).
- Supportive care may include non-invasive ventilation and tube-feeding depending on patient preference and appropriateness.
- Multidisciplinary input is important, with roles for physiotherapists, occupational therapists, and speech and language therapists. Emotional support for both the patient and their family is vital.
- Other issues which should be addressed include advance directives or living wills.
- End of life care should be centred on comfort and dignity and may be provided at home, in hospital, or in a hospice depending on patient and family preference.

## Prognosis

- MND is inevitably fatal, usually secondary to respiratory failure.
- On average, patients survive for 2 years after diagnosis (3–4 years after symptom onset) although longer survival than this has been reported (20% of patients survive for >5 years; 10% for >10 years).
- Longer survival is associated with:
  - ♂ patients.
  - Younger age of onset.
  - Limb, rather than bulbar involvement—primary lateral sclerosis particularly is associated with longer-term survival, up to 25 years or more.
- Death is usually as a result of hypoventilation or infection.

## Background

- Peripheral neuropathy affects 2–8% of the population.
- The peripheral nerve lies between the nerve root proximally, and the neuromuscular junction or skin distally.
- Cranial neuropathies are part of peripheral nerve disease, but will be discussed elsewhere unless directly relevant.

## Terminology and abbreviations

| | |
|---|---|
| Dysaesthesia | Discomfort or pain from nerve damage or irritation (e.g. burning, tight, cold, achy). |
| Dysautonomia | Autonomic nerve dysfunction. |
| NCS/EMG | Nerve conduction studies/electromyography. |
| Paraesthesia | 'Pins and needles' or tingling. |
| Pes cavus | Inability to flatten arches fully (Fig. 14.29). |
| Radiculopathy | Nerve root disease. |

## Clues to a diagnosis of neuropathy

- From history:
  - Slowly progressive.
  - Symmetrical and starting in feet.
- From examination:
  - Hyporeflexia/areflexia.
  - Distal wasting/numbness.
  - High arches/pes cavus.

If all absent, neuromuscular and CNS disease must be excluded.

## A neuropathy key

Only a few neuropathies are life threatening. The simplest approach to spotting them is to establish disease tempo:

- Acute/subacute (days to weeks).
- Chronic (months to years).

### Acute neuropathies

- Focal (i.e. mononeuropathies).
- Diffuse (i.e. polyneuropathies).

Acute diffuse are the most dangerous.

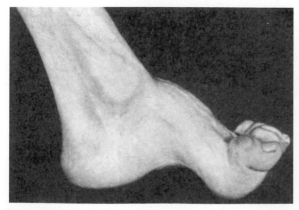

**Fig. 14.29** Pes cavus.

### Box 14.4 Causes of peripheral nerve disorders

*Acute focal*
- Entrapment:
  - Carpal tunnel syndrome
  - Ulnar neuropathy
  - Wrist drop
  - Meralgia paraesthetica
  - Foot drop
- Mononeuritis multiplex
- Brachial neuritis
- Diabetic amyotrophy
- Infective.

*Acute diffuse*
- Infective
- Postinfective.

*Chronic acquired*
- Drugs
- Diabetes
- Vitamin $B_{12}$ deficiency
- Pure sensory
- Autoimmune and/or paraproteinemia
- Infective.

*Chronic hereditary*
- Charcot–Marie–Tooth disease (aka HMSN)
- Familial amyloidosis.

### Chronic neuropathies

- Acquired.
- Hereditary.

Chronic are almost always diffuse.

See Box 14.4 for causes of peripheral nerve disorders.

## Acute focal

### Carpal tunnel syndrome (median nerve)

- Symptoms (Sx): paraesthesia in lateral 3½ fingers.
- On examination (O/E): weak thumb abduction, numbness of thumb and index, middle and (lateral half of) ring fingers.
- Cause: compression at wrist (pregnancy, endocrinopathies).
- Differential diagnosis (DDx): C6–7 radiculopathies.
- Investigation (Ix): NCS—not highly sensitive though.
- Treatment (Rx): conservative (wrist splints), steroid injections, decompressive surgery (most effective).
- Prognosis (Px): usually recovers fully if treated early.

### Ulnar neuropathy

- Sx: paraesthesia of medial forearm into little and ring fingers.
- O/E: numbness of little and ring finger (medial half), weakness of finger abduction (interossei) and finger extension (lumbricals) causing 'clawing' of the little and ring fingers (Fig. 14.30), and flexion of the thumb's interphalangeal joint when performing a pinch grip (Froment's sign).
- Cause: compression (e.g. during surgery, resting on elbows, rheumatoid nodules, long distance cycling).
- DDx: C8 radiculopathy.

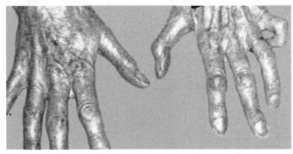

Fig. 14.30 Clawing of fingers due to ulnar neuropathy.
Image reprinted with permission from Donald R. Gore, MD, published by Medscape (http://www.medscape.com/), 2013, available at: http://www.medscape.com/viewarticle/408540.

- Ix: NCS—if normal consider MRI C-spine.
- Rx: avoid compression postures, decompressive surgery.
- Px: recovers fully if caught early.

### Wrist drop (radial nerve)
- O/E: loss of all finger extension and wrist extension, numbness of dorsum of hand and forearm:
  - **If lesion above elbow:** loss of supinator jerk.
  - **If lesion in axilla:** loss of triceps jerk + weak triceps.
- Cause: compression or trauma (falling asleep with arm hanging over chair compresses spiral groove of humerus; poorly used crutches compress axilla).
- DDx: C7 radiculopathy (spares supinator jerk).
- Ix: NCS ± imaging axilla or elbow.
- Rx: conservative if distal; may need exploration of nerve if no recovery after 3 months.
- Px: usually recovers fully.

### Meralgia paraesthetica (lateral cutaneous nerve of thigh)
- Sx: painful paraesthesia, exacerbated by walking.
- O/E: numbness of anterolateral thigh (Fig. 14.31).
- Causes: compression at inguinal ligament (obesity, pregnancy, tight clothing, rarely tumours).
- DDx: L1–2 radiculopathy (but causes weakness).
- Ix: rarely required.

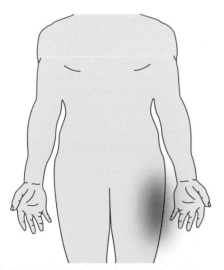

Fig. 14.31 Distribution of pain and sensory loss in meralgia paraesthetica.

- Rx: conservative, treat cause.
- Px: pain settles, numbness may remain.

### Foot drop (common peroneal nerve)
- Sx: falls, especially on uneven ground.
- O/E: weak ankle dorsiflexion and eversion ± numb dorsum of foot and shin.
- Cause: compression at fibula head (trauma, tumour).
- DDx: L5 radiculopathy (clue: inversion also weak), motor neurone disease, multiple sclerosis, stroke.
- Ix: NCS ± lumbar MRI ± brain MRI.
- Rx: ankle splint, treat cause.
- Px: usually recovers fully.

### Mononeuritis multiplex
- Stepwise or simultaneous multifocal symptoms.
- Any peripheral and cranial nerve can be affected.
- Reflexes often initially preserved.
- May be an emergency (e.g. vasculitis) requiring urgent treatment.
- Cause: diabetes, vasculitis (PAN, Churg-Strauss syndrome, RA), infiltrative (sarcoid, amyloid, carcinoma, lymphoma), infective (Lyme disease, HIV, leprosy).
- DDx: polyneuropathy (e.g. CIDP), hereditary neuropathy and liability to pressure palsies (HNPP).
- Ix: directed at identifying cause.
- Rx: of underlying cause; IV steroids; cyclophosphamide for vasculitis.
- Px: depends on early Rx and causes.
NB: for recurrent focal neuropathies only at entrapment sites, consider HNPP, for which there is a blood test (*PMP22* gene deletion).

### Brachial neuritis
- Sx: severe, often nocturnal, shoulder and axillary pain progressing over days → followed by flaccid limb weakness and numbness.
- O/E: proximal >distal multiple root involvement (as it affects the brachial plexus).
- Causes: post infection/vaccine, surgery, trauma, malignancy (especially if prolonged or intractable pain).
- DDx: C5/6 radiculopathy.
- Ix: NCS/EMG, consider MRI C-spine/brachial plexus.
- Treatment: analgesia, physiotherapy. High-dose oral steroids are often given (though minimal evidence).
- Px: good for idiopathic cases—occasionally complicated by phrenic nerve palsy.

### Diabetic amyotrophy
- Sx: acute pain and weakness, excessive weight loss.
- O/E: wasting of one or both quadriceps.
- DDx: pelvic malignancy, lumbosacral neuritis.
- Cause: microvasculitis of lumbosacral plexus.
- Rx: pain and diabetes control, physiotherapy.
- Px: good if diabetic control optimized.

## Acute diffuse

### Guillain–Barré syndrome (GBS)
- Sx: initial tingling of hands and feet followed by progressive weakness over hours to days; later dysautonomia (constipation, arrhythmias).
- Often ascending symptoms, but not always!
- O/E:
  - Areflexia in weak muscles **required**.
  - Weakness: symmetrical limb and face; if bulbar muscles involved (respiratory, swallowing), may require ITU.
  - Sensory loss is usually minimal.

- DDx: botulism, myelitis, brainstem lesion.
- Ix: LP shows raised protein but normal cell count (protein can also be normal in 1st week); NCS after 1st week should confirm a demyelinating neuropathy.
- Cause: 50% within 2 weeks of diarrhoeal/viral illness; glycolipid antibody +ve in >50%.
- Rx: IVIGs, plasma exchange; DVT prophylaxis; monitor heart and breathing (four times daily FVC—**not** PEFR—if FVC <1.5, call ITU); SLT input.
- Px: most recover fully; can be fatal if bulbar involved.

### GBS variant—Miller Fisher syndrome (MFS)

- Sx: unsteadiness, diplopia, dysarthria over a few days.
- O/E triad: ataxia–ophthalmoplegia–areflexia.
- DDx: Wernicke, myasthenia, brainstem encephalitis.
- Ix: LP and NCS as for GBS.
- Cause: post infective; 99% have positive glycolipid antibody (GQ1b).
- Px: better than GBS, often no treatment required.

### Acute infective

- Lyme disease (*Borrelia burgdorferi*):
  - Stage 1: rash (erythema migrans).
  - Stage 2: cranial neuropathies, root pain, arthritis.
  - Stage 3: encephalomyelitis, paraparesis.
  - Ix: positive *Borrelia* serology confirms previous exposure; active CSF supports recent infection.
  - Cause: tick bite (*Ixodes*)—from woodland/deer.
  - Rx: stage 1 or 2: 30 days oral doxycycline; stage 3: 30 days of IV ceftriaxone.
  - Px: good if identified and treated early.
- HIV:
  - Sx and O/E: same as GBS but more dysaesthesia.
  - DDx: GBS, retroviral drug side effects.
  - Ix: LP—raised protein **and** white cell count; NCS—demyelinating neuropathy.
  - Rx and Px: of the HIV.

## Chronic acquired

### Drugs

- E.g. chemotherapy, antiepileptics, amiodarone, statins, antibiotics and most commonly alcohol.
- Stopping drug **may** arrest ± reverse neuropathy.

### Diabetes

Any focal/multifocal cranial or limb neuropathy, especially:

- Distal symmetrical sensory lower limb (LL).
- Painful amyotrophy (see earlier in section).
- Recurrent cranial mononeuropathies especially IIIrd nerve (pupil sparing).

### Vitamin B₁₂ deficiency

- Sensory >motor axonal neuropathy.
- Often begins with upper extremity tingling.
- Causes: intrinsic factor or parietal cell antibodies, coeliac disease, rarely dietary.
- Upper motor neurone signs imply cord also affected.
- Reversible if caught early (<12 months).

### Pure sensory neuropathies

- Especially affecting proprioception → pseudoathetosis of outstretched hands.
- Produces 'sensory weakness' and 'sensory ataxia.'

- Cause: Sjögren syndrome (Ro/La antibodies), paraneoplastic (Hu antibodies), paraprotein (MAG antibodies).

### Autoimmune and/or paraproteinaemias

*Chronic inflammatory demyelinating polyneuropathy (CIDP)*

- Sx: paraesthesia and limb weakness progressing for >8 weeks (vs. GBS which peaks in <4 weeks).
- O/E: usually symmetrical, numbness, weakness, areflexic, rarely affects face or bulbar muscles.
- DDx: Charcot–Marie–Tooth disease, paraprotein-related.
- Ix: NCS—demyelinating neuropathy.
- Cause: ganglioside antibodies in ~50% (e.g. GD1b).
- Rx: oral steroids, IVIGs.
- Px: may require regular top-up immunoglobulin courses to keep symptoms controlled.

*Multifocal motor neuropathy (MMN)*

- Pure motor CIDP-like illness, rare.
- Main DDx: motor neurone disease, but no UMN signs.

*IgM paraproteinemic neuropathies*

- MAG antibody: pure sensory neuropathy + tremor.
- GM1 antibody: pure motor neuropathy.

*IgG or IgA paraproteinemic neuropathies*

POEMS syndrome (**required features; *major criteria):

- **P**olyneuropathy: sensory, motor, autonomic (profuse sweating); demyelinating and/or axonal.
- **O**rganomegaly: spleen, liver, lymph nodes.
- **E**ndocrinopathy: gonadal, pituitary, adrenal.
- **M**onoclonal paraprotein: IgG or IgA (especially myeloma).
- **S**kin changes: hypopigmentation typical:
  - Sx: painless peripheral neuropathy + weight loss.
  - O/E: febrile, papilloedema, areflexia, distal numbness.
  - Ix: **bloods**—Hb and platelets often raised, protein electrophoresis, endocrine screen, *vascular endothelial growth factor (**VEGF**) raised; **urine**—light chains; CSF—protein often raised; **skeletal survey**—*osteosclerotic lesions (myeloma is usually osteolytic); **abdominal CT**—organomegaly; **lymph node biopsy**—*Castleman disease (lymphoma-like disease, but not cancerous)

## Chronic hereditary

### Charcot–Marie–Tooth (CMT) disease or hereditary motor and sensory neuropathy (HMSN)

- Onset: teens to 20, poor at sports, family history of 'funny feet' and clumsiness.
- Sx: difficulty running, unsteady, falls.
- O/E: initially LL only—very symmetrical, distal weakness, wasting and numbness, pes cavus/high arches, hammer toes and areflexia. Later there are upper limb motor and sensory changes and areflexia.
- DDx: CIDP, muscular dystrophy.
- Ix: NCS—distinguishes between demyelinating (CMT1) or axonal (CMT2) subtypes; selective gene testing (*PMP22* mutations in some CMT1 cases; same gene as HNPP).
- Rx: physiotherapy, orthoses, foot care.
- Px: degenerative, life expectancy not affected.

### Familial amyloid

- Bimodal onset: 20s or 60s. ♂ >♀.
- Sx: distal dysaesthesia, dysautonomia.
- O/E: mainly pain and temperature loss (small fibres); painless ulcers, Charcot joints.

- DDx: diabetes, AL amyloid.
- Ix: autonomic function tests, nerve biopsy.
- Rx: pacemaker for cardiac arrhythmia. Early liver transplant in a specific subtype (transthyretin).
- Px: mean survival 11 years after symptom onset (cardiac, sepsis).

## Standard investigations

### Neurophysiology

*Nerve conduction studies (NCS)*
- Measurement of speed and size of nerve impulses.
- Categorises neuropathy into mainly demyelinating or axonal, and into sensory, motor or both.
- Slow conduction implies demyelination (i.e. GBS, CIDP, CMT1, most paraprotein, some drugs, e.g. amiodarone).
- Small action potentials (reduced nerve impulse amplitude) imply an axonal neuropathy.

*Electromyography (EMG)*
- Measures muscle activity at rest and on exertion.
- Distinguishes neurogenic vs. myopathic weakness.

*Lumbar puncture (LP)*
- Normal protein, glucose, cells in axonal neuropathies.
- High protein (often ++) but normal cells in demyelination.
- Abnormally high white cells implies infection.

### Nerve biopsy
- Reserved for the diagnosis of vasculitis and amyloid.
- Sometimes combined with muscle biopsy to increase yield in suspected vasculitis.

## Management approach

1. Rule out acute reversible neuropathies.
2. Look for treatable causes of chronic neuropathies.
2. If no treatable cause is found, concentrate on:
   a. Meticulous footcare (chiropody if necessary).
   b. Palliative treatments (drugs*, physiotherapy, speech therapy, occupational therapy, orthotics or rehabilitation team).
   c. Patient education and support (<http://www.neurocentre.com>).

*Typical neuropathic analgesics (maximum daily doses): gabapentin (2.7g or 2700mg, as preferred) or pregabalin (600mg), amitriptyline (100mg)

## Mitochondrial neurological disease

- Mitochondria contain the respiratory chain or energy-producing (ATP) machinery of each cell.
- Clinically heterogeneous disorders, typically multisystem (Table 14.14).
- Brain and skeletal muscle often affected due to high energy demand; endocrinopathies and cardiopathies also common, e.g. hypertrophic cardiomyopathy and diabetes mellitus.
- Mitochondrial DNA either mitochondrial encoded (maternal inheritance) or nuclear encoded, although most significant mutations are of mitochondrial-encoded DNA.

### Assessment

- Full history including obstetric, neonatal, and developmental details should be recorded.
- Note maternal lineage in the family history.
- Full systemic and neurological examination should be performed.
- Presence of short stature, deafness, diabetes mellitus, migraine, or premature exercise-induced fatigue may be clues.

### Investigations

- Blood tests: lactic acidosis (in about 50%) and CK (usually normal or mildly elevated).
- Genetic tests: numerous genetic mutations identified but a negative test may not exclude mitochondrial disease.
- CSF: may show elevated protein and lactate (even with normal serum lactate).
- EEG/EMG: non-specific changes of seizures/myopathy.
- ECG/Echo/CXR: if cardiac involvement suspected.
- Imaging: CT may show basal ganglia changes and proton MR spectroscopy may show lactic acid peaks in MELAS.
- Muscle biopsy: ragged red fibres (mitochondrial aggregates) in skeletal muscle; characteristic cytochrome oxidase staining is seen depending on the type of myopathy.

### Treatment

Primarily symptomatic and supportive (e.g. treatment of cardiac and endocrine defects). Supplements and antioxidants, e.g. vitamins A, C, E, coenzyme Q10, creatine are recommended by some clinicians but no robust evidence. Future possibilities include genetic treatment.

## Channelopathies

- Group of conditions characterized by either abnormal muscle relaxation (myotonia) or episodic weakness.

- Caused by ion gene mutations (voltage-gated sodium, calcium, chloride, and potassium ion channels).
- Several other conditions with underlying channelopathy include familial hemiplegic migraine, episodic ataxias, congenital myasthenic syndromes, and acquired neuromyotonia, are not covered here.

### Chloride channelopathies—myotonia congenita

- Thomsen disease—autosomal dominant; usually presents in childhood or adolescence; mild myotonia that improves with exercise (warm-up phenomenon).
- Becker disease—autosomal recessive, similar to but more common and severe than Thomsen; often with fixed or episodic limb weakness; ♂ predominance.

### Calcium channelopathies

- **Hypo**kalaemic periodic paralysis—autosomal dominant condition; 1/3 are sporadic mutations; weakness following a fall in serum K⁺ (e.g. after carbohydrate ingestion or when resting post-exertion).
- Malignant hyperthermia—most common cause of death during anaesthesia; due to a massive Ca⁺ release with volatile anaesthetic agents or suxamethonium; less severe following strenuous exercise or infections; muscle spasm, rigidity and rhabdomyolysis leading to myoglobinuria ± renal failure, hyperthermia, tachycardia, lactic acidosis; treat with active cooling, dantrolene, intubation + hyperventilation. Susceptibility tests in family members.

### Sodium channelopathies

- **Hyper**kalaemic periodic paralysis—autosomal dominant; episodic flaccid weakness, localized or generalized, (up to several hours); triggered by rest or after exercise; terminated by carbohydrates or inhaled salbutamol to lower serum K⁺.
- Paramytonia congenita—autosomal dominant; episodic myotonia and weakness; induced by cold and worsen with continued activity.

### Potassium channelopathies

- Anderson syndrome—autosomal dominant, dysmorphic faceis/hands, cardiomyopathy, periodic paralysis, limb weakness; short stature.
- Normokalaemic periodic paralysis—autosomal dominant; weakness with rest after exercise.

### Investigations

- Bloods: K⁺ levels; exclude secondary cause of hypo- or hyperkalaemia; TFT (thyrotoxicosis possible in hypokalaemic paralysis).
- ECG: to exclude arrhythmia.
- EMG: may show myotonia.

### Treatment

Symptomatic; directed either to myotonia, e.g. phenytoin, carbamazepine, mexiletine, or periodic weakness, e.g. acetazolamide.

| Table 14.14 Clinical features of some of the classical mitochondrial syndromes | |
| --- | --- |
| Syndrome | Clinical characteristics |
| Chronic progressive external ophthalmoplegia (CPEO) | Classic presentation—3rd or 4th decade—ptosis, then proximal muscle weakness, fatigue. May see progressive ophthalmoplegia, cardiomyopathy, deafness, ataxia, peripheral neuropathy |
| Kearns–Sayre syndrome | Ophthalmoplegia and pigmentary retinopathy <20 years. May also see cerebellar ataxia, proximal myopathy, complete heart block |
| Mitochondrial encephalopathy, lactic acidosis, and stroke-like syndrome (MELAS) | Intermittent encephalopathic episodes with high plasma and CSF lactate. Dementia, vomiting, migraine, epilepsy. Stroke-like episodes in young patients not localized to specific vascular territory |
| Myoclonic epilepsy and ragged red fibres (MERRF) | Myoclonic epilepsy, muscle weakness/wasting, dementia, cerebellar ataxia, deafness, cardiomyopathy |
| Neuropathy, ataxia and retinitis pigmentosa (NARP) | Peripheral neuropathy, cerebellar ataxia, pigmentary retinopathy. May see developmental delay, dementia, proximal weakness (Leigh syndrome) |
| Leber hereditary optic neuropathy | Usually young ♂—progressive painless central visual loss, often one eye initially, spreads to affect other in a few months. May see dystonia, cardiac conduction defects |

## Myasthenia gravis

This condition is characterized by fluctuating weakness of ocular, bulbar, limb, and respiratory muscles.

### Pathophysiology

Myasthenia gravis (MG) is an autoimmune disease arising due to antibody-mediated attack of acetylcholine (ACh) receptors at the neuromuscular junction.

### Epidemiology

- Prevalence: 1–2/10,000; all ethnic groups.
- Bimodal distribution: ♀ 20–30 years, ♂ 50–70 years.

### Clinical evaluation

- Look for evidence of a characteristic pattern of weakness with evidence of fatigability and fluctuation in severity.
- Consider other associated autoimmune conditions.
- Ensure you assess respiratory muscle function to exclude myasthenic crisis (severe MG endangering life).

*History and examination*

- Early in MG, symptoms are often intermittent.
- Ocular symptoms (50–70% with ocular symptoms develop generalized MG; 15% have purely ocular MG).
- Ptosis—may be asymmetrical. Pupil always spared.
- Diplopia—horizontal or vertical, not fitting with single cranial nerve lesion.
- Dysarthria and dysphagia—worst with liquids, ask about choking or nasal regurgitation.
- Dyspnoea and orthopnoea.
- Limb weakness—typically proximal >distal, and arms >legs.
- Fatigable—reduction in strength of a muscle after sustained use rather than a patient's sense of tiredness.
- Fluctuation—often symptoms worst in the evening and after exercise, improving after a period of rest.
- Reflexes preserved.

*Investigations*
*Making the diagnosis*

- Serum ACh receptor antibody test—85% sensitive (50% in purely ocular MG). Almost 100% specific to MG.
- Anti-MuSK (muscle specific kinase) or antibody to clustered AChRs if AChR antibody –ve.
- Neurophysiology (stop ACh-esterase 24 hours beforehand).
- Repetitive stimulation is 75% sensitive.
- Single-fibre EMG—95% sensitive but less widely available.
- Tensilon (edrophonium) test—used in those who cannot be otherwise diagnosed. Full resuscitation facilities must be available, contraindicated in cardiac disease.

*Looking for associated conditions*

- CT chest—thymoma in 10%.
- TFT—Graves disease coexists in 3–8%.
- ANA or rheumatoid factor if history suggestive.

### Differential diagnoses

- Ocular symptoms—hyperthyroidism, mitochondrial disease (chronic progressive external ophthalmoplegia), botulism.
- Bulbar symptoms—MND, brainstem lesion, oculo-pharyngeal muscular dystrophy (rarely).
- Limb symptoms—MND, motor neuropathy, myopathy, Lambert–Eaton myasthenic syndrome (LEMS).
- Acute presentations—botulism, GBS.

### Management
*Medical*

- Anticholinesterase drugs (symptomatic)—pyridostigmine. Propantheline can reduce cholinergic side effects.
- Corticosteroids (disease-modifying)—start cautiously at low dose
- Azathioprine/mycophenolate/ciclosporin used as steroid-sparing agents, rituximab for refractory cases.
- IVIG or plasma exchange used in myasthenic crisis or perioperatively (rapid onset but short duration of action).
- Aminoglycosides and β-blockers may worsen myasthenia.

*Surgical*

- Thymectomy—improvement in MG symptoms seen in 1/3 of younger patients with or without thymoma. If found, thymoma should be removed as risk of local invasion.

*Managing myasthenic crisis*

- Can be precipitated by infection, systemic upset, or drugs. Patients often require artificial ventilation and feeding.
- Check FVC in all MG patients:
  - If FVC <1.5L, check ABG; if FVC <1L involve ITU immediately.
- Assess adequacy of airway protection (swallow and cough).

### Prognosis

Patients have a near-normal life expectancy but many will require lifelong therapy for symptoms. Respiratory failure may be life-threatening.

## Lambert–Eaton myasthenic syndrome (LEMS)

This condition has many features in common with MG but is much less common. Certain features are used to discriminate the two (see Table 14.15).

### Pathophysiology

Also autoimmune in nature, 50–60% of cases are paraneoplastic in origin (typically small cell lung cancer (SCLC)). Antibodies to

**Table 14.15** Differentiating neuropathy, MG, LEMS, and myopathy

| | Motor neuropathy | MG | LEMS | Myopathy |
|---|---|---|---|---|
| Predominant distribution of weakness | Distal | Ocular/bulbar/proximal arms, respiratory | Proximal legs | Symmetrical proximal arms and legs |
| Other features | Fasciculation Wasting | Fatigability | Fatigability Autonomic | |
| Reflexes | Reduced | Normal | May be decreased but return after exercise | Normal |
| Neurophysiology | Reduced velocity or amplitude of nerve conduction | Repetitive stimulation decrement in motor action potential causes | Repetitive stimulation causes increment in motor action potential | Myopathic EMG |

pre-synaptic voltage-gated calcium channels (VGCC) are found in many cases. Like MG, association is seen with other autoimmune conditions such as insulin dependent diabetes and thyroid disease.

### Diagnosis and management

- Paraneoplastic and idiopathic LEMS very similar.
- Limb weakness—proximal >distal and legs >arms.
- Autonomic dysfunction—dry mouth, impotence.
- Bulbar/respiratory features—typically less common and less severe than in MG.
- Ocular symptoms—rare.
- Reflexes often depressed but improve after exercise.
- VGCC antibodies—highly sensitive in paraneoplastic LEMS (75–100%) but also found in other autoimmune conditions.
- Neurophysiology—increment with rapid repetitive stimulation.
- Imaging to investigate for underlying SCLC is essential.
- Anticholinesterase drugs and 3,4-diaminopyridine as well as immunomodulation may help.
- If paraneoplastic, treating the underlying malignancy may induce neurological remission.

## Myopathy

This term refers to any structural or functional abnormality of the muscle. Many of these conditions share common features in history, examination, and initial investigation.

### Aetiology

Conditions can be helpfully categorized by aetiology, e.g. inflammatory, endocrine, inherited muscular dystrophies, metabolic, drug-related and other causes (Table 14.16).

### Clinical evaluation

*History*

- Most primary disorders of the muscle cause weakness that is persistent and progressive. Delay in reaching motor milestones during childhood might suggest muscular dystrophy.
- Metabolic myopathies refer to conditions where inborn errors of metabolism cause abnormality of skeletal muscle function, and often simultaneously cause abnormalities in other organs such as liver, brain, and heart. Symptoms may vary over time.

| Table 14.16 Causes of myopathy | |
|---|---|
| Category of myopathy | Condition |
| Inflammatory | Poly/dermatomyositis |
| | Inclusion body myositis |
| Endocrine | Hypothyroidism |
| | Cushing disease |
| | Osteomalacia |
| Drugs/toxins | Corticosteroids |
| | Statins |
| | Alcohol excess |
| Inherited muscular dystrophy (MD) | Duchenne/Becker MD |
| | Myotonic dystrophy |
| | Limb-girdle MD |
| | Fascio-scapulo-humeral MD |
| Metabolic myopathies | Glycogen storage diseases |
| | Disorders of lipid metabolism |
| | Mitochondrial myopathy |
| Other causes | Infection, e.g. CMV, HIV |

- Muscle pain—may occur in inflammatory myopathy but if severe, consider PMR/fibromyalgia. Disorders of carbohydrate or lipid metabolism may cause muscle cramps during exercise or, in extreme cases, rhabdomyolysis.
- Myopathic weakness tends to affect proximal limbs symmetrically (often sparing facial/ocular/bulbar muscles).
- Family history—may suggest inherited muscular dystrophy, mitochondrial disease, or other metabolic myopathy.
- Drug and alcohol history.

*Examination*

- Wasting is usually absent until late in myopathy.
- Pattern of weakness—detecting exceptions to the usual proximal limb weakness pattern may suggest particular diagnoses.
- Finger flexion and quadriceps weakness typical of inclusion body myositis.
- Extraocular muscle weakness in mitochondrial myopathy.
- Ptosis suggests inherited muscular dystrophy/mitochondrial myopathy.
- Reflexes should be preserved.
- Sensory examination will be normal.

*Investigations*

- Bloods tests: muscle enzymes—particularly CK (MM)—are raised in many myopathies. Screening for endocrine or metabolic derangement.
- Neurophysiology—helpful in distinguishing myopathy from disease affecting the neuromuscluar junction or motor nerves. However, myopathic features seen on EMG are not helpful in distinguishing causes of myopathy.
- Gene testing—can identify certain muscular dystrophies.
- Muscle biopsy—helpful in the diagnosis of many causes of myopathy (Fig. 14.32).
- MRI is likely to become increasingly useful in distinguishing myopathies and detecting subclinical muscle abnormalities.

### Management

This will depend in the underlying cause (reversing endocrine/drug aetiologies, treating inflammation).

## Polymyositis and dermatomyositis

- Inflammatory muscle diseases usually affecting age groups 40–60 years.
- Both thought to be autoimmune although the exact auto-antigens are unknown.
- Associated with mildly increased risk of malignancy and may also overlap with other connective tissue diseases, e.g. SLE.

### Clinical features

- Systemic upset (malaise, fever, weight loss) commonly accompanies weakness at onset.
- Limb weakness is usually proximal.
- Involvement of bulbar, cardiac and respiratory muscles is well-recognized.
- Involvement of the extraocular muscles/ptosis is rare.
- Dermatomyositis has the same muscle features as polymyositis but is also associated with several skin manifestations: heliotrope rash (violaceous periorbital), photosensitive erythematous rash, Gottron papules, nailbed infarcts, and cuticle changes.

*Investigation*

- ESR often elevated.
- Antinuclear antibodies present in 80% of cases.
- Muscle biopsy reveals inflammation.

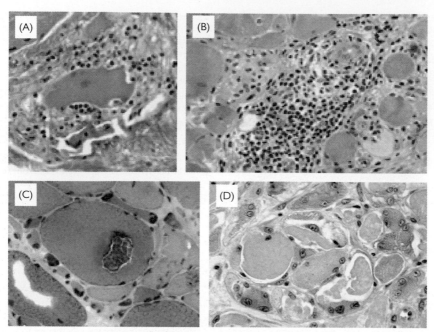

**Fig. 14.32** Muscle biopsy appearance of myopathy. (A) Polymyositis—lymphocytic infiltrate. (B) Dermatomyositis—vasculitis affecting muscle capillaries. (C) IBM—vacuoles filled with basophilic granules. (D) Duchenne muscluar dystrophy.

### Treatment

Oral prednisolone is the mainstay of treatment. Steroid-sparing agents (e.g. azathioprine) are commonly required.

### Prognosis

While few patients recover completely, mortality is low and disease often becomes gradually less active over time.

## Inclusion body myositis (IBM)

- Inflammatory myopathy; more common in ♂.
- Gradual onset. Rarely seen <50 years.
- Like poly/dermatomyositis, IBM can cause limb girdle weakness but also causes distal weakness, particularly affecting the finger flexors. Forearm and quadriceps wasting can be profound.
- CK elevation can be mild but muscle biopsy is characteristic (Fig. 13.32).
- Immunosuppressive therapy is not beneficial and prognosis is that of steady progression of weakness.

## Inherited muscular dystrophies

The abnormal gene in muscular dystrophy (MD) usually results in absence or abnormality of muscle protein resulting in muscle necrosis and fibrosis leading to progressive weakness. Current treatment is supportive including physiotherapy, orthoses, and other aids to mobility. Monitoring cardiac and respiratory function is important because of the incidence of cardiomyopathy and ventilatory failure (including sleep apnoea) requiring pacemaker and/or ventilatory support in some muscular dystrophies like Duchenne. As with many inherited conditions, genetic counselling is an important component of management.

### Duchenne muscular dystrophy

- **X-linked** condition arising in 1/3000 ♂ births and results in absence of the dystrophin protein.
- Onset in infancy with death usually occurring before 30 years.
- Delayed motor milestones and pseudohypertrophy of muscles.
- CK very elevated.
- ECG abnormal in 80% (conduction abnormalities).
- Gene testing often reveals a mutation.
- Muscle biopsy performed if genetic test inconclusive.

### Becker muscular dystrophy

- An **autosomal recessive** condition causing abnormal dystrophin.
- 10× less common than Duchenne MD.
- Milder clinical picture with onset in young adulthood with a near-normal life expectancy.

### Myotonic dystrophy

- This rare **autosomal dominant** condition arises due to a tri-nucleotide repeat on chromosome 19 which exhibits genetic anticipation, i.e. lengthening of the repeat with phenotypic worsening in successive generations.
- Distal limb weakness, facial and bulbar weakness, and ptosis begin in adulthood.
- Cardiac, respiratory, gut, and bladder muscles may be affected.

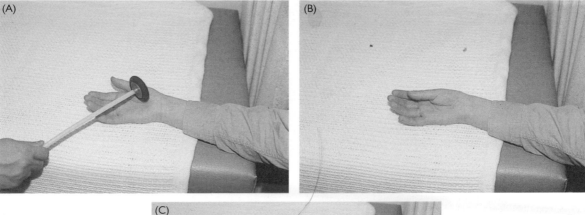

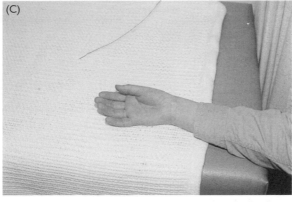

**Fig. 14.33** Percussion myotonia: following a sharp tap, the thenar eminence muscles contract and then relax slowly. (photographs taken at 3-s intervals).

Reproduced from Warrell et al., *Oxford Textbook of Medicine*, 2012, Figure 24.24.3.2, with permission from Oxford University Press, www. oxfordmedicine.com

- Myotonia (failure to relax a muscle after voluntary contraction has ceased) is best demonstrated in the hands (Fig. 14.33).
- Also associated are frontal balding, cataracts, gynaecomastia, and testicular atrophy (♂), diabetes mellitus.

- DNA testing for number of triplet repeats is diagnostic.
- Patients often die in their 50s from cardiac/respiratory disease.
- General anaesthesia should be avoided if possible because of the high risk of respiratory/cardiac complications.

# 14.29 Sleep disorders

## Background

Sleep is a natural, universal, circadian period of unconsciousness. Roughly 1/3 of our lives is taken up in this (in)activity, and yet we still do not know why we sleep. Nonetheless, it is intuitive to assume that regular, restful sleep is a prerequisite of physical and psychological health. This section provides an overview of disorders affecting sleep.

## Sleep stages

Sleep is divided into phases with and without rapid eye movement (REM vs. non-REM sleep). Non-REM sleep consists of four distinct stages (stage 1 to 4). Each stage has its behavioural and EEG characteristics, and is affected by its own different set of sleep disorders (see Table 14.17). Sleep consists of cyclical progression through non-REM and REM sleep, typically four to five cycles a night.

## Epidemiology of sleep disorders

Disorders affecting sleep are common:
- Occasional insomnia reported in 33% of adults.
- Alcohol or hypnotics used by up to 25% of adults to aid sleep.
- Sleep apnoea in 2–4% of the Western population.
- Sleep disorders increase with age.
- Sleep dysfunction can be secondary to other illness, both neurological (MS, PD) or others (heart failure, obesity).

## Classification of sleep disorders

See Table 14.18.

## Taking a sleep history

A good history is the cornerstone of the clinical approach to a sleep disorder. Encourage the patient to keep a sleep log, where patterns and quantity of sleep are recorded.

### 1. Quality, quantity, and timing of sleep
- What time do they (and partner) go to bed?
- What times do they (and partner) wake up?
- Do they wake up during the night and, if so, why?

### 2. Lifestyle, comfort, and medical factors
- Amount and timing of last meal, caffeine, alcohol, tobacco?
- Noise and light levels? Mattress quality?
- Types and timing of medication?
- Any pain, breathlessness, anxiety, depression or stress?

### 3. Daytime sleepiness
- Do they fall asleep in the day? Are naps appropriate?
- Time and duration of daytime naps? Specific circumstances?
- Daytime atonia with preserved awareness (cataplexy)?

### 4. Symptoms on falling asleep or waking up
- Strange feelings? Hallucinations? Paralysis?

### 5. History from bed partner
- Movements and behaviour in sleep.
- Breathing patterns and snoring during sleep.

## Specific sleep disorders

### Obstructive sleep apnoea (OSA)
- 100× more common than narcolepsy! Mainly in 40–50s. Narrowing/occlusion of airway in sleep cause brief periods of apnoea and awakenings—disruptive to sleep architecture.
- Associations: obesity (50%), acromegaly, jaw problems.
- Snoring and excessive daytime sleepiness.
- Complications of OSA: traffic accidents, hypertension, heart disease, polycythaemia.
- Polysomnography: periodic increased respiratory effort and $CO_2$.
- Central sleep apnoea (brainstem lesions).
- Treatment: weight loss, reduce alcohol intake, CPAP.

### Narcolepsy
- Recurrent attacks of irresistible sleepiness with refreshing naps of 15–20 minutes (3–6×/day).
- Modal onset is in 20s: onset after 50 is unusual.
- Occurs with (70%) and without cataplexy—muscle atonia (i.e. jaw drops open or collapses to ground)—typically triggered by strong emotion (e.g. laughing, excitement, grief).
- Diagnosed with multiple sleep latency tests (by EEG): time from falling sleep to onset of REM is pathologically brief.
- Orexin (a hormone involved in maintaining wakefulness and appetite) is reduced in narcolepsy with cataplexy.
- Treatment:
  - Optimize nocturnal sleep and daytime naps (just after meals).
  - CNS stimulants (e.g. modafinil 100–400mg, amphetamines, methylphenidate) for excessive sleepiness.
  - Clomipramine or venlafaxine very effective for cataplexy.

Table 14.17 Sleep stages

| Stage | EEG | Motor and cognitive features and comments | 'Abnormal' activities |
|---|---|---|---|
| 1 | $\alpha \to \tau$ waves | Some awareness Roving eye movements | Hypnic jerks Hypnogogic hallucinations |
| 2 | Sleep spindles K complexes | Little or no awareness | |
| 3 | $\delta$ waves | Transition to stage 4 | Sleepwalking Sleeptalking Night terrors |
| 4 | $\delta$ waves | Deep sleep | |
| REM | Mixed frequency Low amplitude | Dream sleep Hypotonia (effective paralysis) Obliterated by certain drugs, e.g. MAOIs | REM sleep disorder (RSD) |

Table 14.18 Classification of sleep disorders

| Category | Examples |
|---|---|
| 1. Dyssomnias—affect amount and timing of sleep | • Insomnia (too little sleep) <br> • Hypersomnia (too much sleep) <br> • Narcolepsy (inappropriate sleepiness) <br> • Circadian disorders (disturbed timing) |
| 2. Parasomnias—abnormal sleep behaviours <br> 3. Sleep/wake interface disturbances | • Non-REM disorders (sleep walking/sleep talking, night terrors) <br> • REM sleep disorders (dream enaction) <br> • Sleep paralysis <br> • Hallucinations |
| 4. Disturbed respiratory pattern | • Obstructive sleep apnoea <br> • Central sleep apnoea |

### Restless legs syndrome

- Irritative or painful feelings in legs whilst in bed or at rest, relieved by walking. Usually worse in evenings.
- Iron deficiency can cause similar symptoms (check ferritin).
- 50% have family history.
- Treatment: L-dopa, dopamine agonists, clonazepam (not tricyclics).

### Parasomnias

- Abnormal behaviour associated with abnormal sleep physiology.
- Categorized into disorders of REM vs. non-REM (NREM).
- NREM sleep disorders tend to occur in the early part of the night and involve younger patients. There is little or no recollection if woken during episodes, e.g. sleepwalking.
- REM sleep disorders—behavioural disturbance during REM sleep (RSD), with loss of the normal (protective) REM atonia. There is dream enacting (shouting, violence). It is more common in Parkinson disease and can precede its onset by decades.

## Background

This section discusses neurological conditions which are unique to pregnancy (e.g. eclampsia), or for which pregnancy is a significant risk factor (e.g. Bell palsy). Pregnancy also presents particular therapeutic challenges for women with other neurological conditions (e.g. epilepsy or headache).

## Eclampsia

Pre-eclampsia (hypertension newly developed in pregnancy) occurs in 5% of pregnancies, usually between 28 weeks of gestation and 1 week postpartum. Eclampsia arises in 0.5% of patients with pre-eclampsia causing seizures and encephalopathy.

### Epidemiology
- Eclampsia is a rare but important cause of maternal mortality.
- It is far more common in developing countries, most likely because of less efficient screening of BP in pregnancy.

### Pathophysiology
Eclampsia is poorly understood but is thought to be related to hypertensive encephalopathy.

### History
- Tonic–clonic seizure in a hypertensive, pregnant patient.
- Other features: headache, blurred vision, epigastric pain.

### On examination
- Hypertension (BP >140/90mmHg) is characteristic but can be mild or occasionally absent (in ~15% cases).
- Pitting oedema and proteinuria commonly associated.
- Altered mental state.
- Less commonly: focal neurological deficit.

### Investigation
- Diagnosis is essentially clinical.
- Cerebral imaging is indicated if there is focal neurology.

### Treatment
- Supportive management of seizures, e.g. oxygen.
- Expedite delivery: labour often induced or caesarean section performed.
- Magnesium sulphate given IV during labour and up to 24 hours postpartum.
- BP lowered to systolic 140–160mmHg.
- Careful attention to fluid balance.

## Stroke

Pregnancy itself carries a comparatively low risk for stroke, certainly when compared with risk factors such as diabetes and hypertension. Risk is highest during the 3rd trimester. Stroke experienced during pregnancy is more likely to be haemorrhagic or due to venous thrombosis than in the non-pregnant individual. The management of stroke in pregnancy does not differ from the non-pregnant female. In particular, the absence of clear risk factors for atherosclerosis should prompt a search for other underlying conditions rather than attributing risk to the pregnant state.

## Conditions affecting cranial and peripheral nerves

### Carpal tunnel syndrome
Pregnancy appears to predispose to carpal tunnel syndrome. Symptoms arise as a result of excess swelling within tissues of the carpal tunnel during pregnancy (due to fluid retention). This explains why symptoms usually disappear after delivery but may recur during subsequent pregnancies. Reassurance plus conservative management (e.g. splinting) is appropriate.

### Bell palsy
This condition is about twice as common in pregnancy than in non-pregnant women. Treatment is identical (see Section 14.9).

## Movement disorders

**Restless leg syndrome** is not uncommon in pregnancy. Sufferers describe the urge to move their legs, associated with unpleasant sensations in the legs, usually worst whilst sitting/lying still and relieved by movement. Iron or folate deficiency should be identified and treated. A hereditary predisposition or, less commonly, uraemia can also underlie symptoms but the condition can also be idiopathic. A conservative approach is favoured rather than dopaminergic agents which are held in reserve for those severely affected.

**Chorea gravidarum** refers to the onset of acute chorea during pregnancy. The syndrome is rare and the underlying causes of chorea do not differ from the non-pregnant individual. Sydenham chorea (associated with rheumatic fever) is now rare but occasionally diseases such as SLE or antiphospholipid syndrome cause chorea in young females.

## Headache

Whilst tension headache and migraine account for most headaches during pregnancy, persistent or severe symptoms might prompt consideration of cerebral venous thrombosis, benign intracranial hypertension, or tumour. Paracetamol is safe throughout pregnancy and NSAIDs during 1st/2nd trimesters (later use carries risk of premature closure of the ductus arteriosus). Migraine sufferers often experience remission of attacks during pregnancy but, nevertheless, migraine may persist or indeed first present during pregnancy. Symptomatic treatment options for severe attacks include NSAIDs (except in 3rd trimester), metoclopramide, chlorpromazine, or steroids. Options for prophylaxis include β-blockers and amitriptyline.

## Epilepsy

See Section 14.15.

# 14.31 The neurology of HIV infection

## Background

Epidemiological surveys in 2013 estimated that there were 107,800 people in the UK infected with the human immunodeficiency virus (HIV), 24% of whom would be unaware of their infection.

Neurological manifestations of HIV are due to:

1. Direct infection (vacuolar myelopathy, AIDS dementia complex).
2. Immune dysfunction, i.e. autoimmunity (GBS, CIDP).
3. Immunodeficiency (opportunistic infections, neoplasms).

Clinical manifestations are frequently dependent on disease staging.

## Early infection (CD4 count >500/mm³)

### Acute seroconversion illness

- 50% of individuals within 6 weeks of seroconversion.
- Features include: fever, headache, myalgia, neck stiffness (rarely an aseptic meningitis), lymphadenopathy, cranial nerve palsies (Bell), and acute GBS.

### Other manifestations

- Occasional HIV meningoencephalitis which can be fatal.

## Intermediate infection (CD4 count 200–500/mm³)

Generally asymptomatic, but may be marked by:

- Mild cognitive impairment (minor cognitive and motor disorder) preceding AIDS dementia complex.
- Multidermatomal herpes zoster.
- Neurosyphilis (greater progression to neurosyphilis in HIV-infected patients than immunocompetent individuals).
- Neuropathies, including mononeuritis multiplex, CIDP.

## Late infection (CD4 count <200/mm³)

The latter stages of HIV infection result in AIDS.

Clinical manifestations result from the following:

### Direct HIV infection

*AIDS dementia complex*

- 5–20% of untreated patients, 60% of children with AIDS.
- Motor involvement (tremor, gait instability, ataxia).
- Cognitive impairment (mental slowing, forgetfulness).
- Behavioural abnormalities (apathy, emotional lability).
- MRI reveals diffuse white matter change, HIV RNA in CSF.

*Vacuolar myelopathy*

- Prevalence of 30% at postmortem in fully developed AIDS.
- Thoracic cord frequently involved.
- Insidious progression (months).
- Myelopathic clinical features (spasticity, bladder involvement, sensory loss in lower limbs).
- Differential diagnoses: vitamin $B_{12}$ deficiency, HTLV-1 infection (check $B_{12}$ levels and CSF for HTLV-1).

*Painful distal sensory polyneuropathy*

- Paraesthesia, gait instability, autonomic dysfunction.
- Peripheral neuropathy can also arise from highly active antiretroviral therapy (HAART) (especially ddI, ddC, d4T).

*Myopathy*

- Polymyositis and dermatomyositis are recognized complications of HIV infection.
- A myopathy may arise from HAART (especially zidovudine (AZT)).

### Immunosuppression

Impaired T-cell immunity in AIDS renders the patient susceptible to various pathogens and mitogens, some of which affect the nervous system:

*Toxoplasmosis*

- *Toxoplasma gondii* found in cat faeces.
- Opportunistic intracerebral infection in the immunosuppressed individual.
- Variable clinical presentation from myoclonus and asterixis to meningoencephalitis, confusion, and coma.
- Imaging reveals multiple ring-enhancing lesions (especially near basal ganglia).
- Serology will reveal an elevated IgG titre (sensitive, but not specific).
- Treatment with pyrimethamine and sulphadiazine.

*Cryptococcal meningitis*

- *Cryptococcus neoformans* found in pigeon droppings.
- Causes subacute or chronic meningitis: look for meningism, confusion, myoclonus, seizures.
- Lymphocytic CSF with +ve cryptococcal Ag and India ink stains.
- Treatment with amphotericin B and flucytosine.

*Progressive multifocal leucoencephalopathy*

- JC virus: commensal papovavirus; 70% of population seropositive.
- Infects oligodendrocytes with widespread demyelination.
- Onset over weeks, mainly involves cerebral hemispheres.
- Aphasia, apraxia, cortical blindness, dementia, death.
- MRI is diagnostic, with multiple, non-enhancing white matter lesions.
- Treatment with HAART and immune reconstitution.

*Cytomegalovirus*

- Herpesvirus family.
- Retinitis and encephalitis in immunosuppressed patients.
- Clinical features: visual loss, confusion, other CN palsies.
- PCR CMV in CSF.
- Treatment with ganciclovir and foscarnet.

*Mycobacterium*

- Two mycobacterial organisms in AIDS: *Mycobacterium tuberculosis* (MTB) and *Mycobacterium avium-intracellulare* (MAI).
- MTB causes chronic meningitis and has a tendency to occur in the intermediate, asymptomatic stage of infection.
- MAI causes pneumonia and disseminated infection in advanced disease.
- Treatment is through multiple antimycobacterial agents.

*Primary CNS lymphomas*

- CNS lymphomas tend to carry a poorer prognosis in AIDS patients than in immunocompetent individuals.
- Poor response to steroids, radiotherapy, or chemotherapy.
- Definitive diagnosis is obtained by histology.
- Imaging appearances can mimic toxoplasma.
- Possible use for PET or SPECT in identifying CNS lymphomas.

## Background

Symptoms and signs never due to a structural cause and of presumed psychological origin.

## Spectrum

- **Reactive symptoms:** transient symptoms immediately after life events.
- **Anxiety symptoms 'plus':** 'fight or flight' symptoms interpreted (by the patient or doctor) as pathology, e.g. tremor, dizziness, palpitations.
- **Functional overlay:** elaboration/exaggeration of physical symptoms.
- **Functional proper:** manifestation of subconscious thoughts and feelings as physical, cognitive or affective disability.

To be distinguished from factitious or malingered disorders:

- Deception (including of self) for emotional or financial gain respectively.
- They are in the differential of all diseases, but harder to separate from functional disorder as few objective 'tests'.

## Symptoms (neurological)

### Common

Fatigue, confusion, forgetfulness, dizziness, disequilibrium, derealization/depersonalization (feeling separated from reality or oneself), unconsciousness, unresponsiveness, headache, slurred speech, effortful speech, aphonia, blurred vision, dysphagia, paresis/paralysis, dystonia, tingling, muscle pain, numbness, jerks, tremor, atonia, convulsions, gait disturbance, urinary incontinence/retention.

### Less common

Paraparesis, facial droop, deafness, ptosis, blepharospasm, hypopnoea/apnoea, bowel incontinence, below-waist anaesthesia, whole body anaesthesia, hallucinations.

## Signs

### General

- Effortful motor and cognitive function during testing.
- Improved function with distraction.
- Abnormalities reflect expectation more than anatomy (e.g. tubular vision, dissociated sternal vibration, non-pyramidal weakness).
- Non-anatomical/physiological combinations (e.g. hemiparesis and ipsilateral blindness, dysarthria and dysphasia, auras and myoclonus).
- Hyperventilating for 1–2 minutes may reproduce their symptoms (jerks, dizziness, imbalance, numbness, coma, atonia, paralysis).

### Specific tests

*Limb paralysis test*
- Unilateral lower limb weakness test (Hoover sign).
- If hip flexion (or extension) appears weak, retest when extending (or flexing) contralateral hip to restore full power.

*Limb or gait ataxia tests*
- Heel–toe walking increases sway without losing balance.
- Finger-to-own-nose testing is worse with eyes shut.

*Visual disturbances*
1. Blindness tests:
   - Unable to sign name despite normal motor function.
   - Intact blink reaction to a visual 'menace'.
2. Tubular vision test:
   - Visual field fails to enlarge despite retreating from patient.
3. Homonymous hemianopia (HH) test:
   - Binocular vision reveals HH; monocular testing reveals tubular vision on 'bad side', intact monocular visual fields on 'good side'.

*Tremor tests*
- **Entrainment:** rhythmic tapping of an unaffected limb at different frequency 'entrains' the tremor to that frequency.
- **Co-activation:** restraining or weighing down a tremulous limb causes a paradoxical increase in tremor amplitude.
- **Distraction:** reduces or stops tremor, rather than exacerbates it.

*Psychogenic non-epileptic seizures (PNES)*
Signs specific for convulsive PNES are:
- Seizure duration >5 minutes.
- Ictal weeping.
- Absence of postictal confusion.

Signs specific for tonic–clonic epileptic seizures are:
- Postictal stertor (rasping breathing or 'snoring').
- Marked peri-ictal acidosis (e.g. pH <7.20).

Gold standard for diagnosis of a seizure type is video telemetry—but the best way to exclude a dual diagnosis is a thorough history.

*Gait disturbances*
- Extremely cautious or slow ('walking on ice').
- Dragging one leg without circumduction.

## A clinical approach

### History

Look out for clues:
- Explosive onset without progression.
- Symptom variability typical for functional problems and atypical for known neurological conditions.
- A history of anxiety, self-harm, or 'breakdown'.
- A history of functional syndromes (irritable bowel, dysfunctional uterine bleeding, multiple chemical sensitivities, chronic fatigue, fibromyalgia, a label of complex regional pain, globus hystericus, atypical facial pain).
- Recurrent admissions with either atypical chest pain, asthma without signs of infection, unexplained abdominal/pelvic pains or apparent epileptic status.

### Examination

Positive signs as already described, inconsistencies between examination on the bed and on general observation.

### Explaining the diagnosis

- This is a **positive** diagnosis based on the history and examination.
- It is a common, recognized condition with a name.
- Acknowledge it as serious, but not sinister.
- Emphasize that it is non-life threatening and potentially reversible.
- Try and give an understandable mechanism.
- You don't need to address causes, unless revealed already.
- Arrange appropriate investigations, but avoid over-investigating.
- Do mention the term 'functional' from the outset, even if you haven't yet excluded organic causes. That way it doesn't seem to be a diagnosis of exclusion if/when the tests prove negative.

## Treatment

- Starts with a clear, positive and sympathetic, explanation.
- Consider Predisposing, Precipitating, and Perpetuating factors:
  - Predisposing—trauma, family dysfunction, neglect, illness.
  - Precipitating—acute illness, injury, stress, new diagnosis.
  - Perpetuating—(a) secondary gain: indirect, subconscious benefits from having (any) visible illness, demotivating for recovery; (b) medical attitudes—cynicism/ disbelief undermines patient engagement with therapy; nihilism/ pessimism are self-fulfilling and increase patient despair.
- Formal treatments
  - Cognitive behavioural therapy (CBT)—modifying unhelpful thought processes exacerbating/driving symptoms.
  - Psychotherapy—exploring primary causes; upsetting.
  - Drugs—anxiolytics (if used cautiously), antidepressants.
  - Physiotherapy can help movement disorders and fatigue.
- Follow them up:
  - Shows them you take their symptoms seriously.
  - Builds a therapeutic relationship.
  - Reinforces functional when undermined by others with less familiarity (family, junior doctors, some GPs).
  - Minimizes fear of 'missing something' (only 4% of functional diagnoses turn out to be wrong)!

# Chapter 15

# Oncology

639

# 15.1 Basic science

## Background

Basic knowledge of molecular biology is necessary to understand the nature of malignant disease. Cancer is a clonal disorder which requires a highly sophisticated system to produce clones of malignant cells able to spread to other organs.

## Cell cycle

The cell cycle is the main mechanism of maintaining the replication of genetically identical cells.

All cells go through:

**S phase**—DNA replication or **synthetic** phase.

**M phase**—cell **division** phase.

**G1 gap**—between M and S.

**G2 gap**—between S and M.

The initial phase of the cell cycle is known as a G1 phase (Fig. 15.1). The cell in G1 is susceptible to mitogenic signals stimulating the cell to enter the cell cycle.

Once the cell enters the S phase, the process of DNA replication continues until the whole DNA is copied. Each sequence is copied only once with the help of enzymes called DNA polymerases. Any mutations are corrected by a DNA mismatch repair mechanism which cuts out unwanted DNA fragments.

### Inefficient DNA repair mechanism is one of the predisposing factors leading to cancer

Following S phase, the cell enters G2 gap, a transition from DNA replication to condensing and segregating its chromosomes.

The whole process is regulated very tightly by cyclin-dependent kinases (CDKs), as well as other proteins involved in the synthesis of enzymes necessary for DNA replication and mismatch repair. Cyclins form complexes with CDKs and activate the latter's protein kinase function. Any abnormality occurring during the cell cycle may lead to carcinogenesis. Recent insights into the control of the cell cycle have led to the development of anti-cancer drugs targeting factors responsible for cell cycle dysregulation.

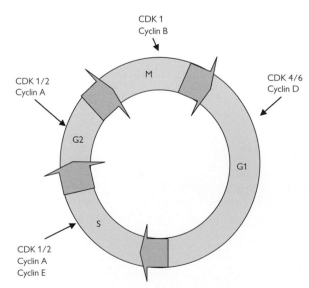

**Fig. 15.1** The cell cycle.

## Mechanisms of oncogenesis

Abnormal cell proliferation that leads to growth and spread of cancer is a result of control failure at multiple levels. The cell cycle is at the centre of this process but the trigger factors can originate at various stages of cellular development.

Abnormalities in the regulation, structure, and function of genes are very important in the pathogenesis of cancer. Genes that once encoded for exogenous proteins within the cells can become overexpressed and cause malignant transformation. These are called **oncogenes**.

Structural alterations that lead to oncogenesis include:

- **Mutation**—usually an exchange of a *single nucleotide* in a regulatory or coding region of a gene. Will lead to loss or gain of function of the protein encoded by the gene.

- **Deletion**—loss of *several nucleotides* will lead to amino acid change and loss or gain of function of the protein encoded by the gene.

- **Amplification**—the number of *copies* of the particular *gene* is multiplied leading to overexpression of the encoded protein.

- **Rearrangement**—result of *chromosomal translocation* and formation of a novel transcript that will lead to expression of a protein with a novel function.

## Oncogenes and tumour suppressor genes

### Oncogenes—mutated genes that result in a *gain* of function

Most known oncogenes were originally identified as tumour-inducing **viruses**. The genes that become altered as a result of viral infection are known as **proto-oncogenes**. Most proto-oncogenes have key regulatory functions in the cells, such as control of cellular proliferation, growth factor signalling, cell cycle progression, and regulation of DNA transcription.

Examples of frequently occurring oncogenes include:

- **Ras**—signal transduction gene, present in ~20% of human tumours-K-*ras* mutation—very common in pancreatic cancer (70–90%).

- **ErbB2**—growth factor receptor, very common in breast (~35%), stomach, and ovarian cancer.

Oncogenes and tumour suppressor genes target several main pathways that affect cell division:

- Signal transduction—accelerates cell proliferation.
- Cell cycle.

### Tumour suppressor genes—mutated genes that result in a *loss* of function

*Retinoblastoma gene (RB1)*

- Acts as a tumour suppressor gene in the familial form of retinoblastoma.

- Also occurs in other cancers.

- A loss-of-function mutation in this gene alters one of the major cyclins involved in cell cycle and leads to dysregulation of the cycle.

Another way that oncogenes and tumour suppressor genes can cause a malignant process is by affecting the cell genome *stability*. All cells have highly sophisticated mechanisms of DNA repair. The mutations that result in impaired ability to repair damaged DNA may result in cancer.

**Table 15.1** Examples of oncogenes and tumour suppressor genes

| Oncogene | Protein properties | Cancer type |
|---|---|---|
| K-ras | Signal transduction Membrane-associated protein | Pancreatic, colorectal, lung, melanoma |
| N-ras | Signal transduction Membrane-associated protein | Melanoma, myeloid, leukaemia |
| H-ras | Signal transduction Membrane-associated protein | Melanoma, bladder |
| ErbB1 | Growth factor receptor (epidermal growth factor receptor, EGFR) | Glioma, squamous cancer |
| ErbB2 | Growth factor receptor (EGFR) | Breast, ovary, colon, stomach |
| Myc | Transcription factor | Burkitt lymphoma, breast, cervix, small-cell lung cancer (SCLC) |
| L-myc | Transcription factor | SCLC |
| N-myc | Transcription factor | Neuroblastoma, SCLC |
| Bcl-2 | Anti-apoptosis protein | B-cell lymphoma |
| **Tumour suppressor gene** | **Protein properties** | **Cancer type** |
| $RB_1$ | Transcriptional regulator | Osteosarcoma, SCLC, retinoblastoma, |
| p53 | Transcriptional regulator | Breast, lung, pancreas, colon |
| BRCA1 | Transcriptional regulator | Breast, ovary |
| BRCA2 | Transcriptional regulator | Breast |
| DCC | Transcriptional regulator | Colorectal, neuroblastoma, germ cell |

Hereditary non-polyposis colon cancer (HNPCC) is an example of a cancer caused by abnormal DNA repair mechanism.

*p53*

- The most common tumour suppressor gene.
- Encodes a protein that is frequently involved in human cancers.
- First identified in cells transformed by SV40 (simian virus 40).
- Plays an important role in cell cycle regulation.
- Loss of *p53* leads to abnormal cell cycle *checkpoints* and allows cells with abnormal DNA to enter the S phase.
- Mutation in one allele of the *p53* gene causes **Li–Fraumeni** syndrome (see Section 15.2).

New oncogenes and tumour suppressor genes are described all the time and the list of mutations involved in carcinogenesis is getting longer. A few examples are listed in Table 15.1, but a comprehensive review is outside the scope of this chapter.

# 15.2 Genetics in oncology

## Background

Most cancers are *sporadic* and not hereditary, but cancer is generally regarded as a genetic disease, as it usually arises from somatic tissue mutations in critical growth regulation genes. Some rare cancers arise from germline mutations or chromosomal rearrangements. To establish whether a specific cancer is 'hereditary', a careful **family history** on both sides is essential, together with elucidating the *age* of affected family members, as well as confirmation of *histological diagnosis* and testing for a specific gene.

## Chromosomal rearrangements

Abnormalities in chromosomal structure (resulting from loss of chromosome or translocation) often lead to altered function of genes responsible for cell growth regulation. There are several groups of such genes:

- Tyrosine kinases
- Cell surface receptors
- Growth factors
- Transcriptional regulating factors

The commonest resulting malignancies are *haematological* such as leukaemia and lymphoma but also some solid tumours.

### Chronic myeloid leukaemia

(See also Section 11.7.) The characteristic chromosomal abnormality in chronic myeloid leukaemia (CML) is the Philadelphia chromosome (a translocation between chromosome 9 and 22) (Fig. 15.2). It is present in about 92% of patients with CML. Patients who do not have the 9;22 translocation usually have a normal karyotype but the disease is more aggressive.

## Lymphoma

8;14 translocation—characteristic in Burkitt lymphoma but can also be present in other aggressive lymphomas.

14;18 translocation—very common, mainly follicular non-Hodgkin lymphoma (NHL); it leads to translocation of the *BCL2* gene from chromosome 18 to the *IGH* gene at chromosome 14; the resulting *BCL2–ICH* gene expresses a protein that blocks apoptosis.

Other frequently occurring chromosomal translocations include:

- 4;11
- 1;19
- 12;21

## Solid tumours

The pattern of chromosomal rearrangements in solid tumours is complex and not consistent.

Most of the tumours have *multiple rearrangements* and the detection of such abnormalities is not helpful in either the diagnosis or the treatment. However, some of the rearrangements have prognostic significance.

## Germline mutations

Germline mutations detectable in hereditary cancer may occur in oncogenes and tumour suppressor genes.

### Retinoblastoma

- A tumour of the eye that affects young children usually between the ages of 2–4 years.
- Usually occurs in one eye but can also be bilateral or multiple.
- Caused by a germline mutation of a tumour suppressor gene—***RB1***. *RB1* is expressed in many different cells and has growth-suppressing

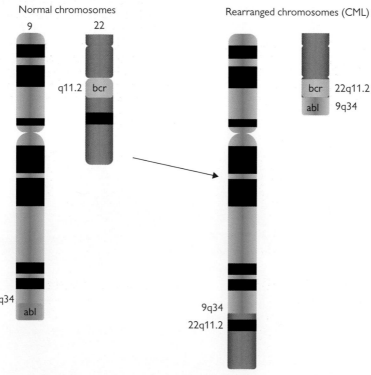

Normal chromosomes

9    22

q11.2  bcr

q34
abl

Rearranged chromosomes (CML)

bcr   22q11.2
abl   9q34

9q34
22q11.2

Fig. 15.2 Chromosomal rearrangement associated with chronic myeloid leukaemia.

**Table 15.2** Conditions associated with MEN syndrome

|  | MEN-I | MEN-II-A | MEN-II-B |
|---|---|---|---|
| Parathyroid adenomas | ~90% | 25% | Rare |
| Pituitary adenomas | 50–60% | – | – |
| Medullary carcinoma of thyroid | – | >90% | >90% |
| Pancreatic islet cell tumours | 30–75% | – | – |
| Phaeochromocytomas | – | 50% | 60% |
| Mucosal neuromas | – | – | 100% |
| Marfanoid features | – | – | 100% |

activity. Inactivation of one copy of *RB1* is probably sufficient to transform cells from normal to malignant. The *RB1* mutation has also been detected in other tumours (breast, lung, and urothelial).

### Multiple endocrine neoplasia (MEN)

(See also Section 7.18.) MEN type I and II are examples of a germline mutation of an oncogene. MEN syndromes are *autosomal dominant* and are characterized by medullary thyroid carcinoma and phaeochromocytoma (Table 15.2). The mutation affects the **RET** gene, which encodes tyrosine kinase, a transmembrane cell receptor very important in cell signalling.

### Li–Fraumeni syndrome

- Rare autosomal dominant disorder predisposing to multiple malignancies.
- Associated with a germline mutation of tumour suppressor gene *p53* on chromosome 17p. This gene is important in cell cycle control, and mutations in *p53* have been identified in ovarian, lung, bowel, breast, and other cancers.

The most common tumours that affect patients with Li–Fraumeni syndrome are:

- Breast
- Soft tissue sarcoma
- Osteosarcoma
- Acute leukaemia
- Brain
- Adrenal (cortical)

# DNA repair defects

DNA repair defects often lead to malignant processes as damaged DNA contains a high number of mutations.

### Xeroderma pigmentosum

- Autosomal recessive disorder.
- Characterized by extreme photosensitivity and skin cancers.
- DNA repair defect.

### Hereditary non-polyposis colon cancer (HNPCC)

- Associated with impaired DNA repair.
- Caused by a mutation in mismatch repair gene *MSH2*.

### Familial breast and ovarian cancer

Familial breast cancer occurs in about 5% of all breast cancer patients. It is attributed to the cancer susceptibility genes *BRCA1* and *BRCA2*.

*BRCA1* and *BRCA2* proteins have a role in DNA repair as they form complexes with a known DNA repair protein RAD51. Carriers of *BRCA* gene mutations have a lifetime risk of breast cancer of around *80%*. Women with *BRCA1* mutations have a 55% risk of developing ovarian cancer compared with 25% risk for *BRCA2* mutation carriers.

Men with mutations in *BRCA1/2* have an increased risk of developing male breast cancer (about 6%) and *prostate* cancer.

Women at high risk of breast cancer should be referred to a specialist genetic clinic and are offered regular surveillance.

Known *BRCA* mutation carriers should have:

- 12-monthly clinical breast examination (in addition to regular self-examination).
- Annual mammography and MRI from the age of 30.
- Annual transvaginal ultrasound from the age of 35 and cancer antigen (CA)-125 test every 4 months.

Treatment options for women who are *BRCA1* mutation carriers include prophylactic mastectomy and oophorectomy.

# 15.3 Screening strategies in oncology

## What is screening?

Screening for medical conditions aims to save lives and improve quality of life by early diagnosis and treatment of illness. Screening is targeted at *healthy* people who are invited to undergo screening tests to detect a specific condition. Effective screening has to be based on good clinical evidence showing that early detection is likely to improve disease outcome. It has set criteria and good quality assurance (see Box 15.1). The screening test is not intended to be diagnostic.

The screening programmes define the population screened, usually by age criteria. Some patients, however, are not within the target screening population, yet can develop the disease earlier or later in life. Although breast cancer screening targets women aged from 50–70 years old, it is known that the most aggressive form of breast cancer often occurs in premenopausal women under 50. Nevertheless, around 80% of breast cancers occur after the age of 50.

Screening in general is only considered for conditions that are a considerable public health problem and that are not possible to prevent by cost-effective interventions.

Screening tests are not 100% sensitive and, therefore, there is a risk that there will be some cancers that are missed ('false negative') and some patients will be recalled unnecessarily as a result of a 'false positive' test. This inevitably leads to distress and anxiety generated by waiting for further results and investigations, not all of which may be conclusive.

There are currently three large-scale cancer screening programmes in the UK.

## UK cancer screening programmes

### NHS Breast Screening Programme (NHS BSP)

- Offered to all women between the ages of 50–70 years.
- Breast cancer screening was recommended 20 years ago by Professor Emeritus Sir Patrick Forrest from the University of Edinburgh.
- The programme was set up in 1998 by the Department of Health.
- Currently the UK NHS BSP is thought to be the best in Europe.
- Around 1.5 million women are screened each year.

Box 15.1 Key features of screening

1. It targets the healthy population and is easy to perform.
2. It is sensitive and specific.
3. It is a simple test that will separate those who may have disease from those who are not affected.
4. Further investigations are available to diagnose the condition screened.
5. An effective intervention is available to treat the condition diagnosed at an early stage.

- It is estimated that breast cancer screening saves around 1400 lives each year.
- There are ~80 screening units throughout the UK and the current budget is ~£75 million.

Women invited for screening have two-view mammography. Those who have suspicious results are recalled to the assessment clinic where they will be offered clinical examination, breast ultrasound, and fine-needle aspiration biopsy.

### NHS Cervical Screening Programme (NHS CSP)

- Offers screening to women aged 25–64 years.
- Tests are offered every 3–5 years.
- Women are offered a smear test or liquid-based cytology (LBC).
- LBC is a new method where instead of using a microscope slide and a direct smear, the diagnostic brush is sent off in a liquid preservative to the laboratory where a cytospin is prepared and examined by a cytologist. This method allows the separation of contaminating material such as mucus or pus.
- Women with atypical cells will be recalled and if there is ongoing concern on a repeat test will then go on to have a colposcopy and biopsy.

An estimated 4 million women/year are screened. The incidence of cervical cancer is substantially reduced by detecting pre-cancerous lesions. The protection from cancer offered by a single negative smear with 3-yearly screening varies from 41% in 20–39-year-old women to 73% in 50–69-year-old women.

### NHS Bowel Cancer Screening Programme (NHS BCSP)

- Currently being rolled out across the country.
- The aim is to detect bowel cancer at an early stage and reduce the mortality associated with this disease.
- The plan is for the programme to be up and running within the next 3 years.
- It is based on testing faecal occult blood (FOB).
- Patients who test positive will be recalled for colonoscopy and, if positive, referral to a specialist centre.
- The screening will be offered every 2 years to people aged 60–69 years.

### Prostate cancer

There is currently no formal screening for prostate cancer in the UK. Patients are, however, offered advice as part of a **Prostate Cancer Risk Management Programme**. Patients receive information packs with an explanation on what a prostate-specific antigen (PSA) test involves and who requires it.

Although prostate cancer is very common in elderly men, only a small percentage of men die from the disease, with most patients being managed with a 'watch and wait' policy.

Inappropriate testing for PSA often leads to anxiety and unnecessary investigations.

Further information on cancer screening programmes in UK can be found at <http://www.cancerscreening.nhs.uk>.

# 15.4 Diagnostic techniques in oncology

## Background

Investigating a patient with a suspected diagnosis of cancer requires thorough examination skills and knowledge of multisystem symptoms and signs. All patients require full history-taking and a physical examination, followed by baseline blood tests and imaging investigations as clinically indicated.

### Baseline investigations
- FBC
- U&E
- LFTs
- Bone profile

### Additional information: tumour markers
- Lactate dehydrogenase (LDH) (useful in Non-Hodgkin lymphoma (NHL)).
- Alpha fetoprotein (AFP): hepatocellular carcinoma.
- Beta human chorionic gonadotropin (βhCG): germ cell tumours.
- PSA: prostate.
- Carcinoembryonic antigen (CEA): colorectal.
- CA19-9: pancreatic and bowel.
- CA125: ovarian.
- CA15.3: breast.

## X-rays

Plain radiographs of the chest and skeleton are still very useful in the diagnosis of lung pathology and bone metastases (Fig. 15.3). The common causes for lesions on the plain radiograph are:
- Myeloma (solitary lytic lesion/plasmacytoma)
- Sclerotic metastases

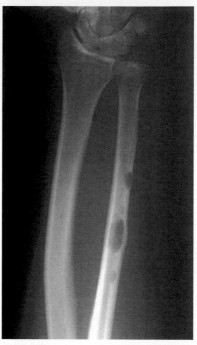

Fig. 15.4 Lytic bone lesions in the ulna in a patient with multiple myeloma.

Always perform plain X-rays where you suspect that a lytic lesion could result in a pathological fracture, particularly in weight-bearing bones such as the neck of femur or shaft of long bones (Fig. 15.4).

## Ultrasound

Uses in oncology include the diagnosis of liver metastases and to determine the cause of obstructive jaundice.

Many invasive procedures can be facilitated under USS guidance, such as drainage of loculated effusions and ascites, and biopsy of liver metastases or retroperitoneal masses.

Endoscopic USS is used in the staging and assessment of lymph node involvement in oesophageal, gastric, rectal, and bronchial malignancies.

## Computed tomography

Used to diagnose and stage cancer in all patients where involvement of internal organs is suspected (Box 15.2).

CT allows more precise detection of disease sites (in particular lymphadenopathy), due to faster and thinner multislice acquisition (Figs 15.5 and 15.6). A higher resolution and multiplanar format is

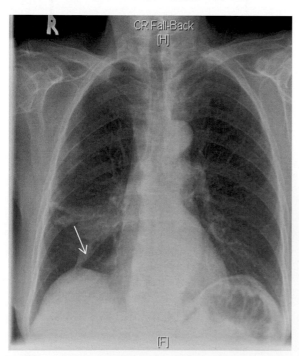

Fig. 15.3 CXR demonstrating opacification in the right lower zone from an underlying malignancy (arrow).

### Box 15.2 Uses of CT
- Diagnosis
- Staging
- Treatment decision
- Assessment of treatment response
- Detection of recurrence
- Facilitate biopsies
- Planning of radiotherapy

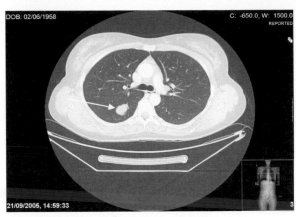

**Fig. 15.5** CT showing a large lung tumour (arrow).

also achieved. Implicit with this improved technology, however, is the potential for higher radiation exposure.

## Magnetic resonance imaging

- Uses magnetic movements of atomic nuclei to delineate tissues.
- Gives a very high-resolution picture and excellent tissue characterization.
- Safe—does not require ionizing radiation, but is more expensive and requires a longer time for image acquisition.
- Used mainly for the detection and characterization of brain lesions, and for staging of prostate and rectal tumours (although its use is extending to other tumour types).
- MRI of the spine is used to diagnose spinal cord compression (Fig. 15.7).

Other uses:

- MR cholangiopancreatography (MRCP)—commonly used to diagnose cholangiocarcinoma.
- MR urography (MRU).
- MR small bowel enema.

## Nuclear medicine investigations

These rely on the use of various radioisotopes. The tests are generally quite sensitive and specific, but there is poor anatomical definition despite whole-body imaging.

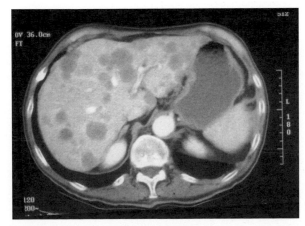

**Fig. 15.6** CT showing multiple liver metastases.

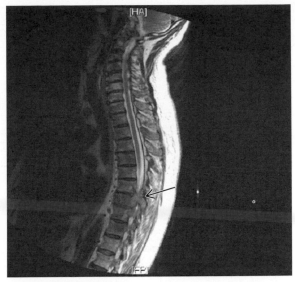

**Fig. 15.7** MRI showing multiple metastases in the thoracic vertebral bodies. There is extensive metastatic disease at T8 with effacement of the cerebrospinal fluid (CSF) spaces and cord compression at this level (arrow).

The most common nuclear medicine investigations are:

**Bone scan** used to detect bone metastases, either as part of the initial staging or to investigate pain (Fig. 15.8). False positive results can be caused by infection or trauma.

**Lung V/Q scan** used to investigate a suspected pulmonary embolism which has a higher incidence in all types of cancer. It relies on the difference between ventilation and perfusion of both lungs visualized using two different radiolabelled tracers.

**MUGA scan** (multichannel uptake gated acquisition) estimates left ventricular ejection fraction with radiolabelled red cells and measurements of cardiac blood pool. A precise assessment of ejection

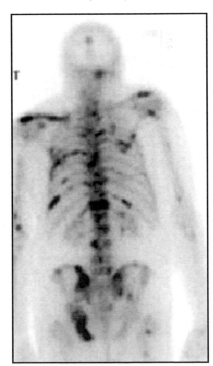

**Fig. 15.8** Technetium bone scan showing multiple 'hot spots' throughout the skeleton indicating metastatic bone cancer.

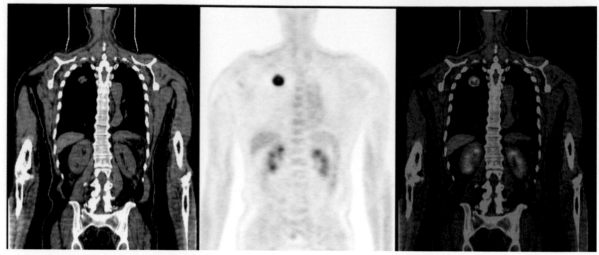

Fig. 15.9 PET scan of a patient with high FDG uptake in the right upper lobe of the lung (primary lung cancer).

fraction is very important when treating patients with cardiotoxic chemotherapy, such as doxorubicin.

**MAG3 renogram** estimates renal function by measuring the excretion of a compound labelled with a short half-life radiotracer such as technetium 99.

## Positron emission tomography

This technology relies on attaching positron-emitting radionuclides to functional molecules to determine the physiological distribution within the body.

The most common tracer used is fluorodeoxyglucose (FDG). PET-CT allows the combination of a functional image with precise anatomy.

Its use helps to discriminate benign from malignant disease.

The areas of proven benefit for using PET/PET-CT are:

- Assessment of pulmonary nodules/staging lung cancer (Fig. 15.9).
- Assessment of recurrent colorectal cancer.
- Lymphoma staging.
- Recurrent disease in head and neck tumours.

Other uses include:

- Assessment of metastatic melanoma.
- Monitoring response to treatment in lung, oesophageal, and colorectal cancer.

A number of conditions will cause high uptake on PET scanning ('false positives'):

- Infection, granulomatous disease (e.g. sarcoid), or reactive lymph nodes.

# 15.5 Oncological emergencies

## Neutropaenic sepsis

### Definition

- Absolute neutrophil count $<1.0 \times 10^9$/L

  +

- Temperature of 38°C for >1 hour **or**
- A single reading of ≥38.5°C

(in the absence of blood product administration)

Most patients on chemotherapy treatment become neutropaenic, but only a minority will develop neutropaenic fever. Neutropaenic sepsis should be suspected in those patients receiving chemotherapy who become feverish, confused, oliguric, hypotensive, or hypoxic.

### Treatment of neutropaenic sepsis

Refer to Fig. 15.10 for a management flowchart and Box 15.3 for possible pathogens causing neutropaenic sepsis.

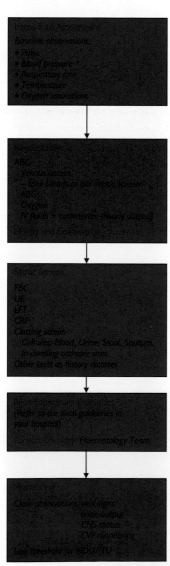

**Fig. 15.10** Management flowchart for the patient presenting with presumed neutropaenic sepsis.

---

**Box 15.3 Possible pathogens**

**Gram-positive bacteria**
  *Staphylococcus aureus/epidermidis*
  *Streptococcus pneumoniae/viridans*
  *Enterococcus*

**Gram-negative bacteria**
  *Escherichia coli*
  *Klebsiella* spp.
  *Proteus* spp.
  *Enterobacter* spp.

**Fungi**
  *Candida* spp.
  *Aspergillus* spp.

---

Continue broad-spectrum intravenous antibiotics and fluids until fever settles. If temperature does not settle within 48 hours consider second-line antibiotics (including antifungals). It is important to work closely with the microbiologist as in many cases blood cultures are negative and the source of sepsis is unknown. Organize appropriate further investigations:

- Atypical serology, viral screen
- Tuberculosis cultures
- CXR
- Bronchoscopy ± bronchoalveolar lavage (BAL)

---

## Superior vena cava obstruction

Superior vena cava obstruction (SVCO) is usually caused by external compression from thoracic tumour disease or by intraluminal thrombus (Fig. 15.11). The most common cancer that causes SVCO is lung, but other malignancies may also be the cause, such as lymphoma or germ cell tumours.

### Symptoms and signs

- Swelling of the face, neck, and arms (worse in the morning).
- Headache.
- Shortness of breath (usually due to associated airway compression).
- Visual disturbance.
- Collateral circulation on the chest wall.
- Engorgement of jugular veins.

### Investigations

- CXR
- CT chest
- Biopsy of obstructing mass
- If no mass visualized, venography may be necessary

### Treatment

- Depends on the cause of SVCO.
- Some malignancies will be treated with urgent chemotherapy (lymphoma, small cell lung cancer).
- Others will require urgent radiotherapy. Radiotherapy does not work immediately and so in severe cases insertion of a stent may be necessary.
- **Steroid** treatment is given to *all* patients as it sometimes alleviates the symptoms.

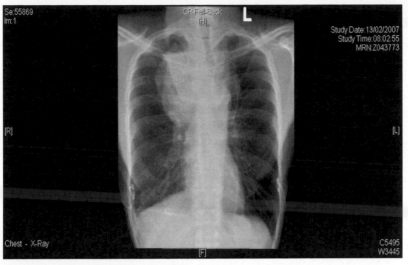

Fig. 15.11 CXR demonstrating a large superior mediastinal mass causing SVCO (SVC stent *in situ*).

# Spinal cord compression

Caused by tumour infiltration of the spinal canal or, more commonly, by crushed vertebrae affected by advanced metastatic disease. Non-oncological causes include trauma and disc prolapse.

## Symptoms and signs

- Back pain, often sudden onset, in 'girdle' or nerve root distribution.
- Weakness in the legs (and arms if a high lesion).
- Urinary and faecal retention.
- Neurological signs may be upper motor neurone (UMN) or, in the case of cauda equine syndrome, lower motor neurone (LMN).

## Investigations

- Spinal X-ray
- MRI spine

## Treatment

- Must commence within hours.
- The treatment of choice is **surgery**, however in advanced malignancy this may not be feasible due to:
  - Patient frailty for general anaesthesia
  - Inoperable disease
  - Multiple spinal deposits
- In these cases the treatment of choice is urgent **radiotherapy** and **steroids**.

# 15.6 Breast cancer and lymphoma

## Breast cancer

### Epidemiology of breast cancer
- Most common female malignancy in Europe, North America, and Australia.
- Most commonly presents after the age of 50 (80%), median age of 60, incidence declines after the age of 80.
- In UK, 42,000 women are diagnosed and 13,000 die every year from breast cancer (<http://www.cruk.org.uk>).
- About 5% will have a genetic abnormality (*BRCA1/BRCA2* mutations) with a lifetime risk of developing breast cancer of around 80%.

### Clinical presentation and staging
- Palpable or visible breast change (breast lump)
- Nipple discharge (watery, bleeding)
- Nipple eczema
- Axillary lymphadenopathy

All patients who present with one of these signs will undergo triple assessment:
- Clinical examination
- Radiological examination (mammography or ultrasound)
- Histological assessment (cytology and core biopsy)

Depending on the results of the triple assessment, the diagnosis will be classified into: benign, uncertain, and cancer. Staging of the breast cancer is based on the TNM—tumour, node, metastases—system.

### Histological types
See Table 15.3.
All breast cancers will be assessed for:
- Type
- Grade
- Size
- Excision margins (postoperative)
- Lymphovascular invasion
- Axillary nodes
- Oestrogen receptors
- HER2 (human epidermal growth factor receptor 2) testing is also becoming standard practice (Fig. 15.12)

### Non-invasive
- Ductal carcinoma *in situ*
- Lobular carcinoma *in situ*

These often present a difficult clinical dilemma.

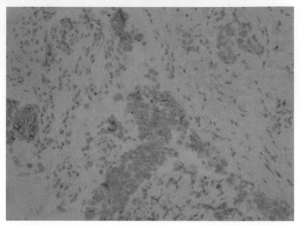

Fig. 15.12 Breast cancer expressing HER2/neu—brown membrane staining.

### Invasive cancer
- Ductal carcinoma
- Lobular carcinoma
- Other rare types, e.g. lymphoma, sarcoma and metastases

A separate type is inflammatory breast cancer. It is diagnosed clinically and usually bears a very poor prognosis.

### Treatment
Early-stage disease is treated with surgical excision, either wide local excision or mastectomy in the case of large or multifocal tumours. All patients have axillary nodes examined, usually by way of a sentinel node biopsy. A sentinel node is a main draining node which is detected by injection of special dye together with a radioactive label near the tumour site. At the time of biopsy it is possible to detect which lymph nodes have taken up the radioactive substance and dye, and these are removed and examined as sentinel nodes. In cases where sentinel nodes contain malignant cells, the patient will have to undergo axillary node resection.

Further treatment (such as postoperative radiotherapy and chemotherapy) depends on the histology (including oestrogen receptor and HER2 status), size, grade, axillary lymph node involvement, and the presence of lymphovascular invasion.

Metastatic disease is treated with systemic chemotherapy and is not curable; radiotherapy is used to palliate symptoms such as painful bone metastases.

## Lymphoma

### Epidemiology of lymphoma
Two types:
- Non-Hodgkin lymphoma (**NHL**):
  Common (>9000 people diagnosed each year in UK).
  3% of all cancers in UK.
  Incidence increases with age.
  Male: female ratio 3:2.
- Hodgkin lymphoma (**HL**):
  Less common.
  1% of all cancers in UK.
  Bimodal peak incidence: 20–30 years and >60 years.
  Male predominance.

| Table 15.3 Pathology of breast carcinoma | |
|---|---|
| No special type | No/<50% special type characteristics present<br>*Commonest* category of invasive breast cancer<br>Often described as **ductal** cancer |
| Pure special type | A classic example showing the hallmark histological features<br>Definitions require 90% purity<br>Types:<br>• **Lobular**—classic, alveolar, solid, tubulo-lobular, lobular-mixed<br>• Tubular<br>• Medullary<br>• Mucinous<br>• Invasive papillary<br>• Invasive cribriform<br>• DCIS—ductal carcinoma *in situ*<br>• LCIS—lobular carcinoma *in situ* |

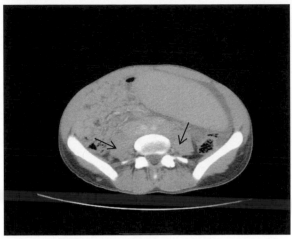

Fig. 15.13 CT scan of patient with lymphoma and extensive para-aortic lymphadenopathy (arrows).

## Clinical presentation
- 'B' symptoms: sweats, fever, weight loss.
- Painless lymphadenopathy (Fig. 15.13).
- Other symptoms and signs may include pain, organomegaly (e.g. palpable spleen), skin lesions, or signs of intracerebral lesion in case of primary CNS lymphoma (often connected with HIV infection).

## Staging
Staging follows the Ann Arbor classification:

Stage **I**—involvement of a single lymph node region or structure.

Stage **II**—involvement of two or more lymph node regions on the same side of the diaphragm.

Stage **III**—involvement of lymph node regions or structures on both sides of the diaphragm.

Stage **IV**—involvement of one or more extranodal sites (e.g. bone marrow, liver).

Letters are added to the stage as follows:

**A**—absence of constitutional symptoms.

**B**—fever, drenching night sweats, weight loss >10% in 6 months.

**X**—bulky disease.

## Histological types
### NHL
Classification is very complex and still evolving:
- Generally divides into B-cell and T-cell neoplasms.
- Each of these subtypes divides further into precursor and mature (peripheral) B- and T-cell lymphoma.
- Indolent versus aggressive lymphomas (although some overlap):
  - Classical **indolent** lymphomas are: follicular NHL, marginal zone lymphoma, small lymphocytic lymphoma, and lymphoplasmacytic lymphoma.
  - **Aggressive** lymphomas comprise: diffuse large B-cell lymphoma, Burkitt lymphoma (Fig. 15.14), peripheral T-cell NHL, mantle cell NHL, angioimmunoblastic, and anaplastic large cell lymphoma.

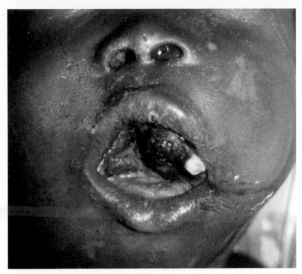

Fig. 15.14 Burkitt lymphoma (caused by 8;14 translocation) From Wikimedia Commons/Mike Blyth. This image is licensed under the Creative Commons Attribution-Share Alike 2.5 Generic (//creativecommons.org/licenses/by-sa/2.5/deed.en) license. http://creativecommons.org/licenses/by-sa/2.5/ (http://commons.wikimedia.org/wiki/File:Burkitt%27s_lymphoma.jpg).

### HL
Classified into:
- Nodular sclerosing (80%)
- Mixed cellularity (17%)
- Lymphocyte depleted (rare)
- Lymphocyte predominant (uncommon)

## Treatment
Depends on the histological type and stage.

**HL** is cured with systemic chemotherapy (often with addition of radiotherapy) in about 80–90% of cases; the success rate depends on stage and presence of poor prognostic factors.

**Indolent NHL** is, by and large, not a curable disease. It is often, however, asymptomatic and patients can survive many years without systemic treatment. The drug of choice is often single-agent chlorambucil, but in the case of progressive, symptomatic illness, combination chemotherapy regimens are used.

**Aggressive NHL** can be cured and the success rate depends on the stage and the histological subtype. A complete response can be achieved in >50% of patients and 2/3 of those patients will remain disease free. Treatment is with systemic chemotherapy often with the addition of radiotherapy. The most commonly used regimen for aggressive NHL is CHOP: cyclophosphamide, doxorubicin, vincristine, and prednisolone.

In recent years a monoclonal antibody targeting the CD20 molecule (expressed on the surface of many lymphoma cells, such as diffuse large B-cell lymphoma or follicular NHL) has become a standard of treatment. It is administered together with chemotherapy and improves response rate and overall survival.

# 15.7 Prostate cancer

## Background

- Sixth most common malignancy in the world.
- ~20% of all new cancer cases in UK.
- High incidence in USA and Western Europe (low in Asia, India, and Far East).
- In USA more common in men of African descent, occurs at an earlier age (55–64 years) and usually more aggressive.
- Risk increases with age.
- ~75% of cases are diagnosed in men >65 years of age.

In the last two decades the incidence has increased partly due to:
- An aging population in the West.
- Greater awareness and screening.

Incidence is also influenced by:
- Genetic factors: epidemiological studies show that the relative risk of prostate cancer increases with the number of affected close family members. Many genes are likely to be involved.
- Environmental factors:
  - Smoking
  - Obesity
  - Red meat and alcohol consumption

## Clinical presentation, histology, and staging

- Often asymptomatic.
- Can present with symptoms of prostatism (urinary frequency, hesitancy, and dribbling).
- Advanced disease can present with bone pain or spinal cord compression.
- Most common histological type is adenocarcinoma.
- Diagnosis is usually made on a prostate biopsy (usually transrectal).
- Graded according to one of five categories on the **Gleason score** (Fig. 15.15).
- Staging is based on the TNM classification.
- Serum PSA is usually elevated (Fig. 15.16)
- It is usually necessary to use MRI to adequately stage the patient.

The **prognostic factors** in prostate cancer are:
1. Gleason score
2. Tumour stage
3. Tumour volume
4. Lymph node involvement
5. Perineural invasion
6. Seminal vesicle involvement
7. Positive margins (indicating incomplete excision).

## Treatment

Depends on the presence/number of prognostic factors and individual patient characteristics.

Although a common cancer, the majority of patients are diagnosed at an advanced age (often due to lack of symptoms), and most die of unrelated causes.

More aggressive 'curative intent' treatments are generally offered to men with a life expectancy >10 years (taking into account comorbidities and 'biological' rather than chronological age).

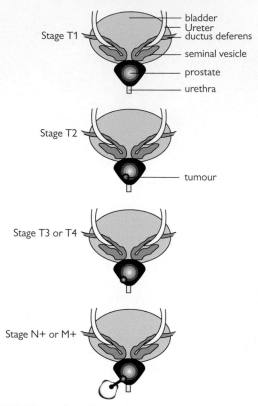

**Fig. 15.15** Gleason Score. Staging of prostate cancer:
T1—clinically impalpable.
T2—confined to the prostate.
T3—tumour breaches the capsule.
T4—tumour invades adjacent structures.
Reproduced from Epstein J et al., 'The 2005 International Society of Urological Pathology (ISUP) Consensus Conference on Gleason Grading of Prostatic Carcinoma', *The American Journal of Surgical Pathology*, 29, 9, copyright 2005, with permission from Wolters Kluwer Health.

In general, the treatment options include:
- Surgery (radical prostatectomy).
- Radiotherapy (external beam, brachytherapy).
- Localized intraprostatic treatment (e.g. laser).
- Hormones:
  - Luteinizing hormone-releasing hormone (LHRH) analogues—goserelin
  - Anti-androgens
  - Non-steroidal (bicalutamide, flutamide), steroidal (cyproterone acetate)
  - Oestrogens—diethylstilbestrol (Stilboestrol®)
- Corticosteroids—used in hormone-refractory patients.
- Palliative chemotherapy (hormone failure).

Localized prostate cancer diagnosed in an elderly man with multiple comorbidities and low Gleason score (<6) is unlikely to be treated with aggressive surgery and radical radiotherapy, as the disease will progress very slowly.

Localized prostate cancer with higher Gleason score can be treated with either radical prostatectomy or radiotherapy.

Radical surgery carries certain risks:

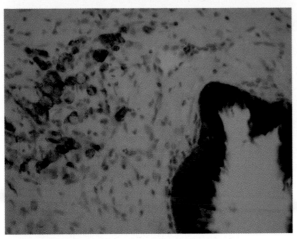

**Fig. 15.16** Prostate cancer showing PSA staining (brown dye).

- Incontinence (15%, falling to ~7% after 1 year).
- Impotence (50%).

As does radical radiotherapy:

- Impotence (40%).
- Rectal stricture (1%).
- Bladder irritation (mainly a short-term problem).

Locally advanced prostate cancer cannot be cured with surgery or radiotherapy. Primary hormone treatment with anti-androgens followed by radiotherapy can give good results.

Metastatic disease is treated with hormonal therapy and palliative radiotherapy to painful bone metastases (Fig. 15.17). Recently, chemotherapy has shown some survival advantage.

## Hormones

Anti-androgens are often used with gonadorelin analogues but can cause:

- Loss of libido and impotence.
- Lack of energy.

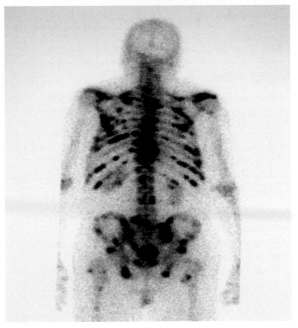

**Fig. 15.17** Bone scan showing multiple bone metastases in prostate cancer.

- Hot flushes.
- Osteoporosis.
- Inability to concentrate.
- Glucose intolerance.

Patients will usually respond to hormonal therapy for 12–18 months and then become 'hormone-resistant'. Further treatment is then aimed at maintaining patients' quality of life and symptom control.

# 15.8 Paraneoplastic syndromes

## Background

Paraneoplastic syndromes are a group of clinical disorders associated with malignancy, but directly related to the *physical effects* of primary or metastatic tumour.

The pathogenesis of paraneoplastic syndromes may be related to the production of active biological substances secreted *by* the malignant tumour, or in *response* to the tumour.

## Endocrine paraneoplastic syndromes

### Ectopic adrenocorticotrophic hormone (ACTH) secretion

- Frequently associated with lung cancer (50%), particularly small cell lung cancer (SCLC).
- Causes ectopic Cushing syndrome.
- Presentation: proximal myopathy, moon facies, hypokalaemia, and hypercalcaemia.
- Active substance is a precursor of ACTH: pro-opiomelanocortin (POMC).
- Some carcinomas may produce higher amounts of POMC and can also convert it to ACTH.

*Treatment*
- Depends on the underlying cause.
- Chest CT will often aid the diagnosis and treatment since bronchial neoplasm is most commonly associated.
- Hypokalaemia and hypercalcaemia need to be corrected first.

### Syndrome of inappropriate antidiuretic hormone secretion (SIADH)

- Caused by release of arginine vasopressin (ADH) by tumour cells.
- Mainly associated with lung cancer.
- Although increased production of ADH is common, the symptoms of SIADH do not occur as frequently:
  - Hyponatraemia.
  - Increased urine osmolality (higher than plasma osmolality).
  - Increased sodium excretion in urine.
- Presentation is with mainly neurological symptoms:
  - Fatigue
  - Anorexia
  - Headaches
  - Confusion
- In more advanced stages:
  - Seizures
  - Coma
- Improves with treatment of the underlying malignancy.
- Other measures:
  - Fluid restriction.
  - Demeclocycline (inhibits the concentrating ability of the distal tubules).

### Hypercalcaemia

May be related to:
- Excessive tumour production such as parathyroid hormone-related peptide (PTHrP).
- Local osteolytic reactions causing increased production of cytokines such as interleukin 6 and tumour necrosis factor.

Clinical features are:
- Fatigue
- Abdominal pain, anorexia
- Constipation
- Confusion
- Polydipsia
- Polyuria
- Dehydration

Hypercalcaemia is an oncological emergency, otherwise acute renal failure may be precipitated

*Treatment*
- Intravenous fluids.
- Bisphosphonates (e.g. IV pamidronate).
- Calcitonin may be used where urgent calcium lowering is required.

Other paraneoplastic phenomena can lead to hypocalcaemia and hypoglycaemia.

## Neurological paraneoplastic syndromes

- Caused by the effects of cancer on the nervous system.
- Extremely rare (occur in about 1% of patients with malignant disease).

Examples include:
- Lambert–Eaton myasthenic syndrome (LEMS):
  - Associated with lung tumours, mainly SCLC.
  - Characterized by proximal muscle weakness and dysphagia.
  - Not always associated with malignancy.
  - Caused by circulating antibodies that result in reduced calcium-dependent acetylcholine release.
  - Usually improves with treatment of the underlying malignancy.
  - Other treatments include steroids and plasma exchange.
- Peripheral neuropathy:
  - Either pure sensory or motor (rare) or combined sensorimotor (more common).
  - Caused by disruption of normal metabolism by the tumour itself, chemotherapy, or malnutrition.

---

**Box 15.4 Haematological paraneoplastic syndromes**

- **Erythrocytosis:**
  - Renal cell carcinoma—often elevated erythropoietin levels
  - Hepatoma
  - Wilms tumour
  - Uterine fibroid
  - Phaeochromocytoma
  - Adrenal tumour
- **Anaemia:**
  - Common presentation of malignancy.
  - Characteristic feature: normochromic, normocytic.
  - Pure red cell aplasia (rare)—leukaemia, lymphoma, thymoma.
- **Granulocytosis:**
  - Common with leukaemia, lymphoma.
  - Sometimes seen in gastric, brain, pancreatic, lung cancers.
- **Granulocytopenia**: some cases of leukaemia and lymphoma.
- **Thrombocytosis**: Hodgkin disease, lymphoma, leukaemia.

**Box 15.5 Dermatological paraneoplastic syndromes**

- **Acanthosis nigricans:** grey-brown hyperpigmented plaque, often on the neck, axilla, or flexor areas, may occur in cancer of the GI tract as well as lung, breast, and some haematological malignancies.
- **Tripe palms**: exaggerated ridges and hyperpigmentation of the hands, associated with lung and gastric cancers.
- **Melanosis**: dark discolouration of the skin, precedes malignant melanoma.
- **Acrokeratosis paraneoplastica (Bazex syndrome)**: psoriasiform acral keratosis, associated with oesophageal and head/neck cancer.
- **Paget disease of the nipple**: hyperkeratosis and discolouration of the skin around the nipple, usually a sign of breast cancer.
- **Sweet syndrome**: painful raised cutaneous plaques, fever, and neutrophilia, may be associated with leukaemia, myelodysplastic syndromes.
- **Erythema gyratum repens**: scaling erythema with a characteristic pattern, associated with lung, breast, and GI tract malignancies.
- **Necrolytic migratory erythema**: circinate erythema of the face, abdomen, and limbs, occurs in glucagonoma.

- Dermatomyositis and polymyositis:
  - Inflammatory myopathies that cause proximal muscle weakness.
  - Can be associated with pain and skin changes.
  - Treatment: usually steroids and immunosuppressive agents.

## Haematological paraneoplastic syndromes

- Common and may often be the first sign of underlying malignancy.
- Most are asymptomatic although can cause tiredness and general malaise (Box 15.4).

## Dermatological paraneoplastic syndromes

- Rare, and can also occur with a variety of benign conditions (Box 15.5).

## Others

- Protein-losing enteropathy (excessive GI loss of protein)—commonly associated with GI cancers.
- Hypertrophic osteoarthropathy (clubbing and periosthosis)—associated with lung and hepatic carcinoma.

# 15.9 Chemotherapy, biological therapy, and targeted therapy

## Principles of chemotherapy

The development of chemotherapy agents dates back to World War II, when an explosion in the harbour in Bari, Italy, caused exposure to mustard gas. This led to the observation that mustard gas caused hypoplasia of bone marrow, and subsequently to its use in treating HL.

Over the last few decades the development of new chemotherapy agents has produced marked improvements in the treatment of many malignancies.

Chemotherapy is usually given in *combination* to target cancer cells at different stages of their development and division. The mechanism of action of most of the currently known cytotoxics is through targeting:

- DNA or RNA structure and chemistry.
- Cell cycle mechanism.

In order for the chemotherapy combination to be effective there are certain rules that are important when choosing different agents:

- Combined chemotherapy drugs should have a different mode of action.
- All drugs should have anticancer activity as a single agent.
- The toxicity profile should be different for the individual drugs.

Other important considerations when administrating drugs together include:

- Route of administration.
- Frequency of administration.
- Possible mechanisms of tumour resistance.

A classification of chemotherapy drugs can be found in Box 15.6.

## Side effects of chemotherapy

Most of the chemotherapy drugs (whether administered orally or intravenously) will cause a variety of side effects. It is important to know and explain the possible toxicity of the treatment, as in some cases the balance between the benefits and risks associated with chemotherapy treatments may be of great importance, especially in patients with poor performance status.

The severity of side effects is assessed according to the WHO toxicity criteria and graded from 0 to 4 (Table 15.4):

- 0 meaning no toxicity.
- 4 indicating a severe reaction.

In case of grade 3 and 4 toxicity, the chemotherapy dose is usually reduced.

Common side effects of chemotherapy include:

- Asthenia
- Hair loss
- Anaemia
- Neutropaenia
- Thrombocytopaenia
- Nausea and vomiting
- Peripheral neuropathy
- Loss of taste
- Diarrhoea

Long-term effects of chemotherapy are important for patients who receive chemotherapy with curative intent or for patients on adjuvant treatment (treatment following curative surgery) to reduce the chance of recurrence.

The main longer-term effects are:

- Cardiac damage (e.g. anthracyclines).
- Pulmonary fibrosis (e.g. bleomycin).
- A second malignancy.

The most common condition seen in the hospital inpatient is neutropaenic fever (see Section 15.5).

---

### Box 15.6 Examples of chemotherapy drugs

- Alkylating agents:
  - Melphalan
  - Chlorambucil
  - Cyclophosphamide
  - Ifosfamide.
- Antitumour antibiotics:
  - Anthracyclins: doxorubicin, daunorubicin, epirubicin
  - Mitoxantrone
  - Mitomycin C.
- Antimetabolites:
  - Antifolates: methotrexate, fluorouracil
  - Antipurines: azathioprine
  - Cytosine analogues: cytosine arabinoside.
- Cisplatin and carboplatin.
- Topoisomerase inhibitors:
  - Topotecan
  - Etoposide.
- Anti-microtubule agents:
  - Vincristine
  - Vinblastine
  - Vinorelbine
  - Paclitaxel
  - Docetaxel.

---

## Biological therapy

### Hormone therapy

Some cancers require hormonal stimuli for their growth, and endocrine manipulation can be an effective treatment.

Two main cancers where hormonal treatment is used routinely are:

- **Breast cancer**:
  - Some breast malignancies are stimulated by oestrogens.
  - Depleting the source of oestrogens by suppressing luteinizing hormone (LH) results in a good response in ~50%.
  - Tamoxifen (an anti-oestrogen) has become the standard treatment for early and metastatic breast cancer.
  - Aromatase inhibitors may prove to be even more effective. These work by inhibiting the enzyme aromatase which metabolizes adrenal androgens to oestrogens.

- **Prostate cancer:**
  - Is stimulated by androgens.
  - Blocking endogenous androgens is an effective anticancer treatment.
  - This can be achieved by chemical castration with the help of LHRH analogues or anti-oestrogens.
  - Used for patients in combination with surgery or radical radiotherapy (in early prostate cancer) and in patients with advanced disease.

### Monoclonal antibody therapy

Monoclonal antibodies (mAbs) are directed against tumour-associated antigens. The first mAbs in human use were of murine (mouse) origin. This led to high rates of immune response, but most agents had

| Table 15.4 Toxicities associated with chemotherapy drugs | | | | | |
|---|---|---|---|---|---|
| Toxicity | 0 | 1 | 2 | 3 | 4 |
| Total WBC | ≥4.0 | 3–4 | 2–3 | 1–2 | ≤1.0 |
| Platelets | Normal | 75–normal | 50–75 | 25–50 | <25 |
| Haemoglobin | Normal | 10–normal | 8–10 | 6.5–8.0 | <6.5 |
| Neutrophils | ≥2.0 | 1.5–2.0 | 1.0–1.5 | 0.5–1.0 | <0.5 |
| Lymphocytes | ≥2.0 | 1.5–2.0 | 1.0–1.5 | 0.5–1.0 | <0.5 |
| Bleeding (clinical) | None | Mild (no transfusion) | Gross (1–2 units transfusion/episode) | Gross (3–4 units transfusion/episode) | Massive (>4 units transfusion/episode) |
| Infection | None | Mild | Moderate | Severe | Life threatening |
| Nausea | None | Able to eat reasonably well | Intake significantly decreased | No significant intake | |
| Vomiting | None | 1 episode in 24 hours | 2–5 episodes in 24 hours | 6–10 episodes in 24 hours | >10 episodes in 24 hours **or** requiring parenteral support |
| Diarrhoea | None | Increase of 2–3 stools/day over pre-Rx | Increase of 4–6 stools/day **or** nocturnal stools **or** moderate cramping | Increase of 7–9 stools/day **or** incontinence **or** severe cramping | Increase of 10 stools/day **or** grossly bloody diarrhoea **or** need for parenteral support |
| Stomatitis | None | Painless ulcers, erythema or mild soreness | Painful erythema, oedema or ulcers | Painful erythema, oedema or ulcers and cannot eat | Requires parenteral or enteral support |

a limited serum half-life and caused re-infusion-related toxicity due to immune rejection reactions. Chimeric (part-murine/part-human) and humanized mAbs show more promise as they have longer half-lives and a lower toxicity profile.

Antibodies commonly used in clinical practice are:

- **Trastuzumab** (Herceptin®):
  - Targets the HER2 receptor and can achieve durable clinical responses even in patients with metastatic breast cancer.
  - HER2 is a member of the EGFR family and overexpression of this receptor is associated with a more aggressive type of breast cancer.
- **Rituximab** (MabThera®):
  - An anti-CD20 antibody, used in lymphoma.
  - CD20 receptor is expressed on many B-cell lymphomas.

There is a whole range of other monoclonal antibodies currently in use in the treatment of both haematological malignancies and solid tumours. Their use is becoming increasingly widespread, and is likely to become standard treatment in the near future.

# Targeted therapy using small molecule inhibitors

Small molecule inhibitors form a new class of drugs that can target specific molecular pathways active in the development and growth of cancer cells. In the last few years there has been an expansion of various new molecular targets and some of the drugs have found their way to the clinic.

Pathways that can be targeted include:

- **EGF** (epidermal growth factor):
  - EGF receptor is a family of transmembrane receptors that can be overexpressed in cancer and are often associated with more aggressive disease.
  - Two new agents targeting this pathway are **gefitinib** and **erlotinib** (non-SCLC).
- **VEGF** (vascular endothelial growth factor):
  - Blocking this pathway results in inhibition of new vessel formation and disrupted tumour blood supply.

# 15.10 Radiotherapy

## Background

- Radiotherapy is a very effective single modality treatment for certain types of cancer.
- In combination with surgery, curative rates of up to 40% can be seen for certain cancer types.
- Is the use of ionizing radiation to eradicate tumour cells.
- A localized treatment that is directed to the site of the tumour and draining lymph node regions.
- Can be used on its own or as part of a combination of treatments with surgery or chemotherapy.
- In combination with surgery, radiotherapy can be given *prior* to surgery to downstage the tumour (making it smaller and safer to resect), or as an adjuvant treatment *after* surgery with the intent of eradicating any microscopic tumour cells that may have been left in the tumour bed (Fig. 15.18).
- Chemotherapy can be given at the same time as radiotherapy to sensitize the cells and thereby enhance the chances of treatment success.

Combinations of treatments are being increasingly used as the evidence for these multimodality regimens accumulates showing improved survival statistics.

## Principles of radiotherapy

Ionizing radiation interacts with tissues leading to DNA damage. Ionization of atomic elements within the DNA structure results in an unstable environment and destructive chemical reactions (such as double/single-strand DNA breaks, free radical formation, and DNA–protein cross linking). If this damage cannot be repaired by normal cellular processes the cell will die.

Radiation can be delivered either using an external source of radiation (**external beam radiotherapy**), or an internal source (**brachytherapy**). The internal administration of radiation is carried out either by the systemic administration of a radioactive drug that is taken up physiologically by a particular tissue or tumour, or the placing of radioactive sources within or adjacent to a tumour following resection.

## External beam radiotherapy

- The most common delivery method of radiation.
- Radiation is produced in a linear accelerator by the acceleration of electrons across a voltage gradient in order to gain energy. These energetic electrons are accelerated towards a target made of tungsten metal, and the ensuing interaction releases photons. The photons produced are directed through the head of the linear accelerator towards the patient's tumour.
- These photon beams can be shaped in 2D or 3D in order to create a dose distribution that matches the volume required to irradiate an individual's tumour.
- Advances in radiotherapy mean that complex tumour shapes can now be treated with minimal radiation exposure to the normal surrounding tissues (reducing radiation toxicity).

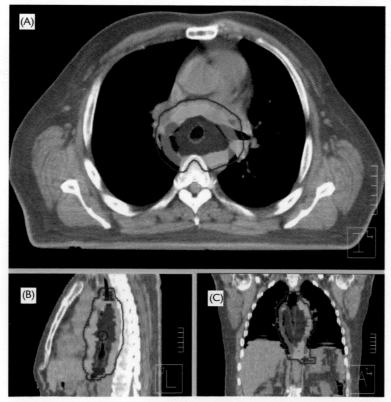

**Fig. 15.18** Radiotherapy dose volume for oesophageal carcinoma. Axial (A), sagittal (B), and coronal (C) images. The red area on each image shows the high-dose region containing the tumour.

Image courtesy of St. Luke's Cancer Centre, Royal Surrey County Hospital, Guildford, UK.

- Electron (rather than photon) beams can also be used; however, electrons are not as penetrating as photons, so they are usually used for the treatment of more superficial tumours.

## Brachytherapy

- The use of radioactive sources that can be placed either directly within or adjacent to a tumour.
- Typically, the sources used emit radioactive particles (beta- and alpha-particles) that are damaging over very short distances (usually millimetres).
- Very tight radiation dose distributions can be achieved with minimal damage to normal tissues beyond the reach of these radioactive particles.
- Higher doses of radiation can be achieved than would ordinarily be feasible using external beam radiotherapy because of the steep fall-off in dose, separating the tumour from normal tissue.
- Types in clinical use:
  - **Interstitial brachytherapy** (implanting radioactive wire or seeds directly into tumour tissue).
  - **Intracavity brachytherapy** (delivery of radioactive sources to a pre-existing cavity adjacent to tumour).
  - **Mould brachytherapy** (placing sources within a custom-made mould that can be placed on top of a superficial tumour).

## Radionuclide therapy

- The use of radionuclides on their own or attached to a biologically active agent that is taken up physiologically by the tissue requiring treatment.
- Agents used are generally beta-particle emitters so that once they are in the target organ the release of radiation is very localized.
- Some radionuclides additionally emit more penetrating gamma rays which traverse the body and permit images of the distribution of the radionuclide to be obtained.
- Example—iodine-131:
  - A radionuclide used in the treatment of differentiated thyroid cancer.
  - Administered systemically.
  - Taken up by malignant thyroid tissue.
  - Has resulted in the curative treatment of both localized and metastatic thyroid cancer.

## Radical radiotherapy

- Definition—radiation given with curative intent.
- Tumours amenable to radical radiotherapy:
  - Head and neck
  - Prostate
  - Bladder
  - Lung
  - Skin.

In cases of head and neck cancer, radiotherapy is often given as an alternative to surgery to prevent the need for laryngectomy. Radical radiotherapy tends to be the treatment of choice in these

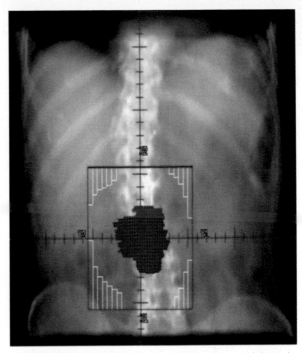

**Fig. 15.19** Palliative radiotherapy volume for a symptomatic abdominal mass (red area represents tumour). Red box is radiotherapy field, white rectangles represent multileaf collimators used to shape the field. Image courtesy of St. Luke's Cancer Centre, Royal Surrey County Hospital, Guildford, UK.

situations, with surgery offered as a salvage treatment should the cancer recur.

- Generally given on a daily basis over the course of several weeks.
- The total dose to be administered is fractionated over the course of the treatment. This means that low daily doses are administered which are toxic to the inherently sensitive tumour cells but which allow normal tissues to undergo repair.

Side effects of radiotherapy are very site specific depending on the organ being irradiated. Most patients experience acute toxicity to some degree, however late side effects can occur 6 weeks or more after a course of treatment.

## Palliative radiotherapy

- The use of radiation to alleviate symptoms of cancer in an identified region, either the primary tumour or a secondary deposit (Fig. 15.19).
- Not given with the intent of cure, permitting lower doses of radiation with concomitant shorter duration of treatment courses and minimization of side effects.
- Uses:
  - Pain
  - Haemoptysis
  - To relieve pressure symptoms.

# 15.11 End of life: the multidisciplinary approach

## The multidisciplinary approach to the end of life

Caring for a dying patient forms an integral part of every hospital doctor's and health professional's work. A holistic approach to the patient's care is paramount. This healthcare approach emphasizes the patient's *total* well-being, including psychological, spiritual, as well as physical aspects.

In practical terms, it means integrating palliative care with good medical care whilst addressing any other needs the patient may have. In many instances, this can be provided by the extended oncology team responsible for the patient's care. Nevertheless, where an individual's problems are more complex (e.g. involving significant physical, social,, or emotional issues), specialist palliative care input should be requested.

In 2002, WHO defined palliative care as: 'an approach that improves the quality of life of patients and their families, facing the problems associated with life-threatening illness'. This is achieved by:

- Providing relief from pain and other distressing symptoms.
- Integrating the psychological and spiritual aspects of patient care.
- Offering a support system to help patients to live as actively as possible until death.

The affirmation of life whilst regarding dying as a natural process is the main philosophy of palliative care.

Members of the patient's family are also given help and support to cope with the patient's illness and their own bereavement. To achieve this, a multidisciplinary team approach is essential. In cancer care, this team generally comprises each of the following:

- Cancer physician (medical or clinical oncologist)
- Palliative care physician
- Palliative care nurse
- Social worker
- Physiotherapist
- Occupational therapist.

Care of terminally ill patients in the community is especially important. Many patients with cancer choose to spend their last hours at home with their family, in familiar surroundings. This situation can be achieved with the help of both a primary care and community palliative care team. The community palliative care team will also have other members such as a community physiotherapist, social worker, and occupational therapist.

*An integral part of holistic patient care in both the community and hospital settings is an appropriate, early referral to the palliative care team.*

The acute medical care and treatment of cancer should be introduced at the same time as the palliative care services. This way the needs of the patient as well as the family will be addressed at multiple levels, not only physical.

Palliative care offers services in hospitals (usually NHS funded) and specialized inpatient units around the country. The majority of hospices are funded by charities.

Hospice care is offered not only to cancer patients but also to any patients suffering from advanced, progressive, disabling illness such as HIV, neurological disease, and end-stage cardiac or renal failure. Some palliative care units specialize in paediatric patients' care.

The vast majority of patients do not require admission to a hospice and are, instead, managed by primary care teams supported by specialist palliative care services (although the organization of community-based care varies between areas). Patients are visited in their own home and given advice regarding symptom control such as pain, nausea, and constipation.

Preparing the patient and their family for a 'good death' is one of the principal tasks of palliative care. Problems that need to be addressed in this situation are not only those concerning symptom control, but also treating the patient 'as a whole' and making clear plans in preparations for death.

The most important part of preparing the patient and the family for the end of life is **effective communication**. Breaking bad news in a sensitive way and telling the truth are difficult tasks, requiring an empathetic approach to the patient and their family.

## Liverpool Care Pathway and current approach to the end-of-life care

In 2003, the Department of Health introduced a new initiative to improve the care of dying patients. One of the components of the new programme was the **Liverpool Care Pathway (LCP)**. The LCP provided an evidence-based framework for the delivery of care for dying patients and their relatives in a variety of care settings such as hospitals, hospices, care homes, and the community. It was developed to transfer the hospice model of care to other settings. The pathway was subsequently criticized and in July 2013, the Department of Health released a statement which stated that the use of the LCP should be 'phased out over the next 6–12 months and replaced with an individual approach to end-of-life care for each patient'.

The individual assessment is multi-disciplinary and in the first stage of the pathway a team caring for the patient needs to agree that all reversible causes for the patient's conditions have been considered and that the patient is in fact 'dying'. The assessment then makes suggestions for the palliative care options to be considered and whether non-essential treatments and medications should be discontinued. The decision not to undertake cardio-pulmonary resuscitation needs to be clearly recorded. It is important to recognize the patient's insight and address their spiritual and religious needs; clear communication with the family is essential. The patient's GP also needs to be notified of the situation.

# 15.12 Symptom control

## Pain

- One of the most common symptoms that patients with cancer experience.
- >80% will suffer pain at some stage of their illness.
- Most causes are as a direct cancer effect.
- Important considerations:
  - Pain is a subjective experience that has physical as well as social, psychological, and spiritual dimensions.
  - Pain is not always due to the cancer itself. It is important to try and identify the cause to manage the pain appropriately.
  - Patients should be informed about the possible source of pain and actively encouraged to take control in pain management.
  - Pain management requires a multidisciplinary approach and regular review by a health professional.
  - Pain management should follow the WHO ladder of analgesics (Fig. 15.20) with introduction of another painkiller from the level above when necessary.
  - Pain may have multiple sources and adequate assessment is necessary to control the pain.

Possible causes of pain include:
- Visceral
- Bone
- Nerve compression
- Soft tissue pressure
- Muscle spasm
- Lymphoedema
- Raised intracranial pressure.

In some patients a combination of factors may be responsible. Factors that can contribute to pain in cancer patients may also include:
- Post-surgical complications (healing wounds, adhesions)

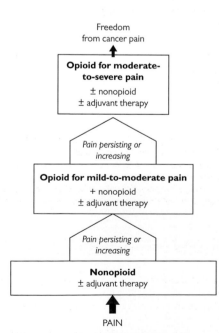

**Fig. 15.20** WHO pain ladder: the escalation of analgesia in cancer-related pain control.

Reproduced with permission of Ogle KS, Lovell K, and Zaluski H. Opioid Management of Pain. (https://www.msu.edu/course/hm/691/Block%20II%20neuromuscular%20domain/)

- Side effects of chemotherapy (neuropathy, infection)
- Side effects of radiotherapy (fibrosis, skin changes, mucositis).

The general medical condition of cancer patients is often very susceptible to minor insults which will exacerbate pain and anxiety. A separate common problem is constipation, which is frequently a side effect of analgesia. It requires careful assessment and administration of laxatives *from the time* the painkillers are started. Other common conditions that exacerbate pain are:
- Pressure sores
- Painful joints
- Muscle spasms
- Fear and anxiety.

Assessment of pain includes:
- A thorough clinical history from the patient (number and sites of pain, intensity, radiation, duration, aggravating and relieving factors).
- Analgesic history.
- Effect of pain on daily activities.
- Examination.
- Appropriate investigations.
- Frequent review and adjustment of prescribed analgesia.

Types of pain include:
- Somatic
- Visceral
- Neuropathic
- Sympathetically mediated
- Mixed.

## Management

1. Anticancer therapy:
   - Usually the best form of pain treatment as it centres on the cause of pain, which in the majority of cases is the cancer itself.
   - The effects of anticancer treatment are not immediate, however, and most patients will also require other measures for pain control.
2. Pharmacological methods:
   - The analgesic ladder starts from mild pain and goes through moderate to severe.
   - It is important to remember breakthrough pain and encourage the patient to take adequate analgesia.
3. Non-pharmacological methods:
   - May be effective for mild pain.
   - Include relaxation techniques, aromatherapy, or massage.
   - Often combined with pharmacological therapy for maximum effect.
4. Anaesthetic techniques:
   - Include nerve blocks/infusions with local anaesthetic or steroids, neuraxial methods (epidural or intrathecal/spinal analgesia).
   - Occasionally neurolysis (nerve destruction) is used.
   - Patients are usually referred when pharmacological methods of pain control are not effective.

Paracetamol ± NSAIDs may be effective alone for *mild* pain and can be used as an adjunct at all steps of the analgesic ladder.

The next step includes weak opioids for *moderate* pain and opioids for *severe* pain.

Treatment should be adjusted from one step to the next according to pain severity, response to analgesics, and side effects.

*Neuropathic* pain may not respond to the standard painkillers and use of tricyclic antidepressants or anticonvulsants may be more effective.

*Bone* pain can also be difficult to control with opioid analgesics and radiotherapy to the affected sites can often bring effective pain relief. In selected cases, orthopaedic interventions may prove helpful.

## Morphine preparations

- Normal release:
  - Onset of action ~20 minutes, peak levels ~60 minutes.
  - Should be administered every 4 hours to maintain plasma levels.
  - Changes to the regular dose should be assessed after about 16–24 hours (steady plasma level).
- Modified release:
  - Twice-daily preparations: slower onset of action ~1–2 hours, peak plasma levels after ~4 hours.
  - Once-daily preparations: plasma peak after ~8.5 hours.

Many patients will require a breakthrough dose of morphine which should be around **1/6** of the total daily dose.

Morphine has some predictable side effects/toxicity:

- Constipation (start laxatives as prophylactic measure).
- Nausea and vomiting (usually wears off after 5–10 days).
- Sedation (usually apparent after the first few days).
- Dry mouth.
- Respiratory depression, delirium, poor concentration, myoclonic jerks (with chronic usage).
- Rarely: hypotension, urinary retention.

Remember that the dose of morphine has to be appropriately reduced in patients with renal impairment as it will accumulate. Safer opioids to use in a patient with significant renal impairment include oxycodone, fentanyl, or buprenorphine.

Subcutaneous morphine infusion is an effective delivery method where patients are unable to take oral medication.

All patients with pain that cannot be relieved by the treating (oncology) team should be referred to the palliative care team.

## Nausea and vomiting

- Experienced by the majority of cancer patients at some stage in their illness.
- Can be caused by the cancer itself or as a result of treatment.
- Causes (may be multiple and complex) include:
  - Drug-induced
  - Radiotherapy-induced
  - Chemotherapy-induced
  - Metabolic (hypercalcaemia)
  - Raised intracranial pressure
  - Gastric outlet obstruction
  - Bowel obstruction.

As some causes are reversible, a careful assessment is required and includes full clinical examination, blood chemistry (renal function, thyroid function tests, bone profile, LFTs), and a plain abdominal X-ray.

CT brain should be considered especially in patients with headache as neurological deficit may be a late presentation of raised intracranial pressure.

### Management

- Emetogenic drugs should be stopped.
- Patients with bowel or gastric outlet obstruction should be referred for a surgical opinion.
- If raised intracranial pressure is caused by tumour (space-occupying lesion), whole-brain radiotherapy may alleviate the symptoms.
- Patients who are not able to swallow tablets due to severe nausea or vomiting, should be prescribed intravenous/subcutaneous or intramuscular anti-emetics.
- All non-essential drugs should be stopped and others converted to parenteral routes of administration.

In cases of vomiting induced by chemotherapy or radiotherapy, the most effective anti-emetics are **5-HT3 antagonists** such as **granisetron** or **ondansetron**. They are usually prescribed along with domperidone. Drug-induced vomiting may respond to haloperidol and levomepromazine, whereas delayed gastric emptying is often helped by **prokinetic drugs** such as metoclopramide.

## Constipation

- A very common symptom, often caused by medication.
- Aggravating factors in cancer patients include poor diet and lack of mobility.
- Untreated, can lead to serious complications such as overflow diarrhoea, bowel obstruction, urinary retention, and severe pain, leading to great distress for patients.

### Causes

- Cancer-related:
  - Immobility
  - Poor nutrition
- Dehydration:
  - Poor fluid intake
  - Loss of fluid (vomiting, polyuria)
- Intestinal obstruction
- Drugs:
  - Opioids
  - Anti-emetics
  - Ferrous sulphate
- Metabolic:
  - Hypercalcaemia
  - Hypokalaemia.

A careful clinical history, including medication, dietary changes, bowel habit, and physical examination, is essential to establish the probable cause of constipation. Some patients may require regular laxatives (e.g. if regular opioid analgesics prescribed).

Most cases respond to a combination of a **stimulant** and **softener**, although suppositories or enemas may be required (Table 15.5).

| Table 15.5 Types of laxatives and faecal softeners | | |
|---|---|---|
| Category | Drugs | Description |
| Osmotic laxatives | Lactulose, Movicol® | Not absorbed from the gut and cause retention of water in the lumen by osmotic action. Can cause abdominal distension |
| Stimulant laxatives | Senna, bisacodyl, docusate sodium (stimulant and softener) | Can cause abdominal cramps, should be avoided in patients with intestinal obstruction |
| Bulk forming laxatives | Ispaghula husk (Fybogel®, Regulan®) | Increase faecal mass which stimulates peristalsis, useful for patients with colostomy, ileostomy, diarrhoea associated with diverticular disease |
| Faecal softeners | Liquid paraffin Arachis oil enema | Useful in the management of haemorrhoids and anal fissure |

## Diarrhoea

- Frequent symptom.
- Common causes include anticancer treatment and inappropriate use of laxatives.
- Definition: the passage of more than three loose stools/day.

### Causes

- Inappropriate use of laxatives
- Drugs (antibiotics, NSAIDS)
- Partial intestinal obstruction
- Faecal impaction ('overflow' diarrhoea)
- Radiotherapy
- Chemotherapy
- Malabsorption (post-gastrectomy, post-bowel surgery, pancreatic cancer).

A careful clinical history, physical examination (including rectal examination), and stool cultures are essential. In many cases an infective cause may be implicated (especially *Clostridium difficile*).

### Treatment

Treatment depends on the cause of diarrhoea:

- If there is any suspicion of pseudomembranous colitis (caused by *C. difficile*), patients must not be given antidiarrhoeal agents. If infection is confirmed, oral **metronidazole** is usually effective.
- Supportive treatment with IV fluids is necessary for some patients.
- In cases of overflow diarrhoea, an appropriate **laxative** is essential.
- Patients who develop diarrhoea as a side effect of chemotherapy or radiotherapy should be given **loperamide** or **codeine phosphate**. These both act via gut opioid receptors to reduce peristalsis and increase sphincter tone.
- Specific causes of diarrhoea such as malabsorption due to pancreatic tumour will require pancreatic enzymes replacement such as **pancreatin**.

## Intestinal obstruction

- Common in patients with bowel or ovarian cancer.
- May be caused by luminal obstruction by tumour bulk (bowel) or, more commonly, as a result of peritoneal disease (ovary) (Fig. 15.21).

Intestinal obstruction can be:

- Intramural.
- Intraluminal.
- Extraluminal (peritoneal disease).
- Functional (motility disorders, metabolic).
- Secondary to constipation.

A surgical opinion should be sought in most cases of mechanical obstruction, with the advantages and disadvantages of operative intervention being carefully assessed.

Patients with proven severe peritoneal disease are unlikely to benefit from surgery. Similarly, rapidly recurrent massive ascites would be a relative contraindication to surgery. In patients with poor performance status, cachexia, or previous radiotherapy to the pelvis, the decision has to be undertaken on an individual basis after careful assessment.

Non-surgical management relies on management of:

- Pain (syringe driver).
- Colic (often responsive to **hyoscine** compounds via their antimuscarinic action).

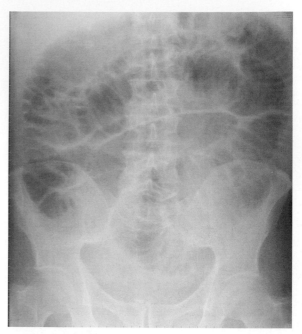

**Fig. 15.21** Plain abdominal X-ray demonstrating intestinal obstruction.

- Nausea and vomiting (e.g. cyclizine, haloperidol, levomepromazine, metoclopramide).
- Steroids may play a role in some patients.

Avoid nasogastric tube placement if at all possible—it causes distress to the patient and does not effectively relieve vomiting.

## Breathlessness

- Common symptom, not always explained by any detectable lung pathology.
- Frequently experienced by patients with lung cancer, but also those with breast, colon, prostate, and other cancers.

### Causes

Cancer-related:

- Primary or secondary tumour in the lungs (obstruction of large airways, infiltration).
- Lymphangitis carcinomatosa.
- Pleural or pericardial effusions.
- SVCO.
- Ascites (splinting of the diaphragm).
- Thoracic wall pain (hypoventilation).

Treatment-related:

- Surgery (pneumonectomy).
- Chemotherapy (lung fibrosis, pneumonitis).
- Radiotherapy (fibrosis).

Other conditions:

- Pulmonary embolism (very common).
- Chest infection.
- Pre-existing pathologies (congestive cardiac failure, chronic obstructive pulmonary disease, asthma).

Breathlessness may be aggravated by other problems such as anaemia, fatigue, or muscle weakness.

### Management

- Careful history and examination.
- Treat reversible causes (e.g. chest infection, anaemia).

- Drain pleural/pericardial effusions for comfort.
- Optimally manage co-existing conditions (cardiac, pulmonary disease).

Breathlessness due to lung cancer or metastases can be managed with a combination of the following:

*Medical treatment*

- Nebulized **salbutamol**:
  - Helpful even though cancer does not usually induce bronchospasm.
- Steroids:
  - May help in cases of widespread metastatic lung disease, lymphangitis, and SVCO.
  - Will decrease production of mucus and reduce inflammatory changes.
  - Good for chemo- and radiotherapy-induced breathlessness.
- Opioids:
  - Slow down the respiratory rate and improve symptoms of anxiety.
- Painkillers:
  - Where dyspnoea is aggravated by pain.
- Benzodiazepines:
  - Alleviate the panic associated with breathlessness.
- Oxygen.

In terminally ill patients, an effective treatment is a syringe driver with morphine, midazolam, and hyoscine (if excessive respiratory secretions) set up over 24 hours for continuous symptom control.

*Surgical treatment*

Bronchoscopy with a view to **stenting**:

- If large airway obstruction present.
- Obstruction usually either extrinsic or caused by a large intrabronchial mass.

# Depression

- Common symptom, often underdiagnosed and, therefore, not treated.
- Associated with poorer quality of life.
- Often leads, indirectly, to a worse response to anticancer treatment and decreased survival.
- An estimated ~50% of cancer patients suffer from some form of depression.

One of the problems with diagnosing depression is that the majority (if not all) of patients will experience sadness when told about the cancer diagnosis, and anxiety during treatment and hospital visits. Their behaviour may, therefore, reflect only a natural reaction to these life-changing events, rather than clinical depression. Psychosocial needs of cancer patients are often not addressed and this will subsequently lead to a delay in the diagnosis of depression.

Assessing patients with depression:

- Severity (presence of suicidal thoughts).
- Duration of symptoms.
- Association with family, social situation.
- Association with alcohol/drug use.

In cases where you suspect severe depression with suicidal thoughts seek urgent advice from a psychiatrist.

Pharmacological treatment of depression includes:

- **Tricyclic** antidepressvants (amitriptyline, imipramine).
- Selective serotonin uptake inhibitors (**SSRIs**) (paroxetine, fluoxetine).

SSRIs are usually the first-line agent as they are less sedative and have a faster onset of action with low side effects profile.

Other treatments that are often very effective include non-pharmacological methods of treatment such as counselling and psychotherapy, relaxation techniques, music therapy, and massage.

# Chapter 16

# Ophthalmology (medical)

# 16.1 Normal ocular structure and function

## Introduction

The eye is a highly developed structure that, in conjunction with the various regions of the brain and their inter-positioned pathways, allows visualization, interpretation, and understanding of the complex world around us. The eye is highly adapted, allowing it to perform its role of light perception.

Conditions affecting the eye may occur in isolation or as part of a systemic disease. Treatments used for the management of ocular conditions may have a systemic effect. Likewise, systemic drugs used for non-ophthalmic conditions may affect visual function.

It is therefore essential for all physicians to have an understanding of basic ocular structure and function.

## Basic ocular anatomy

The eye is approximately a spherical structure:
- Diameter 2.5cm
- Average axial length 2.4cm.

Consists of three layers (Fig. 16.1):
1. Corneoscleral (fibrous) layer
2. Uveal layer (iris, ciliary body, choroid)
3. Neural layer (retina).

### Corneoscleral layer

#### Cornea
- Responsible for most of the light refraction that occurs in the eye, i.e. acts as the main lens of the eye.
- Dimensions:
  - Vertical diameter 10.6mm
  - Horizontal diameter 11.7mm
  - Corneal thickness 0.67mm periphery, 0.52mm centrally.
- Provides a strong, transparent, physical barrier.
- Transparency due to:
  - Regularity of stratified, non-keratinized squamous epithelium.
  - Extra- and intracellular structure of the stroma, e.g. uniform diameter collagen fibrils.
  - Lower than normal stromal hydration level.
- Endothelium:
  - Essential for controlling hydration.
  - Damage leads to corneal oedema with stromal swelling and loss of transparency.

#### Sclera
- Protects and maintains shape of globe.

- Dense irregular collagen fibres present a barrier to light transmission and results in its opacification.

### Uveal layer

#### Trabecular meshwork
- Situated at the iridocorneal angle.
- Majority of aqueous humour drains from the anterior chamber via the trabecular meshwork and canal of Schlemm.

#### Uveal tract
- Consists of iris, ciliary body, and choroid.

#### Iris
- Situated anterior to lens and ciliary body.
- Acts as aperture to control amount of light entering eye.
- Separates anterior and posterior chambers of the eye.
- Diameter 12mm.

#### Ciliary body
- 5–6mm wide ring of tissue located anterior to ora serrate.
- Divided into two areas, the pars plicata (anterior) and pars plana (adjacent to retina).
- Pars plicata arranged into radial folds (ciliary processes).

Ciliary muscle makes up the anterior 2/3 of the ciliary body. In combination with lens zonules and the lens capsule the ciliary muscle functions to change the refractive power of the eye required for accommodation.

#### Aqueous humour
- Clear, colourless fluid
- Secreted by ciliary processes.

Functions
- Delivery of nutrients to, and removal of waste products from the avascular anterior chamber tissue.
- Provides high levels of ascorbate to the anterior chamber, at concentrations approximately ×25 those found in the plasma, though its actual role remains uncertain.
- Involvement in local immune responses.
- Maintenance of the shape of the globe to allow it to perform as an optical apparatus.

#### Choroid
- Posterior extension of uveal tract situated between the sclera and the retina.
- Main function is to provide blood supply to outer layers of the retina.
- Thermoregulatory role.
- Choroidal pigments absorb unwanted light.
- Affects perfusion rate of ciliary processes and therefore has an effect on intraocular pressure.

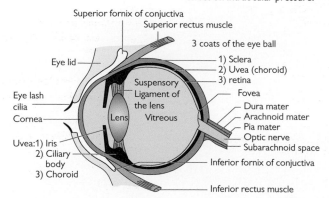

**Fig. 16.1** Horizontal section of eye.

Reproduced from Collier J. et al., Oxford Handbook of Clinical Specialties, 2013, Figure 16.1, page 433, with permission from Oxford University Press.

- Bruch's membrane, a modified collagenous layer, separates the choriocapillaris from the retinal pigment epithelium.
- Choriocapillaris:
  - Extensive layer of fenestrated capillaries.
  - Provides nutrition to the outer retina, including the photoreceptors.
  A vascular layer is present external to the choriocapillaris, consisting of both supplying arteries and draining veins. Ultimately these drain into four large vortex veins, one in each quadrant of the globe.

### Neural layer

- Retina is inner layer of eye.
- Consists of outer retinal pigment epithelium (RPE) and inner neurosensory retina (Fig. 16.2).
- Converts information regarding the image on the retina into neural impulses that subsequently are transmitted to the brain for processing and interpretation.
- Retina is enclosed on its outer aspect by Bruch's membrane, in contact with the choricapillaris, and on its inner surface by the vitreous body (gel).

*Retinal pigment epithelium*
- Critical single layer of terminally differentiated pigmented cuboidal/columnar epithelial cells.
- Role of RPE:
  - Maintains apposition of overlying neurosensory retina.
  - Selectively permeable barrier between choroid and neurosensory retina (blood–retinal barrier).
  - Phagocytosis of shed tips of used photoreceptor outer segments.
  - Synthesizes photoreceptor matrix.

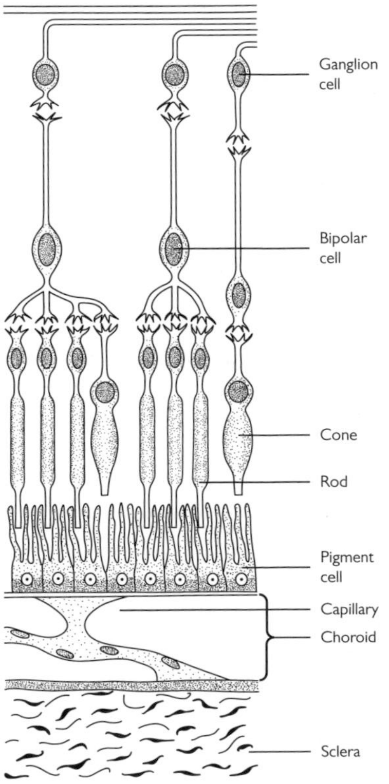

**Fig. 16.2** Low-power micrograph of retina.
Reproduced from *Oxford Concise Medical Dictionary*, 2002, page 597, with permission from Oxford University Press.

- Reduces light scatter by absorption of light.
- Transports and stores vitamins (especially vitamin A) and metabolites.

*Neurosensory retina*
- Consists of neural cells, glial cells, microglia, pericytes, and some blood vessels.
- Converts light into neural impulses.
- Some signal modification occurs in the neurosensory retina before the impulse is transmitted onward to the brain.
- Main neuronal cells are:
  - Photoreceptors
  - Bipolar cells
  - Ganglion cells.
Their impulses are modified by horizontal and amacrine cells that have a role in retinal processing.

*Photoreceptors*
Two types:
- Rods, detect:
  - Contrast
  - Brightness
  - Motion
- Cones, detect:
  - Fine resolution
  - Spatial resolution
  - Colour vision.
Density of rods and cones dependent on region of retina with the periphery predominantly rods and the fovea only cones.
   Three types of spectrally distinct cones:
- Blue
- Green
- Red.

*Bipolar cells*
- Transmit signal from photoreceptors to ganglion cells.
- At fovea, one bipolar cell provides the connect between one cone and one ganglion cell.
- In periphery, one bipolar cell receives input from up to 100 rods.
- This improves the sensitivity of rods in low levels of illumination.

*Ganglion cells*
- Found in inner layer of retina.
- Axons form nerve fibre layer and eventually optic nerve.
- Synapse with cells in the lateral geniculate nucleus in thalamus.

*Astrocytes*
- Provide structural support to vessels and neural cells within retina.
- Separate neurons in retina, preventing effect on nearby neural cells.

*Muller cells*
- Supporting glial cell in retina.
- Provide nutrition to outer retina.

*Microglia*
- Derived from mononuclear phagocyte system.
- May act as antigen presenting cells in the retina but mostly scavenging role.

*Vitreous*
- Transparent viscoelastic collagen gel (98% water).
- Viscosity dependent on sodium hyaluronate contained within a type II collagen matrix.
- Attached at peripheral retina and pars plana, posterior lens capsule, optic disc margin and retinal inner limiting membrane along retinal vessels.

# 16.2 The red eye

## Introduction

The red eye is a generic description for a multitude of potential diagnoses as a result of a large spectrum of underlying conditions. A patient with a red eye may have pain, visual acuity may be affected, or they may be asymptomatic.

Diagnoses range from a self-limiting viral conjunctivitis to sight-threatening necrotizing scleritis for instance, as part of granulomatosis with polyangitis. To ensure an accurate diagnosis, it is essential to have a systematic and logical approach to both the history and examination when such a patient presents.

## History

- What was the patient doing prior to/at the time of onset?
- Rate of onset and duration.
- Associated symptoms:
  - Nausea or vomiting
  - Systemic upset.
- Discharge:
  - Purulent
  - Clear
  - None.
- Pain:
  - Important to identify type—scratchy, foreign body sensation suggestive of ocular surface problem. A dull ache/pain may be suggestive of an ocular inflammatory or infective process or an elevated intraocular pressure. Deep boring pain present in scleritis.
  - Constant, intermittent, keeping them awake at night?
- Photophobia:
  - Important, but not specific. May indicate corneal problem or an anterior uveitis, though can occur in conjunctivitis. Important symptom of sympathetic ophthalmia and corneal graft rejection.
- Visual dysfunction:
  - How long has the vision been blurred?
  - Is it getting worse?
  - What is the temporal association with the redness and/or pain?
- Is there any diplopia?
- Past ocular and medical history.
- Known amblyopia/squint?
- Contact lens wearer?

## Examination

Always remember to think about the whole patient and not just their eyes! Initially when the patient enters the room have an overall general view; this can be difficult once the patient sits down, hidden by the slit lamp. Does the patient appear unwell?

Always examine the periorbital region in detail, otherwise you may miss an important sign, for example, vesicles on the forehead of a patient with uveitis, consistent with a herpes zoster aetiology.

### Examine the eye in an organized manner

- Visual acuity:
  - Reduced acuity is concerning and may suggest a serious eye condition such as infectious keratitis, iritis, or angle-closure glaucoma.
  - Measure each eye separately, either with a Snellen chart at 20 feet (if available) or by assessing near vision with a book/magazine held at a comfortable distance.
- Eye movements (if diplopia).
- Assess pupils:
  - Equal and reactive.
  - Relative afferent pupillary defect?

- Where is the redness?
  - Conjunctival?
  - Episcleral?
  - Scleral?
- Conjunctival appearance:
  - Follicles?
  - Papillae?
  - Forniceal shortening?
- Assess tear film:
  - Tear break-up time (performed by measuring tear clearance time and osmolality after instillation of fluorescein).
  - Schirmer test (sterile filter paper is placed at outer 1/3 of lower eyelid and extent of wetting in a given time is measured; <5mm in 5 minutes is abnormal).
- Discharge:
  - Serous?
  - Mucous?
  - Purulent?
- Corneal appearance:
  - Foreign body?
  - Clear/hazy?
  - Ulceration?
  - Infiltrate?
  - Thinning?
  - Old scarring?
- Anterior chamber:
  - Cells?
  - Flare?
  - Hypopyon?
  - Hyphaema?

## Differential diagnosis

See Table 16.1.

### Conjunctival causes

- Conjunctivitis, may be infectious, allergic, chemical, or medication-related
- Conjunctival foreign body
- Subconjunctival haemorrhage
- Cicatricial pemphigoid
- Stevens–Johnson syndrome
- Conjunctival neoplasia.

### Adnexal causes

- Ingrowing eyelashes (trichiasis)
- Entropion/ectropion
- Lagophthalmos (incomplete eyelid closure)
- Blepharitis
- Meibomianitis
- Acne rosacea
- Dacryocystitis.

### Corneal causes

- Keratitis, may be infectious or inflammatory (Fig. 16.3)
- Recurrent corneal erosion
- Contact lens-related problems
- Corneal foreign body
- Dry-eye syndrome.

Table 16.1 Differential diagnosis of the red eye—based on five parameters: redness plus any of pain, corneal haze, discharge, and loss of vision

| Redness/injection | Pain | Corneal haze | Discharge | Vision | Diagnosis |
|---|---|---|---|---|---|
| Pericorneal, none | None-->mild | Minimal | No | Blurred | Uveitis |
| Peripheral/diffuse | None-->FB sensation/itch | No | Yellow | Normal | Conjunctivitis (bacterial) |
| Peripheral/diffuse | | No | Watery | Normal | Conjunctivitis (viral) |
| Peripheral/diffuse | | No | No | Normal | Conjunctivitis (allergic) |
| Sectoral/diffuse | Severe/boring | No | No | Normal | Scleritis |
| Pericorneal | Severe/headache | Yes | No | Lost | Acute glaucoma |
| Pericorneal | Severe/eye closing | Yes | No | Lost | Keratitis/corneal ulcer |
| None | Severe/periocular | No | No/Yes | normal | Orbital cellulitis |

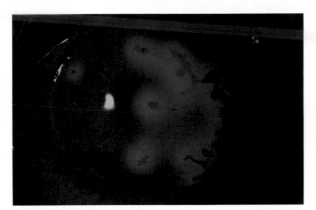

Fig. 16.3 Dendritic ulcer.

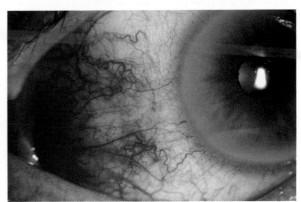

Fig. 16.4 Scleritis.

## Other causes
- Anterior uveitis
- Episcleritis
- Scleritis (Fig. 16.4)
- Angle-closure glaucoma
- Migraine
- Trauma
- Postoperative
- Endophthalmitis
- Pharmacological/iatrogenic.

# Specific conditions

### Blepharitis
- Very common.
- May be staphylococcal related, eyelash crusting commonly occurs.
- May be seborrhoeic, often with coexistent aural and scalp disease.

### Infectious keratitis
- Pain, redness, and reduced visual acuity.
- Usually underlying susceptibility, e.g. trauma or contact lens wear.
- Ulcer seen with surrounding white infiltrate.

### Conjunctivitis
- Associated with redness and discharge.
- May be irritation, generally not painful.
- Bacterial infection causes a purulent discharge, whereas viral infection tends be either serous or mucopurulent.
- Lymph node enlargement suggestive of viral infection.
- Allergy-related disease tends to be itchy, with a serous, often stringy discharge. There may be a history of atopy.

### Episcleritis
- Mild irritation and photophobia.
- Increased lacrimation.

- Visual acuity normal.
- May be diffuse or sectoral redness, occasionally a nodular appearance.

### Anterior scleritis
- Severe pain, tenderness.
- Deep bluish red discolouration.
- May be associated corneal thinning/ulceration or uveitis.
- May be associated with underlying systemic condition, e.g. rheumatoid arthritis, granulomatosis with polyangitis, relapsing polychondritis.
- Sometimes infectious cause, e.g. herpes zoster.

### Uveitis
- Term used to describe intraocular inflammation.
- Sudden-onset pain, photophobia, blurred vision.
- Circumlimbal injection.
- May be tenderness on palpation.
- Pupil may be miosed (spasm of ciliary muscle—very painful).
- Cells and flare present in anterior chamber.
- Intraocular pressure may be affected (high or low).
- May be associated with underlying systemic condition, e.g. HLA-B27.

### Acute angle-closure glaucoma
- Severe ocular pain, nausea, and vomiting.
- Decreased vision.
- Patient may see coloured haloes around lights.
- May be minimal ocular pain.
- Headache.
- Pupil fixed and mid-dilated.
- Cornea hazy.
- Intraocular pressure significantly raised.

# 16.3 Uveitis

## Introduction

Uveitis is a general term used to describe intraocular inflammation involving the uveal tract, retina, and vitreous to various degrees. It is a significant, but largely unrecognized, cause of visual impairment in the UK. Incidences of uveitis in the Western world vary between 38 and 200 per 100,000. Significant visual loss may be as high as 35%. As the highest incidence of uveitis occurs in the working population, there are important socioeconomic consequences.

## Classification of uveitis

Generally accepted classification is based on anatomical position of the inflammation within the eye:

- Anterior uveitis—involving anterior chamber.
- Intermediate uveitis—centred on the pars plana, choroid, and peripheral retina.
- Posterior uveitis—affecting any structure in posterior fundus, i.e. retina and optic nerve, and/or vitreous and/or choroid.
- Panuveitis.

## Anterior uveitis

### Symptoms
- May last several days to several weeks.
- Recurrence common.
- May alternate between eyes.
- Uncommonly bilateral.
- Pain/ache.
- Photophobia.
- Reduction in visual acuity.
- Red eye.

### Signs
- Circumlimbal injection.
- Flare/cells in anterior chamber.
- Keratic precipitates (inflammatory cells on endothelium).
- Hypopyon (settling out of inflammatory cells inferiorly in anterior chamber; Fig. 16.5).
- Synechiae (iris adhesions):
  - Posterior to lens
  - Anterior to cornea.
- Iris atrophy.
- Intraocular pressure may be affected—low pressure is sign of chronic uveitis in children.
- Occasionally cystoid macular oedema (Fig. 16.6).

## Intermediate uveitis

### Symptoms
- Usually bilateral.
- Generally good long-term visual outcome.
- Often asymptomatic.
- Floaters.
- Blurred or reduced vision.
- Flashing lights.
- Occasionally presents with photophobia and pain.

### Signs
- Diagnosis made by the presence of vitritis in absence of focal retinal or choroidal disease.
- Eye usually white.
- Anterior segment quiet or low-grade inflammation.
- Vitritis (vitreous cellular infiltrate).
- Snowballs (inflammatory cell aggregation inferiorly).
- Snowbanking (inflammatory cell aggregation on pars plana).
- Occasionally cystoid macular oedema (Fig. 16.6).
- Optic disc swelling.
- Sheathing of peripheral retinal vessels.
- Neovascularization.

## Posterior uveitis

### Symptoms
- Blurred or reduced vision.
- Floaters.
- Flashing lights.
- Occasionally presents with photophobia and pain.
- Untreated long-term visual outcome poor.

### Signs
- Vitreous cells
- Vitreous inflammatory exudates
- Retinal vasculitis
- Retinitis
- Retinal pigmentary disturbance

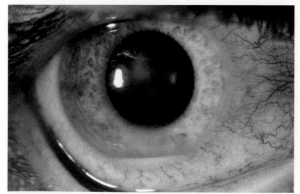

Fig. 16.5 *Hypopyon.*

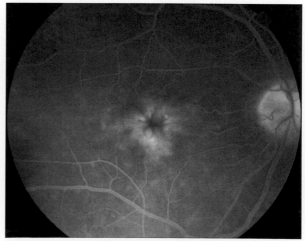

Fig. 16.6 Fluorescein angiogram of cystoid macular oedema.

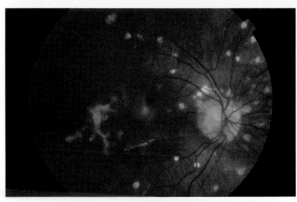

**Fig. 16.7** Punctate inner choroidopathy with inflammatory subretinal neovascular membrane.

- Choroiditis (Fig. 16.7)
- Macular oedema
- Optic disc swelling
- Neovascularization:
  - Retinal
  - Subretinal.

## Complications

- Cataract
- Glaucoma
- Vitreous haemorrhage
- Macular oedema
- Glaucoma
- Retinal tears/retinal detachment
- Retinoschisis (abnormal splitting of retina's neurosensory layer)
- Epiretinal membrane
- Neovascularization.

## Aetiology

Uveitis may be infectious, autoimmune, neoplastic, or post-traumatic. In >50% cases, the cause remains unknown (idiopathic):
- Idiopathic
- Infectious:
  - Bacterial (inc. tuberculosis)
  - Viral (inc. herpes simplex/zoster, HIV, cytomegalovirus (CMV))
  - Fungal (inc. candidiasis)
  - Protozoal (toxoplasmosis)
  - Helminths (toxocariasis)
  - Nematodes (onchocerciasis)
  - Spirochete (Lyme disease, syphilis)
- Medication-related:
  - Rifabutin
  - Cidofovir
  - Pamidronate
  - Sulphonamides
- Associated with systemic disease
- Juvenile idiopathic arthritis
- HLA-B27 associated:
  - Ankylosing spondylitis
  - Reiter syndrome
  - Inflammatory bowel disease
  - Psoriatic arthritis

- Sarcoidosis
- Behçet disease
- Multiple sclerosis
- HIV
- Tubulointerstitial nephritis and uveitis syndrome (TINU)
- Specific uveitic entities:
  - Birdshot chorioretinopathy
  - Serpiginous choroidopathy
  - Sympathetic ophthalmia
  - Vogt–Koyanagi–Harada syndrome
  - Fuchs heterochromic cyclitis
  - Pars planitis
  - Presumed ocular histoplasmosis syndrome
- Masquerade syndromes (neoplastic):
  - Non-Hodgkin lymphoma
  - Choroidal melanoma
  - Metastatic disease.

## Investigation

It is essential when seeing a patient with uveitis to take a full systemic history. This should include joint and skin, gastrointestinal tract, respiratory, neurological, and haematological problems, infections (current and past), medications, and a full sexual history. In patients with recurrent, bilateral, or atypical uveitis a full systemic examination should be performed and further investigations performed to identify or exclude an underlying cause.

## Treatment

Management will depend upon the underlying cause. Infectious and neoplastic causes need to be either excluded or treated appropriately.

The mainstay of treatment is *steroids*. By controlling inflammation uveal damage is reduced. In general, topical steroids (prednisolone, dexamethasone) are effective for the majority of patients with non-sight threatening acute anterior uveitis. In patients with complicated anterior or intermediate uveitis and all forms of posterior uveitis, topical therapy is ineffective and an alternative route of delivery needs to be considered. This could be subconjunctivally, periocularly, intraocularly, or systemically. In the presence of anterior chamber inflammation, *mydriatics* (cyclopentolate or atropine) should be given. They help prevent synechiae and reduce the pain caused by ciliary spasm.

Corticosteroids remain the mainstay of treatment in sight-threatening uveitis. Additional systemic immunosuppression may be required in patients with sight-threatening uveitis to allow disease control and a reduction in the steroid dosage.

### Second-line immunosuppressive agents include:

- Antimetabolites:
  - Azathioprine
  - Mycophenolate mofetil
  - Methotrexate.
- T-cell inhibitors/calcineurin inhibitors:
  - Ciclosporin
  - Tacrolimus.
- Alkylating agents:
  - Cyclophosphamide.
- Biological agents:
  - Anti-TNF therapy (e.g. Infliximab, Adalimumab)
  - Rituximab
  - Anakinra
  - Campath.

Although all these medications are licensed for other indications none are currently licensed for the treatment of ocular inflammatory disease and are used at the discretion of the prescribing consultant.

# 16.4 Retinal vein occlusion

## Introduction

Central retinal vein occlusion is characterized by:

- Tortuous, dilated retinal veins
- Extensive superficial and deep retinal haemorrhages
- Cotton wool spots
- Retinal oedema
- Frequently disc oedema.

The appearances of a branch retinal vein occlusion are as described for central retinal vein occlusion, but involving only a segment of the retina (Fig. 16.8). **Branch** retinal vein occlusion is two to three times more common than **central** retinal vein occlusion.

## Pathophysiology

Retinal vein occlusion is due to thrombosis of retinal veins. Depending where the obstruction occurs this may result in either a central, hemi-, or branch retinal vein occlusion.

It may result from any of the following processes:

1. Compression of the vein:
   - Raised intraocular pressure
   - Compression by crossing artery (hypertension or arteriosclerosis).
2. Disease of the vein wall:
   - Inflammation.
3. There may be a hypercoagulable state:
   - Increased viscosity (polycythaemia, dehydration, hyperviscosity states)
   - Thrombophilia.

## Risk factors

Established risk factors for both central and branch vein occlusions include:

- Hypertension
- Hyperlipidaemia
- Diabetes mellitus
- Glaucoma
- Thrombophilia
- Migraine
- Oral contraceptive pill
- Chronic renal failure
- Myeloproliferative disorders

- Vascular disease:
  - Carotid artery disease
  - Peripheral vascular disease
- Retinal vasculitis in association with:
  - Behçet disease
  - Polyarteritis nodosa
  - Granulomatosis with polyangitis
  - Sarcoidosis
  - Goodpasture syndrome
- Endocrine disease:
  - Acromegaly
  - Cushing syndrome
  - Hypothyroidism.

## Investigations

### All patients

- Full blood count and ESR
- U&E
- Random blood glucose
- Random total and HDL cholesterol
- CRP
- Plasma protein electrophoresis
- ECG
- Thyroid function
- BP
- Urinalysis.

### In patients <50 years consider:

- Serum ACE
- Auto-antibodies: rheumatoid factor/antinuclear antibodies (ANAs)/anti-dsDNA antibodies/antineutrophil cytoplasmic antibodies (ANCAs)
- CXR
- Fluorescein angiogram to look for vasculitis
- Thrombophilia screen including:
  - Antiphospholipid antibodies
  - Anticardiolipin antibody
  - Antithrombin III
  - Lupus anticoagulant
  - Activated protein C resistance
  - Factor V Leiden

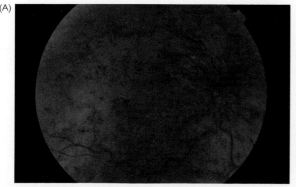
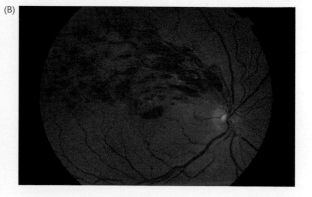

**Fig. 16.8** Central (A) and branch (B) retinal vein occlusion.

- Prothrombin
- Protein S deficiency
- Protein C deficiency
- Fasting homocysteine level.

## Treatment

Studies have shown that patients with retinal vascular disease have an increased mortality and morbidity from both stroke and cardio-vascular disease. When managing patients with retinal vein occlusion it is important to treat any underlying risk factors as well as sight-threatening complications.

### Medical management

- Any underlying condition identified should be managed appropriately.
- Lower intraocular pressure if elevated (consider topical β-blocker or prostaglandin analogue).
- BP <140/85mmHg.
- Cholesterol <5.0 mmol/L.
- Control diabetes if present.
- Consider systemic steroids if inflammation suspected.
- If presentation acute with incomplete central retinal vein occlusion consider IV streptokinase.

There is a 15% risk of second eye involvement and currently available data suggest that treatment of underlying cardiovascular risk factors reduces recurrence of retinal vein occlusion. Therefore, provided there are no significant contraindications, both aspirin and a statin should be commenced.

### Ophthalmic management

*Central retinal vein occlusion*

It is important to differentiate ischaemic from non-ischaemic central retinal vein occlusion. Patients with ischaemic central retinal vein occlusion are at risk of developing neovascular glaucoma (rubeosis, see Fig. 16.9) which may respond to laser photocoagulation. This is a serious condition, leading to a painful blind eye sometimes requiring removal of the eye for relief of pain. Up to 1/3 of patients with non-ischaemic central retinal vein occlusion will become ischaemic. The patient is often aware of a further sudden deterioration in vision in this situation.

   Characteristics suggestive of ischaemic central retinal vein occlusion include:

- Significantly reduced visual acuity (~50% of eyes with visual acuity (VA) <6/60 will develop rubeosis).
- Relative afferent pupillary defect.
- Multiple deep intraretinal haemorrhages.
- Multiple cotton wool spots.
- Evidence of >10 disc areas of retinal capillary non-perfusion on fluorescein angiography.

*Pan-retinal laser photocoagulation*

- Should be applied as soon as iris or angle new vessels are identified.

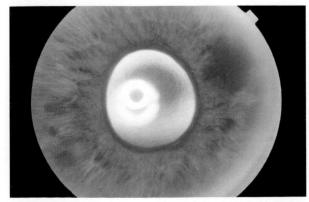

**Fig. 16.9** Rubeosis.

- May sometimes be applied prophylactically if severe ischaemia without new vessels.

*Management of established neovascular glaucoma*

- If possible apply further laser.
- If visual potential remains, aim to control intraocular pressure with topical pressure-lowering agents (consider topical β-blocker, e.g. timolol or prostaglandin analogue, e.g. latanoprost) or cyclo-ablative procedures (diode laser cyclophotocoagulation).
- Aim to keep eye comfortable using topical steroids and atropine

*Management of macular oedema*

- Laser not effective.
- Anti-vascular endothelial growth factor (VEGF) intravitreal injections are beneficial in some patients.
- Intravitreal steroid implants are effective in a proportion of patients.

*Experimental treatments*

- Laser-assisted chorioretinal venous anastomosis.
- Radial optic neurotomy with pars plana vitrectomy.
- Thrombolytic therapies.

*Branch retinal vein occlusion*

- 50% of untreated eyes will retain visual acuity 6/12 or better.
- 25% will have vision <6/60.
- 30% with >5 disc areas of retinal capillary non-perfusion on fluorescein angiography will develop retinal neovascularization.

*Retinal laser photocoagulation*

- Apply to the area of ischaemic retina (sector photocoagulation) in the presence of neovascularization at either the disc or elsewhere.

*Laser treatment for macular oedema*

- May be beneficial.
- Only consider 3–18 months after initial event.
- Vision 20/40 or worse due to macular oedema.
- No retinal haemorrhage preventing fluorescein angiography or laser.
- No foveal haemorrhage.
- Fluorescein angiography should be performed prior to treatment.
- 2/3 treated will have VA 20/40 or better at 3 years, compared to 1/3 untreated.
- Anti-VEGF intravitreal injections are beneficial in some patients.
- Intravitreal steroid implants are effective in a proportion of patients.

*Experimental treatments*

- Vitrectomy and sheathotomy (optic nerve).

*Management of younger patients (<50 years of age)*

*Branch retinal vein occlusion*

- Usually underlying systemic condition such as hypertension or hyperlipidaemia.

*Central retinal vein occlusion*

- Often no identifiable cause despite extensive investigation.
- Consider recent period of acute dehydration.
- Combined oral contraceptive pill most common association in females.
- Identified inflammatory disease should be treated as appropriate to the condition.
- 20% of patients have poor visual outcome with severe neovascular complications.
- Better visual outcome in a greater proportion of patients when compared to an older age group.
- Spontaneous resolution may occur.
- Use of oral steroid therapy may be effective in some patients.

# 16.5 Retinal artery occlusion

## Introduction

Retinal arterial occlusion may be either central or branch depending on the anatomical location of the obstruction.

Central retinal artery occlusion is characterized by:

- Sudden, painless loss of vision.
- Retinal oedema secondary to ischaemia with pallor of the posterior pole.
- Cherry-red spot.
- Segmentation of blood column within the retinal vessels ("cattle-trucking").
- 10% have had a recent preceding episode of amaurosis fugax.
- Visual acuity generally poor (counting fingers or worse).
- Rarely, normal central visual acuity is retained if a patent cilioretinal artery present.
- Relative afferent pupillary defect is present.
- Retinal neovascularization may occur.

Branch retinal artery occlusion (Fig. 16.10) is characterized by:

- Retinal pallor only occurs in the region supplied by the occluded artery.
- Embolus may be identified within an occluded artery.
- Visual field defect occurs corresponding to the area of occlusion.
- Central acuity often intact.
- 80% recover 6/12 or better central acuity.
- >75% are secondary to emboli.
- Emboli are often seen in the arterial tree.
- In presence of underlying carotid artery disease, amaurosis fugax occurs in ~25% patients prior to definitive obstruction.
- Relative afferent pupillary defect is common, and is determined by the extent of retinal involvement.
- Retinal neovascularization may occur (though uncommon).

## Pathophysiology

- Central retinal artery, an end artery, supplies the inner retina.
- Outer retina supplied by the choroidal circulation.
- Only *inner* retina is affected by retinal artery occlusion.

### Histology

*Initially*

- Intracellular oedema affecting the inner retinal tissue due to obstructed axoplasmic flow.

- Coagulative necrosis of the inner layers of the neural retina occurs early.

*Long term*

- Outer retina well preserved.
- Loss of the nerve fibre layer, ganglion cell layer and inner plexiform layer.
- Inner retina becomes an acellular layer containing retinal blood vessels.
- Sections of occluded artery show embolus, thrombus or recanalization.

## Risk factors

Majority of both central and branch retinal arterial occlusions are either thrombotic or embolic in nature:

- 65% of branch retinal artery occlusions are caused by emboli.
- 30% of central retinal artery occlusions are caused by emboli.

Established risk factors for retinal artery occlusion include:

- Hypertension
- Hyperlipidaemia
- Cigarette smoking
- Diabetes mellitus
- Thrombophilia
- Vascular disease:
  - Carotid artery disease
  - Peripheral vascular disease
- Retinal vasculitis in association with:
  - Behçet disease (Fig. 16.11)
  - Polyarteritis nodosa
  - Granulomatosis with polyangitis
  - Sarcoidoisis
  - Goodpasture syndrome
- Cardiac disease:
  - Arrhythmias (common)
  - Subacute bacterial endocarditis
  - Cardiac arrhythmias
  - Valvular heart disease
  - Bacterial endocarditis

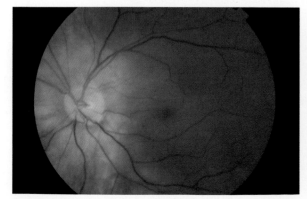

Fig. 16.10 Inferotemporal branch retinal artery occlusion.

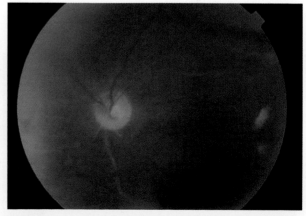

Fig. 16.11 Ocular Behçet syndrome with mixed arterial and venous occlusion.

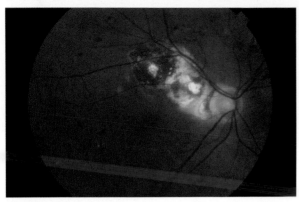

**Fig. 16.12** Chorioretinal scar secondary to ocular toxoplasmosis.

- Coagulopathy
- Malignancy
- Medical procedures including angiography and angioplasty
- Systemic vasculitis (esp. giant cell arteritis)
- Systemic infections
- Pregnancy
- Oral contraceptives
- Cocaine abuse
- IV drug use
- Inflammatory eye disease:
  - Toxoplasmosis (Fig. 16.12)
  - Acute retinal necrosis
  - Retinal vasculitis.

## Investigations

As there is a strong association with systemic disease, all patients who suffer retinal artery obstructions should undergo a systemic evaluation.
- Systemic evaluation reveals no definite cause for the obstruction in >50% of affected patients.
- Potential embolic sources are found in <40% of cases.
- Significant ipsilateral carotid artery disease is found in ~30%.
- Cardiac embolic source found in <10% of patients.

*All patients*
- Full blood count and ESR
- U&E
- Random blood glucose
- Random total and HDL cholesterol
- CRP
- Plasma protein electrophoresis
- ECG
- Thyroid function
- BP
- Urinalysis
- Carotid Doppler ultrasound
- Echocardiogram.

*In patients <50 years consider:*
- Serum ACE
- Auto-antibodies: rheumatoid factor/ANA/anti-dsDNA/ANCA

- CXR
- Fluorescein angiogram to look for vasculitis
- Thrombophilia screen.

## Treatment

Studies have shown that patients with retinal vascular disease have an increased mortality and morbidity from both stroke and cardiovascular disease. When managing patients with retinal artery occlusion it is important to treat any underlying risk factors as well as sight-threatening complications.
  Aims of treatment are to:
- Improve oxygen supply to retina.
- Increase retinal arterial blood flow.
- Remove arterial obstruction.
- Reduce retinal damage due to hypoxia.

### Medical management
- BP <140/85mmHg.
- Cholesterol <5.0mmol/L.
- Control diabetes if present.
- Consider systemic steroids if inflammation suspected.
- Any other underlying condition identified should be managed appropriately.

### Ophthalmic management

*Central retinal artery occlusion*
- Lowering intraocular pressure with resultant increase in retinal blood flow.
- Ocular massage.
- Paracentesis.
- Ocular antihypertensive medications.
- Hypotensive agents (glyceryl trinitrate (GTN), β-blockers) have been used to dilate retinal arteries and block vascular spasm though there is no evidence for their efficacy.

*Experimental treatments*
- Antioxidant medications, to reduce hypoxic damage are currently under investigation.
- Thrombolytic therapies:
  - IV infusion of recombinant tissue plasminogen activator (rTPA).
  - Selective ophthalmic artery catheterization with infusion of rTPA.
- Vitrectomy and sheathotomy (optic nerve).
- Hyperbaric oxygen.

*Giant cell arteritis*
- ESR is most important single investigation in all patients >50 years with central retinal artery obstruction.
- Underlying cause in ~5% central retinal artery occlusions.
- Check ESR, CRP, and platelet count.
- If strong suspicion, commence systemic therapy immediately and organize temporal artery biopsy.
- Treat immediately with high-dose steroids.
- Rarely any recovery in vision in the affected eye. The main reason for treatment is to reduce the risk to the other eye.

# Chapter 17

# Renal medicine

# 17.1 Renal basic science

## Background

The main roles of the kidneys are regulation of:
- Water excretion.
- Electrolyte balance.
- Acid–base balance.
- Blood pressure.

They also have important endocrine functions, secreting erythropoietin and activating vitamin D.

## Structure and function of the kidney

The kidneys lie retroperitoneally on either side of the vertebral column. Each is ~11cm long, 6cm wide, and 3cm in thickness. They consist of an outer cortex and an inner medulla. The medulla is divided

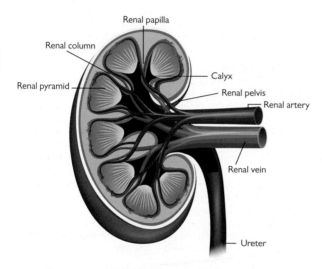

**Fig. 17.1** A schematic diagram of the anatomical components of the kidney.

into 8–18 conical masses, the renal pyramids. The base of each pyramid originates at the corticomedullary junction, whilst the apex, or papilla, extends into the pelvic space. The renal pelvis is an extension of the ureter, allowing collection of the urine excreted from the medulla. The pelvis divides into two or three open-ended pouches, the major calyces, which in turn divide into minor calyces—these collect urine from each papilla (Fig. 17.1).

### The renal blood supply

The renal artery enters the kidney alongside the ureter, then divides into the interlobular arteries. These cross the renal medulla and then further divide into arcuate arteries at the junction of the cortex and the medulla. These then branch to form cortical radial arteries, then afferent glomerular arteries that supply the glomeruli. Efferent glomerular arteries drain the glomeruli and supply the peritubular capillaries of the cortex and medulla. Efferent arteries from the cortical region closest to the medulla form the descending vasa recta, the blood supply to the medulla. The medulla is drained by the ascending vasa recta, which join the cortical radial veins to form the arcuate veins, then the interlobular veins, and finally the renal vein, which runs next to the renal artery (Fig. 17.2).

### The nephron

The nephron is the functional unit of the kidney. It is comprised of:
- The glomerulus.
- The proximal tubule.
- The loop of Henle.
- The distal tubule and collecting duct.

#### The glomerulus

The glomerulus consists of a network of capillaries supplied by the afferent arteriole and drained by the efferent arteriole, sitting within Bowman capsule at the proximal end of the nephron. The capillaries are supported by the mesangium, consisting of mesangial cells and the matrix they secrete. The main job of the glomerulus is to act as a filter. The walls of the glomerular capillaries form a filtration barrier, comprising:

- **Endothelium:** this is fenestrated but as the gaps are relatively large (70nm), it acts as a filtration barrier only to cells.
- **Basement membrane:** this is the main filtration barrier to plasma proteins >7–9nm (60–70 kilodaltons) (Fig. 17.3).

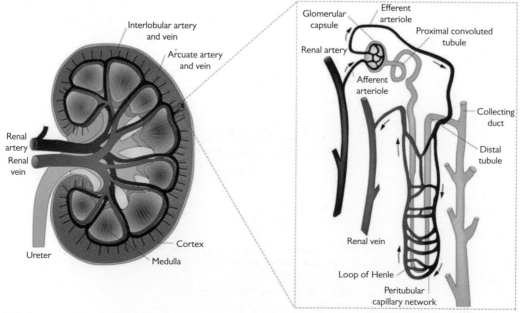

**Fig. 17.2** Details of the renal vasculature.

Reprinted by permission from Macmillan Publishers Ltd: *Nat. Rev. Nephrol.* Mimura, I. & Nangaku, M. (2010) The suffocating kidney: tubulointerstitial hypoxia in end-stage renal disease. doi:10.1038/nrneph.2010.124 copyright (2010).

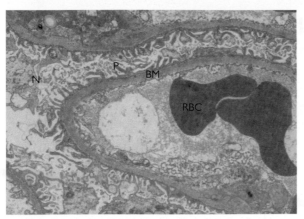

**Fig. 17.3** Electron micrograph of the glomerular basement membrane (×7,000) demonstrating the basement membrane (BM), the foot processes of the podocytes (P) within the nephron space (N), and a red cell within the capillary lumen (RBC).
Courtesy of Cambridge University Hospitals NHS Foundation Trust's Histopathology dept.

- **Podocytes:** these phagocytic cells have long finger-like processes that encircle the capillaries and interdigitate to cover the basement membrane. Tiny gaps called filtration slits between the foot processes allow small molecules to be filtered.

All three structures contain negatively charged glycoproteins, thus filtration occurs according to charge as well as according to size. So although albumin, for example, has a molecular weight of 60kDa, relatively little albumin is filtered because of its negative charge.

*Glomerular filtration rate*
The blood flow to the two kidneys is equal to 25% of the cardiac output in resting subjects (1.25L/min). All of this passes through the glomeruli for filtration. Filtration occurs passively, and depends on the permeability of the glomerular capillary walls, the net hydrostatic pressure across them, and the oncotic pressure within the capillaries. Although average values for healthy young adults are 130mL/min/1.73m² for a man and 120mL/min/1.73m² for a woman, the range seen in normal individuals is large: 70–140mL/min/1.73m². In general, GFR declines from the age of 40 by 1mL/min/1.73m² per year—so by the age of 80, it is usual to have a GFR that is approximately half that of a young adult. See Box 17.1 for calculation of the GFR.

*The proximal tubule*
The proximal tubule reabsorbs 50% of the filtered sodium. The Na⁺ K⁺ ATPase in the basolateral membrane of the cells lining the proximal tubule actively pumps sodium out of the proximal tubular cells, allowing passive transport across the apical membrane of glucose, chloride, bicarbonate, potassium, calcium, magnesium, phosphate, and amino acids (via sodium co-transporters) and hydrogen ions via a sodium anti-porter. Water follows solute transport down an osmotic gradient via both a transcellular and a paracellular route. Proximal tubule cells also secrete substances into the tubular lumen—endogenous substances include creatinine and urate; exogenous substances include thiazide and loop diuretics, trimethoprim, and penicillins.

*Loop of Henle*
This is a long loop of tubule that passes into the inner medulla, as the descending limb, before doing a U-turn and returning as the ascending limb. The descending limb has numerous aquaporins (water channels), and therefore is very water permeable, but is impermeable to sodium. The thick ascending limb is impermeable to water, and pumps sodium and chloride into the interstitium. This creates a very high peritubular osmolarity at the apex of the tubule, the medullary concentration gradient, that creates the potential for a large amount of water to be reabsorbed in the medulla. About 20% of filtered sodium and water are reabsorbed here. It is also the site of action of loop diuretics.

*Distal tubule and collecting duct*
These segments reabsorb about 15% of the filtered sodium, chloride, and water, and secrete potassium and protons. They are able to fine-tune reabsorption of salt and water to maintain homeostasis by:
- Antidiuretic hormone (ADH)—increases water reabsorption in the collecting duct by stimulation of receptors on the basolateral (non-luminal) membrane, leading to insertion of aquaporins in the apical (luminal) membrane. The aquaporins then allow uptake of water from the luminal fluid.
- Aldosterone-sensitive sodium channels are responsible for 2% of all sodium reabsorption, hence regulation of sodium retention by the renin–angiotensin–aldosterone (RAA) system.

Spironolactone antagonizes the aldosterone receptors in both the distal tubule and the collecting duct, blocking sodium and water reabsorption and preventing potassium excretion.

---

**Box 17.1 Calculating glomerular filtration rate (GFR)**

*From plasma creatinine*
Creatinine is released at a constant rate by muscle, freely filtered by the glomeruli and not reabsorbed by the tubules, so the amount of plasma creatinine can be used to estimate GFR.
   Two formulas are commonly used for this:
1. Cockcroft and Gault equation:

$$GFR = \frac{(140 - age) \times weight\ (kg) \times 1.23\ (\male)\ or\ 1.04\ (\female)}{Plasma\ creatinine\ (\mu mol/L)}$$

This formula tends to overestimate GFR in people with low GFRs, women, and the elderly.
2. MDRD (Modification of Diet in Renal Disease) study equation:

$$GFR = 170 \times (P_{Cr}/88.4)^{-0.999} \times (age)^{-0.176} \times 0.762\ (if\ \female) \times 1.18\ (if\ black) \times (urea \times 2.8)^{-0.170} \times (alb/10)^{+0.318}$$

where $P_{Cr}$ is serum creatinine concentration in µmol/L, urea is serum urea nitrogen concentration in mmol/L and alb is serum albumin concentration in g/L.
This formula is more accurate in advanced renal failure.

*From urinary creatinine*
A 24-hour urine collection can be used to calculate creatinine clearance:

$$CrCl = \frac{U_{Cr} \times U_V \times 1000mL/min}{P_{Cr}}$$

where $U_{Cr}$ = urine creatinine concentration (µmol/L), $U_V$ = urine volume (L) and $P_{Cr}$ = plasma creatinine concentration (µmol/L).
   This formula will overestimate GFR (particularly in advanced renal impairment) as creatinine is secreted into the tubules.

*By measurement of inulin clearance*
This small molecule is freely filtered by glomeruli, and not secreted or absorbed by the tubules.

*By chromium-labelled EDTA*
This radio-isotope is also freely filtered in the glomerulus, allowing an accurate measurement of GFR.

### Acute kidney injury

- The majority of cases of acute kidney injury (AKI) are due to acute tubular necrosis (ATN) following a prolonged period of renal hypoperfusion and consequent renal ischaemia.
- During the ischaemic insult, vasoconstrictors are released, including endothelin, and levels of intrinsic vasodilators (e.g. nitric oxide and prostaglandin $I_2$).
- The renal blood flow decreases and GFR falls.
- This results in hypoxic injury to the energy-consuming cells of the proximal tubule and the ascending limb of the loop of Henle.
- Necrosis occurs and the cells are shed from and into the tubular lumen.
- Casts may then form which block urine flow.
- With resolution of adequate renal perfusion, tubular cells may regenerate. Renal recovery, however, is variable.

### Chronic kidney disease/renal failure

- When irreversible renal injury occurs, the kidney adapts to nephron loss by an increase in the function of residual nephrons.
- This allows life-sustaining renal excretory and homeostatic functions to continue until the GFR has fallen to <10mL/min/1.73m$^2$.
- However, the subsequent rise in single nephron GFR and glomerular pressure further damages the remaining glomeruli.
- The damaged kidney is particularly susceptible to the hypertension that results from fluid retention as the preglomerular arterial vessels become damaged and dilated with consequent loss of autoregulation.
- Thus because of the maladaptive response to nephron loss, chronic kidney disease is likely to progress if not managed adequately.
- Reduction of nephron numbers leads to impaired exocrine function (sodium/water retention with hypertension and oedema, phosphate retention) and endocrine function (reduced synthesis of erythropoietin and calcitriol).

### Immunopathology in renal disease

The immune system plays an important role in a number of renal diseases. There are several mechanisms underlying this immunopathology:

- **Autoantibodies to renal components**: e.g. in antiglomerular basement membrane (GBM) disease, IgG targets the GBM, causing inflammation.
- **Immune complex deposition**: e.g. in a number of types of glomerulonephritis (GN), immune complexes form in the blood and are then deposited in the glomeruli, where they cause inflammation via complement activation and Fc receptor leucocyte recruitment. These immune complexes may be composed of IgG reactive to either pathogenic antigen (from infectious organisms e.g. hepatitis C), or to self antigen (e.g. components of cell nuclei in systemic lupus erythematosus).
- **Leucocyte recruitment without antibody deposition**: e.g. in small vessel vasculitidies, neutrophils infiltrate glomeruli and small blood vessels, causing inflammation. These lesions are 'pauci-immune' with scanty IgG deposits. The factors controlling this leucocyte recruitment have not been well defined.

# 17.3 The kidney as an 'endocrine' organ

## Erythropoietin

- Erythropoietin (EPO) is responsible for maintaining the proliferation and differentiation of erythroid progenitor cells in the bone marrow.
- About 90% of the circulating levels of this hormone are produced by the kidney.
- Erythropoietin is synthesized by interstitial, peritubular cells in the renal cortex through the actions of HIF (hypoxia inducible factor)-2α.
- During chronic renal failure, erythropoietin production is variably altered depending on the cause of kidney destruction.
- In CKD stages 4 and 5, treatment with recombinant erythropoietin is usually required (see Section 17.6).

## Calcitriol

- The kidney plays a central role in calcium and phosphate homeostasis not only by controlling ion reabsorption but also by synthesizing 1,25-dihydroxyvitamin $D_3$ (1,25(OH)$_2$D$_3$), the most active metabolite of vitamin D.
- Vitamin $D_3$ is obtained from 7-dehydrocholesterol by action of sunlight on the skin or is derived from the diet, then is hydroxylated in the liver into 25-hydroxyvitamin.
- The final hydroxylation to the active form, 1,25(OH)$_2$D$_3$, by the enzyme 1α-hydroxylase occurs in the renal proximal tubule.
- The activity of the 1α-hydroxylase is regulated by parathyroid hormone (PTH) and plasma phosphate concentration.
- While low serum calcium concentrations and high levels of PTH and hypophosphataemia stimulate 1,25(OH)$_2$D$_3$ production; hypoparathyroidism and hyperphosphataemia blunt renal 1α-hydroxylase activity even in the presence of hypocalcaemia. As numbers of nephrons decline with worsening chronic kidney disease, less 1α-hydroxylase is available to convert vitamin D into the active form.
- Thus low circulating concentration of 1,25(OH)$_2$D$_3$ may be due to low vitamin D storage, hypoparathyroidism, hyperphosphataemia, or advanced renal insufficiency.
- Increased levels of 1,25(OH)$_2$D$_3$ are observed in granulomatous disorders (sarcoidosis, tuberculosis, etc.) because of the expression of extra-renal non-regulated 1α-hydroxylase.

## Renin

- The renin–angiotensin–aldosterone (RAA) system has a central role in maintaining circulating blood volume.
- Renin, the primary determinant of activity of the renin–angiotensin system, converts angiotensinogen to angiotensin. ACE (angiotensin converting enzyme) in the lung (principally) converts angiotensin I to angiotensin II, the active form. Angiotensin II increases circulating volume by:
  - Releasing aldosterone from the adrenal glands.
  - Inducing thirst.
  - Inducing vasoconstriction.
- Renin is secreted by the juxtaglomerular apparatus of the kidney.
- Renin production is controlled by the renal vascular baroreceptor in the afferent arteriole, the delivery of sodium chloride at the macula densa, the renal sympathetic nerve activity, and various humoral agents including angiotensin II, nitric oxide, adenosine, atrial natriuretic peptide, and prostaglandins.
- Thus renal hypoperfusion, hyponatraemia and increased sympathetic drive all lead to activation of the RAA system and a rise in blood pressure.
- Activation of the RAA in CKD is the major cause of secondary renal hypertension.

# 17.4 Renal investigations

## Urinalysis

Standard dipsticks assess the presence of blood, protein, glucose, leucocytes, and nitrites, and the pH and specific gravity of the urine. They are useful screening tests for renal and urological pathology which are widely used in both hospital and general practice.

**Nitrites and leucocytes** with or without blood and protein, suggest a urinary tract infection.

**Specific gravity** is rarely helpful, but dilute urine first thing in the morning may indicate diabetes insipidus.

**Urinary pH** varies widely in health, but should be acidic first thing in the morning. If not, renal tubular acidosis is possible (or systemic alkalosis, in which case alkaline urine is appropriate). Alkaline urine may also indicate infection with a urea-splitting organism (e.g. *Proteus* spp.).

**Glycosuria** should be followed with measurement of the fasting blood glucose, and a formal glucose tolerance test if appropriate. Glycosuria may occur without elevation of the blood glucose if there is a reduced renal 'threshold' for glucose excretion (e.g. in pregnancy), or because of renal damage leading to glucose leakage.

**Haematuria** on dipstick testing may reflect erythrocytes, haemoglobin, or myoglobin in the urine. Dipstick tests are highly sensitive and can give a positive result in the presence of a normal number of red cells (as few as $1–2 \times 10^{12}$/L urine). A test positive for blood should always be followed by urine microscopy looking for red cell casts (see 'Casts'). However, microscopy need not be performed simply to confirm the dipstick finding of 'haematuria'.

**Proteinuria** on dipstick is a sign of glomerular damage and requires further investigation. Standard dipsticks do not detect Bence Jones protein.

### Further investigation of proteinuria

Normal urinary protein loss is <150mg/day.

*Microalbuminuria*

- 30–300mg albumin loss per day.
- Standard urine dipsticks will detect >0.5g/L protein, but may not detect microalbuminuria. Specific dipsticks are, however, able to detect albumin loss within this range.
- Albumin:creatinine ratio (ACR) is often used to quantify proteinuria in clinical practice:
  - Normal ACR <2.5mg/mmol.
  - Microalbuminuria = 2.5–33mg/mmol.
  - Nephrotic range >400mg/mmol.
- Key finding in early diabetic nephropathy.
- Poor prognostic indicator in patients with hypertension or ischaemic cardiovascular disease.

*Non-nephrotic range proteinuria*

- Protein:creatinine ratio 33–400.
- Dipstick + to +++.
- 0.3–3.5g per 24 hours on a 24-hour urine collection. Although this had been the gold standard in quantification of proteinuria, protein:creatinine ratios are now preferred as an alternative.
- This degree of proteinuria usually indicates renal parenchymal disease.
- Non-renal causes of proteinuria:
  - Fever
  - Extreme exercise
  - Cystitis.

*Nephrotic range proteinuria*

- Proteinuria >3.5g/24 hours, dipstick ++++, ACR >400.
- Always due to glomerular disease.

*Orthostatic proteinuria*

- Proteinuria detectable only after several hours in the upright position.
- Early morning urine should be negative.
- Usually <1g per 24 hours.
- Renal biopsy usually normal.
- Excellent prognosis—generally thought to be a benign condition.

## Urine microscopy

See Fig. 17.4.

*Red blood cells (RBCs)*

- $>12 \times 10^6$ RBCs/L urine (>5 RBCs/high-power field) without a red discoloration is termed non-visible haematuria.
- Non-visible haematuria:
  - Is found in 4–13% of the general population.
  - Is associated with a serious underlying condition in 2–22% cases.
- Dysmorphic red cells suggest glomerular haematuria, whereas smooth, uniform cells tend to originate from more distal sites in the urinary tract.
- The significance varies according to age and sex—in men >50 years with non-visible haematuria, ~13% will have neoplasia of the urinary tract. Thus in older patients with haematuria with normal looking red cells on microscopy, and with low levels of proteinuria (ACR <70mg/mmol), urological investigations should precede a renal biopsy.

*White blood cells (WBCs)*

- Up to 2 million WBCs are excreted in the urine every day.
- >4 WBCs per high power field is abnormal.
- Commonest cause of pyuria is infection.
- Sterile pyuria may be seen in association with stones, analgesic nephropathy and renal tuberculosis.
- Eosinophils in the urine may be indicative of an allergic interstitial nephritis.

*Epithelial cells*

- Found in normal urine.
- Shed from the bladder and urethra.
- Large numbers suggest perineal contamination—therefore any associated bacteriuria may not be significant.

*Casts*

- Cylinder structures several times larger than blood cells, and formed from Tamm–Horsfall protein in the renal tubule.
- Occasional hyaline casts are seen in normal urine, but frequency is increased in renal diseases.
- Granular casts are formed when serum proteins are trapped in a matrix of Tamm–Horsfall proteins. These are frequently seen in renal disease.
- Acute tubular necrosis often leads to red-brown granular casts.
- Red cell casts (hyaline casts with dysmorphic red cells stuck to them) are typically found in acute glomerulonephritis.
- White cell casts are found in acute inflammation of the kidney, e.g. pyelonephritis, acute interstitial nephritis and rapidly progressive glomerulonephritis.
- Tubular epithelial casts are found where there is tubular damage, e.g. acute tubular necrosis.

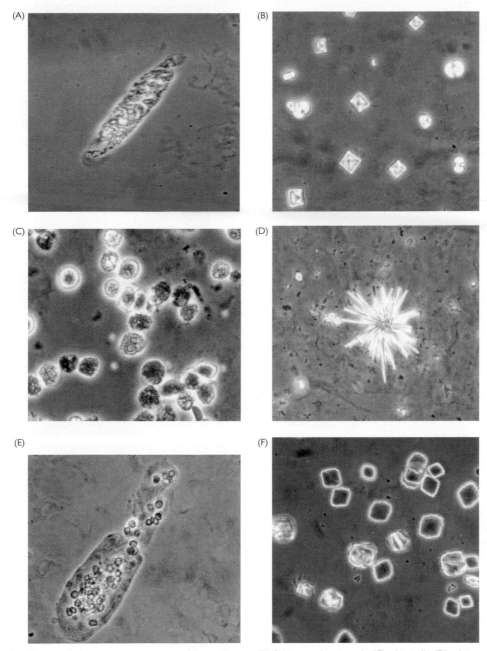

**Fig. 17.4** Examples of various findings on urine microscopy. (A) granular cast. (B) Calcium oxalate crystals. (C) white cells. (D) calcium phosphate crystals. (E) red cell cast. (F) uric acid crystals.

Reproduced from Davison *et al.*, *Oxford Textbook of Clinical Nephrology*, 2005, pp. 35–40, with permission from Oxford University Press.

*Crystals*

- Common but rarely significant. Calcium phosphate, calcium oxalate, and uric acid crystals are most common, and suggest concentrated urine.
- Cystine crystals, if found, are a sign of cystinuria.

---

# Laboratory investigations

## Immunological investigations

A number of immunological tests are used in the diagnosis of renal disease, and also in monitoring disease activity in some disorders.

*Immunoglobulins, serum, and urine electrophoresis*

The detection of a serum paraprotein or a monoclonal light chain in the urine raises the possibility of a diagnosis of myeloma or of amyloid.

However, screening of renal patients may simply bring to light an incidental finding of MGUS—'monoclonal gammopathy of uncertain significance'. Patients with IgA nephropathy may have an elevated serum IgA titre.

*Complement*

- Low complement levels are seen in lupus nephritis, where immune complex-mediated glomerulonephritis results in activation of the classical pathway.
- Low complement levels are also seen in cryoglobulinaemia.
- Activation of the alternative pathway in type II mesangiocapillary glomerulonephritis (MCGN) (by stabilization of C3bBb by C3 nephritic factor) results in a low C3 but a normal C4.

*Antinuclear antibody (ANA)*

Antibodies to components of the cell nucleus are present in the majority (>95%) of patients with systemic lupus erythematosus.

ANA are not very specific, and may be seen other connective tissue diseases. Anti-double-stranded DNA (anti-dsDNA) antibodies and anti-Sm antibodies are much more specific but less sensitive.

### Antineutrophil cytoplasmic antibodies (ANCA)

These are frequently found in the sera of patients with small vessel renal vasculitis. Two patterns of staining are found: perinuclear staining (pANCA) is typical in patients with microscopic polyangiitis (MPA), and granular cytoplasmic staining (cANCA) is seen in patients with granulomatosis with polyangiitis (GPA, Wegener granulomatosis).

### Cryoglobulinaemia

There are three types of cold precipitable immunoglobulins:

- Type I—monoclonal product of a B-cell clone, usually IgM. It may occur in the setting of any disorder associated with paraprotein production.
- Type II—a monoclonal component, usually an IgM, with rheumatoid factor activity which binds polyclonal IgG. It is found in association with lymphoproliferative disorders, infectious diseases, and autoimmune diseases.
- Type III is composed only of polyclonal immunoglobulins and is found in association with a mixture of autoimmune disorders and infections.
- Hepatitis C is a common cause of both type II and type III cryoglobulins.

## Renal imaging

See Fig. 17.5.

### Plain radiography

- Useful for assessing renal tract calcification and the bony skeleton.
- Relatively inexpensive, widely available.
- Relatively limited soft tissue contrast can make the detection of renal outlines and subtle renal calcification difficult.

### Contrast radiography

- The intravenous urogram (IVU)—this provides an overview of the renal collecting system.
- Detects lesions of the renal pelvis and ureter, and large lesions of the bladder.
- Basic assessment of the renal parenchyma and a crude overview of renal function.
- However, has been largely replaced as a method of assessing renal parenchyma by ultrasound, CT, and MRI.

### Ultrasound

- Provides good soft tissue contrast based on differential tissue acoustic impedance.
- Allows measurement of renal size (should be >9cm) as well as identification of lesions within the kidney, thickness of the renal cortex, hydronephrosis, and calcification.
- Pulse wave and colour Doppler methods allow assessment of renal vasculature.
- Widely available, portable, relatively quick to perform, and without the risk of IV contrast media used in CT, angiography, and MRI

### X-ray angiography

- This remains the primary technique for demonstrating renal artery stenosis and permits therapeutic techniques such as angioplasty and stenting.

### CT

- Provides an excellent overview of the renal tract and its relationship with other internal organs and their abnormalities.
- Both CT and radiographic procedures involve ionizing radiation and IV contrast—the associated risks need to be balanced against the diagnostic benefits.

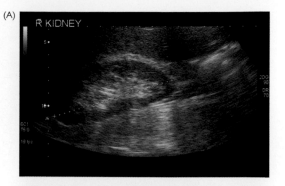

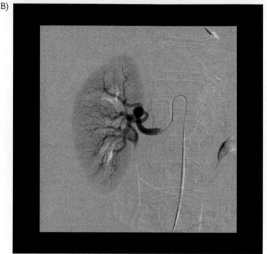

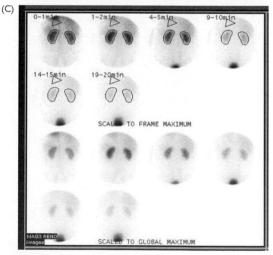

**Fig. 17.5** Examples of a normal renal ultrasound scan (A), a normal renal angiogram (B) and a normal $^{99m}$Tc-MAG3 scan (C). The bottom panel demonstrated prompt uptake and excretion over time of tracer by both kidneys.

Courtesy of Cambridge University Hospitals NHS Foundation Trust's Radiology dept.

### MRI

- Uses static and dynamic magnetic fields combined with pulse radiofrequency energy to generate images with excellent soft tissue contrast.
- MR angiography can be used to investigate renal artery stenosis, with a sensitivity comparable to that of angiography (but with a lower specificity). However, to obtain this degree of sensitivity, intravenous gadolinium is required. This is now contraindicated

in moderate to severe renal impairment (concerns regarding nephrogenic fibrosing dermopathy).

*Nuclear medicine*

- **Static renal scanning** uses technetium-99m-dimercaptosuccinic acid ($^{99m}$Tc-DMSA), which binds to proximal renal tubules. The kidneys are imaged 3 hours post injection, when about 15% of the tracer has been excreted, and about 20% is retained in each kidney. It is used mainly to identify renal scarring.
- **Dynamic renography** uses radiolabelled tracers that are excreted rapidly by the kidneys—their arrival, uptake and elimination over a 30-minute period are imaged using a gamma camera. Commonly used isotopes are $^{99m}$Tc-DTPA and $^{99m}$Tc-MAG3. This test gives useful information on degree of obstruction, relative renal function, and renal artery stenosis and is also used in assessment of the perfusion, filtration, and drainage of renal transplants.

# Renal biopsy

## Indications for renal biopsy
When deciding on whether to perform a renal biopsy, the benefits in terms of diagnosis and informing management must be weighed against the potential risks for that patient. In general, indications are

- Acute kidney injury (except in the context of multi-organ failure and/or prolonged hypotension, where ATN is the most common diagnosis).
- Persistent proteinuria >1g per 24 hours.
- Nephrotic syndrome in adults.
- Steroid-resistant nephrotic syndrome in children.
- Acute nephritic syndrome (constellation of haematuria (with or without red cell casts), hypertension, variable degree of proteinuria with renal insufficiency and oliguria).
- Renal involvement in systemic disorders.
- Chronic progressive renal impairment (except in diabetes with a typical course).
- Non-visible haematuria with >0.5g proteinuria per 24 hours.
- Renal transplant management.

## Contraindications to biopsy

*Absolute contraindications*

- Uncorrected bleeding diathesis.
- Uncorrected hypertension (>160/90mmHg).

*Relative contraindications*

- Single functioning kidney.
- Small kidneys <9cm (histology from small kidneys often just shows chronic damage with no identifiable cause, and the risks are considerably higher).
- Infection (risk of abscess formation).
- Renal mass or cysts.
- Uncooperative patient, when, if deemed essential, a biopsy may need to be undertaken under general anaesthetic

## Complications of renal biopsy

- Inadequate tissue (5–10%).
- Adjacent organ trauma (1%).
- Bleeding (non-visible haematuria 100%; gross haematuria 5–10%; perinephric haematoma).
- Arteriovenous fistula (15–18%; 1% require intervention).
- Nephrectomy and/or death.

## Procedure
The biopsy is performed under local anaesthesia and sedation is not usually required. With the patient lying prone, one kidney is localized with ultrasound. A needle biopsy (usually 16 gauge) is taken from the lower pole of the kidney with the patient holding their breath in exhalation (prevents the kidney moving). The patient is asked to lie supine for 4–6 hours after the procedure. Increasingly this procedure is now undertaken as a day case in those patients with otherwise uncomplicated histories/comorbidities.

# 17.5 Acute kidney injury

## Background

The terms acute kidney injury (AKI) and acute renal failure are often used interchangeably although AKI is now the preferred term. This is a significant cause of in-hospital morbidity and mortality and has multiple aetiologies (see Section 1.11).

Early recognition and management is essential to prevent life-threatening biochemical and volume derangement.

## Definition

- Rapid fall in GFR.
- May be accompanied by oliguria (<300mL urine/day) or anuria.
- Rises in serum urea and creatinine occur only once GFR has fallen by 50%—these are insensitive and late indicators.
- Studies are underway trying to identify **biomarkers** (serum or urine) that are **early** predictors of AKI.

Candidate biomarkers identified to date include:
- Kidney injury molecule-1 (KIM-1).
- Neutrophil gelatinase-associated lipocalin (NGAL).
- Interleukin-18 (IL-18).
- Fatty-acid binding proteins (FABPs).
- Cystatin C.

## Classification

Research publications define AKI in differing ways (including a >50µmol/L or >25% increase in baseline serum creatinine) leading to difficulty in comparing studies, as the inclusion criteria are not identical between groups.

A lack of standard definition for AKI has led to the development of a new classification system—**RIFLE**:
- **R**isk of renal dysfunction.
- **I**njury to the kidney.
- **F**ailure of kidney function.
- **L**oss of kidney function.
- **E**SRF (end-stage renal failure).

## Epidemiology

- Increased incidence of AKI with increasing age.
- Increased risk with underlying chronic renal impairment.
- AKI complicates 13–18% of hospital admissions and is often iatrogenic (drugs, contrast medium, inadequate hydration/resuscitation).
- High mortality if renal replacement therapy is required.
- However, 60% of survivors regain normal renal function.

## Aetiology

The cause of AKI is often accurately identified by thinking of the anatomy and function of the kidney in four distinct stages:
1. Vascular: blood flows to the glomeruli (via the renal artery).
2. Glomerular: the glomeruli form an ultrafiltrate (free of protein and blood) which goes to the tubules.
3. Tubules and interstitium: the ultrafiltrate undergoes both reabsorption and secretion of solute and fluid.
4. Drainage: the final filtrate (urine) drains from the kidney via the ureters to the bladder where it is voided via the urethra.

Decreased blood flow (often called pre-renal AKI), occurs due to interruption at stage 1 and accounts for the majority of cases (~**60%**). Intrinsic renal disease (stages 2 and 3) accounts for a further **30%**, and obstruction to urine flow (post-renal AKI, stage 4) occurs in ~**10%**. Also see Table 17.1.

### Pre-renal AKI

- Autoregulation within the renal vasculature usually protects the glomeruli from variations in systemic blood pressure.
- At persisting low extremes of blood pressure (SBP usually <70mmHg), autoregulation is impaired and leading to poor perfusion and glomerular dysfunction
- Exacerbating factors include:
  - NSAIDs (reduce prostaglandin levels/afferent vasodilatation).
  - ACE inhibitors/ARBs (reduce angiotensin II/efferent vasoconstriction).
  - Renal artery stenosis or severe atherosclerotic disease.
  - Volume depletion.

| Table 17.1 Causes of acute kidney injury | | | |
|---|---|---|---|
| **Pre-renal** | **Hypovolaemia**<br>• Gastrointestinal losses<br>• Haemorrhage<br>• Excessive diuresis<br>• Extensive burns | **Hypotension**<br>• Sepsis<br>• Cardiogenic shock/failure | | |
| **Intrinsic** | **Glomerular**<br>• Autoimmune (e.g. SLE, Goodpasture disease)<br>• Drugs<br>• Infections (e.g. post-streptococcal GN<br>• Henoch–Schönlein Purpura/IgA nephropathy | **Tubular**<br>• ATN<br>• Drugs, contrast media<br>• Myoglobin (rhabdomyolysis)<br>• Crystals (ethylene glycol, urate)<br>• Hypercalcaemia<br>• Light chains/cast nephropathy (myeloma) | **Interstitial nephritis**<br>• Drugs (NSAIDs, antibiotics)<br>• Lymphoma<br>• Granulomatous (tuberculosis, sarcoid)<br>• Infection (pyelonephritis)<br>• Acute phosphate nephropathy (following phosphate-containing bowel prep.)<br>• Tumour lysis syndrome (following chemotherapy) | **Vascular**<br>• Vasculitis (e.g. granulomatosis with polyangiitis (GPA))<br>• Thromboembolic disease (including cholesterol emboli)<br>• Haemolytic uraemic syndrome/thrombotic microangiopathy<br>• Malignant hypertension<br>• Scleroderma<br>• Cryoglobulinaemia<br>• Large vessel occlusion (dissection, thrombosis) |
| **Post-renal** | **Intraluminal**<br>• Calculus (e.g. staghorn)<br>• Blood clot<br>• Sloughed papilla | **Intramural**<br>• Ureteric stricture/neoplasm<br>• Prostatic hypertrophy/carcinoma<br>• Bladder carcinoma | **Extrinsic**<br>• Retroperitoneal fibrosis and periaortitis<br>• Pelvic malignancy | |

- There may be a suggestive preceding history of hypotensive episodes, new drugs, or excessive fluid losses (e.g. ileostomy, diarrhoea, vomiting).
- Clinically features of volume depletion, e.g. postural hypotension.
- Urine dipstick is usually bland.

### Intrinsic AKI
- Caused by damage to glomeruli, tubules, intrarenal vessels, or interstitium.
- Most common cause is ATN, which is the end result of a prolonged pre-renal insult.
- Enquire about drugs (including long-term medication), recent contrast medium exposure, multisystem illness, e.g. systemic lupus erythematosus, recent symptoms of infection.
- Clinically there may be signs of an underlying systemic illness.
- Urine dipstick is usually positive for varying degrees of protein, blood, and leucocytes.

### Post-renal AKI
- Although this is the least common cause of AKI, it is important not to miss as it will often be reversible.
- Obstruction can occur at any site from the renal pelvis down to the urethra.
- Urgent KUB USS (kidneys/ureter/bladder ultrasound scan) is the investigation of choice.
- Be aware of a postobstruction diuresis after the obstruction has been relieved so as to avoid an additional pre-renal injury.

## Prevention

This is essential since neither the incidence nor the outcome (morbidity/mortality) have improved significantly in recent years.
- Identify factors contributing to an 'at-risk' patient:
  - Elderly.
  - Diabetic patients.
  - Hypertension/general vascular disease.
  - Underlying chronic kidney disease.
  - Polypharmacy.
  - Dehydration.
- Good fluid management and avoidance of nephrotoxic agents are the mainstay of preventive management.
- Diuretics can be useful in hypervolaemic, oliguric AKI but do not improve renal recovery or mortality.
- There is no role for 'renal-dose' dopamine.

### Radiocontrast nephropathy
Preventative measures for the avoidance of contrast-induced nephropathy (CIN) include:
- Use of an alternative (non-contrast) investigation where possible, particularly in 'at risk' patients.
- Use of low/iso-osmolar contrast.
- Good hydration periprocedure (beneficial effect in many trials).
- The type of fluid is probably not critical but isotonic sodium bicarbonate may be better than normal saline.

- N-acetyl cysteine (NAC) has been shown in meta-analysis to be of benefit in certain subgroups of patients and some units have a policy of prescribing usually 600mg twice daily orally on day before and day of procedure.
- Renal function must be closely monitored for a few days post procedure as the time-course for development for CIN is 48–72 hours after contrast administration.

## Assessment of the patient with AKI

- **AKI is a medical emergency and so assessment should commence with ABC.**
- As part of **C**, make a volume status assessment with:
  - BP (including postural).
  - Pulse rate/volume/character.
  - Capillary refill time (should be <2 seconds).
  - Central venous pressure (JVP).
  - Urine output (catheterize).
  - Analyse fluid balance charts and daily weights (if available).

Metabolic derangement is life threatening and urgent blood samples for potassium and bicarbonate should be sent immediately.

If the patient is fluid deplete then start fluid replacement with normal saline at a rate titrated to the clinical signs and urine output. If needed, insert a central venous catheter to aid fluid replacement decisions and facilitate inotropic/vasopressor support as required in an ITU setting.

Indications for emergency dialysis:
- Persistent hyperkalaemia (K+ >7mmol/L).
- Fluid overload unresponsive to diuretic challenge.
- Pericarditis (risk of tamponade).
- Acidosis (pH <7.1, serum bicarbonate <12mmol/L).
- Symptomatic uraemia (twitching, cognitive impairment, seizures, coma, urea usually >45mmol/L).

### How acute is the renal failure?
Compare current results with historical (contact GP if necessary).

History may be suggestive of pre-existing renal disease (e.g. long-standing diabetes or vascular disease)

Chronicity **may** be indicated by:
- ↑ phosphate.
- ↓ calcium.
- ↓ haemoglobin.
- Small kidneys on USS (exception is diabetic nephropathy where renal size is usually preserved).
- ↓ corticomedullary differentiation on USS.

### Search for the aetiology
- History (especially drugs, prescribed and over-the-counter).
- Examination (e.g. fluid balance, underlying systemic disease).
- Urinalysis (microscopy for casts (GN), eosinophils (tubulointerstitial nephritis)).
- Laboratory tests as indicated (immunology screen).
- Renal USS.
- Consider renal biopsy for histopathological diagnosis.

Chronic kidney disease (CKD) is staged according to GFR:

- **Stage 1**: loss of renal reserve—GFR >90mL/min/1.73m², with evidence of renal disease, e.g. abnormal imaging or urinalysis.
- **Stage 2**: mild renal impairment—GFR 60–89mL/min/1.73m². Creatinine may be at the top end of the normal range.
- **Stage 3**: moderate renal impairment—serum creatinine and urea are out of the normal range. Stage 3A GFR 45–59mL/min/1.73m²; stage 3B GFR 30–44mL/min/1.73m²
- **Stage 4**: severe renal impairment—GFR 15–29mL/min/1.73m². Symptoms of uraemia may start during this stage. Planning for renal replacement therapy (or conservative management) should start, in particular establishing dialysis access and work up for a transplant if appropriate.
- **Stage 5**: established renal failure—GFR <15mL/min/1.73m². Renal replacement therapy (or a planned conservative management strategy) should start.

Adverse systemic effects of worsening renal function, including the development of anaemia and dysregulation of calcium metabolism, may be detected as early as CKD stage 3. The term 'chronic renal failure' should probably be reserved for stage 5 CKD, where the GFR <15mL/min/1.73m². It is at this stage that severe symptoms related to uraemia tend to occur, requiring renal replacement therapy (RRT). When RRT has been started, patients are said to have reached end-stage renal failure (ESRF).

## Epidemiology

CKD is very common, with a prevalence thought to be at least 2000 patients per million. Exact numbers are uncertain. However, national and international registries provide data on the demographics of patients on RRT. These reflect the numbers of patients with ESRF accepted for dialysis, but not the numbers of patients with CKD stage 5. Acceptance rates have been rising rapidly to:

- UK: 108/million/year in 2005 (US: 317/million/year).
- M:F = 1.5:1.
- Incidence 3–5× higher in Asian and Afro-Caribbean populations.
- 50% >65 years.

## Aetiology

- **Diabetic mellitus (DM) nephropathy:**
  - Most common cause of ESRF in developed countries—20% ESRF in the UK, 43% in the USA.
  - Even greater percentage of ESRF patients have DM—27%.
  - Ratio of type 2 DM patients to type 1 is now 4:1
- **Glomerulonephritis:**
  - Most common diagnosis in patients on RRT, despite the higher incidence of diabetic nephropathy. This difference reflects the reduced survival rates in patients with DM as a cause of their renal failure.
  - IgA nephropathy is the most common diagnosis, but other common glomerulonephritides include focal segmental glomerulosclerosis, membranous nephropathy, and mesangiocapillary glomerulonephritis.
- **Diagnosis uncertain:**
  - In 20% of patients starting on RRT in the UK (and 30% in the >65 age group), the cause of the renal therapy is unknown. This may reflect late presentation, when kidneys are small and shrunken and a biopsy is both more challenging and less informative.
  - Other common causes of ESRF include pyelonephritis, polycystic kidney disease, and hypertension (Table 17.2).

Table 17.2 Causes of end-stage renal failure in the UK (2013)

| Diagnosis | UK < 65 | UK ≥ 65 | UK all | M:F |
|---|---|---|---|---|
| Aetiology uncertain | 13.9% | 19.5% | 16% | 1:1.6 |
| Glomerulonephritis | 21.6% | 14.5% | 19% | 1:2.1 |
| Pyelonephritis | 12.8% | 7.8% | 11% | 1:1.1 |
| Diabetes | 14.8% | 17.9% | 15.9% | 1:1.6 |
| Polycystic kidney | 10.25% | 9.4% | 9.9% | 1:1.1 |
| Hypertension | 5.2% | 7.6% | 6.1% | 1:2.4 |
| Renovascular | 1% | 6.7% | 3% | 1:2.0 |
| Other | 17.8% | 13.5% | 16.2% | 1:1.3 |

- Less common causes of CKD include obstructive uropathy, chronic interstitial nephritis, e.g. sarcoidosis, and myeloma, amyloidosis and post-acute kidney injury.

## Clinical evaluation

5% patients with ESRF present as uraemic emergencies with features that may include:

- Drowsiness/coma.
- Seizures.
- Abnormal biochemistry—elevated urea (often >50mmol/L), elevated creatinine (often >1000μmol/L), hyperkalaemia, hyperphosphataemia, hypocalcaemia, and a partially compensated metabolic acidosis.
- Abnormal haematology—normochromic, normocytic anaemia, normal white cell count, low platelet count.

### History

- **Time course of illness**: often a gradual deterioration over a number of months, with fatigue, anorexia, nausea, and pruritus.
- **Possible causes**: diabetes, hypertension, obstructive uropathy, renovascular disease—these may all cause a gradual onset of renal failure. There may also be an additional factor causing an acute deterioration precipitating admission to hospital, for example:
  - Hypovolaemia, from vomiting/diarrhoea, or iatrogenic from surgery or diuretics.
  - Drugs, e.g. NSAIDS and ACE inhibitors, which may cause an acute reduction in GFR. Several drugs can cause a tubulointerstitial nephritis.
  - Infection.

### Examination

- Signs of chronic renal impairment:
  - Pruritic rash.
  - Pericardial rub.
  - Asterixis.
  - Ammoniacal smell to the breath.
- Signs of the underlying disease, e.g.:
  - Generalized vascular disease.
  - Vasculitic rash.
  - Palpable kidneys (polycystic kidneys).
  - Palpable bladder (outflow obstruction).

### Investigations

In a newly diagnosed patient with CKD, investigations are partly diagnostic and partly designed to help assess the stage and degree of complications of CKD:

- Biochemical:

- eGFR (calculated 'estimated' GFR).
- Calcium, phosphate, and PTH levels.
- Cholesterol and triglyceride levels.
- Haematological:
  - Haemoglobin.
  - Iron status (ferritin, transferrin saturation).
- Radiological:
  - Ultrasound renal tract.
  - Chest radiograph (to assess cardiothoracic ratio and lung fields).
- Immunological:
  - If clinically indicated.
- Cardiological:
  - Electrocardiogram—a routine but insensitive marker of left ventricular hypertrophy and ischaemia.
  - Echocardiography—a more sensitive test of left ventricular dysfunction.
- Virological:
  - Prior to RRT, hepatitis B and C status should be ascertained. Hepatitis surface antigen requires the patient to be haemodialysed in isolation, and the presence of hepatitis C antibodies or RNA will signal a requirement for a dedicated machine. HIV status will also be checked in view of a potential risk to staff and other patients.

# Management of CKD

As patients progress from CKD stage 3 to ESRF, they require careful supervision by a renal physician to both slow progression as much as possible and to manage the complications of CKD.

- **Reduction of proteinuria:** heavy protein losses (>1g/day) are associated with an increased rate of progression in many cases of CKD. Reduction of proteinuria with ACE inhibitors and angiotensin II receptor blockers can slow progression.
- **Control of blood pressure** can slow progression of CKD. For example, diabetic patients with optimal control lose GFR at a rate of 1–2mL/min/1.73m$^2$ per year, compared to a GFR loss of 8–16mL/min/1.73m$^2$ per year in those with poor blood pressure and glycaemic control.
- **Cardiovascular disease prevention:** cardiac disease is the leading cause of death in patients with ESRF, the relative risk being highest in the young. There are two likely processes underlying the cardiac disease:
  - **Uraemic vasculopathy:** stiffening of the vascular wall, probably due to medial calcium deposition, results in a widened pulse pressure with systolic hypertension.
  - **Uraemic cardiomyopathy:** pressure and volume overload lead to thickening of the left ventricular wall and increase in cavity volume. Although these are initially reversible, in the long term they result in irreversible myocardial fibrosis, compounded by calcification of the myocardium, the valves, and the conducting system. Clinically, this manifests as arrhythmias, a reduced ejection fraction, and intolerance of both fluid overload and fluid removal during dialysis.
- Prevention of these complications requires correction of recognized cardiovascular risk factors, some of which are specific to patients with CKD 4 and 5:
  - Cessation of smoking and other healthy lifestyle modifications.
  - Treatment of hypertension and limiting interdialytic fluid gains.
  - Treatment of lipid abnormalities—the Study of Heart and Renal Protection (SHARP) showed that simvastatin with ezetimibe reduced the risk of major athersclerotic events by 17%.

---

- Treatment of anaemia.
- Tight glycaemic control in patients with diabetes.
- Control of plasma calcium, phosphate and PTH levels.
- **Water and electrolyte balance:**
  - Patients with oliguric ESRF will need to restrict their daily fluid intake to 500mL (for insensible losses) plus a volume equivalent to their daily urine output. Pre-dialysis patients with CKD stages 4 and 5 generally pass normal amounts of urine, but may have an impaired ability to concentrate their urine, so need to take extra care in hot weather or during episodes of diarrhoea and vomiting.
  - Both sodium and potassium may accumulate in CKD 4 and 5. Dietary sources of both should be restricted, and appropriate dietary advice given. Both electrolytes should be monitored monthly in ESRF. See Boxes 17.2 and 17.3 for the common causes of and the management of hyperkalaemia.
- **Metabolic acidosis:** acidosis is more common in patients with interstitial renal disease who may have an acquired renal tubular acidosis. The main symptom is effort dyspnoea not explained by pulmonary oedema or anaemia. Chronic acidosis will aggravate hyperkalaemia, inhibit protein anabolism, and accelerate calcium loss from bone. Those patients who can bear an additional sodium load (i.e. not fluid overloaded) can be treated with sodium bicarbonate.

---

# Anaemia

Anaemia may occur in stage 3 CKD, but is common when GFR <30mL/min. Contributory factors are:
- Lack of endogenous erythropoietin production by the damaged kidneys.
- Uraemia has a toxic effect on bone marrow erythropoiesis.
- Hyperparathyroidism with marrow fibrosis.
- Impaired intestinal absorption of iron.

- Anorexia may result in both iron and folate deficiency.
- Reduced red cell survival as a result of haemolysis or hypersplenism.

Patients with polycystic kidney disease are less likely to be anaemic as they tend to have preserved renal production of erythropoietin.

### Erythropoietin therapy

Recombinant erythropoietin is used to treat anaemia in patients with CKD stages 3 and 4, as well as those receiving dialysis. Erythropoietin is a large glycoprotein that is inactive when given by mouth, so is given subcutaneously (or sometimes intravenously in those receiving haemodialysis). The three most common forms are:

- α-Erythropoietin, currently only given IV because of the risk of pure red cell aplasia.
- ß-Erythropoietin.
- Darbopoietin, a novel erythrocyte-stimulating protein with a long duration of action, such that it can be given weekly or even fortnightly.

Current recommendations suggest that erythropoietin should be commenced when the haemoglobin falls below 10g/dL, and the recommended target haemoglobin in dialysis patients is 11–12g/dL. Maintaining a higher haemoglobin may be associated with higher cardiovascular mortality. Iron status needs to be monitored for possible iron deficiency (serum ferritin should be at least 100ng/mL).

### Efficacy

Erythropoietin is effective in improving haemoglobin in 90–95% of patients with renal failure. The benefits include amelioration of the symptoms of anaemia, reduction in cardiac output, improved myocardial ischaemia, and reduced left ventricular mass, as well as improvements in quality of life, cognitive, and sexual function.

### Side effects

Hypertension is common, but rarely severe (when it can result in cerebrovascular disease). Other side effects include thrombosis of vascular access, clotting of dialysis lines, and hyperkalaemia. α-Erythropoietin given subcutaneously has been associated with pure red cell aplasia, thought to be caused by defective packaging and storage of the erythropoietin. In this rare condition, antibodies to both endogenous and recombinant erythropoietin result in an unresponsive, progressive anaemia requiring repeated transfusions.

---

## Renal bone disease

Both high and low bone turnover states may develop in CKD. Histological analysis may show several different conditions.

**Osteomalacia**: defective 1-α-hydroxylation in the damaged kidneys results in a functional vitamin D deficiency, which in turn leads to inadequate mineralization of the osteoid.

**Secondary hyperparathyroidism**: lack of 1-α-calcidol also leads to hypocalcaemia as a result of reduced intestinal calcium absorption, compounded by the effects of high serum phosphate as renal excretion of phosphate falls. The low serum calcium, high phosphate and low levels of 1-α-calcidol all act as triggers for the release of PTH. Elevated PTH not only has a resorptive effect on bone, but also can contribute to left ventricular hypertrophy and resistance to erythropoietin. The bone resorption with accelerated bone turnover and marrow fibrosis is called 'osteitis fibrosis cystica'. In extreme cases, proliferation of osteoclasts results in cyst formation within bone, called a Brown tumour.

- **Adynamic bone disease** is characterized by reduced trabecular bone formation and resorption. It is associated with the use of calcitriol.
- **Osteoporosis** is common in renal patients, particularly as many have been treated with corticosteroids.
- **Aluminium bone disease** is now very rare, as aluminium-containing phosphate binders are used sparingly, and water supplies for dialysis are carefully monitored.

### Management

- Directed at controlling serum calcium, phosphate, and PTH levels.
- Early monitoring of secondary hyperparathyroidism is needed and factors relevant to bone mineral metabolism should be measured regularly when the GFR drops below 30mL/minute (calcium, phosphate, albumin, alkaline phosphate monthly, PTH 3-monthly in patients with ESRF).
- **Low phosphate diet** with adequate calcium intake may suffice initially, and should be continued thereafter—patient education and compliance are critical at all stages of renal bone disease.
- **Phosphate binders** are required, taken with meals with the dose being adjusted according to the anticipated phosphate load of the meal. Calcium carbonate and calcium acetate are the most common binders in use, but the total amount of calcium ingested should be restricted to 3g/day—greater amounts may contribute to vascular calcification. Sevelamer hydrochloride is a non-calcium containing binder that binds phosphate through ion exchange. Lanthanum carbonate is a new, recently licensed phosphate binder that may also prove useful. Serum phosphate should be maintained at <1.8mmol/L
- **Suppression of PTH:** vitamin D analogues such as calcitriol and 1α-calcidol are used to treat secondary hyperparathyroidism. However, over-enthusiastic suppression of PTH should be avoided as this may result in reduced bone turnover and adynamic bone disease. The target PTH should be up to 4× the upper limit of the normal range, and serum calcium (corrected for albumin levels) should be maintained between 2.2–2.4mmol/L.

# 17.7 Renal replacement therapy

## Introduction to renal replacement therapy

Renal replacement therapy (RRT) refers to those treatments which can keep a patient alive when their own kidneys have failed and cannot remove sufficient solute, water and uraemic toxins from their bodies.

There are three modalities:

- Renal transplantation
- Haemodialysis
- Peritoneal dialysis.

At the end of 2013, there were 56,940 patients in the UK receiving RRT, of whom 52% had a functioning renal transplant, 41.6% were receiving haemodialysis and 6.4% peritoneal dialysis.

Though dialysis is a life-saving treatment it can at best provide 10–15% of normal renal excretory function. Hence the majority of patients with advanced chronic kidney disease will only commence dialysis once their GFR has fallen to <10mL/minute.

Transplantation should be considered for patients with progressive renal failure in whom it is anticipated that dialysis will commence within 6 months. It is the optimal treatment for ESRF for a number of reasons:

- It allows greater clearance of solute, water, and uraemic toxins when compared to dialysis.
- It replaces all kidney functions, including the endocrine processes of erythropoietin production and the hydroxylation of 25-hydroxy cholecalciferol.
- Patients with a functioning transplant can expect greater life expectancy and quality of life compared to those who are maintained on dialysis.

However, kidney transplantation is a major undertaking involving an operation, as well as a lifelong burden of immunosuppression. It is not a treatment that can be offered to all patients with ESRF; the elderly, the frail, and those with multiple comorbidities are unlikely to withstand the rigours of this therapy.

# 17.8 Renal transplantation

## Epidemiology

- At the end of 2013 there were ~29,600 patients in the UK with a functioning renal transplant.
- The median age of this population is 52.8 years with a ♂:♀ ratio of 1.6:1.
- There are approximately a further 9000 patients on the renal transplant waiting list.
- Unfortunately the supply of donor kidneys for transplantation is insufficient to meet the demand; in 2013, there were 3,257 kidney or kidney plus other organ transplants performed.
- Consequently the average time patients spend on the waiting list has been increasing and currently stands at 3 years.

## Principles

- Kidney transplantation is the optimal treatment for ESRF as it completely restores renal function.
- Patient survival following renal transplantation is better compared to age-matched controls who are on the transplant waiting list.
- The key understanding that has made transplantation possible is the recognition that the immune system will reject tissue it recognizes as non-self—i.e. an allograft. In order to prevent this event several measures are undertaken:
  1. Preoperatively:
     - The donor and recipient are matched for histocompatibility antigens, to reduce the immune response to the graft.
     - Recipient serum is mixed with donor lymphocytes. This is known as the complement-dependent cytotoxic cross-match and will detect pre-formed antibodies which would precipitate hyperacute rejection of the graft.
  2. Peri/postoperatively: the immune system is suppressed with drugs.

## Evaluation of recipients

Potential recipients undergo careful assessment to determine if they are suitable candidates for renal transplantation. Special attention is given to looking for cardiovascular disease as 50% of deaths occurring within 30 days of transplantation are due to ischaemic heart disease. Coronary artery disease must be treated before a patient can be listed.

Conditions which are considered absolute contraindications to transplantation are:
- Active malignancy.
- Active systemic infection.
- Any condition with a life expectancy <2 years.

## Timing of transplantation

Patients can be placed on the transplant waiting list once they are within 6 months of needing to start dialysis. Ideally patients should receive a kidney before they need to start dialysis (pre-emptive transplantation) as this leads to better outcomes (graft survival) compared to individuals who spend >2 years on dialysis before receiving an organ.

## Donor kidneys

There are three potential sources of donor organs
- Live donors (33.8% (2013) of kidney transplants). They may be genetically related (e.g. siblings/parents) or unrelated

(e.g. spouse) to the patient. Altruistic donation is now also available in the UK (early stages).
- Cadaveric heart beating donors (41.8% (2013) of kidney transplants). The organs are retrieved from patients who fulfil the criteria for brain death.
- Cadaveric non-heart beating donors (24.4% (2013) of kidney transplants). Organs taken from these patients have higher rates of delayed graft function and primary non-function.

## Surgery

The transplant kidney is placed extraperitoneally in the iliac fossa. The renal artery and vein are anastomosed to the external iliac vessels. The donor ureter is implanted into the recipient's bladder.

## Immunosuppression

Drugs are given in two stages to prevent graft rejection:
- **Induction therapy:** basiliximab and daclizumab are monoclonal antibodies which block the IL-2 receptor. This prevents IL-2-dependent T-cell activation and proliferation.
- **Maintenance therapy** (see Table 17.3): this often utilizes a combination of a calcineurin inhibitor (CNI, ciclosporin, or tacrolimus), an antimetabolite (azathioprine or mycophenolate) and steroids. However, there is wide variation in the immunosuppressive protocols used by different transplant units.

When possible, immunosuppression should be tailored for individual patients with the aim of minimizing side effects whilst still providing protection against rejection.

## Complications

### Early (<3 months post transplantation)
- **Graft thrombosis:**
  - Usually due to anatomical problems such as a stenosis at the venous or arterial anastomosis.
  - Presents with graft tenderness and reduced urine output. Usually requires graft nephrectomy.
- **Obstruction:**
  - May be due to ischaemia of the distal donor ureter leading to fibrosis and stenosis.
  - Can also occur as a consequence of fluid collections (e.g. lymphocoele) causing extrinsic compression or kinking of the ureter.
- **Acute rejection:**
  - Occurs in 20–25% cases (Fig. 17.6).
  - A diagnosis of rejection can only be made on the basis of a renal biopsy.
  - The first-line treatment is three pulses of intravenous methylprednisolone. 90% of cases will respond to this.
  - Steroid-resistant rejection requires treatment either with equine polyclonal antibodies—antithymocyte globulin (ATG), or murine anti–CD3 monoclonal antibodies (OKT3).
- **Infection:**
  - There is a significant risk of opportunistic infection as a consequence of immunosuppression.
  - The most common organism is *Cytomegalovirus* (CMV). This can present simply with fever or with invasive disease including pneumonitis, colitis and retinitis. Treatment is with a prolonged course of intravenous ganciclovir for severe cases, or oral valganciclovir for less seriously ill patients.

Table 17.3 Immunosuppressive agents frequently used in the field of renal transplantation and their common side effects

| Drug | Mechanism of action | Side effects | Important drug interactions |
|---|---|---|---|
| Steroids | Multiple immunosuppressive and anti-inflammatory effects, including blockade of cytokine gene expression. | Hypertension Diabetogenic Hyperlipidaemia Osteoporosis Avascular necrosis Cataracts | |
| Ciclosporin | Calcineurin inhibitor Blocks IL-2 production preventing T-cell activation and proliferation. | Nephrotoxic Hypertension Diabetogenic Gum hypertrophy Hirsutism | Both calcineurin inhibitors are metabolized by the cytochrome P450 IIIA pathway.<br>  P450 inducers reduce CNI levels<br>    ● Rifampicin, rifabutin<br>    ● Barbiturates, phenytoin, carbamazepine<br>  P450 inhibitors increase CNI levels<br>    ● Calcium channel blockers<br>    ● Antifungal agents<br>    ● Macrolide antibiotics<br>Grapefruit juice increases absorption of CNIs<br>Statins in conjunction with ciclosporin increase the risk of myopathy and rhabdomyolysis. |
| Tacrolimus | Calcineurin inhibitor Blocks IL-2 production preventing T-cell activation and proliferation. | Nephrotoxic Tremor Hypertension Diabetogenic | |
| Sirolimus | Inhibits molecular target of rapamycin (mTOR) which is a kinase involved in cell proliferation. | Impaired wound healing Leucopaenia Thrombocytopaenia Hyperlipidaemia Mouth ulcers Pneumonitis | Similar interactions to CNIs Sirolimus can potentiate CNI-induced nephrotoxicity |
| Azathioprine | Acts as a purine analogue. Inhibits nucleic acid synthesis and so prevents lymphocyte proliferation. | Myelosuppression Hepatotoxicity | Allopurinol inhibits xanthine oxidase leading to higher functional levels of azathioprine causing severe bone marrow suppression. |
| Mycophenolate mofetil | Inhibits inosine monophosphate dehydrogenase preventing purine synthesis by lymphocytes. | Myelosuppression Diarrhoea Gastritis/oesophagitis | Absorption reduced by iron sulphate and antacids. Ciclosporin reduces mycophenolic acid levels. |

697

- *Pneumocystis* pneumonia is less common but is associated with high morbidity and mortality (Fig. 17.7). All patients should receive co-trimoxazole prophylaxis for the first 6 months post transplant.

### Late (>3 months post transplantation)

- **Cardiovascular disease:** cardiac disease is responsible for 16% of deaths in renal transplant recipients. The use of CNIs contributes to cardiovascular risk by causing hypertension and dyslipidaemia.
- **Malignancy:** the burden of immunosuppression predisposes to two cancers in particular:
  - Skin: patients should be advised to minimize sunlight exposure, and use sun protection factor.
  - Post-transplant lymphoproliferative disease (PTLD): this may be associated with Epstein–Barr virus (EBV). Treatment usually involves a reduction in immunosuppression and referral to haematology to start chemotherapy.

- **Infection:** this is the most common cause of death in renal transplant recipients.
- **New-onset diabetes after transplantation (NODAT):** up to 15% of renal transplant recipients will develop diabetes. This is particularly related to steroid use and CNIs (which are toxic to pancreatic islet cells).
- **Progressive renal failure:** the 10-year graft survival for a kidney transplant is 50%. Grafts fail for a number of reasons:
  - CNI toxicity.
  - Chronic allograft nephropathy (chronic rejection).

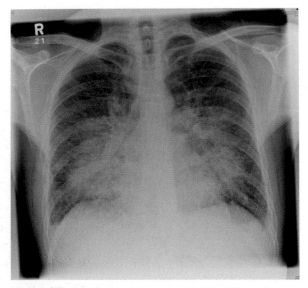

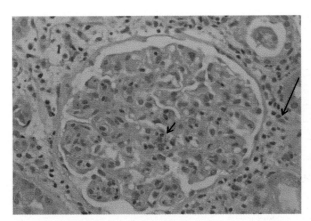

**Fig. 17.6** Acute rejection in a renal allograft. There is stasis of mononuclear cells in the glomerular capillary lumens (small arrow) and several neutrophils are seen. Capillaritis is present in the surrounding interstitium (long arrow).

**Fig. 17.7** A chest x-ray demonstrating the typical 'bats-wing' appearance of *Pneumocystis* pneumonia in a renal transplant recipient. Courtesy of Cambridge University Hospitals NHS Foundation Trust's Radiology dept.

| Table 17.4 1- and 5-year survival rates for deceased donor renal transplantation in the UK (2013) | | | |
|---|---|---|---|
| 1-year survival % | | 5-year survival % | |
| Patient | Graft | Patient | Graft |
| 96 | 93 | 89 | 85 |

- Infection (e.g. BK virus).
- Recurrence of original disease.
- The complications of chronic kidney disease must be addressed, and the patient prepared for either dialysis or another transplant once their own graft fails.

## Outcomes

- Table 17.4 shows outcomes of renal transplantation in the UK.
- On average a kidney from a deceased donor will last 10 years, and a kidney from a live donor will last 13 years.

# 17.9 Haemodialysis

## Epidemiology

- Haemodialysis is the most common form of RRT worldwide.
- In 2012, > 2 million patients worldwide were maintained on this life-saving treatment.
- In the UK there are currently ~24,000 patients receiving regular haemodialysis.
- The median age of this population is 65 years with a ♂:♀ ratio of 1.5:1.

## Principles

- The aim of haemodialysis is to remove excess solute, fluid, and uraemic toxins from patients with acute kidney injury or ESRF.
- Blood from the patient passes through an extra-corporeal circuit into one compartment of a dialyser.
- Flowing countercurrent to this in a separate compartment is dialysis fluid (dialysate).
- The two compartments are separated by a semipermeable membrane, and movement of molecules across this is governed by two transport mechanisms:
  - **Diffusion:** small-molecular-weight molecules move across the membrane from areas of high concentration to low concentration. The use of countercurrent flow within the dialyser maintains the concentration gradient which drives this process. As the dialysate does not contain metabolic waste products, these are rapidly removed from the bloodstream. Furthermore, by adjusting the chemical composition of the dialysate, the patient's electrolytes can be corrected.

- **Ultrafiltration:** water is driven across the membrane from the blood compartment to the dialysate compartment through a combination of hydrostatic and osmotic forces. This creates a convection current which drags solute and larger-molecular-weight molecules across the membrane.

## Technical aspects

Haemodialysis is a technology-dependent treatment that requires careful monitoring. Consequently most haemodialysis occurs in a hospital setting although home dialysis is increasingly being undertaken after suitable training.

### Access

Haemodialysis requires blood flows of 300–400mL/min through the dialyser. Hence reliable vascular access is a pre-requisite and may take the form of:

- Arteriovenous fistula (AVF)—created by anastomosing an artery with a vein, usually at the forearm (radiocephalic AVF) or antecubital fossa (brachiocephalic AVF) (Fig. 17.8). The vein arterializes, providing adequate blood flow and allowing repeated puncture with large-bore dialysis needles.
- Double-lumen dialysis catheters. These may be tunnelled (permanent) or non-tunnelled (temporary) and can be placed in internal jugular, subclavian, or femoral veins (Fig. 17.9).
- Synthetic grafts—plastic tubes placed between an artery and a vein.

It is well recognized that AVFs are the most reliable form of long-term access. They are associated with the lowest morbidity and mortality, largely because of a lower risk of infection.

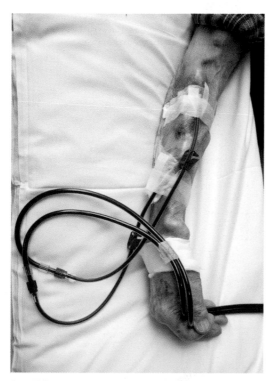
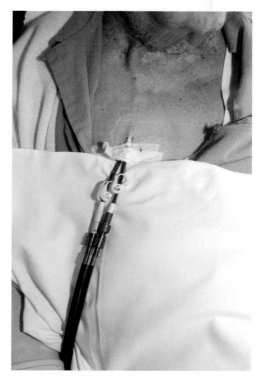

**Figs. 17.8 (left) and 17.9 (right):** A dialysis radiocephalic arteriovenous fistula and a tunnelled right internal jugular permacath, respectively, in use during intermittent haemodialysis.
Reproduced with permission from Cambridge University Hospitals NHS Foundation Trust.

### Dialysis machine

The chief purpose of the dialysis machine is to ensure patient safety. It incorporates a series of blood pump controllers, pressure alarms, blood leak detectors, and air leak detectors.

### Dialyser

This consists of two compartments for blood and dialysate separated by the dialysis membrane. The membrane may be composed of cellulose or synthetic material such as polysulfone. When choosing a dialyser, consideration is given to its biocompatibility and transport properties.

## Dialysis prescription

The standard dialysis prescription has three parameters:

- **Duration and frequency of sessions**: in most UK centres, patients have three haemodialysis sessions per week, each lasting 4 hours.
- **Fluid removal**: all dialysis patients have a prescribed 'target weight' at which they are considered to be euvolaemic. Over the course of a dialysis session, up to 4L of water can be taken off a patient to achieve this.
- **Anticoagulation**: heparin is used to prevent clotting of the extracorporeal blood circuit. A common prescription is a bolus of 1000 units at the start of dialysis, followed by a maintenance infusion of 1000 units/hour; although, increasingly, low-molecular weight heparin (LMWH) is replacing heparin infusions.

## Dialysis adequacy

To determine whether a patient is receiving adequate haemodialysis relies upon two assessments:

- **Clinical**: patients who are under-dialysed may have a constellation of symptoms including fatigue, anorexia, nausea, vomiting, pruritus, restless legs, peripheral neuropathy, and pericarditis. These arise due to the accumulation of uraemic toxins.
- **Biochemical**: this uses mathematical formulae to calculate the amount of urea removed during each session. The simplest formula is the urea reduction ratio (URR):

$$\text{URR} = (\text{Urea pre} - \text{Urea post})/\text{Urea pre} \times 100\%$$

A ratio consistently >65% is considered satisfactory for those dialysing 3× per week. There is an increased mortality rate for patients who fail to achieve this target. As with peritoneal dialysis (see Section 17.10) adequacy may also be assessed by measuring urea clearance (Kt/V).

If the dialysis dose is considered inadequate, it can be increased either by prolonging the length of time spent on haemodialysis each week, or by improving dialysis efficiency (through increased blood flow, or using a larger dialyser).

## Clinical management

Dialysis patients are prone to intercurrent illnesses and have higher hospitalization rates than the general population. There are a number of factors that should be considered when caring for them:

- Avoid damaging potential sites for dialysis access. As a general rule, only use veins on the back of the hand for cannulation.
- Anaemia is common amongst dialysis patients. If they require a blood transfusion, this should ideally be given during dialysis to avoid hyperkalaemia (from red cell haemolysis), and to prevent precipitation of pulmonary oedema.
- Many patients on dialysis will be anuric. Careful management of fluid balance is mandatory to prevent fluid overload. This requires careful clinical examination, daily weights, and review of input/output charts. Most haemodialysis patients will not require maintenance intravenous fluids.

## Complications

### Intradialytic

- **Dialysis associated hypotension:**
  - This is common occurring in up to 25% of dialysis procedures.
  - It arises due to fluid removal on dialysis being either excessive or too rapid, leading to intravascular volume depletion and tissue hypoperfusion.
  - Symptoms include muscle cramps, vomiting, chest pain, and confusion.
  - Treatment involves stopping further fluid removal and giving a bolus of normal saline.
  - Hypotension can be prevented by encouraging greater adherence to prescribed fluid intake, resetting the patient's target weight, reducing the rate of fluid removal (longer sessions), and omitting antihypertensive drugs on dialysis days.
- **Dialyser reactions:**
  - Type A: rare but life-threatening anaphylactic reactions to ethylene oxide which is used to sterilize dialysers. Patients must be taken off dialysis and treated with steroids and antihistamines. Adrenaline intramuscularly may be required.
  - Type B: more common but less severe reactions to the dialyser membrane. These are characterized by chest pain and back pain occurring 30–60 minutes into the dialysis session. They can be alleviated by using more biocompatible membranes (synthetic rather than cellulose).
- **Disequilibrium syndrome:**
  - Occurs if blood urea levels are reduced too quickly leading to an osmotic imbalance across the blood–brain barrier and hence cerebral oedema.
  - Patients complain of headaches, blurred vision, and nausea. Seizures or coma may occur in severe cases.
  - Usually only a problem for patients who are starting haemodialysis, and can be avoided by aiming for only a 30% reduction in serum urea levels for the first few sessions.
- **Air embolism** (rare).

### Long term

- **Cardiovascular disease:** this is the most common cause of death (25%) in dialysis patients. There are a number of factors which promote cardiac disease:
  - Traditional atherogenic risk factors.
  - Chronic inflammation.
  - Vascular calcification as a consequence of abnormal mineral metabolism.
  - Left ventricular hypertrophy due to hypertension and fluid overload.
- **Infection:** 20% of deaths in dialysis patients occur due to infection. Many of these are a direct complication of intravascular catheter use. Bacteria may spread haematogeneously to cause:
  - Endocarditis.
  - Discitis.
- **Amyloidosis:**
  - β2 microglobulin is a protein which is not removed by most conventional methods of haemodialysis. As it accumulates it polymerizes, resulting in deposits of amyloid.
  - Patients may present with polyarthropathy, nerve compression syndromes, polyneuropathy, and subcutaneous deposits.

# 17.10 Peritoneal dialysis

## Epidemiology

- Currently there are ~3,600 patients on peritoneal dialysis (PD) in the UK.
- The median age of this population is 60 years with a ♂:♀ ratio of 1.5:1.
- There has been a steady fall in the proportion of patients with ESRF maintained on peritoneal dialysis in the UK over the last decade. The cause for this in part relates to increased provision of haemodialysis, as well as concerns over the long-term safety of peritoneal dialysis.

## Principles

- As with haemodialysis, the purpose of peritoneal dialysis is to remove solute, toxins and water from the body.
- In this technique the peritoneum is used as the semipermeable membrane.
- It separates blood within peritoneal membrane capillaries from dialysis fluid within the peritoneal space.
- A silicone catheter placed into the peritoneal cavity is used to instil dialysis fluid.
- Molecules move from blood to the dialysate through the following mechanisms:
  - **Osmosis**: water removal occurs through a process of osmosis. The peritoneal dialysis fluid is hypertonic due to a high dextrose concentration. This exerts an osmotic pressure gradient which draws water from the capillary space into the peritoneal space. A number of dextrose concentrations are available (e.g. 1.36%, 2.27% and 3.86%) and other non-glucose based fluids are also available (e.g. icodextrin). Greater fluid removal can be achieved through the use of more hypertonic solutions.
  - **Convection**: the movement of water creates a current which 'drags' both small and large molecules across the peritoneum into the dialysate.
  - **Diffusion**: small solutes such as sodium, potassium, urea and creatinine move across the membrane due to the concentration gradient that exists between blood and dialysis fluid.

## Technical aspects

Peritoneal dialysis is a simple, low technology process compared to haemodialysis. The patient is responsible for performing the treatment themselves giving them a sense of autonomy and control. Peritoneal dialysis can be performed at home or work, hence providing flexibility and allowing the patient to fit the treatment around their lifestyle.

## Access

- The peritoneal dialysis catheter (Tenckhoff catheter) may be inserted surgically, laparoscopically or using the Seldinger technique.
- It lies in the peritoneal cavity with the tip sited in the pelvis. It leaves the peritoneal cavity in the midline and runs in a subcutaneous tunnel, exiting from the anterior abdominal wall (Fig. 17.10).
- There are two Dacron cuffs; the deep one lies over the rectus sheath, and the superficial one lies 2–3cm from the exit site. These cuffs have the dual role of securing the catheter in place and preventing infection by blocking migration of bacteria along the tunnel.

## Modalities

PD can be performed in two ways:

### Continuous ambulatory peritoneal dialysis (CAPD)

- Dialysis fluid is constantly present within the peritoneal cavity.
- The patient performs four or five manual exchanges each day using gravity to drain fluid into and out of the abdomen.

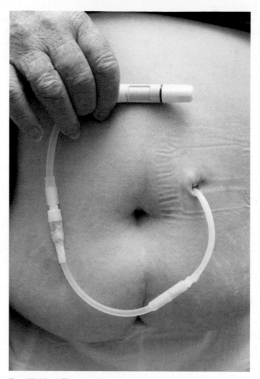

**Fig. 17.10** A Tenckhoff peritoneal dialysis catheter *in situ*. Reproduced with permission from Cambridge University Hospitals NHS Foundation Trust.

- The volume of fluid used varies between 1.5L and 3L.
- The duration of each dwell is 4–5 hours, with a longer period overnight.

### Automated peritoneal dialysis (APD)

- This utilizes a cycler machine which automatically exchanges between 1.5 and 2.5L of fluid into and out of the peritoneal cavity overnight.
- Normally between 4 and 6 exchanges occur with short dwell times.
- After the last cycle, fluid is left in situ until the patient goes back onto the machine the next evening.
- This frees them from having to perform daytime exchanges of dialysis fluid.

## Peritoneal membrane

The transport characteristics of the peritoneum will vary from patient to patient. This has implications for which PD modality is most appropriate for a given patient.

- 'High transporters' have more permeable membranes:
  - Solute and toxins will move rapidly into dialysate.
  - However, the osmotic gradient driving fluid removal dissipates rapidly in these patients due to the absorption of glucose into the bloodstream. Hence fluid removal can be an issue.
  - Patients with this membrane type are more suited to short frequent fluid dwells, i.e. APD
- 'Low transporters' have less permeable membranes:
  - Hence solute and toxin clearance requires long fluid dwells.
  - These patients will perform better on CAPD.

## Contraindications to PD

*Absolute*

- Previous extensive abdominal surgery.
- Presence of colostomy or ileostomy.
- Documented loss of peritoneal membrane function.

*Relative*

- Abdominal hernias.
- Diverticular disease.
- Severe COPD.
- Inability to perform technique.

## Dialysis adequacy

- Two biochemical indices are measured to assess if patients on PD are receiving sufficient dialysis: Creatinine clearance and urea clearance (Kt/V).
- Failure to achieve a minimum threshold is associated with increased morbidity and mortality. Under-dialysed patients require changes to their peritoneal dialysis prescription to improve solute clearance.
- This can be done either by changing the modality of PD, or increasing dwell volumes and times.
- If patients cannot achieve adequate clearance despite optimization of their prescription, they need to switch to haemodialysis.

## Complications

*Infection*

- **Peritonitis:**
  - This is the most common complication of PD with an average occurrence rate of one per 24 patient months.
  - Patients usually present with abdominal pain, fever and cloudy bags of dialysis fluid.
  - The diagnosis is confirmed by the finding of a white blood cell count >100/mm³ with >50% neutrophils in the PD effluent, or a positive culture from the dialysis fluid.
  - Gram-positive organisms (*Staphylococcus epidermidis* and *Staphylococcus aureus*) account for 70% of cases. Gram-negative organisms are responsible in 25% and fungi in 2–3%.
  - Treatment involves antibiotics for 2 weeks given intraperitoneally. Failure to respond within 5 days (or the presence of fungal peritonitis) warrants removal of the PD catheter and switching to haemodialysis.
- **Exit site infections:**
  - Characterized by erythema and purulent discharge from the catheter exit site.
  - *Staphylococcus aureus* and *Pseudomonas aeruginosa* are the most common organisms involved. Treatment is with appropriate oral antibiotics.
  - Prevention of infection is achieved by intensive training of patients, emphasizing the importance of catheter care. The application of topical antibiotics (e.g. mupirocin or gentamicin) to the exit site reduces the frequency of infective complications.

*Mechanical*

- **Poor dialysis fluid drainage:**
  - Often due to constipation which can be treated with laxatives.

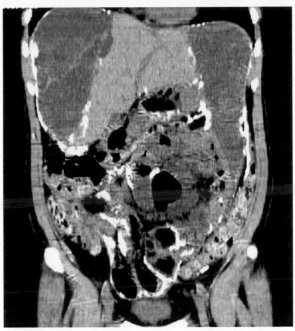

**Fig. 17.11** A coronal section CT scan of the abdomen in a patient with encapsulating peritoneal sclerosis demonstrating extensive peritoneal calcification.

- If the catheter is incorrectly sited, laparoscopic repositioning or catheter replacement may be required.
- **Hernias**: these arise due to raised intraperitoneal pressure and require surgical correction.
- **Dialysis fluid leaks**: these may cause pleural effusions (diaphragmatic leaks), abdominal wall oedema (fluid leak through the peritoneal exit site) or scrotal oedema (inguinal leaks).

*Ultrafiltration failure*

- If the peritoneal membrane becomes too permeable, an osmotic gradient cannot be maintained to allow sufficient fluid removal. The consequences to the patient are refractory hypertension and chronic volume overload.

*Encapsulating peritoneal sclerosis (EPS)*

- This is a life-threatening complication of PD.
- There is progressive inflammation of the peritoneum resulting in sheets of fibrous tissue which encase, bind and constrict the bowel, thereby compromising intestinal motility and function (Fig. 17.11).
- The aetiology remains unclear, but EPS is associated with a prolonged duration of treatment with PD.
- Patients may present with abdominal pain, bloodstained dialysis fluid or bowel obstruction.
- Treatment involves switching from PD to HD and resting the bowel. The use of tamoxifen can be considered. Surgery may be required.
- The mortality rate is >30%.

# 17.11 Nephrotic syndrome

## Background

Nephrotic syndrome (NS) is a common renal problem necessitating referral to a nephrologist. There are many different aetiologies and often significant complications. Most patients will require a renal biopsy for histopathological confirmation of the underlying renal disorder as this will affect treatment decisions.

## Definition

- Heavy proteinuria (>3.5g/day or >350mg/mmol on spot urine protein/creatinine ratio (PCR)).
- Hypoalbuminaemia (usually <25g/L).
- Oedema.

## Pathophysiology

Glomerular proteinuria is responsible for the loss of urinary protein in the nephrotic syndrome. This occurs due to increased filtration across the glomerular capillary wall caused (mainly) by podocyte pathology. The principal plasma protein lost is albumin although others (including clotting inhibitors) also contribute to the clinical picture which can include increased thrombotic risk. An immune aetiology for the glomerular injury is often implicated in primary glomerular disease.

### Oedema

The pathophysiology is not fully understood and there are broadly two prevailing theories:

1. Low plasma oncotic pressure caused by the urinary loss of proteins causes intravascular volume depletion activating the RAA system and sympathetic nervous system promoting sodium and water retention.
2. Primary intrarenal processes alone cause sodium retention and oedema without a significant transcapillary oncotic pressure gradient.

## Aetiology

The frequency of the various aetiologies depends on race and age (e.g. a Caucasian man >50 years old is likely to have membranous disease, whereas patients of African descent are more likely to have focal segmental glomerulosclerosis (FSGS)). See Table 17.5.

## Presentation

- Asymptomatic (identified on routine urinalysis).
- Oedema (peripheral, periorbital).

- 'Frothy' urine due to high protein content.
- Complication (e.g. thromboembolism).
- Symptoms/signs of underlying disease, e.g. diabetes.

## History

- Symptoms of underlying disease.
- Risk factors for hepatitis/HIV.
- Drug history (including 'over the counter' medication).
- Travel history.
- Family history (important for FSGS).

## Diagnosis

- Laboratory tests usually confirm the presence of NS but do not usually identify the aetiology.
- Laboratory investigations:
  - U&E, LFT, albumin, calcium/phosphate, CRP.
  - Lipids, glucose.
  - FBC, coagulation, ESR.
  - ANA, dsDNA. ANCA.
  - Complement levels (C3/C4).
  - Immunoglobulins, serum protein electrophoresis, serum light chains, urinary Bence Jones protein.
  - Hepatitis B/C, HIV (informed consent essential).
  - Quantify the proteinuria with a spot urine sample for PCR.
  - Urine dipstick—the presence of haematuria suggests a glomerulonephritis. Send a MSU to exclude infection.
- USS kidneys:
  - Assess renal size.
  - Exclude renal vein thrombosis (known complication) although a CT scan is more sensitive.
- CXR (may detect a neoplasm—possible cause of a secondary membranous nephropathy).
- Renal biopsy is usually mandatory (the exception being childhood NS where the diagnosis is likely to be minimal change disease and a trial of steroids is undertaken with biopsy reserved for steroid-unresponsive disease).

## Treatment

Treat the underlying disease (if identified), e.g.:
- Immunosuppressants in SLE.
- Antivirals in hepatitis/HIV.
- Surgery/chemotherapy/radiotherapy (neoplasms).

Primary glomerular disease is currently the subject of intense research and a number of clinical trials. Please see the following sections for glomerular disease-specific therapies.

## Complications of nephrotic syndrome (and their management)

- Oedema:
  - Salt/water restriction.
  - Diuretics (furosemide—IV if absorption is poor secondary to gut oedema, bumetanide, or metolazone).
- Hypercholesterolaemia: statins.

Table 17.5 Primary and secondary causes of nephrotic syndrome

| Primary glomerular disease | Secondary causes |
| --- | --- |
| <ul><li>Minimal change disease</li><li>Membranous nephropathy</li><li>Focal segmental glomerulosclerosis (FSGS)</li><li>Mesangiocapillary (membranoproliferative) glomerulonephritis</li><li>IgA nephropathy</li></ul> | <ul><li>Diabetes mellitus</li><li>Amyloid</li><li>Drugs (including NSAIDs, ACE inhibitors, gold, antibiotics)</li><li>Infections (including hepatitis B & C, HIV, malaria)</li><li>Systemic lupus erythematosus</li><li>Malignancy (e.g. lymphoproliferative disorders and breast, lung, gastric, and colon cancer)</li></ul> |

- Prothrombotic tendency:
  - Significant cause of morbidity and mortality.
  - Risk varies depending on the aetiology (high risk with membranous disease and amyloid; lower risk with steroid-responsive minimal change disease).
  - Give aspirin and consider warfarin (usually if albumin <20g/L).
- Infection (increased risk due to loss of IgG): consider vaccination (especially pneumoncoccal—capsular organism).
- Malnutrition: nutritional support.

- Acute kidney injury: this is uncommon but can be induced by excessive diuresis, renal vein thrombosis, interstitial nephritis, or severe sepsis; may require RRT.

*Proteinuria*

- Persistent proteinuria is a predictor of progression to renal failure.
- ACE inhibitors and ARBs both reduce proteinuria and should be used to minimize proteinuria.
- Indapamide and diltiazem/verapamil can also be helpful in reducing proteinuria.

## Minimal change disease

- Major cause of nephrotic syndrome both in adult and paediatric practice.
- ~90% of nephrotic syndrome occurring in children <10 years old is caused by minimal change disease (MCD) (accounts for ~15% of adult-onset NS).
- As the name suggests, there are no abnormalities on light microscopy of kidney biopsy specimens (Fig. 17.12) but on electron microscopy, foot process fusion/effacement is the characteristic pathology seen (Fig. 17.13).
- Severe deficit in glomerular selective permeability leads to massive proteinuria.

### Aetiology

*Idiopathic (primary)*

- Possible immune basis (although there is an absence of immune deposits on biopsy).
- The search for an elusive 'glomerular permeability factor' is an area of ongoing intense research.

*Secondary*

- **Drugs:** e.g. NSAIDs, antibiotics, lithium, bisphosphonates.
- **Malignancy:** especially haematological, although solid tumours can also be associated.
- **Infection:** rarely associated with tuberculosis, HIV, *Mycoplasma*, hepatitis C.
- **Allergy:** associated atopy in up to 1/3 of patients; MCD may be triggered by an allergic reaction, e.g. bee sting.
- Other glomerular diseases, e.g. SLE, IgA, diabetic nephropathy.

### Clinical presentation

- Sudden-onset of nephrotic-range proteinuria, profound hypoalbuminaemia, and massive oedema.

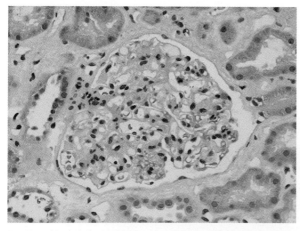

Fig. 17.12 Minimal change disease—this glomerulus shows no abnormality by light microscopy.

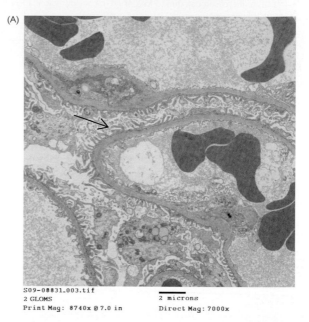

(A)

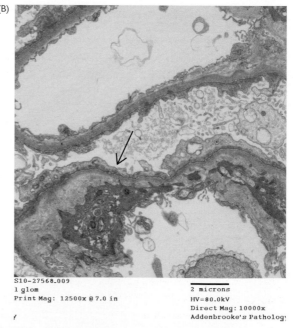

(B)

Fig. 17.13 (A) Electron microscopy of a capillary loop within a glomerulus demonstrating normal epithelial foot processes (arrow) (EM ×7000). (B) EM shows a single capillary loop with fused epithelial foot processes (arrow) (EM ×10,000).

- Non-visible haematuria is often present.
- May follow an upper respiratory tract infection.
- Renal function is usually normal unless massive proteinuria or diuretic therapy leads to pre-renal AKI.
- Patients may be hypertensive at presentation which requires controlling prior to biopsy.

## Diagnosis

- Presumptive in children—empirical steroids used.
- Adults usually require a renal biopsy to exclude other glomerular pathologies.

## Treatment/prognosis

### Idiopathic (primary)

- High-dose corticosteroids (e.g. prednisolone 60mg once daily) leads to remission of proteinuria in 80–90% of cases. The dose can then be weaned and eventually discontinued. Treatment duration may be from a few months to several years.
- Response to steroid therapy correlates directly with prognosis although relapse requiring re-treatment is relatively common (~50% will have a single relapse, ~15% will be frequent relapsers).
- Steroid-resistant disease or frequently-relapsing steroid-responsive disease where a steroid-sparing agent is required can be treated with:
  - Cyclophosphamide.
  - Azathioprine or mycophenolate mofetil (MMF).
  - Calcineurin inhibitors (e.g. ciclosporin/tacrolimus).
  - Rituximab (anti-CD20 monoclonal antibody targeting B cells).

### Secondary

- Usually responds to successful management of the precipitating cause

# Membranous nephropathy

- Diagnosis in up to 1/3 of adult NS.
- Histological diagnosis on renal biopsy demonstrating glomerular basement membrane thickening and immune-dense deposits of IgG and C3 (Fig. 17.14).

## Aetiology

### Idiopathic (primary)

- Accounts for up to 75% of cases.
- Unknown aetiology, but again a possible immune basis. Autoantibodies to PLA2R (phospholipase A2 receptor) are detectable in ~75% of patients with idiopathic MN and may correlate with disease activity.

### Secondary

- **Infection** (especially hepatitis B).
- **Malignancy** (especially in patients >65 years, mainly solid tumours, e.g. lung, breast, gastrointestinal).
- **Drugs** (classically penicillamine, gold for RA).
- **Autoimmune disease** (especially SLE).

## Clinical presentation

- Usually gradual-onset NS (80%).
- Occasionally an incidental finding of proteinuria in an otherwise asymptomatic patient.
- Degree of proteinuria can vary widely.
- Non-visible haematuria present in ~50%.
- Blood pressure and renal function are usually normal at presentation.

## Diagnosis

- Exclude secondary causes with viral serology (hepatitis B and C) and a SLE screen (ANA/dsDNA and C3/4). Anti-PLA2R antibodies suggest primary MN.
- A renal biopsy is required.

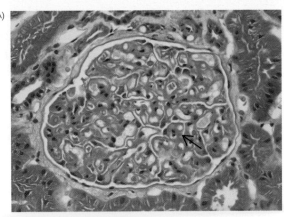

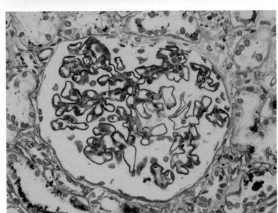

Fig. 17.14 Membranous nephropathy. (A) The glomerular cellularity is normal but the capillary walls have a uniform, thickened, 'rigid' appearance (arrow). Staining for IgG (B) shows uniform, granular staining on the capillary basement membrane indicating immune deposits.

- If MN confirmed, in patients >50 years old an occult malignancy should be considered and appropriate screening and diagnostic tests performed (e.g. CXR/CT chest, mammography, colonoscopy, PSA, etc.).

## Treatment

### Idiopathic MN

Treatment decisions need to bear in mind the natural progression of disease in view of treatment toxicity:

- Up to 1/3 of patients will have a spontaneous complete remission.
- A further 1/3 will have a spontaneous partial remission (<2g proteinuria/day).
- Only 1/3 will progress to ESRF after 10 years.
- **Good** prognostic indicators at diagnosis include:
  - Non-nephrotic range proteinuria.
  - Preserved renal function.
  - Absence of clinical oedema.
- **Poor** prognostic findings associated with progression to ESRF include:
  - Older age at diagnosis (especially >50 years old).
  - ♂ gender.
  - Nephrotic-range proteinuria (especially 8–10g/day).
  - Raised serum creatinine at diagnosis.

### Non-immunosuppression-based treatment

- RAS blockade with ACE inhibitors/ARBs.
- Lipid-lowering with a statin.
- Anticoagulation with aspirin or warfarin.

*Immunosuppression regimens*

- Treatment is usually reserved for those patients most at risk of disease progression.
- No single established optimal treatment regimen exists. This has led to a variety of trials, including one UK-based trial coordinated through the Renal Association and published in the *Lancet* in 2013.
- Options include:
  - Cyclophosphamide with steroids.
  - 'Ponticelli' regimen (chlorambucil and steroids, named after the Italian first author of the trial).
  - Calcineurin inhibitors.
  - Rituximab (for resistant disease).
  - As can be appreciated, all of these options (but particularly the first two) carry significant treatment-related morbidity.
- Side effects include:
  - Severe bone marrow suppression.
  - Infection.
  - Potential subfertility.
  - Increased risk of malignancy.
- The choice of agent is influenced by individual patient characteristics, as well as by clinician preference.

*Secondary MN*

- Treatment of the underlying condition or removal of offending drug often leads to remission of the proteinuria.

**Prognosis**

- Patients who experience spontaneous or drug-related remission have an excellent prognosis with only ~10% risk of progressive renal dysfunction.
- Relapses requiring re-treatment may, however, occur.
- Conversely, patients with high proteinuria (8–10g/day), raised creatinine and poor response to treatment, have a 75% risk of progressive renal dysfunction over 5 years.

# Focal segmental glomerulosclerosis

- There is some debate as to whether MCD and primary focal segmental glomerulosclerosis (FSGS) are part of the same spectrum of disorder as some patients with biopsy-proven MCD may progress to FSGS over time.
- ~20% of adults with nephrotic syndrome have FSGS (increases to ~50% with black ethnicity).
- Various histological variants may be predictive of renal prognosis (Figs 17.15–17.17).

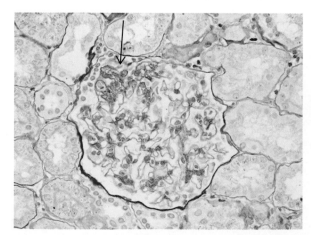

**Fig. 17.15** One segment of the glomerulus is sclerosed (arrow) with normal appearance to the others.

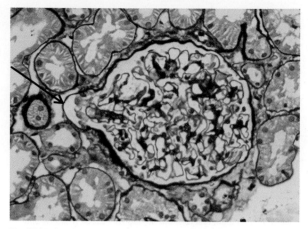

**Fig. 17.16** Silver stain demonstrating a 'tip' lesion of FSGS with the sclerosed segment at the origin of the proximal tubule (arrow). The glomerular tip lesion may be associated with a better renal prognosis.

**Aetiology**

*Idiopathic (primary)*

- No identifiable cause but possible immune mechanism.

*Secondary*

- Previous **glomerular injury** (e.g. renal vasculitis/SLE leading to sclerosis).
- Glomerular **hypertension or hypertrophy/hyperfiltration** (often caused by reduced renal mass, e.g. unilateral renal agenesis; may also be seen in obesity (see later)).

(A)

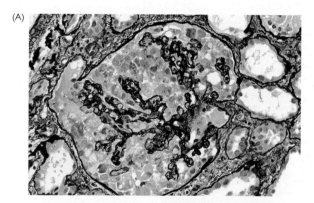

(B)

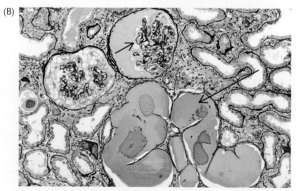

**Fig. 17.17** (Silver stain): both images (A and B) demonstrate collapse of the glomerular capillary tuft (small arrow) and hypertrophy of podocytes. Protein retention is clearly seen within the podocyte cytoplasm and there is associated cystic dilatation of protein-filled tubules (long arrow).

*Other causes*

- **Genetic** (especially in childhood-onset, steroid-resistant FSGS; variable genetic inheritance patterns—genes encoding podocyte proteins are particularly implicated).
- **Toxins/drugs** (e.g. heroin, pamidronate).
- **Infections** (including HIV which causes a characteristic 'collapsing' FSGS on renal biopsy).
- **Malignancy** (especially lymphomas).
- **Obesity**—haemodynamic factors, such as increased renal blood flow, with activation of the RAA system likely play a role here. These patients tend to have elevated glomerular filtration rates and increased glomerular size consistent with intra-glomerular hypertension. These changes can be reversed by weight loss.

## Clinical presentation

- Primary FSGS usually presents in a similar way to MCD whereas secondary FSGS appears to be a more indolent disease with often only asymptomatic proteinuria and some degree of renal dysfunction.
- Hypertension and non-visible haematuria are often present.

## Diagnosis

- Requires a renal biopsy although the focal nature of lesions may lead to missed diagnoses due to sampling variation.
- Presence of interstitial fibrosis on biopsy predicts progression to ESRF.

## Treatment/prognosis

*Primary FSGS*

There are no randomized trials to guide treatment but observational studies indicate a rationale for a trial of high-dose corticosteroids.

- Usually prednisolone 60mg/day for at least 8–12 weeks is used for nephrotic-range primary FSGS.
- FSGS is less responsive than MCD to remission-induction with steroids.
- ~40–80% patients will achieve remission of proteinuria with steroids.
- Often a prolonged course of steroids is necessary.
- It is not possible to determine an individual patient's likelihood of steroid-responsiveness pre-treatment.
- Steroid-resistant or frequently-relapsing disease can be treated similarly to MCD with:
  - Calcineurin inhibitors
  - Cyclophosphamide
  - MMF
  - Sirolimus

*Secondary FSGS*

- Immunosuppression is not usually indicated.
- Treatment of underlying disorder indicated (e.g. HAART for HIV, chemotherapy for lymphoma).

*All types*

- ACE inhibitors or ARBs: blockade of the RAA system is beneficial in reducing proteinuria and slowing the progression of proteinuric kidney disease.
- Statin: hypercholesterolaemia is generally present.
- NSAIDs: occasionally heavy proteinuria is so severe with rapid progression of renal impairment, unresponsive to therapies outlined earlier, that high-dose NSAIDs are administered (sometimes combined with an ACE inhibitor) in an attempt to induce a 'medical nephrectomy'.

## Recurrent FSGS post-transplantation

- Occurs in ~20% of all patients with FSGS as a native renal diagnosis pre-transplantation.
- Higher incidence likely in those with primary FSGS.
- Histology usually of the same variant as pre-transplant.

*Aetiology*

Debate continues—basic and clinical research indicate a possible role for a circulating permeability factor, or for the absence of a normal plasma protein.

*Clinical presentation*

- Often rapid proteinuria develops post-transplant (may be only a few weeks later) with subsequent progressive renal impairment.

*Diagnosis*

- Transplant renal biopsy required if post-transplant proteinuria exceeds 1g/day.
- Exclude viral infection (PCR for parvovirus B19, CMV, EBV, BK, and hepatitis C).

*Treatment*

- Current practice relies on the results of small case series of patients.
- Plasma exchange or protein adsorption columns reduce proteinuria (at least whilst exchange therapy continues) and can be useful in combination with other immunomodulatory therapy (e.g. cyclophosphamide or rituximab).
- IVIg may be useful in the setting of viral infection or severe hypogammaglobulinaemia.
- ACE inhibitors/ARBs and statin used as in native disease.

*Prognosis*

- Recurrent disease may lead to allograft loss (12% at 10 years in one large retrospective analysis from Australia and New Zealand transplant registry data).
- Living-related donor transplantation is not advised as the disease is likely to recur again.

# 17.13  Rapidly progressive glomerulonephritis

## Background

A number of diseases can cause rapidly progressive glomerulonephritis (RPGN). As these are potentially treatable provided that diagnosis and therapy are initiated soon enough after onset, it is therefore critical that a patient with rapidly worsening renal failure is referred to an in-patient nephrology service as soon as possible.

## Epidemiology

- Incidence is 2–5% of renal biopsies (in England, France, USA, India, China).
- ♂:♀ = 2:1.
- Increased incidence in the elderly.
- Afro-Caribbeans less commonly affected, except for RPGN secondary to lupus nephritis, which is more common in this ethnic group.

## Aetiology

There are three broad groups of diseases causing RPGN:

- Immune complex glomerulonephritis (30%)—a heterogeneous group associated with granular deposits of immunoglobulin, in which crescent formation complicates an identifiable form of nephritis.
- Renal-related vasculitidies (60%)—characterized by circulating ANCA and scanty glomerular deposits of immunoglobulin (pauci-immune).
- Anti-GBM disease (10%)—characterized by circulating antibodies to GBM.

## Immune complex glomerulonephritis

### Post-infectious glomerulonephritis

This is relatively rare, but can happen 1–3 weeks after an acute group A streptococcal infection (e.g. pharyngitis, impetigo, or cellulitis) or a staphylococcal infection.

*Pathogenesis*

- Immune complex deposition causes an inflammatory infiltrate, and may result in an RPGN.

- Renal biopsy shows a diffuse proliferative glomerulonephritis. See Fig. 17.18.

*Clinical evaluation*

- Renal impairment with oedema and an active urine sediment occurs 1–3 weeks after an acute infection.
- Throat swab may identify a causative *Streptococcus*, but the infection may have cleared by the time of presentation.
- Complement levels remains low for 6–8 weeks, and antibodies to bacterial antigens (e.g. streptolysin) may be detectable.

*Differential diagnosis*

Both endocarditis and chronically infected ventriculo-atrial shunts can cause an immune complex-mediated GN.

*Management and prognosis*

Renal failure may necessitate dialysis but neither steroids nor antibiotics have any effect on the natural history of the disease. Spontaneous resolution of renal impairment within 2–4 weeks is usual.

### Systemic lupus erythematosus

This multisystem autoimmune disease is characterized by autoantibodies against many circulating antigens. Immune complex deposition may be seen in many organs and is a feature of lupus nephritis. Renal involvement is common in SLE, and can present in a number of ways

- RPGN.
- Nephrotic syndrome.
- Chronic progressive renal impairment.
- Mild renal abnormalities and a benign course.

*Epidemiology*

- Prevalence 10–50 per 100,000 in a Caucasian population.
- ♀:♂ = 10:1.
- Higher in African Americans and Afro-Caribbeans in the USA and UK, and in Southeast Asians.
- Incidence appears to be increasing.

*Aetiology and pathogenesis*

- Genetic studies, including two genome-wide association studies, have identified multiple genetic loci where mutations are thought to contribute to loss of tolerance to self.
- Autoreactive T and B cells result in autoantibody and immune complex formation which deposit in the glomeruli

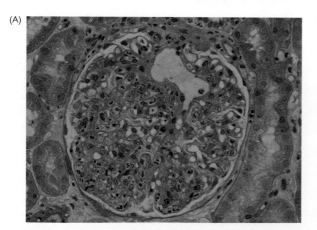
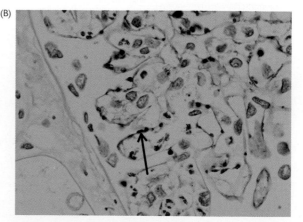

**Fig. 17.18** (A) Haematoxylin & Eosin (H&E): an enlarged, hypercellular glomerulus containing many neutrophil polymorphs in the glomerular tuft. (B) Immunostain for complement C3 shows large 'humps' (arrowed) on the epithelial side of the basement membrane. These are immune complexes. Courtesy of Dr. Moira Finlay, Royal Melbourne Hospital.

## Box 17.4 Modified WHO classification of lupus nephritis (abbreviated)

| Class 0: | Normal. |
|---|---|
| Class 1: | Light microscopy normal, immune deposits on immunofluorescence. |
| Class 2: | A—mesangial deposits. |
| | B—mesangial hypercellularity. |
| Class 3: | Focal proliferative glomerulonephritis with <50% glomeruli affected. |
| | Leucocyte infiltration and immune complex deposition. |
| Class 4: | Diffuse proliferative glomerulonephritis with >50% glomeruli affected (Fig. 17.19). |
| | May also have crescents and fibrinoid necrosis. |
| Class 5: | Membranous nephropathy with uniform thickening of the capillary walls and subepithelial immune complex deposition. |
| Class 6: | Glomerulosclerosis. |

Reproduced with permission from World Health Organization.

and mesangium. These contain IgG, IgM, IgA, and complement components C3, C1q, and C4 (so-called 'full-house' immunofluorescence).

- An inflammatory reaction results in leucocyte infiltration and mesangial proliferation which may progress to fibrinoid necrosis and crescent formation

### Clinical evaluation

- SLE is a multisystem disease and diagnosis requires four of 11 clinical or serological criteria as defined by the American College of Rheumatology (see Box 19.15 in Section 19.11).
- Renal assessment should include urinalysis, quantification of proteinuria, and assessment of GFR.
  - For 25% of patients, renal disease is the first manifestation of SLE.
  - If the GFR is deteriorating, or proteinuria is >1g per 24 hours, renal biopsy should be considered as histological classification aids with prognostic and treatment decisions.

### Management

The therapy is usually guided by the histological class (Box 17.4):

- Class 1: treatment guided by extra-renal lesions.
- Class 2: corticosteroids may be used if renal function deteriorates but generally this has a benign course and treatment is often not required.
- Class 3 and 4: pulsed IV cyclophosphamide with corticosteroids for 3–6 months, followed by maintenance treatment with

azathioprine is widely used. Mycophenolate mofetil is also being used increasingly, both as induction and maintenance therapy. More recently B-cell depletion therapy with rituximab (an anti-CD20 monoclonal antibody) is also proving to be an effective treatment (Fig. 17.9).

- Class 5: corticosteroids tend to be the treatment of choice. If renal function continues to decline, most clinicians would consider treating with cyclophosphamide or MMF.
- Class 6: at this stage, the chronic damage is irreversible, and supportive management, rather than immunosuppression, is instituted.

### Prognosis

- Renal function and histology at presentation predicts likelihood of ESRF.
- Following treatment, normalization of proteinuria and a relapse-free disease course are the best predictors of a good outcome.
- Negative prognostic factors include ♂ gender, black race, and haematological features of SLE.
- ESRF develops in about 20% of patients with lupus nephritis (mainly class 4 and 5). The mean interval between onset of renal symptoms and ESRF is 5 years. Kidney transplantation is generally successful, with a low relapse rate of lupus nephritis post-transplant.

## Renal-related vasculitides

'Vasculitis' refers to a collection of diseases that cause inflammation of the blood vessel wall. These diseases frequently affect blood vessels in more than one organ. Vasculitis that affects small vessels—i.e. capillaries, arterioles, or venules—is often associated with glomerulonephritis.

### Classification

The vasculitides are classified according to the size of the smallest vessels affected (see Table 17.6). The most common vasculitides seen are the ANCA-associated systemic vasculitis (AASV) where ANCA are (usually) detectable in the serum The AASV comprise:

- **Granulomatosis with polyangiitis (GPA; formerly known as Wegener granulomatosis)** characteristically has ENT and/or respiratory involvement. Necrotizing granuloma may cause sinusitis, nasal discharge, damage to the nasal septum, hearing loss, and/or haemoptysis. ~70% of patients are cANCA positive and 25% pANCA positive.
- **Microscopic polyangiitis (MPA)** is a very similar small vessel, pauci-immune vasculitis without evidence of granulomata and upper respiratory tract involvement. 50% are pANCA positive, 40% cANCA positive.

(A)

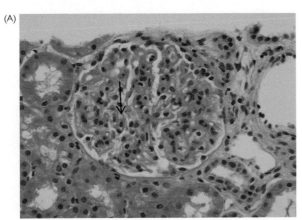

(B)

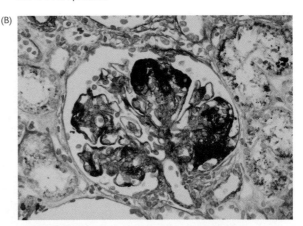

**Fig. 17.19** Class 4 lupus nephritis. (A) There is diffuse, mesangial hypercellularity which includes several neutrophils. There are characteristic 'wire-loop' lesions of thickened capillary walls (arrow). (B) IgG staining reveals dense, irregular immune complex deposition mainly in subendothelial and mesangial positions.

**Table 17.6** Classification of vasculitides by vessel size and (usual) ANCA status

| Vessel size | ANCA positive | ANCA negative |
|---|---|---|
| Small | Granulomatosis with polyangiitis<br>Microscopic polyangiitis<br>Renal-limited vasculitis | Henoch–Schönlein purpura<br>Cryoglobulinaemia |
| Medium | Churg–Strauss syndrome | Polyarteritis nodosa<br>Kawasaki disease |
| Large | | Giant cell arteritis<br>Takayasu arteritis |

- Eosinophilic granulomatosis with polyangiitis (Churg–Strauss syndrome) is a form of vasculitis associated with asthma and eosinophilia. 60% are pANCA positive, 30% are ANCA negative. It is less common than GPA and MPA.

### Epidemiology

Although rare, the incidence of systemic vasculitis appears to be rising, and is now ~20 new cases per million population (pmp) per year in Southern England. This increases with age, to 60pmp in the 65–75 year age group. Men are more commonly affected than women. African Americans seem less susceptible than Caucasians.

### Aetiology

The aetiology of AASV is multifactorial:

- Genetic factors affect susceptibility. There are reports of siblings being affected by the disease, and several genetic polymorphisms have been associated with increased incidence of AASV.
- Environmental factors have also been implicated—hypersensitivity to hydralazine, rifampicin, and minocycline can cause AASV. Penicillamine can cause pANCA-associated crescentic glomerulonephritis with or without pulmonary haemorrhage. Case controlled studies indicate that silica predisposes to ANCA-associated crescentic nephritis and GPA.

### Pathogenesis and histopathology

- The exact pathogenetic mechanisms are not fully understood but are thought to be mediated by abnormal neutrophil function, triggered by ANCA and/or autoreactive leucocytes.
- Renal biopsies show focal (some glomeruli affected), segmental necrotizing glomerulonephritis with 'crescent' formation (Fig. 17.20).
- As the disease progresses crescents in all stages of their evolution are seen.
- Immunohistology shows that the glomeruli contain scanty deposits of immunoglobulins and complement—so-called pauci-immune glomerulonephritis.
- Small vessels may contain inflammatory infiltrates and necrosis of the vessel wall.

### Clinical evaluation

Disease manifestations include:

- Non-specific symptoms and signs that include muscle pains, night sweats, and weight loss.
- Arthralgia due to synovitis, which is symmetrical, relatively mild, and often affects the hands and feet. Some patients have frank arthritis.
- Purpuric rash (cutaneous vasculitis)—may have nail fold infarcts or splinter haemorrhages.
- Red eyes or blurred vision—eye involvement can cause episcleritis, uveitis, or retinal vasculitis.
- Cranial nerve palsies, mononeuritis multiplex, symmetrical polyneuropathies, and cerebral vasculitis.
- Mouth ulcers or abdominal pain as a result of gastrointestinal vasculitis.
- Renal disease typically presents with deteriorating renal function over weeks to months, an active urinary sediment (blood and protein on urinalysis), and proteinuria of 1–3g/24 hours (but not generally with nephrosis).

### Features limited to granulomatosis with polyangiitis

- >90% of patients with granulomatosis with polyangiitis have obvious upper airways disease. This includes nasal crusting, rhinorrhoea, epistaxis, and longer-term complications such as saddle-nose deformity and subglottic stenoses.
- Granulomatous lung disease is common, and may be accompanied by alveolar capillaritis/pulmonary haemorrhage and bronchial tree stenoses (Fig. 17.21).
- Granulomatous inflammation at other sites has been reported in the kidney, in the orbit of the eye, causing exophthalmos, and also in the brain, pituitary, salivary glands, prostate, gingiva, and vertebrae.

### Differential diagnosis

This is wide, given the range of clinical features that may be seen, and includes infection, neoplasia, connective tissue diseases, SLE, and anti-GBM disease.

In addition, other, rarer, causes of renal vasculitis include:

- **Henoch–Schönlein purpura:** in this vasculitis, IgA-containing immune complexes deposit in the small vessels of the skin, joints, gut, and kidney. It usually affects children, causing a purpuric rash on the lower limbs and buttocks, colicky abdominal pain, arthralgia of the large joints, and an active urinary sediment. The disease usually responds to treatment with steroids alone, but in adults the renal disease may be more aggressive, and requires therapy as for AASV with renal involvement.

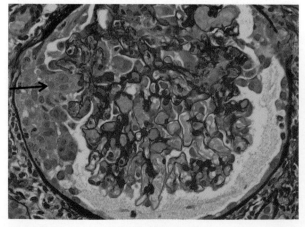

**Fig. 17.20** Segmental necrosis affecting two segments in the upper half of the glomerulus with associated cellular crescent formation (arrow). The capillary tuft in the lower half is unaffected.

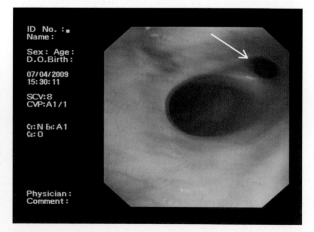

**Fig. 17.21** Bronchoscopic examination demonstrating a severe stenosis of the right main bronchus (arrow) at the carina.
Courtesy of Cambridge University Hospitals NHS Foundation Trust (Dr Sivasothy, Respiratory Dept)

- **Polyarteritis nodosa:** this non-granulomatous vasculitis of medium-sized vessels is uncommon in the UK. It has been associated with hepatitis B infection, which is thought to be causative in a proportion of cases. The vasculitic lesions affect arterial branch points and may lead to aneurysm formation (Fig. 17.22). Clinical features include renal involvement (renal infarcts leading to hypertension and renal failure), peripheral neuropathy, gastrointestinal involvement (haemorrhage, perforation, infarction), and cardiac involvement (angina, myocardial infarction). ANCA is positive in ~10% cases.

### Management

Treatment of AASV with RPGN is divided into two phases (see Section 19.19):

- **Induction therapy:** for the first 3 months, patients are treated with cyclophosphamide (either a daily oral dose or intermittent pulsed intravenous therapy) and high-dose corticosteroids to induce remission. Plasma exchange may be beneficial for those who present with acute kidney injury requiring dialysis.
- **Maintenance therapy** is used in almost all patients with AASV, as without it 50% will relapse. After 3 months of induction therapy the disease is usually quiescent, and patients are then treated with azathioprine (or similar agents including mycophenolate) and low-dose prednisolone for 1–2 years.

Immunosuppressive therapy has risks and side effects, and patients undergoing treatment for AASV may need prophylaxis against infections including *Candida* and *Pneumocystis jirovecii*, gastric ulcers, osteoporosis, as well as monitoring for bone marrow suppression, CMV, diabetes, dyslipidaemias, hypertension, and cancers.

### Outcome and prognosis

- Untreated, the 1-year mortality of AASV is 80%, the main causes of death being renal and respiratory failure.
- With treatment, 5-year survival rates are 60%.
- ~10% die of uncontrolled disease—the majority, however, die of treatment complications, mostly infection.
- Most of those who require dialysis at presentation recover renal function to some extent.
- Those with persistent severe renal failure have the worst prognosis.

# Antiglomerular basement membrane (Goodpasture) disease

Here, patients develop pathogenic autoantibodies against their own glomerular basement membrane. These antibodies may target the lung as well as the kidney, and can cause pulmonary haemorrhage with RPGN—or RPGN alone.

### Epidemiology

- The incidence is thought to be 0.5–1 new case per million of the population per year. It is found in 1–2% of renal biopsies.
- Incidence peaks in the 3rd and 6th decades, and there is a slight excess of ♂.

### Aetiology and pathogenesis

- Essentially all patients with anti-GBM disease have circulating antibodies that bind the α3 chain of type IV collagen. Type IV collagen is found in all basement membranes, but the α3, α4, and α5 chains are found primarily in GBM and alveolar basement membranes.
- These antibodies are pathogenic—there is a correlation between antibody levels and disease activity, and the disease recurs immediately in renal transplants when the recipient still has circulating antibodies.
- Alveolar haemorrhage generally requires a second insult, either local to the lungs (e.g. cigarette smoking or pulmonary oedema), or systemic with activation of cytokines and inflammatory mediators (e.g. sepsis) (Fig. 17.23).
- There is a genetic predisposition. The class II HLA type DRB1*1501 is carried by >85% of patients with anti-GBM disease, compared with 30% of controls.
- Environmental factors may trigger disease presentation in those who have developed GBM antibodies.

### Clinical evaluation

- Most patients present with RPGN or lung haemorrhage, or both. Some patients have isolated lung haemorrhage and never develop renal failure.
- General malaise, fatigue, weight loss, and anaemia are the most common systemic features, whilst other signs and symptoms are much rarer than in patients with systemic vasculitis.

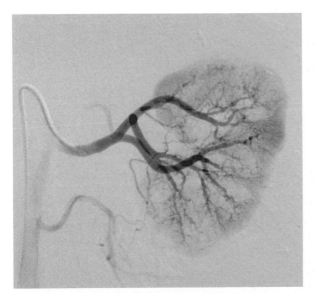

**Fig. 17.22** A renal angiogram demonstrating multiple aneurysms consistent with a diagnosis of polyarteritis nodosa.
Courtesy of Cambridge University Hospitals NHS Foundation Trust's Radiology dept.

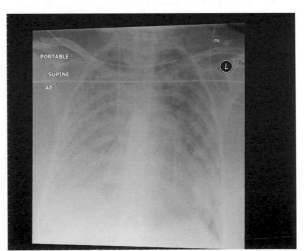

**Fig. 17.23** A chest X-ray demonstrating diffuse bilateral patchy consolidation in a patient with pulmonary haemorrhage secondary to anti-glomerular basement membrane disease.
Courtesy of Cambridge University Hospitals NHS Foundation Trust's Radiology dept.

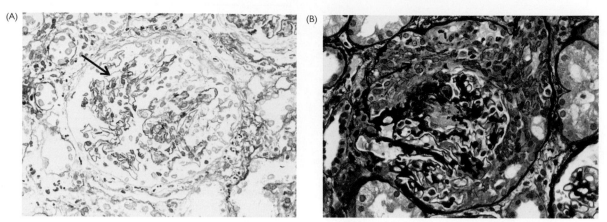

Fig. 17.24 Anti-glomerular basement membrane disease. (A) Linear IgG staining (arrowed) on the GBM indicates anti-GBM antibody deposition. (B) Silver stain demonstrates tuft necrosis and almost circumferential cellular crescent formation (arrow).

- Serology reveals anti-GBM antibodies, and renal biopsy typically shows an RPGN with crescents all of the same age with linear deposition of antibody along the GBM (Fig. 17.24).

### Differential diagnosis

- It is important to distinguish anti-GBM disease from other cause of RPGN, and especially AASV.
- All patients with suspected RPGN, acute kidney injury of unknown cause, or lung haemorrhage and urinary abnormalities, should have both anti-GBM antibody and ANCA assays performed urgently.
- Up to 30% of patients with anti-GBM antibodies are also positive for pANCA but <8% with AASV also have anti-GBM antibodies. These 'double positive' patients tend to behave more like those with anti-GBM disease than those with systemic vasculitis, and should therefore be treated as such.

- Other differential diagnoses to consider include SLE, cryoglobulinaemia, and haemolytic uraemic syndrome.

### Management and prognosis

- Untreated anti-GBM disease is usually fatal, and renal function never recovers.
- Both mortality and renal function have improved dramatically with the widespread use of the plasma exchange, cyclophosphamide, and corticosteroids. Plasma exchange is performed daily for 2 weeks, cyclophosphamide is continued for 2–3 months, and prednisolone for ~6 months.
- This treatment allows up to 90% of patients to survive, but only ~40% of survivors will recover renal function.
- Of those presenting with dialysis-dependent renal failure, <10% will recover independent renal function.

## 17.14 IgA nephropathy

### Background

Primary IgA nephropathy (IgAN), or Berger disease, is the most common primary glomerular disease worldwide. It is characterized by recurrent episodes of macroscopic haematuria associated with infections, and persistent non-visible haematuria.

### Epidemiology

- The frequency of IgA nephropathy varies considerably amongst different countries, although this may, in part, reflect differing practices for both urinary screening and renal biopsy.
- The highest prevalence rates are found in Asia, Australia, and southern Europe, whilst the disease is less common in North America and the UK.
- Prevalence rates are 30–50% of primary glomerulonephritis in Asia and 10–20% in Northern Europe.
- ♂:♀ ratios also vary amongst countries, but are at least 2:1.
- Ethnicity affects susceptibility—IgAN is uncommon in Afro-Caribbeans. It is also less common in Polynesians than in Caucasians in Australasia—a particularly striking finding given the exaggerated susceptibility of Polynesians to most forms of renal disease.

### Aetiology and pathogenesis

- The great majority of cases are sporadic, although it is occasionally familial in nature (e.g. one very large kindred having been described in Kentucky, in the United States).
- The existence of these familial forms, together with the ethnicity differences, points to the existence of genetic susceptibility factors, but despite a number of linkage and genetic association studies, no risk alleles have been consistently identified.
- An abnormal IgA immune response is thought to be causative:
  - Circulating IgA levels, IgA levels in mucosal secretions, and the percentage of plasma cells secreting IgA in both bone marrow and mucosa are increased in patients with IgAN.
  - These levels rise excessively after antigenic stimulation (e.g. influenza vaccination).
- Disease flares are often precipitated by mucosal infections, predominantly of the upper respiratory tract (where IgA levels rise as part of the mucosal immune response).
- It is not clear whether the glomerular mesangial proliferation is caused by IgA immune complexes or by IgA binding directly to glomerular components (Fig.17.25).
- No antigen has consistently been identified, which may indicate that the IgA complexes are a common response to different antigens, or that the initiating antigen has disappeared by the time of the renal biopsy.

### Clinical evaluation

- Most patients present in the 2nd or 3rd decade of life with either:
  - Macroscopic haematuria in the context of an infectious illness, typically pharyngitis or tonsillitis. The haematuria usually occurs within 24–72 hours of the infection, and is red or brown ('Coke'-coloured). It usually persists for 1–3 days, and is associated with loin pain in 1/3 of cases.
  - An incidental finding of non-visible haematuria detected at routine screening. 40% of individuals with IgAN have non-visible haematuria, although it may be intermittent.
- 3–13% of patients present with asymptomatic proteinuria. Nephrotic syndrome is rare, but is a more common presentation in children.
- ~3% of IgAN patients present with acute kidney injury, and about 20% of these will require dialysis.

### Differential diagnosis

- Post-infectious glomerulonephritis:
  - This may present with renal dysfunction, an abnormal urinary sediment, and sometimes macroscopic haematuria, 1–3 weeks after an infection.
  - Hypocomplementaemia is present and renal biopsy early in this disease shows endocapillary proliferative lesions with a mononuclear cell infiltrate and subepithelial deposits of IgG (sometimes IgM and/or IgA).

(A) 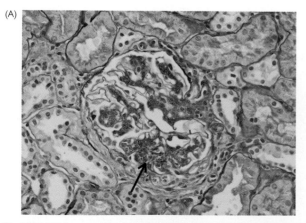 (B)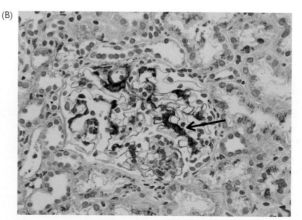

Fig. 17.25  (A) A segmental increase in mesangial matrix and cellularity is observed (arrow) with (B) positive IgA staining (arrow) in a mesangial distribution throughout the glomerulus diagnostic for IgA nephropathy.

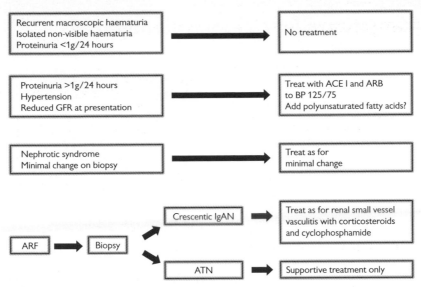

**Fig. 17.26** Suggested management algorithm for patients with IgA nephropathy.
Courtesy of Cambridge University Hospitals NHS Foundation Trust's Nephrology dept.

- Renal biopsy performed later may reveal a mesangial proliferative glomerulonephritis without IgA deposits.
- The disease usually resolves spontaneously, although non-visible haematuria may persist.
- Thin basement membrane nephropathy may cause non-visible haematuria, occasionally with proteinuria. This disease is caused by heterozygous mutations in type IV collagen and has a good prognosis.
- Henoch–Schönlein purpura (HSP) is characterized by a vasculitic skin rash and is more common in children, where it may present as nephrotic or nephritic syndrome. The renal biopsy appearance of HSP and IgAN are often indistinguishable, although endocapillary and extracapillary lesions and fibrin deposits are more frequent in HSP.

# Management and prognosis

- The prognosis is variable.
- The disease is usually slowly progressive and 20–50% reach ESRF 20 years after diagnosis.
- Risk factors for a more rapid decline are:
  - Proteinuria >1g/day.
  - Hypertension at presentation or a family history of hypertension.
  - Serum creatinine >120μmol/L at presentation.
  - More severe glomerular lesions or tubulointerstitial disease on renal biopsy.
  - ♂ gender.
  - Elevated BMI.
  - Age >50 years.
  - High numbers of erythrocytes in the urine.
- There are no treatments that modify mesangial IgA deposition and there is insufficient evidence for the additional use of immunosuppressive agents, antiplatelet agents, or anticoagulants.
- Historical studies suggesting a beneficial effect for the use of fish oils are not applicable to current-day practice (such trials were not conducted using therapies such as ACE inhibitors/ARBs).
- There is also a relative lack of randomized controlled trials in the treatment of IgAN.
- A suggested algorithm is shown in Fig. 17.26.

## Background

Mesangiocapillary glomerulonephritis (MCGN, also known as membranoproliferative glomerulonephritis) is a histological diagnosis in which there is:

- Uniform enlargement of the glomeruli, with lobular glomerular hypercellularity.
- Increased mesangial matrix and mesangial deposition within the glomerular capillary walls leading to thickening of the walls and splitting of the GBM on electron microscopy (Fig. 17.27).

## Classification

MCGN may be classified by histological appearance into:

- **Type I:**
  - Most common.
  - Characterized by subendothelial deposits and activation of the classical complement pathway.
  - Secondary MCGN causes a type I MCGN.
- **Type II:**
  - Also known as 'dense deposit disease'.
  - Differs in that the alternative pathway of complement is activated with the presence of intramembranous dense deposits. It is an example of a C3 glomerulopathy.
- **Type III:**
  - Morphological variant of type I characterized by the presence of additional subepithelial deposits and complex GBM alterations.
  - Clinically, the affected patients are older, less often hypocomplementaemic, and have a more favourable prognosis.

## Epidemiology

- In adults in the developed world, MCGN causes 2–6% of cases of primary glomerulonephritis.
- The incidence of type I MCGN has fallen dramatically in the last 30 years, but it is still the most common variant, found in 80% of cases.
- In the developing world, the disease is much more common. For example, it accounts for 40% of nephrosis in Mexico.
- In children, MCGN accounts for 7–16% of idiopathic NS.
- Type I most commonly presents between the ages of 5–40; type II from 3–20, whilst type III, the least common, typically affects older patients.

---

**Box 17.5 Causes of secondary mesangiocapillary glomerulonephritis**

- Infections:
  - Streptococcal (serological), infective endocarditis (mainly streptococcal), shunt nephritis (staphylococcal), abscesses.
  - Tuberculosis, leprosy.
  - Hepatitis B, C, G, HIV.
  - Filariasis, malaria, schistosomiasis.
  - Candidiasis.
- Autoimmunity:
  - Systemic lupus erythematosus.
  - Systemic sclerosis.
  - Mixed cryoglobulinaemia.
  - Sjögren syndrome.
- Neoplasia/dysproteinaemia:
  - Lymphoma, leukaemia, myeloma, light-chain nephropathy, Waldenström macroglobulinaemia.
- Miscellaneous:
  - Sickle cell disease, cyanotic heart disease, sarcoidosis, partial lipodystrophy, ulcerative colitis, Down syndrome.

---

- ♂:♀ is 1:1.
- Caucasians are the most commonly affected racial group.

---

## Aetiology and pathogenesis

- MCGN may be primary or secondary (see Box 17.5) in origin. Immune complex deposition is the principal feature of MCGN.
- Circulating immune complexes can be identified in the serum of about 50% of cases of primary type I MCGN.
- Secondary type I MCGN occurs in patients with known immune complex diseases, such as SLE, cryoglobulinaemia, shunt nephritis, chronic bacteraemia, and chronic hepatitis B or C infections.
- Complement abnormalities occur in both type I and type II MCGN.
  - In type I, immune complexes activate the classical pathway, resulting in low C3 and C4 levels (see Fig. 17.28).
  - Type II and III are characterized by low C3 but normal C4. This is caused by nephritic factors, IgG autoantibodies that stabilize the C3bBb complex that converts C3 to C3b, driving the terminal complement pathway (see Fig. 17.28).

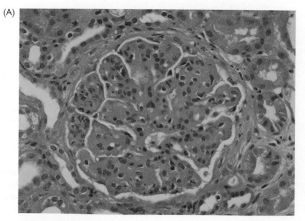

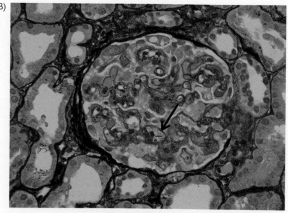

**Fig. 17.27** (A) The glomerulus has a globally 'solid' appearance due to an increase in mesangial substance and cellularity. (B) The silver stain shows double contours (arrowed) to the basement membrane enclosing immune complex deposits. This 'double contouring' is classical for MCGN.

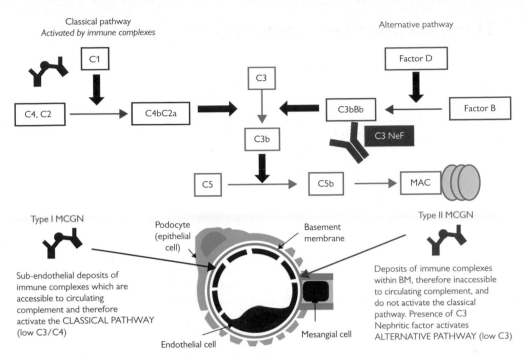

**Fig. 17.28** Complement dysregulation in mesangiocapillary glomerulonephritis.
Reproduced with permission from Clatworthy M, *Nephrology: Clinical Cases Uncovered*, Figure 18.2, page 136, Copyright Wiley 2010.

- One of these autoantibodies may also be found in partial lipod-ystrophy, which is associated with MCGN type II.
- The extent to which complement deficiencies drive the patho-genesis of MCGN is debated.
- Genetic deficiencies of Clq, C2, C3, C6, C7, C8, factor B, and the complement degradation inhibitor factors H and I are frequently, but not invariably, associated with the disease.
- However, complement depletion may cause an immune deficiency state that predisposes the individual to chronic bacterial and viral infections and subsequent immune complex formation.
- It is also possible that complement deficiency impairs the solu-bilization, disaggregation, and clearance of deposited immune complexes.

## Clinical presentation

- MCGN may present with a nephritic syndrome, with nephrotic syndrome or with both.
- Proteinuria is present in almost all patients, with nephrotic-range proteinuria in >50% patients in most series.
- Non-visible haematuria is present in 20–30% patients.
- Macroscopic haematuria is reported by a minority, mostly children.
- 10–20% of patients with MCGN present with an RPGN.
- Hypertension is often present but mild.
- MCGN may present as asymptomatic renal impairment.
- Diagnosis is usually histological, as described earlier.
- Immunofluorescence is strongly positive for C3 in a granular pat-tern along the glomerular capillaries. C1q is present in 50–66%, IgG in 66%, IgM in 60–80%.
- Other investigations should include serum complement compo-nents as most patients develop hypocomplementaemia at some point during their disease. However only ~60% have low levels of C3 at presentation.
- Patients should also be investigated for causes of secondary MCGN (see Box 17.5).

## Differential diagnosis

These include other causes of glomerulonephritis, including mem-branous nephropathy and small vessel vasculitis.

## Management and prognosis

### Natural history

- ESRF develops in 50% of patients at 11 years.
- Clinical remission occurs in 5–20%.
- Nephritic syndrome is a poor prognostic indicator.
- Children tend to have a more acute presentation but a slower progression to ESRF.

### Treatment

- Primary MCGN:
  - There have been no large randomized trials on the treatment of primary MCGN in adults.
  - As with other glomerulonephritides, hypertension in patients with MCGN should be treated aggressively. ACE inhibitors should be the agents of first choice because of their renopro-tective effects.
  - In children there is evidence for the use of corticosteroids, where renal survival increases to 82% at 10 years from diagnosis.
  - Alkylating agents have only been used in small sized studies, e.g. in one study, 15 of 19 patients treated with prednisolone and cyclophosphamide achieved a partial remission.
  - Aspirin with dipyridamole may have a beneficial effect on pro-teinuria but there is conflicting evidence of any beneficial effect on renal function.
  - There is anecdotal evidence that plasma exchange may be of benefit in patients with rapidly deteriorating renal function.
- Secondary MCGN may improve with treatment of the underlying condition. For example, in hepatitis C-associated MCGN, renal disease improves in patients whose viraemia responds to ribavirin and Interferon-α treatment.

# 17.16 Tubulointerstitial nephritis

## Background

Tubulointerstitial atrophy and fibrosis are universal in chronic kidney disease, regardless of cause. In glomerulonephritis, the degree of tubular atrophy is a better prognostic predictor than the degree of glomerular inflammation. The tubulo-interstitial nephritides, however, comprise a heterogeneous group of diseases in which inflammation and fibrosis mainly and initially affect the renal interstitium and tubules. These diseases can be divided into acute and chronic according to their mode of presentation.

## Acute interstitial nephritis

### Epidemiology
- Acute interstitial nephritis (ATIN) accounts for 1.7% of all cases of AKI.
- In several studies of patients with AKI undergoing a renal biopsy, ATIN was seen in 11–24%.

### Aetiology and pathogenesis
Common causes of ATIN include (also see Box 17.6):
- **Drugs:** an idiosyncratic drug reaction is the most common cause of ATIN. It is wise to suspect drug-induced interstitial nephritis in anyone who develops AKI after starting a new drug.
- **Infection:** many infections can cause an inflammatory response within the interstitium. Note that infection-induced TIN is a separate diagnosis from pyelonephritis.
- **Multisystem inflammatory diseases:** several autoimmune diseases may cause an acute or chronic TIN. These include:
  - Sarcoid—a granulomatous TIN which usually responds to steroids. Associated hypercalcaemia is a more frequent cause of renal impairment.
  - Sjögren syndrome can cause a TIN which may manifest as a renal tubular acidosis.
  - Vasculitis—rarely, both SLE and ANCA-associated vasculitis may cause predominantly TIN rather than glomerulonephritis.
  - TIN with uveitis (TINU) is a syndrome in which uveitis generally coincides with or follows TIN.

---

**Box 17.6 Causes of acute tubulointerstitial nephritis**

*Drug causes*
- Antibiotics:
  - Penicillins, cephalosporins.
  - Sulphonamides, rifampicin, quinolones.
- Non-steroidal anti-inflammatory drugs.
- Anticonvulsants: phenytoin, valproate, lamotrigine.
- Diuretics: thiazides, furosemide.
- Other: e.g. allopurinol, omeprazole, cimetidine.

*Infectious causes*
- Bacteria:
  - *Streptococcus, Legionella, Brucella.*
  - *Mycoplasma, Chlamydia, Salmonella, Campylobacter.*
  - Tuberculosis.
- Viruses:
  - Epstein–Barr virus, hantaviruses.
  - Measles, adenovirus, HIV.
  - *Cytomegalovirus*, polyomavirus.
- Spirochaetes: leptospirosis, syphilis
- Others: *Toxoplasma, Leishmania*

---

## Clinical evaluation

*Presentation*
- Usually with mild renal impairment.
- A careful history should be taken to identify any recent infections or changes in medication.
- Hypertension and oliguria are uncommon.
- Proteinuria is generally not in the nephrotic range, and may be below the limit of detection of conventional dipstick urinalysis.
- Non-visible haematuria is common, but red cell casts and macroscopic haematuria are both rare.
- White cells/casts may be seen.
- There may be evidence of tubular dysfunction, including renal tubular acidosis (RTA), aminoaciduria, glycosuria and impaired sodium concentrating and urinary concentrating ability.
- Allergic interstitial nephritis, commonly seen in drug-induced TIN, may cause additional symptoms including fever, rash, eosinophilia, and, rarely, eosinophiluria.

### Investigations
- Renal ultrasonography and autoantibody screens are usually normal. The diagnosis is made on renal biopsy (Fig. 17.29).

### Management and prognosis
- Identification and removal/treatment of the underlying cause usually results in renal recovery.
- Some cases may require treatment with corticosteroids. If there is no improvement in renal function within a week of cessation of the precipitating cause, a 4-week course of prednisolone at a dose of 1mg/kg is often given.
- Most patients will regain the majority of their renal function when evaluated at the end of a year.
- Negative prognostic indicators include:
  - Persistent renal impairment (>3 weeks).
  - Oliguria.
  - Advanced patient age.
  - Extensive tubular involvement and severe cellular infiltrates.

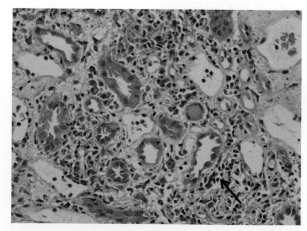

**Fig. 17.29** There is interstitial oedema and a mixed inflammatory infiltrate in the interstitium and tubules, including lymphocytes, plasma cells, and eosinophils (arrow). The presence of eosinophils is typically characteristic of acute TIN of allergic type.

# Chronic interstitial nephritis

A wide variety of diseases, both systemic and localized to the kidneys, can result in chronic inflammation within the interstitium.

## Epidemiology

- Chronic interstitial nephritis (CIN) in association with macroscopically abnormal kidneys is common—e.g. in reflux nephropathy and obstructive and cystic renal disease.
- CIN with macroscopically normal kidneys accounts for about 3% of all causes of ESRF in the UK.
- Analgesic nephropathy is the cause of about 1% of ESRF in the UK, but the prevalence of this disease varies widely.

## Aetiology and pathogenesis

Common causes include (also see Box 17.7):

*Analgesic nephropathy*

- Previously the most common cause of both AKI and CKD in many countries (in the 1950s–1970s).
- NSAIDs are the most common causative agents.
- Women are more affected than men (4:1).

---

**Box 17.7 Causes of chronic interstitial nephritis**

- Drugs:
  - NSAIDs, lithium.
  - Calcineurin inhibitors (e.g. ciclosporin).
  - Cisplatin, iron.
- Heavy metals and toxins:
  - Cadmium, lead.
  - Chinese herb nephropathy.
  - Balkan nephropathy.
- Metabolic disorders:
  - Hyperuricaemia, hypercalcaemia.
- Autoimmune diseases:
  - Systemic lupus erythematosus, Sjögren syndrome.
  - Rheumatoid arthritis.
  - ANCA positive vasculitis.
- Infections:
  - Chronic pyelonephritis.
  - Tuberculosis.
- Haematological disease:
  - Myeloma, light-chain nephropathy.
  - Sickle cell disease.

---

- Clinical features:
  - History of long-term analgesic usage.
  - May have renal pain due to papillary necrosis.
  - Possible lower urinary tract symptoms of dysuria, nocturia, and polyuria.
  - May be asymptomatic, and thus present late, with CKD.
- Investigation:
  - Urinalysis—sterile pyuria, non-visible haematuria, and low-grade proteinuria.
  - Ultrasound—irregular shaped kidneys, which may be small. Classical radiological appearance on IVU of 'cup and spill' calyces due to papillary necrosis with renal scarring.
  - Renal biopsy shows a CIN.
- Patients with analgesic nephropathy have an increased risk of atherosclerosis, and the most common cause of death is acute myocardial infarction.

*Urate nephropathy*

- The incidence of chronic crystal-related interstitial nephropathy in middle-aged men with gout has decreased dramatically over the last 30 years due to lower intake of dietary purines and earlier treatment of gout with allopurinol.
- Inherited disorders of purine metabolism can cause hyperuricaemic nephropathy. These include familial juvenile gout, glycogen storage disease type 1, deficiency of adenine phosphoribosyl synthetase, and hereditary xanthinuria.

*Balkan nephropathy, Chinese herb nephropathy*

- These conditions are caused by a combination of aristolochic acid and a susceptible genetic background.
- Renal scarring occurs with progressive failure.
- There is an increased risk of uroepithelial malignancy.

*Iatrogenic TIN*

- Lithium may cause nephrogenic diabetes insipidus, ATN, and, in the long term, CIN.
- Cisplatin causes AKI in at least 25% of patients, and a minority of these will develop CIN.
- Radiation can cause an acute thrombotic microangiopathy as well as a CIN.
- Calcineurin inhibitors, e.g. ciclosporin often cause nephrotoxicity with vascular and tubulointerstitial damage.

## Management

Treatment/removal of the precipitant is key. However, CIN often presents late when renal recovery is limited. At this point, the management is as for generic CKD.

### Fanconi Syndrome

- Generalised proximal tubular dysfunction, with a failure of re-uptake of amino acids, glucose, phosphate and bicarbonate (and hence their loss in the urine).
- Dehydration, acidosis (proximal RTA), electrolyte imbalance, bone disease (rickets/osteomalacia) and growth retardation result.

| Inherited causes | Acquired causes |
|---|---|
| <ul><li>Idiopathic Fanconi syndrome (sporadic, or AD/AR/X-linked inheritance)</li><li>Inborn errors of metabolism:<br>  Cystinosis (below)    Wilson disease<br>  Tyrosinaemia        Hereditary fructose intolerance<br>  Lowe syndrome (oculocerebral dystrophy)</li></ul> | <ul><li>Heavy metal poisoning (lead, cadmium, mercury)</li><li>Drugs (gentamicin, cisplatin, ifosfamide, sodium valproate)</li><li>Organic compounds (toluene: glue-sniffing)</li><li>Multiple myeloma</li><li>Sjögren syndrome</li></ul> |

- Treatment is directed at the underlying cause wherever possible.
- Phosphate, bicarbonate and electrolyte supplementation, adequate hydration, and vitamin D are all often required.

### Cystinosis (Cystine Storage Disease)

- Autosomal recessive (CTNS gene, chromosome 17)
- Defective cystine export from lysosome → accumulation → intracellular accumulation and toxicity
- Adult form: corneal and bone marrow crystals–benign.
- Infantile form: Fanconi syndrome and end-stage renal failure by late childhood, progressive visual impairment, hypothyroidism, hepatosplenomegaly
- Treatment: cysteamine reduces tissue cystine deposition and slows disease progression

### Aminoacidurias

Specific carrier proteins in the membranes of proximal tubular cells are responsible for the reabsorption of filtered amino acids. Inherited defects in these proteins can cause loss of this specific re-uptake.

Cystinuria

- Autosomal recessive (chromosome 2)
- Loss of re-uptake of cystine plus other di-basic amino acids (COAL: Cystine, Ornithine, Arginine, Lysine)
- Cystine is the least soluble, and easily forms renal calculi.
- Patients present with recurrent renal calculi in their second and third decade of life.
- The calculi are radio-opaque (but less so than calcium-containing stones)
- Treatment involves: increased fluid intake (2-4 l/day); penicillamine reduces renal excretion of cystine and increases its solubility; captopril increases solubility of cystine

### Dent Disease

- X-linked -affected patients develop rickets and renal failure
- Aminoaciduria, glycosuria, phosphaturia (Fanconi syndrome)
- Inactivating mutations in chloride channel (ClC-5) prevent normal uptake by proximal tubular cells.
- Hypercalcaemia, nephrocalcinosis and kidney stones also result.

### Disorders of Phosphate Metabolism

Hypophosphataemia

  X-linked hypophosphataemic rickets:

- Most common inherited form of isolated renal phosphate wasting
- Defect in *PHEX* gene, encoding a Zn metalloproteinase. It is unclear as to how this causes the phenotype.
- Hypophosphataemia + osteoblast defect = abnormal mineralisation of growing bone
- Present in early childhood with growth retardation, bone pain, and, later, rickets.
- All investigations normal except for low serum phosphate and phosphaturia
- Treat with phosphate supplements and vitamin D, plus growth hormone.

Hyperphosphataemia

- Usually a result of chronic renal failure or hypoparathyroidism

### Proximal Renal Tubular Acidosis (RTA type II)

- Failure of bicarbonate reabsorption by the proximal tubule; able to acidify urine (pH < 5.5)
- Mild–moderate metabolic acidosis (normal anion gap/hyperchloraemic) with hypokalaemia
- Most commonly secondary in association with Fanconi syndrome (see above)
- Inherited form is autosomal recessive: mutations in the gene encoding the sodium-bicarbonate co-transporter NBC1. Associated with ocular defects (band keratopathy, cataracts, glaucoma), short stature, intellectual impairment. Affected individuals present in childhood.
- Treatment: large amounts of oral alkali (bicarbonate)

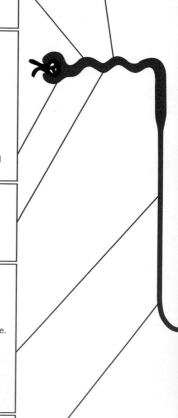

**Bartter Syndrome**
- Failure of sodium and chloride reabsorption by cells of the thick ascending limb of the Loop of Henle.
- Inactivating mutations in NKCC2 -the site of action of *LOOP* diuretics
- Also mutations in other closely-associated ion-channels: ROMK (potassium) plus ClC-Kb (chloride-) and its subunit Barttin
- Hypokalaemia with hyperchloraemic metabolic acidosis
- Hypercalciuria (may lead to nephrocalcinosis and renal failure)
- Present in neonatal period/infancy/childhood with failure to thrive, polyuria, vomiting, dehydration (sodium losses)
- Treatment: correct fluid and electrolyte abnormalities. Prostaglandin synthesis inhibitors (e.g. indomethacin) reduce renal cortical perfusion and hence delivery of sodium and chloride to the nephron, successfully treating the condition.

**Gitelman Syndrome**
- Inactivating mutations in NCCT: the sodium-chloride co-transporter also blocked by *THIAZIDE* diuretics. Autosomal recessive.
- Hypokalaemic metabolic acidosis: similar to Bartter, but…
- Hypocalciuria and hypomagnesaemia
- Present in adulthood with muscle cramps, weakness and low blood pressure
- Treat with magnesium supplements: often enough to correct hypokalaemia but potassium supplements may also be needed

**Liddle Syndrome (pseudohyperaldosteronism)**
- Autosomal dominant: mutations activate the sodium channel ENaC in collecting duct (normally under the control of aldosterone)
- Severe hypertension and metabolic alkalosis (similar to hyperaldosteronism, but with **low** aldosterone levels)
- Presents in childhood–early adulthood
- Treatment: sodium restrict, triamterene/amiloride (inhibit ENaC)

**Classic Distal Renal Tubular Acidosis (RTA type I)**
- Failure of distal urinary acidification
- Moderate-severe metabolic acidosis (normal anion gap/hyperchloraemic) with **hypo**kalaemia
- Hypercalciuria, nephrolithiasis and nephrocalcinosis
- Rickets and growth retardation in affected children, osteomalacia and bone pain in adults
- Diagnose by high urine pH (> 5.5) in presence of systemic metabolic acidosis
- Treat with moderate doses oralalkali
- 

ACQUIRED CAUSES:
- Autoimmune disease: Sjögren syndrome, SLE
- Drugs: amphotericin
- Nephrocalcinosis: hyperparathyroidism

AUTOSOMAL DOMINANT (AD):
- Mutations in gene encoding sodium/bicarbonate exchanger AE1
- Present in teens/adulthood with moderate acidosis

AUTOSOMAL RECESSIVE (AR):
- Mutations in genes encoding proton pump subunits (which have tissue-specific expression)
- Present in infancy with severe acidosis
- Associated with sensorineural hearing loss (the kidney and inner ear share the same protonpump subunits)

**Hyperkalaemic Distal Renal Tubular Acidosis (RTA type IV)**
- Acquired forms only, associated with a deficiency of aldosterone, or a failure of the distal nephron to respond to it appropriately
- Mild metabolic acidosis with **hyper**kalaemia
- Mild to moderate renal impairment invariably present, urine pH can be normal when acidotic
- Causes: Addison disease, diabetes mellitus, renal interstitial disease (chronic obstructive nephropathy, SLE), drugs (ciclosporin, β-blockers, NSAIDs, spironolactone)
- Treatment: stop offending drugs, monitor, consider fludrocortisone/alkali therapy

**Combined Proximal and Distal Renal Tubular Acidosis (RTA type III)**
- Caused by inherited mutations in carbonic anhydrase II (CA II)
- This enzyme is essential for normal acid/base handling by both proximal and distal nephron
- CA II defect also affects osteoclasts and *osteopetrosis* results: defective bone formation (dense but increased fragility) with intracerebral calcification and intellectual impairment.

# 17.18 Urinary tract obstruction

## Background

Chronic urinary tract obstruction is a common cause of CKD, and should be excluded in every patient that presents with acute or chronic renal impairment. Obstruction may occur at any point from the pelvis of the kidney to the distal end of the urethra.

## Epidemiology

- 5% of ESRF is caused by obstruction.
- Urinary tract obstruction has been found in 3.8% of a large series of routine autopsies and 25% of autopsies carried out upon uraemic patients.
- Hydronephrosis is the most common cause of an abdominal mass in neonates, and obstruction, usually due to congenital abnormalities, is also relatively common in children.
- Incidence declines after the age of 10 and is at its lowest in middle age.
- Rises in incidence after the age of 60, particularly in ♂, in whom the most common cause is prostatic enlargement.

## Aetiology

There are many possible causes of obstruction—the most common are:

- **Benign prostatic hyperplasia**—is a major cause of renal failure in men over the age of 60, and frequently presents late. 25% of men >60 years have lower urinary tract symptoms, usually caused by a mixture of obstruction and bladder dysfunction.
- **Prostatic malignancy**—may cause bladder outflow obstruction, and occasionally can cause bilateral ureteric obstruction by occluding both ureters where they enter the bladder.
- **Transitional cell carcinoma of the bladder/ureter**—usually presents with macroscopic haematuria, but may also occlude one or (for bladder cancer) both ureters at the level of entry to the bladder.
- **Neuropathic bladder**—in childhood, is commonly caused by spina bifida, which affects 1–5 per 1000 births. Urinary tract outflow problems are present at birth in 15%, and develop in 50%, often over many years. Urethral sphincter dysnergesia results in incomplete bladder emptying, and those with a less severe neurological deficit may have the swiftest onset of renal impairment as they may generate very high bladder pressure.

- **Stones**—these may cause unilateral ureteric obstruction e.g. a staghorn calculus in the pelviureteric junction (PUJ).
- **Retroperitoneal fibrosis (RPF)**—is a rare cause of bilateral mid-ureteric obstruction. It follows peri-aortic inflammation, which is often autoimmune, and may respond to treatment with steroids. Other causes include an inflammatory aortic aneurysm, retroperitoneal malignancy, drugs (e.g. methysergide) and granulomatous disease (e.g. tuberculosis or sarcoid). Symptoms often include malaise, non-specific back pain and low grade fever, and there is usually an acute phase response.
- **PUJ (pelvicalyceal ureteric junction) obstruction**—which be caused by a stone, a fibrous band or which may be congenital, at the junction of the pelvis and ureter. This condition may present as loin pain, or may be asymptomatic and eventually result in an incidental finding of a grossly hydronephrotic kidney.
- **Posterior urethral valves**—occur in ♂ infants and account for 10% of childhood hydronephrosis. The valves are mucosal diaphragms in the posterior urethra at the level of the prostate. 50% present before the age of one with poor stream, distended bladder and failure to thrive secondary to uraemia. Some are detected antenatally on ultrasound. Treatment is usually with intermittent catheterization, but about 20% will progress to ESRF, often following a late presentation.
- **Pregnancy**—hormonal changes leading to smooth muscle relaxation and physical compression of the ureter by the gravid uterus (more marked on the right than the left) may cause ureteric outflow obstruction.
- In the **elderly**, constipation and medication may also contribute to the development of bladder outflow obstruction.

Prolonged obstruction will result in permanent renal damage from a combination of parenchymal compression and renal ischaemia. Histology in severe cases shows tubular loss, interstitial fibrosis and cortical atrophy (which may result in marked cortical thinning).

## Clinical evaluation

### History and examination

- Urinary tract outflow symptoms in the case of prostatic hypertrophy.
- Macroscopic haematuria may indicate malignancy.
- Loin pain or tenderness is suggestive of PUJ or ureteric obstruction, and there may also be a history of renal stone disease.

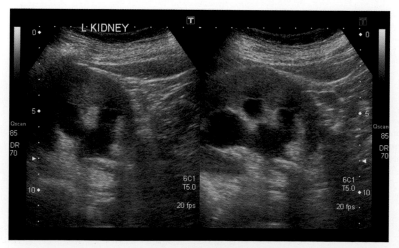

Fig. 17.30 An ultrasound scan of a kidney demonstrating hydronephrosis and pelvicalyceal dilatation in a transverse (left) and longitudinal (right) section.
Courtesy of Cambridge University Hospitals NHS Foundation Trust's Radiology dept.

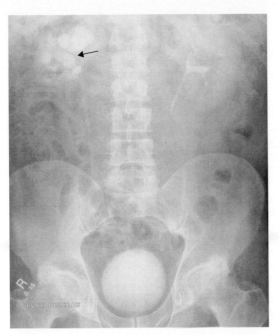

**Fig. 17.31** An intravenous urogram demonstrating excretion of contrast material by the left kidney into the bladder. There is some excretion of contrast from the right kidney along with multiple large round radio-opaque lesions in the kidney consistent with multiple renal calculi (arrow).

Courtesy of Cambridge University Hospitals NHS Foundation Trust's Radiology dept.

### Investigations

- **Urine:**
  - Urinalysis is often normal in obstructive uropathy, but non-visible haematuria may be indicative of malignancy or calculi.
  - Urine cytology should be performed if malignancy is suspected.

- **Radiology:**
  - Ultrasound scan (Fig. 17.30). Hydronephrosis (often with ureteric dilatation) strongly suggests obstruction. However, after the relief of the obstruction the system may remain dilated. Renal transplants may have a dilated renal pelvis without obstruction. Conversely, obstruction may be present without dilation, e.g. if there is peri-renal fibrosis as a result of malignancy or infection (such as tuberculosis).
  - Intravenous urogram (Fig. 17.31). Although this will also show hydronephrosis and may demonstrate the site of ureteric obstruction, it is not a good test if the renal function is poor as little contrast medium may be excreted. In addition the contrast may further impair residual renal function.
  - Dynamic renography with $^{99}$Tc-MAG3 (Fig.17.32). Delay in isotope excretion indicates current, rather than historic, obstruction.
  - Pyelography—either retrograde via cystoscopy and ureteroscopy, or antegrade via a percutaneous nephrostomy, may be required to diagnose both the cause and the site of the obstruction.

## Management and prognosis

Relief of urinary tract obstruction depends on the cause of the obstruction, and may require either:

- Urinary catheter.
- Percutaneous nephrostomy followed by antegrade stenting.
- Ureteroscopy and retrograde stenting.

Patients with urinary tract obstruction should be discussed with the urology team.

The degree of renal recovery following obstruction depends on the duration and degree of the obstruction. After long-standing complete or near complete obstruction, the renal cortex thins, and may disappear entirely, precluding any recovery of renal function in this kidney, now effectively an empty sack. After acute obstruction, relieved promptly, complete renal recovery should be expected.

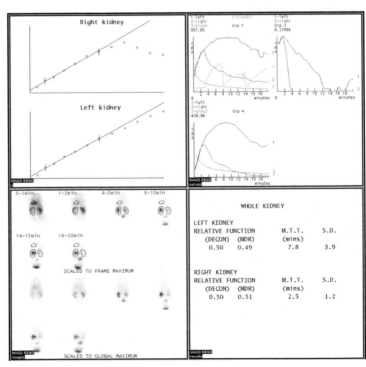

**Fig. 17.32** A $^{99m}$Tc-MAG3 scan demonstrating prompt tracer excretion by the right kidney with delayed excretion by the left kidney. In the upper panel, at 19–20 minutes, trace is still seen in the left kidney (viewed from behind, arrow), whilst virtually none is seen in the right kidney. Similarly in the lower panel tracer is seen to remain in the left kidney over time.

Courtesy of Cambridge University Hospitals NHS Foundation Trust's Radiology dept.

## Background

Stones can form at any level within the urinary tract; the majority, however, form within the renal pelvicalyceal system.

## Epidemiology

- 10% of men, 5% of women.
- 50% of patients will have a further episode within 10 years.

## Risk/predisposing factors

See Table 17.7.

## Pathology

Calcium stones (70–80%):
- Formed of calcium oxalate ± phosphate.
- Usually associated with hypercalcaemia or -calciuria, but 25% of calcium stone-formers have neither.
- Radio-opaque.

Infection (struvite or triple phosphate) stones (15%):
- Caused by infection with urea-splitting bacteria.
- May form staghorn calculi, filling the renal pelvis.
- Radio-opaque.

Urate stones (5–10%):
- Favoured by hyperuricaemic disorders, e.g. leukaemia, gout.
- Radiolucent.

Cystine stones (2%):
- Patients with cystinuria.
- Weakly radio-opaque.

Other:
- Xanthine stones (xanthinuria).
- Drugs, e.g. indinavir.

All stones also contain an organic matrix of mucoprotein (<5% by weight).

## Pathogenesis

All of the following can be important:
1. Supersaturation of urine with stone constituents.
2. Changes in urinary pH (especially alkaline urine).
3. Reduced urine volume (aids point (1)).
4. Infection.

However, stones can form in the absence of these factors, and are usually only unilateral. Therefore local factors favouring precipitation are also important, as may be the concentration of inhibitors of stone formation, such as citrate.

## Presentation

- Asymptomatic haematuria or the passage of small stone(s).
- Acute renal colic; pain radiating from flank to groin.
- May be accompanied by systemic upset with nausea and vomiting, plus fevers if infection present.

## Investigations

- Send stone for composition analysis (if available).
- Urinalysis, urine pH, microscopy and culture.
- U&E.
- Serum calcium, phosphate, bicarbonate, urate.
- PTH if calcium elevated.
- If diagnostic doubt during an acute episode, unenhanced computed tomography is the investigation of choice (99% diagnostic accuracy).
- Plain abdominal radiographs (KUB) may help, particularly to follow stone growth or response to treatment (Figs 17.33 and 17.34).

| Table 17.7  Risk/predisposing factors for the development of renal calculi | |
|---|---|
| **Anatomical** | **Metabolic** |
| • Congenital renal abnormality (horseshoe kidneys) <br> • Urinary stasis (any cause of hydronephrosis, calyceal diverticulae, medullary sponge kidney*) <br> • Vesicoureteric reflux | • Causes of hyper-calcaemia and -calciuria; primary hyperparathyroidism, sarcoidosis <br> • Tubular defects; renal tubular acidosis, cystinuria, medullary sponge kidney* <br> • Hyperoxaluria |
| **Drugs** | **Other** |
| • Carbonic anhydrase inhibitors (e.g. topiramate) <br> • Indinavir <br> • Calcium and vitamin D supplements | • Urinary tract infections <br> • Family history <br> • Diabetes mellitus |

*Medullary sponge kidney is a relatively common disorder that is characterized by malformation of the terminal collecting ducts in the pericalyceal region of the renal pyramids. This is associated with the formation of both small (microscopic) and large medullary cysts that are generally diffuse but do not involve the cortex.

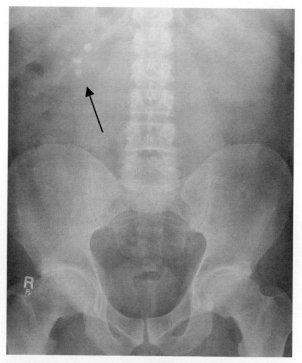

**Fig. 17.33** An abdominal X-ray demonstrating multiple round radio-opaque lesions in the right kidney consistent with multiple renal calculi (arrow). Courtesy of Cambridge University Hospitals NHS Foundation Trust's Radiology dept.

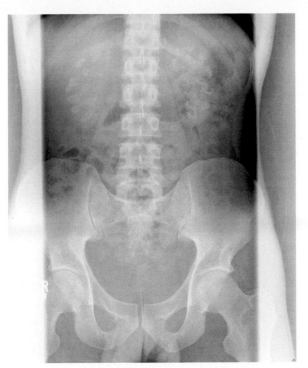

**Fig. 17.34** An abdominal X-ray demonstrating bilateral nephrocalcinosis in a pelvicalyceal distribution.
Courtesy of Cambridge University Hospitals NHS Foundation Trust's Radiology dept.

In **recurrent stone formers, stone disease in childhood, or if an underlying metabolic cause is suspected** a metabolic screen should be performed (after the acute episode) including:

- 24-hour urine collection for urine volume and excretion of calcium and oxalate (in an acidified container), urate (plain container), plus sodium and citrate (either type).
- Urine cystine ('spot' urine; then 24-hour collection if positive).

## Management

The majority of stones <5mm diameter will pass spontaneously, so a conservative approach is sensible:

- Analgesia and anti-emetics.
- Intravenous fluid therapy if required.
- Antibiotics if evidence of infection.

Indications for a more aggressive approach include:

- Obstruction.
- Urosepsis.
- Acute kidney injury.
- Uncontrolled pain.

Urinary tract obstruction may be relieved by insertion of a retrograde ureteric stent or by percutaneous nephrostomy. Ureteroscopy and direct stone retrieval or external shock-wave lithotripsy to shatter the stone may be employed at this point or subsequently.

## Prevention

- All patients should increase their fluid intake, aiming for a urine output of 2–3L/day (reduces urinary concentration of stone constituents).
- Reduce salt intake (urinary calcium excretion correlates with that of sodium).
- Reduce protein intake (leads to lower calcium excretion).
- Treat any underlying metabolic cause.
- Eradicate any chronic urinary infection.
- Avoid foods high in oxalate: rhubarb, tea, chocolate.

## Acute uncomplicated urinary tract infection

One of the most frequent infections in developed countries with 150 million cases per year worldwide and in excess of £4 billion of direct health costs

### Incidence

- Gender (♀ >♂).
- Age (bimodal distribution—the young and old have increased prevalence).
- Sexual activity and spermicide use.
- Predisposing factors (anatomical, functional, urinary stasis, history of diabetes or immunosuppressants).
- Postmenopausal: cystocoele, urinary incontinence or post-micturition residual urine.
- Bacterial virulence factors (fimbriae, siderophores, toxins, protectins).
- 25–30% of patients have recurrent infections.

### Symptoms

- Dysuria.
- Frequency.
- Urgency.
- Suprapubic pain.
- **Note**: the elderly may not present with classic symptoms/signs and may demonstrate:
  - Gastrointestinal complaints (nausea/vomiting).
  - Mental status changes (confusion, delirium).

Differential diagnoses include urethritis and vaginitis.

### Diagnosis

- >$10^5$ organisms per mL **and** white cells in mid-stream specimen of urine (MSSU).
- Common organisms (see Box 17.8).
- Urology evaluation if indicated.

### Treatment

- 3-day course of oral antibiotics.
- Single dose schedule may be useful (improves compliance, reduces antibiotic resistance and side effects).
- Beware resistance (geographical and individual) (Fig. 17.35).
- Early 'recurrence' probably reflects incomplete eradication.
- Longer duration of therapy indicated if there is fever, loin pain or haematuria.

### Prevention

- Increasing fluid intake.
- Voiding post-coitus.
- Cranberry juice:
  - Inhibits adherence of uropathogens to the urothelium
  - A placebo-controlled trial giving cranberry juice to elderly women significantly reduced the incidence of bacteriuria and

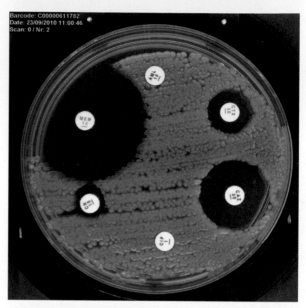

**Fig. 17.35** Microbiological bacterial growth plate (from a mid-stream urine specimen) demonstrating antibiotic resistance testing using drug-impregnated discs. A clear zone around an antibiotic disc reflects bacterial sensitivity to the antibiotic. The larger the zone the more sensitive the bacteria is to the antibiotic.
Courtesy of Cambridge University Hospitals NHS Foundation Trust's Microbiology dept.

pyuria. A non-significant trend towards reduced incidence of symptomatic UTI was observed.
- Antibiotic prophylaxis (post-coital, continuous).
- 'Self-start' regimens (patients have supply of appropriate antibiotic at home to start if symptoms occur).
- Avoid urinary catheterization if possible.

## Complicated UTI

- Usually caused by Gram-negative bacteria.
- Can involve indwelling catheter/stent (frequently requires removal or change).
- Commonly hospital or institution-acquired.
- Incidence increases with advancing age (prostatic disease, neurological conditions, reduced oestrogen levels in postmenopausal women).
- May be associated structural abnormalities of the urinary tract.
- Special consideration of antibiotic choice with renal disease (ciprofloxacin has better cyst penetration in patients with autosomal dominant polycystic kidney disease, ADPKD).

## Asymptomatic bacteriuria

- **Two** separate MSSUs positive for bacterial culture but without symptoms.
- More common in older age group (may not require antibiotics) or those taking immunosuppressants (usually do require antibiotics).
- Affects 2–10% women during pregnancy:
  - If untreated can lead to serious complications (e.g. acute pyelonephritis, premature delivery).
  - **Always treat asymptomatic bacteriuria in pregnancy.**

---

**Box 17.8 Common organisms in acute uncomplicated UTIs**

- *Escherichia coli* (70–95%).
- *Staphylococcus saprophyticus* (5–20%).
- *Proteus mirabilis*.
- *Klebsiella*.
- *Enterococcus*.

## Sterile pyuria

- Leucocytes in urine without apparent bacterial infection.
- Causes include:
  - Recently treated UTI (especially self-treated episodes).
  - Contamination (vaginal flora, sterilizing solution).
  - Chronic interstitial nephritis.
  - Renal stone disease.
  - Urothelial malignancy.
  - Atypical infections—*Mycobacterium tuberculosis*, *Chlamydia*, or *Ureaplasma*.

## Acute pyelonephritis

### Symptoms
- Fevers/rigors.
- Flank, abdominal, or pelvic pain.
- Increased inflammatory markers (WBC, CRP).
- Leucocytes in urine.
- Systemic upset (nausea, vomiting, dehydration).
- Shock with multi-organ involvement including AKI.

### Diagnosis
- Urine culture or blood cultures demonstrating bacterial growth.
- USS—exclude obstruction, renal calculi.

### Treatment
- Hospital admission often required.
- 2-week antibiotic course usually required (although 7 days may be sufficient if it is a mild–moderate infection with an organism susceptible to chosen antibiotic **and** there is clinical improvement following the commencement of antibiotics).
- Parenteral antibiotics may be necessary (at least for first 24–48 hours).
- Supportive rehydration with IV fluids.
- Consider thromboprophylaxis if appropriate.

## Emphysematous pyelonephritis

- Gas-forming organisms (especially *Escherichia coli*) cause a fulminating, necrotizing acute pyelonephritis.
- Diabetes is a significant risk factor (high tissue glucose environment may be favourable to gas-forming organisms).
- Urinary tract obstruction is also a risk factor (especially that caused by papillary necrosis/renal calculi).
- Diagnosed by plain X-ray or CT abdomen/pelvis (Fig. 17.36).
- Clinical features indistinguishable from severe, acute pyelonephritis—systemic antibiotics are essential.
- Sometimes percutaneous drainage of gas/purulent material is required.
- Obstruction, if present, must be relieved.

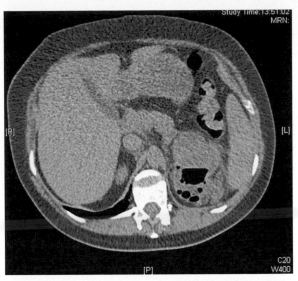

**Fig. 17.36** A CT scan demonstrating free gas in parenchyma of the left kidney secondary to emphysematous pyelonephritis.
Courtesy of Cambridge University Hospitals NHS Foundation Trust's Histopathology dept.

## Xanthogranulomatous pyelonephritis

- Chronic renal infection associated with obstruction and induced by infected renal stones.
- Renal parenchyma replaced by dense infiltrate of lipid-rich macrophages.
- Most common clinical presentation is that of a middle-aged ♀ with a past history of recurrent UTIs.
- A unilateral renal mass can often be palpated.
- Massive destruction of the kidney may occur, requiring nephrectomy.

## Renal abscess

- Rare.
- Two routes of infection:
  - **Ascending:** usually occurs in the setting of an obstructed system and is caused by Gram-negative bacilli—75%.
  - **Bacteraemia:** haematogenous spread—less common, but may be seen in injecting drug user with *Staphylococcus aureus* infective endocarditis.
- Predisposing factors: diabetes, urinary tract abnormalities (e.g. calculi, reflux, obstruction, polycystic kidney disease, neuropathic bladder).
- Treatment includes antimicrobials and drainage.
- Obstruction, if present, must be relieved.

# 17.21 Renovascular disease

## Background

This is usually a consequence of atherosclerosis of the renal arteries; occasionally due to fibromuscular hyperplasia (see Box 17.9).

## Atherosclerotic renovascular disease

- Tends to involve the proximal 1/3 of the renal artery.
- May also be an ostial stenosis (of the renal artery) secondary to encroachment from aortic atherosclerotic plaques.
- Associated with intrarenal atherosclerosis and distal embolism to the kidney (Fig. 17.37).
- Increasing prevalence with increasing age.
- Present in 1/3 of elderly patients with heart failure, 1/3 of patients at coronary angiography, and 2/3 of patients with peripheral vascular disease.
- Accounts for 5–10% of ESRF patients starting dialysis in the UK (the majority of which are aged >65 years).

## Presentation

- Hypertension.
- Chronic renal impairment (ischaemic nephropathy as a result of impaired renal perfusion).
- ACE inhibitor/ARB-related acute renal impairment.
- 'Flash' pulmonary oedema: sudden-onset pulmonary oedema, generally in the presence of normal ventricular function and no evidence of an acute cardiac event.

## Clinical evaluation

### History
- Risk factors for cardiovascular disease.

### Clinical examination
- Blood pressure.
- Evidence of vascular disease elsewhere, e.g. absent peripheral pulses, carotid bruits.
- Renal arterial bruits.

### Investigation
- Inactive urinary sediment.
- U&E.

### Radiology
- Ultrasonography: unequal renal size can provide a clue (implies ischaemic damage, scarring and shrinking of one kidney—the other may be less advanced with the same process).
- Gadolinium-enhanced MRA of the renal arteries is an excellent screening tool, but should be used with caution in those with renal impairment (concerns regarding nephrogenic fibrosing dermopathy).
- Captopril-enhanced renography is a useful screening tool (but not applicable if renal impairment present).
- Angiography of the renal vessels remains the gold standard, and can be combined with treatment (Fig. 17.38).

> ### Box 17.9 Fibromuscular hyperplasia (FMH)
> - Occurs in young females.
> - Presents with difficult-to-control hypertension secondary to hyperplasia of the arterial media.
> - Gives rise to a 'beaded' appearance of the renal artery (mid to distal portions) at angiography.
> - Responds well to angioplasty.

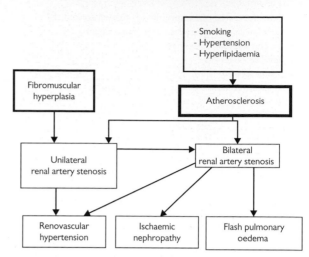

Fig. 17.37 Reduced renal perfusion activates the renin–angiotensin system causing hypertension. The presence of an arterial stenosis means that the affected kidney is unable to mount a pressure natriuresis, so exacerbating the hypertension.

## Treatment

### Medical therapy
- Stop smoking, dietary and lifestyle modification—as for any other atherosclerotic condition.
- Control of hypertension. Because of renin-angiotensin-aldosterone activation, ACEI and ARB are often very effective, but renal function must be monitored after initiation of therapy or dose increases.
- Treat atherosclerotic risk factors, e.g. statins for hyperlipidaemia, aspirin.
- Regular follow-up to monitor renal function

### Radiological intervention: renal revascularization
- Percutaneous angioplasty and stenting is possible in patients with proximal stenoses, generally >70% of the vessel diameter.
- Indications include flash pulmonary oedema and refractory hypertension not controlled by three or more agents. Revascularizing patients with hypertension secondary to renal artery stenosis can provide excellent results, but overall experience from clinical trials has been variable.
- The role of revascularization in patients with renovascular disease causing progressive renal impairment is also unclear. Procedural success rates are high, but long-term renal function may demonstrate little or no benefit.
- Surgical revascularization is possible, and may be necessary if a coexisting aortic aneurysm also requires repair.

## Prognosis
- Prognosis is poor, especially with renal impairment, as a consequence of associated vascular comorbidity.
- <20% 5-year survival on dialysis

## Cholesterol emboli

A systemic disorder with renal impairment that can mimic a systemic vasculitis. Other important differentials include contrast nephropathy, infection, and interstitial nephritis.

### Epidemiology
- Increases with age.

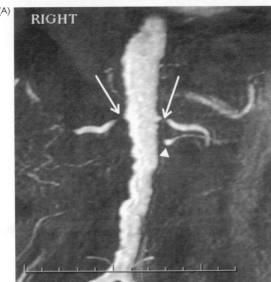

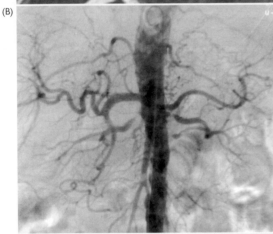

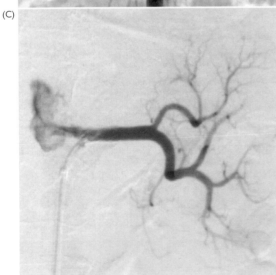

**Fig. 17.38** (A) MR angiogram of a 76-year-old male with bilateral renal artery stenosis (arrowed). Note also the atherosclerotic abdominal aorta. An accessory left renal artery is present, also with origin stenosis (arrowhead). (B & C) Angiographic views of the same patient, with the stenosis clearly evident pre-treatment in (B), and successfully treated post-angioplasty in (C).

Courtesy of Cambridge University Hospitals NHS Foundation Trust's Histopathology dept.

- Caucasians >Afro-Caribbeans.
- ♂ >♀.
- Patients with overt vascular disease.

**Risk factors**
- Hypertension.
- Diabetes.
- Vascular disease.
- Aortic aneurysm.

Often combined with:

**Precipitating factors**
- Interventional procedures: angiography, angioplasty.
- (Cardio)Vascular surgery.
- Anticoagulation, thrombolysis.

**Pathogenesis**
See Fig. 17.39.

**Presentation**
- Stepwise, progressive decline in renal function.
- Typically weeks, occasionally several months between insult and presentation—this obscures the diagnosis (differentiates this from contrast nephropathy which occurs over a few days).
- Classical triad of:
  1. AKI.
  2. Eosinophilia (in 70%).
  3. Skin lesions: blue toes, livedo reticularis.
- Foot pulses palpable (despite signs of distal ischaemia).
- Bruits elsewhere (signs of vascular disease).
- Fever, myalgia.
- Abdominal pain, bowel ischaemia/bleeding, hepatitis.
- Focal neurological deficits.
- Retinal cholesterol emboli (Hollenhorst plaques).

**Investigations**
- Elevated ESR.
- Leucocytosis: eosinophilia.
- Mild proteinuria.
- Hypocomplementaemia.
- Renal biopsy: cholesterol clefts in vessel lumen, surrounded by inflammatory reaction. Biopsy of affected skin may also occasionally demonstrate the same effect.

**Management and prognosis**
- Prevention where possible—use brachial or radial approach to cardiac catheterization in susceptible patients.
- Supportive care.
- Statin therapy may help (stabilizes friable plaques).
- Avoid anticoagulation where possible (may prevent thrombus formation and plaque stabilization).
- Prognosis poor due to general atherosclerotic burden.

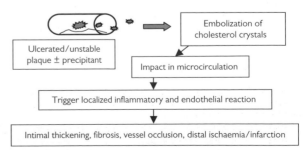

**Fig. 17.39** Pathogenesis of cholesterol emboli.

## Background

Benign renal tumours are relatively common; adenomas (incidental finding in 15% of autopsies) and hamartomas/fibromas. Of malignant tumours, secondary malignancy is statistically more common, but rarely symptomatic. Primary malignancies are predominantly renal cell or transitional cell carcinomas.

## Renal cell carcinoma

### Epidemiology

- 2% adult visceral cancers.
- 90% of adult primary renal malignancy.
- Mean age at presentation = 55 years.
- ♂:♀ = 2:1.

### Aetiology

- 2% are familial: familial renal cell carcinoma (RCC) and von Hippel–Lindau syndrome (see Box 17.10).
- Consider an inherited cause if there is a family history, if patients present before the age of 50 years, or if multiple tumours are present.
- Risk factors: smoking, obesity, hypertension.
- Increased risk in patients with end-stage renal disease.

### Pathology

- Predominantly clear cell type (90%): large cells with clear cytoplasm (Fig. 17.40). Originate from tubular epithelium. Minority described as papillary.
- Highly vascular tumours: invade renal vein early, spread to inferior vena cava and metastasize widely.

### Presentation

- Classic presenting triad:
  1. Haematuria
  2. Loin pain
  3. Abdominal (flank) mass.
- Increasingly an incidental finding during radiological investigation.
- Fever in 20% (cause of a 'pyrexia of unknown origin').
- Due to the 'silent' origin—and tumour biology—of RCC, metastases are seen in 25% at presentation.

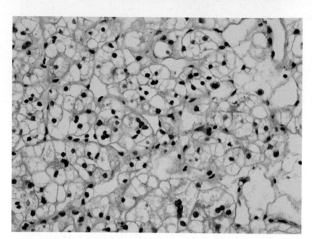

**Fig. 17.40** The carcinoma is characteristically composed of sheets of a fairly uniform population of 'plant-like' cells with clear cytoplasm. The appearance is clear due to the presence of abundant intracytoplasmic lipid which is dissolved out during processing for histology.

- Left-sided RCC invading the renal vein can cause a left varicocoele (the left testicular vein drains into the left renal vein, whereas the right testicular vein drains directly into the inferior vena cava (IVC)).
- Paraneoplastic syndrome (see Box 17.11).

### Investigation

- Renal ultrasonography—solid lesion.
- Enhancing renal mass on CT (with contrast) (Fig.17.41)
- CT and/or MRI to investigate metastatic spread and invasion of the renal vein and IVC.
- Radioisotope imaging (e.g. MAG-3) to determine proportion of overall function contributed by each kidney (important when contemplating surgery).

### Management

Curative surgical treatment for stage I or II disease:
- Radical nephrectomy (can be laparoscopic).
- Partial (or nephron-sparing) nephrectomy: indicated for small (<4cm) tumours, or in patients with single kidney or pre-existing renal impairment.
- Occasionally, surgical resection of advanced disease (e.g. extending into renal vein) may offer a survival advantage.

Medical management for locally invasive or metastatic disease:
- Immunomodulatory therapy with interferon alpha or interleukin-2.
- Emerging therapies target the angiogenesis pathways in RCC (sunitinib and sorafenib), or inhibit the mammalian target of rapamycin—mTOR (temsirolimus)—which activates HIF (see Box 17.10).

---

**Box 17.10 Von Hippel–Lindau (VHL) syndrome**

- Autosomal dominant.
- Incidence = 1/36,000.
- Characterized by:
  - Cerebellar haemangioblastomas.
  - Retinal vascular malformations.
  - Renal, liver, and pancreatic cysts.
  - Phaeochromocytomas.
  - Pancreatic islet cell tumours.
  - 2/3 of patients with VHL develop renal cell carcinoma, often bilateral or multiple.

The underlying cause is a loss-of-function mutation in the tumour suppressor gene *VHL*, located on chromosome 3p25–26. Close to this region (at 3p14) is the gene implicated in familial RCC. 60% of sporadic RCC also contain *VHL* mutations.

The VHL protein normally inhibits hypoxia-inducible factor (HIF). Released from this inhibition, HIF activates expression of pro-angiogenic cytokines. Tumour angiogenesis—and thus growth—is enhanced. mTOR (mammailian target of rapamycin) activates HIF.

---

**Box 17.11 Paraneoplastic syndromes and renal cell carcinoma**

Common, and include:
- Polycythaemia in 2%, due to erythropoietin.
- Hypertension ± hypokalaemia (renin).
- Hypercalcaemia (parathyroid hormone related peptide (PTHrP)).
- Non-metastatic hepatic dysfunction (Stauffer syndrome).
- Cushing syndrome.

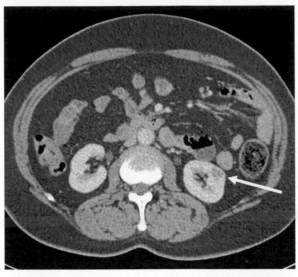

**Fig. 17.41** A CT scan of the abdomen demonstrating a small peripheral lesion in the cortex of the left kidney (arrow) which was subsequently found to be a renal cell carcinoma at nephrectomy.

Courtesy of Cambridge University Hospitals NHS Foundation Trust's Radiology dept.

### Staging and prognosis
See Table 17.8.

---

# Transitional cell carcinoma

- Carcinoma of the urothelium (lining the urogenital tract from renal pelvis to bladder).

### Epidemiology
- 5–10% of adult primary renal malignancy.
- Relatively uncommon in the renal pelvis (bladder:renal pelvis/ureter = 50:1).
- Age at presentation = 50–70 years.
- ♂:♀ = 2:1.

### Risk factors
- Smoking.
- Exposure to industrial carcinogens: arylamines in the paint, rubber and plastics industries.
- Drugs: cyclophosphamide.
- Schistosomiasis (*Schistosoma haematobium*) found in Africa and the Middle East; also predisposes to squamous cell carcinoma of the urothelium.

### Presentation
- Haematuria.
- Obstruction of renal pelvis and flank pain.
- Renal colic due to passage of blood clots.

| Tumour stage | Extent | 5-year survival |
|---|---|---|
| Table 17.8 Staging of RCC | | |
| Stage I | Confined within kidney | 95% |
| Stage II | Extends outside renal capsule, but still within surrounding (Gerota) fascia | 85% |
| Stage 3 | Invading renal vein, IVC or regional lymph nodes | 60% |
| Stage 4 | Invading adjacent viscera ± distant metastases | ≤20% |

### Investigation
- Urine cytology for malignant cells.
- Imaging: intravenous urography and/or CT (Fig. 17.42).
- Ureteroscopy.

### Management
- Radical nephroureterectomy.
- Endoscopic tumour resection if low-grade tumour or patient unsuitable for more aggressive approach.
- Chemotherapy may benefit.
- After surgery, continued surveillance is required to detect tumours arising in the remaining urothelium.

### Prognosis
- 70–90% 5-year survival for lower grade.
- 10% 5-year survival in high-grade tumours.

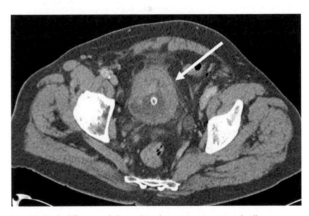

**Fig. 17.42** A CT scan of the pelvis demonstrating a markedly asymmetrical thickening of the bladder wall (arrow) which on histology was seen to be a transitional cell carcinoma. A urinary catheter is *in situ*.

Courtesy of Cambridge University Hospitals NHS Foundation Trust's Radiology dept.

## Polycystic kidney disease

Adult polycystic kidney disease is an autosomal dominant genetic disorder and is the most common inherited renal disease. It is often referred to as **ADPKD**: **A**utosomal **D**ominant **P**olycystic **K**idney **D**isease.

Normal kidney tissue is gradually replaced by cysts leading to renal enlargement and eventually renal failure. Cysts may also occur in other organs. There is an increased risk of intracranial aneurysms (and subarachnoid haemorrhage) in some families.

### Epidemiology
- 5–10% of patients with ESRF.
- Prevalence 1:1000.
- There is considerable phenotypic variability within families, even though the mutation is identical.

### Genetics
- **ADPKD-1** on **chromosome 16**: 85% of cases; encodes polycystin 1, a large transmembrane molecule.
- **ADPKD-2** on **chromosome 4**: 15% of cases; encodes polycystin 2.
- Polycystin 1 and 2 associate to form an ion channel that controls the function of the primary cilium of renal tubular epithelial cells. How this leads to cyst formation is not clearly understood.
- 10% represent new mutations with no family history

### Clinical presentation
- Patients are increasingly likely to be discovered through screening of an affected family (see Box 17.12).

Patients may also present with:
- **Acute abdominal pain** (due to bleeding into a cyst, or cyst infection—as in Fig. 17.43).
- **Hypertension** (present in 80%).
- **Gross haematuria**.
- **Urinary tract infection**—more common in women.
- Incidental discovery of abdominal mass.
- Incidental discovery of renal impairment.

### Physical signs
- Palpable enlarged kidneys.
- Hepatomegaly.
- 'Old' abnormal neurology (if previous subarachnoid haemorrhage).
- Murmur of mitral valve prolapse (associated with ADPKD).

### Diagnosis
- Ultrasound—see Box 17.13.
- Cyst bleeds and infection are essentially a clinical diagnosis. Differentiating cysts containing infection or haemorrhage (from the mass of other cysts) is often very difficult, even with CT or MRI.

### Complications
These are more severe, and occur earlier, in ADPKD-1 than in ADPKD-2.

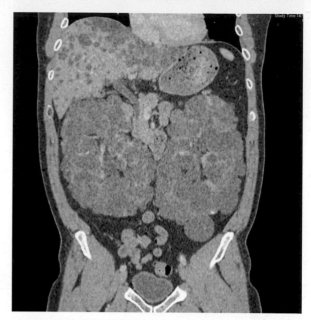

**Fig. 17.43** A coronal CT image of the abdomen in a patient with ADPKD-1. This demonstrates the grossly enlarged kidneys with normal renal tissue replaced by cysts. There are also a few hepatic cysts (top left). This dialysis-dependent patient had been admitted for a nephrectomy in order to create space for a subsequent renal transplant. Courtesy of Cambridge University Hospitals NHS Foundation Trust's Radiology dept.

- ESRF in about 75%:
  - ADPKD-1: at about 50–60 years of age
  - ADPKD-2: at about 65–75 years of age.
- Cardiovascular disease associated with hypertension and CKD.
- Cyst and urinary tract infection
- Bleed into a cyst.
- Chronic back and abdominal discomfort and pain due to the sheer size and weight of the enlarged organs.
- Ruptured intracranial aneurysm. This complicates 5–10% of patients with ADPKD and is much more common in some families than others (Fig. 17.44).
- 70% of patients will have hepatic cysts and although these also enlarge with time, and can produce symptoms through size or internal haemorrhage impairment of liver function is exceedingly rare.

### Treatment
- Hypertension: controlling blood pressure is the best method to retard progression (aim <130/80mmHg). ACE inhibitors **may** be the optimal agent.
- Analgesia (not NSAIDs) for painful symptoms; antibiotics for infection.
- Monitor progression of renal impairment and plan for eventual renal replacement therapy.

---

**Box 17.12 Autosomal recessive polycystic kidney disease**

- Presents in early childhood (can be screened for using antenatal ultrasound).
- Associated with hepatic fibrosis.
- Affected children normally develop end-stage renal failure by the age of 8 years.

**Box 17.13 Differential diagnosis of ADPKD**

- Tuberous sclerosis
- Von–Hippel Lindau
- Oro-facial-digital syndrome
- Acquired cystic disease.

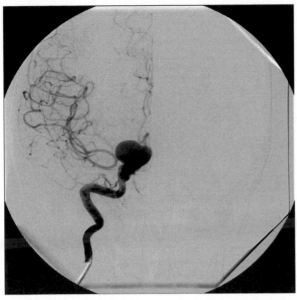

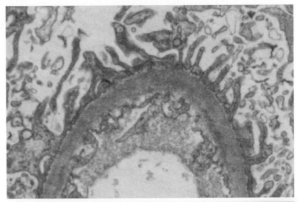

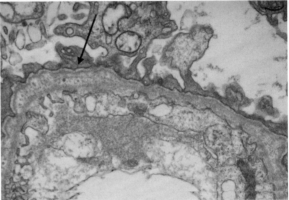

**Fig. 17.44** An intracerebral digital subtraction angiogram demonstrating a cerebral aneurysm in a patient with ADPKD-1.
Courtesy of Cambridge University Hospitals NHS Foundation Trust's Radiology dept.

### Screening for ADPKD

Although genetic testing may become more important in the future, at present ultrasound remains the key diagnostic tool.

The number and size of renal cysts increase with age, and are detectable by ultrasound in most patients from late teens onwards. If cysts are not present in a patient aged <30 years, then the scan should be repeated when they reach this point as a normal ultrasound at age 30 effectively excludes the diagnosis.

Patients wishing to undergo screening should be offered genetic counselling beforehand, as awareness of the diagnosis has implications for financial planning, life insurance, etc.

We normally advocate screening for our patients on the basis that confirming the diagnosis allows planning for the future, closer monitoring of progression and stricter blood pressure control.

#### ADPKD and anaemia

The increased renal mass can result in increased erythropoietin (EPO) production and polycythaemia.

EPO production may be maintained as renal function declines and ADPKD patients often have less problems with anaemia than other patients with ESRF.

### Intracerebral aneurysms (ICA) and ADPKD screening

This is a difficult topic with no definite guidelines—a common approach is:
- Discuss screening for ICA in families who have been affected by this complication, and where it is thus much more likely.
- Cerebral MRA is the current best imaging modality.
- Before imaging the patient, discuss the treatment for ICA if found, i.e. risks of neurosurgery. Because of the difficult nature of such discussions, it may be best to refer the patient to a local neurosurgeon with appropriate expertise before proceeding with screening.
- Unresolved problems with screening include deciding when to start, and whether to repeat imaging in high-risk individuals, (if so, at what interval).

---

# Alport syndrome

Mutations in the genes encoding type IV collagen result in abnormal basement membranes (Fig. 17.45). This is evident in the:

**Fig. 17.45** Electron microscopy (×20,000) demonstrates the classical lamination of the glomerular basement membrane with particles between laminations (arrowed). In other places, the basement membrane thins out. A normal-thickness basement membrane is shown above for comparison.

- **Kidney:** haematuria and progressive renal impairment.
- **Ear:** sensorineural deafness (in 2/3).
- **Eye:** lens abnormalities (in 1/3).

Each type IV collagen molecule is composed of a heterotrimer of three α-chains. Six genes make up the collagen type IV family, encoding chains α1–6, designated COL4A1–6. Although disease results from a variety of mutations in different genes, the common pattern of kidney, eye, and ear pathology persists as mutations in one α-chain prevent normal integration of the other chains into the basement membrane. ~1% of European ESRF patients have Alport syndrome.

### X-linked Alport syndrome
- 80–90% of cases.
- Mutations in COL4A5 encoding α5 chain.
- Different mutations produce different disease phenotypes, hence the pattern of disease is similar within affected families.
- All affected ♂ develop haematuria in childhood, then progressive renal insufficiency, usually reaching ESRF by 15–30 years of age.
- ♀ heterozygotes may have haematuria, but their prognosis is generally benign. Only a few develop renal impairment, late in life.
- Sensorineural deafness affects 2/3. Like the kidney disease, it develops during childhood and early adulthood.
- Ocular defects affect 1/3, classically bilateral anterior lenticonus, or protrusion of the lens into the anterior chamber. Cataracts may develop.

### Autosomal recessive Alport syndrome
- 10% of cases.
- Mutations in COL4A3 or COL4A4 (both on chromosome 2).

- Similar features to X-linked disease. Affected individuals develop ESRF and sensorineural deafness by the age of 30 years, regardless of gender.

## Autosomal dominant Alport syndrome

- Rare, result of various mutations.

## Rare associations of Alport syndrome

- Maculopathy.
- Leiomyomata.
- Thrombocytopaenia (Epstein syndrome).

## Pathophysiology (renal)

Mutation in *COL4* gene

↓

Abnormal collagen type IV in glomerular basement membrane (GBM)—absence or altered structure of one or more α-chains

↓

Abnormal, irregular structure of GBM

↓

Proteinuria

↓ ↑

Progressive renal insufficiency

## Presentation

- Non-visible haematuria in childhood/early adulthood.
- Occasionally macroscopic haematuria (may follow upper respiratory tract infection—like IgA nephropathy).
- Proteinuria and nephrotic syndrome.
- Renal impairment.
- Hearing loss.

## Investigations

- Urinalysis.
- Audiometry.
- Slit-lamp examination of the eye.
- Renal biopsy:
  1. Electron microscopy: ultrastructural abnormalities of the GBM.
  2. Immunohistochemistry: absence of one or more collagen type IV α-chains in basement membranes.
- Genetic mutation identification (occasionally).

## Treatment

- No specific treatment is available.

## Kidney transplantation in Alport syndrome

- The disease does not recur post-transplantation, but…
- Transplantation introduces a kidney expressing normal collagen type IV, and individuals (particularly those with large mutations and absent—rather than truncated—protein) are at increased risk of developing anti-GBM (Goodpasture) disease with subsequent

loss of the transplant. Autoantibodies are produced against the now novel collagen chains in the donor organ GBM.

- This is a problem in 2–3% of cases.

## Primary hyperoxaluria

Oxalate is an organic anion formed in the human body from a combination of dietary ingestion/absorption and biosynthesis. There are three types of primary hyperoxaluria; types I and II are autosomal recessive and indistinguishable clinically.

- **Type I** (the most common): hepatic alanine:glyoxylate aminotransferase deficiency.
- **Type II:** hepatic glyoxylate reductase deficiency.
- **Type III:** intestinal hyperabsorption.

Secondary hyperoxaluria may result from small intestinal disease such as Crohn disease, blind loops, and jejunoileal bypass.

## Pathogenesis

- Normally oxalate is excreted by the kidney.
- In hyperoxaluria, calcium oxalate stones and oxalate deposition in the renal interstitium (nephrocalcinosis) combine to cause progressive renal failure.
- As the GFR falls (especially below 25mL/min) plasma oxalate levels rise and oxalate becomes deposited in many other tissues, particularly vascular and bone.

## Clinical features

- ESRF by age of 20 years.
- Cardiomyopathy, painful osteodystrophy, neuropathy.

## Diagnosis

- Increased 24-hour urinary oxalate excretion (crystals may be seen in the urine—see Section 17.4).
- Decreased enzymatic activity on liver biopsy.

## Treatment

- High fluid intake and low oxalate diet.
- Pyridoxine reduces oxalate production (effective in 2/3 of patients).
- As ESRF approaches, dialyse early and aggressively (GFR <25mL/min) to minimize tissue oxalate deposition.
- Combined liver and kidney transplantation reverses the hepatic enzyme deficiency and renal failure.

## Fabry disease

- Also known as Anderson–Fabry disease.
- An X-linked recessive lysosomal storage disorder.
- Deficiency of lysosomal α-galactosidase A.
- Ceramide trihexoside (a glycosphingolipid) is deposited in the kidneys, skin and vasculature.
- Affected ♂ die in their 4th or 5th decade (secondary to cardiac or renal pathology).
- ♀ heterozygotes are usually asymptomatic, but occasionally have mild manifestations.

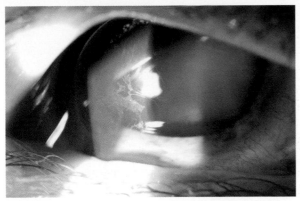

**Fig. 17.46** Cornea verticillata in an individual with Fabry's disease. Reproduced with permission from Cambridge University Hospitals NHS Foundation Trust.

### Clinical features

- Angiokeratoma corporis diffusum—red-black telangiectatic macules and papules over the lower trunk and thighs which appear at puberty.
- Progressive renal failure (ESRF by age 40 years).
- Cardiac sequelae: ischaemic heart disease, cardiac valvular defects, arrhythmias, restrictive cardiomyopathy.
- Autonomic neuropathy.
- Painful peripheral neuropathy with pain and paraesthesiae provoked by temperature change and exercise.
- Cerebrovascular disease.
- Superficial corneal dystrophy—cornea verticillata, whorl-like corneal pattern of lipid (glycosphingolipid) deposits (Fig. 17.46).

### Treatment

Recombinant human α-galactosidase A should reverse the accumulation of glycosphingolipid in affected tissues. It has been demonstrated to reduce the progression of renal disease in patients with Fabry Disease.

# 17.24 Renal disease and pregnancy

## Background

The assessment and management of renal disease in pregnancy is complicated by a number of normal anatomical and physiological changes which take place. Renal biopsy is often avoided in the later stages of pregnancy, whilst many medications used in the treatment of renal disease need to be reviewed because of their risk to the fetus.

## Monitoring renal function in pregnancy

- Renal blood flow, and therefore GFR, rises in pregnancy and this, combined with an expansion in plasma volume, leads to a fall in serum creatinine and urea.
- MDRD and Cockcroft–Gault formulae for the calculation of creatinine clearance are unreliable in pregnant women and have not been properly validated.
- Creatinine clearance by 24-hour urine collection has been shown to correlate well with inulin clearance, and is therefore a more accurate measure of renal function in pregnancy.
- Proteinuria increases—this is predominantly aminoaciduria, although there may also be an increase in albuminuria. Protein loss does not generally exceed 300mg per day in an uncomplicated pregnancy.
- Renal anatomy changes, with an increase in kidney size caused by increased renal vascular and interstitial volume. The collecting system also dilates in 80% of pregnant women by the start of the 2nd trimester, as a result of progesterone-induced reductions in ureteric tone and peristalsis. These changes increase the risk of urinary infection and bacteriuria in a pregnant woman should therefore always be treated. The hydronephrosis usually resolves within a few weeks of parturition.

## Impact of pre-eclampsia on renal function

- Renal blood flow and GFR fall in pre-eclampsia. However, serum creatinine and urea may remain in the normal range, despite a reduction in GFR of 30–40% from the usual high level seen in pregnant women.
- Glomerular capillary lumen size reduces as endothelial cells hypertrophy—a process known as 'glomerular endotheliosis'.
- These changes are associated with a loss of size and charge selectivity of the glomerular barrier, resulting in the proteinuria which is the hallmark of pre-eclampsia. Protein loss can range from 300mg to 10g per day.
- Both the glomerular changes and the proteinuria usually disappear within 2 months of delivery.
- Pre-eclampsia can result in acute tubular necrosis and even renal cortical necrosis. The incidence of AKI requiring renal replacement therapy is unclear, but small studies have found that 20–50% of acute renal failure in pregnant women followed pre-eclampsia.
- Pre-eclampsia is associated with the development of chronic hypertension in the future which has been attributed to subtle renal injury. Pre-eclampsia has also been associated with the development of chronic kidney disease in postmenopausal women, although studies of women between 3 months and 6 years post pregnancy found no difference in renal function between women with or without a history of pre-eclampsia

or HELLP (haemolysis, elevated liver enzymes, low platelets) syndrome.

## Chronic kidney disease and pregnancy

- Women with a creatinine <130μmol/L, without hypertension or proteinuria, have good maternal and fetal outcomes.
- The degree of renal impairment, rather than the nature of the underlying renal disease, is thought to be the principal determinant of outcome.
- Women with serum creatinine between 130 and 250μmol/L tend to have a fall in creatinine in the 1st trimester, which may then rise above the previous baseline as the pregnancy progresses.
- A woman who becomes pregnant with a creatinine >220μmol/L is estimated to have a 70% chance of delivering early, and a 40% chance of pre-eclampsia.
- In addition, women with a GFR <40mL/minute and proteinuria >1g/day are at risk of accelerated renal loss both during and after pregnancy.
- Women with nephrotic range proteinuria have an increased risks of pre-eclampsia, spontaneous abortion, preterm delivery, and intrauterine growth restriction.
- Hypertension is also a risk factor for pre-eclampsia, which occurs in 30% of women with hypertension pre-pregnancy, compared with an incidence of 8% in the general population.

## Pregnancy in transplant recipients

- >14,000 renal transplant recipients have given birth since the first report of a successful pregnancy 18 months after a renal transplant in 1956.
- As in CKD, the risks of pregnancy to both the fetus and the renal allograft depend on the level of renal function and proteinuria.
- Renal transplant recipients with creatinine levels >130μmol/L and proteinuria >500mg/day are significantly more likely to develop accelerated allograft failure.
- It is generally recommended that women should be advised to wait at least 1 year post transplantation before trying to conceive, and that they should be on a stable immunosuppressive regimen.

## Medications in pregnancy

- Ciclosporin, tacrolimus, azathioprine, and corticosteroids are considered the safest immunosuppressants to use in pregnancy.
- Mycophenolate mofetil (MMF) and sirolimus are teratogenic in animals and teratogenicity has also been described with MMF in humans.
- Drugs which inhibit the renin–angiotensin–aldosterone system, including both ACE inhibitors and ARBs, are teratogenic and should be stopped prior to pregnancy.
- If used in the 2nd and 3rd trimesters, these drugs may cause fetal hypotension, anuria-oligohydramnios, growth restriction, pulmonary hypoplasia, renal tubular dysplasia, neonatal renal failure, and hypocalvaria.

# Chapter 18

# Respiratory medicine

# 18.1 An introduction to the respiratory system

## Relevance

Diseases of the respiratory system account for major healthcare burdens in both the developed and developing world. The mortality due to respiratory illnesses varies widely across the different diagnostic categories and ages.

Acute respiratory infection deaths are still common in the developing world; respiratory infections in the UK are a common cause of GP visits. Cigarette smoking advertising is now focused on developing nations and associated illnesses such as chronic obstructive pulmonary disease (COPD) will become a 'top five' cause of death worldwide by 2020 as estimated by the World Health Organization.

## Pulmonary anatomy—an overview

The respiratory tract starts at the nose and ends at the alveoli. The upper airways and sinuses will not be discussed further.

The structure of the lungs is adapted to the functions of
- Gas transport in the airways.
- Gas mixing in the alveoli.
- Gas transfer across the alveolar–capillary membrane.

## Airways

The **trachea** starts immediately below the larynx. It is 'D' shaped in cross-section and only half of it lies within the thorax; the remainder being in the neck. An average adult trachea is approximately 10cm in length.

At the **main carina** (or bifurcation), the trachea divides into the left and right main bronchus (Fig. 18.1). The carina lies at the level of the 'angle of Louis' anteriorly or the 5th/6th thoracic vertebra posteriorly. It is surrounded by pulmonary blood vessels, lymph nodes, and the left atrium sits just inferior to this. The right main bronchus

is less sharply angled from the trachea than the left, making aspirated material more likely to enter the right lung. During intubation, e.g. for general anaesthesia, if the intubation airway is advanced too far it will preferentially enter the right main bronchus and the left lung may not be ventilated. **Bronchi** are conducting airways lined with cilia that have a wave-like motion. The bronchial walls contain smooth muscle and elastic tissue as well as cartilage in the larger airways. In the large airways, gas movement occurs by tidal flow. By contrast, in the small airways (division 17 and smaller) it results from diffusion only. The smallest subdivisions of the bronchi are called **bronchioles**, at the ends of which are the alveoli.

## Alveolar–capillary unit

**Alveoli** are the very small air sacs where gas exchange occurs. The pulmonary capillaries are embedded in the walls of the alveoli. The **pulmonary arteries** supply the alveolar capillaries with deoxygenated blood with the lungs receiving 100% of the right ventricular cardiac output. While in the **pulmonary capillaries** the blood discharges carbon dioxide into the alveoli and takes up oxygen from the air in the alveoli. After gas exchange at the **alveolar–capillary membrane** re-oxygenated blood is taken by the pulmonary veins to the left atrium.

## Other components

The **diaphragm** is the major inspiratory muscle that separates the chest cavity from the abdominal cavity. Although often referred to as a single unit the left and right hemi-diaphragms are separately innervated by the respective **phrenic nerve**. A diaphragmatic palsy can occur after phrenic nerve damage, e.g. after neck surgery or trauma. Healthy diaphragmatic contraction results in downward movement creating negative intrathoracic pressure that draws in the air and expands the lungs. The **pleura** are a double layer of membranes surrounding the lungs—the visceral pleura enveloping the lung itself

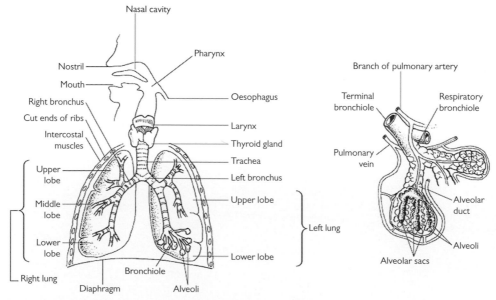

**Fig. 18.1** The lungs and main air passages (left panel) with details of the alveoli (right panel).
Reproduced from *Oxford Concise Medical Dictionary*, 2002, page 401, with permission from Oxford University Press.

and the parietal pleura lining the thoracic cavity. Under normal circumstances the interpleural space between these layers contains only a tiny amount of lubricating fluid. The pleura extend from just above the clavicle down to the 8th rib anteriorly, the 10th rib laterally, and the level of T12 posteriorly. In disease states this volume can increase causing a significant pleural effusion.

## Right and left lung surface markings

**Apex**: both lung apices sit in their respective supraclavicular fossa—this explains the vulnerability of the lungs to iatrogenic pneumothorax when central venous lines (jugular or subclavian) are inserted.

**Bases**: in a normal adult the lungs will extend anteriorly to the level of the 8th thoracic vertebra and posteriorly to the level of the 10th thoracic vertebra.

## Upper, lower, and middle lobes

The right lung is divided into three lobes (upper, middle, and lower) whereas the left has only two (upper and lower), with further division into the broncho-pulmonary segments (10 on the right, 9 on the left). In total there are up to 23 airway divisions between trachea and alveoli.

- The upper lobes sit in the apex and extend to account for **most** of the anterior aspect of the chest.
- The lower lobes lie along the diaphragms and account for **most** of the posterior aspect of the chest.
- The right middle lobe and the left-sided lingula lobe have small surface markings and are found in a small area under the axilla laterally.
- To examine the chest properly and auscultate all lobes you must therefore listen anteriorly, laterally, and posteriorly.

## Respiratory defence

The average person breathes about 20,000 litres of air per day containing potentially harmful particles and gases. Larger particles, fungi, bacteria, and viruses are often trapped in the upper airway whilst small particles <3–5 microns in size can penetrate to the deep parts of the lung.

### Non-specific defence mechanisms

- **Cationic antimicrobial peptides** (CAMPS): highly positively charged peptides secreted into the airways which bind/damage bacterial cell walls. Complement and mannose binding lectin are also present in airway secretions.
- **Mucociliary escalator:** the airways are covered by liquid multilayered mucus that is propelled by the cilia at about 1cm per minute. Particles and pathogens trapped here are cleared to the mouth and swallowed. The alveoli are not protected in this manner.
- **Alveolar macrophages** 'ingest' and remove deposited particles. Injured epithelial cells may release chemokines that recruit additional leucocytes, especially neutrophils, from the bloodstream.

### Specific defence mechanisms

- Antibody production: although the precise site of antibody production may not be clear, patients deficient in antibody secretion, e.g. those with common variable immune deficiency, have much higher rates of respiratory infections. The lung is normally rich in secretory IgA (sIgA)
- Cellular-mediated immunity: memory T and B cells are believed to traffic throughout the body and some may reside in the bronchus-associated lymphoid tissue. Often pathogens are intracellular, e.g. tuberculosis.

## Physiology

The normal respiratory rate is 12–16 breaths per minute. Breathing is controlled by the brainstem which is regulated mainly by the input from chemoreceptors located both centrally and peripherally. Normally control is exercised by the central receptors located in the medulla, which respond to the cerebrospinal fluid (CSF) hydrogen ion concentration, in turn determined by carbon dioxide ($CO_2$), which diffuses freely across the blood–brain barrier from the arterial blood. The response is rapid and sensitive to small changes in arterial $CO_2$ ($PaCO_2$). Peripheral chemoreceptors located in the carotid and aortic bodies mostly respond to a fall in arterial oxygen ($PaO_2$), but some also respond to a rise in $PaCO_2$.

A pressure gradient is required to generate flow in the airways. In spontaneous respiration inspiratory flow is achieved by creating a sub-atmospheric pressure in the alveoli (around −5cm of water pressure during quiet breathing) by increasing the volume of the thoracic cavity under the action of the inspiratory muscles. During expiration the intra-alveolar pressure becomes slightly higher than atmospheric pressure and gas flow to the mouth results.

- The main inspiratory muscles are the diaphragm and inspiration is active.
- Normal expiration is predominantly passive.
- Each breath in a normal adult is around 500mL (tidal volume). All respiratory lung volumes are, however, dictated by height, age, sex, and racial origins.

The alveoli–capillary interface provides a huge surface area for gas exchange with pulmonary blood (between 50–100m²).

- Oxygen ($O_2$) uptake is active and is driven by the oxygen binding affinity of haemoglobin (Hb).
- 1g of Hb can carry 1.34mL of oxygen if fully saturated. At a $PaO_2$ of 13.3kPa, Hb is normally about 97% saturated with $O_2$. If the Hb concentration is 15g/100mL, arterial blood will hold approximately 200mL/L $O_2$. At a cardiac output of 5L/min, the amount of $O_2$ available in the circulation is 1000mL/minute. Of this, approximately 250mL/minute is used at rest, the Hb in venous blood being about 75% saturated.
- Normal Hb saturations in adults are 96–97%. The Hb–$O_2$ dissociation curve means that any fall in $PaO_2$ from the normal arterial value will have little effect on the Hb saturation (and $O_2$ content) until the steep part of the curve is reached, normally around 8kPa. Once the $PaO_2$ has fallen to this level, however, any further decrease in will result in a dramatic fall in the Hb saturation. $O_2$ saturations of 95% or below are abnormal; saturations of 95% are equivalent to an arterial $O_2$ partial pressure of 9.5kPa.
- At sea level air $O_2$ has a partial pressure of 21kPa. Oxygenated blood in the pulmonary veins has a partial pressure of around 14kPa whilst normal adult systemic arterial $O_2$ partial pressures are 12kPa. Hypoxia occurs when $PaO_2$ is <10kPa.
- $CO_2$ excretion is passive and relies on passive diffusion from the blood to the alveoli (negligible concentrations).

### Ventilation/perfusion matching

In contrast to the rest of the body the pulmonary arteries carry deoxygenated blood and the pulmonary veins carry oxygenated blood. The arteries are able to constrict in the presence of low $O_2$ content (hypoxic vasoconstriction) whereas systemic arteries passively dilate in the presence of low $O_2$/high $CO_2$ content (hypoxic vasodilatation). This unique phenomenon in the lung maximizes air to blood mixing and gas exchange. This is called **ventilation/perfusion (V/Q) matching**. Processes disrupting ventilation perfusion matching, e.g. pulmonary emboli, COPD will cause hypoxia.

### Hypoxia

**Hypoxic hypoxia**—defined as an inadequate $PaO_2$ in arterial blood. This occurs when the $PaO_2$ is <10kPa and can result from an inadequate $PO_2$ in the inspired air (e.g. altitude), hypoventilation (from central or peripheral causes), or from inadequate alveolar–capillary transfer (such as an arteriovenous shunt or V/Q mismatch).

**Anaemic hypoxia**—the $O_2$ content of arterial blood is almost all bound to Hb. With severe anaemia, the $O_2$ content falls in proportion to the reduction in Hb, even though the $PO_2$ is normal. When the normal compensatory mechanism of an increase in cardiac output can no longer be sustained, tissue hypoxia results.

**Circulatory or stagnant hypoxia**—in circulatory failure even though the $O_2$ content of arterial blood may be adequate, delivery to the tissues is not. Initially tissue oxygenation is maintained by increasing the degree of $O_2$ extraction from the blood, but as tissue perfusion worsens this becomes insufficient and tissue hypoxia develops.

**Histotoxic hypoxia**—here there is an inability of the tissues to use $O_2$ even though $O_2$ delivery to the tissues is normal. The best known cause of histotoxic hypoxia is cyanide poisoning, which inhibits the intracellular respiratory chain. Carbon monoxide poisoning can also contribute to this form of hypoxia where the $O_2$ is delivered to the tissues but the carboxy-haemoglobin does not release it once there.

# 18.3 Respiratory investigations

## An overview

The respiratory system can be tested functionally or radiologically. 'Simple' chest radiography is the focus of other texts and will not be specifically discussed. CT scanning allows the 2D or 3D assessment of more dense structures such as the mediastinum/blood vessels and less dense structures such as the lungs. The test does require patients to lie flat and is often unhelpful in very tachypnoeic patients. CT pulmonary angiograms (CTPA) are increasingly replacing ventilation/perfusion (V/Q) scans as a means to identify pulmonary emboli.

## Pulmonary function

Pulmonary function tests offer several useful functions in patients with respiratory disease:
- Defining the respiratory disorder.
- Quantifying the severity of any deficit.
- Monitoring the course of a disease.

Normal values depend on the patient's height, age, and sex.

Simple tests such as spirometry or measurement of peak expiratory flow may be performed at the bedside; more complex tests require a lung function laboratory (Fig. 18.2).

## Lung volumes

- Tidal volume is the volume of air which enters and leaves the lungs during normal breathing ($V_T$).
- The functional residual capacity (FRC) is the volume of gas within the lungs at the end of a normal expiration.
- The volume of gas in the lungs after a full inspiration is the total lung capacity (TLC).
- After full expiration there is still some gas in the lungs called the residual volume (RV).
- Vital capacity (VC) is the volume of air expelled by maximal expiration after full inspiration.

## Spirometry

Spirometry measures changes in lung volume by recording the volume of air exhaled through the airway opening (Fig. 18.3). One common technique is to plot the volume of air exhaled from a patient's lungs against time following a forced expiratory manoeuvre—a forced expiratory spirogram.

### Vital capacity

- Vital capacity is the volume of air expelled by maximum expiration after full inspiration. This is often derived from a forced expiratory spirogram—the forced vital capacity (FVC). If measured by a slow exhalation it is slow vital capacity. The slow VC and FVC are very similar but in patients with airflow obstruction, e.g. COPD, the FVC may be significantly smaller than the slow VC.
- Reduced vital capacity is seen in:
  - Reduced lung compliance, e.g. lung fibrosis and loss of lung volume.
  - Chest deformities, e.g. kyphoscoliosis.
  - Muscle weakness, e.g. myopathy, myasthenia.
  - Airflow obstruction, e.g. COPD.

### Forced expiratory volume in 1 second ($FEV_1$)

- The volume of air expelled in the first second of maximal forced expiration from full inspiration.
- Reduced in any condition that reduces the VC.
- Particularly reduced where there is airflow obstruction (defined as $FEV_1$/VC below 0.75).
- A restrictive defect is defined by a proportional reduction in both VC and in $FEV_1$ so that the $FEV_1$/VC ratio is normal.

### Peak expiratory flow rate (PEFR)

- Peak expiratory flow is the maximum rate of airflow achieved during a sudden forced expiration from a full inspiration. The best of three attempts is usually accepted. It is effort dependent and mainly determined by the resistance of the major airways.

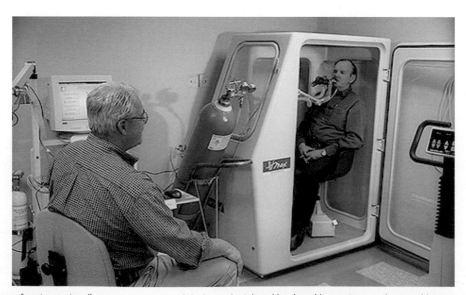

**Fig. 18.2** Respiratory function testing allows many measures of the lungs physiology. Very breathless patients or those unable to sit within a body plethysmograph, e.g., severe kyphoscoliosis, spinal fixation may be unable to perform many of the tests.

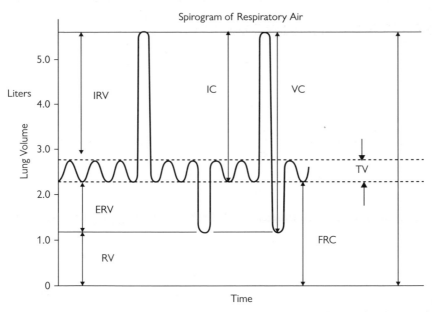

Spirogram of Respiratory Air

**Fig. 18.3** A spirogram demonstrating static lung volumes. TV represents tidal volume (adult normal ~500mL). VC vital capacity (adult normal 4–5L). RV represents residual volume (adult normal <1.5L). The predicted values differ based on age, sex, height, and race.

Reproduced from Weatherall DJ, Ledingham JGG, Warrell DA. *Oxford Textbook of Medicine, Second Edition*, 1987, Figure 15.25, with permission from Oxford University Press.

## Flow volume loop

- Forced ventilatory manoeuvres may be displayed by plotting flow against volume during both expiration and inspiration. Normal and abnormal flow volume curves are shown (Fig. 18.4). Peak expiratory flow is reached early in expiration and flows faster than peak inspiratory flow. There is a steady fall in flow as expiration progresses due to narrowing of the airways as a consequence of loss of lung volume.
- Flow volume loops are useful in suggesting causes of central airflow obstruction where there is loss of both expiratory and inspiratory peaks with a plateau indicating fixed flow over the change in lung volume.

## Total lung capacity (TLC)

- TLC is measured via a body plethysmograph and less reliably using helium dilution. The body plethysmograph is a large airtight container that allows the simultaneous determination of the pressure volume relationship of the thorax of a patient placed inside the box. When the plethysmograph is sealed, changes in lung volume are reflected by an increase in pressure within the plethysmograph. Standard recordings are made of TLC, RV, and FRC. In general, the volumes are increased in diseases associated with airflow obstruction, e.g. COPD, and reduced in diseases associated with restriction such as pulmonary fibrosis.

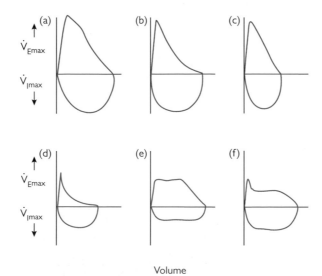

Volume

**Fig. 18.4** Schematic maximum expiratory and inspiratory flow–volume curves in: (a) normal young adult; (b) normal older adult; (c) patient with pulmonary fibrosis and reduced FVC; (d) patient with moderately severe chronic obstructive pulmonary disease showing overall reduction in maximal flow but particularly in $\dot{V}_{Emax}$, at lower lung volumes; (e) patient with subglottic (extrathoracic) tracheal stenosis showing markedly reduced $\dot{V}_{Imax}$ at all volumes and reduced $\dot{V}_{Emax}$ at higher volumes; (f) patient with central intrathoracic (carinal) tracheal narrowing showing similar plateau of flow to (e) but greater reduction of $\dot{V}_{Emax}$ than of $\dot{V}_{Imax}$.

Reproduced from Warrell. *Oxford Textbook of Medicine*, 2012, Figure 18.3.1.3, with permission from Oxford University Press, www.oxfordmedicine.com

### Transfer factor of carbon monoxide

- The rate at which gas passes from the alveoli to the bloodstream is measured using a low concentration of carbon monoxide which binds to haemoglobin and gives a measure of diffusion across the alveolar capillary membrane. It is also known as the transfer factor, TLCO. The transfer coefficient (KCO) is the gas transfer standardized for the alveolar volume (VA).
- A reduced TLCO is a strong indicator of a parenchymal lung disorder involving the alveoli blood supply such as emphysema, fibrosing alveolitis, or pulmonary arterial hypertension assuming normal haemoglobin levels.
- Increased TLCO is seen in patients with well-controlled asthma because of improved distribution of ventilation and perfusion, polycythaemia, and alveolar haemorrhage because extravasated blood binds carbon monoxide. Adjusting the TLCO for alveolar volume giving the transfer coefficient is useful in assessing if the reducing transfer factor is due to a true loss of surface area for diffusion or due to a mild re-distribution of ventilation alone.

## Other respiratory muscle function tests

Weakness of the respiratory muscles causes a restrictive ventilatory defect reducing TLC and VC. Comparison of the VC in the erect and supine position may demonstrate a significant fall (>30% suggests diaphragmatic weakness). Global respiratory muscle function may be assessed by measuring inspiratory and expiratory pressures at the mouth. The negative pressure associated with a sniff correlates well with the measurement of transdiaphragmatic pressure.

## Arterial blood gases

Blood gas analysis provides a useful adjunct to the management of many patients with respiratory disease.
- Arterial puncture should only be undertaken from vessels with adequate collateral circulation (check Allen's test at the wrist for adequate ulnar supply).
- Risk of spasm, bleeding, or haematoma formation.
- Sample taken into a pre-heparinized syringe from which all of the air has previously been expelled. It should be analysed promptly or otherwise cooled to 4°C where it may be stored for up to 1 hour.

## Sputum culture

Sputum culture may be invaluable in the diagnosis and management of patients, particularly those with chronic respiratory disease.
- Sputum may be obtained by expectoration, induction with saline, endotracheal suction, or bronchoalveolar lavage.
- It is then sent in a sterile container for microbiological analysis including Gram (and other specific) stains followed by culture in various types of media.
- This may allow for the identification of bacteria, viral, or fungal infections. It is important though that adequate clinical information is provided to the laboratory to ensure that the appropriate cultures are setup especially if fastidious organisms are to be identified. Organisms such as mycobacteria may take up to 6 weeks to grow satisfactorily.
- A positive growth can then be used to ascertain antimicrobial sensitivities. Remember that a negative growth does not absolutely rule out a suspected organism, particularly in an immuno-compromised individual.

## Lung biopsy

A better understanding of lung pathology can be gained by biopsy. There are a number of ways to approach this dependent on:
- The size of lesion.

- The likely underlying process (e.g. localized or widespread).
- Site of lesion (intrapulmonary peripheral vs. central or pleural).

Better diagnostic rates are generally achieved if direct vision or radiological guidance is used.

Options for biopsying the lung therefore include;
- Flexible bronchoscopy with bronchial brushing, endobronchial biopsy (biopsy of bronchial mucosa), and bronchoalveolar lavage.
- Flexible bronchoscopy with transbronchial biopsy (biopsy of lung parenchyma including blood vessels).
- Flexible bronchoscopy with endobronchial ultrasound and lymph node sampling.
- CT-guided fine needle aspiration.
- Pleural biopsy (pleural biopsy needle or thoracoscopic guided).
- Video-assisted thoracoscopic (VATS) biopsy.
- Open lung biopsy.

Most of these procedures are performed with fully conscious or sedated patient (open lung biopsy performed under general anaesthetic).

## Flexible bronchoscopy

Flexible bronchoscopy (Fig. 18.5) is a safe and well tolerated procedure in experienced hands. Its features are:
- It allows direct vision of central parts of the lung, e.g. trachea, major and some smaller bronchi.
- Mortality rates are generally quoted at around 1/100,000 procedures.
- Most procedures are performed with local anaesthesia (e.g. throat spray) and sedation.
- Patients with high oxygen requirements, unable to lie flat or unable to protect their airway, e.g. unconscious should not have this procedure done without intubation and an anaesthetist present.
- The bronchoscope is inserted through either the nose or mouth into the trachea and lungs.
- Endobronchial biopsy: direct vision biopsy approximately 3–5mm from the bronchial wall may be used to diagnose cancer but may also confirm asthma and other conditions affecting the bronchi.

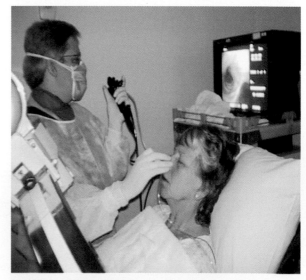

Fig. 18.5 Respiratory investigations: bronchoscopy. A sedated patient is undergoing flexible bronchoscopy. Oxygen is administered during the procedure and oxygen saturation and ECG monitoring is undertaken. The screen shows the bifurcation of the trachea. Bronchial lavage brushing and biopsy can be undertaken to identify malignancy, respiratory infections and can be therapeutic, e.g. removal of smaller inhaled foreign bodies.

- Endobronchial ultrasound (EBUS)-guided lymph node sampling: a method of sampling abnormal mediastinal lymph nodes, e.g. in suspected cancer/cancer staging.
- Transbronchial biopsy: the bronchoscope is introduced and a biopsy forceps is passed deeper into the lung beyond direct vision. Biopsy here can help with the diagnosis of certain interstitial lung processes but the blind nature of the biopsy and the patchy nature of some lung conditions means non-diagnostic biopsies scan occur. The bleeding rates are higher than with endobronchial biopsy.

## Fine-needle aspiration (FNA) biopsy of the lung

This involves removal of tissue or fluid from the lung using a thin needle.
- Abnormal tissue (or fluid) usually localized by CT although ultrasound or fluoroscopy may also be used.
- The biopsy needle is inserted after local anaesthesia through surrounding skin and normal lung tissue into the abnormal tissue or fluid.
- Development of a small pneumothorax is a risk, thus a chest X-ray (CXR) is always required afterwards.

## Pleural biopsy and thoracoscopy

Pleural biopsy is often carried out if pleural fluid aspiration (thoracentesis, see Section 18.9) and other investigations have not revealed the cause of a pleural effusion. It is usually only necessary with an exudative pleural effusion rather than with a transudative one.

Biopsies taken from a random area of pleura 'blind biopsy' have a fairly low diagnostic yield. These are therefore now not widely used; the yield is considerably better with image-guided pleural biopsy or thoracoscopy. For the latter, a rigid thoracoscope and biopsy forceps are passed into the pleural space similar to laparoscopic surgery. VATS has also been used for thoracic malignancy resection, to treat empyema and obtain lung biopsies in diffuse parenchymal disease.

Possible complications
- Pneumothorax.
- Extravasation of pleural fluid.
- Haemorrhage with haemothorax occurs very rarely.
- Empyema due to subsequent infection is possible but rare.
- Tumour seeding may occur; it occurs relatively commonly with mesothelioma and can be a distressing and painful complication. When mesothelioma is the suspected diagnosis, it may be better to use open or thoracoscopic biopsy.

# 18.4 Respiratory failure

The respiratory system supplies the body with oxygen for aerobic metabolism and removes the major metabolic waste gas, carbon dioxide. Respiratory failure develops when the body's metabolic demands outstrip the rate of gas exchange between the atmosphere and blood.

Respiratory failure is diagnosed when the patient develops isolated hypoxaemia $PaO_2$ below 8kPA (type I respiratory failure) or when the patient is unable to ventilate adequately and develops hypercapnia and hypoxaemia (type II respiratory failure), $PaO_2$ below 8kPA and $PaCO_2$ above 6.5kPa.

## Classification of respiratory failure

Respiratory failure can be classified on the basis of pathophysiological mechanisms that lead to hypoxaemia and/or hypercarbia. Acute respiratory failure can occur when hypoxaemia is caused by any or a combination of the following abnormalities:

- Alveolar ventilation (V) and pulmonary perfusion (Q) mismatching 'V/Q mismatch'.
- Intrapulmonary shunt (anatomical, e.g. arteriovenous malformation or functional shunt, e.g. acute respiratory distress syndrome).
- Hypoventilation, e.g. acute: opioid overdose; chronic: neuromuscular conditions.
- Abnormal diffusion of gases at the alveolar–capillary interface, e.g. pulmonary oedema or pulmonary fibrosis.
- Reduction in inspired oxygen concentration, e.g. high altitude.
- Increased venous de-saturation with cardiac dysfunction plus one or more of the above five factors.

The three most important abnormalities in gas exchange that lead to respiratory failure are V/Q mismatch, an intrapulmonary shunt, and hypoventilation.

- The V/Q ratio determines the adequacy of gas exchange in the lung. When alveolar ventilation matches pulmonary blood flow, $CO_2$ is eliminated and the blood becomes fully saturated with oxygen.
- Gravitational forces affect the regional blood flow and hence V/Q ratio. Erect the V/Q ratio is >1 at the apex of the lung (ventilation exceeds perfusion) and <1 at the base (less ventilation with more perfusion). In healthy lungs, the V/Q ratio is assumed to be ideal and = 1.
- A V/Q mismatch is the most common cause of hypoxaemia. If the V/Q ratio is <1 throughout the lung, arterial hypoxaemia results.
- As V/Q mismatch worsens, the respiratory rate (and thus minute ventilation) increases producing either a low or normal arterial partial pressure of $CO_2$ ($PaCO_2$). The hypoxaemia caused by low V/Q areas will respond to oxygen administration.

When the V/Q ratio = 0, pulmonary blood flow does not participate in gas exchange because the perfused lung unit receives no ventilation; this is intrapulmonary shunting. A normal intrapulmonary shunt level is <10%. If shunting is >30%, the resultant hypoxaemia cannot respond to supplemental oxygen as the shunted blood bypasses the alveoli. Treatment therefore consists of alveolar recruitment (e.g. with positive end expiratory pressure (PEEP)) and maximizing lung volume with positive pressure. $PaO_2$ falls proportionally as the shunt increases.

$PaCO_2$ remains constant until the shunt fraction exceeds 50%. Hypoxic pulmonary vasoconstriction (HPV) is a protective reflex that reduces the degree of intrapulmonary shunting. Here alveolar hypoxia leads to vasoconstriction of the perfusing vessel. This increases pulmonary vascular resistance but partially corrects the regional V/Q mismatch. Long term this will lead to right heart strain, pulmonary hypertension, and cor pulmonale.

When ventilation is in excess of the capillary blood flow, the V/Q ratio is >1. Some areas of ventilated lung receive almost no perfusion; here the V/Q ratio approaches infinity. This is referred to as alveolar dead-space ventilation. The alveolar dead space, plus anatomical dead space is the volume of air that cannot participate in gas exchange. Combined, the alveolar and anatomic dead-space volumes are referred to as 'physiological dead space,' which normally accounts for 30% of total ventilation.

Increased dead-space ventilation results in hypoxaemia and hypercapnia. This increase can be caused by decreased pulmonary perfusion due to pulmonary embolism or alveolar over-distension during mechanical ventilation. The ratio of dead-space to tidal-gas volume can be calculated on the basis of the difference between $CO_2$ in the arterial blood and the exhaled gas.

Generally, $PaCO_2$ is inversely proportional to alveolar ventilation (VA). When VA decreases, $PaCO_2$ increases.

## Type I and type II respiratory failure

Respiratory failure can also be classified based on two patterns of blood-gas abnormalities.

- **Type I respiratory failure** results from poor matching of pulmonary ventilation to perfusion; this leads to non-cardiac mixing of venous blood with arterial blood. As a result, type I respiratory failure is characterized by arterial hypoxaemia with normal or low arterial $CO_2$. Hypoxaemic respiratory failure (type I) is characterized by a $PaO_2$ of <8kPa (60mmHg) with a normal or low $PaCO_2$. This is caused by V/Q mismatch with under-ventilated alveoli (e.g. pulmonary oedema, pneumonia, or acute asthma) or venous blood bypasses ventilated alveoli (e.g. right-to-left cardiac shunts). Hyperventilation increases $CO_2$ removal but does not

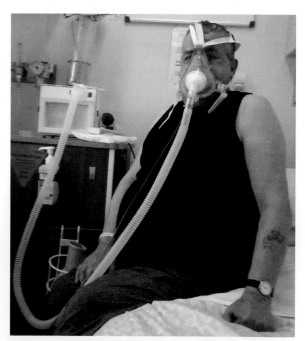

**Fig. 18.6** Respiratory failure due to advanced COPD is being treated with non-invasive ventilation. The patients arterial blood gases were $PaCO_2$ 8.4kPa and $PaO_2$ 7kPA consistent with type II respiratory failure. The bedside ventilator is visible as is the supplemental oxygen administered.

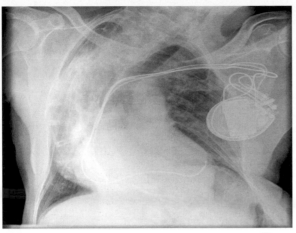

**Fig. 18.7** Thoracic deformity can impair respiratory mechanics. In this case severe kyphoscoliosis caused type II respiratory failure and the patient was established on home nasal ventilation similar to that seen in Fig. 18.6. The patient has an incidental finding of a cardiac pacemaker.

increase oxygenation as blood leaving unaffected alveoli is almost fully saturated.

- **Type II respiratory failure** results from inadequate alveolar ventilation. Hypercapnic respiratory failure (type II) is characterized by a raised $PaCO_2$ of >50mmHg (6.5kPa). Any ventilation/perfusion mismatch will affect $PaO_2$ and therefore hypoxaemia is also common. Hypercapnia due to alveolar hypoventilation is the hallmark of diseases involving the respiratory 'pump'. In clinical practice the most common cause is severe COPD (Fig. 18.6); other causes include obesity-hypoventilation syndrome, opioid toxicity, thoracic wall deformities (Fig. 18.7), and neuromuscular diseases.

# 18.5 Pneumonia

## Community-acquired pneumonia

### Epidemiology

- Worldwide—strong association with poverty, malnutrition, and overcrowding.
- A common cause of infant mortality in developing countries.
- Increasing rates are noted in winter and during influenza outbreaks.

### Pathogenesis

- Bacterial and viral causes are common
- Preceding upper respiratory tract infection is commonly reported.
- Gram-positive organisms more common in community acquired pneumonia than Gram-negative ones.
- Alveolar filling with inflammatory exudates and resulting impaired gas exchange.

### Clinical presentation

- Usually recent onset.
- Shortness of breath, cough, sputum, haemoptysis.
- Confusion.
- Chest pain or pleurisy.
- Septic shock, collapse.

### Physical signs

- Pyrexial.
- Confused, tachypnoea.
- *Herpes* labialis.
- Dull note on percussion, increased (bronchial) breath sounds.
- Signs of a pleural effusion can be noted in 10–20% cases.
- Hypotension suggests possible septic shock.

### Diagnosis

- Many cases are diagnosed clinically and treated in the community without tests.
- Raised CRP and white cell count.
- Raised urea or abnormal liver function tests (not diagnostic but important for management and or prognosis).
- Sputum and blood culture.
- Cold agglutinins may be seen with *Mycoplasma*.
- Pneumoccocal and *Legionella* antigen testing in urine.
- ABGs may show hypoxaemia, respiratory acidosis, or metabolic acidosis.
- X-ray—opacification of the affected lung (Fig. 18.8):
  - Diffuse bronchopneumonia.
  - Well-defined area of consolidation—lobar pneumonia.
  - Cavities are more common in staphylococcal pneumonia or with *Klebsiella*.

### Complications

- Death—~10% death rate.
- Septic shock and multi-organ failure.
- Respiratory failure.
- Pericarditis, pericardial effusion, cardiac tamponade.
- Post-pneumonic lung abscess or bronchiectasis (Figs 18.9–18.11).
- Pleural disease:
  - Pleural effusion.
  - Empyema (pus in pleural cavity).
  - Pleurisy or pneumothorax.
- Meningitis.
- Biochemical abnormalities: hyponatraemia, hepatitis.
- Haematological abnormalities:
  - Disseminated intravascular coagulation (DIC).
  - Intravascular haemolysis.
  - Leucocytosis or leucopenia.
  - Thrombocytosis is common.

### Pathogens

- *Streptococcus pneumoniae* is the commonest bacterial cause isolated.
- Other common pathogens include influenza virus, *Mycoplasma pneumoniae*, *Haemophilus pneumoniae*, *Legionella pneumophila*.
- Culture-negative pneumonia is common, ~40–60%.
- Methicillin-resistant *Staphylococcus aureus* (MRSA) pneumonia is rare in the community.

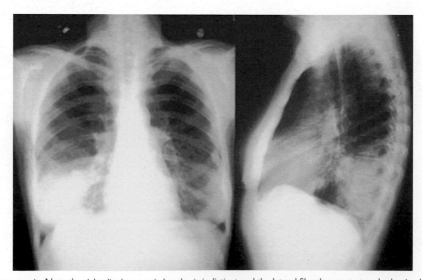

**Fig. 18.8** Right basal pneumonia. Note the right diaphragmatic border is indistinct and the lateral film demonstrates shadowing below the oblique fissure confirming lower lobe disease. The right middle lobe is not affected as the right heart border is clearly defined on the PA film.

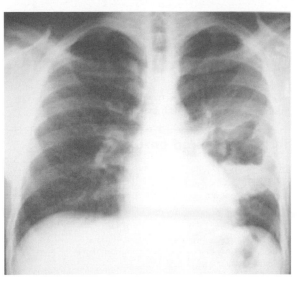

Fig. 18.9 Post-pneumonic lung abscess at left mid-zone. Note the flat air fluid level and the thinner upper aspect to the abscess.

### Typical and atypical pneumonia

- Previously it was felt possible to predict which pathogen was causative based on the clinical presentation.
- Typical—acute febrile illness with lobar pattern and lack of extra pulmonary features.
- Atypical—more insidious process associated with non-lobar pattern and many extrapulmonary features (e.g. hepatitis).
- More recent data suggests that **this distinction is not discriminatory** and there is a move away from these terms.

### Specific syndromes

- *Streptococcus pneumoniae* is more commonly associated with lobar pneumonia, local complications such as pericarditis, and there is often *Herpes* labialis.
- *Mycoplasma* pneumonia is often associated with extrapulmonary complications such as hepatitis and hyponatraemia. It has a cyclical incidence peaking every 4 years. There is a high prevalence of cold agglutinins in the blood.

- *Legionella* pneumonia is more common in elderly male smokers and is associated with contaminated water. About 70% have recently travelled abroad. No person-to-person transfer has been recorded. 25% of cases in the UK are **not** associated with travel.
- Influenza pneumonia is difficult to distinguish from bacterial pneumonia clinically:
  - Onset in the midst of an outbreak helps diagnosis.
  - Secondary streptococcal pneumonia is common but greater than expected rates of staphylococcal pneumonia are also seen.

### Vaccination

- Pneumoccocal polysaccharide and, more recently, peptide-based antigen vaccines have become available.
- They appear to be reducing rates of pneumonia in those vaccinated as well as in those who are not vaccinated raising the possibility of herd immunity.

### Prognostic scoring

- At least three major scoring systems exist.
- They are most widely validated in community acquired pneumonia—CURB-65 is the most widely used.
- **CURB-65** score:
  - **C**onfusion.
  - **U**rea >7mmol/L.
  - **R**espiratory rate >30 per minute.
  - **BP** <90mmHg systolic or <60mmHg diastolic.
  - Age >**65** years.
  - Score >3 suggests consideration for high dependency treatment/monitoring.
  - Score of 1 or less—outpatient treatment likely to be safe.
  - Score of 5—mortality ~40%.

### Treatment

- High-flow oxygen.
- Antibiotic therapy (see later).
- Fluid resuscitation.
- Analgesia.
- Deep vein thrombosis (DVT) prophylaxis.
- Oral steroids and nebulized bronchodilators are rarely indicated.

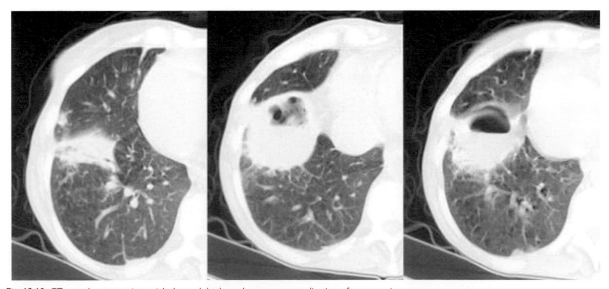

Fig. 18.10 CT scan demonstrating a right lower lobe lung abscess as a complication of pneumonia.

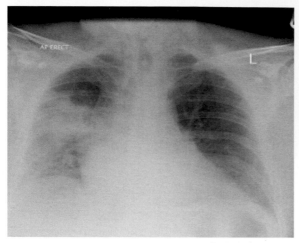

**Fig. 18.11** Right upper lobe pneumonia. There is ill-defined consolidation in the right upper. Blood cultures grew *Pneumococcus*. Despite treatment the patient deteriorated and developed ARDS (see Fig. 18.21).

- Severe pneumonia is one of the commonest reasons for admission to ICU. It is also one of the most common reasons to have activated protein C treatment whilst in ICU.

*Antibiotic treatment for community-acquired pneumonia*

- Treatment is usually empirical whilst awaiting microbiological diagnosis.
- There will be local protocols for antibiotic treatment of pneumonia which reflect differences in pathogen frequencies and resistance rates.
- Antibacterial cover is aimed against the most common pathogens:
  - Amoxicillin (*Streptococcus* cover) **and** usually
  - Macrolide (*Mycoplasma* cover.)
- If *Legionella* is diagnosed, rifampicin therapy may be considered.

- If there has been a recent influenza outbreak, antibiotic cover often includes flucloxacillin cover for *Staphylococcus*.
- Consider anaerobic cover if there is suspicion of aspiration.
- It is common to give antibiotic therapy intravenously for the first 24–48 hours.
- Perhaps more important than the route of administration (intravenous vs. oral) is administering therapy quickly. A delay to first dose may be associated with an increased mortality.

## Hospital-acquired pneumonia

- This is defined as pneumonia occurring 48 hours **after** a hospital admission.
- The pathogens are very different to those of community-acquired pneumonia.
- Gram-negative organisms predominate (*Escherichia coli*, *Klebsiella*, *Pseudomonas*).
- MRSA pneumonia is much more common than in community-acquired pneumonia.
- Mortality rates are much higher than community-acquired pneumonia:
  - The patients usually have another illness requiring their admission.
  - Comorbidities are commonly age, other cardiorespiratory disease, and poor mobility.
- Mortality rates of 40% are reported.
- Prognostic scoring systems for community-acquired pneumonia are not appropriate.
- Sputum culture and blood culture should be sent where possible.
- Supportive measures should not be forgotten: oxygen supplementation, thromboprophylaxis against DVT, antipyrexial treatment, and good fluid balance should be initiated.
- There will be local protocols for antibiotic treatment of hospital-acquired pneumonia.
- Antibacterial cover is aimed against the most common pathogens and should include anti-*Pseudomonas* and anti-MRSA cover, e.g. piperacillin/tazobactam plus vancomycin.

# 18.6 Tuberculosis

## Aetiology and epidemiology

- *Mycobacterium tuberculosis* is an obligate aerobic bacterium.
- Increasingly associated with immigration (see later in list) though recrudescence in elderly Caucasians can predominate, dependent on local ethnic mixes.
- Associated with poverty, HIV infection, alcoholism.
- Immigration from high-risk countries (Eastern Europe, Africa, Indian subcontinent).
- This is one of the commonest causes of death worldwide (7% annual deaths worldwide).
- 8 million new cases per year worldwide.
- There are increasing concerns over multidrug-resistant tuberculosis (MDR-TB).

## Pathophysiology

- Person-to-person transmission (droplet).
- The organism is slow growing *in vitro* and *in vivo* (subacute infection).
- Organism engulfed by macrophage but survives and replicates within macrophage (giant cells may form).
- Intracellular component to the infection.
- As the macrophage ruptures lymphatic and blood spread occurs.
- Bacteria then grow in oxygen-rich areas (lung, kidneys, brain, bone).
- Cell-mediated immunity (T lymphocytes and primed macrophages) may cause disease containment.
- Clusters of immune cells form granulomas and central caseous necrosis can occur
- Calcification in areas of granulomas.
- Bacterial growth is slow with scope for the rapid development of resistance.
- Treatment requires prolonged and multidrug regimens (expert help required).

## Clinical presentation

- Only 10% infected develop tuberculous disease.
- Potential long period of dormancy.
- Generally three syndrome clusters.

### Primary pulmonary TB

- Often resolves spontaneously.
- Fever and non-productive cough.
- CXR may show an inflammatory infiltrate in lower and middle lung fields (unilateral).
- Sputum culture usually negative at this point.
- Tuberculous pleurisy is seen in 10%.
- A Ghon focus is a calcified granuloma usually seen in the lateral mid to lower zone on X-ray.
- Latent infection is common with 50–60% of patients at risk of reactivation at later point.

### Reactivation TB

- Most common clinical form of TB.
- Reactivation of latent disease occurs insidiously.
- Fevers, sweats, and weight loss common. Haemoptysis can also occur.

- Physical signs can be absent but may include lymphadenopathy, cachexia, and focal respiratory signs.
- Radiology—bilateral or unilateral infiltrates with cavity formation usually involving the apical segments of the lung.

*Miliary TB*

- Can occur as part of primary or reactivation TB.
- Reflects unhindered blood-borne spread of TB usually where there is a defect in cell-mediated immunity (children, elderly, alcoholism, HIV disease).
- Multiple small rice grain-sized opacities seen on CXR.

### Extrapulmonary TB

- ~15% of active TB is extrapulmonary.
- Lymph nodes, genitourinary, bone, meningeal, breast, and gastrointestinal tract are all recognized sites of TB infection.
- TB lymphadenitis is the commonest site. The importance of culture of excised lymph nodes cannot be overemphasized as TB organisms are rarely seen in staining.
- TB osteomyelitis of the spine used to be common—'Pott disease'.

## Diagnosis (Figs 18.12 and 18.13)

- CXR may show cavities, Ghon focus, mediastinal lymphadenopathy (enlarged nodes).
- Miliary TB may show multiple small nodules.
- Sputum may stain with Ziehl–Neelsen (ZN) stain showing alcohol acid-fast bacilli (AAFB).
- Sputum, pleural biopsy, or lymph node culture (including more recent rapid culture techniques).

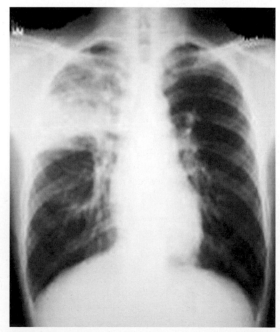

Fig. 18.12 Right upper lobe shadowing noted after 3 months of cough sputum and minor haemoptysis. Sputum analysis revealed alcohol acid-fast bacilli with subsequent culture revealing *Mycobacterium tuberculosis*. The CXR abnormalities could be caused by a simple pneumonia reinforcing the need to correlate clinical history with radiological findings.

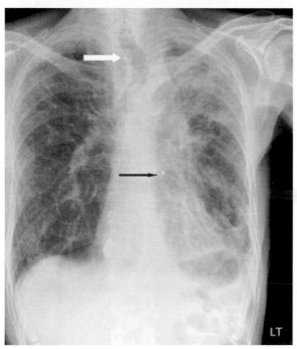

**Fig. 18.13** Post-tuberculous scarring demonstrating volume loss of the left upper lobe. These scarred areas can develop secondary infection, e.g. aspergilloma or secondary bacterial bronchiectasis. The patient has undergone arterial embolization for haemoptysis—the embolization coil is noted by the smaller black arrow. The trachea is deviated to the left (larger white arrow).

- Skin testing (Mantoux) may be useful.
- Recently whole blood immunological testing for 'latent TB', e.g. QuantiFERON® gold.
- Raised ESR and normochromic anaemia can occur.
- HIV testing should be undertaken in at-risk groups.

## Complications

- Spread (household members at greatest risk).
- Haemoptysis (rupture of a Rasmussen aneurysm).
- Death—10% mortality.
- Pleural effusion (can be haemorrhagic).
- Lobar collapse—'Brock syndrome', right middle lobe collapse.
- Post-tuberculous bronchiectasis.
- Extrapulmonary TB.
- Complications of therapy (see later topic in this section).

## Treatment

- Expert help required.
- Try to avoid hospital admission if the patient is well (reduces exposure risk).
- Treatment is dictated by a number of factors:
  - Need for blind treatment vs. obtaining culture results (treatment is usually started after positive smear with ZN stain).
  - In some patients with underlying chest disease other mycobacterial infections can occur.
  - Comorbidity (liver disease or renal disease mean altered drug regimens).
  - Drug contraindications.
  - Likelihood of resistance.

## Drug treatment

Treatment is prolonged and usually at least 6 months in duration. In some cases treatment is extended to 9 months. Multidrug regimens are used to prevent resistance occurring. Typically oral triple or quadruple therapy is used.

- Rifampicin
- Isoniazid
- Pyrazinamide
- Ethambutol

## Complications of therapy

### Drug treatment

- Hepatitis—common and can occur with pyrazinamide or rifampicin (usually reversible).
- Autoimmune hepatitis—rare (due to isoniazid if it occurs).
- Optic nerve toxicity (ethambutol).
- Haematological dyscrasia (low platelets, immune haemolysis).
- Renal failure.
- Gout (pyrazinamide or ethambutol).
- Peripheral neuropathy (isoniazid—may be prevented by pyridoxine (vitamin B6) therapy).
- Treatment failure (often associated with poor compliance).
- Treatment errors—a number of single-agent and combined-agent preparations exist that sound similar but are different, e.g. Rifater® vs. Rifinah®.

### Surgery

- Thoracoplasty patients can develop respiratory failure many years after the thoracic wall surgery.

## Multidrug resistant TB

- Increasing problem worldwide.
- Often Eastern Europe or developing world-associated TB.
- Poverty and partial compliance in areas where medical treatment is not easily available are the commonest causes.
- Patients are isolated as soon as possible where possible within a specialist or infectious diseases unit.

## Public health issues

- Tuberculosis is a notifiable disease and must be notified under the Public Health Act 1984.
- Notification helps to provide surveillance data and initiate contact tracing.
- Contact tracing aims to detect those who are infected but who do not have clinical evidence of disease (10% of all cases).
- Screening is recommended only for those contacts identified since the index case developed respiratory symptoms. Otherwise contacts during the 3 months prior to diagnosis are screened.

## Prophylaxis

- Increasingly a complex area with scanty evidence base.
- Recommend seek expert help.
- Usually isoniazid monotherapy in at-risk groups.
- At-risk groups include:
  - Children with positive skin tests who are household contacts of known TB cases.
  - Adults with positive skin test, on immunosuppressive therapy.

# 18.7 Cystic fibrosis

## Aetiology and epidemiology

- The most common, lethal, single gene disorder in the Western hemisphere.
- Molecular defect in the cystic fibrosis trans-membrane regulator (CFTR) sodium/chloride ion channel.
- Autosomal recessive (two defective genes required).
- Affects 1/2000 live births, ♂ = ♀.
- Carriers are asymptomatic and are seen in 1/20 of the population.

## Pathogenesis

- Cystic fibrosis (CF) is a multisystem disease.
- Thick viscid mucus causes pancreatic duct, bronchiolar, biliary, and vas deferens obstruction.
- Excessive inflammation and recurrent bacterial infections affect the lungs causing bronchiectasis.
- Other respiratory diseases include nasal polyps, sinusitis, pneumothorax, allergic bronchopulmonary aspergillosis (ABPA).
- Gastrointestinal disease—peptic ulcers, intestinal obstruction 'meconium ileus', rectal prolapse.
- Pancreatic disease—chronic pancreatitis, malabsorption, diabetes mellitus.
- Liver disease—gallstones, cirrhosis, portal hypertension and varices.

## Clinical presentation

- Perinatal diagnosis (screening programme).
- Recurrent lower respiratory tract infections.
- Failure to thrive and malabsorption.
- Cough, sputum, and wheeze.
- Acute exacerbation/acute respiratory failure.
- Pneumothorax.
- Atypical CF may present with sinus disease, infertility, pancreatitis, etc.

## Physical signs

- Low body weight, failure to thrive, short stature.
- Delayed puberty/secondary sexual characteristics.
- Cough, large volumes of sputum, hyperinflation, and crackles on respiratory examination.
- Signs of respiratory failure.
- Hepatomegaly.

## Diagnosis

- Clinical diagnosis.
- Genetic testing (DF508 commonest mutation in West).
- Hyperinflation on CXR with bronchial wall thickening (Fig. 18.14).
- Sweat test characterized by excessively high sodium and chloride in sweat.
- Spirometry—obstructive in pattern.

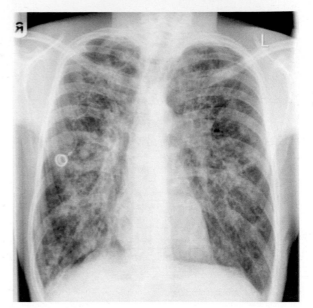

**Fig. 18.14** A CXR of cystic fibrosis. There is widespread peribronchial shadowing with predominance at the apices. The opacity in the right upper zone is an implantable device used for administering anti-pseudomonal antibiotics.

## Complications

- Premature death—survival to age 40–45 years is the current prediction for a CF child (increasing survival noted since 1980s). Massive haemoptysis is sometimes the cause.
- Respiratory failure.
- Pneumothorax.
- Osteoporosis.
- Infertility in ♂.
- Renal disease (antibiotic related or renal amyloid).
- ABPA.
- Rectal prolapse and urinary incontinence (excessive coughing).

## Treatment

- Nutritional support (pancreatic enzyme replacement, gastrostomy feeding).
- Pancreatic enzyme replacement, e.g. Creon®.
- Inhaled bronchodilators.
- Nebulized antibiotics—colomycin or tobramycin.
- Nebulized DNAse (sputum is rich in DNA which increases sputum viscosity).
- Prompt treatment of respiratory exacerbations.
- Insulin for CF-associated diabetes.
- Treatment of respiratory failure may include long-term oxygen therapy and/or overnight non-invasive ventilation.

- Lung transplantation—CF is one of the commonest reasons for bilateral lung transplantation worldwide.
- Liver transplantation—occasionally required.

## Pathogens in cystic fibrosis

- Cystic fibrosis pathogens include *Staphylococcus aureus*, *Haemophilus influenzae*, *Pseudomonas aeruginosa*.
- Less common pathogens include *Burkholderia cepacia* complex, *Stenotrophomonas*, *Mycobacterium abscessus*.
- Fungi include *Aspergillus*, *Scedosporium*.

## Antibiotics in cystic fibrosis

- Usually close liaison with microbiology required.
- Patients eventually graduate from pathogens that can be treated with oral antibiotics to those requiring intravenous treatment.

- Early detection of *Pseudomonas aeruginosa* infection may offer a window of opportunity for eradication therapy (e.g. high-dose oral ciprofloxacin plus nebulized antibiotics).
- Established *Pseudomonas aeruginosa* infection often becomes resistant to ciprofloxacin and alternative intravenous antibiotics are required.
- Common combinations include ceftazidime and tobramycin, or meropenem and tazobactam.
- Care should be taken with aminoglycoside antibiotics as there is a clear risk of renal and ototoxicity.

# 18.8 Bronchiectasis

## Background

Bronchiectasis is an abnormal dilation of the proximal and medium-sized bronchi (>2mm in diameter) caused by destruction of the muscular and elastic components of the bronchial walls. Congenital bronchiectasis usually affects infants and children. It results from a problem in the development of the lungs in the fetus. Acquired bronchiectasis occurs in adults and older children. It is much more common than the congenital form of the condition.

## Aetiology and epidemiology

The prevalence is unclear. The causes of bronchiectasis may be classified into five main groups:
- Defective host defences, e.g. immotile cilia, hypogammaglobulinaemia.
- Post-infectious, e.g. post-TB or post pneumonic.
- Localized bronchial obstruction.
- Inflammatory (systemic) disorders, e.g. rheumatoid arthritis.
- Miscellaneous, e.g. COPD, alpha-1 antitrypsin deficiency.
- Idiopathic bronchiectasis (unknown cause) is still the predominant form.

## Pathophysiology and prognosis

- Airway inflammation, scarring, and mucus hypersecretion can be found. Distal areas of lung are damaged secondary to persistent infection and/or collapse. Neovascularization forms bronchial vessels.
- Pathogens include *Staphylococcus aureus, Pseudomonas, Haemophilus influenza*, and *Mycobacteria* spp.
- Prognosis is generally very good although a small proportion gets severe disease with *Pseudomonas* infection and respiratory failure.

## Clinical presentation

- Large volume sputum production is mostly limited to severe cases.
- Cough, wheeze, and occasional sputum are more common.
- Haemoptysis.
- Sinusitis, recurrent infections.
- ♂ infertility (suggests a ciliary defect or CF).

## Diagnosis

Radiological studies confirm diagnosis, the remainder provide management or aetiology designation benefits.
- CXR to exclude localized bronchiectasis—~50% of patients with bronchiectasis have characteristic features of thickened bronchial walls (seen as parallel 'tramlines', ring lesions, and hyperinflation; Fig. 18.15).
- A normal CXR does **not** exclude bronchiectasis.
- High-resolution CT (HRCT) scan—peribronchial thickening, ring shadows, including signet ring sign. High sensitivity and specificity—90% and 89% respectively.
- Sputum culture including tests for *Mycobacteria*.

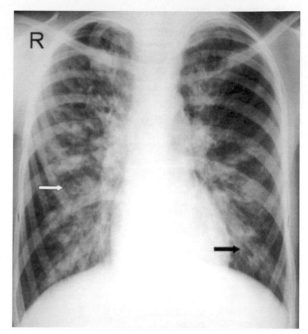

**Fig. 18.15** Widespread idiopathic adult bronchiectasis. There is some tramlining (longitudinal peribronchial wall thickening) at the left base (black arrow). Cystic or ring shadows are seen throughout both mid zones (white arrow).

- Lung function tests—functional severity assessment, usually airflow obstruction noted.
- Serum immunoglobulin and subclass levels (IgG4).
- Specific antibody titres to *Haemophilus influenza*e and pneumococcal vaccines (functional antibodies).
- Autoantibodies.
- CF genotype and sweat test, to exclude/confirm CF.
- Skin prick tests for *Aspergillus*.
- Ciliary studies—electron microscopy

## Syndromes in bronchiectasis

Most cases of bronchiectasis are idiopathic or post-infectious. Severe asthma particularly with ABPA and severe COPD are associated with secondary bronchiectasis.
- CF is a common genetic cause of bronchiectasis.
- Kartegener syndrome—immotile cilia, sino-pulmonary disease, and dextrocardia.
- Williams–Campbell syndrome (congenital cartilage deficiency).
- Mounier–Kuhn syndrome (tracheo-bronchomegaly).
- Alpha-1 antitrypsin deficiency.
- Autoimmune diseases—bronchiectasis is seen in patients with rheumatoid arthritis, Sjögren syndrome, and ankylosing spondylitis.
- Inflammatory bowel disease, both ulcerative colitis and Crohn disease. The onset of aggressive lung disease can occur after colectomy.

## Complications

- Recurrent pneumonia requiring hospitalization.
- Pneumothorax.
- Empyema and lung abscess.
- Urinary incontinence (excessive coughing).
- Haemoptysis (bronchial arterial bleeds from neo-vascularization).
- Progressive respiratory failure/cor pulmonale.
- Renal amyloidosis (increasingly rare).

## Treatment

Antibiotics and chest physiotherapy are the mainstay modalities. Influenza and pneumococcal vaccination is recommended as is smoking cessation. Others (excluding those for specific bronchiectasis syndromes) include:

- Physiotherapy
- Bronchodilators.
- Inhaled and oral corticosteroid therapy in subgroups.
- Nebulized antibiotics (aminoglycosides or colistin).
- Long-term, low-dose macrolide antibiotics are increasingly used as anti-inflammatory agents
- Mucolytics including nebulized hypertonic saline.
- Oxygen.
- Surgical therapies (bilateral lung transplantation for severe diffuse disease; lobectomy for localized disease).
- Bronchial artery embolization may be attempted to control haemoptysis.

# 18.9 Pleural effusion

Pleural effusions occur when pleural fluid forms quicker than it is absorbed.

## Pathogenesis

The following mechanisms play a role in the formation of pleural effusion:

- Changed pleural membrane integrity, e.g. inflammatory process, neoplastic disease, pulmonary embolus.
- Increased capillary hydrostatic pressure in the systemic circulation, e.g. congestive heart failure.
- Reduced intravascular oncotic pressure, e.g. hypoalbuminaemia, hepatic cirrhosis.
- Increased capillary permeability or vascular disruption, e.g. trauma, neoplastic disease, inflammatory process, infection, pulmonary infarction, drug hypersensitivity.
- Decreased lymphatic drainage or complete blockage, including thoracic duct obstruction or rupture, e.g. malignancy, surgery.
- Increased fluid in the peritoneal cavity—increased permeability/transdiaphragmatic migration, e.g. hepatic cirrhosis, peritoneal dialysis.

## Clinical presentation

- Pleuritic or dull chest pain, chest tightness.
- Dyspnoea and cough.
- Physical findings may be detectable when the effusion is >500mL.
- Quiet/absent breath sounds.
- Dullness to percussion—'stony dull'.

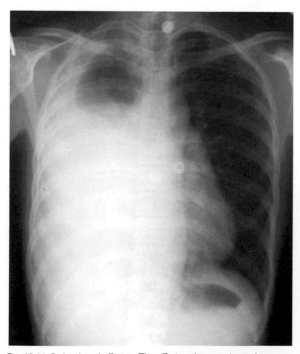

Fig. 18.16 Right pleural effusion. The effusion shows a classical meniscus. The diaphragm is obscured throughout its length. The trachea remains central suggesting no mediastinal shift has occurred. Large unilateral effusions are often malignant in this case mesothelioma was diagnosed.

- Reduced tactile and vocal fremitus, and occasionally a pleural friction rub.

## Diagnosis

- If a pleural effusion is suspected on examination, a CXR is required. With a subpulmonic effusion (collects below the lung but above the hemidiaphragm), a lateral decubitus film usually confirms the presence of fluid (Figs 18.16–18.18).
- Pleural space ultrasound is extremely helpful to locate small amounts or isolated loculated pockets of fluid. Pleural tap/thoracentesis can be performed simultaneously using ultrasound guidance.

## Thoracentesis and pleural fluid analysis

Not all effusions need be tapped. If a patient has no obvious clinical cause for the effusion, is pyrexial, or is in respiratory distress, then a thoracentesis (fluid tap) is mandatory as this frequently helps establish the aetiology. 50–100mL of fluid are usually removed and sent for analysis.

Pleural fluid pH, glucose, protein, lactate dehydrogenase (LDH), and fluid culture are sent. Other tests may include amylase, adenosine deaminase, and fluid cytology.

Transudative effusions are more likely to be bilateral due to systemic factors (e.g. low serum proteins and increased pulmonary venous pressure).

Exudative effusions are more commonly unilateral but can be bilateral. They occur when local factors are altered (e.g. infection and malignancy).

Exudates must meet one or more of the following criteria, whereas transudates meet none:

- Pleural fluid/serum protein ratio >0.5 or absolute value >30g/L.
- Pleural fluid/serum LDH ratio >0.6 or absolute value >0.45 upper normal serum limit.

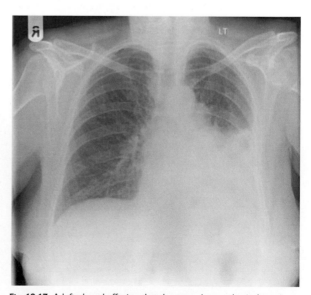

Fig. 18.17 A left pleural effusion that does not show a classical meniscus. The diaphragm is obscured throughout its length. The effusion was tapped and was blood stained. Small cell lung cancer was diagnosed based on fluid cytology.

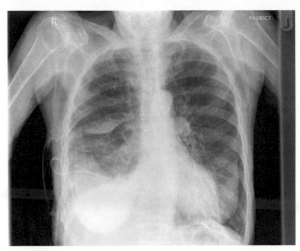

**Fig. 18.18** An encysted pleural effusion with right chest drain. This patient had a right-sided haemorrhagic effusion. Cytology revealed adenocarcinoma of the lung. After chest tube placement fluid in the fissure was present for many days suggesting an encysted effusion. Occasionally an encysted effusion occurs without fluid collecting inferiorly. This may appear as a mass or 'pseudotumour'.

## Aetiology of pleural effusions

**Transudates**—the causes of transudative pleural effusions include:
- Congestive heart failure: probably the most common cause of pleural effusion. This is bilateral in 75% of cases and the fluid is usually straw coloured.
- Cirrhosis, nephrotic syndrome, and hepatic hydrothorax.

**Exudates**—the causes of exudative pleural effusions are legion. Common causes are parapneumonic (associated with pneumonia), malignancy, pulmonary embolism, tuberculosis, trauma, collagen vascular disease (especially rheumatoid arthritis), and post-cardiac injury (including myocardial infarction and cardiac surgery).

## Parapneumonic effusion and empyema

Half of all bacterial pneumonias have associated pleural effusions which require drainage if they become 'complicated'. Complicated parapneumonic effusions include empyema (pus in the pleural space), those with positive pleural fluid cultures or Gram stains, and those with a low fluid pH (anaerobic metabolism). Drainage is by chest drain placement—'tube thoracostomy'.

Empyema is often culture negative but *Streptococcus milleri* or MRSA are common underlying causes. Prompt sampling and drainage is necessary. Ultrasound may show loculation due to fibrin strands walling of areas within the effusion. This will prevent a single chest drain successfully treating the empyema. Recent trials suggesting the practice of adding streptokinase to the pleural space via the drain for fibrinolytic effect have not been clearly beneficial. Surgical intervention is often required.

## Malignant effusions

Malignancy is the second most common cause of exudative pleural effusions with lung cancer (36%), and breast cancer (25%) frequent causes. Neoplastic effusions occasionally exhibit anaerobic metabolism and have a low pH and a low glucose level. This indicates a poorer prognosis.

## Tuberculous effusion

The glucose may be low and adenosine deaminase levels are usually elevated (>70IU/L). Pleural fluid smears and cultures are rarely positive (25% or less). If TB is suspected, pleural biopsy culture in addition to a pleural tap is required. This yields the diagnosis in 80% of cases.

## Pleural biopsy and thoracoscopy

Pleural biopsies (see Section 18.3) may be performed using closed guided techniques (ultrasound/CT) or via direct vision using thoracoscopic techniques.

## Patient safety

Increasingly ultrasound should be used prior to the insertion of a chest drain. The National Patient Safety Agency has noted a number of deaths due to incorrect placement of drains.

## Management

- Primary treatment of a pleural effusion should be to deal with the underlying cause.
- Recurrent effusions (which may recur even when the underlying cause is treated) may be treated with intermittent thoracentesis or pleurodesis.
- Rarely, an indwelling pleural catheter for intermittent drainage or a pleural-peritoneal shunt are performed.
- Pleurodesis obliterates the pleural space to prevent recurrence of the effusion following the installation of a fibrosis-inducing chemical irritant into the pleural space, e.g. talc, tetracycline (historical), minocycline, doxycycline or bleomycin.

# 18.10 Chronic obstructive pulmonary disease

## Aetiology and epidemiology

- COPD is predominantly a disease of smokers.
- It is a preventable disease.
- Worldwide there are greatly increasing rates in developing countries.
- Increasingly recognized in ♀ though still has a ♂ preponderance.
- 1 in 10–20 smokers develop COPD.

## Pathophysiology

- Disease occurs in 'susceptible smokers'.
- Occupational exposure and air pollution may also be relevant.
- Excessive inflammation, oxidant levels, and protease activity after smoking.
- Alpha-1 antitrypsin (a key anti-protease) deficiency, an autosomal dominant trait, is responsible for <10% of COPD (Fig. 18.19).
- Smoking cessation prevents disease occurrence and in established disease reduces progression.

## Clinical presentation

- Cough and sputum.
- Wheeze and/or breathlessness.
- Recurrent lower respiratory tract infections.
- 'Chronic bronchitis' (cough with sputum production for at least 3 months over 2 years).
- Leg oedema (as part of cor pulmonale).
- Acute exacerbation and/or acute respiratory failure.
- Pneumothorax.

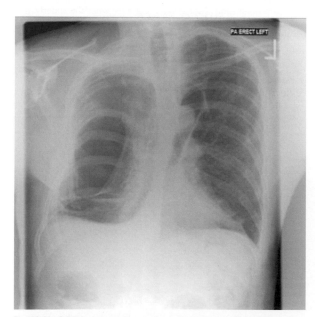

**Fig. 18.19** COPD variant with massive bullous disease. This male smoker had no family history of COPD and had normal alpha-1 antitrypsin levels. His X-ray may confuse admitting teams into thinking there is a large right-sided pneumothorax.

## Physical signs

- Features of nicotine use—tar staining of fingers and hair.
- Cyanosis in some patients.
- Finger clubbing is **not** a sign of COPD.
- Hyperinflation (barrel-shaped chest, reduced cricosternal distance, poor expansion, breath sounds over the praecordium, low-lying liver) (Fig. 18.20).
- Commonest sign is likely to be poor air entry/quiet breath sounds.
- Raised jugular venous pulse with peripheral oedema in cor pulmonale.

## Diagnosis

- Spirometry—obstructive in pattern, reduced $FEV_1/FVC$ ratio i.e. <70%.
- Reduced $FEV_1$ <80% (a normal $FEV_1$ excludes COPD).
- Hyperinflation on CXR.
- CT scanning may show emphysema or bullae.

## Complications

- Acute exacerbations (viral/bacterial/air pollution).
- Respiratory failure (type I or type II).
- Cor pulmonale—'blue bloater'.
- De-conditioning with muscle wasting.
- Pneumothorax.
- Development of secondary bronchiectasis (in 30% of severe COPD patients).
- Cachexia—'pink puffer'.
- Polycythaemia.

## Treatment

- Smoking cessation.
- Pulmonary rehabilitation.
- Inhaled bronchodilators, e.g. salbutamol, terbutaline, salmeterol, formoterol, vilanterol, and indacaterol.
- Long-acting anticholinergics, e.g. tiotropium, aclidinium bromide, umeclidinium, and glycopyrronium bromide.
- Inhaled corticosteroids with long-acting beta agonist for more severe disease with recurrent exacerbations.
- Oral mucolytics.
- Nebulizers—rarely needed in chronic stable patients.
- Oral steroids are used in acute exacerbations.
- Antibiotics in exacerbations include amoxicillin, doxycycline, or quinolones.

## Surgery

- Rarely indicated for the majority of patients.
- Lung volume reduction surgery used in those with large heterogeneous areas of emphysema but with well-preserved gas transfer. Recent endobronchial valve therapy is being developed to reduce hyperinflation without surgery
- Lung transplantation (this is a common indication for single-lung transplantation).

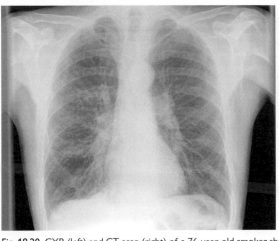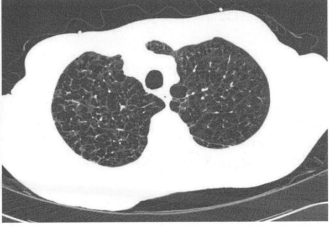

Fig. 18.20 CXR (left) and CT scan (right) of a 76-year-old smoker shows widespread emphysema. The plain CXR shows marked hyperinflation with flattened diaphragms. The patient's $FEV_1$ was 0.6 and FVC was 2.6L confirming obstructive lung physiology.

## Associated conditions

- Head and neck cancer and lung cancer.
- Ischaemic heart disease (common smoking aetiology).
- Peripheral vascular disease.

## NICE 2010 severity grading

- $FEV_1$ >80% predicted but $FEV_1$/FVC ratio <70%—stage 1 mild COPD
- $FEV_1$ ≤80% predicted but ≥50%—stage 2 moderate COPD.
- $FEV_1$ <50% predicted but ≥30%—stage 3 severe COPD.
- $FEV_1$ <30%—stage 4 very severe COPD.

## Oxygen and stable COPD

- Should only be prescribed with expert guidance.
- Commonly viewed as contraindicated in current smokers.
- Criteria suggest a minimum 6-week period of stability before deciding upon long-term oxygen.
- Resting $PaO_2$ of <7.3kPa, or
- Resting $PaO_2$ of <8.0kPa with right heart failure or $FEV_1$ <1.5 litres.

## Oxygen and acute exacerbations of COPD

- A small proportion of COPD patients are sensitive to the effects of uncontrolled oxygen. This exacerbates hypercapnia.
- ABGs should be checked as soon as possible in COPD patients who are receiving oxygen.
- For those with a raised $PaCO_2$ controlled oxygen (via Venturi mask, e.g. 24% or 28%) should be considered.
- Often lower than usual oxygen saturations levels are accepted in this setting, e.g. saturations of 88–93%.
- Seek help if unsure.

## Non-invasive ventilation (NIV)

- This may be lifesaving in those with acidotic (type II) respiratory failure.
- Indicated where pH <7.30 and $PaCO_2$ >6kPa.
- Reduces mortality by 45%.
- Audit data suggests this is grossly **underused**.

# 18.11 Acute respiratory distress syndrome

Acute respiratory distress syndrome (ARDS) is a syndrome rather than a diagnosis. It is characterized by diffuse parenchymal injury associated with non-cardiogenic pulmonary oedema. This results in hypoxaemic respiratory failure.

## Pathophysiology

The hallmark is diffuse alveolar damage (DAD). As lung tissue is rarely available for pathological diagnosis a clinical scoring system exists. Acute lung injury (ALI) is a milder lung injury that may or may not progress to ARDS. The American-European Consensus Conference criteria for a diagnosis of ARDS are:

- Acute onset.
- Bilateral infiltrates.
- Pulmonary artery wedge pressure <19mmHg on Swan–Ganz catheter (or no clinical signs of congestive heart failure).
- Arterial oxygen ($PaO_2$)/inspired oxygen ($FiO_2$) ratio <200 (ARDS) or <300 (ALI).

## Causes of ARDS

- Direct pulmonary injury, e.g. pneumonia, aspiration, near drowning, and toxic inhalation.
- Indirect injury, e.g. pancreatitis, multiple trauma, cardiac bypass, and fat embolization.
- Massive blood transfusion.
- Drug ingestion, e.g. heroin and other opioids, barbiturates, and salicylates.
- Often ARDS develops alongside other organ dysfunction; the multi-organ dysfunction syndrome (MODS).

## Pathology of ARDS

Abnormalities in cytokine regulatory, complement, and coagulation pathways are found. Endotoxin, free radicals, proteolytic enzymes, and surfactant depletion may also be involved in disease processes.

- Alveolar–capillary barrier disruption with transudation of protein-rich fluid across the barrier, alveolar oedema occurs.
- Surfactant deficiency causes alveolar collapse and atelectasis.
- Hypoxaemia from intrapulmonary shunting occurs.

## Clinicopathological phases of ARDS

Three phases of ARDS have been described:
- **Exudative phase** with injury to the endothelium and epithelium, inflammation, and fluid exudation.
- **Fibro-proliferative phase** follows with influx and proliferation of fibroblasts and other cells. This phase may resolve or become persistent.
- **Fibrosis phase** of healing follows with varying degrees of pulmonary fibrosis in those who recover.

## Clinical features

- Features of the precipitant, e.g. pancreatitis, sepsis.
- Confusion/agitation.
- Cyanosis and moist skin.
- Tachycardia, tachypnoea—'air hunger'.
- Scattered crackles.
- Increased work of breathing.

## Diagnosis

- ABG analysis documents hypoxaemic respiratory failure.
- This is usually type I respiratory failure initially but as fatigue ensues hypercapnia occurs (type II respiratory failure). $PaO_2$ <8kPa (60mmHg) with a $FiO_2$ >0.6 (60% inhaled oxygen).
- The chest radiograph reveals characteristic diffuse alveolar-interstitial infiltrates throughout (Fig. 18.21).
- Focal CXR changes may be present if the precipitant was pneumonia.
- Echocardiography or Swan–Ganz catheter to exclude a cardiogenic aetiology for pulmonary oedema.

## Differential diagnosis

- Cardiac failure and pulmonary oedema.
- Pneumonia (aspiration, bacterial, viral).
- Pneumocystis pneumonia
- Fat embolism.

## Treatment

- High-flow oxygen. Extremely careful fluid balance.
- Seek senior help.
- Admit all patients to the ICU.
- Patients with early ARDS can deteriorate rapidly.

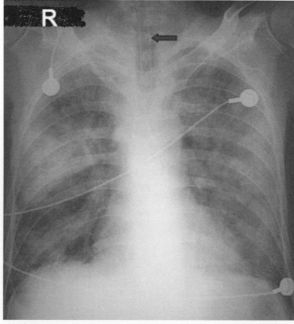

**Fig. 18.21** Acute respiratory distress syndrome. Note the bilateral infiltrates and the endotracheal tube (indicated by black arrow). The patient is being mechanically ventilated.

- Supportive care for any precipitating event.
- Invasive mechanical ventilation is almost universally required.
- Low-pressure ventilation with permissive hypercapnia is a strategy now employed (i.e. preserve lung tissue by preventing barotrauma even if this means allowing the $CO_2$ levels to rise). This is because pulmonary barotrauma due to previous high pressure/volume ventilatory strategies has been identified as a cause of increased mortality.

## Prognosis

- Mortality rates are high: 40–70%.
- Most survivors, however, have few long-term functional or respiratory sequelae.
- Radiologically visible pulmonary fibrosis may occur.

- Morbidity related to prolonged stays in intensive care is common, however.

## Complications

- Complications are usually related to the primary insult.
- Death—usually secondary sepsis related.
- Second organ or multiple organ failure.
- Ventilator-associated pneumonia.
- Ventilator-associated pneumothorax.
- Pulmonary embolism.
- Barotrauma.
- Post intensive care neuropathy, myopathy, psychological problems.

### Aetiology and epidemiology

- Asthma is a multifactorial inflammatory airways disease.
- Allergic and non-allergic syndromes exist.
- Genetic and environmental aspects to the disease.
- Occurs worldwide with high rates in developed countries.
- Less common in the developing world but greatly increasing rates.
- 7–10% of the adult UK population have asthma.
- Asthmatics who smoke have more symptoms.

### Pathophysiology

- Genetic factors.
- Trigger factors, e.g. infections, air pollution, drugs.
- Structural changes—airway remodelling, basement membrane thickening.
- Cellular component—airway mast cells, eosinophils and in some cases neutrophils.
- Lymphocytes more commonly have Th2 phenotype.
- Cytokine elevation especially IL-4, IL5, IL-13.
- Inflammatory mediators released, e.g. leukotrienes.
- All of these factors contribute to airway obstruction.

### Clinical presentation

- Cough, especially nocturnal.
- Wheeze and/or breathlessness.
- Acute exacerbation/acute respiratory failure.
- Pneumothorax.
- Death (sudden acute severe asthma still occurs).

### Subtypes

- Episodic asthma.
- Exercise-induced asthma.

- Occupational asthma (5% of asthma—many causes, commonly paint sprayers, bakers, soldering).
- Drug-induced asthma (beta-blockers, contrast media).
- Brittle asthma (rare and severe, sudden attacks).

### Physical signs

- Commonest sign is likely to be wheeze, reduced peak flow.
- Signs of atopy—nasal polyps, dermatitis.
- Severe childhood asthma is associated with chest wall deformities (Harrison sulci and 'pigeon chest' deformity).

### Diagnosis

- History, examination, and lung function tests can all be normal whilst the patient is well.
- Spirometry—obstructive in pattern.
- Acute bronchodilator reversibility testing, e.g. after salbutamol 200mcg inhaled.
- Reduced $FEV_1$ with reduced $FEV_1$/ FVC ratio, i.e. <70%.
- Diurnal variation in PEFR (worse in morning and higher in after-noon (Fig. 17.22)).
- Raised IgE or eosinophils can be seen in a proportion of asthmatics (sputum eosinophilia is possibly more common).
- Bronchial provocation tests, e.g. methacholine or adenosine challenges.
- Hyperinflation on CXR is relatively rare.
- Skin prick testing—supporting evidence only.

### Complications

- Acute exacerbations (viral/bacterial/air pollution).
- Pneumothorax.
- ABPA.
- Fixed airflow obstruction—loss of reversibility.

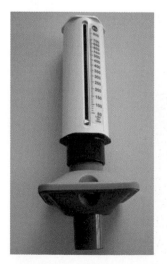

Height: 49°        Predicted norm: 240        Patient's personal best: 280

Instructions

| Date | Jan 18 | | Jan 19 | | Jan 20 | | Jan 21 | | Jan 22 | | Jan 23 | | Jan 24 | |
|---|---|---|---|---|---|---|---|---|---|---|---|---|---|---|
| Drugs | | | | | | | | | | | | | | |
| | 7 a.m. | 7 p.m. | 7 a.m. | 7 p.m. | 7 a.m. | 7 p.m. | 7 a.m. | 7 p.m. | 7 a.m. | 7 p.m. | 7 a.m. | 7 p.m. | 7 a.m. | 7 p.m. |
| Time | | | | | | | | | | | | | | |

**Fig. 18.22** Asthma. Peak flow meter (left) and peak flow chart demonstrating characteristic diurnal variation (right).

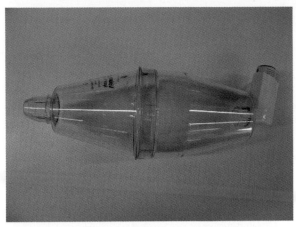

**Fig. 18.23** Asthma therapy. A volume-spacing device. Generally manufactures have tried to use colour coding: blue inhalers are short-acting beta agonists (e.g. salbutamol, terbutaline) and brown inhalers are inhaled corticosteroids (e.g. beclometasone, fluticasone, budesonide).

## Treatment

- Smoking cessation.
- National and international guidelines are available: <http://www.brit-thoracic.org.uk>, <http://www.ginasthma.com>.
- Emphasis is on stepwise treatment.
- Focus on checking compliance and inhaler technique (Fig.18.23).
- **Step 1:** inhaled bronchodilators.
- **Step 2:** inhaled corticosteroids (beclometasone, fluticasone, budesonide—adult dose often around 200–400mcg twice a day).
- **Step 3:** long-acting beta agonist if symptoms persist (formoterol or salmeterol).

- Combination inhalers are often prescribed these contain salmeterol + fluticasone or budesonide + formoterol.
- More severe disease may need specialist input, e.g. theophyllines, anti-IgE therapy, long-term steroids.
- Nebulizers; rarely needed in chronic stable patients.
- Oral steroids are used in acute exacerbations.

## Acute asthma

- **Moderate attack**—increasing symptoms, PEFR >50–75% best or predicted, no features of acute severe asthma.
- **Acute severe**—PEFR 33–50% best or predicted, respiratory rate 25 breaths/minute or faster, heart rate 110bpm or faster.
- **Life threatening**—PEFR 33% best or predicted or less, unable to speak sentences, normal or rising $PaCO_2$, drowsiness, bradycardia, silent chest.

## Acute severe asthma

- A medical emergency (see Section 1.8). Get senior help.
- Do not move the patient from a closely observed area till stable.
- Do **not** send the patient to the radiology department. If an X-ray is felt necessary a portable film should be requested. Notably the incidence of pneumothorax in acute severe asthma is very low.
- ABGs, high-flow oxygen, repeated PEFR, respiratory rate, and cardiac monitoring.
- Continuous nebulized salbutamol (and ipratropium) give this 'back-to-back' and not 2-hourly.
- Oral steroids (40mg prednisolone) or 200mg intravenous hydrocortisone.
- Intravenous magnesium sulphate (1.4–2g slow IV push in adults; with cardiac monitoring).

# 18.13 Fungal lung diseases

Fungal diseases of the lung are relatively rare despite worldwide endemic exposure to fungi. The type of pathogen and disease spectrum are influenced by local geography and the immunocompetency of the patient.

## Allergic bronchopulmonary aspergillosis (ABPA)

This occurs in people with an apparently exaggerated immune response to *Aspergillus*.

- An allergic response to the spores of the *Aspergillus* moulds (type III delayed hypersensitivity reaction).
- Patients often have eosinophilia, skin prick test, and serum evidence of allergy (positive precipitins) to *Aspergillus*.
- Between 0.2% and 4% of adult asthmatics are affected; it is also common in CF patients (7% of patients).
- ABPA is defined by several abnormalities, including asthma, eosinophilia, a positive skin test result for *Aspergillus*, marked elevation of the serum immunoglobulin E (IgE) level > 1000IU/dL, fleeting pulmonary infiltrates, central bronchiectasis, mucoid impaction, and positive test results for *Aspergillus* precipitins.
- Symptoms include: intermittent episodes of feeling unwell, cough, wheeze, and coughing mucus plugs.
- In the long term, ABPA can lead to permanent lung damage (fibrosis) if untreated.
- The treatment is with inhaled or oral steroids.
- Itraconazole (an oral antifungal drug) may be useful as a steroid-sparing agent.

## Aspergilloma and chronic pulmonary aspergillosis

This occurs in people with an apparently normal immune response but where local factors favour *Aspergillus* growth.

- This is a very different disease also caused by the *Aspergillus* mould.
- The fungus grows within a cavity of the lung, which was previously damaged during an illness such as tuberculosis, sarcoidosis, silicosis, or any other condition leaving a cavity.

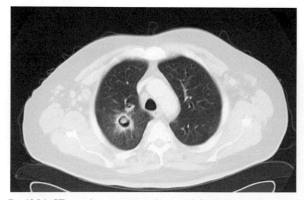

**Fig. 18.24** CT scan demonstrating right upper lobe mycetoma/aspergilloma. Note the scarring in the contralateral lung. Aspergillomas usually occur in already damaged lung. In this case the underlying disease was a haematological disorder with reduced immunity.

- The fungus grows within the cavity as a fungal ball (mycetoma) called an aspergilloma (Fig. 18.24).
- Symptoms—general malaise, weight loss, chronic cough, feeling rundown, and haemoptysis (in 50–80% of affected patients). Haemoptysis, may be severe and life threatening. Asymptomatic cases have been noted after 'routine' X-rays.
- X-rays and CT demonstrate a ball within the prior cavity sometimes with an air rim or 'halo'. Excluding a cavitating carcinoma is often difficult. The thickness of the cavity wall on CT may aid separating these diagnoses.
- Treatment may include:
  - Oral itraconazole or voriconazole.
  - Surgical removal has also been reported with some success.
  - Bronchial embolization for haemoptysis may be needed.

## Invasive aspergillosis

This occurs in patients with very impaired systemic immunity, e.g. bone marrow transplants, neutropaenic patients, or those with AIDS. It occurs in 5–13% of bone marrow transplant recipients.

Patients usually have a fever and symptoms from the lungs (cough, chest pain, or dyspnoea) which do not respond to antibacterials. The infection is characterized by invasion of blood vessels, resulting in multifocal infiltrates, which are often wedge-shaped, pleural-based, and may cavitate. Haematogenous spread to other organs, including the eye, the brain, the kidneys, and the skin is common. Cultures and blood tests may confirm the disease but it is usually a clinical diagnosis. Treatment is often started before microbiological confirmation with systemic antifungal drugs such as voriconazole, caspofungin, or amphotericin B.

## Other *Aspergillus*-related lung disease

Chronic necrotizing pulmonary aspergillosis (CNPA) is a subacute process usually found in patients with a lesser degree of immunosuppression, e.g. underlying lung disease, alcoholism, or chronic corticosteroid therapy. Because it is uncommon, CNPA often remains unrecognized for weeks or months and causes a progressive cavitatory pulmonary infiltrate. CNPA has a reported mortality rate of 10–40%. Patients have often received prolonged courses of antibiotic therapy and even empiric anti-tuberculous therapy without response prior to diagnosis via biopsy or culture. Chronic necrotizing pulmonary aspergillosis is rare and frequently undetected prior to autopsy.

Bronchocentric granulomatosis and malt worker's lung are two hypersensitivity lung diseases that are caused by *Aspergillus* species. Both are rare.

## Pulmonary candidiasis

Despite the ubiquity of *Candida albicans* and the high frequency of oral-pharyngeal candidiasis, clinically important pulmonary infection with *Candida* is uncommon. It is rarer than systemic candidaemia even in those with severe immunodeficiency. Bone marrow transplant recipients and neonates are the most common groups affected. The disease spreads via the airways; CXRs are characterized by bilateral, diffuse, and poorly marginated areas. Pulmonary parenchymal densities are common. Other non-specific findings include air bronchograms and obscure cardiac and hemidiaphragm borders. If the means of spread of the infection is haematogenous then a miliary nodular pattern is seen.

## Other fungal lung diseases

Histoplasmosis—this disease is endemic in the Mississippi delta but is unreported in the UK. It often causes a skin infection but may affect the lungs. The acute respiratory disease is characterized by fever, chest pains, and a dry or non-productive cough. Chronic lung disease resembles tuberculosis and can worsen over months or years. It is due to *Histoplasma capsulatum*.

Histoplasmosis is the most common cause of fibrosing mediastinitis, itself a rare disease. Pulmonary lesions have a tendency to calcify as they heal.

Other fungal infections that are uncommon in the UK but have been reported in North and South America and South-East Asia include blastomycosis, coccidioidomycosis, paracoccidioidomycosis, actinomycosis, and nocardiosis.

# 18.14 Pulmonary embolism

## Case history

A 45-year-old man, currently an inpatient, collapses with chest pain, breathlessness, and haemoptysis 5 days after sigmoid colectomy for colorectal cancer.

See also Section 1.9.

## Aetiology and epidemiology

- Third most common cause of death in the US.
- Present in >30% of hospital postmortem examinations (and often unsuspected by attending clinicians).
- Genetic factors—relatively rare but familial tendency and specific gene defects well recognized (antithrombin III deficiency, factor V Leiden mutation).
- Previous pulmonary embolus (PE) is a strong risk factor for further events.
- ~1/3 of patients who survive an initial PE die of a future embolic episode.
- Massive PE is one of the most common causes of unexpected death second only to coronary artery disease as a cause of sudden unexpected natural death at any age.
- Increasingly common with age.

## Pathophysiology

- Trigger factors 'Virchow triad of thrombosis':
  - Changes in vessel wall (endothelial injury).
  - Changes in flow (circulatory stasis).
  - Changes in blood characteristics/composition (hypercoagulable state).
- Situations associated with high risk include:
  - Cancer, pregnancy, recent major surgery, recent hospitalization, prolonged immobility.
  - Travel and attendant immobility widely accepted as risk factor for pulmonary embolism though not as high risk as above.
- Thromboembolism is due to clot formation by the intrinsic or extrinsic pathway. Platelets inhibition therefore has a minimal effect.
- Most cases are due to thromboembolism of a DVT to the pulmonary circulation.
- Complete RV outflow obstruction causes sudden death.
- Moderate sized PE probably cause less symptoms than smaller PE with hypoxia and hypotension.
- Smaller PE causes peripheral lung infarction and are associated with the above clinical history.
- Infarcted tissue is inflammatory, and so fevers and raised inflammatory markers are common.

## Clinical presentation

- Suspect PE in any patient who has chest symptoms that cannot be explained otherwise.
- Unfortunately PE is common in those with coexistent cardiorespiratory disease (COPD, pneumonia, etc.).
- Chest pain (pleuritic), haemoptysis, fever, dyspnoea.
- Collapse, hypotension, death.
- Many patients with PE are initially completely asymptomatic.

- Of patients who go on to die from massive PE, only 60% have dyspnoea, 17% have chest pain, and 3% have haemoptysis.

## Differential diagnosis

- Acute coronary syndrome/myocardial infarction.
- Aortic dissection.
- Oesophageal rupture.
- Pericarditis and cardiac tamponade.
- Pneumonia, pneumothorax.
- Sepsis.

## Physical signs

- Tachycardia, isolated hypoxia, crackles.
- Raised JVP, hypotension, cool peripheries, poor capillary refill, and oliguria all suggest life threatening event.
- Pleural rubs are relatively uncommon.
- Non-specific chest wall tenderness is common in those with acute PE and does **not** exclude PE.

## Diagnosis

- Have a high index of suspicion.
- Abnormalities on a CXR are relatively rare; Westermark sign, a dilatation of the pulmonary vessels proximal to an embolism.
- Pulse oximetry is extremely insensitive and is normal in the majority of patients with PE.
- ABGs are often misleading and can be normal.
- ECG—the commonest abnormality is sinus tachycardia (20% of patients have normal ECG).
- S1–Q3–T3 pattern on ECG has low sensitivity and specificity (seen in 25% of PE).
- A raised troponin suggests myocardial strain related to pulmonary embolism and should prompt consideration for thrombolytic therapy and high intensity monitoring.

## D-dimer

- D-dimer is a unique degradation product produced by plasmin-mediated proteolysis of cross-linked fibrin.
- D-dimer is a useful test at excluding pulmonary embolism in low-risk groups.
- A low-risk patient with a negative D-dimer does not need further imaging.
- D-dimer should **not** be used in high-risk groups where imaging is mandatory.
- At least three commercially assays are available including agglutination and ELISA-based types. There is considerable variation in the sensitivity and specificity profiles between the different types of tests.

## Imaging studies

- If you suspect PE the consensus is to commence treatment with heparin and then arrange investigations. The investigations are dependent on patients presentation (acute massive vs. sub-massive), comorbidities, and availability of tests locally.

## Ventilation/perfusion scanning (V/Q scans)

- PE shows mismatched defect (ventilation present, perfusion absent). This is unlikely to be helpful in patients with other significant cardiorespiratory disease where there may be other effects on ventilation and/or perfusion.
- Higher sensitivity than specificity; possible outcomes:
  - Negative scan—stop therapy if low risk; investigate further if high risk.
  - Indeterminate scan—further tests are required.
  - Positive scan—continue therapy.

## Computed tomography pulmonary angiogram (CTPA)

- Can be performed in relatively sick patients as only a short breath-hold manoeuvre required.
- Does involve modest intravenous contrast load (caution in renal failure).
- High sensitivity and specificity.
- Often demonstrates alternate diagnosis where PE is excluded, e.g. basal pneumonia, oesophageal rupture. See Fig. 18.25.

## Direct pulmonary angiogram

- Catheter studies of the pulmonary vascular bed are now becoming much less common.
- Does involve modest intravenous contrast load (caution in renal failure).
- The test is invasive but offers high sensitivity and specificity in experienced hands.
- Often patients are too breathless to tolerate the procedure.

## Transthoracic echocardiography

- Of limited role except in sub-massive PE where circulatory stress may allow right ventricular dysfunction and ventricular septal bowing to be seen.

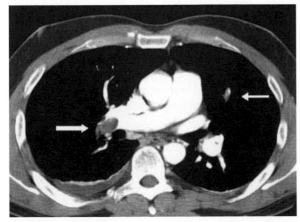

**Fig. 18.25** Computerised Tomographic Pulmonary Angiogram (CTPA). This demonstrates a large right-sided central pulmonary embolus (large arrow). A smaller and more peripheral embolus is shown as a filling defect with the smaller arrow. Note there is also a small pleural effusion on the right.

- The test is, however, rapid and available at the bedside.
- Helps exclude some of the differential diagnoses.

## Doppler ultrasound

- The majority of PE arise from DVTs of the leg.
- Colour ultrasound of the legs may be useful in confirming the DVT.
- A negative scan for DVT is seen in 40–50% of patients who have had a confirmed pulmonary embolism.
- Negative leg scans should not be used to refute a diagnosis of PE.

## Treatment

### Anticoagulants

- Heparin augments the activity of antithrombin III.
- Heparin or heparinoids should be started as soon as a diagnosis is suspected.
- Heparin is given as a continuous intravenous infusion and needs monitoring with coagulation studies (APTT)
- Low-molecular-weight (LMW) heparinoids (tinzaparin, enoxaparin) are given subcutaneously once or twice daily. Dosing is based on the patient's weight and no monitoring is routinely undertaken. Monitoring will be needed in those with substantial renal failure and in those who are pregnant.
- Trials in PE without haemodynamic compromise demonstrate that LMW heparinoids are at least as efficacious as intravenous unfractionated heparin infusions.
- Once a diagnosis is confirmed warfarin therapy can be commenced.

### Thrombolytics

- In sub-massive pulmonary embolism fibrinolytic therapy is given when there are signs of imminent circulatory collapse (hypotension and tachycardia).
- Various agents have been used including streptokinase, urokinase, and alteplase.
- In one study, a 2-hour infusion of alteplase was more effective (and more rapidly effective) than urokinase or streptokinase over a 12-hour period.
- Alteplase usually is given as a front-loaded infusion over 90 or 120 minutes.
- Alteplase is licensed by the US FDA for sub-massive pulmonary embolism.

### Surgery

- Surgical embolectomy has been described but very few patients are suitable for this reflecting either the severity of the illness and proximity to cardiothoracic surgical services,

## Complications

- Collapse, acute renal failure.
- Recurrence, further embolic event.
- Septic complications—secondary pneumonia.
- Pleural effusion (often bloody).
- Paradoxical embolus (in the presence of an abnormal right-to-left shunt).
- Chronic thromboembolic pulmonary hypertension.

# 18.15 Lung cancer

Secondary deposits (metastases) are common in the lung from breast, colon, renal, ovary, testis, thyroid and melanoma. Primary lung cancer arises in the lung and will be discussed here.

## Epidemiology

- Lung cancer is the leading fatal cancer in both men and women.
- About 14% of all people who develop lung cancer survive for 5 years.
- Tobacco smoke contains >40 carcinogens.
- 86% of lung cancer is diagnosed in current or past smokers (non-smokers still account for ~14% of lung cancer).
- Passive smoking—living with a smoker doubles the risk of lung cancer.
- Asbestos exposure and cigarette smoking compounds the risk by 50-fold.
- A person with COPD has a 4–6× greater risk of lung cancer even when the effect of cigarette smoking is excluded.
- Radon is a by-product of naturally occurring radium that increases the risk of lung cancer.

## Clinical presentation

- New-onset cough, chest pain, haemoptysis.
- Dyspnoea, pleural effusion.
- Stridor—indicates compression of a major airway.
- Incidental finding on CXR performed for other reasons (10–20%).
- 25% present with symptoms related to metastasis.
- Hoarse voice (due to compression of the intrathoracic part of the left recurrent laryngeal nerve).

- Horner syndrome—small pupil with ptosis due to sympathetic chain compression.
- SVCO—superior vena cava obstruction—flushed upper extremities, fixed raised JVP, and headache are all due to obstruction of the SVC. This can occur with any lung cancer but small cell lung cancer (SCLC) with extensive mediastinal lymphadenopathy is often the cause.

## Diagnosis

- CXR (Figs 18.26–18.28).
- Sputum cytology—40–60% diagnostic rate for central tumours.
- Bronchoscopy—this has a diagnostic rate for central tumours of 90% or higher.
- Percutaneous transthoracic needle biopsy of the primary lesion or metastasis.
- Pleural fluid or lymph node cytology (60–90% diagnostic rate).
- Thoracoscopy or mediastinoscopy and lymph node sampling.

## Staging

- TNM—Tumour Node Metastasis scheme.
- CT scanning of head (if neurological symptoms), chest, and abdomen.
- Positron emission tomography (PET) scanning increasingly used in early stage non-SCLC (NSCLC) to exclude occult metastasis.
- Bone scans are often required.

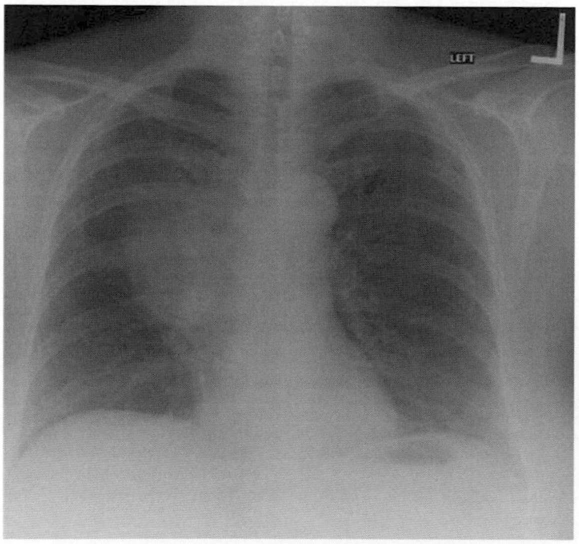

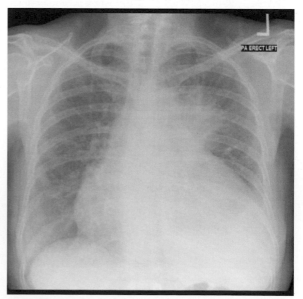

**Fig. 18.26** This demonstrates a large right upper zone mass. The diagnosis was non-small cell lung cancer diagnosed on histology of bronchoscopic biopsies. The tumour was not resectable surgically due to mediastinal disease noted on staging CT scan. Chemotherapy or radiotherapy may be potential treatments.

**Fig. 18.27** CXR demonstrating an inoperable lung cancer. This patient presented with increasing breathlessness. The plain CXR film shows a left upper zone mass and cardiomegaly. The cardiomegaly was found on echocardiogram to be due to a pericardial effusion. This was drained and fluid cytology revealed non-small cell lung cancer.

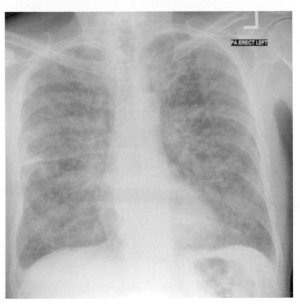

**Fig. 18.28** This CXR demonstrates multiple pulmonary metastases. Note the multiple rounded nodules that are poorly defined.

## Subtypes of lung cancer

Primary lung cancers are usually divided into two groups that account for about 95% of all cases. They are called small cell lung cancer and non-small cell lung cancer. NSCLC includes several more types of cancer.

- SCLCs are less common, but grow rapidly and are more likely to metastasize than NSCLCs.
- SCLCs have often metastasized by the time of diagnosis.
- NSCLC includes adenocarcinoma, squamous cell carcinoma, large cell, and bronchoalveolar cell tumours.

Treatment and prognosis depend upon the histological type of cancer, the stage (degree of spread), and the patient's performance status. Treatments include surgery, chemotherapy, radiotherapy, and best supportive care (symptom-based therapy).

## Surgery

- This is the preferred treatment for patients with early-stage NSCLC.
- It offers curative intent.
- 60–80% of all patients have advanced or metastatic disease and are therefore not suitable for surgery (Figs 18.26–18.28).
- Late (inoperable) presentation is common.
- Coexistent COPD further reduces the number of operable cases. Pneumonectomy usually requires a preoperative $FEV_1$ of 2L or greater. Lobectomy can be performed with an $FEV_1$ of approximately 1.5L.

## Other treatments

- Radiotherapy—this is usually given with palliative intent. Small NSCLC tumours in those too frail for surgery may be cured. Useful for pain or haemoptysis. Radical radiotherapy and combined chemoradiation regimens do exist for those with inoperable but localized disease.
- Chemotherapy—specific regimens exist for SCLC or NSCLC. They are given with palliative intent.
- SVC stents are placed radiologically and relieve SVCO rapidly.
- Endobronchial stents can be placed to prevent major airway collapse due to tumour compression.

## Screening

- Low-dose CT scans have potential in detecting early-stage lung cancer and therefore increasing rates of surgical cure.
- These are still being evaluated in research studies. No national guidelines currently exist on this area pending further studies.

# 18.16 Pulmonary fibrosis

## Background

Localized pulmonary fibrosis can occur after any injurious insult to the lungs, e.g. post infectious, inflammatory, radiotherapy, or drug related. These causes will not be discussed further. Diffuse idiopathic pulmonary fibrosis (IPF) and cryptogenic fibrosing alveolitis (CFA) are deemed synonymous for this chapter.

## Epidemiology and aetiology

- IPF affects elderly persons, with an average age of onset of ~60 years.
- Prevalence 175 cases per 100,000 in people >75 years.
- IPF affects more ♂ than ♀.
- There is no racial predilection. Most cases are sporadic, but a familial variant has been reported.
- Wood or metal dust exposure and smoking are more common in patients with IPF.
- Gastro-oesophageal reflux and chronic aspiration has been implicated in the development of pulmonary fibrosis.

## Mortality/morbidity

- The course of IPF is variable and unpredictable.
- A rapidly progressive fatal course over several weeks or months is recognized, Others demonstrate deterioration in lung function over a longer period.
- Median survival is 3–5 years from the onset of symptoms.

## Clinical presentation

- Dyspnoea.
- Dry unproductive cough.
- Chest tightness.

## Clinical findings

- Tachypnoea, panting breaths.
- Clubbing of the fingers is noted in 20–50% of cases.
- Fixed end-inspiratory crackles can be heard at the lung bases (fixed—crackles do not change with coughing).
- Signs of pulmonary hypertension and right-sided heart failure (e.g. a loud second heart sound, right ventricular heave) develop as disease progresses.

## Diagnosis

No specific diagnostic test exists. Clinicopathological-radiological correlation required. Many patients never undergo a lung biopsy.

- Elevated ESR in 40–50%.
- Restrictive impairment (reduced $FEV_1$ with high or normal $FEV_1/FVC$ ratio) does not distinguish between alveolitis and fibrosis.
- Serologic tests—non-specific (low titres of antinuclear antibodies or rheumatoid factor are common). The presence of high titres suggests the presence of connective-tissue diseases.
- ABGs reveal hypoxia with an increased alveolar–arterial partial pressure of oxygen gradient.

## Pulmonary function tests

- Restrictive impairment (see earlier).
- Single-breath diffusing capacity for carbon monoxide.
- A diffusing capacity for carbon monoxide <45% predicted or a FVC <50% predicted correlates with higher mortality. It forms part of the referral criteria for lung transplantation.

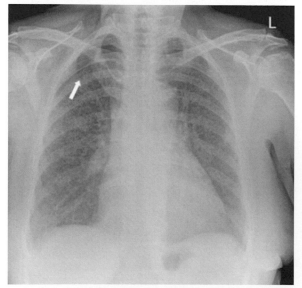

**Fig. 18.29** This patient has an idiopathic interstitial lung disease—note the widespread fine nodularity. There is a right pneumothorax indicated by the arrow. There is also some subcutaneous emphysema in the soft tissues.

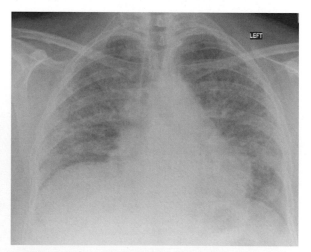

**Fig. 18.30** CXR of another case of idiopathic interstitial lung disease with a presumptive diagnosis of cryptogenic fibrosing alveolitis. This condition is also known as idiopathic pulmonary fibrosis. Note the diffuse fine linear scars throughout and the low lung volumes (small lungs due to restrictive physiology).

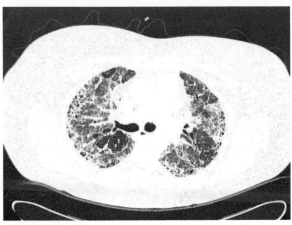

**Fig. 18.31** A CT scan of interstitial lung disease (same case as 18.30). Note the widespread increased density of the parenchyma with peripheral honeycombing.

## Imaging studies

- CXR—abnormal in 95% of patients but no pathognomonic features are recognized.
- Bilateral diffuse reticular or reticulonodular infiltrates seen at the periphery and the bases (Figs 18.29–18.31).
- HRCT scan has better resolution and pick-up rate than CXR or conventional CT scan images.
- Scattered mediastinal lymph nodes are relatively common.
- A pattern of coarse, reticular shadows, especially subpleurally, suggests a fibrotic histopathological process.
- Ground-glass opacities predict a good response to corticosteroids or immunosuppressive agents.
- The presence of pleural effusions, hilar lymphadenopathy, and localized densities suggests an alternate diagnosis should be sought.

## Treatment

To date, most treatments for pulmonary fibrosis have been disappointing. This probably reflects the fact that by presentation significant irreversible scarring has occurred.

- 15% respond to oral steroids.
- Early steroid withdrawal is recommended in non-responders. In responders azathioprine can be used as a steroid-sparing agent.
- Acetylcysteine, an antioxidant, has recently been shown to have benefits in combination with steroids and azathioprine. (Newer agents in use include pirfenidone and nintedanib.)
- Cyclophosphamide has benefits in scleroderma-associated pulmonary fibrosis but no clear role in idiopathic pulmonary fibrosis.
- Oxygen therapy including long-term treatment.
- Influenza vaccination and other supportive measures.
- Lung transplantation in younger patients (often single-lung transplantation).

## Differential diagnosis

Upper zone (predominantly):
- Collagen vascular-associated pulmonary fibrosis.
- Drug-related interstitial lung diseases (amiodarone, nitrofurantoin, methotrexate, etc.).
- Sarcoidosis, eosinophilic granuloma (pulmonary Langerhans cell histiocytosis/histiocytosis X).
- Extrinsic allergic alveolitis/hypersensitivity pneumonitis.
- Chronic infection, e.g. tuberculosis, *Histoplasma*.
- Occupational-related fibrosis (see later).

Lower zone (predominantly):
- Asbestosis
- Rheumatoid arthritis
- Idiopathic
- Pulmonary oedema.

## Occupational causes of pulmonary fibrosis

A number of occupational exposures may lead to pulmonary fibrosis (predominantly upper zone)
- Inorganic dusts—silica (silicosis), asbestos (asbestosis), beryllium (berylliosis).
- Progressive massive fibrosis is seen in those exposed to either coal or silica dust where large masses of confluent fibrosis occur.
- Organic dusts—hypersensitivity pneumonitis.

# 18.17 Extrinsic allergic alveolitis

## Background

Extrinsic allergic alveolitis (EAA) is also known as hypersensitivity pneumonitis.

## Pathogenesis

This is a hypersensitivity immune reaction to the repeated inhalation or ingestion of various antigens or irritants. Antigens are often related to the patient's occupation. The most common diseases seen are farmer's lung and bird fancier's lung.

- Two clinical phases or syndromes are identified: acute and subacute/chronic. Most affected patients present acutely with flu-like illness with cough.
- Patients can also present subacutely with recurrent pneumonia or chronically with exertional dyspnoea, productive cough, and weight loss.
- Most patients have circulating IgG antibodies that are antigen specific.
- Antibodies may be non-specific and seen in ~50% of asymptomatic people exposed to the sensitizing antigen.

## Epidemiology/prognosis

- Hypersensitivity pneumonitis affects 0.5–6% of the farming population.
- Prevalence in bird fanciers is estimated to be 20–20,000 cases per 100,000 persons at risk. Pigeons and budgies are recognized causes of EAA.

## Mortality/morbidity

The mortality and morbidity of hypersensitivity pneumonitis is variable and depends on the type and length of antigen exposure. Most patients recover completely after removal of the offending antigen.

- Many farmers develop mild chronic lung impairment and obstructive airflow disease associated with mild emphysematous changes.
- Most patients experience total recovery of lung function, but this may take several years.
- Bird fancier's lung carries a prognosis worse than that of farmer's lung.
- The poorer prognosis has been linked to higher antigenic exposure and the persistence of exposure to avian antigen, e.g. continued bird-handling, even after birds are removed.
- The 5-year mortality rate is ~30%.

## Clinical presentation

- Patients with hypersensitivity pneumonitis may present acutely with a flu-like illness or with fevers with a cough.
- The presentation is usually a few hours after exposure (e.g. in the evening after a work exposure).
- Subacute presentation with recurrent pneumonia.
- Chronic presentation with exertional dyspnoea, productive cough, and weight loss.
- Often the diagnosis is made after repeated episodes of what has been treated as a community-acquired pneumonia.

## Examples of EAA

- Farmer's lung—mouldy hay.
- Bird fanciers lung—pigeon or budgie bloom.
- Bagassosis—mouldy sugar cane.
- Hot tub lung—*Mycobacterium avium*.

## Diagnosis

- A good history covering occupational and hobby-related exposures often raises the suspicion of EAA.
- Antigen-specific antibodies can be seen.
- Pulmonary function tests can show a restrictive defect in early disease.
- In late disease a restrictive, obstructive, or mixed pattern can be seen in the pulmonary function tests.
- Conventional chest radiography is the examination of choice (abnormal in most patients with hypersensitivity pneumonitis).
- HRCT is commonly performed to confirm the diagnosis and to rule out other possibilities (Fig. 18.32).
- A normal HRCT scan does not exclude hypersensitivity pneumonitis (seen in up to 50% of patients).
- Lung biopsy is occasionally performed to confirm the diagnosis and exclude other causes of interstitial disease.

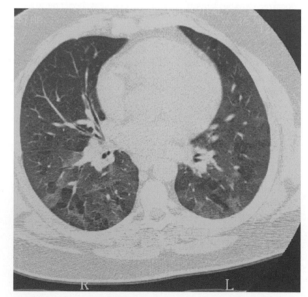

**Fig. 18.32** Acute extrinsic allergic alveolitis showing airway centred nodules and ground-glass shadowing with areas of hyperlucency.
Reproduced from Maskell N and Millar A. *Oxford Desk Reference, Respiratory Medicine*, 2009, Figure 7.8.2, page 149, with permission from Oxford University Press.

# 18.18 Occupational lung diseases

## Background

Occupational lung diseases are a result of exposure to dusts, gases, fumes, and vapours at work. There are many lung diseases that are associated with industrial exposure including:

- Occupational asthma—paint sprayer's asthma, baker's asthma, platinum mining.
- Extrinsic allergic alveolitis, e.g. farmer's lung.
- Pulmonary fibrosis due to exposure to mineral dust, e.g. silicosis, asbestos. Exposure to iron or barium can lead to dense nodular shadowing but minimal fibrosis.
- Lung cancer—exposure to second-hand smoke, asbestos, radon, heavy metals, e.g. arsenic, ionizing radiation, silica (see later), and polycyclic aromatic hydrocarbons are all risk factors.
- Exposure to particulate matter, dusts, and noxious gases may also be a risk factor for COPD.
- In the UK those diagnosed with occupational lung disease may be able to claim financial compensation either: (1) Industrial Injuries Disablement Benefit if the disease is a so-called 'prescribed disease' (recognized by the Department for Work and Pensions as an industrial disease), or (2) by suing for damages.

## Asbestos-related lung disease

There are many manifestations of asbestos exposure including the following:

- Pleural plaques are the most common. They consist of acellular collagen bundles on the parietal pleura. They are not premalignant. Asbestosis is rarely seen in the absence of plaques but plaques commonly occur in isolation.
- Diffuse pleural thickening is not specific for asbestos exposure (also seen with tuberculous pleuritis and empyema). It leads to breathless due to extrapulmonary restriction (Fig. 18.33).
- Benign asbestos-related pleural effusions are exudative or occasionally haemorrhagic. Diffuse pleural thickening occur as a sequelae to the effusion.

- Asbestosis—a diffuse interstitial pulmonary fibrosis is seen in heavily exposed workers. Latency is around 30 years. Presents insidiously with cough and exertional dyspnoea. Physical signs are exactly the same as for idiopathic pulmonary fibrosis. No satisfactory treatment is available.
- Rounded atelectasis ('folded lung' or Blesovsky syndrome) is an area of atelectatic lung adjacent to pleural thickening, with characteristic in-drawing of bronchi and vessels—'comet sign' on CT. It is strongly associated with asbestos exposure but can be seen with any infective organizing pleural exudate. The lingula is the most common site, followed by the middle lobes.
- Malignant pleural mesothelioma is a rare neoplasm (<5% of pleural malignancies). It is strongly associated with asbestos exposure but can occur after minor environmental or household exposure. 20% of patients have no identifiable asbestos exposure. A long latent period of 30–40 years is classical. 80% arise in the pleura and 20% from the abdominal peritoneum. They can metastasize but most symptoms are due to the primary tumour. A major differential is pleural metastases especially with adenocarcinoma.
- Bronchogenic carcinoma occurs in 25% of heavily exposed asbestos workers. Smoking increases the risk of lung cancer 90-fold. Bronchoalveolar cell carcinoma predominates.

### Radiology of asbestos-related diseases

- **Benign pleural plaques** may be seen in profile or 'en face'. In profile, plaques appear as dense focal smooth opacities, usually <1cm thick, paralleling the chest wall. Appearances 'en face' are ill-defined opacity with irregular margins—'holly leaf calcification'. Most pleural plaques are multiple and bilateral on the diaphragm or in the mid zones. CT is more sensitive than CXR (Fig. 18.34).
- **Asbestosis**—plain X-ray usually shows coexistent pleural plaques or diffuse pleural thickening. With advanced disease the heart borders become indistinct—'shaggy heart'. HRCT shows subpleural nodularity with traction bronchiectasis and honeycombing in severe cases.
- **Malignant mesothelioma**—CT is the test of choice. Irregular nodular pleural thickening (92%) is seen, particularly involving the mediastinal pleura with or without pleural effusion. Chest wall invasion is seen in ~20%. Pleural thickening is typically nodular, >1cm thick. In contrast to the common perception, malignant mesothelioma does metastasize though and most symptoms relate to the primary tumour. Abdominal cavity mesothelioma may occur.

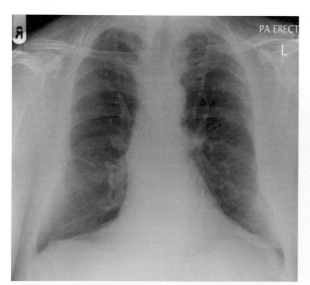

**Fig. 18.33** Asbestos-related pleural thickening. Compare the thick blurred line at the lung edges to other X-rays in this chapter.

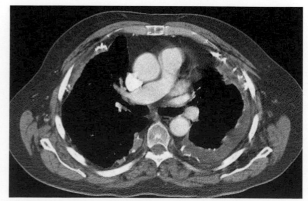

**Fig. 18.34** Industrial lung disease. This CT scan demonstrates asbestos-related pleural disease. There is a small left pleural effusion. There is dense calcification throughout the pleura on pleural plaques.

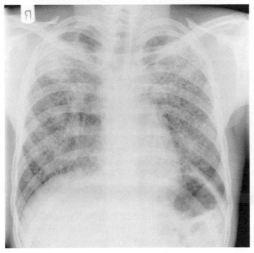
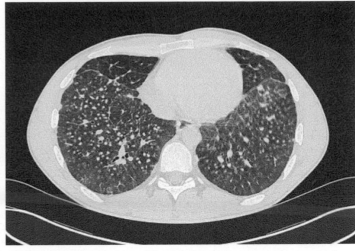

**Fig. 18.35** Industrial lung disease. Silicosis was diagnosed due to widespread fine nodularity in a sandblaster (radiological appearances in an exposed individual with occupational risks). The CT scan (right) shows multiple nodular areas within the lung fields. This patient required lung transplantation due to respiratory failure.

# Silicosis

Silicosis is an occupational lung disease that develops over time when dust-containing silica is inhaled into the lungs. It is preventable and <100 new cases of silicosis are diagnosed each year in the UK. Occupations at risk include any occupation where fine dust from concrete, masonry, sandstone, rock, paint, and other abrasives are produced, e.g. miners, tunnellers, and sandblasters.

## Symptoms
- Tachypnoea after physical exertion.
- Dry or severe cough, often persistent and accompanied by hoarseness of the throat.
- Fatigue or tiredness.
- Loss of appetite/weight loss.
- Chest pain/fever.

## Chronic silicosis
This is the most common type of silicosis. It develops after 20 years or longer of exposure to low levels of silica dust. Chronic silicosis itself is further subdivided into simple and complicated silicoses (also called progressive massive fibrosis) (Fig. 18.35).

## Acute silicosis
This is lung disease that develops after 1–3 years of exposure to very high concentration of silica dust. It does not necessarily progress to chronic disease if dust avoidance is followed. Alveolar filling on CXR is characteristic.

## Accelerated silicosis
Silicosis that develops after an average of 10 years of exposure to high concentration of silica dust.

## Complications
- Respiratory failure.
- Tuberculosis is particularly common in silicosis.
- Cavitation and mycetoma/fungal infection.
- Caplan syndrome (also seen in coal workers) is characterized by pulmonary nodules with cavitation with seropositive rheumatoid arthritis in silica workers.
- Silica is a known carcinogen and is associated with the development of lung cancer.

## Background

Sarcoidosis is an idiopathic multisystem disorder of variable presentation, outcome, and disease pattern characterized by non-caseating granulomas.

## Pathogenesis

- Dysregulation of immunity with non-caseating epithelioid granulomas that may affect any organ system.
- An increase in B-cell activity with hypergammaglobulinaemia is seen in 50%.
- Increased Th1 response, e.g. induced by therapeutic interferon, can trigger or exacerbate sarcoidosis.
- Persistent antigenic stimulation by *Mycobacterium*, other bacteria, heavy metals or auto-antigens has been proposed.

## Epidemiology and risk groups

Sarcoidosis affects people worldwide with incidence varying dramatically. In Europe, the disease affects whites more commonly than other races (Western more than Eastern Europe). In the US, Afro-Caribbeans are more likely to be affected than whites. Sarcoidosis affects both men and women.

- Bimodal distribution peaks at ages 25–35 and 45–65 years.
- Higher incidence in people of Asian, Irish, and Scandinavian origin.
- Higher incidence in healthcare workers and non-smokers.

## Prognosis

This is variable, from a self-limiting syndrome to a chronic debilitating disease causing death. Spontaneous remission occurs in 2/3. The remainder have a more chronic or progressive course.

The mortality rate is 1–6%. Causes of death are pulmonary fibrosis, respiratory failure and a consequence of myocardial involvement (arrhythmias and cardiac failure). CNS involvement, renal failure, and liver disease can cause significant morbidity. Disease patterns appear to vary from country to country, e.g. cardiac sarcoid is more common in Japan.

## Clinical presentation

- Onset is usually insidious—1/3 have fatigue and weight loss.
- Asymptomatic cases can be discovered on routine CXR.
- Cutaneous involvement seen in 25% of patients. Erythema nodosum is the main non-specific cutaneous disease.
- Lupus pernio is a striking manifestation of sarcoid skin lesions (raised purple lesions on the face).
- Lungs are affected in 90%, e.g. dyspnoea, dry cough, and chest tightness or pain. The disease can progress to irreversible fibrosis.
- Nodal disease—1/3 have palpable lymph nodes.
- Ocular involvement—an anterior uveitis is the most common finding. Any part of the eye may be affected, however.
- Neurosarcoidosis—this is rare (<10% of patients). A VIIth cranial nerve palsy is the most frequent finding.

## Clinical syndromes

Cutaneous involvement is either specific (lupus pernio) or non-specific (erythema nodosum) (Fig. 18.36). Lymphadenopathy can be found.

- Löfgren syndrome is erythema nodosum in conjunction with unilateral or bilateral hilar and/or right paratracheal lymphadenopathy, with anterior uveitis. It usually resolves spontaneously in 6–8 weeks.
- Uveoparotid fever—an uveitis associated with fever and parotid swelling (Heerfordt syndrome).
- Sarcoid infiltration of scars may occur. Scars from previous trauma or surgery become infiltrated and show a red or purple colour. These lesions may be tender.

## Differential diagnosis

- Stage IV disease—idiopathic pulmonary fibrosis can be an alternative diagnosis.
- Lymphoma.
- Tuberculosis.
- Other interstitial lung diseases especially berylliosis.

## Diagnosis

- FBC—non-specific abnormalities are common, e.g. leucopenia, thrombocytopenia, eosinophilia, and anaemia.
- Hypercalciuria and hypercalcaemia are due to increased vitamin D metabolism by granulomas.
- Serum angiotensin-converting enzyme level is non-specific and is not sensitive in diagnosing sarcoidosis.
- CXR—this is abnormal in almost 90% of patients (Fig. 18.37):
  - Stage I disease—bilateral hilar lymphadenopathy (BHL).
  - Stage II disease—BHL plus pulmonary infiltrates.
  - Stage III disease—pulmonary infiltrates without BHL.
  - Stage IV disease—pulmonary fibrosis.

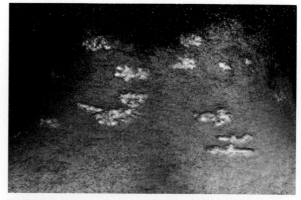

**Fig. 18.36** Typical sarcoid cutaneous lesions on nape of neck.
Reproduced from Maskell N and Millar A. *Oxford Desk Reference, Respiratory Medicine*, 2009, Figure 7.9.1, with permission from Oxford University Press.

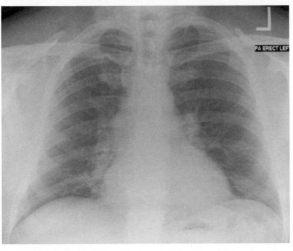

**Fig. 18.37** Sarcoidosis. This patient presented with malaise and sweats. The CXR demonstrates bilateral hilar lymphadenopathy and right paratracheal lymphadenopathy. This in conjunction with a raised calcium was strongly suggestive of sarcoidosis.

- HRCT may show lymphadenopathy or granulomatous infiltration. Honeycombing, bronchiectasis, and alveolar consolidation are seen in more severe cases.
- Kveim test—this is now outmoded as it carries cross-infection risks.
- Pulmonary function tests may show defects in diffusing capacity and vital capacity (obstructive, restrictive, or mixed spirometry can be seen).
- ECG can demonstrate unsuspected or symptomatic arrhythmias and/or heart block.
- Skin or endo-/transbronchial lung biopsy can be used. Any lymph node excised must be cultured for mycobacterial infections.

## Treatment

Watchful waiting is often all that is required. Hydroxychloroquine seems useful in some cases especially for fatigue.

Prednisolone (30–40mg of prednisone daily for 2–3 months, with a gradual taper over 1 year) for patients with:

- Symptomatic stage II and all stage III pulmonary disease.
- Neurological, cardiac, or refractory ocular disease.
- Hypercalcaemia.

# 18.20 Cor pulmonale and pulmonary hypertension

## Background

- Pulmonary hypertension is defined by a mean pulmonary artery pressure of >25mmHg with a low pulmonary capillary wedge pressure (PCWP) of <15mmHg and a raised pulmonary vascular resistance (PVR) of >240 dynes/sec/cm$^5$.
- Onset is usually insidious—1/3 have fatigue and weight loss.
- Pulmonary arterial hypertension (PAH) is most commonly associated with hypoxic lung disease and left heart disorders.
- There are a wide number of other causes including idiopathic pulmonary arterial hypertension, pulmonary hypertension secondary to connective tissue disease, portal hypertension, HIV, systemic-to-pulmonary shunts, and chronic thromboembolic disease.

## Epidemiology and aetiology

- Cor pulmonale is a term used to describe pulmonary hypertension and right ventricular hypertrophy secondary to pulmonary disease. This is a common syndrome.
- Hypoxaemia is a powerful stimulus of pulmonary vasoconstriction and this is the most common mechanism. Treatment is usually supplemental oxygen to maintain oxygen saturations >90%.
- Idiopathic pulmonary arterial hypertension (IPAH) is an orphan disease with an incidence of 3–5 per million. It has a familial form associated with mutation of a gene called bone morphogenetic protein receptor type II (BMPR2).
- Up to 20% of sporadic IPAH may be associated with a mutation in BMPR2. Other mutations, e.g. serotonin transporter gene and ALK1 (associated with hereditary haemorrhagic telangiectasia) may play a role.
- Chronic thromboembolic pulmonary hypertension and sickle cell disease may also lead to pulmonary hypertension. ~4% of patients with idiopathic pulmonary emboli may develop chronic thromboembolic pulmonary hypertension.
- Congenital cardiac anomalies are also associated with PAH.

## Clinical presentation

- Patients present with exertional dyspnoea accompanied by chest pain and syncope. Patients may present late with right heart failure.
- Diagnosis is often delayed due to the non-specific nature of symptoms and the subtle signs which comprise a loud split pulmonary component of the second heart sound, a right ventricular heave, and increased 'a' and 'v' waves in the JVP.

## Investigations

Investigations of suspected pulmonary hypertension can be divided into:
- Confirming the presence of pulmonary hypertension.
- Investigating the cause of pulmonary hypertension.
- Investigating the severity of pulmonary hypertension.

Echocardiography is used to suggest the presence of pulmonary hypertension but this must be confirmed on right heart catheterization The CXR may be normal but see Fig. 18.38.

The diagnosis of idiopathic PAH is one of exclusion—all patients are tested to exclude underlying cardiorespiratory disease, connective tissue disease, portal hypertension, HIV infection, sickle cell disease, and chronic thromboembolic pulmonary hypertension.

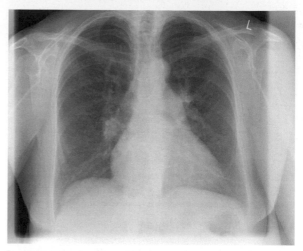

**Fig. 18.38** CXR of a patient with pulmonary hypertension demonstrating bilaterally enlarged pulmonary arteries.
Reproduced with permission from Dr Karen Sheares and Dr Deepa Gopalan, Pulmonary Vascular Diseases Unit, Papworth Hospital, UK.

Prior ingestion of anorexigens (diet aids), e.g. phenchloramine, have been associated with the development of IPAH.

All patients require ventilation perfusion imaging or CTPA (Figs 18.39 and 18.40) to exclude chronic thromboembolic pulmonary hypertension. This condition can be cured by pulmonary thromboendarterectomy.

A 6-minute walk test is often used to determine functional capacity/exercise induced desaturation.

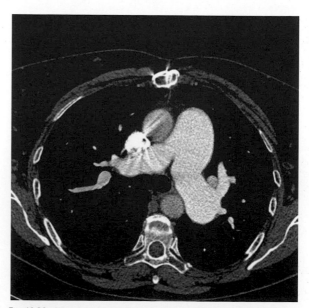

**Fig. 18.39** CT pulmonary angiogram demonstrating an enlarged main pulmonary artery.
Reproduced with permission from Dr Karen Sheares and Dr Deepa Gopalan, Pulmonary Vascular Diseases Unit, Papworth Hospital, UK.

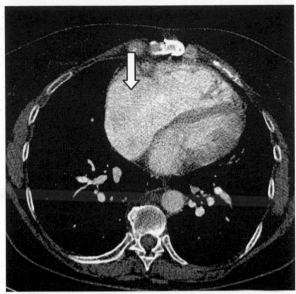

**Fig. 18.40** CT pulmonary angiogram from the patient in Fig. 18.39 demonstrating an enlarged right ventricular chamber (arrow).

Reproduced with permission from Dr Karen Sheares and Dr Deepa Gopalan, Pulmonary Vascular Diseases Unit, Papworth Hospital, UK.

## Severity grading

The severity of the disease can be characterized by exercise testing and right heart catheterization. Severe disease is identified by:

- High right atrial pressure (>50mmHg)

- Low cardiac output ($<2L/min/m^2$) with a low, mixed venous oxygen (<63%).

A WHO functional class of III or greater and a 6-minute walking distances of <350 metres identify patients with a poor prognosis.

## Pathophysiology and treatment

Most cases are treated in specialist centres. IPAH is associated with pulmonary arterial wall remodelling and not simple vasoconstriction. The proliferative events in the vessel wall are associated with the effects in three pathways including reductions in endogenous prostacyclin, decreases in nitric oxygen, and increases in endothelin 1.

Targeted therapy towards the treatment of pulmonary hypertension includes:

- The use of continuous intravenous prostanoids given by Hickman catheter, e.g. epoprostenol.

- Nebulized prostanoid, e.g. iloprost.

- Oral phosphodiesterase V inhibitors, e.g. sildenafil.

- Oral endothelin antagonists, e.g. bosentan, macitsenatan, and ambrisentan.

The prognosis for patients with severe IPAH has improved dramatically from a median survival of 18–24 months before the introduction of these treatments although cure is still not possible. Heart–lung or lung transplantation still needs to be considered.

The disease-targeted therapies for IPAH mentioned have also been shown to be effective in pulmonary hypertension relating to connective tissue disease, portal hypertension, HIV, and in those with gentle systemic to pulmonary shunts including Eisenmenger syndrome and peripheral chronic thromboembolic disease not amenable to treatment with thromboendarterectomy.

## Epidemiology

Primary pneumothoraces arise in otherwise healthy people without any lung disease. Secondary pneumothoraces arise in subjects with underlying lung disease.

- Primary pneumothorax has a reported incidence of 18–28/100,000 per year per men and 1.6–6/100,000 per year for women.
- Subpleural blebs and bullae are likely to play a role in the pathogenesis of primary pneumothorax and these are seen in up to 30% of cases who undergo CT scanning.
- A strong association between the occurrence of a pneumothorax and smoking exists. The lifetime risk of developing a pneumothorax in healthy smoking men may be as much as 12% compared with 0.1% in non-smoking men.
- Risk of recurrence of primary pneumothorax is 54% within the first 4 years.
- Secondary spontaneous pneumothoraces are most commonly caused by COPD. Rarer underlying lung conditions include CF, Langerhan cell histiocytosis, and lymphangioleiomyomatosis.

## Clinical presentation and evaluation

Presenting symptoms are:
- Dyspnoea (80–90%).
- Chest pain (75–90%).

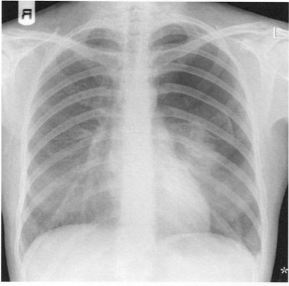

**Fig. 18.41** Left-sided pneumothorax. The radiographer has placed a warning star on the film indicating likely important abnormality (lateral to the left diaphragm). Note the absence of lung markings at the left apex extending down to the 4th interspace posteriorly. The edge of the lung can then be identified.

- Cough (25–35%).
- Signs include hyper-resonance and reduced air entry on the side of the pneumothorax. Subcutaneous emphysema may also be present.
- The size of a pneumothorax is based upon CXR appearances into small or large depending on the presence of a visible rim of <2cm or >2cm between the lung margin and the chest wall. (A 2cm gap implies a 50% reduction in lung volume.) (See Fig. 18.41: large pneumothorax.)

## Tension pneumothorax

- This is a medical emergency that can lead to death rapidly.
- Occurs when the interpleural pressure exceeds the atmospheric pressure throughout inspiration as well as expiration probably due to a one-way valve effect.
- The development of tension pneumothorax leads to rapid respiratory distress, cyanosis, sweating, and tachycardia. The deterioration in cardiopulmonary status is related to impaired venous return, reduced cardiac output, and hypoxaemia.
- This should be particularly suspected in those on mechanical ventilators or nasal NIV who suddenly deteriorate.

## Management of pneumothorax

British Thoracic Society guidelines are available at <http://www.brit-thoracic.org.uk>.

- Observation is the treatment of choice for small closed pneumothoraces without significant breathlessness.
- Breathless patients should have intervention regardless of the size of the pneumothorax on a CXR.
- For a tension pneumothorax:
  - Give high-flow oxygen.
  - Emergency insertion of a large-bore IV cannula (14–16 G) in the mid-clavicular line, 2nd intercostal space can be lifesaving—air flowing out confirms the diagnosis.
  - After this, insert a chest drain and arrange CXR.
- Simply aspiration is recommended as first-line treatment for all small pneumothoraces (defined earlier).
- Repeated aspiration is reasonable for primary pneumothorax when the first aspiration has been unsuccessful and a volume of <2.5L was aspirated on the first attempt.
- Intercostal tube drainage—'chest drain'—is recommended in patients with large primary pneumothoraces and all secondary pneumothoraces except in patients who are not breathless and have a very small (<1cm or apical) pneumothorax.
- There is no evidence that large tubes (20–24 F) are any better than small 'Seldinger' tubes (10–14 F) in the management of pneumothorax.

## Chemical pleurodesis

This is the process of fusing visceral and parietal pleura using an agent usually introduced to the pleural space via the chest drain (Fig. 18.42). It can control difficult/recurrent pneumothoraces. Many

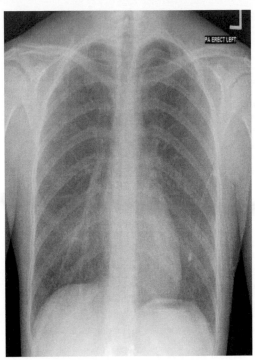

**Fig. 18.42** Left-sided pneumothorax treated with a chest drain (same case as Fig. 18.36). This was the second recurrence of the pneumothorax in a young female smoker. Operative intervention (pleurectomy) was undertaken.

sclerosing agents have been used including tetracycline (or more recently, minocycline or doxycycline) and talc.

## Surgical pleurodesis

Thoracic surgical opinion should be sought in patients with a persistent air leak or failure of the lung to re-expand after 5 days. Indications for surgical pleurodesis including talc abrasion or pleurectomy are:

- Second ipsilateral pneumothorax.
- Post-contralateral pneumothorax.
- Bilateral spontaneous pneumothorax.
- Persistent air leak but >5 days' acute drainage.
- Spontaneous haemothorax.
- Professions at risk, e.g. pilots.

## Risk of recurrence

The risk of recurrent pneumothorax after two primary spontaneous pneumothoraces is 83%. The risk of recurrent secondary pneumothorax after two pneumothoraces is 90%.

Smoking greatly increases the risk of recurrence.

Patients are advised not to fly for 6 weeks after a pneumothorax. Though little evidence supports this statement it seems prudent to avoid situations where a recurrence could leave the patient away from medical services and thus be particularly dangerous, e.g. diving, flying.

## Cough

### Diagnosis

Cough can be classified into two categories: acute and chronic. An acute cough is one that been present for <3 weeks while chronic coughs have been present for longer.

Acute coughs can be divided into infectious and non-infectious causes.

- Infectious causes include viral upper respiratory infections (the common cold), sinus infections, whooping cough, and pneumonia.
- Non-infectious causes can be secondary to many chronic conditions, e.g. COPD, asthma, and environmental allergies. Cigarette smoke is a common environmental irritant causing chronic cough. Dusts, pollens, pet dander, industrial chemicals, and pollution can contribute to cough. Underlying parenchymal disease, e.g. lung cancer or interstitial lung diseases can cause cough. Drugs are also important, e.g. ACE inhibitors causes cough in 10%. Cough is well recognized in heart failure.

Cryptic cough, present for >3 weeks with a normal CXR and examination, often remains idiopathic in nature despite investigation. Three underlying causes are important and commonly identified:

- Gastro-oesophageal reflux disease (GORD) is a commonly identified cause of cough and occurs when gastric contents enter the oesophagus. This can cause irritation of the oesophagus resulting in a reflex cough.
- Asthma can present with cough well before wheeze and dyspnoea. A peak flow diary and occasionally allergy testing/bronchial provocation is required.
- Post nasal drip—patients give a history of excessive nasal mucous, nasal blockage sinusitis, and a morning cough. Ear, nose, and throat examination may reveal erythematous vocal cords. Nasal inhaled steroids may help.

The listed causes are often identified by a positive response to a therapeutic trial, e.g. cough improves after proton pump inhibitor with GORD.

### Investigations

- Detailed history (include occupation, hobbies).
- Careful examination.
- CXR.
- Pulmonary function tests including peak flow diary, flow volume curves, and gas transfer.
- Tests for oesophageal reflux.
- Bronchoscopy and CT scanning are often held in reserve.

### Treatment

- Post nasal drip and other upper airway disease. In the US the first-line approach is with a sedating antihistamine/decongestant combination (not available in the UK). Topical nasal steroids given for 2 months are effective. Actual sinusitis should be considered in patients who fail to respond.
- Asthma syndromes. Cough variant asthma responds to treatment with inhaled corticosteroids.
- GORD. Proton pump inhibitors such as omeprazole 20–40mg twice daily or equivalent should be taken before meals for at least 8 weeks. Prokinetic agents, e.g. metoclopramide 10mg three times a day were popular but note recent safety concerns.

## Haemoptysis

Haemoptysis is a common alarming symptom leading to medical consultation. The vast majority (95%) is minor with major haemoptysis defined as >200–600mL of fresh blood per 24 hours.

### Aetiology and pathogenesis

- The majority of haemoptysis originates from bleeding from bronchial arteries.
- Common causes (Table 18.1) comprise carcinoma, bronchiectasis, acute bronchitis, pneumonia, tuberculosis, lung abscess, and pulmonary embolism.
- Rarer causes include bleeding from pulmonary circulation including vasculitic disease (granulomatosis with polyangiitis (Wegener), microscopic polyarteritis, Goodpasture disease), left heart disease, and pulmonary arteriovenous malformations.

### Clinical evaluation and management

- The primary goal in minor haemoptysis is to diagnose the underlying cause.
- The primary goal of massive haemoptysis is to secure the airway and stop the bleeding.
- Haemoptysis should be confirmed and bleeding from upper respiratory tract or gastrointestinal tract excluded.
- CXR will demonstrate abnormality or localize the cause by demonstrating a mass/cavity/infiltrate or atelectasis in 60% of cases.
- Fibreoptic bronchoscopy can be performed to identify the bronchial lesions and take specimens for diagnosis. It can also help localize the site of bleeding but is not a therapeutic intervention.
- CT scanning is needed in patients who present with haemoptysis but with no diagnostic features on CXR. CT will diagnose a specific condition in 50% of such patients, most commonly bronchiectasis or a cavity.
- Massive haemoptysis is a medical emergency; it is most commonly associated with bronchiectasis, lung cancer, aspergilloma, or tuberculosis.
- The primary goal is to protect the airway until locating and controlling bleeding. Patients should be admitted to a HDU. Control of the airway may demand intubation.
- Once the side is localized and the airway secure, patients should undergo bronchial embolization. Over 90% of such cases will bleed from a bronchial artery, and embolization is successful in 85% of cases.

| Table 18.1 Causes of haemoptysis | |
| --- | --- |
| **Final diagnosis** | **% of cases** |
| Malignancy | 25 |
| Bronchiectasis | 18 |
| Acute bronchitis | 13 |
| Cryptogenic | 20 |
| Miscellaneous | 14 |
| Pneumonia | 5 |
| Tuberculosis | 5 |

## Pulmonary eosinophilia

### Epidemiology

Pulmonary eosinophilia occurs worldwide. Outside of the developed world parasites are the most common cause including *Strongyloides stercoralis*, *Ascaris lumbricoides*, *Toxicara canis*, and *Ancylostoma duodenale*.

### Diagnoses to consider

- Loeffler syndrome. This is characterized by migrating infiltrate peripheral blood eosinophilia and minimal pulmonary symptoms.
- Chronic eosinophilic pneumonia. This is characterized by constitutional symptoms, progressive shortness of breath, and cough over a period of several months.
- Acute eosinophilic pneumonia which comprises of an acute illness over 1–5 days leading to extreme shortness of breath, diffuse alveolar infiltrates, and crackles on auscultation of the lungs. Severe hypoxaemia is common.
- ABPA which occurs in patients with asthma and CF. This is typified by constitutional upset, mucus plugging of airways, soft migratory infiltrates, and the development of central bronchiectasis.
- Eosinophilic granulomatosis with polyangiitis (Churg-Strauss syndrome) (EGPA) which occurs in asthmatic patients with sinusitis and is characterized by the development of systemic vasculitis. The p-ANCA is positive in 50% of such patients.
- Drug-induced eosinophilic pneumonia. Drug-induced eosinophilic infiltrate are reported in a wide number of drugs, common causes include nitrofurantoin, bleomycin, carbamazepine, dantrolene, imipramine methotrexate, minocycline, naproxen, penicillins, phenytoin, sotalol, tetracycline, and venlafaxine.

### Treatment

- Oral corticosteroids—prednisolone 40–60mg per day comprises the basic treatment. Prolonged courses may be required for chronic eosinophilic pneumonia, EGPA, and ABPA.
- Discontinue causative drugs if responsible.
- Specific treatments for parasites.
- Oral antifungal agents such as itraconazole may have a role in the management of ABPA in addition to normal asthma therapy.

## Obstructive sleep apnoea (OSA)

A condition typified by day time sleepiness due to recurrent episodes of upper airway occlusion during sleep leading to diminution (hypopnoea) or cessation (apnoea) of airflow in the pharynx provoking arousals and sleep fragmentation/disruption.

### Epidemiology and pathogenesis

- ~4% of middle-aged men have obstructive sleep apnoea syndrome.
- Pharyngeal dilator muscles maintain patency of the upper airway. During sleep there is a reduced muscle tone leading to a potential collapse of the airway especially during rapid eye movement (REM) sleep.
- Use of sedatives/alcohol may cause further loss of muscle tone.
- Obesity with fat deposition in the neck is the commonest predisposing factor (other factors include bone morphology, e.g. micrognathia, soft tissue deposition, e.g. hypothyroidism

and acromegaly, enlargement of tonsils or adenoids may be important).
- Negative pressure in the airway acts as a force sucking in or collapsing the upper airway.
- Syndrome characterized by recurrent episodes of airway obstruction leading to a fall in oxygen saturation depending on the degree, frequency, and duration of collapse.
- Inspiratory effort increases as the diaphragm and intercostals muscles try to overcome the closed upper airway and the apnoea is terminated by brief arousal from deep sleep associated with a burst of sympathetic nerve activity, release of catecholamines, and fluctuations in pulse rate and blood pressure.
- The resumption of pharyngeal airflow is accompanied by loud snoring. These events can occur 60 times per hour of sleep.

### Clinical presentation

- Obesity with increased neck circumference and anatomical abnormalities reducing pharyngeal calibre.
- Daytime symptoms of sleepiness, poor concentration, irritability, and morning headaches. The sleepiness results in road traffic accidents (threefold increase).
- Nocturia is common.
- The patient may be unaware of night-time symptoms but the bed partner reports loud snoring, witnessed apnoeas, and restless sleep.
- Obstructive sleep apnoea syndrome is associated with an increased incidence of cardiovascular disease such as hypertension, myocardial infarction and stroke.

### Diagnosis

- The Epworth sleepiness score allows excessive sleepiness to be identified.
- The 'gold' standard for the investigation of obstructive sleep apnoea syndrome is polysomnography although many cases are diagnosed using more limited sleep studies. This involves the recording of signals related to oxygenation and airflow, heart rate, chest wall movement, and sleep stage.
- Diagnosis based upon the frequency of respiratory events during sleep and the presence or absence of symptoms:
  - >15 apnoeas or hypopnoeas per hour of sleep if asymptomatic, or
  - >5 apnoeas or hypopnoeas per hour of sleep if symptomatic (e.g. sleepiness, fatigue, and inattention) or signs of disturbed sleep.

### Treatment

- Weight loss is the most important treatment though difficult to achieve.
- Aggravating factors should be removed, e.g. alcohol.
- Nasal continuous positive airway pressure (CPAP) applied by a tight-fitting nasal mask has become the standard treatment for OSA. This is very effective and acts by splinting the pharyngeal airway open counteracting the tendency to airway collapse.
- Surgical correction of bone abnormalities such as mandibular advancement or micrognathia may also be effective in selected cases.
- **Driving**—patients must stop driving until symptoms have been satisfactorily controlled (confirmed by medical opinion). Particularly important for commercial goods vehicles.

# Chapter 19

# Rheumatology

# 19.1 Basic science

## Normal structure and function of joints

Synovial joints are the most common joints in the human body. Other types of joints include fibrous joints where articulating bones are joined by flexible fibrocartilage and cartilaginous joints. Apart from structural classification, joints can also be classified functionally (see later).

## Synovial joint components

These joints are cushioned by hyaline cartilage which are nourished and lubricated by synovial tissue. They are stabilized by ligaments and driven by tendons and muscles (Fig. 19.1).

### Hyaline cartilage

- This is a living tissue mainly composed of water, collagen, and proteoglycans including chondroitin sulphate and keratan sulphate.
- Chondrocytes are involved in continual turnover and renewal of the matrix in cartilage.
- Normal hyaline cartilage lacks blood vessels and nerves. Nutritional needs of chondrocytes are supplied by synovial fluid and adjacent tissues.
- Acts as a biological 'shock absorber' and lines the articulating surfaces of synovial joints.
- Cartilage loss is fundamental to the development of osteoarthritis and other 'degenerative' joint diseases.

### Synovium

- A very thin structure (25–35μm) covering all intra-articular surfaces except the articulating areas of cartilage.
- Composed of a well-organized matrix of proteoglycans, microfibrils and synovial cells, mast cells, and leucocytes.

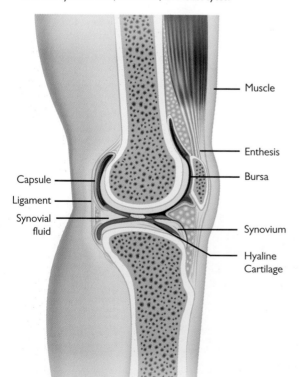

**Fig. 19.1** Diagram of a synovial joint.

- The source of inflammation in most inflammatory joint diseases—synovitis (see Section 19.2).

### Ligaments

- Composed of type 1 collagen fibres.
- Links bone to bone, the insertion points being the entheses.
- Ligaments passively limit the range of joint movement and prevent inappropriate movements.
- Entheses are the sites of inflammation for spondyloarthritides and various 'soft tissue' musculoskeletal disorders (e.g. 'tennis elbow').

### Bursae

- Fluid sacs of synovium with a thin film of synovial fluid inside.
- They lubricate and protect areas of potential friction between ligaments, bone prominences, and overlying skin.

### Capsule

- Completely envelops the joint.
- Consists of two layers—the outer fibrous capsule and the inner synovial membrane.

### Synovial fluid

- Consists mainly of water, hyaluronan (which contributes to its elastic and viscous properties), and lubricin (glycoprotein that provides lubrication).
- Normal joints have a microscopic film of synovial fluid at subatmospheric pressure.
- Roles include hydrodynamic lubrication between cartilage and cushioning synovial lining.
- In inflammatory joint diseases, effusions may occur and due to the binding of water by hyaluronan, the effusion may persist despite subsequent adequate control of the inflammation.

### Nerve supply

- The nerve supply to a joint also supplies the muscles moving the joint and the overlying skin.
- Pain fibres are numerous in the fibrous capsule and associated ligaments.
- The main joint sensation is proprioception.

## Functional classification of joints

See Table 19.1 for examples of physiological range of joint movement.

### Synarthrosis

- Permits little or no mobility.
- Examples include:
  - Skull sutures.
  - Synchondrosis (temporary cartilaginous joint), e.g. epiphyseal plate.

### Amphiarthrosis

- Permits slight mobility.
- Examples include:
  - Syndesmosis (interosseous ligaments), e.g. distal tibiofibular joint.
  - Symphysis (fibrocartilage separates bones), e.g. symphysis pubis.

### Diarthrosis

- Freely movable joint. All are synovial joints.
- Stability depends upon three factors:

| Table 19.1 Physiological range of joint movement | |
|---|---|
| Joint type | Movement range |
| **Hip:** | |
| Abduction | 25° |
| Adduction | 40° |
| Flexion | 120° |
| Extension | 5–20° |
| Internal rotation | 30° |
| External rotation | 60° |
| **Ankle:** | |
| Dorsiflexion | 15° |
| Plantar flexion | 55° |
| Knee flexion | 135° |
| **Wrist:** | |
| Flexion | 60–90° |
| Extension | 60–90° |
| Elbow flexion | 145° |
| **Cervical spine:** | |
| Rotation | 60–90° |
| Flexion | 60–90° |
| Extension | 60–90° |
| Lateral flexion | 30–60° |
| Thoracic spine rotation | 45–75° |
| **Lumbar spine:** | |
| Extension | 30° |
| Lateral flexion | 30° |

True lumbar flexion ≥+5cm on modified Schober test.

| Table 19.2 Subtypes of diarthroses | |
|---|---|
| Subtype | Example of joint |
| Ball and socket | Shoulder and hip |
| Condyloid | Radio-carpal, metacarpophalangeal |
| Saddle | Thumb carpometacarpal |
| Hinge | Elbow |
| Pivot | Radioulnar |
| Gliding | Facet joints |

1. Shape of bone components.
2. Strength of ligaments, capsule, and tendons surrounding joint.
3. Muscles that span the joint.
- There are six subtypes of diarthroses (Table 19.2).

## 19.2 The synovium

### Immunopathology

Soft tissue lining the non-cartilaginous surfaces of synovial joints, ten-don sheaths, and bursae. Key area for inflammation in inflammatory arthritis.

### Structure

- A thin structure of 25–35μm in thickness. It consists of an intima and subintima.
- Synovium can be divided into three main types based upon the structure of the subintima:
  - Areolar—subintima of loose connective tissue (Fig. 19.2).
  - Adipose—subintima rich in adipose tissue. Intra-articular fat pads.
  - Fibrous—indistinct structure with a subintima of denser collagen.
- The intimal layer contains two main cell types:
  - Fibroblasts—secrete hyaluronan and lubricin into synovial fluid.
  - Macrophages—involved with immune reactions.

### Normal function of synovium

- Maintaining a non-adherent surface for continued movement. Also produces hyaluronan and lubricin to aid movement.
- Provides nutrition to avascular cartilage via vascular network and synovial fluid.
- Control of synovial fluid volume and composition.

### Synovium in disease states

- The vast majority of inflammatory arthritides, including rheu-matoid arthritis (RA), systemic lupus erythematosus (SLE), and seronegative spondyloarthritis involve the synovium as the source of joint inflammation.
- In inflammatory arthritis the synovium becomes markedly hyperplastic and infiltrated with T cells, B cells, macrophages, and plasma cells.

- Angiogenesis within synovium is increased due to relative hypoxia and angiogenic factors such as vascular endothelial growth factor (VEGF) are abundant.
- Critical cytokines which mediate inflammation include tumour necrosis factor alpha (TNFα) and interleukin (IL)-1 which are produced by macrophages and fibroblasts in the synovium.
- The inflamed synovium forms an inflammatory granulation tissue called a pannus in RA (Fig.19.3). This invades and destroys carti-lage and underlying subchondral bone.
- Current available biological treatments for synovitis are aimed at targeting cytokines such as TNFα and IL-1 which are crucial in the formation of inflammatory synovial tissue.

Autoimmune diseases occur when the adaptive immune system mounts a response against self-antigens. Unlike the action on foreign antigens, the response to self-antigens is unable to clear the antigen completely and the response is sustained, resulting in chronic inflam-matory injury.

### Major histocompatibility complex

- The association of MHC genotype with autoimmune disease is unsurprising as the MHC is expressed on almost all cells and is normally involved in antigen presentation to T lymphocytes.
- MHC genotype is significantly influenced by other genetic and environmental factors before disease expression.

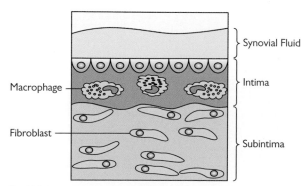

**Fig. 19.2** Diagram of areolar synovium.

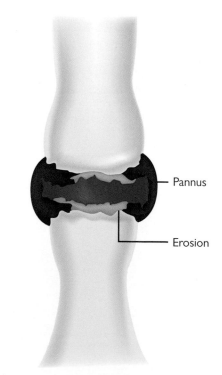

**Fig. 19.3** Diagram of pannus in rheumatoid arthritis.

## Role of infection

Infectious micro-organisms have been linked to the development of arthritis in genetically susceptible individuals, e.g. reactive arthritis in a HLA-B27 positive individual infected with *Salmonella*. Theoretical mechanisms for disease induction include:

1. Superantigens—microbial structures which are able to bind MHC class II molecules as well as stimulate T cells without undergoing antigen processing in immune cells.

2. Molecular mimicry—a microbial antigen which has structural similarities to host antigens and may trigger an immune response to self, e.g. group A Streptococci and rheumatic fever.

## Role of pregnancy (microchimerism)

There is increasing evidence that fetal cells in maternal tissue (micro-chimerism) may trigger rheumatological disorders such as juvenile inflammatory myositis, dermatomyositis, Sjögren syndrome, and systemic sclerosis.

## Role of apoptosis

Impaired apoptosis (programmed cell death) has been implicated in the development of SLE:

- Reduced clearance of apoptotic blebs full of nuclear autoantigens may allow the formation of ANA.
- Immunological tolerance is dependent on early apoptosis of potential autoreactive T and B cells which may be impaired in SLE.

# 19.3 Autoantibodies

## Background

Autoantibodies are immunoglobulins which bind to antigens originating in the same individual.

## Types of autoantibodies

Autoantibodies and their association with diseases are shown in Table 19.3.

- **Rheumatoid factor (RF)**—autoantibodies directed to the Fc portion of IgG. High titre is associated with severe RA. IgM-RF may be present years before RA onset.
- **Anti-cyclic citrullinated peptide (Anti-CCP)**—has the highest specificity for RA (98%) and is associated with severe RA.

Table 19.3 Autoimmune diseases and autoantibodies

| Autoantibody | Disease | Frequency |
|---|---|---|
| RF | RA | 60–90% |
| ANA | SLE | 95–100% |
| | Scleroderma | 60–80% |
| Anti-dsDNA | SLE | 30–70% |
| Anti-Ro/La | 1° Sjögren 75%/40–50% | |
| | 2° Sjögren | 10–15% |
| ACA | LCSS | 20–40% |
| Anti-SCL-70 | DCSS | 20–40% |
| CANCA | WG | 90% |
| PANCA | MPA | 50–70% |
| | CSS | 70–85% |
| ACL | APS | 80% |
| Anti-Jo-1 | Polymyositis | 20–30% |

APS: antiphospholipid syndrome; CSS: Churg–Strauss syndrome; DCSS: diffuse cutaneous systemic sclerosis; LCSS: limited cutaneous systemic sclerosis; MPA: microscopic polyangiitis; WG: Wegener granulomatosis.

- **Antinuclear antibody (ANA)**—high sensitivity/low specificity for SLE. False positives commonly found in normal women, elderly patients (usually low titres), infectious diseases, and may be drug-induced.
- **Anti-dsDNA**—are specific (95%) but not sensitive for SLE. Titres of anti-dsDNA are associated with disease activity especially lupus nephritis.
- **Anti-Ro**—more common in primary than secondary Sjögren. High titres are associated with greater incidence of extraglandular features in Sjögren, neonatal lupus, congenital heart block, and photosensitivity in SLE.
- **Anticentromere antibody (ACA)**—found almost exclusively in limited cutaneous systemic sclerosis.
- **Anti-Scl-70**—appears to increase the risk for pulmonary fibrosis in scleroderma.
- **Antineutrophil cytoplasmic antibody (ANCA)**—typically occurs in two forms. Cytoplasmic ANCA (cANCA) directed against proteinase 3 (PR3) and perinuclear ANCA (pANCA) directed against myeloperoxidase (MPO). The presence of ANA on indirect immunofluorescence (IIF) may lead to a false positive pANCA. Combination testing of IIF and ELISA testing for PR3 and MPO are more accurate. cANCA is specific (98%) for granulomatosis with polyangiitis (Wegener).
- **Anticardiolipin antibody (ACL) and lupus anticoagulant (LA)**—both are associated with antiphospholipid syndrome (APS). In their presence, a false positive serological test for syphilis may occur.
  - ACL can be IgG or IgM but IgG ACL is more commonly associated with clinical APS.
  - LA is demonstrated by a prolongation of the activated partial thromboplastin time (aPTT) and a dilute Russell viper venom time that is not correctable by normal plasma.
  - Both ACL and LA have to be repeated at least 6 weeks apart in the presence of a positive test result to be considered truly positive.
- **Anti-Jo-1**—autoantibody found in a subgroup of inflammatory myositis called anti-synthetase syndrome. This is characterized by myositis, interstitial lung disease, arthritis, fever.

# 19.4 Osteoarthritis

## Background

Osteoarthritis (OA) is the most common articular disease world-wide and, with a growing elderly population, is a significant cost to society. It is confined to joints and has no systemic component.

## Epidemiology

- OA affects up to 8.5 million people in the UK.
- At least 4.4 million people have moderate to severe hand OA on X-rays. Over 0.5 and 0.2 million people have moderate to severe knee and hip OA respectively.
- ♀:♂ ratio is 1:1 at age 45–55 years. The prevalence in ♀ is greater after age 55 years, and in OA of the hands and knees.
- Prevalence rises with age.

## Aetiology

- OA is joint failure due not only to the destruction of articular cartilage but subchondral bone and synovium as well.
- Risk factors for OA:
  - Age.
  - Obesity (associated with knee OA).
  - Family history (associated with hand OA).
  - Trauma.
  - High bone density (osteopetrosis).
  - Hypermobility.
- OA initially involves cartilage breakdown and the cartilage fragments induce an inflammatory response by the secretion of metalloproteinases, IL-1 and TNFα in joints. Subchondral bone also releases peptides such as substance P from its nerve endings contributing to pain. Compensatory bone growth occurs as a result of architectural joint changes.
- In primary generalized OA, first-degree relatives of patients are at three times greater risk of developing generalized OA compared to the normal population. The genetic influence is most likely polygenic.

## Clinical evaluation

OA tends to present late and there may be referred pain (e.g. knee pain in ipsilateral hip OA).

### History

- Pain—insidious in onset, exacerbated by exertion.
- Stiffness—after inactivity ('gelling'). Stiffness in OA usually lasts only a few minutes, in contrast to inflammatory arthritis.
- Joint swelling and deformity.
- Loss of function and subsequently weakness.

### Examination

- Gait abnormalities—in lower limb joints.
- Joint:
  - Tenderness.
  - Effusion—usually cool to touch.
  - Deformities—Heberden (distal interphalangeal joints) and Bouchard (proximal interphalangeal joints) nodes (Fig. 19.4), classically varus knee.
  - Crepitus.
- Limitation of range of movement.

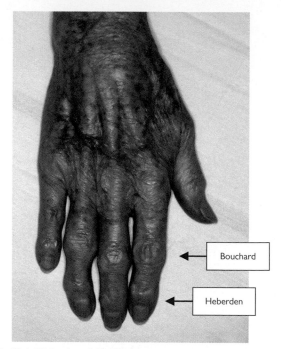

Bouchard

Heberden

**Fig. 19.4** OA hands with Bouchard and Heberden nodes.

## Investigations

- No laboratory tests are diagnostic—minor elevation of inflammatory markers occasionally.
- Synovial fluid—calcium pyrophosphate and calcium hydroxyapatite crystals may be present in up to 40% of OA synovial fluid.
- Radiographic changes—osteophytes, subchondral bone sclerosis, joint space narrowing, subchondral cysts (geode) (Fig. 19.5).
- Ultrasonography—increasingly being used. Real-time imaging with no radiation. Can visualize soft tissue (synovium, tendons, Baker cyst). Operator dependent.
- MRI/CT scan—for visualising soft tissue structures, cartilage and bone lesions.
- Arthroscopy—direct view of intra-articular structures and can deliver treatment. However, it is invasive and deep chondral lesions are not visualized.

## Management

- Symptomatic treatments:
  - Topical agents, e.g. capsaicin, NSAID gel.
  - Oral analgesics/NSAIDs.
  - Intra-articular steroids (risk of infection or crystalline synovitis).
  - Viscosupplementation—intra-articular hyaluronan.
- Adjunctive therapies:
  - Tricyclic antidepressants—potentiate analgesic effects and improves sleep.
- Disease-modifying agents:
  - Glucosamine sulphate—shown to reduce progression of knee OA and provide mild pain relief in one study (Pavelká et al., 2003) but several other studies have **not** confirmed this.
  - Chondroitin sulphate—may reduce pain in knee OA.

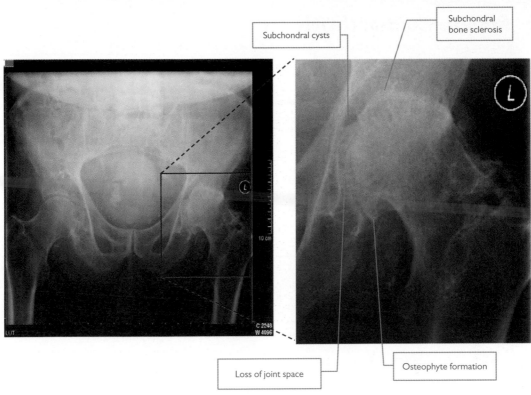

Subchondral cysts

Subchondral bone sclerosis

Loss of joint space

Osteophyte formation

**Fig. 19.5** Pelvic radiograph demonstrating OA left hip with incidental Paget disease in right pubic rami.

- Patient education:
  - Weight loss.
  - Exercise—e.g. swimming, walking.
- Maintain function—physiotherapy, occupational therapy.
- Support devices—cane, walking frames, orthotics.
- Self-management and pain management programmes.
- Surgery—in uncontrolled pain and/or limited function (independent of pain).

# Reference

Pavelká K, Gatterová J, Olejarová M, *et al*. Glucosamine sulfate use and delay of progression of knee osteoarthritis: a 3-year, randomized, placebo-controlled, double-blind study. *Arch Intern Med* 2003; 162(18): 2113–23.

# 19.5 Rheumatoid arthritis

## Background

Rheumatoid arthritis (RA) is a chronic systemic inflammatory disease characterized by symmetrical polyarthritis (Fig. 19.6).

## Epidemiology

- Prevalence rate estimated to be 0.5–2.0%. Rare in rural African populations with a greater prevalence in North American Indians. Prevalence also increases with age.
- ♀:♂ ratio 3:1.
- Can present at any age but most often presents between 40–50 years of age.

## Aetiology

- Unknown cause. Twin studies show a concordance for RA of 12–15% in monozygotic twins compared to 4% in dizygotic pairs.
- HLA-DR4 and other HLA-DRB1 alleles encode a common amino acid sequence ('shared epitope') which is associated with severe RA (Box 19.1).
- Genetic factors account for up to 60% of disease susceptibility. Hormonal and reproductive factors have also been linked to RA.

## Clinical evaluation

Most RA cases have a gradual onset although an acute arthritis is a presenting feature in 10–25% of cases.

### History

- Fatigue and weight loss.

---

**Box 19.1 Markers of disease severity (on presentation)**

- Autoantibodies—RF, anti-CCP.
- Genetic factors—'shared epitope'.
- Elevated CRP/ESR.
- Total number of swollen/tender joints.
- Radiological damage: erosion on X-ray, ultrasound, MRI.

---

- Symmetrical joint pains (especially in feet, wrists, and small joints of hands).
- Early morning stiffness lasting >1 hour.

### Examination

- Symmetrical synovitis in hands (with sparing of distal interphalangeal joints), wrists, feet, and knee joints in a majority of cases.
- Rheumatoid nodules in 30% of cases—mainly on pressure points, e.g. elbows, finger joints.
- Deformities: 'Swan-neck', Boutonniere, 'Z' thumb, ulnar deviation of metacarpophalangeal joints (Fig 19.7).
- Extra-articular features—disease in pulmonary, cardiac (pericarditis), ocular, and gastrointestinal systems occur in 40% of patients during the course of the disease.

### Investigations

- FBC—anaemia of chronic disease, thrombocytosis in active disease, neutropaenia in Felty syndrome.
- ESR/CRP—elevated in active disease.
- Autoantibodies—RF is present in 60–80% of RA patients but has low specificity. (RF is usually a IgM autoantibody against self-IgG.) ANA is present in 20% of patients. Anti-cyclic citrullinated peptide (anti-CCP)—see Box 19.2.

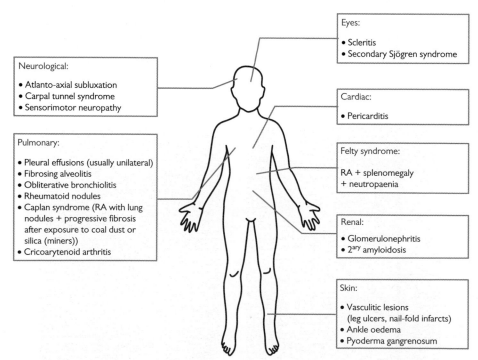

Neurological:
- Atlanto-axial subluxation
- Carpal tunnel syndrome
- Sensorimotor neuropathy

Pulmonary:
- Pleural effusions (usually unilateral)
- Fibrosing alveolitis
- Obliterative bronchiolitis
- Rheumatoid nodules
- Caplan syndrome (RA with lung nodules + progressive fibrosis after exposure to coal dust or silica (miners))
- Cricoarytenoid arthritis

Eyes:
- Scleritis
- Secondary Sjögren syndrome

Cardiac:
- Pericarditis

Felty syndrome:
RA + splenomegaly + neutropaenia

Renal:
- Glomerulonephritis
- 2$^{ary}$ amyloidosis

Skin:
- Vasculitic lesions (leg ulcers, nail-fold infarcts)
- Ankle oedema
- Pyoderma gangrenosum

**Fig. 19.6** Systemic features of RA.

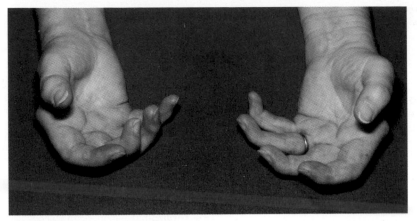

**Fig. 19.7** RA hands showing deformities.

**Box 19.2 Anti-cyclic citrullinated peptide (anti-CCP)**

- Higher specificity (98%) for RA than RF. Sensitivity 50–70%.
- Also found to be positive in RF-negative patients who later develop RA. Can be positive years before development of clinical RA.
- Anti-CCP is associated with severe erosive RA.
- Combining RF and anti-CCP gives a positive predictive value for RA of 91% and a negative predictive value of 78%.

- Imaging:
  - Radiographs—of hands, wrists, and feet. Erosions, joint space loss, periarticular osteopenia may be seen. Used for disease monitoring but may be negative in early disease (Fig. 19.8).
  - Ultrasound (with colour Doppler)—increasingly used in detecting subclinical synovitis and early RA.
  - MRI—can detect early joint changes such as bone oedema.

## Management

There is considerable evidence that adequate immunosuppression during early disease, i.e. 3–6 months after onset (the 'window of opportunity'), is associated with a better long-term prognosis. The main therapeutic aim is to prevent the development and progression of erosions/permanent joint damage.

- Interdisciplinary management—involving physiotherapy, occupational therapy, psychologist, vocational counsellor, self-management programmes.
- NSAIDS/COX-II (cyclo-oxygenase II) inhibitors—for symptom control. Consider cardiovascular (Box 19.3) and gastrointestinal risk with long-term use.

**Box 19.3 Cardiovascular risk in RA**

- The commonest cause of death in RA is cardiovascular disease (CVD).
- Standardized mortality rates in RA range from 1.13–5.25.
- Traditional cardiovascular risk factors alone do not explain the increased CVD risk.
- Persistent inflammation is an independent risk factor and methotrexate has been shown to be cardioprotective in RA.
- Both selective (COX-II inhibitors) and non-selective NSAIDS have been linked to increased CVD. NSAIDs may reduce the antiplatelet effects of aspirin as well.
- European Medicines Agency (EMA) guidelines state that:
  - COX-II inhibitors are contraindicated in patients with CVD, stroke, or peripheral vascular disease.
  - Caution should be exercised when prescribing COX-II inhibitors in patients at risk of CVD.
  - The lowest dose and shortest duration should be used.

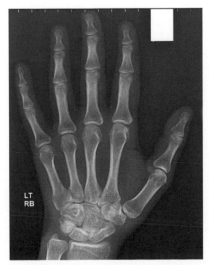
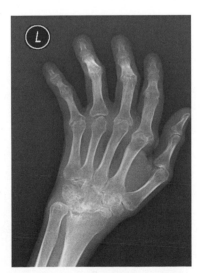

**Fig. 19.8** Radiographs of left hand taken 2 years apart in an untreated RA patient showing extensive joint damage.

---

**Box 19.4 DMARDS considered safe in pregnancy**

- Azathioprine.
- Sulphasalazine.
- Hydroxychloroquine.
- Corticosteroids.
  - None of the medications used in RA are absolutely safe during pregnancy. However, the listed drugs have not been shown to cause an increase in fetal morbidity or mortality.
  - There is too little information regarding the safety of anti-TNFα and rituximab during pregnancy.
  - Methotrexate and leflunomide are absolutely contraindicated in pregnancy.

---

- Corticosteroids—intra-articular, intramuscular, and oral steroids are used in flare-ups and early control. Oral steroids also used in pregnancy and poorly controlled disease.

## Disease-modifying anti-rheumatic drugs (DMARDs)

- Methotrexate—drug of choice. Usual dose range 15–25mg/week.
- Sulphasalazine—usual dose 2–3g/day.
- Leflunomide—usual dose 10–20mg/day.
- Hydroxychloroquine—usual dose 200–400mg/day. Usually in combination with others.
- Other DMARDS—gold salts, D-penicillamine, azathioprine, ciclosporin.

- Evidence supports better response and side effect profiles with combination DMARD therapy compared to monotherapy.
- Most DMARDS require regular blood monitoring.
- See Box 19.4 for use of DMARDs in pregnancy.

### Biological agents

- **Anti-TNFα**—infliximab, etanercept, certolizumab, and adalimumab are approved for RA not controlled on traditional DMARDs (Lipsky, 2000).
- **Rituximab**—anti-CD20 antibodies against B cells. Good evidence, in combination with methotrexate, for control of disease resistant to DMARDs (Edwards, 2004).
- **Abatacept**—selective costimulation modulator binding to CD80/86 on antigen presenting cells. Trials show evidence of its role in RA uncontrolled on DMARDS or anti-TNFα.
- **Tocilizumab**—monoclonal antibody against the IL-6 receptor.

---

## References

Edwards JC, Szczepanski L, Szechinski J. Efficacy of B-cell-targeted therapy with rituximab in patients with RA. *N Eng J Med* 2004; 350(25): 2572–81.

Lipsky P, van der Heijde DMFM, St Clair EW. Infliximab and methotrexate in the treatment of RA. *N Eng J Med* 2000; 343: 1594–602.

# 19.6 Septic arthritis

## Background

Septic arthritis remains the **main diagnosis to exclude when presented with an acute monoarthritis**, with a case fatality rate of 11%.

## Epidemiology

- Annual incidence in UK is 2–10 per 100,000.
- Incidence is higher in patients with RA or joint prostheses (30–70 per 100 000).
- ♀:♂ ratio 1:1.
- Can present in all age groups, 45% of cases occur in patients over 65 years of age.

## Aetiology

Fig. 19.9 shows how bacteria may reach the affected joint. Organisms involved:
- *Staphylococcus aureus* (commonest cause).
- *Neisseria gonorrhoeae* (especially in young adults) (Figs 19.10 and 19.11).
- Streptococci spp.
- *Haemophilus influenzae B* (common in children in some parts of the world).

## Clinical evaluation

### History
- Short history of hot, swollen painful joint.
- Often a large joint monoarthritis (*N. gonorrhoea* may be a migratory polyarthralgia and tends to affect upper limbs).
- Recent penetrating joint trauma or invasive procedure.
- Recent sepsis, or remote infectious focus.
- Past history of joint prosthesis surgery.
- High-risk sexual history.

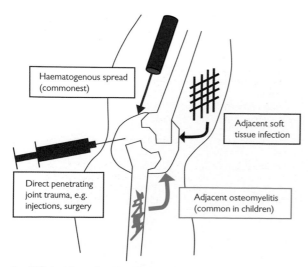

Fig. 19.9 Aetiology of septic arthritis.

(Diagram labels:)
- Haematogenous spread (commonest)
- Adjacent soft tissue infection
- Direct penetrating joint trauma, e.g. injections, surgery
- Adjacent osteomyelitis (common in children)

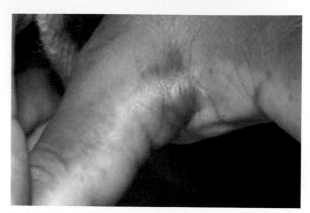

Fig. 19.10 Gonococcal pustule in disseminated gonococcal infection.

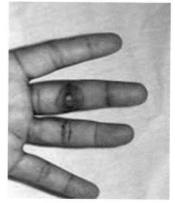

Fig. 19.11 Gonococcal septic arthritis.

- Increased risk in those taking immunosuppressive therapy including anti-TNFα drugs.
- Consider alternative cause if there is a history of spondyloarthropathy related diseases, podagra, etc.

### Examination
- Fever ± sepsis.
- Red, swollen, tender affected joint with marked restriction of movement. Often monoarthritis in lower limb (22% of cases involve more than one joint).
- Skin: pustules/blisters in gonococcal arthritis (tophi, psoriatic plaques may suggest an alternative non-septic arthritis) (Fig. 19.12).

## Investigations

- Joint aspiration (Figs 19.12 and 19.13):
  - **Should be performed before antibiotic treatment is commenced**.
  - Synovial fluid—urgent microscopy for crystals and gram stain for organisms. Culture.
  - Avoid aspiration through cellulitic skin (risk of introducing infection into joint).

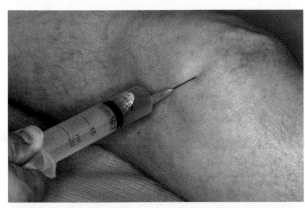

**Fig. 19.12** Knee joint aspiration.

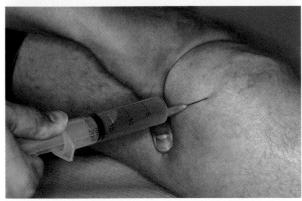

**Fig. 19.13** Knee joint aspiration.

1. Knee should be in full extension.
2. Mark position of entry—just under the patella at the medial edge, at the midpoint between the upper and lower poles.
3. Clean aspiration area with alcohol swab and leave for at least 1 minute to dry.
4. Insert needle, without touching cleaned area, at marked position and advance under patella while aspirating.
5. Fluid in the suprapatellar bursa may be compressed to aid aspiration of entire knee effusion.
6. Send off knee aspirate for microscopy including cell count, Gram staining for organisms, crystals, and culture.
7. Note: infection may coexist with crystals especially in joints previously injected with corticosteroids (corticosteroid crystals).

- Prosthetic joints—absolute contraindication to needle aspiration outside theatres. Should be reviewed by an orthopaedic team.
- Hip joints—require ultrasound guidance for needle aspiration.
- **Absence of organisms on Gram stain or culture does not exclude the diagnosis of septic arthritis** (especially if antibiotics were started before aspiration). Repeat aspiration if culture negative but suspicion of infection high.
- Blood cultures (repeated if suspicion high but results negative), swabs, MSU (and three early morning urine samples if TB suspected), sputum.

- FBC, ESR/CRP, U&E, LFTs. (Serum urate may not be of diagnostic value in acute sepsis or gout.)
- Imaging:
  - X-ray—as a baseline. Not urgent but may be helpful for alternative diagnoses (e.g. chondrocalcinosis in pseudogout).
  - MRI—most appropriate imaging. May detect osteomyelitis.

## Management

- Antibiotics:
  - See Box 19.5 for empirical treatments.
  - Conventionally, IV antibiotics are given for 2 weeks or until signs improve, and oral antibiotics are given for a further 4 weeks or until symptoms, signs, and inflammatory markers return to normal.
- Aspirate joint to dryness repeatedly if necessary (seek a senior opinion if needed and consider urgent orthopaedic referral). This may be done via closed-needle approach or surgically. However, if the closed-needle approach is unsatisfactory, then a surgical route should be used.
- Hip joint sepsis requires orthopaedic intervention for surgical washout.
- Affected joint should be rested and weight-bearing avoided until inflammation subsides enough for passive mobilization.
- Clinical signs, symptoms, and inflammatory markers should be reviewed regularly during treatment to determine satisfactory progress.

---

**Box 19.5 Initial empirical antibiotic treatments**

- **No risk of atypical organisms:**
  - Flucloxacillin 2g four times daily IV (local policy may add IV gentamicin).
  - If penicillin allergic, clindamycin 450–600mg four times daily IV or second- or third-generation cephalosporin IV.
- **High risk of Gram-negative sepsis** (elderly, frail, recurrent UTI, recent abdominal surgery):
  - Second- or third-generation cephalosporin, e.g. cefuroxime 1.5g three times daily IV (local policy may add flucloxacillin IV to third-generation cephalosporin).
  - Discuss allergic patients with microbiology.
- **MRSA risk:**
  - Vancomycin IV plus second- or third-generation cephalosporin IV.
- **Suspected Gonococcus** or Meningococcus:
  - Ceftriaxone IV or similar (dependent on local policy or resistance).
- **IV drug user:**
  - Discuss with microbiologist.
- **ITU patients, known colonization of other organisms**
  (e.g. cystic fibrosis):
  - Discuss with microbiologist.

Antibiotic choice needs to be modified in light of Gram stain and culture results.

Reproduced from Coakley G et al., 'BSR & BHPR, BOA, RCGP, and BSAC guidelines for the management of the hot swollen joint in adults', *Rheumatology*, 2006, 45, pp. 1039–1041, by permission of Oxford University Press and British Society for Rheumatology.

# 19.7 Crystal arthropathies

## Background

This is a group of disorders characterized by the deposition of various minerals in joints and soft tissues leading to inflammation. Common examples include gout and pseudogout.

## Epidemiology

|  | Gout | Pseudogout |
|---|---|---|
| Prevalence | 1% of ♂ aged 30–50 | 8% rising with age |
| ♂:♀ ratios | 7:1 | 1:2 |
| Peak age of onset (years) | ♀: 30–50♀: >60 | 65–75 |

## Aetiology

### Gout

Caused by urate crystal deposition. Hyperuricaemia may be due to:
- Urate underexcretion—renal impairment.
- High purine intake—alcohol, purine-rich foods.
- Malignancy—myeloproliferative disorder, leukaemia, chemotherapy.
- Psoriasis.
- Drugs—diuretics, calcineurin inhibitors, aspirin.

### Pseudogout

Caused by calcium pyrophosphate dihydrate crystal deposition. May be secondary to:
- Age.
- Osteoarthritis.
- Metabolic syndromes—haemochromatosis, hyperparathyroidism, Wilson disease, hypomagnesaemia, hypophosphatasia.

## Clinical evaluation

### Gout

- An acute self-limiting monoarthritis; rapid onset of joint pain over 6–18 hours.
- Almost all cases will have foot involvement at some time, particularly at the first metatarsophalangeal joint (podagra).
- There may be a fever, bursitis (e.g. olecranon, prepatellar) and polyarticular involvement.
- Chronic tophaceous gout (e.g. ear pinna, elbow, digits, Achilles tendon) can develop with persistent hyperuricaemia (Fig. 19.14).
- Urate nephropathy may develop with chronic gout (a chronic tubulointerstitial nephritis, with uric acid crystals often seen in tubules and interstitium).

### Calcium pyrophosphate dihydrate

- Usually presents as an acute monoarthritis (pseudogout) affecting the knee, wrist, shoulder, or ankle.
- May present with fever but concurrent involvement of more than one joint is rare.
- Chronic pyrophosphate arthropathy often affects joints already affected by OA and chondrocalcinosis.
- Rarely presents with tenosynovitis, tendinitis, bursitis, and odontoid peg involvement (crowned dens syndrome).

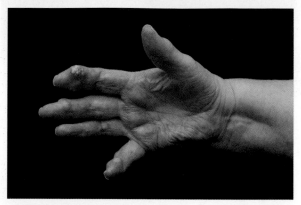

Fig. 19.14 Chronic tophaceous gout.

## Investigations

- **Synovial fluid analysis**—essential in all acute monoarthritis (except for obvious podagra in gout) to **exclude infection** and confirm diagnosis:
  - Gout—needle-shaped negatively birefringent crystals seen with polarizing light microscopy. May be found in joint and bursa fluid and tophi.
  - Pseudogout—weakly positive birefringent rhomboid crystals seen with polarizing light microscopy.
- **Blood tests:**
  - Gout—hyperuricaemia is usually found between acute attacks. 1/3 of patients are normouricaemic during attacks. Elevated CRP and ESR may occur. Elevated urea and creatinine in urate nephropathy.
  - Pseudogout—screening for a metabolic cause is warranted in young patients (<55 years), polyarticular involvement, and recurrent attacks. This includes calcium, alkaline phosphatase, magnesium, ferritin, iron, iron binding capacity.
- **Imaging:**
  - Gout—usually normal but may show 'punched out' erosions (Fig. 19.15).
  - Pseudogout—changes of osteoarthritis and chondrocalcinosis (calcification of fibro- and hyaline cartilage) (Fig. 19.16). Chondrocalcinosis is a common finding in the elderly and may be incidental.

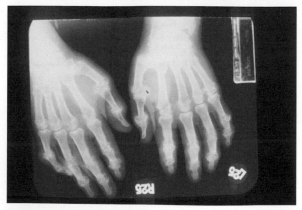

Fig. 19.15 Gouty erosions in hands.

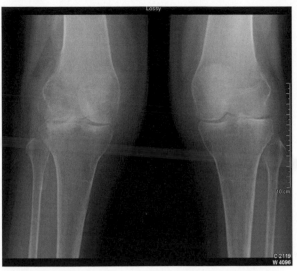

**Fig. 19.16** Knee chondrocalcinosis; more marked in the right knee cartilage.

---

**Box 19.6 Lifestyle modification for gout**

- Weight loss can significantly reduce hyperuricaemia.
- Reduce alcohol intake (especially beer).
- Reduce intake of fructose-rich soft drinks.
- Restrict foods high in purines, e.g.:
  - Shellfish
  - Fish: herring, sardines
  - Meat
  - Offal including heart, liver.
- Often difficult to maintain.
- Also treat hypertension, if present, and stop diuretics, if possible.

---

## Management

### Gout

- Acute attacks:
  - Local application of ice.
  - Short course of NSAIDs (etoricoxib, indomethacin).
  - Colchicine (0.5mg, 6–12-hourly; lower than the traditional dose but as efficacious and less likely to cause diarrhoea).
  - Systemic steroids for the duration of the attack (high doses needed).
  - Intra-articular steroid injection (inject steroids at same time as aspirating for diagnosis and excluding infection).
- Lifestyle modification: please refer to Box 19.6.

**Box 19.7 Correction of hyperuricaemia**

- Indications:
  - Recurrent attacks of gout.
  - Tophaceous gout.
  - Urate nephropathy.
  - Anticipated severe hyperuricaemia (tumour lysis syndrome).
- Should not be given for asymptomatic hyperuricaemia or during an acute attack of gout.
- Correct underlying cause if possible.
- The intention to treat is **lifelong**.

Reduce uric acid production
- Allopurinol—xanthine oxidase inhibitor.
- Major adverse effect is allopurinol hypersensitivity manifesting as a severe skin rash but this is generally rare.
- In patients with renal impairment, and the elderly, start at a low dose of 100mg once a day.
- Dose of allopurinol should gradually be increased to therapeutic levels (check urate levels 4 weeks after change in dose). Aim for a plasma urate <250–350μmol/L to achieve 'cure'.
- The introduction of allopurinol can be covered by low-dose colchicine (0.5mg twice daily), NSAIDs (for at least 1 month) or low-dose steroids (10–20mg once daily), especially in the setting of an acute attack; but this is less of a problem when starting at a low dose and titrating up.

Increase uric acid excretion (uricosuric agents)
- Probenecid, sulphinpyrazone. Unsuitable in renal disease.
- Benzbromarone. Safe in mild–moderate renal impairment, but named-patient availability only.
- In patients intolerant of other medications, long-term colchicine 500mcg twice daily may prevent further attacks.
- Losartan (angiotensin-II receptor blocker) lowers uric acid levels and is a good antihypertensive choice.

Newer agents
- Rasburicase (recombinant uricase): currently only licensed for tumour lysis syndrome.
- Febuxostat: a novel xanthine oxidase inhibitor which is now NICE approved for the treatment of gout in patients who are allopurinol intolerant.

- Pharmacological correction of hyperuricaemia: please refer to Box 19.7.

### Pseudogout

- Acute attack—aspiration and injection of monoarthritis with intra-articular corticosteroids is usually preferable. May benefit from oral NSAIDS, colchicine, or corticosteroids.
- Recurrent attacks may be prevented by low-dose NSAIDs or colchicine.

# 19.8 Spondyloarthritides

## Background

The spondyloarthritides (or seronegative spondyloarthropathies) are a family of interrelated diseases (Box 19.8). They share similarities in clinical presentation and genetic associations (Box 19.9).

## Epidemiology

- Overall estimated prevalence rate: 2%.
- Prevalence rates (♀:♂):
  - Ankylosing spondylitis: 1% (1:3).
  - Reactive arthritis: 0.1% (1:5).
  - Enteropathic arthritis: 0.1% (1:1).
  - Psoriatic arthritis: <0.1% (1:1).
- Age at presentation: 20–40 years.

## Aetiology

- Significant association with HLA-B27:
  - Ankylosing spondylitis: 95%.
  - Reactive arthritis: 40–80%.
- HLA-B27 is a class I HLA molecule involved with antigen presentation to CD8+ T cells.
- Spondyloarthritides, especially reactive arthritis, may be associated with bacterial infection (including *Chlamydia* trachomatis, *Klebsiella*).
- There are several hypotheses linking HLA-B27 to infection and autoimmune disease (e.g. molecular mimicry).

## Clinical features

### Ankylosing spondylitis (AS)

- Chronic systemic inflammation particularly in axial skeleton and entheses.
- Low back/buttock pain (often alternating sides) and early morning stiffness.
- Limitation of spinal movement and chest expansion.
- Other features:
  - Anterior uveitis (25–40% of cases).
  - Aortitis, aortic valve incompetence, cardiac conduction defects.
  - Restrictive lung disease, **apical** pulmonary fibrosis (1–2%).
  - Spinal osteoporosis, spondylodiscitis, spinal fractures.
  - Chronic adhesive arachnoiditis.
  - Peripheral large joint arthritis.
  - Secondary amyloidosis.

### Reactive arthritis (ReA)

- Sterile synovitis developing after a distant infection (usually urogenital, e.g. *Chlamydia* or enteric, e.g. *Yersinia, Campylobacter, Shigella,* or *Salmonella,* occurring up to 1 month before arthritis).

---

**Box 19.8 Spondyloarthropathy diseases**

- Ankylosing spondylitis.
- Reactive arthritis.
- Psoriatic arthritis.
- Enteropathic arthritis (Crohn disease, ulcerative colitis).
- Undifferentiated spondyloarthropathy.
- Juvenile-onset ankylosing spondylitis.

---

**Box 19.9 Characteristics of spondyloarthropathies**

- Absent rheumatoid factor.
- Sacroiliitis.
- Asymmetric mono- or oligoarthritis.
- Anterior uveitis.
- Familial aggregation.
- Association with HLA-B27.
- Enthesopathy.

---

- Monoarthritis or oligoarthritis—usually involving lower limb joints.
- Other features—enthesitis, conjunctivitis, keratoderma blenorragicum, circinate balanitis.

### Psoriatic arthritis

See Section 19.9.

### Enteropathic arthritis

- Monoarthritis and oligoarthritis are associated with Crohn disease and ulcerative colitis (2–20% of patients in each group).
- Peripheral joint arthritis is closely associated with bowel exacerbations (surgical removal of colon in ulcerative colitis has been shown to be curative for joint symptoms).
- Sacroiliitis may precede bowel disease by many years—activity here is independent of gut activity.
- Lower limb joints frequently affected.

---

## Investigations

- ESR, CRP—elevated in most active arthritis. May not correlate with disease activity in AS.
- Blood, stool, and urine culture, vaginal/urethral swab—for ReA.
- Serology—for *Salmonella, Yersinia, Campylobacter, Chlamydia* in ReA.
- Joint aspirate—to exclude infection, crystal arthropathy.
- Radiology—tends to be the most useful investigative modality for diagnosing AS:
  - Plain radiographs—sacroiliitis (Fig. 19.17), syndesmophytes (Fig. 19.18).
  - MRI—useful for early sacroiliitis and spinal inflammation.
  - CT—useful for spinal disease.
- HLA-B27—this is not recommended as a diagnostic test since 8% of the normal population are positive and not all spondyloarthropathies have strong associations. However, it may be useful in some clinical situations.

---

## Management

- Patient education and exercise programme including hydrotherapy for spinal involvement. Physical and occupational therapy, plus posture advice (Fig. 19.19).
- NSAIDs—mainstay of symptomatic therapy—continuous use has been shown to slow radiographic progression in AS.
- Sulphasalazine, methotrexate—effective for peripheral joint arthritis. No clear evidence of benefit for spinal disease.
- Local steroid joint injections—for peripheral mono/oligoarthritis and sacroiliitis.

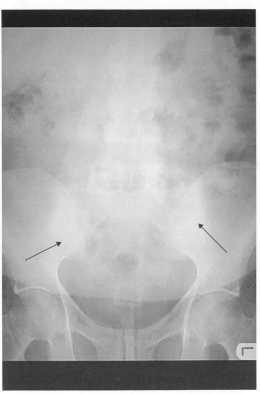

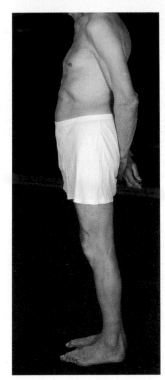

Fig. 19.19 Patient with AS: note accentuated thoracic kyphosis and loss of lumbar lordosis, with extension of cervical spine: the 'question mark' posture.

Fig. 19.17 Radiograph demonstrating bilateral sacroiliitis, which is usually symmetrical. There is loss of joint space and bony sclerosis around the sacroiliac joints (arrows).

(A)
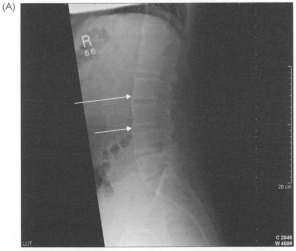

(B)
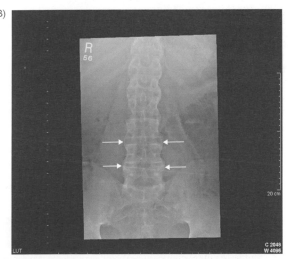

Fig. 19.18 Lateral (A) and anteroposterior (right) spinal radiographs showing syndesmophytes (arrows). These represent ossification of the outer fibres of the annulus fibrosis, with a 'flowing' appearance as new bone extends across the disc space. Eventually this can produce the appearance termed 'bamboo spine'.

- Anti-TNFα therapy—infliximab, etanercept, and adalimumab have been shown to be effective for: (1) AS (Braun et al., 2002), although not yet confirmed to slow radiographic progression, and (2) psoriatic arthritis (peripheral and spinal disease).
- Pamidronate—open label studies showing benefit for AS (Maksymowych et al., 1998).
- Thalidomide—open-label studies show benefit in AS.
- Stop smoking (especially in AS).

## References

Braun J, Brandt J, Listing J, et al. Treatment of active ankylosing spondylitis with infliximab: a randomised controlled multicentre trial. *Lancet* 2002; *359*(9313): 1187–93.

Maksymowych WP, Jhangri GS, Leclercq S, et al. An open study of pamidronate in the treatment of refractory ankylosing spondylitis. *J Rheumatol* 1998; *25*: 714–17.

# 19.9 Psoriatic arthritis

## Background

Psoriatic arthritis (PsA) is an inflammatory arthritis associated with a personal or family history of psoriasis which is usually negative for rheumatoid factor. It also belongs to the spondyloarthritis group of disorders.

## Epidemiology

- Prevalence: ≤0.3%.
- ♀:♂ ratio 1:1.
- Age of onset typically 30–55 years.
- 67% of patients develop psoriasis before arthritis.

## Aetiology

- Although the exact aetiology in PsA is unknown, it is thought to be multifactorial involving the immune system, genetics, and the environment.
- 40–50% of PsA patients are HLA-B27 positive. Other HLA associations: HLA-B13, HLA-B17, and HLA-Cw6.
- The role of environmental triggers including infection, trauma, and psychological stress is still unclear.

## Clinical evaluation

- PsA can be classified into five clinical subtypes according to Moll and Wright (see Box 19.10).
- The pattern of arthritis may, however, change over time in 60% of cases.

### History

- Significant early morning stiffness (>1 hour) in peripheral joints and/or lower back.
- Joint swelling/pain depending on subtype.
- Personal and/or family history of psoriasis (Box 19.11).

### Examination

- Psoriatic plaques—extensor surfaces, scalp, umbilicus, natal cleft, ears (skin disease activity does not correlate with joint disease activity).

- 60–80% of PsA patients have psoriatic nail changes, e.g. pitting, onycholysis (however, nail changes occur in only 20–40% of patients with uncomplicated psoriasis) (Fig. 19.20)
- Arthritis (Fig. 19.21)—digital telescoping, subluxation in arthritis mutilans.
- Dactylitis (particularly in feet).
- Enthesitis, tendonitis, plantar fasciitis.
- Iritis.

## Investigations

- ESR, CRP—correlates with disease activity.
- FBC—anaemia of chronic disease.
- Rheumatoid factor—positive in 10% of cases.
- Uric acid—elevated in active psoriasis (20% PsA). It is important to exclude crystal arthropathy, as a result.
- Radiographic changes:
  - Erosive changes (depending on joint involved; Fig. 19.22).
  - Absence of juxta-articular osteoporosis.
  - 'Pencil in cup' deformities.
  - Acro-osteolysis.
  - Ankylosis.

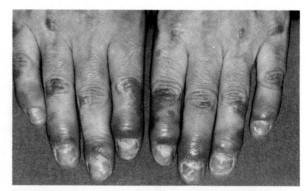

**Fig. 19.20** Hands with psoriatic arthritis: distal interphalangeal joint involvement, multiple well-demarcated 'salmon-pink' skin plaques, and extensive nail involvement.

> **Box 19.10  Moll and Wright classification of psoriatic arthritis**
>
> - Arthritis with distal interphalangeal joint involvement (similar to osteoarthritis).
> - Asymmetric (usually large joint) oligoarticular arthritis.
> - Symmetric polyarthritis (indistinguishable from rheumatoid arthritis).
> - Spondyloarthropathy (similar to ankylosing spondylitis).
> - Arthritis mutilans.

> **Box 19.11  Risk factors for joint disease in psoriatic patients**
>
> - Extensive psoriasis.
> - Nail involvement.
> - Family history of psoriasis.

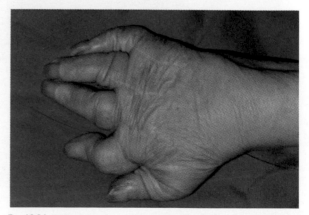

**Fig. 19.21** Arthritis mutilans: telescoping of the digits (especially 3rd and 4th), sometimes referred to as 'opera-glass hand'.

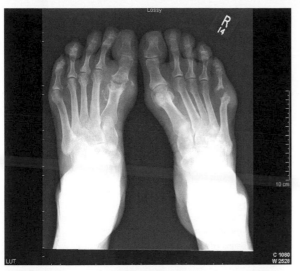

**Fig. 19.22** Radiograph of foot demonstrating destructive changes of psoriatic arthropathy, particularly distal interphalangeal joints, left great toe and right 5th toe.

- Periostitis.
- Sacroiliitis (often asymmetric as opposed to ankylosing spondylitis).
- MRI—demonstrates involvement of ligaments, soft tissue, tendon sheath, bone.
- Ultrasound.
- Bone scintigraphy—demonstrates extent of disease (Fig. 19.23).

## Management

- Patient education.
- Physiotherapy and occupational therapy.
- NSAIDs—symptomatic treatment for peripheral arthritis.
- Corticosteroids—topical use for psoriasis. Intra-articular and tendon sheath injections. Systemic use should be limited as psoriasis may flare on withdrawal of steroids.
- Disease-modifying agents: methotrexate, sulphasalazine, ciclosporin, leflunomide.
- All are effective for both skin and joint involvement.
- Biologics:
  - Infliximab (Antoni et al., 2005), etanercept (Mease et al., 2004), adalimumab, and golimumab.
  - All have been shown to be highly effective for skin and joint disease unresponsive to other disease-modifying agents.
  - All are NICE approved for PsA.

## References

Antoni CE, Kavanaugh A, Kirkham B, *et al*. Sustained benefits of infliximab therapy for dermatologic and articular manifestations of psoriatic arthritis: results from the infliximab multinational psoriatic arthritis controlled trial (IMPACT). *Arthritis Rheum* 2005; 52(4): 1227–36.

Mease PJ, Kivitz AJ, Burch FX, *et al*. Etanercept treatment of psoriatic arthritis: safety, efficacy, and effect on disease progression. *Arthritis Rheum* 2004; 50(7): 2264–72.

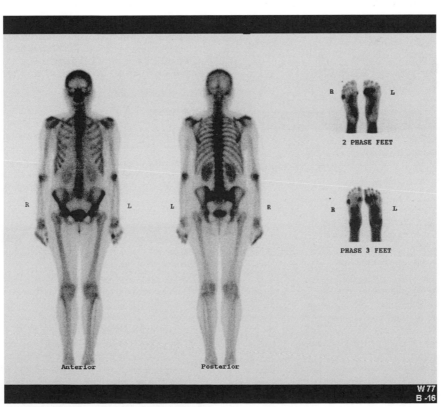

**Fig. 19.23** Bone scan in psoriatic arthritis. Increased uptake in feet.

# 19.10 Low back pain

## Background

Low back pain is one of the most frequently encountered medical complaints and >80% of people will suffer from it during their lifetime.

## Epidemiology

- Lifetime prevalence of low back pain is 84%.
- Prevalence of chronic (>12 weeks) non-specific low back pain is estimated at 23% in general population.
- ♀:♂ ratio 1:1.
- Peak age incidence: 35–55 years.
- Estimated 52 million working days lost in the UK annually due to low back pain.

## Aetiology

- 90% of back pain is due to 'mechanical' factors. However, the precise source of the 'mechanical' factor is often not identifiable.
- The remaining 10% have back pain as a manifestation of a systemic illness and need to be identified early.

## Clinical evaluation

Low back pain may be triaged into three categories based on clinical evaluation:

1. Serious spinal pathology—requires investigation.
2. Radicular pain—initial conservative management; may require investigation if persists.
3. Non-specific low back pain—conservative measures.

### Box 19.12 ❗ 'Red flags' of 'serious spinal pathology'

1. Age of onset <20 years or >55 years.
2. Recent history of violent trauma.
3. Constant, progressive, non-mechanical back pain (no relief with bed rest).
4. Thoracic pain.
5. Night pain.
6. Past medical history of malignant tumour.
7. Prolonged use of corticosteroids.
8. Drug abuse, immunosuppression, HIV.
9. Systemically unwell, fever, weight loss.
10. Widespread neurological symptoms.
11. Progressive neurological deficit.
12. Structural deformity.
13. Symptoms/signs of cauda equina syndrome require immediate investigation:
    - Sphincter disturbance.
    - Gait disturbance.
    - Saddle anaesthesia.

If any of these are present, further investigations may be required to exclude serious spinal pathology.

From Waddell G, McIntosh A, Hutchinson A, Feder G, Lewis M, (1999) *Low Back Pain Evidence Review* London: Royal College of General Practitioners.

## History

- **Mechanical pain:** often acute in onset. Worsens with certain movements and eases at night/rest.
- **Inflammatory pain:** insidious in onset. Patients report early morning stiffness eased by movement.
- **Infection/malignancy:** often focal, severe, unremitting pain. Night pain is prominent.
- **Radicular pain:** sharp, shooting pain radiating from the back to the lower limbs.
- **'Red flags'** (Box 19.12)—symptoms which require further investigation to exclude serious spinal pathology should be identified from the history.
- **'Yellow flags'** (Box 19.13) identify psychological/social factors that may predispose to chronicity of symptoms.
- Family history of spondyloarthopathies may be significant. Past medical history of malignancy, spondyloarthropathy, metabolic bone disease, including osteoporosis/fracture should be identified.
- Occupational and social history may identify risk factors for low back pain and any claim for compensation which may influence response to treatment and prognosis.

## Examination

- General observation—observe for kyphosis or scoliosis and gait.
- Regional back examination—spinal point tenderness may suggest infection/fracture/malignancy. Observe range of movement.
- Neurological examination—look for lower limb sensory, motor, and reflex deficits.
- Sciatic nerve tension—Laseague sign is positive for sciatic nerve irritation when pain is experienced radiating down to the foot between 30° to 70° of straight leg raise (SLR). Contralateral pain on SLR is suggestive of a large central disc protrusion.

## Prognosis

- 90% of non-specific back pain improves after 6 weeks with conservative measures alone.
- The longer a person is off work due to back pain, the lower their chance of returning to work. After 6 months, there's a 50% chance of returning to work, decreasing to 10% after 2 years.

### Box 19.13 'Yellow flags'

1. Negative attitude that back pain is harmful or potentially severely disabling.
2. Fear avoidance behaviour or reduced activity levels.
3. An expectation that passive, rather than active, treatment will be beneficial.
4. A tendency to depression, low morale, and social withdrawal.
5. Social or work-related problems, or compensation issues:
   - The yellow flags are psychosocial factors that increase the risk of developing chronic pain and long-term disability.
   - Identification of yellow flags should lead to appropriate cognitive and behavioural therapy. Assess for signs of depression.

Reproduced from *The BMJ*, Chronic low back pain, Jo Samanta, Julia Kendall, and Ash Samanta, 326, 2003, with permission from BMJ Publishing Group Ltd.

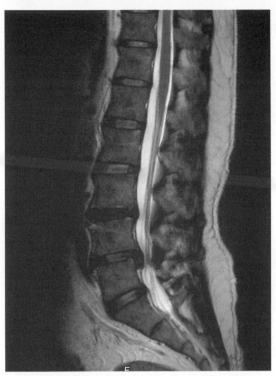

**Fig. 19.24** MRI (T2-weighted) image of lumbosacral disc prolapse.

## Investigations

- Blood investigations—elevated ESR/CRP may indicate an inflammatory/malignant cause.
- Diagnostic imaging is not routinely indicated for non-specific back pain.

- Radiographs—may show structural abnormalities, but changes may be incidental and not the cause of pain.
- Bone scintigraphy—sensitive but non-specific method for demonstrating infection or malignancy. May demonstrate a recent fracture—'hot' lesion.
- MRI—good for demonstrating disc lesions (Fig. 19.24), infection, or malignancy.
- CT—better demonstrates bony lesions (e.g. pars defects).
- Bone densitometry—if vertebral wedging/collapse is identified.

## Management

- Further investigation if 'red flags' are present. Immediate imaging if cauda equina syndrome or cord compression suspected.
- Radicular pain is usually managed conservatively (as for non-specific low back pain) for 6–8 weeks. This is normally effective. Specialist opinion may be warranted if the problem persists.
- In acute non-specific low back pain:
  - Give adequate information and reassure patient that >90% recover in 6 weeks.
  - Bed rest should **not** be prescribed. Advise patients to stay active and return to work
  - Regular analgesics if necessary: paracetamol first choice followed by NSAIDs or weak opioids.
  - Consider short course of muscle relaxants if analgesia inadequate.
  - Multidisciplinary (bio-psycho-social) treatment programme if low back pain is subacute or chronic and if 'yellow flags' identified.

# 19.11 Systemic lupus erythematosus

## Background

Systemic lupus erythematosus (SLE) is a complex inflammatory disorder affecting most of the body's systems with a variable course and prognosis. SLE is often associated with other autoimmune disorders including antiphospholipid and Sjögren syndromes.

## Epidemiology

- Prevalence varies between different racial groups with rates highest for African American ♀ (280 per 100,000).
- Age at presentation commonly 14–50 years.
- ♀:♂ ratio 9:1.

## Aetiology/pathogenesis

- Unknown—associated with cellular immune system abnormalities leading to defective B-cell tolerance, autoantibody secretion, immune complex production, and immunologically mediated disease.
- ANA positive in 95% of cases. Anti-dsDNA and anti-Sm have high specificity for SLE but only found in 60% and 30% of patients respectively.
- Other associated antibodies: anti-Ro (30%), anti-La (15%), anti-cardiolipin (30%), rheumatoid factor (25%).

## Clinical evaluation

### History

- Fever.
- Lethargy and fatigue.
- Photosensitive rash.
- Increased hair loss and mouth ulcers.
- Myalgia, arthralgia, arthritis.
- Pleuro-pericarditic chest pain (serositis).
- Raynaud phenomenon.
- Dry eyes/mouth.
- Neurological symptoms—migraines, psychiatric disease, seizures.

### Examination

- Butterfly facial rash in 1/3 of cases (see Fig. 19.25).
- Alopecia.
- Lymphadenopathy, splenomegaly.
- Jaccoud arthropathy (deforming but non-erosive arthritis).
- Myopathy—myalgia, myositis (may also be secondary to antimalarials and corticosteroids).
- Cardiac—pericardial rub, Libman–Sacks endocarditis (fibrinous deposits on mitral valve leaflets—no inflammatory cell infiltrate).
- Lung—pleural effusion, late inspiratory basal crepitations.

### Investigations

- FBC, Coomb test, U&E, LFT.
- ESR, CRP (see Box 19.14).
- Complement—C3, C4.
- Autoantibodies—ANA, anti-dsDNA, anti-ENA (Ro, La, Sm), anti-cardiolipin antibodies.
- Urine—dipstick for proteinuria ± haematuria (evidence of renal involvement). If present: microscopy for casts, urinary ACR, and creatinine clearance.

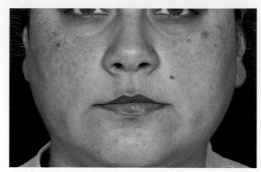

Fig. 19.25 Image of butterfly malar rash in a patient with SLE.

- Histology—characteristic histological and immunological abnormalities in renal and skin biopsies (lupus 'band' test).
- MRI/EEG—may be useful in SLE neurological involvement.

## Management

- Avoid overexposure to sunlight (use suncreams of >factor 50+).
- NSAIDs—arthralgia, serositis.
- Hydroxychloroquine—arthralgia, myalgia, hair loss, rash.
- Corticosteroids—for acute flares, severe disease, major organ involvement.
- Azathioprine/methotrexate—for steroid-sparing effects, maintenance therapy.
- Cyclophosphamide/immunoglobulins/mycophenolate—for major organ involvement (e.g. renal, pulmonary)—see Section 19.19.

---

**Box 19.14 1997 Revised American College of Rheumatology criteria for classification of SLE**

1. Malar rash
2. Discoid rash
3. Photosensitivity
4. Oral ulcers
5. Arthritis
6. Serositis: pleuritis or pericarditis
7. Renal disorder: proteinuria or cellular casts
8. Neurological disorders: seizures or psychosis
9. Haematological disorders:
   - Haemolytic anaemia or
   - Leucopenia or
   - Lymphopenia or
   - Thrombocytopaenia
10. Immunological disorders:
    - Anti-DNA antibody or
    - Anti-Sm antibody or
    - Positive antiphospholipid antibody
11. Positive ANA.

   SLE may be diagnosed if four or more criteria are present serially or simultaneously.

Reproduced with permission from Hochberg MC, Updating the American college of rheumatology revised criteria for the classification of systemic lupus erythematosus, *Arthritis & Rheumatology*, Copyright Wiley 2005

> **Box 19.15** ❗ SLE and cardiovascular disease
>
> - SLE, as well as other inflammatory rheumatic diseases, is associated with a higher risk of cardiovascular disease.
> - Manzi et al. (1997) found that the incidence of acute myocardial infarction in women with SLE aged 35–44 years was 50× greater than age-matched controls.
> - This excess risk is independent of classical cardiovascular risk factors. (Esdaile et al., 2001)
> - All patients with SLE should have cardiovascular risk factors monitored and treated aggressively.
>
> Data from Manzi S et al., 'Age-specific incidence rates of myocardial infarction and angina in women with systemic lupus ery-thematosus: comparison with the Framingham Study', *Am J Epidemiol*, 1997, 145, pp. 408–415; and Esdaile JM, et al., 'Traditional risk factors fail to fully account for accelerated atherosclerosis in systemic lupus erythematosus', *Arthritis Rheum*, 2001, 44, pp. 2331–2337.

- Anti-CD20 (rituximab)—mixed results for SLE—may be of value in those with cytopenias.
- Belimumab—this targets the cytokine BLyS, a member of the TNF family and acts as a B-lymphocyte stimulator protein inhibitor. It is not yet recommended for severe active nephritis or CNS disease.

## Monitoring disease

Involves separate consideration of active disease and end-organ damage.

### Activity
- ESR—elevated in active disease.
- C3, C4—both reduced in active SLE.
- FBC—anaemia (chronic disease, renal disease, drugs, or haemolytic), lymphopenia and leucopenia, and thrombocytopaenia in active disease.
- Anti-dsDNA—rising titres correlate with renal disease activity.

### Damage
- Radiographs (relevant to organ-specific problems).
- U&E, 24-hour creatinine clearance and proteinuria.

## Prognosis

- Mortality rates are 3–5× greater than normal population.
- Bimodal mortality curve—early mortality due to active disease. Late mortality due to cardiovascular (Box 19.15), renal disease, and infection (often as a consequence of prolonged immunosuppressive treatment).
- Poor prognostic markers:
  - Renal involvement.
  - Central nervous system disease.
  - Race (e.g. African Americans have a more severe disease than Caucasian Americans).
  - Older age onset (>50 years).
  - Low socioeconomic status.

### Inflammatory markers in SLE
- In active SLE, ESR is usually elevated while CRP is frequently normal.
- CRP usually normal but may be elevated in:
  - Infection.
  - Arthritis.
  - Serositis (i.e. pericarditis, pleuritis).
- Infection may sometimes be differentiated from a disease flare by a raised CRP.

## References

Esdaile JM, Abrahamowicz M, Grodzicky T, *et al*. Traditional risk factors fail to fully account for accelerated atherosclerosis in systemic lupus erythematosus. *Arthritis Rheum* 2001; 44: 2331–7.

Manzi S, Meilahn EN, Rairie JE, *et al*. Age-specific incidence rates of myocardial infarction and angina in women with systemic lupus erythematosus: comparison with the Framingham Study. *Am J Epidemiol* 1997; 145: 408–15.

# 19.12 Systemic sclerosis

## Background

Disease characterized by overproduction of connective tissue, widespread microvascular damage, and inflammation. This condition is also known as scleroderma.

## Epidemiology

- Prevalence: 8.2 patients per 100,000.
- ♀:♂ ratio 5:1.
- Age of onset 30–60 years.
- African Americans show an earlier age of onset and more severe disease.

## Clinical features

### Limited cutaneous systemic sclerosis (LCSS)

- Skin thickening present distal to elbow and knees. Perioral furrowing (Fig. 19.26).
- **C**alcinosis, **R**aynaud, o**E**sophageal dysmotility, **S**clerodactyly (Fig. 19.27), **T**elangiectasia (LCSS was previously known as CREST).
- Pulmonary hypertension occurs in 10% of cases and is the leading cause of mortality.
- Prognosis—5-year survival is 80–85%.

### Diffuse cutaneous systemic sclerosis (DCSS)

- Skin thickening extends proximal to elbow and knees.
- Secondary Raynaud phenomenon may be differentiated from primary Raynaud phenomenon by older age of onset, severity with ulceration/gangrene, nailfold capillary abnormalities, and presence of ANA/ACA/anti-Scl-70.
- Tendon friction rubs—in 30% of cases and is a predictor of worse disease.
- Early internal organ involvement:
  - Interstitial lung disease.
  - Renal failure (including renal hypertensive crisis).
  - Gastrointestinal disease (dysmotility → bacterial overgrowth).
  - Myopathy, myositis (overlap syndrome).
- Prognosis—5-year survival is 75%.

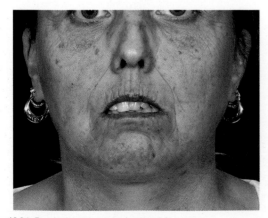

Fig. 19.26 Facial telangiectasia and perioral furrowing.

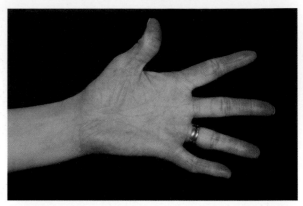

Fig. 19.27 Sclerodactyly: tight, shiny skin with tapering of the fingers. Raynaud phenomenon may be visible.

## Management

Current management involves organ-specific treatments:

- Severe Raynaud phenomenon—calcium channel blockers, serotonin antagonists, ACE inhibitors, iloprost, PDE 5 inhibitors, e.g. tadalafil.
- Interstitial pulmonary fibrosis—cyclophosphamide ± corticosteroids in active alveolitis.
- Pulmonary hypertension—anticoagulation, prostacyclin, endothelin receptor antagonist (bosentan), sildenafil.
- Renal crisis—ACE inhibitor, iloprost. Temporary dialysis may be required as recovery may be slow.
- Gastrointestinal disease—proton-pump inhibitors and metoclopramide for oesophageal disease. Antibiotics for bacterial overgrowth.
- Diffuse skin disease—limited evidence for methotrexate, D-penicillamine, ciclosporin, mycophenolate mofetil.
- High-dose corticosteroids should be avoided where possible—predispose to scleroderma renal crisis.

### Monitoring lung function in systemic sclerosis

- Annual pulmonary function tests and echocardiography are recommended for follow-up of scleroderma patients.
- **Pulmonary hypertension:**
  - Isolated reduction in transfer factor on pulmonary function test.
  - Echocardiography may show elevated pulmonary artery pressures.
  - May be followed by pulmonary angiography: exclude thromboembolic disease and confirmatory right heart catheterization.
- **Interstitial pulmonary fibrosis:**
  - Reduction in transfer factor **and** lung volumes on pulmonary function test.
  - Chest radiographs can be insensitive for detecting fibrosing alveolitis.
  - Echocardiography may show secondary pulmonary hypertension.
  - HRCT chest.
  - Bronchoalveolar lavage and transbronchial biopsy to define histological subtype of lung disease.

# 19.13 Polymyositis/dermatomyositis

## Background

The two most common forms of **idiopathic inflammatory myopathy**, with the latter distinguished by a characteristic rash. The Bohan and Peter classification (Box 19.16) is still useful for epidemiological and diagnostic purposes.

## Epidemiology

- Incidence: 2–10 new cases per million annually.
- ♀:♂ ratio 2.5:1. Ratio higher with coexisting connective tissue disease (10:1) and lower with malignancy (1:1) (Box 19.17).
- Peak age of onset: 40–60 years.
- African Americans have a higher incidence and younger age of onset compared to Caucasians.

## Clinical features

- Usually presents as an insidious onset of proximal symmetrical muscle weakness. Muscles may be tender.
- Dysphagia may occur with regurgitation of food or aspiration—indicates severe disease.
- Rash—occurs in dermatomyositis; heliotrope facial rash, Gottron papules (Fig. 19.28), and 'shawl sign'.
- Periorbital oedema.
- Antisynthetase syndrome—a subtype characterized by erosive arthritis, fever, interstitial pulmonary disease, 'mechanic's hands' (cracked and fissured palmar skin) and anti-Jo-1 antibody positivity.
- Respiratory—non-pulmonary (diaphragmatic and intercostal muscle weakness) or interstitial pulmonary disease.

## Investigations

- Blood investigations—muscle CK usually elevated in active myositis although may be normal (especially dermatomyositis, chronic muscle atrophy). ANA and anti-Jo-1 antibodies. ESR/CRP poorly reflect activity.

> **Box 19.16** Bohan and Peter modified criteria for polymyositis and dermatomyositis
>
> Individual criteria
> 1. Symmetric proximal muscle weakness.
> 2. Muscle biopsy evidence of myositis.
> 3. Increase in serum skeletal muscle enzymes.
> 4. Characteristic EMG pattern.
> 5. Typical rash of dermatomyositis.
> Diagnostic criteria
> - Polymyositis:
> - Definite:   all of 1–4.
> - Probable:   any 3 of 1–4.
> - Possible:   any 2 of 1–4.
> Dermatomyositis:
> - Definite:   5 plus any 3 of 1–4.
> - Probable:   5 plus any 2 of 1–4.
> - Possible:   5 plus any 1 of 1–4.
> Reproduced from Bohan A et al., 'A computer-assisted analysis of 153 patients with polymyositis and dermatomyositis', *Medicine*, 56, 4, pp. 255–286, copyright 1977, with permission from Wolters Kluwer Health.

> **Box 19.17** Malignancy in inflammatory muscle disease
>
> - There is an increased risk of malignancy with dermatomyositis (3–12× increased risk).
> - Associated malignancies: ovarian, lung, pancreatic, stomach, colon, lymphoma.
> - Continued surveillance is required throughout the follow-up of disease since the increased risk of malignancy persists (highest in first 3 years of diagnosis).
> - The presence of an associated connective tissue disease decreases the risk of malignancy with myositis.
> - Suggested screening of patients with dermatomyositis:
>   - Physical examination including rectal, pelvic, and breast.
>   - CXR, CT scan (chest, abdomen, pelvis).
>   - Mammography.
>   - PSA, CA-125.

- Electromyography—>90% of active myositis will have positive results. Useful for detecting myositis in presence of a normal CK, weakness in chronic damaged muscle.
- MRI—useful in directing site of biopsy, differentiating active myositis from chronic damage.
- Muscle biopsy—remains the gold standard to confirm diagnosis. However, false negatives can result from sampling error.

**Note**: biopsy the **contralateral** weak muscle (after abnormal EMG) to avoid artefacts in histology due to EMG needle trauma.

## Management

- Myositis—oral corticosteroids, ± methotrexate, ± azathioprine.
- Dysphagia, cardiac involvement, alveolitis—pulsed methylprednisolone, ± intravenous gammaglobulin, ± treatments for vasculitis.
- Rash—hydroxychloroquine, topical corticosteroids.
- Osteoporosis and gastric protection therapies also.

## Prognosis

Variable illness course. Most commonly slowly progressive, but occasionally either fluctuating with spontaneous remissions and relapses, or rapidly deteriorating. Treatment can achieve a cure in 50%.

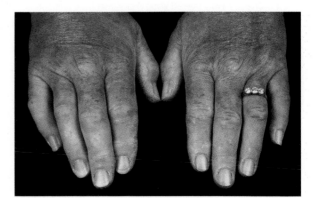

Fig. 19.28 Gottron papules in dermatomyositis: purple rash on the hands, especially the knuckles. Ragged cuticles and nail-fold telangiectasia may also be present. The purple rash is often referred to as 'heliotrope', after the colour of the flowers of the shrub *Heliotropium*.

# 19.14 Sjögren syndrome

## Background

A chronic autoimmune disease primarily affecting the exocrine glands. May be either primary Sjögren syndrome (SS) or secondary to other autoimmune diseases (RA, SLE).

## Epidemiology

- Prevalence: 3–4% of adult population.
- ♀:♂ ratio 9:1.
- Peak age of onset 40–50 years of age.

## Clinical evaluation

### History

- Ocular involvement (95%)—burning, gritty sensation under eyelids.
- Oropharyngeal involvement (90%)—difficulty swallowing dry food, dry mouth, increase in dental caries.
- Other symptoms—vaginal dryness, hoarseness. Arthritis (50%), Raynaud phenomenon (35%).

### Examination

- Parotid gland enlargement (45%), mononeuritis multiplex, isolated cranial nerve neuropathy.
- Lymphoproliferative disease (see Box 19.18).
- Pulmonary fibrosis, vasculitic skin rash.

## Investigations

- Blood investigations—ESR elevated, normal CRP. Leucopenia, hypergammaglobulinaemia (80%) in 1° SS.

---

**Box 19.18 Lymphoproliferative disease and Sjögren syndrome**

- Patients with 1° SS have a 44× higher risk of developing lymphoma.
- Most lymphomas are of B-cell origin.
- The disease location is mainly extranodal and in salivary glands in 55% of cases.
- Risk factors for lymphoma:
  - Persistent, painful parotid gland enlargement.
  - Splenomegaly and lymphadenopathy.
  - Type II mixed cryoglobulinaemia.
  - Persistent active disease: vasculitis, neuropathy, fever, anaemia, lymphopenia.
- In such situations, a biopsy may be warranted.
- Patients should be routinely asked about fever, weight loss, and night sweats.

---

- Autoantibodies—RF (60%), ANA (90%), anti-Ro (60%), anti-La (40%) in SS.
- Schirmer test—Fig. 19.29.
- Sialometry—unstimulated whole salivary flow rate measurement involves collecting saliva over 15 minutes. A volume <1.5mL is considered abnormal.
- Minor salivary gland biopsy—cornerstone in diagnosis of SS, e.g. lip.
- The following are occasional investigations for diagnosis of SS:
  - Rose Bengal staining—demonstrates damaged corneal epithelium.
  - Sialography—may show sialectasis.
  - Scintigraphy—a functional evaluation of all salivary glands.

## Management

- Dry eyes—artificial tears. Smoking and drugs with anticholinergic side effects should be avoided. May benefit from lateral tarsorrhaphy
- Dry mouth—stimulation of saliva production with sugar-free lozenges. Good oral hygiene to avoid dental caries. Artificial saliva or pilocarpine in severe cases. Regular dental review.
- Vaginal dryness—lubricant jellies.
- Arthralgia/rash—hydroxychloroquine.
- Interstitial lung disease, vasculitis—see Section 19.19.

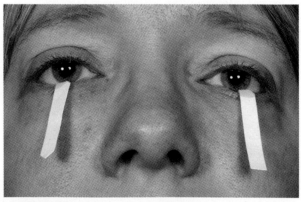

**Fig. 19.29** Schirmer test:
1. Bend the Schirmer test strip at the indentation and place it under the lower eyelid.
2. Leave test strip in place for 5 minutes.
3. Measure how much of the test strip is wet from the indentation.
4. A healthy person wets 15mm or more after 5 minutes. A positive test occurs when <5mm is wet.

# 19.15 Giant cell arteritis/polymyalgia rheumatica

## Background

**Giant cell arteritis** (GCA) is a granulomatous arteritis of the aorta and its major branches frequently involving the temporal arteries. **Polymyalgia rheumatica** (PMR) is an inflammatory disease with periarticular bursitis and synovitis in proximal joints which is closely associated with GCA.

## Epidemiology

- Most GCA reports originate from Northern Europe and USA. Although it occurs worldwide, it affects mainly Caucasians.
- PMR and GCA affect the elderly and are rare in patients younger than 50 years. Mean age of onset is ~70 years.
- PMR has a prevalence of 1 per 1000 people aged over 50 years.
- ♀:♂ ratio 2:1.
- 50% of GCA patients have symptoms of PMR while 20% of PMR patients also have a diagnosis of GCA.
- Positive temporal biopsies for GCA are also found in 10–15% of PMR cases who have no symptoms or signs of GCA.

## Aetiology

- Unknown cause. Studies linking infection with PMR and GCA have been inconclusive.
- GCA is associated with HLA-DRB1*04.
- Predominance of CD4 T cells in arteritic lesions with clonal expansion suggests an antigen-driven disease.

## Clinical evaluation

General symptoms such as fever, fatigue, weight loss, and depression are present in the majority of patients (see Boxes 19.19 and 19.20 for diagnostic criteria).

### History and examination (GCA)

- Headache/scalp tenderness ('pain on brushing/washing hair')— occurs in 70% of patients and often localizes around temporal or occipital regions.
- Visual disturbance—in 25–30% of cases (amaurosis fugax, blurred vision, transient or permanent blindness). Most common lesion is anterior ischaemic optic neuropathy.
- Jaw claudication—in 67% of cases ('pain on chewing food'), tongue pain, and ischaemia (lingual artery).

> **Box 19.19  American College of Rheumatology criteria for GCA**
>
> 1. Age of onset >50 years.
> 2. New headache.
> 3. Temporal artery tenderness or decreased pulsation.
> 4. ESR >50mm/hour.
> 5. Temporal artery biopsy showing vasculitis characterized by mononuclear cell infiltration or granulomatous infiltration.
> Diagnosis requires three out of five criteria.
>   Sensitivity 94% and specificity 91%.
> Reproduced from Hunder GG et al. 'The American College of Rheumatology 1990 criteria for the classification of giant cell arteritis', *Arthritis and Rheumatology*, 33, pp. 1122–1128, copyright 1990, with permission from American College of Rheumatology.

> **Box 19.20  Bird et al. criteria for PMR**
>
> 1. Age > 65 years
> 2. ESR > 40mm/hr
> 3. Bilateral upper arm tenderness
> 4. Morning stiffness >1 hour
> 5. Onset of illness within 2 weeks
> 6. Depression or weight loss, or both
> Diagnosis requires three of the seven listed features.
>   Sensitivity 92% and specificity 80%.
> Reproduced from *Annals of the Rheumatic Diseases*, H A Bird, W Esselinckx, A S Dixon, A G Mowat, P H Wood, 38, Copyright 1979, with permission from BMJ Publishing Group Ltd.

- Less common features—stroke, myocardial ischaemia, limb claudication.
- Large vessel vasculitis—in 10–15% of cases. May present as limb ischaemia, bruits over large arteries, tenderness, or aortic dissection.

### History and examination (PMR)

- Symptoms are usually bilateral and symmetric.
- Proximal pain in the shoulders, neck, and pelvic girdles.
- Early morning stiffness in proximal joints.
- Signs of subacromial bursitis (restricted shoulder abduction).
- Distal synovitis—usually transient and non-erosive.
- See Box 19.21 for differential diagnosis of PMR.

### Investigations

- FBC—anaemia of chronic disease.
- LFTs—elevated ALP with active PMR.
- Inflammatory markers—ESR and CRP are often markedly elevated in active disease (ESR >100mm/hour (Box 19.22); consider if >40mm/hour).
- Temporal artery biopsy:
  - Useful for confirming diagnosis.
  - Skip lesions—occur in 67% of biopsies. False negatives are found in 9–45% of biopsies.

> **Box 19.21  Differential diagnosis for PMR**
>
> - RA
> - SLE
> - OA
> - Spondyloarthritis
> - Inflammatory myopathy
> - Hypo/hyperthyroidism
> - Neoplastic disease including myeloma
> - Bilateral shoulder capsulitis
> - Parkinsonism
> - Sepsis.

> **Box 19.22  Causes of an ESR >100mm/hour**
>
> - GCA/PMR
> - Multiple myeloma
> - Sepsis
> - Occult malignancy
> - SLE.

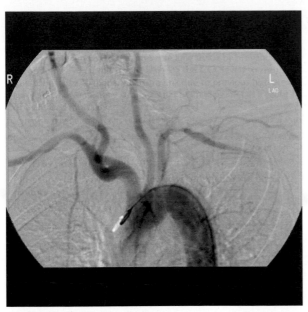

**Fig. 19.30** Angiogram showing left subclavian artery stenosis due to giant cell arteritis. Note the collateral vessels.

- Biopsy most useful within 24 hours of starting steroids—however, do **not** delay treatment for sake of biopsy.
- Negative biopsy result does **not** exclude GCA.
- Usually performed by ophthalmologists or vascular surgeons—local practices vary.
- Newer diagnostic tools:
  - Colour Doppler ultrasound—of temporal arteries.
  - MR angiogram—for large vessels (Fig. 19.30).
  - 18-FDG-PET scanning—for large vessel involvement (Fig. 19.31).

## Management

Rapid initiation of steroid therapy is vital in GCA to prevent blindness—start treatment *then* arrange biopsy.
- Corticosteroids:
  - Oral prednisolone remains the mainstay of treatment.
  - Dramatic response within 24 hours.
  - Patients usually need steroids for at least 1–2 years.
    - Initial dose varies:
    - 60mg once daily in GCA with visual symptoms.
    - 40mg once daily in GCA without visual involvement.
    - 10–15mg once daily in PMR.
- Dose tapering (see Box 19.23):
  - Start to reduce high doses in GCA after 4 weeks; aim for <10mg/day by 1 year.
  - Gradually reduce dose in PMR, i.e. by 1mg/month.
  - Clinical response and inflammatory markers should be used to guide treatment.
  - Methylprednisolone (MP)—trial of regular intramuscular MP for PMR showed reduced adverse effects (Dasgupta et al., 1998). Intravenous MP also used in GCA and impending visual loss.

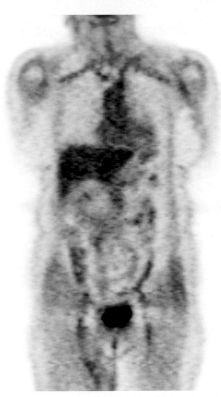

**Fig. 19.31** PET scan showing inflammation in all large vessels due to giant cell arteritis.

> ### Box 19.23 Relapse during/after treatment
>
> - Mainly clinical diagnosis.
> - Increased ESR, CRP—but not always.
> - Relapse usually occurs due to rapid tapering of steroids.
> - Prednisolone should be increased to the dose used before relapse or higher and tapered at a slower rate thereafter (e.g. reduce prednisolone by 0.5–1mg every 4–8 weeks when <10mg once daily).

- Methotrexate/azathioprine—useful for steroid-sparing effects in prolonged steroid use.
- Aspirin—reduces cerebral ischaemia in GCA.
- Bone prophylaxis—osteoporosis risk assessment needed and calcium and vitamin D supplementation as a minimum—consider a bisphosphonate.
- Gastroprotection—proton-pump inhibitors with high-dose oral steroid doses.
- Newer therapies—anecdotal reports involving successful anti-TNFα and rituximab use in steroid-resistant cases.

## Reference

Dasgupta B, Dolan AL, Panayi GS, *et al*. An initially double-blind controlled 96 week trial of depot methylprednisolone against oral prednisolone in the treatment of PMR. *Br J Rheumatol* 1998; 37(2): 189–95.

# 19.16 Polyarteritis nodosa

## Background

Polyarteritis nodosa (PAN) is a necrotizing inflammation of medium or small arteries with a predilection for microaneurysms without glomerulonephritis or vasculitis in arterioles, capillaries, or venules.

## Epidemiology

- Incidence: 2.4/million people in the UK.
- ♀:♂ ratio 1:2.
- Peak age of onset: 40–60 years.
- The prevalence of PAN reflects that of hepatitis B in the population although the exact link is not understood.

## Clinical features

- Spectrum of disease ranging from limited disease (single organ involvement) to progressive systemic disease.
- Non-specific symptoms—most patients experience fever, malaise, weight loss, and myalgia.
- Cutaneous lesions (25–60% of patients)—palpable purpura, infarctions, livedo reticularis, ischaemia of distal digits.
- Musculoskeletal—arthralgia/arthritis and myalgias occur in 50% of cases each. May also present like polymyalgia rheumatica.
- Mononeuritis multiplex or peripheral neuropathy in 70% of cases.
- Renal—in PAN, there is no glomerulonephritis. Vascular nephropathy and renal infarctions are the usual renal lesions.

- Gastrointestinal—involvement of the gastrointestinal tract, abnormal liver enzymes, mesenteric thrombosis. Rarely localized appendiceal or gallbladder involvement.
- Other systems—orchitis, temporal arteritis.

## Investigations

- Blood results—elevated ESR, CRP. Anaemia of chronic disease and thrombocytosis.
- Hepatitis B serology—hepatitis B surface antigen is found in 7–54% cases. Associated with gastrointestinal involvement.
- Mesenteric angiography—mesenteric microaneurysms occur in 60% of cases, mostly at the coeliac and renal arteries.
- Biopsy—of abdominal viscera or affected tissue may show the presence of granulocytes and mononuclear leucocytes in the arterial wall.

## Treatment

- No visceral organ involvement (except gallbladder or appendix)—corticosteroids.
- Rapidly progressive disease or organ involvement—see Section 19.19.
- Hepatitis B positive cases—must be identified before immuno-suppressive therapy. Antiviral therapy (interferon-alpha) should be given.

# 19.17 Churg–Strauss syndrome (eosinophilic granulomatosis with polyangiitis)

## Background

Eosinophilic granulomatosis with polyangiitis (EGPA) is an eosinophil-rich and granulomatous inflammatory disorder involving the respiratory tract with necrotizing vasculitis affecting small to medium-sized vessels. It is also associated with asthma and blood eosinophilia.

## Epidemiology

- Incidence: 3.1/million adults in the UK.
- ♀:♂ ratio 1:1.
- Age of onset: 10–75 years (mean 40 years).

## Clinical features

- Asthma usually precedes the systemic features for many years and is unusual in EGPA in that it begins late in life. Associated with rhinitis and nasal polyps.
- Pulmonary—pulmonary infiltrates in 60–80% of cases.
- Skin—cutaneous lesions including purpura, nodules, occur in 70% of cases.
- Neurological—mononeuritis multiplex in 60–80% of patients, peripheral neuropathy (frequently painful).
- Cardiomyopathy—major cause of mortality.
- Renal—focal segmental glomerulonephritis in 20–50% of cases.
- Others—mesenteric vasculitis, gastrointestinal bleeding, polyarthralgia, myalgia.

## Investigations

- Blood results—eosinophilia (> 1 × 10⁹/L), elevated IgE, ESR. pANCA and anti-MPO are positive in 70% of cases.
- Radiology—CT chest or CXR may demonstrate pulmonary infiltration (in 30–80%), pleural effusion.
- Biopsy—of sural nerve, muscle, lung, or renal tissue may show an eosinophilic rich granulomatous vasculitis.

## Treatment

- Corticosteroids—remains first-line treatment for CSS, either oral or as pulsed intravenous therapy in severe systemic vasculitis.
- Cyclophosphamide—indicated in severe organ involvement. See Treating Systemic Vascullitis.
- Prognosis—is associated with cumulative organ involvement (eg. renal insuffiency, cardiomyopathy, CNS and GI involvement) and may guide choice of treatments (Guillevin et al. 1996).

## Reference

Guillevin L, Lhote F, Casassus P, et al. Prognostic factors in polyarteritis nodosa and Churg–Strauss syndrome. A prospective study in 342 patients. *Medicine* 1996; 75: 17–28.

# 19.18 Granulomatosis with polyangiitis (Wegener)

## Background

Granulomatosis with polyangiitis (GPA) is a granulomatous inflammatory disorder of the respiratory tract with necrotizing vasculitis affecting small to medium-sized vessels including glomerulonephritis.

## Epidemiology

- Incidence: 9 per million people in the UK.
- ♀:♂ ratio 1:1 (slight ♂ predominance).
- Peak age of onset: 40–50 years.

## Clinical features

- Classic triad of upper airway, lung, and renal disease is often described. GPA should be suspected in all cases of persistent otitis, rhinitis, or sinusitis; destructive upper respiratory tract changes or severe glomerulonephritis.
- Upper respiratory tract/ears (>90% of cases)—rhinitis, epistaxis, persistent crusting, 'saddle nose deformity'. Sinusitis; both conductive (middle ear involvement) and sensorineural hearing loss may occur. Subglottic stenosis may present as hoarseness, stridor.
- Eyes—retro-orbital mass leading to proptosis; necrotizing scleritis, episcleritis, keratitis.
- Lung—pulmonary nodules, fleeting infiltrates, alveolar haemorrhage.
- Renal (80% show renal involvement)—rapidly progressive glomerulonephritis.
- Others—arthralgias/non-destructive arthritis in 50% cases. Mononeuritis multiplex or polyneuropathy in 30% of cases.
- Limited GPA—this is a subgroup of GPA that tends to involve the upper respiratory tract but does not involve the renal system. May mimic granulomatous infections, malignancy, or illicit drug use.

## Investigations

- Blood results—elevated ESR, CRP. Normochromic, normocytic anaemia, leucocytosis.
- Urinalysis and urine microscopy for cellular casts (active urine sediment), assessment of proteinuria.
- U&E.
- cANCA with positive anti-proteinase-3 antibodies is highly specific (98%) for GPA. Found in 90% of generalized GPA and 60% of limited GPA. Titres may correlate with disease activity in some patients (serial measurements over time).

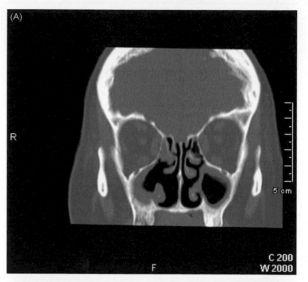

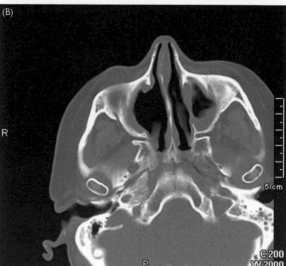

**Fig. 19.32** CT (A and B) sinus showing inflamed mucosa in granulomatosis with polyangiitis (Wegener) and loss of the medial wall of the right maxillary sinus.

- CT sinus and orbits—demonstrate sinus involvement (Fig. 19.32).
- CXR—may show cavitating lung lesions (Fig. 19.33).
- Biopsy—sinus/nasal mucosa, renal, lung.

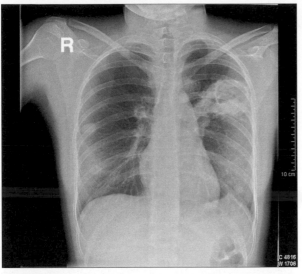

**Fig. 19.33** CXR showing left lung cavity in granulomatosis with polyangiitis (Wegener).

## Treatment

- See Section 19.19.
- Co-trimoxazole (trimethoprim/sulfamethoxazole)—to treat chronic nasal bacterial carriage and thus reduce upper airway flares of disease.

## Background

The treatment of vasculitis is dependent on the type of vasculitis (e.g. large or small vessel), organ involvement (particularly renal), and disease activity:

- Corticosteroids—play a critical role in the management of almost all forms of vasculitis as a lone agent as well as part of a combination treatment.
- Large vessel vasculitides (e.g. GCA, Takayasu arteritis)—corticosteroids remains the primary treatment. Methotrexate, azathioprine, and leflunomide can be used to help reduce the total dose of corticosteroids (EULAR, 2009a).
- Small and medium vessel vasculitides (e.g. ANCA-associated vasculitis (AASV): GPA, MPA, EGPA), inflammatory lung disease, and lupus nephritis—the combination of cyclophosphamide and corticosteroids has revolutionized the treatment of these life-threatening diseases (EULAR, 2009b).
- The principle behind treating severe vasculitides involves initial **remission induction** followed by long-term **remission maintenance**.

## Remission induction

- The National Institutes of Health (NIH) regimen of cyclophosphamide and corticosteroids has been the gold standard for induction.
- Use of oral cyclophosphamide was associated with a high incidence of infections, urothelial malignancies, haemorrhagic cystitis, and infertility. As a result, IV pulsed cyclophosphamide is increasingly used to lower the cumulative dose.
- The CYCLOPS trial was designed to compare the efficacy and toxicity of pulsed IV vs. oral cyclophosphamide and they were found to be equally effective with less side effects and lower cumulative doses with IV cyclophosphamide (de Groot et al., 2009). Recommended regimen:
  - IV cyclophosphamide (15mg/kg, or less if in renal failure or elderly, maximum 1.2g) initially 2-weekly for three doses and 3-weekly for further seven doses (i.e. total 6 months).
  - Oral prednisolone (1mg/kg/day initially) to be reduced progressively to maintenance of 5mg once daily.
- Anti-emetics and mesna should be administered with above regimen to prevent nausea and haemorrhagic cystitis.
- Co-trimoxazole (trimethoprim/sulfamethoxazole) 480mg twice a day may be given three times a week for *Pneumocystis jirovecii* prophylaxis and bisphosphonates for osteoporosis risk reduction.

- Rituximab—the RITUXVAS trial has shown rituximab to be equally effective as cyclophosphamide in remission induction for AASV (Jones et al., 2010).
- Methotrexate—in the NORAM trial, methotrexate has been shown to be as effective as cyclophosphamide in the treatment of early AASV without critical organ involvement (de Groot et al., 2005).
- Plasma exchange—useful in severe renal vasculitis (MEPEX trial) or pulmonary haemorrhage.

## Remission maintenance

Following remission induction, low-dose corticosteroids are continued and cyclophosphamide replaced with the following drugs for maintenance of remission:

- Azathioprine (2mg/kg/day)—has been shown to be effective for AASV in the CYCAZAREM trial (Jayne et al., 2003).
- Methotrexate—effective in case series and open label studies.
- Mycophenolate mofetil (2g/day)—the IMPROVE trial concluded that among patients with AAV, mycophenolate mofetil was less effective than azathioprine for maintaining disease remission. Both treatments had similar adverse event rates. However, this drug may still have a role in azathioprine intolerance or failure.

## References

de Groot K, Harper L, Jayne DR, et al. Pulse versus daily oral cyclophosphamide for induction of remission in antineutrophil cytoplasmic antibody-associated vasculitis: a randomized trial. *Ann Intern Med* 2009; 150(10): 670–80.

de Groot K, Rasmussen N, Bacon PA, et al. Randomized trial of cyclophosphamide versus methotrexate for induction of remission in early systemic antineutrophil cytoplasmic antibody-associated vasculitis. *Arthritis Rheum* 2005; 52(8): 2461–9.

EULAR recommendations for the management of large vessel vasculitis. *Ann Rheum Dis* 2009; 68: 318–23.

EULAR recommendations for the management of primary small and medium vessel vasculitis. *Ann Rheum Dis* 2009; 68: 310–17.

Jayne D, Rasmussen N, Andrassy K, et al. A randomized trial of maintenance therapy for vasculitis associated with antineutrophil cytoplasmic autoantibodies. *N Engl J Med* 2003; 349(1): 36–44.

Jones RB, Tervaert JW, Hauser T, et al. Rituximab versus cyclophosphamide in ANCA-associated renal vasculitis. *N Engl J Med* 2010; 363(3): 211–20.

# 19.20 Relapsing polychondritis

## Background

Rare autoimmune disease producing inflammation in cartilaginous structures throughout the body.

## Epidemiology

- Incidence: 3.5 per million population (USA).
- ♀:♂ ratio 1:1.
- Peak age of onset: 40–50 years.
- 30% associated with autoimmune/haematological disorder.

### Associated conditions

- Rheumatoid arthritis
- Myelodysplasia
- Ankylosing spondylitis
- Rheumatoid arthritis
- Lymphoma
- Eosinophilic granulomatosis with polyangiitis
- Behçet disease
- Granulomatosis with polyangiitis (Wegener)
- Polyarteritis nodosa
- Systemic lupus erythematosus
- Inflammatory bowel disease.

## Clinical features

- Ear involvement in 80%:
  - Acute unilateral or bilateral auricular chondritis (Fig. 19.34).
- Hearing loss in 30%—conductive or neurosensory (due to vasculitis).
- Saddle-nose deformity in 30%.
- Tracheobronchial tree involvement—localized or diffuse obstruction due to cartilage ring damage.
- Arthritis in 70%—non-deforming, non-erosive, asymmetric oligo- or polyarticular arthritis.
- Ocular involvement in 50%—episcleritis, scleritis, and periorbital oedema.
- Cardiac involvement—aortitis, valvular incompetence.

## Investigations

- Blood—elevated ESR, leucocytes, platelets. Anaemia.
- Anti-cartilage antibodies (to type II collagen) found in 50% of cases during a disease flare.
- Autoimmune serology—for associated conditions.
- Biopsy of auricular chondritis rarely needed to confirm diagnosis, occasionally required to exclude infection.
- Lung function test (flow–volume loop)—**essential** to exclude laryngotracheal involvement.
- MRI of laryngotracheal tree—inflammation, fibrosis.

## Management

- Corticosteroids.
- Steroid-sparing agents, e.g. dapsone, azathioprine.
- Nasal CPAP/tracheostomy may be required in laryngotracheal involvement.

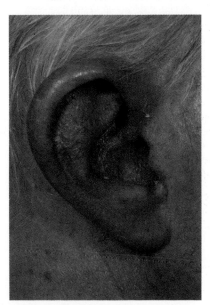

Fig. 19.34 Auricular chondritis: inflamed pinna but sparing of earlobe.

# 19.21 Behçet disease

## Background

A systemic vasculitis of unknown cause involving both veins and arteries.

## Epidemiology

- Most common in Mediterranean, Turkey, Iran, and Japan.
- ♂:♀ ratio 2:1, with more severe disease in young men.
- Peak age of onset: 30–45 years of age.
- HLA-B51 association: mainly in Japan and Turkey.

## Clinical features

- Skin and mucosal involvement:
  - Recurrent oral ulceration occurs (>90%).
  - Genital ulceration (85%) including the scrotum or labia with scarring.
  - Erythema nodosum, acneiform, or vasculitic rash, and pathergy reaction.
- Eye involvement (50%)—bilateral recurrent pan-uveitis is a major complication. Associated with retinal vasculitis
- Musculoskeletal (50%)—non-erosive oligoarthritis.
- Venous/arterial involvement (35%):
  - Thrombophlebitis, DVT, Budd–Chiari syndrome. Embolism is rare.
  - Aneurysms or occlusion anywhere in arterial tree.
- CNS involvement (5%)—usually brainstem (pyramidal and cerebellar signs). Psychiatric symptoms, dural sinus thrombosis, peripheral neuropathy.
- GI—common in Japan, rare in the Mediterranean. Mucosal ulceration, bowel perforation.

826

---

Box 19.24 Pathergy test—pustular reaction to sterile subcutaneous puncture

1. Use a 20–22G sterile needle, puncture skin obliquely to a depth of 5mm and read at 48 hours.
2. An erythematous papule/sterile pustule >2mm at the trauma site after 48 hours = positive test result:
   - Due to neutrophil accumulation along needle track.
   - Common finding in those from Japan and Turkey but rare in Northern Europe and USA.
   - May also be positive in those with:
     - Pyoderma gangrenosum.
     - Hairy cell leukaemia, non-Hodgkin lymphoma.
     - Chronic myeloid leukaemia treated with interferon-alpha.

## Investigations

- Diagnosis is mainly based on clinical findings:
  - Recurrent oral ulcers (three or more times per year).
  - Two or more of: recurrent genital ulcers, ocular lesions, skin lesions positive pathergy test (Box 19.24).
- Blood tests—non-specific results. May show elevated ESR, CRP, leucocytosis, or anaemia.

## Management

- Topical steroids /colchicine for mucocutaneous and joint involvement.
- Thalidomide in resistant orogenital ulceration.
- Prednisolone/azathioprine/sulphasalazine/cyclophosphamide—for severe disease and DVT (+ anticoagulation).
- Anti-TNFα—some success in resistant cases.

# Chapter 20

## Epidemiology and evidence-based medicine

# 20.1 Introduction

## Introduction to chapter

The first step to any research study is stating the problem, and answering the question 'What is the main purpose of the study?'. This question may be based on clinical expertise, gaps in the literature, or an extension of ongoing or previous research. The characteristics of a good research question are that it is relevant, original, answerable, clear and simple, and manageable in terms of time and cost.

Once the main research question is a fully formed, clearly stated research question, the primary outcome measure needs to be determined. The primary outcome measure will either be qualitative or quantitative, and this in turn will determine what statistical analysis should be undertaken. Another important consideration for statistical analysis is the study design. The following section in this chapter will discuss the main types of study, and the advantages and disadvantages of each. The next section will outline the main types of data and ways to describe the data. This will be followed by a section on analysis for estimation from samples to populations. Separate sections will follow with an introduction to regression, odds ratios and relative risk, survival analysis, sample size calculations, diagnostic tests, and meta-analysis. The final section will discuss how to read a paper from a statistical point of view

# 20.2 Study design

## Types of study

This section will discuss the main types of study design. There are two types of study: observational and experimental.

### Observational studies

These are studies where the investigator does not intervene. The goal is to observe. Observational designs vary from weak studies like descriptive or ecological studies, to stronger study designs like case–control and cohort studies.

### Experimental studies

These are where the investigator has control over the experiment and the participants are allocated to a group. These studies tend to be trials, whereby participants are randomly allocated to a treatment/intervention or to a control group.

## Definitions of common study designs

The following will outline the most common study designs. Fig. 20.1 shows the timeline for each study design.

### Case report

A description of a single case which displays interesting features. This is used to generate ideas and raise questions, rather than to answer them.

### Case series

A case series is a description of a series of cases, usually consecutive cases of a condition in one place. This is usually descriptive.

### Cohort studies

A cohort study is an observational study in which participants are identified and followed up over time. The selection of the participants occurs at the point of entry—the cohort. Selection is usually based upon demographic criteria or exposure to an environmental or medical event. This design may be used to investigate the causes of disease or the prognosis of people who have a disease.

### Case–control studies

A case–control study is an observational study in which the cases are compared with controls. The cases and controls may be matched for factors other than that under investigation, e.g. age and sex. The selection of participants is usually based upon the presence of a certain condition, outcome, or medical endpoint. This can be epidemiological, where we look back at possible causes of the disease, or clinical, where we look now at features of the disease.

### Cross-sectional study

A cross-sectional study is an observational study which occurs where a population or sample of participants is studied at a particular point in time, such as a sample survey or a prevalence study. Studies of observer variation and measurement error are usually of this type. It may be descriptive or analytical. This may be in the form of a retrospective observational study.

### Ecological study

This is an observational design where each observation is a community of people, such as a city or a country. For example, we might ask whether infant mortality for a country is related to the proportion of mothers who breastfed exclusively in the first 3 months.

### Randomized controlled trial

This is an experimental study. Different treatments are given to participants and the effects compared. This is the design for testing new treatments for a disease. There are two types of controlled trial: parallel and crossover.

The most common design is the parallel design. This is where participants are randomized so that the groups are comparable at the beginning of the study. There may be two groups or several groups. There is generally a control group who receive no treatment/intervention, a placebo (an inactive treatment/intervention that will not improve the condition under study), or current standard treatment. This enables the effects of the treatment/intervention to be compared with the control group.

In a crossover design, participants are randomly allocated to the intervention or control group. Then at a certain time point in the study they are crossed over into the other group. The participants then acts as their own control.

In a cluster randomized trial, groups of participants, such as primary care practices, are allocated to a treatment together.

More complex designs may incorporate features of more than one of these designs, e.g. nested case–control study within a cohort study.

## Advantages and disadvantages of each type of study design

Table 20.1 outlines the advantages and disadvantages of the different types of study design (Centre for Evidence-Based Medicine, 2007). It should be noted that case studies and case series are to ask questions rather than answer them, so there is usually little problem with these limited studies.

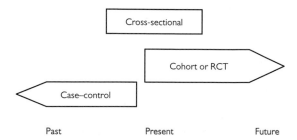

**Fig. 20.1** Study designs and time.

**Table 20.1** Advantages and disadvantages of the common study designs

| Study type | Advantages | Disadvantages |
|---|---|---|
| Cohort study | • Ethically safe | • Exposure may be linked to a hidden confounder |
| | • Eligibility criteria and outcome assessments can be standardized | • Blinding is difficult |
| | | • Randomisation is not present |
| | | • For rare disease, large sample sizes or long follow-up |
| Case-control study | • Quick and cheap | • Reliance on recall or records to determine exposure status |
| | • Only feasible method for very rare disorders or those with long lag between exposure and outcome | • Confounders |
| | • Fewer participants needed than cross-sectional studies | • Selection of control groups is difficult |
| | | • Potential bias: recall, selection |
| Cross-sectional study | • Cheap and simple | • Establishes association at most, not causality |
| | • Ethically safe | • Recall bias susceptibility |
| | | • Confounders may be unequally distributed |
| | | • Group sizes may be unequal |
| Ecological study | • Can use readily available data | • Difficult to draw conclusions about relationships at the person level |
| Randomized controlled trial: Parallel design | • Unbiased distribution of confounders | • Expensive: time and money |
| | • Blinding more likely | • Volunteer bias; ethically problematic at times |
| | • Randomisation facilitates statistical analysis | |
| Randomized controlled trial: Cross-over design | • All participants serve as own controls and error variance is reduced thus reducing sample size needed<br>• All participants receive treatment (at least some of the time) | |
| | • Statistical tests assuming randomisation can be used | • All participants receive placebo or alternative treatment at some point |
| | • Blinding can be maintained | • Washout period lengthy or unknown |
| | | • Cannot be used for treatments with permanent effects |
| | | • No long-term follow-up |
| Randomized controlled trial: cluster randomized design | • Avoids contamination between treatment groups | • Must take clusters into account in the analysis |
| | • Can evaluate community level interventions | • Needs very large samples |

# Reference

Centre for Evidence-Based Medicine. *Study design*. Oxford: CEBM, 2007. Available at:<http://www.cebm.net/index.aspx?o=1039>

# 20.3 Types of data and descriptive statistics

## Background

In statistics, the term variable is used to mean a quality or quantity which varies from one member of a sample or population to another. Systolic blood pressure is a variable, which varies both from person to person and from measurement to measurement within the same person. Sex is a variable, people being either male or female.

It is useful to think of data as being of several different types, as the type of data is important in deciding which methods of presentation and analysis we should adopt. Data are summarized to help reveal information that they contain.

## Types of data

### Qualitative data

These arise when participants fall into separate classes, such as diagnosis or sex. A qualitative variable is also termed a nominal categorical variable or a classification variable.

### Quantitative data

These are numerical, arising from counts or measurements. Wound area is a quantitative variable, as is the length of time until the wound heals.

### Discrete data

These are observations where the values of the measurements can only take a few separate values, often integers, e.g. parity, the number of previous pregnancies which an expectant mother has had.

### Continuous data

These are observations where the values of the measurements can take any number in a range, e.g. wound area, height, or weight. Measurements are often made to within some degree of precision when reading off a scale so although there are many possible values, only a finite number can be recorded in a discrete way, e.g. height to the nearest centimetre. However, if the underlying variable is continuous, we can usually ignore the limitations introduced by practical measurement and treat the measurement as continuous.

### Main types of data

*Nominal*

These are observations where participants fall into separate categories. These categories have no numerical relationship between them. For example: sex: male, female; marital status: single, married, divorced, widowed; absence or presence of a disease; alive or dead.

*Ordinal*

These are observations where one can say that the observation for one participant exceeds that for another, but the size of the difference may not be meaningful. Generally ordinal data are derived from a scale or a subjective measure. For example: a visual analogue scale measuring pain; a quality of life score; a Likert scale measuring satisfaction.

*Interval*

These are observations the size of the difference between two observations is meaningful. Interval data can either be continuous or discrete.

## Histograms

A histogram is a graph showing a frequency distribution and is primarily used to summarize interval data. Fig. 20.2 shows a histogram of serum cholesterol (Markus et al., 1995). The variable 'serum cholesterol' in stroke patients is shown along the horizontal axis and the frequency on the vertical axis. Each interval has a rectangular bar

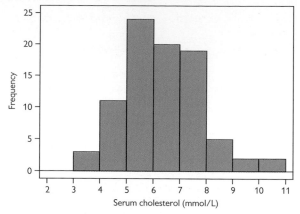

**Fig. 20.2** Histogram of serum cholesterol.

Data from Markus HS, Barley J, Lunt R, et al. Angiotensin-converting enzyme gene deletion polymorphism: a new risk factor for lacunar stroke but not carotid atheroma. *Stroke* 1995; 26: 1329–33.

over it, the height of which represents the frequency, the number of observations which fall in that interval.

Fig. 20.3 shows an other histogram for the same data. The interval width is 0.5 mmol/L, with the starting point changed from 3.0 to 3.25.

Although the frequencies are different, the shapes of the two histograms are similar. Both have low frequencies for small cholesterols, bigger frequencies as we move along the axis, peaking between 5 and 6, and then declining as cholesterol increases, with no observations beyond 11 mmol/L. As we shall see, it is the shape of the distribution which is important. However, Fig. 20.2 is more even than Fig. 20.3, which is quite 'bumpy' by comparison. This is because the intervals are smaller and so the frequencies in them are smaller, which makes them more prone to random fluctuations. It is usual to try to choose an interval size which makes the shape of the distribution most clear.

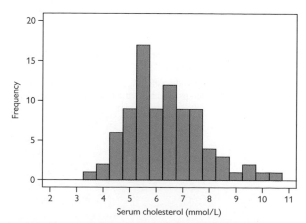

**Fig. 20.3** Histogram of serum cholesterol using a starting point of 3.25mmol/L.

Data from Markus HS, Barley J, Lunt R, et al. Angiotensin-converting enzyme gene deletion polymorphism: a new risk factor for lacunar stroke but not carotid atheroma. *Stroke* 1995; 26: 1329–33.

# Describing data

There are two ways to describe data (Table 20.2):
- Measures of central tendency to give a summary measure for the data.
- Measures of variability, which allow you to describe the variation in the data.

## Measures of central tendency (Fig. 20.4)

### Median

The central value where half the data points are less than or equal to it and half are greater than or equal to it. It is also referred to as the second quartile.

### Mean

The arithmetic mean (or average) is usually referred to as the mean. It is found by taking the sum of the observations and dividing by their number.

*Advantages of the mean over the median*

- The mean uses all the data equally, that is, each observation carries equal weight in its calculation. For the median, observations at the extremes have very little effect on the median and can be changed quite a lot without the median being changed.
- The mean uses the information more efficiently than the median and so it varies less from sample to sample than does the median.
- The mean has more convenient mathematical properties thus it is easier to compare the means of different groups than it is to compare the medians of different groups.

*Advantages of the median over the mean*

- The lack of effect of extreme observations on the median makes it preferable to the mean sometimes as a summary statistic to describe data, especially when there are extreme observations. The median is a very useful descriptive statistic, but not much used for other purposes.

## Measures of variability

### Range

The range is the simplest measurement of variability and is the difference between the smallest and largest observation. It is often presented as the lowest and highest observation, rather than the difference between them.

### Interquartile range

The interquartile range is the difference between the lower and upper quartile of the distribution:

- The first quartile is the value for which a quarter of the data points are less than or equal to it.
- The third quartile is the value for which a quarter of the data points are greater than or equal to it.
- The interquartile range is the difference between the first and third quartile. It is often presented as the first and third quartile, rather than the difference between them.

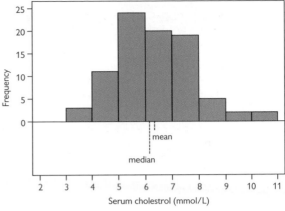

**Fig. 20.4** Histogram of serum cholesterol in stroke patients, showing position of median and mean.

Data from Markus HS, Barley J, Lunt R, et al. Angiotensin-converting enzyme gene deletion polymorphism: a new risk factor for lacunar stroke but not carotid atheroma. *Stroke* 1995; 26: 1329–33.

*Variance and standard deviation*

These both measure how far observations are from the mean of the distribution.

If we subtract the mean from each observation, we get a new set of numbers which we call the deviations from the mean. By adding the squares of these deviations we get a positive number which we call the sum of squares about the mean. We often abbreviate this to 'sum of squares'. This will be large for highly variable data and small for data with little variability.

**Variance**—the average squared difference from the mean—the sum of squares about the mean divided by the number of observations minus one.

**Standard deviation**—the square root of the variance, usually denoted by s or SD. This is quite a good descriptive statistic.

For most distributions:
- Usually about 2/3 of observations fall within one SD of mean.
- Usually about 95% fall within about two SD of mean.

For example, Fig. 20.5 shows the heights of women in the VenUS I trial (Nelson et al., 2004), with the positions of the mean, the mean ± one standard deviation, and the mean ± two standard deviation marked. About 2/3 of the observations lie within one standard deviation on either side of the mean (in fact, 65% here) and most of the heights appear to fall within two standard deviations of the

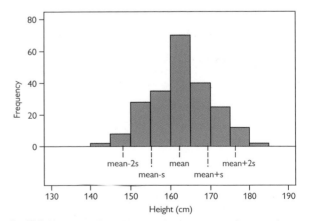

**Fig. 20.5** Histogram of female height showing position of mean and mean ± 2 standard deviations.

Data from Nelson EA, Iglesias CP, Cullum N, et al. Randomized clinical trial of four-layer and short-stretch compression bandages for venous leg ulcers (VenUS I). *Br J Surg* 2004; 91: 1292–9.

| Table 20.2 The appropriate measure of central tendency and variability, by study type | | |
|---|---|---|
| **Type of data** | **Measure of central tendency** | **Measure of variability** |
| Nominal | Number (%) | None |
| Ordinal | Median | Range<br>Interquartile range |
| Interval | Mean<br>Median | Range<br>Interquartile range<br>Variance<br>Standard deviation |

mean (in fact, 94% here). The mean minus two standard deviations is 148.1 cm, which is very close to the 2.5 centile, 148.6 cm. Similarly, the mean plus two standard deviations is 176.3 cm, very close to the 97.5 centile, which is 177.8 cm.

Variance and standard deviation use all the data equally, unlike ranges, and so use the data most efficiently. This is why we use them as our first choice methods of measuring variability.

## Skewness

The parts of the histogram at the far left and far right are called the tails. If one tail is roughly a mirror image of the other, then the distribution is symmetrical; if one tail is longer than the other then it is skew.

If the longer tail is:

- on the right, the distribution is skew to the right or positively skew,
- on the left, the distribution is skew to the left or negatively skew.

In a skew distribution the mean and the median will usually be different because the values in the tails affect the mean but not the median. Consequently a substantial difference between the median and mean is an indicator that there is skewness present.

If the distribution is:

- skew to the right, usually mean > median,
- skew to the left, usually median > mean.

Even in a positively skew distribution, we usually find that about 95% of observations are within two standard deviations from the mean, but the 5% outside the limits tend to be at the high end. The mean minus two standard deviations is therefore a negative number. If the variable cannot be negative then the upper tail must be longer than the lower. We can use this as a handy check for skewness in a published paper.

Fig. 20.6 shows a positively skew distribution, for the duration of venous leg ulcers prior to admission to the VenUS I trial (Nelson et al., 2004). Here the standard deviation, 14.0 months, is actually bigger than the mean, 9.4 months. The mean minus one standard deviation is therefore a negative number and no observations can be below it. The 87% observations within one standard deviation from the mean therefore include the smallest. There are 7% of observations more than two standard deviations above the mean.

These rules of thumb for skewness only work one way, e.g. the mean may exceed two standard deviations and the distribution may still be positively skew. Fig. 20.7 shows the same thing for the negatively skew gestational age (Brooke et al., 1989). This time the observations more than two standard deviations from the mean are nearly all small. Only 2

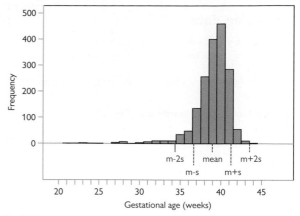

Fig. 20.7 Histogram of gestational age at birth showing position of mean and mean ± 2 standard deviations.

Data from Brooke OG, Anderson HR, Bland JM, Peacock JL, Stewart CM. Effects on birth weight of smoking, alcohol, caffeine, socioeconomic factors, and psychosocial stress. *British Medical Journal* 1989;298:795–801.

out of 1749 observations are more than two standard deviations above the mean.

To sum up, the majority of observations (usually about 2/3) are expected to be within one standard deviation from the mean. Almost all observations (usually about 95%) are expected to be within about two standard deviations from the mean, but those outside may all be at one end. This is often the case when the data are skewed.

## The Normal distribution

Many statistical methods are only valid if we can assume that our data follow a distribution of a particular type, called the Normal distribution. Many naturally occurring biological variables follow distributions which are very similar to the Normal. For example, Fig. 20.8 shows the distribution of birthweight in 1603 singleton term births (37 weeks' gestation or more) to Caucasian mothers at St George's Hospital, London, with the curve which represents the Normal distribution (Brooke et al., 1989). Fig. 20.9 shows a Normal distribution superimposed on the distribution of height in women with venous ulcers (Nelson et al., 2004).

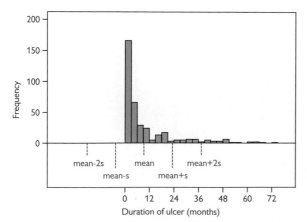

Fig. 20.6 Histogram of duration of venous ulcer showing position of mean and mean ± 2 standard deviations.

Data from Nelson EA, Iglesias CP, Cullum N, et al. Randomized clinical trial of four-layer and short-stretch compression bandages for venous leg ulcers (VenUS I). *Br J Surg* 2004; 91: 1292–9.

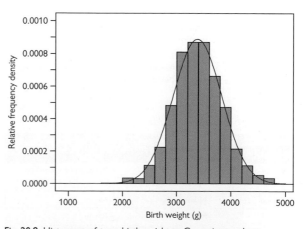

Fig. 20.8 Histogram of term birth weight to Caucasian mothers.

Data from Brooke OG, Anderson HR, Bland JM, Peacock JL, Stewart CM. Effects on birth weight of smoking, alcohol, caffeine, socioeconomic factors, and psychosocial stress. *British Medical Journal* 1989;298:795–801.

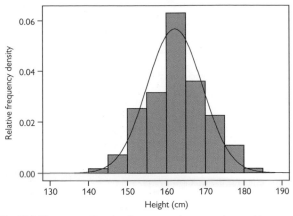

**Fig. 20.9** Histogram of height of women with venous ulcers, with corresponding Normal distribution curve.

Data from Nelson EA, Iglesias CP, Cullum N, et al. Randomized clinical trial of four-layer and short-stretch compression bandages for venous leg ulcers (VenUS I). *Br J Surg* 2004; 91: 1292–9.

The curves in Figs 20.8 and 20.9 have similar shapes, but they are not identical. In Fig. 20.8 the middle of the curve is at 3384 g and in Fig. 20.9 the middle of the curve is at 162.2 cm, for example. The Normal distribution is not just one distribution, but a family of distributions.

The Normal distribution is important because:
- Many natural variables follow it quite closely, certainly sufficiently closely for us to use statistical methods which require this.
- Even when we have a variable which does not follow a Normal distribution, if we then take the means of several samples of observations, such means will follow a Normal distribution.

For all Normal distributions, whatever the mean, variance, and standard deviation:
- 68% of observations lie within one standard deviation from the mean.
- 95% lie within 1.96 standard deviations from the mean.

Therefore if we can assume that our observations follow a Normal distribution, we can estimate the 95% range from the mean minus 1.96 standard deviations to the mean plus 1.96 standard deviations.

## References

Brooke OG, Anderson HR, Bland JM, et al. Effects on birth weight of smoking, alcohol, caffeine, socioeconomic factors, and psychosocial stress. *BMJ* 1989; 298: 795–801.

Markus HS, Barley J, Lunt R, et al. Angiotensin-converting enzyme gene deletion polymorphism: a new risk factor for lacunar stroke but not carotid atheroma. *Stroke* 1995; 26: 1329–33.

Nelson EA, Iglesias CP, Cullum N, et al. Randomized clinical trial of four-layer and short-stretch compression bandages for venous leg ulcers (VenUS I). *Br J Surg* 2004; 91: 1292–9.

## The sampling distribution

Most research data come from participants we think of as samples drawn from a larger population. The notion of sampling is familiar in healthcare. For example, we use the concentration of glucose in a pin-prick sample to give us an estimate for the blood in the entire body. The problem is that not all samples produce the same estimate. Multiple blood samples will give many, possibly differing measurements. They are all estimates of the same quantity, but we do not know whether any of them is exactly right. The estimates which we might obtain from all the possible samples drawn in the same way as ours have a distribution—the sampling distribution.

## Standard errors

Standard error is one measure used to describe how accurate an estimate is. The standard deviation of the sampling distribution tells us how accurate our sample statistic is as an estimate of the population value. This standard deviation is the standard error of the estimate and it tells us how variable estimates would be if obtained from other samples drawn in the same way as the one being considered.

Use the term:

- 'standard deviation'—when talking about distributions, either of a sample or a population,
- 'standard error'—when talking about an estimate found from a sample.

## Confidence intervals

Confidence intervals are another way to think about the closeness of estimates from samples to the quantity we wish to estimate. A confidence interval is a plausible range within which we are fairly confident that the true value lies.

Some, but not all, confidence intervals are calculated from standard errors. Confidence intervals are called 'interval estimates', because we estimate a range with a lower and an upper limit which we hope will contain the true values. An estimate which is a single number, such as the treatment difference we observed from a trial, is called a point estimate.

*Confidence interval calculation*

- It is not possible to calculate useful interval estimates which always contain the unknown population value.
- There is always a very small probability that a sample will be very extreme and contain a lot of either very small or very large observations.
- Therefore the aim is that most of the intervals calculated will contain the population value we want to estimate.
- For example, a 95% confidence interval is calculated so that 95% of intervals from such samples would contain the true population value.

Confidence intervals do not always include the population value. If 95% of 95% confidence intervals include it, it follows that 5% must exclude it. In practice, we cannot tell whether our confidence interval is one of the 95% or the 5%.

A trial compared elastic and inelastic bandages for the treatment of venous leg ulcers (Northeast et al., 1990).

Ulcer healing:

- 63% in the elastic bandage group.
- 50% in the inelastic bandage group.
- Estimated difference—13 percentage points.

Sampling distribution:

- Approximately Normal.
- Mean equal to the unknown population difference.
- Standard deviation equal to the standard error (estimated to be 10).

We know:

- 95% of observations from a Normal distribution are closer than 1.96 standard deviations to the mean.
- So 95% of possible samples will have their estimated difference closer than $1.96 \times 10$ percentage points to the unknown population mean.

If we estimate the unknown population value to be between the observed sample value $\pm$ 1.96 standard errors, then that range of values will include the population value for 95% of possible samples.

The 95% confidence interval is therefore between:

- $13 - 1.96 \times 10 = -7$, and
- $13 + 1.96 \times 10 = 33$ percentage points.

Hence we estimate that the true difference in the population lies between $-7$ and $+33$ percentage points.

## Significance tests

Significance tests provide a different way to draw conclusions from samples. The following sections will discuss each of the general principles of significance tests in detail (Box 20.1).

### Step 1: set up the hypotheses

To carry out a test of significance, suppose that, in the population, there would be no difference or no effect—the null hypothesis. This then is compared with the alternative hypothesis that there is a difference or effect.

For example, in a study comparing partnership caseload midwifery care with conventional team midwifery, the primary outcome measure was epidural rate (Benjamin et al., 2001). The null hypothesis is that there is no difference in the epidural rate between women given the partnership caseload midwifery care and women given the conventional team midwifery care. The alternative hypothesis is that there is a difference in the epidural rate.

### Step 2: choose the test and check assumptions

Choosing the statistical test to be used involves decisions about:

- the number of groups you want to compare,
- whether or not the groups are independent,
- the type of data,
- the distribution of the data.

Table 20.3 outlines the most commonly used statistical tests.

*Different types of data*

For interval data like height and weight, the measurements can be treated as actual numbers. Mean and standard deviation can be calculated. This is not the case for either nominal or ordinal data even if numerical codes (e.g. 1=male, 2=female) are used.

*Parametric/non-parametric tests*

- Parametric tests—assume the data are sampled from a particular form of distribution, such as a Normal distribution. Non-normal

---

**Box 20.1 General principles of significance tests**

1. Set up the null hypothesis and its alternative.
2. Choose the test and check any assumptions of the test.
3. Find the value of the test statistic and find the probability of a value of the test statistic arising which is as or more extreme than that observed, if the null hypothesis were true.
4. Conclude that the data are consistent or inconsistent with the null hypothesis.

| Table 20.3 Commonly used statistical tests | | |
|---|---|---|
| **Purpose of test** | **Data from a Normal distribution** | **Data from a non-Normal distribution** |
| Compares two independent samples | Two-sample (unpaired or independent) *t*-test | Mann–Whitney U test |
| Compares two sets of observations on a single sample | One-sample (paired) *t*-test | Wilcoxon matched pairs test, sign test |
| Compares three or more independent samples | One way analysis of variance (*F* test) using total sum of squares | Kruskal–Wallis analysis of variance by ranks |
| Compares three or more sets of observations made on a single sample | Two-way analysis of variance | Friedman two-way analysis of variance by ranks |
| Tests for presence of a straight line association between two continuous variables | Product moment correlation coefficient (Pearson *r*) | Spearman rank correlation coefficient ($\rho$), Kendall rank correlation coefficient ($\tau$) |
| **Purpose of test** | **Large sample** | **Sample of any size** |
| Tests for a relationship between two categorical variables | $\chi^2$ (chi-squared) test | Fisher exact test |

(skewed) data can sometimes be transformed to give a distribution which is approximately Normal in shape by performing some mathematical transformation (such as using the variable's logarithm, square root, or reciprocal). Some data, however, cannot be transformed to a Normal distribution.

- Non-parametric tests—no assumptions about the exact distribution sampled, but some tests have assumptions such as differences must have a symmetrical distribution.
- Parametric tests are generally more powerful than non-parametric ones when the assumptions of the parametric test are met.
- Some non-parametric tests look at the rank order of the values (which one is the smallest, which one comes next, and so on) and ignore the absolute differences between them.
- Statistical significance is more difficult to show with non-parametric tests.

Whether or not data are normally distributed determines what type of statistical tests to use. Transforming data to achieve a normal distribution is not cheating: it simply ensures that data values are given appropriate emphasis in assessing the overall effect. Using parametric tests to analyse non-normally distributed data can be misleading.

### Step 3: test statistic and p value

Whichever statistical test is used, a test statistic is calculated from the data which can then be used to test the null hypothesis. The test statistic is referred to a known distribution which it would follow if the null hypothesis were true. We find the probability of a value of the test statistic arising which is as or more extreme than that observed, if the null hypothesis were true.

In the same midwifery study (Benjamin et al., 2001), 20.1% of the women who had partnership caseload care had an epidural, compared to 31.8% of the women who had conventional team midwifery. A chi-squared test was used to compare the two groups. The probability of a difference as far as that observed from what would be expected if the null hypothesis were true was 0.001.

### Step 4: conclude that the data are consistent or inconsistent with the null hypothesis

If the significance test probability is small, we have observed something unlikely and the data are not consistent with the null hypothesis—the difference is said to be statistically significant.

*The p value*

- The probability of such an extreme value of the test statistic occurring if the null hypothesis were true.
- It indicates the probability that the result you got would happen if there were really no difference.
- It is **not** the probability that the null hypothesis is true. The null hypothesis is either true or it is not; it is not random and has no probability. The p value is the probability that, if the null

hypothesis were true, we would get data as far from expectation as those we observed.

In the midwifery study (Benjamin et al., 2001), the p value was 0.001. Hence, we can conclude that there is a statistically significance difference in the epidural rate between partnership caseload care and conventional team midwifery.

*How should we interpret the p value?*

Suppose we take a probability of 0.01 or less as constituting reasonable evidence against the null hypothesis. If the null hypothesis is true, we shall make a wrong decision one in a hundred times (Table 20.4).

- Deciding against a true null hypothesis is called an error of the first kind, type I error, or $\alpha$ (alpha) error.

Sometimes there is a difference in the population, but our sample will not produce a small enough probability for us to conclude that there is evidence for a difference in the population.

- Deciding in favour of a null hypothesis which is in fact false is called an error of the second kind, type II error, or $\beta$ (beta) error.

The smaller we demand the probability be before we decide against the null hypothesis:

- the larger the observed difference must be,
- the more likely we are to miss real differences,
- so by reducing the risk of a type I error we increase the risk of a type II error.

Conversely, allowing the critical probability to increase:

- reduces the risk of a type II error,
- but increases the risk of a type I error.

The conventional compromise is to say that differences are significant if the probability is less than 0.05. This is a reasonable guideline, but should not be taken as some kind of absolute demarcation. For some purposes, we might want to take a smaller probability as the critical one, usually 0.01. For example, in a major clinical trial we might think it is very important to avoid a type I error because after we have done the trial the preferred treatment will be adopted and it would be ethically impossible to replicate the trial. For other purposes, we might want to take a larger probability as the critical one, usually 0.1. For example, if we are screening possible new drugs for biological

| Table 20.4 p value interpretation | |
|---|---|
| **p value** | **Evidence for a difference or relationship** |
| Greater than 0.1 | Little or no evidence |
| Between 0.05 and 0.1 | Weak evidence |
| Between 0.01 and 0.05 (<0.05) | Evidence |
| Less than 0.01 (<0.01) | Strong evidence |
| Less than 0.001 (<0.001) | Very strong evidence |

activity, we might want to avoid type II errors, because potentially active compounds will receive more rigorous testing but those producing no significant biological activity will not be investigated further.

## Is the difference important?

If a difference is statistically significant, then it may well be real, but it is not necessarily important.

For example, the UK Prospective Diabetes Study Group compared atenolol and captopril in reducing the risk of complications in type 2 diabetes. 1148 hypertensive diabetic patients were randomized. The authors reported that 'captopril and atenolol were equally effective in reducing blood pressure to a mean of 144/83mmHg and 143/81mmHg respectively' (UKPDS, 1998). However, the difference in diastolic pressure was statistically significant, p= 0.02, despite being clinically unimportant.

Conversely just because a difference is not statistically significant, it does not mean that it is not real. We may simply have too small a sample to show that a difference exists. Furthermore, the difference may still be important.

*'Not significant' does not imply that there is no effect. It means that we have failed to demonstrate the existence of one.*

**Remember** that tests of significance will be wrong sometimes, with both type I and type II errors, and we must always be cautious in our interpretation.

## Significance tests and confidence intervals

Significance tests and confidence intervals often involve similar calculations and have a close relationship. Where a null hypothesis is about some population value, such as the difference between two means or two proportions, we can use the confidence interval as a test of significance. If the 95% confidence interval does not include the null hypothesis value, the difference is significant.

In the midwifery study (Benjamin et al., 2001), the difference between the epidural rates was 11.7%. The 95% confidence interval for the difference was 4.8% to 18.3%. The p value was 0.001.

For the difference between two proportions, the null hypothesis value is zero. Zero is not contained within the confidence interval and the difference is significant for this trial.

## Multiple significance tests

If we test a null hypothesis which is in fact true, using 0.05 as the critical significance level, the probability that we will come to a 'significant' conclusion (i.e. false) is 0.05. If we test 20 such true null hypotheses the probability that none will be significant is $0.95 \times 0.95 \times 0.95 \times \ldots \times 0.95$ twenty times, or $0.95^{20} = 0.36$. The probability of getting at least one significant result is therefore $1.00 - 0.36 = 0.64$. We are more likely to get one than not.

*Problem*

- When using 0.05 as the critical significance level, on average we will get one significant result, i.e. one type I error, every time we do 20 tests of null hypotheses which are true.

- If we go on testing long enough we can expect to find something which is 'significant', even when all the null hypotheses we test are true and there is nothing to find.

*Solution*

- One way (of many) to deal with the problem of many significance tests is the Bonferroni correction. We multiply all the P values by the number tests. If any of the tests is significant after this, the test of the overall composite null hypothesis is significant.

- Researchers sometimes panic about the problem of multiple testing and wonder whether they should apply the correction to all the tests in a paper, or to all the tests in all the papers they have ever written. There is no need for this and we should only use the correction when making more than one test of the same hypothesis, such as that two treatment groups differ.

## References

Benjamin P, Walsh D, Taub N. A comparison of partnership caseload midwifery care with conventional team midwifery care: labour and birth outcomes. *Midwifery* 2001; 17: 234–40.

Northeast ADR, Layer GT, Wilson NM, et al. Increased compression expedites venous ulcer healing. *Royal Society of Medicine Venous Forum* 1990. London: Royal Society of Medicine.

UKPDS Group. Efficacy of atenolol and captopril in reducing risk of macrovascular and microvascular complications in type 2 diabetes. *BMJ* 1998; 317: 713–20.

## 20.5 Relationships

## Background

This section will outline correlation, which is used to measure the strength of the relationship between quantitative variables. We give an overview of regression and multiple regression, which are methods for predicting one variable from another.

## The correlation coefficient

The correlation coefficient:

- is used to measure the **strength** of the relationship or association between two quantitative variables,
- is usually denoted by $r$,
- maximum value = 1.00; minimum value = –1.00,
- is positive when large values of one variable are associated with large values of the other,
- is negative when large values of one variable are associated with small values of the other,
- is also known as Pearson correlation coefficient and the product moment correlation coefficient.

There are other correlation coefficients as well, such as Spearman and Kendall, but if it is described simply as 'the correlation coefficient' or just 'the correlation', then Pearson is the one intended.

Fig. 20.10 shows a plot of strength against height (Hickish, 1989). This is a scatter diagram where each point represents one participant. It is fairly easy to see that taller men tend to be stronger than shorter men, or, looking at it the other way round, that stronger men tend to be taller than weaker men. It is only a tendency though, the tallest man is not the strongest nor is the shortest man the weakest. Correlation enables us to measure how close this association is. Here, $r = 0.42$. This is a positive correlation of fairly low strength.

Fig. 20.11 shows the correlations between several simulated variables. Each pair of variables was generated to have the correlation shown above it and the size of the correlation coefficient clearly reflects the degree of closeness on the scatter diagram. The first panel in Fig. 20.11 shows a perfect correlation ($r = +1.00$) where the points lie exactly on a straight line and we could calculate Y exactly from X. Other panels show varying degrees of both positive and negative correlation.

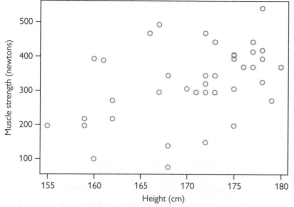

**Fig. 20.10** Scatter diagram showing muscle strength and height for 41 male alcoholics.

Data from Hickish T, Colston K, Bland JM, et al. Vitamin D deficiency and muscle strength in male alcoholics. *Clin Sci* 1989; 77: 171–6.

## Regression

Regression is the name given to a set of methods for **predicting** one variable from another.

For an example, a student project (Savage, 1999) aimed at estimating body mass index (BMI) using only a tape measure with abdominal circumference, mid upper arm circumference, and sex as possible predictors. Starting with the female participants only and looking at abdominal circumference—can we predict BMI from abdominal circumference? Fig. 20.12 shows a scatter plot of BMI against abdominal circumference and there is clearly a strong relationship between them. We could draw many lines on the scatter diagram, as shown, which would represent the relationship between the two variables and which might enable us to predict one from the other, but which line should we choose? The method to be used here is simple linear regression, which is a method to predict the mean value of one variable from the observed value of another. In our example we shall estimate the mean BMI for women of any given abdominal circumference measurement.

Note: we do not treat the two variables, BMI and abdominal circumference, as being of equal importance, as we did for correlation coefficients. We are predicting BMI from abdominal circumference and BMI is the outcome, dependent, y, or left-hand side variable. Abdominal circumference is the predictor, explanatory, independent, x, or right-hand side variable.

- The outcome variable is predicted from the observed value of the predictor variable.
- The relationship to be estimated is linear, because it makes a straight line on the graph.
- This linear relationship takes the form

    BMI = intercept + slope × abdominal circumference

- The intercept is the value of the outcome variable, BMI, when the predictor, abdominal circumference, is zero.
- The slope is the increase in the outcome variable associated with an increase of one unit in the predictor.

To find a line which gives the best prediction, we need some criterion for what constitutes 'best'. One method is to choose the line which makes the distance from the points to the line *in the y direction* a minimum. These are the differences between the observed BMI and the predicted BMI. As when estimating variation using the variance and standard deviations we square the differences to get rid of the minus signs and choose the line which will minimize the sum of the squares of these differences. This is the principle of least squares; the estimates that we obtain are the least squares line/equation. This is also called estimation by ordinary least squares (OLS).

There are many computer programs which will estimate the least squares equation and for the example data:

    BMI = –1.45 + 0.35 × abdominal circumference

The regression coefficient:

- is the estimate of the slope, here 0.35,
- unlike the correlation coefficient is not a dimensionless number; it has dimensions and units depending on those of the variables,
- here it is the increase in BMI per unit increase in abdominal circumference—dimensions are kg per square metre per cm (BMI being in $kg/m^2$ and abdominal circumference in cm),
- will change if the units of measurement are changed—if abdominal circumference is measured in metres, the regression coefficient would be $35 kg/m^2/m$.

In this example, the intercept is negative, which means that when abdominal circumference is zero the BMI is negative. This is impossible, of course, but so is a zero abdominal circumference. Be wary of attributing any meaning to an intercept which is outside the range of the data. It is just a convenience for drawing the best line within the range of data that we have.

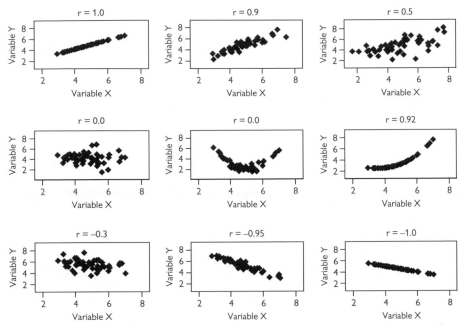

**Fig. 20.11** Simulated data from populations with different relationships between the two variables, and the population correlation coefficient.

### Confidence intervals and p values in regression

We can find confidence intervals and p values—for the BMI data:

- The estimated slope = 0.35kg/m²/cm.
- 95% confidence interval is 0.31 to 0.40kg/m²/cm.
- p <0.001—the p value tests the null hypothesis that in the population from which these women come, the slope is zero.

### Testing the assumptions of regression

For our confidence intervals and p values to be valid, the data must conform to the following assumptions:

- the deviations from line should have a Normal distribution with uniform variance,
- the observations must be independent,
- our model of the data is that the line is straight, not curved, and we can check how well the data match this.

We can check the assumptions about the deviations by calculating the residuals and plotting these graphically.

- Calculate the differences between the observed value of the outcome variable and the value predicted by the regression, the regression estimate.
- These deviations from the regression line are called the residuals about the line, or simply residuals.
- Residuals should have a Normal distribution and uniform variance, that is, their variability should be unrelated to the value of the predictor.

Fig. 20.13 shows a histogram and a Normal plot for the residuals for the BMI data. In a Normal plot, the points should lie close to the straight line if the data follow a Normal distribution. Curvature indicates a departure from the Normal. The distribution is a fairly good fit to the Normal. Fig. 20.14 assesses the uniformity of the variance by simple inspection of residual against the predictor variable. It also shows a plot of the residual against the regression estimate, the value predicted by the regression. The two plots are identical, only the horizontal scale is changed. The plot of residual against predictor should show no relationship between mean residual and predictor

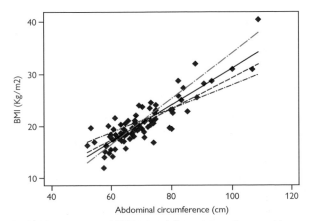

**Fig. 20.12** Scatter plot of BMI against abdominal circumference with possible lines to represent the relationship.

Data from Savage M. MBBS at St George's Hospital Medical School, University of London, 1999.

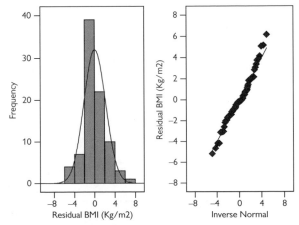

**Fig. 20.13** Histogram and Normal plot for residuals for the BMI and abdominal circumference data.

Data from Savage M. MBBS at St George's Hospital Medical School, University of London, 1999.

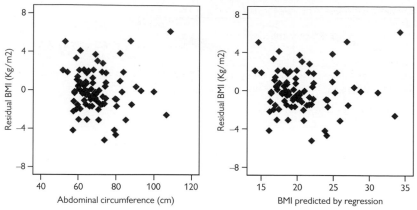

**Fig. 20.14** Scatter plot of residual BMI against abdominal circumference and against the regression estimate. Data from Savage M. MBBS at St George's Hospital Medical School, University of London, 1999.

if the relationship is actually a straight line. If there is a relationship, usually that the residuals are higher or lower at the extremes of the plot than they are in the middle, this suggests that a straight line is not a good way to look at the data. A curve might be better..

## Multiple regression

By expanding the ideas of regression, multiple regression is used to describe relationships using **more than one predictor variable**.

Simple linear regression was illustrated using the prediction of body mass index (BMI) from abdominal circumference in a population of adult women. Fig. 20.15 shows scatter diagrams of BMI against abdominal circumference and of BMI against mid upper arm circumference. This time both men and women are included in the sample.

The regression equations predicting BMI from abdominal circumference and from mid upper arm circumference are:

$$BMI = -1.35 + 0.31 \times abdomen$$
$$BMI = -4.59 + 1.09 \times arm$$

Both abdominal and arm circumference are highly significant predictors of BMI ($p < 0.001$).

Could we get an even better prediction if we used both of them? Multiple regression enables us to do this. We can fit a regression equation with more than one predictor:

$$BMI = -5.94 + 0.18 \times abdomen + 0.59 \times arm$$

This multiple regression equation predicts BMI better than either of the simple linear regressions. The regression equation was found

by an extension of the least squares method (OLS regression) described for simple linear regression.

Although both variables are highly significant ($p < 0.001$), the coefficient of each has changed. Both coefficients have got closer to zero, going from 0.31 to 0.18 for abdomen and from 1.09 to 0.58 for arm circumference. This is because abdominal and arm circumferences are themselves related. The correlation is $r = 0.77$, $p < 0.001$. Abdominal circumference and arm circumference each explains some of the relationship between BMI and the other. When we have only one of them in the regression, it will include some of the relationship of BMI with the other. When both are in the regression, each appears to have a relationship which is less strong than it really is.

Each predictor also reduces the significance of the other because they are related to one another as well as to BMI.

There is another possible predictor variable in the data, sex. If we include sex in the regression, using the variable 'male' = 1 if male and = 0 if female, we get

$$BMI = -6.44 + 0.18 \times abdomen + 0.64 \times arm - 1.39 \times male$$

This time the coefficients for abdomen and arm are hardly changed. This is because neither is closely related to sex, the new variable in the regression. Sex is not a significant predictor when considered alone ($p = 0.49$) but in multiple regression it has become significant ($p < 0.001$). This is because including abdominal and arm circumference as predictors removes so much of the variation in BMI that the relationship with sex becomes significant. When we have continuous and categorical predictor variables together, regression is also called analysis of covariance or ANCOVA, for historical reasons.

We have to make the same assumptions for multiple linear regression as for simple linear regression.

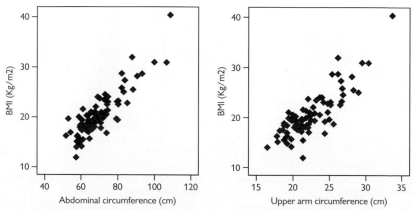

**Fig. 20.15** Scatter diagrams of BMI against abdominal circumference and of BMI against mid upper arm circumference.

For our confidence intervals and P values to be valid the data must conform to the assumptions that:

- Deviations from the line should have a Normal distribution with uniform variance.
- The observations must be independent.

Finally, our model of the data is that the relationship with each of our predictors is adequately represented by a straight line rather than a curve.

We can check these assumptions in the same way as we did for simple linear regression.

## References

Hickish T, Colston K, Bland JM, et al. Vitamin D deficiency and muscle strength in male alcoholics. *Clin Sci* 1989; 77: 171–6.

Savage, M. *MBBS at St George's Hospital Medical School*, University of London, 1999.

# 20.6 Relative risk, odds ratios, and 'number needed to treat'

## Background

This section will discuss how to determine estimates of the strength of relationships. There are different ways of doing this for different kinds of data and sizes of table, but two are particularly important in health research: the risk ratio or relative risk and the odds ratio.

## Risk ratio or relative risk

In Table 20.5 the question is: do children with bronchitis in infancy get more respiratory symptoms in later life than others (Bland et al., 1974)?

Considering the data in the form of proportions:

- 9.5% of children with a history of bronchitis before the age of 5 years are reported to have day or night cough at the age of 14 (26/273 = 0.095 = 9.5%). The risk of cough here is 9.5%.
- 4.2% of children with no history of bronchitis before the age of 5 years are reported to have day or night cough at the age of 14 (44/1046 = 0.042 = 4.2%). The risk of cough here is 4.25%.
- The difference between them is 0.095 − 0.042 = 0.053 (called 5.3 percentage points) and the standard error is 0.019. The 95% confidence interval for the difference is:

$$0.053 - 1.96 \times 0.019 \text{ to } 0.053 + 1.96 \times 0.019$$
$$= 0.016 \text{ to } 0.090.$$

- **This difference is the absolute risk difference or absolute risk reduction.**
- The ratio of the proportion with cough at age 14 for bronchitis before age 5 to the proportion with cough at age 14 for those without bronchitis before age 5 is 0.095/0.042 = 2.26.
- **This ratio is the risk ratio or relative risk (RR).**
- The standard error for this ratio is complex as the ratio itself does not approximate well to a Normal distribution. It is therefore calculated using the logarithm of the ratio. For the example the log ratio = 0.817 and the standard error = 0.238.

The 95% confidence interval for the log ratio is:

$$0.817 - 1.96 \times 0.238 \text{ to } 0.817 + 1.96 \times 0.238$$
$$= 0.351 \text{ to } 1.283.$$

The 95% confidence interval for the ratio of proportions is the antilog of this, 1.42 to 3.61. Thus we estimate that the proportion of children reported to cough during the day or at night among those with a history of bronchitis is between 1.4 to 3.6 times the proportion among those without a history of bronchitis.

## The odds ratio

- The probability or risk of an event is the number experiencing the event divided by the number who could experience it.

- The odds of an event is the number experiencing the event divided by the number who do not experience it.

In the example:

- The probability of cough for children with a history of bronchitis is 26/273 = 0.095. For every 100 children who do not cough, 9.5 cough.
- The odds of cough for children with a history of bronchitis is 26/247 = 0.105. For every 100 children, 10.5 cough.
- The probability of cough for children without a history of bronchitis is 44/1046 = 0.042.
- The odds of cough for children without a history of bronchitis is 44/1002 = 0.044.

**The odds ratio (OR)**:

- Is another way to compare the two groups. The OR and RR are **not** the same.
- This is (26/247)/(44/1002) = 0.105/0.044 = 2.40.
- Thus the odds of cough in children with a history of bronchitis is 2.4 times the odds of cough in children without a history of bronchitis. This is not the same as the relative risk.

Like RR, OR has an awkward distribution. We use the log OR, which will follow an approximately Normal distribution provided the frequencies are not too small, and which has a simple standard error. In the example:

- The log OR = 0.874, with standard error = 0.257.
- The approximate 95% confidence interval is:

$$0.874 - 1.96 \times 0.257 \text{ to } 0.874 + 1.96 \times 0.257 = 0.370 \text{ to } 1.379.$$

- To get a confidence interval for the OR itself we must antilog, giving 1.45 to 3.97.

**Note**: it does not matter which way round the calculation is. This is **not** true for RR.

- The OR for cough given a history of bronchitis = (26/247)/(44/1002) = 2.397.
- The OR for a history of bronchitis given a current cough = (26/44)/(247/1002) = 2.397.
- The OR is therefore called the ratio of cross products.
- Switching the rows or columns inverts the OR. For example, the OR for no cough given a history of bronchitis = (247/26)/(1002/44) = 0.417 = 1/2.397. This is the reciprocal of the OR for cough.

The odds ratio is extensively used in medical research. Odds ratios can be calculated for case–control studies, where they can be used to approximate the relative risk, even though risks could be estimated directly. Other analysis methods, such as logistic regression, can be used to correct for confounding factors, allowing adjusted odds ratios to be calculated allowing for the simultaneous effect of other variables.

## 'Number needed to treat' (NNT)

- The NNT is the number of patients that need to be treated to prevent one additional adverse outcome (e.g. death, stroke, etc.).
- The 'best' NNT is a value of 1, where all patients given treatment recover and none recover when given control agent (e.g. treating susceptible bacterial infections with antibiotics produces NNTs close to 1).
- The higher the NNT the less good the treatment is when comparing two similar treatments.
- Prophylactic therapies which may have only small effects when given to large numbers of patients will have high NNTs but this

| Cough at age 14 | Bronchitis at age 5 | | Total |
|---|---|---|---|
| | Yes | No | |
| Yes | 26 | 44 | 70 |
| No | 247 | 1002 | 1249 |
| Total | 273 | 1046 | 1319 |

Table 20.5 Cough during the day or at night at age 14 and bronchitis before the age of 5 years

Source: Bland JM, Holland WW, Elliott A. The development of respiratory symptoms in a cohort of Kent schoolchildren. *Bull Physiopathol Respir* 1974; 10: 699–716.

not mean that they are not useful therapies especially if the adverse events which they prevent are very severe.

- The NNT is the inverse of the absolute risk reduction (ARR) in an interventional trial (NNT = 1/ARR).
- In the ASCOT-LLA study (Sever et al., 2003) looking at the effect of atorvastatin as primary prevention in patients with hypertension, the rate of total cardiovascular events was 9.5% (0.095) in the control group and 7.5% (0.075) in the treatment group.
- The ARR is 0.095 − 0.075 = 0.02.
- The NNT is then 1/0.02 = 50. Therefore 50 patients with hypertension need to be treated with atorvastatin as primary prevention for 3.3 years (the duration of the study) to prevent one adverse cardiovascular event.

## References

Bland JM, Holland WW, Elliott A. The development of respiratory symptoms in a cohort of Kent schoolchildren. *Bull Physiopathol Respir* 1974; 10: 699–716.

Sever PS, Dahlöf B, Poulter NR, et al. Prevention of coronary and stroke events with atorvastatin in hypertensive patients who have average or lower-than-average cholesterol concentrations, in the Anglo-Scandinavian Cardiac Outcomes Trial—Lipid Lowering Arm (ASCOT-LLA): a multicentre randomised controlled trial. *Lancet* 2003; 361 (9364): 1149–58.

# 20.7 Survival analysis

## Background

In this section we will look at data which are the time to an event, such as death or healing. The main problem with such data is that participants are usually observed for differing lengths of time. We can:

- estimate the proportion who are still free of the event at any time, using the Kaplan–Meier survival curve method,
- do a test of significance between different groups using the log-rank test,
- get an estimate of the difference in survival between two groups using the hazard ratio,
- estimate the effects of quantitative variables and of several different variables on survival using a regression method called Cox regression or proportional hazards regression.

## Time to event data

In healthcare research we often measure the time which elapses until some event occurs. This might be the time from diagnosis to death of cancer patients, the time to metastasis or to local recurrence of a tumour, the time to readmission to hospital after discharge, the age at which breastfeeding ceased, the time to healing of a wound, etc.

- Such data are called time to event or survival data.
- The terminal event, death, healing, etc., is called the endpoint.
- The statistical techniques developed to deal with them are known collectively as survival analysis.

The analysis of time to event data would be straightforward if we knew the time to event of every participant. What makes time to event data difficult to analyse is that often we do not know the exact survival times of all cases.

- Some participants will still be surviving when we want to analyse the data.
- For some events, such as conception or readmission to hospital, the event may never happen for some participants.
- When cases have entered the study at different times, some of the recent entrants may be surviving, but have been observed for a short time only. Their observed survival time may be less than those participants admitted early in the study and who have since experienced the event. When we know for some participants only that the time to the event is greater than some value, we say that the data are censored. This occurs when a participant is withdrawn from follow-up.
- All of these factors must be considered when designing the analysis.

Fig. 20.16 shows the recruitment, time to event, and time to censoring of 10 participants recruited into a hypothetical study.

- Participants 1, 2, and 3 are recruited at the beginning of the study. participant 1 experiences the event, but participants 2 and 3 do not. When we want to analyse the data, they have yet to experience the event.
- Participants 4 and 6 are recruited after the start of the study and do not experience the event before the analysis point.
- Participant 5 is recruited after the start and does experience the event.
- Participant 7 is recruited after the start and is censored before the analysis point. There are many reasons why this might be. In a wound healing trial, the participant many be transferred to another treatment centre for clinical reasons. In a conception study, the participant might decide not to make any further attempt to conceive. In the study of Luthra et al. (1982), who compared the incidence of pregnancy in attendees at a subfertility clinic before and after laparoscopy and hydrotubation, one of the couples in the

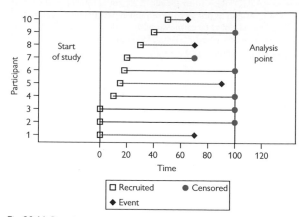

**Fig. 20.16** Recruitment, time to event, and time to censoring of 10 participants recruited into a study.

sample decided to divorce and cease trying for a family, another decided to adopt.

- Participant 7 is observed for a shorter time than participants 1 and 5 take to experience the event.
- We cannot therefore simply say that we will look at whether participants have experienced the event within the shortest observation time for a participant who has not experienced it, because we will lose most of our data.

## Kaplan–Meier survival estimates

Sometimes some censored times may be shorter than some times to events. We overcome this difficulty by the construction of a life table. A life table was originally a table showing what would happen to a cohort of hypothetical individuals from birth to death if the current death rates operated throughout their lives. It showed how many would still be alive at each age. Now we use the term to describe following a hypothetical cohort from any time point onwards.

Here is an example to illustrate the methodology. The time to event data is the time to healing of venous ulcers for patients recruited to the VenUS I trial (Nelson et al., 2004):

- a randomized trial of two types of bandage for treating venous leg ulcers,
- test treatment, a four layer bandage (4LB), which gave elastic compression,
- control treatment, a short-stretch bandage (SSB), which gave inelastic compression,
- endpoint—complete healing of the index ulcer. Time to healing is measured in days.

For each patient, the information which is available is either the time at which the ulcer healed, e.g. the patient healed at day 7, or, alternatively, the time at which there was the last contact for a patient not known to have healed. If the patient has not healed, we have censored data, e.g. for a patient who at day 8 had not healed, but this is the last known information.

By combining the data from all of the patients, we calculate the life table for presentation in the form of a Kaplan–Meier survival curve. The Kaplan–Meier estimates are the proportions which we would expect to remain at each follow-up time if they had experienced the event rates of those in the sample. For example, in the SSB group we estimate that the proportion unhealed after one year is 0.26, or 26%. We can find a confidence interval for this estimate, called the Greenwood interval, in this case 0.20 to 0.33, or 20% to 33%.

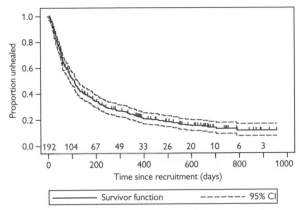

Fig. 20.17 Kaplan–Meier survival curve for the SSB group in the VenUS I trial with ticks added to show where censoring took place and the number at risk shown at 100-day intervals and Greenwood confidence limits added.

Data from Nelson EA, Iglesias CP, Cullum N, et al. Randomized clinical trial of four-layer and short-stretch compression bandages for venous leg ulcers (VenUS I). *Br J Surg* 2004; 91: 1292–9.

## The Kaplan–Meier survival curve

A table with tens or even hundreds of survival estimates is quite cumbersome and so Kaplan–Meier survival analyses are usually presented graphically.

Fig. 20.17 shows the Kaplan–Meier survival curve for the SSB data. Although it is called a curve, it is usually shown as a series of steps, changing sharply at each time when an event takes place. The steps get larger as we move from left to right, because as we get to longer survival times more observations have been censored and there are fewer participants at risk. This makes the proportions surviving following each event smaller and so the steps are larger.

Fig. 20.17 also shows:

- The size of the sample used.
- Where people were censored—ticks are added to indicate the times where there were censored observations.
- The number remaining at risk is displayed along the bottom of the graph. This has been done at intervals of 100 days. The number remaining falls not only because of censoring but because ulcers have healed.
- 95% confidence intervals for the survival estimate, called Greenwood bounds, are present. The bounds get further apart as we move from left to right because as participants have been censored, there is less and less information on which to base the estimate.

## The log-rank test

Greenwood standard errors and confidence intervals for the survival probabilities (Fig. 20.18) are useful for estimates such as 5-year survival rate. They are not a good method for comparing survival curves, as they do not include all the data and the comparison would depend on the time chosen.

To compare survival curves we need a method which makes use of the full survival data. There are several significance tests which we can use for this, of which the best known is the log-rank test. This is a non-parametric test which makes use of the full survival data without making any assumptions about the shape of the survival curve.

- The null hypothesis is that at every time the chance of a member of a group experiencing an event is the same for all groups, though the chance of an event may change over time in any way.
- The alternative hypothesis is that at some time the chance of an event is different in different groups.

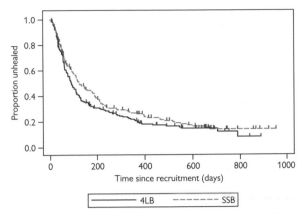

Fig. 20.18 Kaplan–Meier survival curves for the treatment arms in the VenUS I trial.

Data from Nelson EA, Iglesias CP, Cullum N, et al. Randomized clinical trial of four-layer and short-stretch compression bandages for venous leg ulcers (VenUS I). *Br J Surg* 2004; 91: 1292–9.

- When an event takes place, we use the numbers at risk in each group to calculate how many we would expect in the group if the null hypothesis were true. We then sum the expected events for each group and compare them with the number actually observed.

Like the Kaplan–Meier survival curve, the log-rank test makes certain assumptions about the data:

- the observations are independent,
- the risk of an event is the same for censored participants as for non-censored participants,
- survival is the same for early and late recruitment.

The log-rank test:

- is much better at detecting differences where the risk is higher in one group than the other throughout,
- is less good at detecting differences where the survival curves cross,
- is a test of significance only and does not provide any estimate of the size of the difference in survival.

For the data shown in Fig. 20.18, the log-rank test gives a P value of 0.1. There is no evidence to reject the null hypothesis.

## The hazard ratio

To produce an estimate of the size of the difference in survival, we have to make some assumptions about the shape of the curve. We have to assume that they are similar in some way, so that we can find some numerical value to compare between them.

One way to estimate the difference between survival curves uses the hazard.

- Hazard is a measure of the chance that a member of the population will have an event at any given time.
- Hazard depends on the survival time, so it may increase or decrease as follow-up goes on.
- If we assume that survival curves follow the same pattern, then we can assume that if hazard is greater in one group than another at one time point, it will also be greater at another time point.
- If this is so, then the hazard in one group is equal to the hazard in the other group multiplied by a constant number, which we will estimate. This is the **hazard ratio**. A ratio of 1.0 means that the risk of an event is the same in the two groups

For the 4LB versus SSB group comparison (Fig. 20.18):

- the hazard ratio is 1.20,
- there is a small increase in the risk of an event in the 4LB group compared to the SSB group,

- here the event is healing, a good thing, so this shows an advantage to the 4LB group.

This is only an estimate and is subject to error in the estimation, so we need a confidence interval. As with other ratios, the hazard ratio is much easier to analyse on the logarithmic scale.

- Log hazard ratio = 0.177, with standard error = 0.115.
- The approximate 95% confidence interval is:

$$0.177 - 1.96 \times 0.115 \text{ to } 0.177 + 1.96 \times 0.115$$
$$= -0.048 \text{ to } 0.402.$$

- To get a confidence interval for the hazard ratio itself we must antilog, giving 0.95 to 1.49.
- This includes 1.00, the null hypothesis value, so it is consistent with the log-rank test above.

## Cox regression

Cox regression (also known as proportional hazards regression) is a method for analysing survival data, very similar to multiple regression by least squares and logistic regression.

- It uses an outcome variable, censored survival time, and some predictor variables with which we hope to predict the survival.
- The great strength of Cox regression compared to log rank tests and simple hazard ratios is that we can have **more than one predictor variable**.
- It predicts the hazard ratio for participants with any given values of the predictor variables compared to participants for whom the predictor variables are all equal to zero:

$$\log \text{ hazard ratio} = \text{slope}_1 \times \text{predictor}_1 + \text{slope}_2 \times$$
$$\text{predictor}_2 + \text{slope}_3 \times \text{predictor}_3 + \cdots$$

- There is no intercept in the Cox method—when all the predictor variables are equal to zero the hazard ratio must be one, and so the log hazard ratio must be zero.
- It assumes that the hazard ratio does not depend on the time of follow-up, just as for the simple hazard ratio described earlier.

In the VenUS I trial, area of the ulcer at randomization was a powerful predictor of healing. If we include this in the regression model, we get:

$$\log \text{ hazard ratio} = 0.0238 \times 4LB - 0.028 \times \text{area(cm}^2)$$

The antilog of 0.238 = 1.27 is the adjusted hazard ratio for 4LB treatment and is statistically significant, p = 0.04.

As with the log-rank test, Cox regression does not need to assume any particular shape for the survival curve. This is why it is the regression method for time to event data which is almost always used in health research.

There are several assumptions we must make about the data for Cox regression:

- the observations are independent,
- as for Kaplan–Meier analysis and the log-rank test, the risk of an event is the same for censored participants as for non-censored participants,
- the proportional hazards model applies,
- there are sufficient data for the maximum likelihood fitting, the large sample z tests, and confidence interval calculations.

There are several ways to check the proportional hazards assumption. We can look at the Kaplan–Meier plots to see whether they look satisfactory, e.g. that they do not cross. However, it is not very easy to see anything other than gross departures. If we look at the survival curves for treatment (Fig. 20.18) they appear to be almost identical for the first 50 days of follow-up, then to diverge, and then to come together again at about 650 days. Whether this means anything is difficult to say, but the hazard ratio may not be uniform. For the last of these assumptions, a rule of thumb is that there should be at least 10 (preferably 20) events for every variable included in the model.

## References

Luthra P, Bland JM, Stanton SL. Incidence of pregnancy after laparoscopy and hydrotubation. *BMJ* 1982; 284: 1013.

Nelson EA, Iglesias CP, Cullum N, et al. Randomized clinical trial of four-layer and short-stretch compression bandages for venous leg ulcers (VenUS I). *Br J Surg* 2004; 91: 1292–9.

# 20.8 Sample size

## Background

One of the most frequently asked questions to a statistician working in healthcare research is 'How big a sample do I need?'. The key question is usually how many participants are required so that a researcher has good chance of detecting a clinically relevant difference *if it exists*. The first thing we need to decide is what is the outcome variable. An outcome variable is one which we hope to change, predict, or estimate in a study. For example, in a trial of a treatment for hypertension the outcome variable might be systolic blood pressure; in an obstetric study it might be whether the participant has a caesarean section; in a cancer trial it might be survival time or recurrence-free survival time; in a patient satisfaction survey it might be a score on a satisfaction scale.

- The primary outcome variable must relate to the main aim of the study.
- For sample size calculations, we must choose a primary variable.

## Sample size for estimation

In some studies, we want to estimate some population quantity, such as a mean or proportion. To decide the sample size for such a study we need to decide how accurate we want the estimate to be. The confidence interval for this estimate will be our measure of accuracy and the width of this will depend on the sample size. We decide the width of the interval we want and work back to the sample size.

For example, suppose we wish to estimate the mean serum cholesterol in a population of apparently healthy adults.

- We know from many studies that serum cholesterol usually lies between 3 and 8 mmol/L.
- We decide that a reasonable accuracy for the mean would be to within 0.2 mmol/L.

*How big a sample would we need for this?*

- The 95% confidence interval for a mean is 1.96, or about 2, standard errors on either side of the sample mean, unless the sample is quite small.
- The standard error should therefore be $0.2/2 = 0.1$.
- Once we know what the standard deviation is going to be, we can calculate the sample size needed.

In this case, it is easy to get an estimate. There are many published studies of cholesterol which can provide this.

If we use the data of Markus et al. (1995), a case–control study of stroke, the 84 people in the control group had mean cholesterol = 5.54 mmol/L with standard deviation 0.95mmol/L. The standard error is 0.1.

Sample size = $0.95^2/0.1^2 = 90.25$, so in this study 90 would be the required sample size to achieve this. A typical estimate might then be 5.5mmol/L with 95% confidence interval 5.3 to 5.7 mmol/L.

Only the researcher can decide whether this accuracy is good enough for the purpose, the statistician cannot.

To summarize, we need to specify the width of the confidence interval and know how this is related to the sample size. We can then calculate the sample size required to give a confidence interval with the desired width.

## Sample sizes for significance tests

Most sample size questions involve a comparison of some sort, such as the difference between two means or between two proportions. There are a lot of free programs available to do this and some very comprehensive commercial ones. There are five key questions to answer regarding the size of the study.

1. What is the main purpose of the study?
2. What is the principal measure of patient outcome?
3. How will the data be analysed to detect a treatment difference?
4. What types of results are anticipated using the 'standard' treatment?
5. How small a treatment difference is it important to detect and with what degree of certainty?

By 'degree of certainty' here we mean statistical power. We do not want to make a type II error, where we miss a real difference.

The **power** of the study is the probability that if in the population there really were a difference of the size we are looking for, a sample of the chosen sample size would give a significant difference. If the power is 90%, then of 100 samples of patients we might choose, 90 would give us a significant difference.

### Test of two means

In some studies, the primary measure of patient outcome takes the form of a quantitative measurement, such as blood pressure. The data collected during the study could then be analysed using a two-sample t-test to compare the mean response in the two groups.

In order to calculate the number of patients per group ($n$), we need to know the following numbers:

- $\mu_1$ = mean 'outcome' for the 'standard' treatment group.
- $\mu_2$ = mean 'outcome' for the new treatment group.
- $\mu_1$ and $\mu_2$ are needed to show the minimum difference between the groups considered clinically relevant.
- $\sigma$ = common standard deviation of 'outcome' for the two groups.
- $\alpha$ = significance level of test.
- $1 - \beta$ = power of study

In planning a trial of an intervention for patients with type 2 diabetes, to compare the two groups of patients we might use $HbA_1c$ as the principal outcome measure. In such a trial, we would want a baseline measurement of $HbA_1c$ and would use this in our analysis. Our plan is to recruit patients with $HbA_1c$ between 53 mmol/mol and 108 mmol/mol and randomize them to usual care or to our innovative support regimen. How many patients do we need?

*'How big a difference do we want our trial to detect?'*

There is no point is saying any difference at all. If the effect of our intervention is to reduce mean $HbA_1c$ by 1 mmol/mol, we would need about 6000 participants in each group to have a good chance of the trial producing a significant difference. To design a practical study, we must set a realistic limit to our ambition. How do we decide how big a difference to look for? Three main approaches are used:

- clinical judgement as to what would be important,
- what the treatment might achieve,
- back calculation from what is feasible.

We can use clinical judgement as to what treatment effect would be important, for example, a difference which would lead us to change our practice and introduce the treatment. We could use own judgement, or to give it more weight we could ask colleagues what they would consider worthwhile. We might formalize this as a focus group of clinicians who would discuss the question.

For a study of the time to treatment of venous ulcers, clinicians were asked how many weeks of reduction in healing would justify their use of the intervention.

We might also ask some potential research participants what they think; what benefit would they need to accept the treatment?

- For a trial, designing the study to detect a clinically important effect is the best approach, but for observational studies it may be less relevant.

We can design our study so that it can detect the size of difference which we think might exist in the population. For example, in a trial this would be the effect which the treatment might achieve. We can get this from pilot studies, or from other trials of similar treatments.

- This approach is good for observational designs like case–control studies.

If we have no idea what to look for, we can start with what is feasible with the number of participants who are likely to be available to us. We then ask what size of difference we can detect with a study of this size. This is acceptable provided we are frank about what we are doing and do not pretend that the difference we can detect is what we wanted to detect from the beginning.

- This is often suitable for exploratory studies, where our main aim is to get some idea of what size of effect might exist.

*Sample size calculation*

- We shall decide that a clinically important difference in $HbA_{1c}$ would be 10 mmol/mol. If our treatment could reduce mean $HbA_1c$ by this amount, it would be worthwhile.

- To calculate the sample size needed to detect this difference, we need to choose the significance level for the two-sample t-test which we would do on the final data. This is usually 0.05, as this is the conventional cut-off for significance.

- We also need to choose the power, the proportion of samples which would produce a significant difference if the difference in the whole population were that hypothesized, i.e. 10 mmol/mol of $HbA_1c$. The usual choice for this is 0.90 = 90%, or 0.80 = 80%. We want a fairly high power, a good chance that the study will produce an answer to the research question. We will choose 0.90.

- The standard error of the difference in mean $HbA_1c$ will depend on two things: the sizes of the two samples and the standard deviation of the final measure of $HbA_1c$. As we are choosing participants to have $HbA_1c$ between 53 mmol/mol and 108 mmol/mol, it is easy to find data on a few patients and calculate the standard deviation. For a sample available to us, this was 16. We intend to choose patients between 53 and 108 mmol/mol, but when we measure them again we expect that some may have $HbA_1c$ below 53 mmol/mol and some above 108 mmol/mol, so the standard deviation might increase a bit. We could allow for this possibility by inflating the standard deviation or by looking at a second measurement from our records. We shall take 18 as the standard deviation.

- Finally, we shall design the trial to have equal numbers in the two patient groups.

- Using computer software, a sample size of 69 in each group will have 90% power to detect a difference in means of 10, assuming that the common standard deviation is 18 using a two-group t-test with a 5% two-sided significance level.

### Test of two proportions

The most common statistical analysis in trials is to focus on a single outcome of patient response, which can be classified as either a 'success' or a 'failure'. For example, death in a year = failure, survival = success. The data collected during the study could then be analysed using a chi-squared test.

In order to calculate the number of patients per group ($n$), we need to know the following numbers:

- $p_1$ = proportion of the 'standard' treatment group with a 'successful' outcome.

- $p_2$ = proportion of the new treatment group with a 'successful' outcome.

- $p_1$ and $p_2$ are needed to show the minimum improvement over 'standard' therapy considered clinically relevant.

- $\alpha$ = significance level of test.

- $1 - \beta$ = power of study.

Let us suppose that we want to do a study to compare the proportions undergoing caesarean section, in two groups of pregnant women.

*Sample size calculation*

- We will have two equal sized groups.

- From clinical records we observe 0.24 = 24% of women have sections and we think that a reduction to 0.20 = 20% would be of clinical interest.

- Using a significance level 0.05 and power 0.90 as before, we want the study to be able to distinguish between, 0.24 and 0.20.

- Using computer software, the required sample size, $n = 2302$ in each group. Such a large sample size is necessary to detect small differences between proportions.

## What should we do if we don't anticipate any difference?

Sometimes we do not wish to detect a difference, because we do not think that there will be one. We might have a trial where we expect or hope to show that two treatments are similar in their effects on the primary outcome. The better treatment would then be decided on the basis of secondary outcomes, such as side effects or cost.

*How do we plan such a study?*

If we were to do a significance test of the null hypothesis that the treatments are the same, we expect that it would be not significant. We can get this because there is no difference in the population, or because the sample is too small. Either way, we cannot interpret it as showing no difference.

*Could a power calculation help us to decide the sample size?*

We could say how far apart would the two groups have to be for us to conclude that we could not accept them as equivalent. Then we can design the sample size to have a high power to detect that difference. There are special tests of significance which have been devised to test the null hypothesis that the effect size is greater than some specified value, called tests of equivalence and **tests of non-inferiority**. A significant result would mean that there is evidence against this null hypothesis, so we think that the difference is less than the specified value. Given the difficulty of the arguments surrounding such studies, we would recommend that you consult a statistician if you are planning one.

## How reliable are sample size calculations?

There are a number of reasons why sample size calculations must be interpreted with a little caution.

Most sample size calculations involve some approximation to the significance test which would be used in the analysis and different sample size programs, tables, and graphical methods do not always use the same ones. As a result, they may give slightly different results.

Sample size calculations involve a guess at what we might find in our study, based on what we know before the study is carried out.

- For example, we may need to estimate the standard deviation of a continuous outcome measurement. The sample we get may be more or less variable than our present data suggests. Furthermore, treatments may increase the variability of a measurement.

- We may need to estimate the proportion of control participants who experience some event, such as caesarean section. When we do the study, the proportion experiencing the event may be reduced. Changes in the population or in other aspects of care may lead to this, or there may be a reluctance to recruit high-risk participants into a trial.

Participants who begin a study may not complete it. They may drop out of treatment or fail to complete questionnaires. The number we start with will exceed the number we finish with.

We can allow for all these problems by increasing the sample size. Researchers usually allow between 10% and 20% increase for potential dropout. We should always err on the side of a larger sample. Whether we can achieve it is another matter.

## Reference

Markus HS, Barley J, Lunt R, et al. Angiotensin-converting enzyme gene deletion polymorphism: a new risk factor for lacunar stroke but not carotid atheroma. *Stroke* 1995; 26: 1329–33.

# 20.9 Diagnostic tests

## Background

One of the main purposes of making clinical measurements is to aid in diagnosis. This may be to identify one of several possible diagnoses in a patient, or to find people with a particular disease in an apparently healthy population. The latter is known as screening.

In either case the measurement provides us with a test, which we may be able to compare later with a true diagnosis. The test may be based on a continuous variable and the disease indicated if it is above or below a given level, or it may be a qualitative observation such as carcinoma *in situ* cells on a cervical smear. In either case we will call the test positive if it indicates the disease and negative if not; and the diagnosis positive if the disease is later confirmed, negative if not.

## How do we measure the effectiveness of the test?

Table 20.6 shows three artificial sets of test and diagnosis data. We could take as an index of test effectiveness the proportion giving the true diagnosis from the test. For Test 1 in the example it is 94%. Now consider Test 2, which always gives a negative result. Test 2 will never detect any cases of the disease. It is, though, correct for 95% of the participants! However, the first test is useful, in that it detects some cases of the disease, whilst the second is not, so this is clearly a poor index. Test 3 is not as good as Test 1 in one respect: it only detects two of the five disease positives, compared to the four detected by Test 1. On the other hand, it is a better test in another way: it does not diagnose as positive any disease negatives.

## Sensitivity and specificity

There is no one simple index which enables us to compare different tests in all the ways we would like. This is because there are two things we need to measure: how good the test is at finding disease positives, i.e. those with the condition, and how good the test is at excluding disease negatives, i.e. those who do not have the condition. The indices conventionally employed to do this are sensitivity and specificity.

- **Sensitivity** is the proportion of patients who are disease positive and who are test positive.
- **Specificity** is the proportion of patients who are disease negative and who are test negative.
- Sensitivity and specificity are often multiplied by 100 to give percentages.

For our three tests (Table 20.6) these values are:

|        | Sensitivity | Specificity |
|--------|-------------|-------------|
| Test 1 | 0.80        | 0.95        |
| Test 2 | 0.00        | 1.00        |
| Test 3 | 0.40        | 1.00        |

Test 2 misses all the disease positives and finds all the disease negatives. The difference between Tests 1 and 3 is brought out by the greater sensitivity of 1 and the greater specificity of 3. We can see that Test 3 is better than Test 2, because its sensitivity is higher and its specificity the same. However, it is more difficult to see whether Test 3 is better than Test 1. We must come to a judgement based on the relative importance of sensitivity and specificity in each particular case.

For a practical example, a remarkable number of alcoholics have evidence at X-ray of past rib fractures (Maxwell et al., 1983). We asked whether this would be of any value in the detection of alcoholism in patients.

Table 20.6 Some artificial test and diagnosis data

|          | Disease diagnosis | | |
|----------|----------|----------|-------|
|          | Positive | Negative | Total |
| **TEST 1** | | | |
| **Positive** | 4 | 5 | 9 |
| **Negative** | 1 | 90 | 91 |
| **Total** | 5 | 95 | 100 |
| **TEST 2** | | | |
| **Positive** | 0 | 0 | 0 |
| **Negative** | 5 | 95 | 100 |
| **Total** | 5 | 95 | 100 |
| **TEST 3** | | | |
| **Positive** | 2 | 0 | 2 |
| **Negative** | 3 | 95 | 98 |
| **Total** | 5 | 95 | 100 |

- Among 74 patients with alcoholic liver disease, 20 had evidence of at least one past fracture on chest X-ray and 11 had evidence of bilateral or multiple fractures.
- In a control group of 181 patients with non-alcoholic liver disease or GI disorders, six had evidence of at least one fracture and two of bilateral or multiple fractures.

For any fractures as a test for alcoholism:
- Sensitivity = 20/74 = 0.27.
- Specificity = (181–6)/181 = 0.97.

For bilateral or multiple fractures:
- Sensitivity = 11/74 = 0.15.
- Specificity = (181–2)/181 = 0.99.

Hence both tests were very specific; very few non-alcoholics would be indicated as alcoholics by them. On the other hand, neither was very sensitive; many alcoholics would be missed. As might be expected, the more stringent test of bilateral or multiple fractures was more specific and less sensitive than the test of any fracture.

## ROC curves

Sometimes a test is based on a continuous variable. For example, Fig. 20.19 shows a scatter plot which shows measurements of creatine kinase (CK) in patients with unstable angina and acute myocardial infarction (AMI) (Frances Boa, personal communication). We wish to detect patients with AMI among patients who may have either condition and this measurement is a potential test, AMI patients tending to have high values.

### How do we choose the cut-off point?

The lowest CK in AMI patients is 90, so a cut-off below this will detect all AMI patients. Using 80, for example, we would detect all AMI patients, sensitivity = 1.00, but would also only have 42% of angina patients below 80, so the specificity = 0.42.

We can alter the sensitivity and specificity by changing the cut-off point. Raising the cut-off point will mean fewer cases will be detected and so the sensitivity will be decreased. However, there will be fewer false positives and the specificity will be increased. For example, if CK ≥100 were the criterion for AMI, sensitivity would be 0.96 and specificity 0.62.

There is a trade-off between sensitivity and specificity. It can be helpful to plot sensitivity against specificity to examine this trade-off.

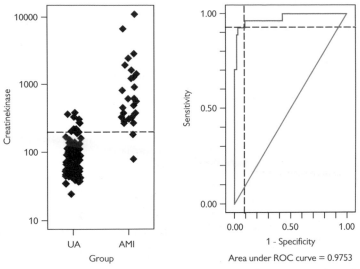

**Fig. 20.19** Scatter diagram and ROC curve for the data showing cut-off at 200 and corresponding sensitivity and specificity. Data from Frances Boa.

This is called a receiver operating characteristic or ROC curve. (The name comes from telecommunications.)

We often plot sensitivity against one minus specificity, as in Fig. 20.19. We can see from Fig. 20.19 that we can get both high sensitivity and high specificity if we choose the right cut-off. With 1 − specificity less than 0.1, i.e. specificity greater than 0.9, we can get sensitivity greater than 0.9 also. In fact, a cut-off of 200 would give sensitivity = 0.93 and specificity = 0.91 in this sample. These estimates will be biased, as we are both estimating the cut-off and testing it in the same sample. We should check the sensitivity and specificity of this cut-off in a different sample to be sure.

The area under the ROC curve is often quoted (here it is 0.9753). It estimates the probability that a member of one population chosen at random will exceed a member of the other population. It can be useful in comparing different tests. In this study another blood test gave us an area under the ROC curve = 0.9825, suggesting that this test may actually be slightly better than the CK test.

## Positive and negative predictive value

We can also estimate the probability that a participant who is test positive will also be a disease positive, called the positive predictive value (PPV). This depends on the prevalence of the condition. If our test and true diagnosis data are from a simple random sample of the population in which we are interested, we can estimate these as simple proportions. If this is not the case, as in the usual situation, we can calculate the PPV for any population prevalence.

Denote the sensitivity by $p_{sens}$, the specificity by $p_{spec}$, and the prevalence by $p_{prev}$.

- Probability of being both disease positive and test positive is $p_{prev} \times p_{sens}$.
- Probability of being disease negative and test positive is $(1-p_{prev}) \times (1-p_{spec})$.

- Total probability of being test positive is the sum of these: $(p_{prev} \times p_{sens}) + ((1-p_{prev}) \times (1-p_{spec}))$.

The **positive predictive value** is the proportion of test positives who are disease positives, and is calculated using the following formula:

$$PPV = \frac{p_{prev} \times p_{sens}}{p_{prev} \times p_{sens} + (1-p_{prev}) \times (1-p_{spec})}$$

In screening situations the disease prevalence is almost always small and the PPV is therefore low. Suppose we have a test which is both sensitive and specific, $p_{sens} = 0.95$ and $p_{spec} = 0.95$, and the disease has prevalence $p_{prev} = 0.01$ (1%). Then, using the above formula only 16% of test positives would be disease positive:

$$PPV = \frac{0.01 \times 0.95}{0.01 \times 0.95 + (1-0.01) \times (1-0.95)} = 0.16$$

The probability that a participant who is test negative will not have the disease is the **negative predictive value** (NPV). This is usually high. The formula for the NPV is:

$$NPV = \frac{(1-p_{prev}) \times p_{spec}}{(1-p_{prev}) \times p_{spec} + p_{prev} \times (1-p_{sens})}$$

PPV and NPV are what we really want to know to interpret a test result, but they are properties of the test in a particular population, not just of the test itself.

## Reference

Maxwell JD, Patel SP, Bland JM, et al. Chest radiography compared to laboratory markers in the detection of alcoholic liver disease. *J R Coll Physicians Lond* 1983; 17: 220–3.

# 20.10 Meta-analysis

## What is a meta-analysis?

Meta-analysis is a set of statistical techniques, for summarization of the results of several studies into a single estimate. Many systematic reviews include a meta-analysis, but not all. Meta-analysis takes data from several different studies and produces a single estimate of the effect, usually of a treatment or risk factor. We improve the precision of an estimate by making use of all available data.

To do a meta-analysis, we must have more than one study which has estimated the effect of an intervention or of a risk factor. The participants, interventions or risk factors, and settings in which the studies were carried out need to be sufficiently similar for us to say that there is something in common for us to investigate. We would not do a meta-analysis of two studies, one of which was in adults and the other in children, for example. We must make a judgement that the studies do not differ in ways which are likely to affect the outcome substantially. We need outcome variables in the different studies which we can somehow get in to a common format, so that they can be combined. Finally, the necessary data must be available. If we have only published papers, we need to get estimates of both the effect and its standard error, for example.

The sort of subjects addressed in meta-analysis include:

- interventions: usually randomized trials to give treatment effect,
- epidemiological: usually case–control and cohort studies to give relative risk,
- diagnostic: combined estimates of sensitivity, specificity, positive predictive value.

A meta-analysis consists of three main parts:

- a pooled estimate and confidence interval for the treatment effect after combining all the studies,
- a test for whether the treatment or risk factor effect is statistically significant or not (i.e. does the effect differ from no effect more than would be expected by chance?),
- a test for heterogeneity of the effect on outcome between the included studies (i.e. does the effect vary across the studies more than would be expected by chance?).

Fig. 20.20 shows the results of a meta-analysis of three clinical trials of metoclopramide compared with placebo in reducing pain from acute migraine (Colman et al., 2004).

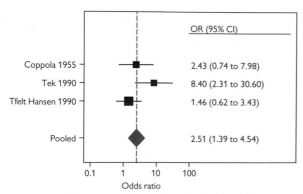

Heterogeneity: chi-squared = 4.91, df = 2, P = 0.086
Test for overall effect: z = −2.05, P = 0.04

**Fig. 20.20** Graphical representation of a meta-analysis of metoclopramide compared with placebo in reducing pain from acute migraine.
Data from Colman I, Brown MD, Innes GD, et al. Parenteral metoclopramide for acute migraine headache: meta-analysis of randomised controlled trials. *BMJ* 2004; 329: 1369–73.

## Individual study estimates

The squares represent the odds ratios for the three individual studies and the horizontal lines their confidence intervals. This is called a forest plot (historically originating from when the confidence intervals were drawn vertically, because the lines were thought to resemble trees in a forest). The size of the squares can represent the amount of information which the study contributes. If they are not all the same size, their area may be proportional to the sample size, the standard error of the estimate, or the variance of the estimate. This means that larger studies appear more important than smaller studies.

## Pooled estimate

The diamond or lozenge shape represents the common meta-analysis estimate. The thickest point is the estimate itself and the width of the diamond is the confidence interval. The choice of the diamond is now widely accepted, but other point symbols may be used for the individual study estimates.

On the right-hand side are the individual trial estimates and the combined meta-analysis estimate in numerical form. The horizontal scale is logarithmic, labelling the scale with the numerical odds ratio. A vertical line is shown at 1.0, the odds ratio for no effect, making it easy to see whether this is included in any of the confidence intervals.

## Significance tests

There are two tests of significance. The first is for heterogeneity, which we deal with later. The second is for the overall effect, testing the null hypothesis that there is no difference between the two treatments. In, this test is significant (0.04). Individually, only one of the three trials gave a significant improvement and pooling the data from all three enables us to draw a more secure conclusion about the existence of a treatment effect and its magnitude.

## Using summary statistics

Most meta-analysis is done using the summary statistics representing the effect and its standard error in each study. We use the estimates of treatment effect for each trial and obtain the common estimate of the effect by averaging the individual study effects. We do not use a simple average of the effect estimates, because this would treat all the studies as if they were of equal value. Some studies have more information than others, e.g. are larger. We therefore weight the trials before we average them.

To get a weighted average we must define weights which reflect the importance of the trial. The usual weight is:

- weight = 1/variance of trial estimate, or
- weight = 1/standard error squared.

We multiply each trial difference by its weight and add, then divide by sum of weights.

- If a study estimate has high variance, this means that the study estimate contains a low amount of information and the study receives low weight in the calculation of the common estimate.
- If a study estimate has low variance, the study estimate contains a high amount of information and the study has high weight in the common estimate.

We can summarize the general framework for pooling results of studies as follows:

- the pooled estimate is a summary measure of the results of the included studies,
- the pooled estimate is a weighted combination of the results from the individual studies,
- the weight given to each trial is the inverse of the variance of the summary measure from each of the individual studies,
- therefore, more precise estimates from larger trials with more events are given more weight,

- then find 95% confidence interval and p value for the pooled difference.

There are several different ways to produce the pooled estimate:

- Inverse-variance weighting, as described earlier.
- Mantel–Haenszel method.
- Peto method.
- DerSimonian and Laird method.

## Heterogeneity

### Clinical heterogeneity

Studies differ in terms of participants, interventions, outcome definitions, and study design. These produce clinical heterogeneity, meaning that the clinical question addressed by these studies is not the same for all of them. We have to consider whether we should be trying to combine them, or whether they differ too much for this to be a sensible thing to do. We detect clinical heterogeneity from the descriptions of the trial populations, treatments, and outcome measurements.

### Statistical heterogeneity

We may also have variation between studies in the true treatment effects or risk ratios, either in magnitude or direction. If this is greater than the variation between individual participants would lead us to expect, we call this statistical heterogeneity. We detect statistical heterogeneity on purely statistical grounds, using the study data.

Statistical heterogeneity may be caused by clinical differences between studies, i.e. by clinical heterogeneity, by methodological differences, or by unknown characteristics of the studies or study populations. Even if studies appear clinically homogeneous there may be statistical heterogeneity.

To identify statistical heterogeneity, we can test the null hypothesis that the studies all have the same treatment (or other) effect in the population. The test looks at the differences between observed treatment effects for the trials and the pooled treatment effect estimate. We square these differences, divide each by variance of the study effect, and then sum them. This gives a chi-squared test with degrees of freedom = number of studies – 1.

If there is significant heterogeneity, then we have evidence that there are differences between the studies. It may therefore be invalid to pool the results and generate a single summary result. We should try to describe the variation between the studies and investigate possible sources of heterogeneity. We should not just ignore it, but try to account for the heterogeneity in some way. If we can explain the heterogeneity, we may be able to produce a final estimate of the effect which adjusts for it. If not, we can also carry out meta-analysis which allows for heterogeneity, called random effects analyses.

If the heterogeneity is not significant, we have little or no statistical evidence for differences between studies. However, the test for heterogeneity has low power. The number of studies is usually low and the test may fail to detect heterogeneity or statistically significant when it exists. As with any significance test, we cannot simply interpret a not significant result as definite evidence of homogeneity. To compensate for the low power of the test some authors accept a larger p value as being significant, often using $p < 0.1$ rather than $p < 0.05$.

In the test for heterogeneity gives $\chi^2 = 4.91$, df = 2, p = 0.086. In light of the earlier discussion some would conclude that there is evidence of statistical heterogeneity here.

## Types of outcome measure

The choice of the measure of treatment or other effect depends on the type of outcome variable used in the study. These might be:

- **dichotomous**—e.g. dead/alive, success/failure, yes/no. We use a relative risk or risk ratio (RR), odds ratio (OR), absolute risk difference,
- **continuous**—e.g. weight loss, blood pressure. We use the mean difference, or standardized mean difference (SMD),
- **time-to-event or survival time**—e.g. time to death, time to recurrence, time to healing. We use the hazard ratio,
- **ordinal** (very rare)—an outcome categorised with ordering applied to the categories, e.g. mild / moderate / severe, score on a scale, which we may dichotomise, treat as continuous, or use advanced methods specially developed for this type of data.

## Publication bias

One of the great problems with systematic review is that not all studies carried out are published. Those which are published may be different from those which are not. Research with statistically significant results is more likely to be submitted and published than work with null or non-significant results. Research with statistically significant results is likely to be published more prominently than work with null or non-significant results, for example in English, in higher impact journals. To make things worse, well-designed and conducted research is less likely to produce statistically significant results than badly designed and conducted research. Combining only published studies may therefore lead to an over-optimistic conclusion and this should be borne in mind when considering the results of meta-analyses.

## Reference

Colman I, Brown MD, Innes GD, et al. Parenteral metoclopramide for acute migraine headache: meta-analysis of randomised controlled trials. *BMJ* 2004; 329: 1369–73.

## Introduction

In reading a medical research paper, several different aspects should be considered: the question being asked, the study design, the sample and controls, if any, the measurement process, the completeness of the data, and the statistical analysis. Few papers are totally satisfactory in every respect. Having considered all these aspects, we must form a judgement on the validity of the conclusions and their value for our own work.

The purpose of critical reading, also called critical appraisal, is to discover

- if the methods used can produce useful information,
- if the conclusion drawn by the authors follow from the results of the study.

Here we shall look at a framework for reading medical papers.

Medical research is a very difficult business. The essence of research is that we are doing something which has not been done before, and so researchers are bound to make mistakes and not do the best study which is possible with hindsight. Also there are often great limitations in terms of resources, such as the number of patients available, which prevent us doing a flawless study.

Researchers are often so close to their project and know it so well that they fail to mention things which are so obvious to them that they forget that the reader does not know them. Finally, the pressure on journal space means that information may be omitted which authors would have included if they could. As a result, the perfect paper is hard to find and most published research has problems. We should not approach appraisal in a hypercritical, nit-picking way, but in an attempt to make a reasonable judgement on the value of the paper as an addition to knowledge and to decide whether this study is relevant to the question in which we ourselves are interested.

The guidelines given here are necessarily abbreviated, and are intended only to get you started (Begg, 1996; Fowkes and Fulton, 1992; Sackett et al., 1991). A useful tool is provided by the *British Medical Journal* (2007) which is a checklist for statistical assessment of randomized controlled trials. Box 20.2 shows the guidelines, which have been printed by kind permission of the *British Medical Journal*.

We will now look at each aspect in turn.

## What are the objectives?

The first step in appraising a paper is to decide what the authors were trying to find out. This should be stated clearly in the Abstract or Summary as well as in the Introduction, but it may not be. It can be helpful while reading the paper to keep asking what the authors are really trying to discover.

---

Box 20.2 BMJ checklist

The guidelines are:
(a) What are the objectives?
(b) Is the study design appropriate?
(c) Is the study sample appropriate?
(d) Are the controls acceptable?
(e) Measurements and outcomes
(f) Completeness
(g) Statistical analysis
(h) Making a judgement.

Reproduced from *The BMJ*, Murphy B, 'Checklists for statisticians', 312, copyright 1996, with permission from BMJ Publishing Group Ltd.

---

## Is the study design appropriate?

The study design should be clearly laid out in the Methods section of the paper, in sufficient detail that the study could be repeated by other researchers. Most medical research takes one of the forms discussed in the section 'Study Design'. We must ask whether the design is appropriate to the objectives. We have already examined the properties of the each of the different study designs.

## Is the study sample appropriate?

(a) Are the participants from the right population?
(b) Is there an adequate description of the sample?
(c) Do they have the appropriate sort of age and sex distribution in which we are interested?
(d) Is the diagnosis the one we want?
(e) Are criteria for including and excluding participants described clearly?
(f) Is the participant group very specialized, e.g. babies born with very low weights?
(g) Is the sample large enough? Authors should give some justification for why the chosen sample size was appropriate. Even when the total sample is large, there may be comparisons made between subgroups of participants which may be too small.
(h) Is the sample one from which we can draw conclusions about a wider population?
(i) What limitations does it impose? For example, many medical studies use non-random samples. Differences between groups in such studies are usually more reliable than absolute estimates of means and proportions.

## Are the controls acceptable?

Not all designs have controls, but if we have them, as in case–control studies or clinical trials, we need to know that they are suitable. In clinical studies looking at the effects of disease, controls may be asked to undergo invasive or stressful tests and measurements. This may make controls hard to find, and we must ask whether those obtained are truly comparable to the patients. Is like being compared with like? If there is lack of comparability between cases and controls, for example, in an unmatched case–control study, is this dealt with in the analysis?

In case–control studies:
- Is the source of controls reasonable?
- Are they really similar to the cases apart from the disease?
- In such studies, controls may be matched to cases. Are the matching criteria sensible?

In clinical trials:
- Participants should be randomized.
- Is the method of randomization described?
- Some medical researchers think that alternate allocation is the same as randomization, which it is **not**.

## Measurements and outcomes

- Measurements should be valid, i.e. should measure what they set out to measure.
- Is the measurement blind? If it is not blind, is this a serious problem?
- If measurements are by patients' recall, is recall itself likely to be related to the treatment or risk factor being investigated?

## Completeness

- Did all participants provide data?
- In treatment studies, did all comply with the treatment? If not, which is quite likely, was an appropriate analysis carried out?
- In treatment studies, this might be analysis by intention to treat.
- In other studies, authors might look at what the effects would have been if drop-outs and refusers differed from the sample who complied.

## Statistical analysis

The methods of statistical analysis used may be set out at the end of the methods section. Given the data, we should be able to reproduce the analysis. Watch out for p values quoted without any method to produce them being named.

- Is the statistical analysis appropriate? For example, if t-tests were used, are the data from Normal distributions with the same variance?
- A great variety of statistical methods are now used in the medical literature. Do you know enough about the one used here to judge whether it is the suitable? If not, look it up.
- Have estimates been given, or have authors relied on p values only? In negative studies in particular, confidence intervals should be given.
- Have the authors calculated many p values and just discussed the one which is significant?
- Was the clinical significance or importance of any differences considered, rather than the statistical significance only?

## Making a judgement

We must form a judgement about whether any deficiencies in the paper are sufficiently severe as to invalidate the study. Judgement is needed, for most studies have some deficiencies, even our own. Readers will not necessarily agree. Their background and experience will make them more sensitive to some types of errors than to others, and may also lead them to attach different importance to these. We, for example, quickly spot errors in statistical analysis which others may not notice, but might miss completely the use of an inappropriate outcome measurement.

If we are happy that the design and analysis are appropriate and that the study has been carried out satisfactorily, we must then decide whether the conclusions follow from the results of the study. We have already looked at the problems and limitations associated with different research designs, and here issues such as whether we can conclude causality are important. We must also look at the plausibility of the results, and how they fit in with other work. This should be covered in the Discussion section.

Finally, having come to a decision on the validity of the conclusions, we must consider whether the paper influences our own work.

## References

Begg C, Cho M, Eastwood S, et al. Improving the quality of reporting of randomized controlled trials: the CONSORT Statement. *JAMA* 1996; 276: 637–9.

*British Medical Journal. Statisticians checklist: checklist for statistical assessment of randomised controlled trials.* 2007. Available at: <http://resources.bmj.com/bmj/authors/checklist–forms/statisticians–checklist>.

Greenhalgh, T. How to read a paper: Statistics for the non–statistician. I: Different types of data need different statistical tests. *British Medical Journal* 1997;315:364–366.

Fowkes FG, Fulton PM. Critical appraisal of published research: introductory guidelines. *BMJ* 1992; 302: 1136–40.

Sackett DL, Haynes RB, Guyatt GH, et al. *Clinical Epidemiology. A Basic Science for Clinical Medicine* 2nd ed. Boston, MA: Little, Brown and Company; 1991.

# Chapter 21

# Professionalism, communication, and ethics

## Introduction

The problem about writing a chapter like this is that it is the only one covering the 'soft' aspects of medicine in an otherwise highly technical and scientific text. Having read books like this myself in the past as a junior doctor, I know only too well that I would have needed some persuasion to start reading such a non-technical chapter. What you may be expecting to read is something which is perhaps a little boring, or perhaps obvious—'motherhood and apple pie', full of buzzwords, and 'pc' statements. For me as the author there is the additional problem that there is little evidence that people learn communication, attitudes, professionalism, or ethical practice from text books. Some form of experiential learning and guided reflection is required to make the subject come alive and change behaviour in the real world.

So my task is to make this chapter worthwhile reading, to offer you and your patients something of practical use rather than a collection of terms to which you cannot relate. Indeed what I want to offer you is a practical approach that will enable all of your hard-earned factual learning and experience to make a difference to your patients. How you communicate with your patients will ultimately determine your clinical excellence. How you are perceived as a professional and how you turn ethical principles into practice are all mediated through the final common pathway of communication.

## Why communication determines your clinical excellence

The medical interview is central to clinical practice. It has been estimated that doctors perform 200,000 consultations in a professional lifetime so it is worth struggling to get it right. To achieve an effective interview, doctors need to be able to integrate four aspects of their work which together determine their overall clinical competence:

- Knowledge.
- Communication skills.
- Problem-solving.
- Physical examination.

These four essential components of clinical competence are inextricably linked: outstanding expertise in any one alone is not sufficient. It is, for example, not good enough to be factually excellent if communication difficulties stand between you and the patient and prevent you from discovering the patient's story or from discussing a plan that the patient can understand and wishes to put into action. It is, however, similarly useless having effective communication skills with deficient knowledge.

### Communication is core to your practice, not an optional extra

How we communicate is just as important as what we say. The prize on offer from effective communication is improved clinical performance.

### More effective consultations

Excellent communication skills can produce more effective consultations for both patients and doctors. However knowledgeable doctors are about the facts of medicine, without appropriate communication skills they may not be able to:

---

**Core benefits of communication**

Communication is not just 'being nice' but produces a more effective consultation for both patient and doctor.
Effective communication significantly improves:
- Accuracy, efficiency, and supportiveness.
- Health outcomes for patients.
- Satisfaction for both patient and doctor.
Communication bridges the gap between evidence-based medicine and working with individual patients.

---

- Efficiently discover the problems or issues that the patient wishes to address.
- Accurately obtain the full history.
- Collaboratively negotiate a mutually acceptable management plan.
- Supportively form a relationship that helps reduce conflicts for both patient and doctor.

*Improved health outcomes*

Communication can significantly improve health outcomes for patients: individual skills can lead to improvements in patient satisfaction, adherence, symptom relief, and physiological outcome. Effective communication makes a difference to patients' health.

Communication can also improve outcomes for doctors. The use of appropriate communication skills not only increases patients' satisfaction with their doctors but also helps doctors to feel less frustrated and more satisfied in their work. Appropriate communication reduces conflict by preventing the misunderstanding which is so often the source of difficulties between doctors and patients.

## Why communication mediates your professionalism and ethical practice

The problem with professionalism is that everyone 'buys' into it apart from those who do not. Very few people on the face of it would disagree with the GMC 'Duties of a Doctor':

Those who get into real trouble through lack of professionalism are a tiny minority—everybody else feels that the principles are blatantly obvious. Surely respect, altruism, probity, responsibility, ethical practice, and self-awareness go without saying?

But there is a genuine problem here. The environment in which we work in medicine often undermines these very qualities. Medical students arrive with appropriate attitudes and commitment. By the time they have been qualified for several years, they may well have been influenced by unsupportive working conditions, poor role models, and cynicism. Changes in the medical system have led to considerable threats to professionalism via fragmentation and reduced continuity of care. Shift working, moves towards maximum bed efficiency, reduction in 'home ward' patients, lack of a continuing relationship between junior and senior staff and between doctors and nurses have all led to a difficult situation for the modern junior doctor. It is all too easy for an unconscious shift to occur from the principles of professionalism as embodied in 'Duties of a Doctor' to a more cynical approach of job survival and a 'them' versus 'us' mentality. The danger is then that unconsciously acquired attitudes will undermine professionalism and be all too apparent to patients and their relatives.

Patients must be able to trust doctors with their lives and health. To justify that trust you must show respect for human life and make sure your practice meets the standards expected of you in four domains.

*Knowledge, skills, and performance*
- Make the care of your patient your first concern.
- Provide a good standard of practice and care.
  - Keep your professional knowledge and skills up to date.
  - Recognise and work within the limits of your competence.

*Safety and quality*
- Take prompt action if you think that patient safety, dignity or comfort is being compromised.
- Protect and promote the health of patients and the public.

*Communication, partnership and teamwork*
- Treat patients as individuals and respect their dignity.
  - Treat patients politely and considerately.
  - Respect patients' right to confidentiality.
- Work in partnership with patients.
  - Listen to, and respond to, their concerns and preferences.
  - Give patients the information they want or need in a way they can understand.
  - Respect patients' right to reach decisions with you about their treatment and care.
  - Support patients in caring for themselves to improve and maintain their health.
- Work with colleagues in the ways that best serve patients' interests.

*Maintaining trust*
- Be honest and open and act with integrity.
- Never discriminate unfairly against patients or colleagues.
- Never abuse your patients' trust in you or the public's trust in the profession.

You are personally accountable for your professional practice and must always be prepared to justify your decisions and actions.

Reproduced from *Good medical practice* with permission of the General Medical Council. © (2013).

## Why communication skills demonstrate your attitudes, values, beliefs, and intent

How though, is your professionalism transmitted to the patient? Professionalism encompasses a set of underlying attitudes, values, beliefs, and intent. Communication is a set of learned behaviours and skills. Yet it is only via your behaviour that patients and other health professionals can ascertain your true professional stance.

Firstly, your non-verbal behaviour will always leak clues to your underlying beliefs and attitudes. Patients will always pick up if there is a mixed message from your verbal and non-verbal communication and will always believe the non-verbal over the verbal. Non-verbal communication transmits more about your inner world of attitudes and emotions than the more cognitive verbal communication and it is very difficult to hide—it leaks out in multiple transmission modes to betray your true feelings. That is why saying 'have a nice day' is not enough in itself, it is whether you mean it and whether that meaning is transmitted non-verbally that will make it appear genuine or not. So saying to an elderly patient 'we will do everything we can to get you home' while sounding bored and avoiding eye contact will not make the patient believe you.

Secondly, it is all too easy for you to become institutionalized and accept some of the work practices you see around you as being appropriate.

- Is it respectful to the patient's right to reach decisions with you about their treatment and care if you talk about the patient at the end of the bed with colleagues without explaining to the patient what you are doing and involving them in any decisions that you make about discharge?

- Can you listen to patients' concerns and preferences if you rush from patient to patient checking their charts without actually asking them if they have any questions for you?
- Can you work with colleagues in the ways that best serve patients' interests if you do not listen to their contributions or provide a forum for this?
- Can you make the patient your first concern unless you find time each day to ask them not only for their current symptoms but also for their questions and concerns about their care?

Thirdly, it is quite possible to have all the appropriate professional attitudes and yet not have the skills to communicate that to the patient. The base from which you as a healthcare provider start is important, for instance, if you believe it is important to be a 'caring' person. But it is equally important to find ways to communicate that caring on an everyday basis as well as in times of extreme crisis. It is fine to recognize in your mind that this elderly patient is extremely distressed by the thought of dying in hospital and would rather be discharged to their home if at all possible. However, without the skills to communicate this understanding to the patient through empathetic statements and non-verbal behaviour, without the ability to pick up cues and explore the patient's concerns, and without the ability to have the skills of negotiation to discuss what is and what is not possible, the patient will not appreciate or benefit from your understanding. On a more cognitive, less emotional, level, it would be very difficult to maintain a good standard of practice and care if an inadequate ability to use open and closed questions, to summarize, to timeframe, and to clarify prevented you from taking an appropriate and full clinical history.

Communication skills and attitudes are both vital: both must be addressed, both demand careful attention. Without communication skills, however, the patient may not know or understand your intent and may misinterpret your professionalism.

## Why communication skills are vital for ethical practice

Similarly, without effective communication skills, how do you actually manage an ethical dilemma? Lectures and discussions about ethical principles enable you to know about ethics and formulate approaches.

You can learn about the Four Principles framework:
- Respect for autonomy.
- Beneficence.
- Non-maleficence.
- Justice.

You can understand the Jonsen Framework:
- Indications for medical intervention—establish a diagnosis, what are the options for treatment, what are the prognoses for each of the options?
- Preferences of patient—is the patient competent?—if so what does he/she want? If not competent, then what is in the patient's best interest?
- Quality of life—will the proposed treatment improve the patient's quality of life?
- Contextual features—do religious, cultural, legal factors have an impact on the decision?

However, these theories can only be turned into a practical discussion between the doctor and the patient or relative through effective communication. If a patient says that they have had enough and could you do something about it to end their life, only communication can turn knowing about the ethical and legal principles to knowing how to discuss this with the patient. Only a keen understanding that you may have to dig deeper to discover what it is the patient is concerned about rather than address the initial statement, plus the practical communication skills to be able to do this, will enable you to help this particular patient to be more settled in their last days. If a patient with a learning disability or dementia refuses an operation, even when you understand the concepts of autonomy, competence, and best interest, you will have to have a discussion with the patient, relatives, and carers about the most appropriate way forward. Even if you understand the duty of confidentiality to a 15-year-old girl, only the communication skills associated with the three-way interview will enable you to handle the situation of seeing both the girl and her angry father in accident and emergency when the father believes she may be having under-age unprotected sex.

## So what are the important principles of effective communication?

To be quite clear, **there are no intrinsically good or bad communication skills**. Communication is only useful as a means of achieving an end and the skills that you employ will depend on where you want to get to. So communication skills are not morally right or wrong, they are only effective (or not) in achieving a certain outcome for you and the patient. For instance, a list of appropriate skills would look very interesting indeed if the underlying ethos of the communication you wished to utilize was paternalistic, controlling, and attempted to retain the mystery of medicine in the face of 50 years of societal changes.

So first we have to **define an outcome**. You will already know that the skills that are normally taught in communication skills programmes to medical students and doctors support a patient-centred or relationship-centred approach, promoting a collaborative partnership between patient and doctor.

The **concept of a collaborative partnership** implies a more equal relationship between patient and doctor than in the past and a shift in the balance of power away from medical paternalism towards mutuality. Modern communication teaching therefore promotes skills that doctors can employ to enhance their patients' ability to become more involved in the consultation and to take part in a more balanced relationship.

This is not because of political dogma, subjective opinion, or personal belief—those teaching communication take this approach because the skills that enable it to be achieved have been shown both in practice and in research to produce better outcomes for both patients and doctors. So perhaps the most important overriding principle of effective communication is that it should be as research-based as other cognitive or technical areas of medicine.

Therefore when you read any text on communication skills in medicine, implicit within it will be the following principles:

- Patient-centeredness.
- Collaboration.
- Partnership (to the extent that the patient wishes to be involved).
- Flexibility to the situation and to the individual patient.
- Respectfulness.

Of course, these ground rules fit perfectly with the ethical and professional principles we have already discussed—both are predicated on the same belief system about the very basis of medical practice. But this is more than belief or attitude, this is an approach which will enable you to maximize your clinical effectiveness and value to the patients you serve.

## So what are the key practical lessons about communication?

What are the communication skills that will enable you to put all of the aforementioned into practice? Here, I am not going to produce a guide to the whole medical interview but instead will look at selective elements that will make a difference to your day-to-day work, to how you are perceived by patients and colleagues alike, and to whether or not you fulfil your professional and ethical commitments.

## Learn to control your non-verbal communication

I have already mentioned the importance of non-verbal communication and how much of our communication is mediated non-verbally. However, although it leaks spontaneously through a myriad of channels (i.e. it is impossible not to communicate non-verbally), it is much more under your control than you would think.

As doctors, as well as recognizing patients' non-verbal cues in their speech patterns, facial expression, affect, and body posture, we also need to be aware of our own non-verbal behaviour and how our use of eye contact, body position and posture, movement, facial expression, and use of voice can all influence the success of the interview. The disparity in power and control between patient and doctor leads patients to be particularly attentive to doctors' non-verbal cues: patients rarely ask for verbal confirmation of cues that they pick up and commonly base their impressions of you primarily on non-verbal messages. If you give the wrong impression non-verbally, that impression will remain. Your attitudes, values, and beliefs will be inferred by the patient and your professional intent may well be undermined.

The number one message is to be very conscious of your non-verbal communication, particularly when you are stressed and under pressure. Learn to recognize your body's characteristics when you are stressed and learn how to revert to your normal non-verbal communication style. For instance, if when you are tense, you always scrunch up your shoulders, learn how to relax your shoulders and improved non-verbal communication will follow—a handy tip for job interviews. If you become aware that when under pressure you tend to talk too much, deliberately slow your pace down and leave bigger gaps. In fact, this is probably the biggest take-home message about non-verbal skills—leave gaps. Slow your communication down enough so that the patient has some opportunity to enter into the conversation when they have questions, queries, or thoughts.

---

### Channels of non-verbal communication

- **Posture**: sitting, standing, erect, relaxed.
- **Proximity**: use of space, physical distance between and positioning of communicators.
- **Touch**: handshake, pat, physical contact during physical examination.
- **Body movements**: hand and arm gestures, fidgeting, nodding, foot and leg movements.
- **Facial expression**: raised eyebrows, frown, smiles, crying.
- **Eye behaviour**: eye contact, gaze, stares.
- **Vocal cues**: pitch, rate, volume, rhythm, silence, pause, intonation, speech errors.
- **Use of time**: early, late, on time, overtime, rushed, slow to respond.
- **Physical presence**: race, gender, body shape, clothing, grooming.
- **Environmental cues**: location, furniture placement, lighting, temperature, colour.

---

## Listen for the first minute

This brings me on to the golden minute, which most readers will have heard about. However rushed you are, prepare yourself to listen to the first minute of any interview. Put your pen down, give the patient eye contact, nod and grunt facilitatively, and bite your tongue! Counter-intuitively, this will save you a lot of time but perhaps more

---

### Active listening

Full attention through active listening allows you to:
- Signal your interest to the patient.
- Hear their story.
- Prevent yourself from making premature hypotheses and chasing down blind alleys.
- Not miss key symptoms and concerns.
- Hear both disease information and the patient's framework.
- Not have to think of the next question (which blocks your listening and renders the patient passive).
- Calibrate the patient's emotional state.
- Observe more carefully and pick up verbal and non-verbal cues.

importantly will increase your efficiency as a diagnostician while simultaneously allowing your professional concern for the patient to become apparent.

A lot goes on in the very first minute of a patient consultation with much of the diagnostic information surfacing. With so much to hear and see at the beginning of the interview, why not consciously set aside this time for the patient and concentrate on listening and facilitating rather than questioning? Listening attentively instead of moving immediately to a series of questions about the history will allow you to achieve more of both your and the patient's objectives. You can get a good feel for the story and the patient can tell you what is on their mind in their own words.

## Learn how to discover the patient's perspective as well as the medical perspective

So how are you going to fulfil the following aspects of modern professionalism: treat patients as individuals, work in partnership with patients, listen to patients and respond to their concerns and preferences, and give patients the information they want or need?

This is at the heart of patient-centred medicine and yet it is so easy in the busy world of junior doctors to get drawn into 'sorting people out' as rapidly as possible to early discharge, considering only the diagnostic and treatment aspects of their care and omitting to focus in on their individual requirements as a person.

Paradoxically though, the key to an effective consultation is to combine both the medical and personal aspects of a medical interview into a seamless whole. You need to do the medical business of course, but research clearly points to the need to discover the patient's ideas, concerns, feelings, and expectations (the 'illness perspective') as well so that you can tailor your explanations to the patient's needs and enable the patient to understand and be involved in their care. This is not just being supportive—it makes a difference to patient understanding, commitment, adherence, and even physiological outcome.

How do you do this? What communication skills will enable you to rapidly discover a whole new set of information as well as the medical facts?

The phrase 'ideas, concerns, and expectations' is one that it is now frequently taught to medical students in this context. However, it is essential that these concepts are not simply followed slavishly. For example, when you hear students in Objective Structured Clinical Examinations (OSCEs) waiting until the end of the station and then asking 'what are your expectations?' it just so clearly does not work. Moreover, when somebody presents with acute central chest pain to emergency admissions, asking them about their ideas may seem somewhat superfluous, if not ridiculous. But most consultations are not undertaken in the acute situation or with an incoherent patient and increasingly in your work as a junior and then senior doctor, you will be seeing patients with chronic illness, patients in outpatients, and patients who are several days in from their acute admission. In these patients, there is no doubt that discovering the issues that they would like answering and keying into their worries and needs is an essential component of modern medicine and your work.

In fact, the key to discovering the patient's ideas, concerns, and expectations is not by asking for them directly but instead is by picking up cues provided by the patient during the course of the interview. If patients are asked a suitably open question at the beginning of an interview they will tell you a story that includes what has been happening medically as well as verbal and non-verbal cues about their thoughts and feelings. A skilled and fluent interviewer often does not need to ask specifically about these areas but can simply pick up these cues, which are woven into the fabric of the story, and reflect them back to the patient.

- 'I sense that you're not quite happy with the explanations you've been given in the past—is that right?'
- 'Am I right in thinking you're quite upset about us not finding a diagnosis for your illness?'

Be especially careful about failing to pick up cues to the patient's framework because you are preferentially listening for cues about disease. If the patient says 'It's been difficult at home and I've been getting a lot more pains lately', it is far easier to pick up the disease rather than the situation cue and say 'Tell me about the pains' without returning to 'You mentioned things have been difficult at home…', even though that might be key to the cause of the pain.

That is not to say that asking directly is not also a good idea. But it has to be done in a very flexible way with a truly appropriate question. Not 'What are your expectations today?' but, for instance, 'Was there something in particular that you hoped I might be able to sort out for you today?'.

## Use summarizing

Underlying all of clinical excellence, professionalism, and ethics is a desire to 'get it right' for the patient. Yet there is one skill used far too infrequently by doctors which aims to do just that. Summarizing is the key skill that brings together all your attempts at accuracy and efficiency as well as being highly supportive.

'Can I just see if I've got this right—you've had indigestion before, but for the last few weeks you've had increasing problems with a sharp pain at the front of your chest, accompanied by wind and acid, it's stopping you from sleeping, it's made worse by alcohol and you were wondering if the painkillers were to blame. Is that right? (Pause…)'

By this quick and easy statement, you have a chance to make sure that you have accurately heard the symptoms, time-framed the illness, and given the patient an opportunity to further elaborate or correct you if you have it wrong.

**This is a key skill in discovering the patient's perspective**. Unless you include what you have heard into your summary, it will send a clear message to the patient that you are not interested in their ideas or concerns and that you are running a solely doctor-centred interview.

The advantages of an internal summary for **the patient** are:
- It clearly demonstrates that you have been listening.
- It demonstrates that you are interested and care about getting things right.
- It offers a collaborative approach to problem-solving.
- It allows the patient to check your understanding and thoughts.
- It gives the patient an opportunity to either confirm or correct your interpretation and to add in missing areas.
- It invites and allows the patient to go further in explaining their problems and thoughts by acting as a facilitative opening.
- It demonstrates your interest in the illness as well as in the disease aspects of the patient's story.

The advantages of an internal summary for **the doctor** are:
- It maximizes accurate information gathering by allowing you to check the accuracy of what you think the patient has said and to

then rectify any misconceptions thus promoting mutually understood common ground.

- It provides a space for you to review what you have already covered.
- It allows you to order your thoughts and clarify in your mind what you are not sure about and what aspect of the story you need to explore next.
- It helps you to recall information later.
- It allows you to distinguish between, and consider, both disease and illness.

## Learn how to use the twin skills of acceptance and empathy

To practise ethically, you need to know where the patient is 'coming from' cognitively as well as emotionally and what they want from you as an autonomous individual. To practise as a professional you need to be able to treat all patients as equals whatever their cultural or social background, to respect patients' views, and to work with the patient in partnership. One of the first steps to enable all of this to happen is, as we have already discussed, discovering the patient's questions, concerns, and wishes.

But then what? What you do with this 'Pandora's box', especially if you disagree with any of the patient's views? It is so easy to provide immediate and rather ill-considered reassurance, rebuttal, or even agreement before you have all the information to hand. Instead, the twin skills of acceptance and empathy are the bridge to a truly patient-centred and sensitive approach.

Exploring the patient's beliefs should be a three-stage process:

1. **Identification**—discover and listen to the patient's ideas, concerns, and expectations.
2. **Acceptance**—acknowledge the patient's views and their right to hold them, without necessarily agreeing with them; pause so the patient can say more if they wish and then 'put on hold'.
3. **Explanation**—explain your understanding of the problem in relation to the patient's understanding and reach a mutually understood common ground.

**Acceptance** provides a practical and specific way of:

- Accepting non-judgementally what the patient says.
- Acknowledging the legitimacy of the patient to hold their own views and feelings.
- Valuing the patient's contributions.

You can use the following set of skills to signal acceptance to the patient. In this example, the patient has expressed his thoughts by saying 'I think I might have cancer doctor; I've been getting an awful lot of wind lately'.

- Acknowledge the patient's thought or feeling by naming, restating, or summarizing—'So, you're worried that the wind might be caused by cancer?'.
- Acknowledge the patient's right to feel or think as he does by using legitimizing comments—'I can understand that you would want to get that checked out'.
- Come to a 'full stop'; using attentive silence and appropriate non-verbal behaviour to make space for the patient to say more—'Yes, doctor, you see my mother died of bowel cancer when she was 40 and I remember she had a lot of wind—I'm terrified of getting it too'.
- Avoid the tendency to counter with 'yes but...'—'I can understand your concern—we'll check that out carefully. Tell me a bit more about your symptoms and then I'll examine you to see if you're OK'.

Here, the patient's concerns are acknowledged and put on hold until they can be incorporated into an explanation later. Evidence clearly shows that the patient's ideas and beliefs, concerns, and expectations need to be built into our explanation of the disease process so that we can cover the questions that are most important from the patient's perspective and together reach some degree of common

ground. It is important to get to a position where our explanations make sense in the patient's world.

**Empathy** is a closely related skill. It is in fact a two-stage process:
1. The understanding and sensitive appreciation of another person's predicament or feelings.
2. The communication of that understanding back to the patient in a supportive way.

The key to empathy is not only being sensitive but overtly demonstrating that sensitivity to the patient so that they appreciate your understanding and support. It's not good enough to think empathically, you must show it too. What then are the building blocks of the empathic response?

### Understanding the patient's predicament and feelings

Many generic skills demonstrate to patients that you are genuinely interested in hearing about their thoughts. Together they provide an atmosphere which facilitates disclosure and enables the first step of empathy—understanding the patient's predicament—to take place:

- Welcoming the patient warmly.
- Clarifying the patient's agenda and expectations.
- Attentive listening.
- Facilitation especially via paraphrasing of content and feelings and repetition.
- Encouraging the expression of feelings and thoughts.
- Picking up cues, checking out our interpretations or assumptions.
- Summary.
- Acceptance.
- Non-judgemental response.
- Use of silence.
- Encouraging the patient to contribute as an equal.

Having set up a climate conducive to patient disclosure, you have to pick up your patients' verbal and non-verbal cues, become aware of their predicament, and consider their feelings and emotions.

### Communicating empathy to the patient

The skills just outlined do not complete the second step of empathy, which is communicating your understanding back to the patient so that they know that you appreciate and are sensitive to their difficulty. Both non-verbal and verbal skills can help us here.

Empathic non-verbal communication can say more than a thousand words. Facial expression, proximity, touch, tone of voice, or use of silence in response to a patient's expression of feelings can clearly signal to the patient that you are sensitive to their situation. But what are the verbal skills that allow us to demonstrate empathy? Empathic statements are supportive comments that specifically link the 'I' of the doctor and the 'you' of the patient. They both name and appreciate the patient's affect or predicament:

- 'I can see that your husband's memory loss has been very difficult for **you** to cope with.'
- 'I can appreciate how difficult it is for **you** to talk about this.'
- 'I can sense how angry **you** have been feeling about your illness.'
- 'I can see that **you** have been very upset by her behaviour.'
- 'I can understand that it must be frightening for **you** to know the pain might keep coming back.'

## Explanation and planning skills

In the GMC's 'Duties of a Doctor', it recommends that you give patients the information they want or need in a way that they can understand, and that you respect patients' right to reach decisions with you about their treatment and care. So how do you do that in practice?

This short chapter could not possibly do justice to the skills of explanation and planning, shared decision-making, and concordance. But here are just a few points:

- Do not give a lecture with all your considerable knowledge: break it up into small pieces, so that you can stop, check for understanding, and use the patient's response as a guide as to how to proceed—be flexible to the patient.

- Always find out what the patient already knows—what is their starting point?
- Ask the patient what other information would be helpful to them.
- Relate explanations to your patient's illness framework—to previously elicited ideas, concerns, and expectations.
- Provide opportunities and encourage your patient to contribute—to ask questions, seek clarification, or express doubts.
- Pick up and respond to your patient's verbal and non-verbal cues, e.g. their need to contribute information or ask questions, information overload, or distress.
- Try to discover your patient's beliefs, reactions, and feelings about the information given.
- Explore all the management options available.
- Involve your patient in decision-making by offering suggestions and choices rather than directives and encouraging the patient to contribute their ideas.
- Discover the level of involvement your patient wishes to have in making the decision at hand.
- Negotiate a mutually acceptable plan that takes into account the patient's preferences.

Moving towards shared decision-making rather than paternalism, towards concordance rather than compliance, implies that you move from only considering the best possible control of the disease (e.g. seizures) to looking at the best outcome from the point of view of the patient and their quality of life. This can be uncomfortable for some doctors. However, the aim of a concordant discussion is to make these differences and difficulties overt rather than covert so that you know if the patient does not wish to take all the medication prescribed. The concept is to have an honest relationship with your patient—doctors in the past simply did not appreciate that their patients were non-compliant—here the aim is to fully understand your patient and what they have decided to take.

## Record all of this in the medical records

One of the major problems of current medical practice is the reduction in continuity of care engendered by the move towards shift working in medicine. This of course has some advantages for doctors and ensures compliance with various external directives. At the same time though we must ensure that patient care is not compromised. Clearly handovers and medical record-keeping need to be a major part of ensuring that patient care is as seamless as possible. However, a brief look at hospital records in the UK will demonstrate that the quality of record-keeping has not caught up with this pressing need. Indeed in many cases progress notes, in particular, are very sub-standard. Yet how are you as a junior doctor going to speak to the relatives of the patient for whom you are cross-covering when you cannot easily glean from the notes what the current management plan is and what the patient has been told?

It is extremely important therefore to include in your progress notes clear information about:

- The nature of the current problems.
- What is being done and why.
- What it is that the patient is concerned about.
- What the patient has already been told
- What plans have been agreed with the patient and/or the relatives.

## Final words

What I have tried to provide you with here are some practical approaches to clinical communication skills which will help make a difference to both you and your patient. The aim has been to encourage the use of exemplary communication enabling you to put your clinical excellence, professionalism, and ethical stance into action. It is clear that such skills, when informed by a greater understanding of the underlying principles and when developed and honed over time with practice, lead to a better healthcare experience for all concerned.